Place-of-Service Codes for Professional

Listed below are place-of-service codes and descriptions. These codes should be used on professional claims to specify the entity where service(s) were rendered. Check with individual payers (eg, Medicare, Medicaid, other private insurance) for reimbursement policies regarding these codes. If you would like to comment on a code(s) or description(s), please send your request to posinfo@cms.hhs.gov.

Place of Service Code(s)	Place of Service Name	Place of Service Description
01	Pharmacy	A facility or location where drugs and other medically related items and services are sold, dispensed, or otherwise provided directly to patients. (effective 10/1/05)
02	Unassigned	N/A
03	School	A facility whose primary purpose is education.
04	Homeless shelter	A facility or location whose primary purpose is to provide temporary housing to homeless individuals (eg, emergency shelters, individual or family shelters).
05	Indian Health Service freestanding facility	A facility or location, owned and operated by the Indian Health Service, that provides diagnostic, therapeutic (surgical and nonsurgical), and rehabilitation services to American Indians and Alaska Natives who do not require hospitalization.
06	Indian Health Service provider-based facility	A facility or location, owned and operated by the Indian Health Service, that provides diagnostic, therapeutic (surgical and nonsurgical), and rehabilitation services rendered by, or under the supervision of, physicians to American Indians and Alaska Natives admitted as inpatients or outpatients.
07	Tribal 638 freestanding facility	A facility or location owned and operated by a federally recognized American Indian or Alaska Native tribe or tribal organization under a 638 agreement that provides diagnostic, therapeutic (surgical and nonsurgical), and rehabilitation services to tribal members who do not require hospitalization.
08	Tribal 638 provider-based facility	A facility or location owned and operated by a federally recognized American Indian or Alaska Native tribe or tribal organization under a 638 agreement that provides diagnostic, therapeutic (surgical and nonsurgical), and rehabilitation services to tribal members admitted as inpatients or outpatients.
09	Prison-Correctional Facility	A prison, jail, reformatory, work farm, detention center, or any other similar facility maintained by either Federal, State, or local authorities for the purpose of confinement or rehabilitation of adult or juvenile criminal offenders. (effective 7/1/06)
10	Unassigned	N/A
11	Office	Location, other than a hospital, skilled nursing facility, military treatment facility, community health center, state or local public health clinic, or intermediate care facility, where the health professional routinely provides health examinations, diagnosis, and treatment of illness or injury on an ambulatory basis.
12	Home	Location, other than a hospital or other facility, where the patient receives care in a private residence.
13	Assisted living facility	Congregate residential facility with self-contained living units providing assessment of each resident's needs and on-site support 24 hours a day, seven days a week, with the capacity to deliver or arrange for services including some health care and other services. (effective 10/1/03)
14	Group home	A residence, with shared living areas, where clients receive supervision and other services such as social and/or behavioral services, custodial service, and minimal services (eg, medication administration) (effective 4/1/04)
15	Mobile unit	A facility or unit that moves from place to place and is equipped to provide preventive, screening, diagnostic, and/or treatment services.
16-19	Unassigned	N/A
20	Urgent care facility	Location, distinct from a hospital emergency department, an office, or a clinic, whose purpose is to diagnose and treat illness or injury for unscheduled, ambulatory patients seeking immediate medical attention.
21	Inpatient hospital	A facility, other than psychiatric, that primarily provides diagnostic, therapeutic (both surgical and nonsurgical), and rehabilitation services by, or under, the supervision of physicians to patients admitted for a variety of medical conditions.
22	Outpatient hospital	A portion of a hospital that provides diagnostic, therapeutic (both surgical and nonsurgical), and rehabilitation services to sick or injured persons who do not require hospitalization or institutionalization.
23	Emergency room—hospital	A portion of a hospital where emergency diagnosis and treatment of illness or injury is provided.
24	Ambulatory surgical center	A freestanding facility, other than a physician's office, where surgical and diagnostic services are provided on an ambulatory basis.
25	Birthing center	A facility, other than a hospital's maternity facilities or a physician's office, that provides a setting for labor, delivery, and immediate postpartum care as well as immediate care of newborn infants.
26	Military treatment facility	A medical facility operated by one or more of the uniformed services. Military treatment facility also refers to certain former US Public Health Service facilities now designated as uniformed service treatment facilities.
27-30	Unassigned	N/A
31	Skilled nursing facility	A facility that primarily provides inpatient skilled nursing care and related services to patients who require medical, nursing, or rehabilitative services but does not provide the level of care or treatment available in a hospital.

32	Nursing facility	A facility that primarily provides to residents skilled nursing care and related services for the rehabilitation of injured, disabled, or sick persons, or, on a regular basis, health-related care services above the level of custodial care to other than mentally retarded individuals.
33	Custodial care facility	A facility that provides room, board, and other personal assistance services, generally on a long-term basis, and does not include a medical component.
34	Hospice	A facility, other than a patient's home, in which palliative and supportive care for terminally ill patients and their families are provided.
35-40	Unassigned	N/A
41	Ambulance—land	A land vehicle specifically designed, equipped, and staffed for lifesaving and transporting the sick or injured.
42	Ambulance—air or water	An air or water vehicle specifically designed, equipped, and staffed for lifesaving and transporting the sick or injured.
43-48	Unassigned	N/A
49	Independent clinic	A location, not part of a hospital and not described by any other place-of-service code, that is organized and operated to provide preventive, diagnostic, therapeutic, rehabilitative, or palliative services to outpatients only. (effective 10/1/03)
50	Federally qualified health center	A facility located in a medically underserved area that provides Medicare beneficiaries preventive primary medical care under the general direction of a physician.
51	Inpatient psychiatric facility	A facility that provides inpatient psychiatric services for the diagnosis and treatment of mental illness on a 24-hour basis, by or under the supervision of a physician.
52	Psychiatric facility—partial hospitalization	A facility for the diagnosis and treatment of mental illness that provides a planned therapeutic program for patients who do not require full-time hospitalization but who need broader programs than are possible from outpatient visits to a hospital-based or hospital-affiliated facility.
53	Community mental health center	A facility that provides the following services: outpatient services, including specialized outpatient services for children, the elderly, individuals who are chronically ill, and residents of the community mental health center's mental health services area who have been discharged from inpatient treatment at a mental health facility; 24-hour-a-day emergency care services; day treatment, other partial hospitalization services, or psychosocial rehabilitation services; screening for patients being considered for admission to state mental health facilities to determine the appropriateness of such admission; and consultation and education services.
54	Intermediate care facility/mentally retarded	A facility that primarily provides health-related care and services above the level of custodial care to mentally retarded individuals but does not provide the level of care or treatment available in a hospital or skilled nursing facility.
55	Residential substance abuse treatment facility	A facility that provides treatment for substance (alcohol and drug) abuse to live-in residents who do not require acute medical care. Services include individual and group therapy and counseling, family counseling, laboratory tests, drugs and supplies, psychological testing, and room and board.
56	Psychiatric residential treatment center	A facility or distinct part of a facility for psychiatric care that provides a total 24-hour therapeutically planned and professionally staffed group living and learning environment.
57	Nonresidential substance abuse treatment facility	A location that provides treatment for substance (alcohol and drug) abuse on an ambulatory basis. Services include individual and group therapy and counseling, family counseling, laboratory tests, drugs and supplies, and psychological testing. (effective 10/1/03)
58-59	Unassigned	N/A
60	Mass immunization center	A location where providers administer pneumococcal pneumonia and influenza virus vaccinations and submit these services as electronic media claims or paper claims or by using the roster billing method. This generally takes place in a mass immunization setting, such as a public health center, pharmacy, or mall but may include a physician office setting.
61	Comprehensive inpatient rehabilitation facility	A facility that provides comprehensive rehabilitation services under the supervision of a physician to inpatients with physical disabilities. Services include physical therapy, occupational therapy, speech pathology, social or psychological services, and orthotics and prosthetics services.
62	Comprehensive outpatient rehabilitation facility	A facility that provides comprehensive rehabilitation services under the supervision of a physician to outpatients with physical disabilities. Services include physical therapy, occupational therapy, and speech pathology services.
63-64	Unassigned	N/A
65	End-stage renal disease treatment facility	A facility, other than a hospital, that provides dialysis treatment, maintenance, and/or training to patients or caregivers on an ambulatory or home-care basis.
66-70	Unassigned	N/A
71	Public health clinic	A facility maintained by either state or local health departments that provides ambulatory primary medical care under the general direction of a physician. (effective 10/1/03)
72	Rural health clinic	A certified facility located in a rural, medically underserved area that provides ambulatory primary medical care under the general direction of a physician.
73-80	Unassigned	N/A
81	Independent laboratory	A laboratory certified to perform diagnostic and/or clinical tests independent of an institution or a physician's office.
82-98	Unassigned	N/A
99	Other place of service	Other place of service not identified above.

CPT® Assistant references within CPT® Professional 2008

When using your *CPT® Professional* codebook you will notice the symbol "➲" located next to many codes throughout the body of the book. This symbol has been included to indicate that the AMA has published in-depth information in *CPT® Assistant* on that particular code.

Example	✚ 34808	Endovascular placement of iliac artery occlusion device (List separately in addition to code for primary procedure) ➲ *CPT Assistant* Dec 00:1

This reference indicates that in the **CPT Assistant** newsletter December 2000 issue, page 1, there is material that will assist you in understanding the application of this code.

As the AMA's official communication tool for circulating accurate information and guidance on CPT codes and issues, this insightful monthly newsletter should be part of every compliance program. Each issue features articles used for answering day-to-day coding questions, appealing insurance denials and validating coding to auditors.

Enhance your coding proficiency—Case studies and clinical examples offer insight into confusing coding situations

Direct link to AMA coding experts— Coding consultation section features a "question and answer" format drawn from the CPT Information Services helpline

Keep informed on critical code changes—Get timely, up-to-date information on code changes and correct code assignment

E-mail **amy.burgess@ama-assn.org** to request a free sample issue, and an issue will be e-mailed to you promptly.

CPT® Assistant Archives 1990-2007

Enjoy convenient access to 18 years of *CPT® Assistant* newsletter articles on your computer desktop. Search past and present issues of the AMA's authoritative coding newsletter by keyword, phrase, CPT code number, newsletter issue, article index or codebook table of contents. Includes a cumulative index of article titles and a complete historical CPT code list that references when a code was added, deleted and/or revised.

CD-ROM, Shipping included
Order #: OP511907CCW (single user license fee)
Price: $320.00   **AMA member price: $240.00**

Subscribe today!

You'll receive 12 or 24 monthly issues, special report bulletins, the frequently asked questions/answers bonus issue and the ability to earn CEU credits toward AAPC and AHIMA certification. Call (800) 621-8335 to order or go online to *www.amabookstore.com*.

Order #: CA500900CCW
Price: $199.00/one year; $299.00/two year
AMA member price: $149.00/one year; $205.00/two years

CPT® Changes references within CPT® Professional 2008

When using your *CPT® Professional* codebook you will notice the symbol "⊃" located next to many codes throughout the body of the book. This symbol has been included to indicate that the AMA has published in-depth information in *CPT® Changes* on that particular code.

Example	✚ 34808	Endovascular placement of iliac artery occlusion device (List separately in addition to code for primary procedure) ⊃ *CPT Changes: An Insider's View* 2001

This reference indicates that in the ***CPT Changes: An Insider's View*** 2001 edition, there is material that will assist you in understanding the application of this code.

Understand the changes to *CPT® 2008* in detail and code accurately

An indispensable guide for CPT® Professional users.
CPT® Changes: An Insider's View provides the official AMA interpretations and explanations for each CPT code and

guideline change in the *CPT 2008* codebook. Every new, revised, or deleted code, text and guideline change is listed along with a detailed rationale for the change.

Organized by CPT® code section and code number, just like the CPT® Professional book.

Detailed rationales provide an explanation as to why the code change(s) occurred.

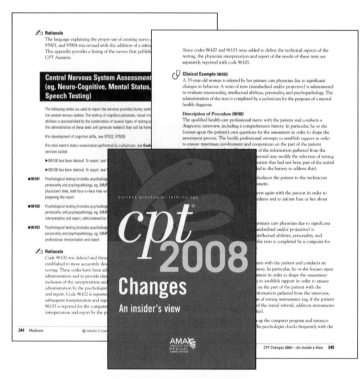

"At-a-glance" tabular review of 2008 code, text and guideline changes.

Useful clinical examples and procedural descriptions are presented to help you understand the practical application for that code.

Order the 2008 edition today! Call (800) 621-8335

Order #: OP512908CCW   Price: $65.95   AMA member price: $46.95

CPT® Changes Archives 2000–2008

Access current and historical CPT® code and guideline changes on your computer desktop. An invaluable electronic library, use it to search past and present editions of the AMA's best-selling *CPT® Changes: An Insider's View* by keyword, phase, CPT code number, edition and CPT codebook table of

contents. Also included is a complete historical CPT code list from 1990–2008, that references when a code was added, deleted, and/or revised.

CD-ROM, Shipping included
Order #: OP133308CCW (single user license fee)
Price: $184.95   AMA member price: $144.95
Purchase includes free *CPT Changes 2008* book!
For system requirements or multi-user pricing call Customer Service at (800) 621-8335.

AMA
AMERICAN
MEDICAL
ASSOCIATION

current procedural terminology

cpt® 2008

Professional Edition

Michael Beebe
Joyce A. Dalton
Martha Espronceda, AAS
Desiree D. Evans, AAS
Rejina L. Glenn
Gloria Green, BA
DeHandro Hayden, BS

Anita Majerowicz, MS, RHIA
Janette Meggs, RHIA
Marie L. Mindeman, BA, RHIT
Karen E. O'Hara, BS, CCS-P
Mary R. O'Heron, RHIA, CCS-P
Danielle Pavloski, BS, RHIT, CCS-P
Dan Reyes

Desiree Rozell, MPA
Lianne Stancik, RHIT
Peggy Thompson, MS, RHIA, CCS
Susan Tracy, MA, RHIT
Jennifer Trajkovski, MJ, RHIT
Ada Walker, CCA

AMA
AMERICAN
MEDICAL
ASSOCIATION

Executive Vice President, Chief Executive Officer: Michael D. Maves, MD, MBA
Chief Operating Officer: Bernard L. Hengesbaugh
Senior Vice President, Publishing and Business Services: Robert A. Musacchio, PhD
Vice President, Business Products: Anthony J. Frankos
Director, Editorial and Operations: Mary Lou White
Senior Acquisitions Editor: Elise Schumacher
Director of Marketing, Business Marketing and Communication: Pam Palmersheim
Director of Sales, Business Products: J.D. Kinney
Director, Production and Manufacturing: Jean Roberts
Manager, Marketing and Strategic Planning: Erin Kalitowski
Developmental Editor: Carol Brockman
Senior Production Coordinator: Rosalyn Carlton
Senior Production Coordinator: Boon Ai Tan
Senior Print Coordinator: Ronnie Summers
Marketing Manager: Leigh Bottiger

Professional ISBN: 1-57947-791-7
Professional ISBN: 978-1-57947-940-4
ISSN: 0276-8283

1st Edition printed 1966
2nd Edition printed 1970
3rd Edition printed 1973
4th Edition printed 1977
Revised: 1978, 1979, 1980, 1981, 1982, 1984, 1985, 1986,
1987, 1988, 1989, 1990, 1991, 1992, 1993, 1994, 1995, 1996,
1997, 1998, 1999, 2000, 2001, 2002, 2003, 2004, 2005, 2006, 2007

To purchase additional CPT products, contact the American Medical Association Customer Service
at 800 621-8335.

To request a license for distribution of products containing or reprinting CPT codes and/or guidelines,
please see our Web site at *www.ama-assn.org/go/cpt* or contact the American Medical Association CPT
Intellectual Property Services, 515 N. State Street, Chicago, Illinois 60610, 312 464-5022.

AC36:EP054108:10/07

Foreword

Current Procedural Terminology, (CPT®) Fourth Edition, is a listing of descriptive terms and identifying codes for reporting medical services and procedures performed by physicians. The purpose of the terminology is to provide a uniform language that will accurately describe medical, surgical, and diagnostic services, and will thereby provide an effective means for reliable nationwide communication among physicians, patients, and third parties. *CPT 2008* is the most recent revision of a work that first appeared in 1966.

CPT descriptive terms and identifying codes currently serve a wide variety of important functions in the field of medical nomenclature. The CPT codebook is useful for administrative management purposes such as claims processing and for the development of guidelines for medical care review. The uniform language is also applicable to medical education and outcomes, health services, and quality research by providing a useful basis for local, regional, and national utilization comparisons. The CPT codebook is the most widely accepted nomenclature for the reporting of physician procedures and services under government and private health insurance programs. In 2000, the CPT code set was designated by the Department of Health and Human Services as the national coding standard for physician and other health care professional services and procedures under the Health Insurance Portability and Accountability Act (HIPAA). This means that for all financial and administrative health care transactions sent electronically, the CPT code set will need to be used.

The changes that appear in this revision have been prepared by the CPT Editorial Panel with the assistance of physicians representing all specialties of medicine, and with important contributions from many third-party payers and governmental agencies.

The American Medical Association trusts that this revision will continue the usefulness of its predecessors in identifying, describing, and coding medical, surgical, and diagnostic services.

Michael D. Maves, MD, MBA
Executive Vice President, CEO

Acknowledgments

Publication of the annual CPT codebook represents many challenges and opportunities. From reconciling the many differences of opinion about the best way to describe a procedure, to the last details on placement of a semicolon, many individuals and organizations devote their energies and expertise to the preparation of this revision.

The editorial staff wishes to express sincere thanks to the many national medical specialty societies, health insurance organizations and agencies, and individual physicians and other health professionals who have made contributions.

Thanks are due to Robert A. Musacchio, PhD, Sr VP, American Medical Association; Claudia Bonnell, Blue Cross and Blue Shield Association; Nelly Leon-Chisen, American Hospital Association; Jeannette Thornton, America's Health Insurance Plans; and Sue Bowman, RHIA, American Health Information Management Association, for their invaluable assistance in enhancing the CPT code set.

For their assistance in development of the CPT Category II codes:

Ronald A. Gabel, MD
Darryl T. Gray, MD, ScD
Peter A. Hollmann, MD
Susan M. Nedza, MD
Gregory Pawlson, MD, MPH
Sylvia Publ, RHIA, MBA
Phil Renner, MBA
Sam J. W. Romeo, MD, MBA
Paul M. Schyve, MD
Sharon Sprenger, RHIA, PHQ, MPA
Sally Turbyville, MA

We recognize the following people for efforts in working with the Physician Consortium for Performance Improvement and other quality measurement organizations:

Karen S. Kmetick, PhD
Mark Antman, DDS, MBA
Heidi Bossley, MSN, MBA
Joseph Gave, MPH
Kendra Hanley, MS, CHE
Erin Kaleba, MPH
Beth Tapper, MA, MPH
Samantha Tierney, MPH

AMA CPT Editorial Panel

Chair
Tracy R. Gordy, MD*
Vice-Chair
William T. Thorwarth, Jr, MD*
Joel F. Bradley, Jr, MD
Kenneth P. Brin, MD, PhD† (6/06)
Patrick J. Cafferty, MPAS, PA-C
Helene M. Fearon, PT*
Robert S. Haskey, MD† (11/06)
Samuel Hassenbusch III, MD, PhD
M. Bradford Henley, MD, MBA
Lee Harold Hilborne, MD, MPH
Peter A. Hollmann, MD
Andrea H. McGuire, MD
Bernard M. Rosof, MD, MACP
Kenneth B. Simon, MD, MBA*
Stanley W. Stead, MD, MBA*
J. Martin Tucker, MD
Richard W. Waguespack, MD

Secretary
Michael Beebe
*Member of the CPT Executive Committee
†New Panel Member June 2006 and November 2006
‡New Advisors

AMA CPT Advisory Committee

American Academy of Allergy, Asthma and Immunology
Donald W. Aaronson, MD, JD, MPH
American Academy of Child & Adolescent Psychiatry
David I. Berland, MD
American Academy of Dermatology Association
Dirk M. Elston, MD
American Academy of Facial Plastic and Reconstructive Surgery
Mark V. Connelly, MD
Edward H. Farrior, MD, FACS‡
American Academy of Family Physicians
David A. Ellington, MD
American Academy of Neurology
Marc Nuwer, MD, PhD
American Academy of Ophthalmology
Michael X. Repka, MD
American Academy of Orthopaedic Surgeons
Richard J. Friedman, MD, FACSC‡
American Academy of Otolaryngic Allergy
Harold R. Wright, Jr, MD
American Academy of Otolaryngology-Head and Neck Surgery
Joseph E. Leonard, MD, FACS
American Academy of Pain Medicine
Eduardo M. Fraifeld, MD
American Academy of Pediatrics
Richard A. Molteni, MD
American Academy of Physical Medicine and Rehabilitation
Francis P. Lagattuta, MD
American Academy of Sleep Medicine
Samuel A. Fleishman, MD
American Association for Clinical Chemistry
Robert L. Murray, JD, PhD‡
American Association for Thoracic Surgery
Kirk R. Kanter, MD
American Association of Clinical Endocrinologists
Eric A. Orzeck, MD, FACP, FACE

American Association of Hip and Knee Surgeons
Richard Iorio, MD‡
American Association of Neurological Surgeons
Jeffrey Cozzens, MD, FACS
American Association of Neuromuscular Electrodiagnostic Medicine
Kyle W. Ruffing, MD
American Association of Public Health Physicians
Arvind K. Goyal, MD, MPH, FAAEP, FACPM
American Clinical Neurophysiology Society
Marc Nuwer, MD, PhD
American College of Allergy, Asthma and Immunology
Gary N. Gross, MD
American College of Cardiology
Diane E. Wallis, MD, FACC
American College of Chest Physicians
Steve G. Peters, MD
American College of Emergency Physicians
Kenneth L. DeHart, MD, FACEP
American College of Gastroenterology
Robert B. Cameron, MD
American College of Medical Genetics
David B. Flannery, MD
American College of Medical Quality
Joel Grossman, MD
American College of Nuclear Physicians
Gary L. Dillehay, MD, FACNP, FACR
American College of Obstetricians and Gynecologists
Jordan G. Pritzker, MD, MBA, FACOG
American College of Occupational and Environmental Medicine
Elizabeth Genovese, MD, MBA
American College of Physicians
H. Christopher Alexander III, MD, MACR, FACP
R. Scott Hanson, MD, MPH‡
American College of Preventive Medicine
Fred T. Nobrega, MD
Ryung Suh, MD, MPP, MBA, MPH‡
American College of Radiation Oncology
Thomas J. Weatherall, Jr, MD
American College of Radiology
Richard Duszak, Jr, MD
American College of Rheumatology
Robert J. Lloyd, MD, FACR
American College of Surgeons
Albert E. Bothe, Jr, MD, FACS
American Dental Association
Anthony M. Spina, DDS, MD‡
American Gastroenterological Association
Joel V. Brill, MD, AGAF, FASGE, FACG, CHCQM
American Geriatric Society
Robert A. Zorowitz, MD, MBA
American Institute of Ultrasound in Medicine
Harvey L. Nisenbaum, MD
American Medical Directors Association
Dennis L. Stone, MD, MBA
American Medical Group Association
David E. Hooper, MD
American Orthopaedic Association
Blair C. Filler, MD
American Orthopaedic Foot and Ankle Society
Walter J. Pedowitz, MD
American Osteopathic Association
Boyd R. Buser, DO, FACOFP
American Pediatric Surgical Association
John P. Crow, MD

American Psychiatric Association
Chester W. Schmidt, Jr, MD
David K. Nace, MD‡
American Society for Aesthetic Plastic Surgery, Inc.
Paul R. Weiss, MD
American Society for Clinical Pathology
Mark S. Synovec, MD
Lee H. Hilborne, MD, MPH‡
American Society for Dermatologic Surgery
Pamela K. Phillips, MD
American Society for Gastrointestinal Endoscopy
Glenn D. Littenberg, MD‡
American Society for Reproductive Medicine
John T. Queenan, Jr, MD
American Society for Surgery of the Hand
Daniel J. Nagle, MD
American Society for Therapeutic Radiology and Oncology
Michael L. Steinberg, MD, FACR
American Society of Abdominal Surgeons
Louis F. Alfano, Jr, MD
American Society of Anesthesiologists
H. J. Przybylo, Jr, MD
Douglas G. Merrill, MD‡
American Society of Bariatric Physicians
Mary C. Vernon, MD
American Society of Cataract and Refractive Surgery
Stephen S. Lane, MD
American Society of Clinical Oncology
William C. Penley, MD
American Society of Colon and Rectal Surgeons
Guy R. Orangio, MD, FACS, FASCRS
American Society of Cytopathology
Patricia A. Gregg, MD, FCAP
American Society of General Surgeons
Charles Drueck III, MD, FACS
American Society of Hematology
Samuel M. Silver, MD, PhD, FACP, FAHA
American Society of Neuroimaging
Mircea A. Morariu, Jr, MD
American Society of Neuroradiology
Robert A. Murray, MD
C. Douglas Phillips, MD, FACR‡
American Society of Ophthalmic Plastic and Reconstructive Surgery
L. Neal Freeman, MD, MBA, CCS-P, FACS
American Society of Plastic Surgeons
Raymond V. Janevicius, MD
American Thoracic Society
Stephen P. Hoffmann, MD
American Urological Association
Jeffrey A. Dann, MD, MBA
Association of University Radiologists
Bob W. Gayler, MD
College of American Pathologists
James P. Almas, MD, FCAP
Congress of Neurological Surgeons
R. Patrick Jacob, MD
Contact Lens Association of Ophthalmologists
Charles B. Slonim, MD, FACS
Infectious Disease Society of America
Lawrence P. Martinelli, MD
International Spinal Injection Society
Claire Tibiletti, MD
National Association of Medical Examiners
Paul A. Raslavicus, MD, MHA, CPE
North American Spine Society
William Mitchell, MD
Radiological Society of North America
Richard E. Fulton, MD

Renal Physicians Association
Richard J. Hamburger, MD
Society for Investigative Dermatology
Stephen P. Stone, MD
Society for Vascular Surgery
Anton N. Sidawy, MD, MPH
Society of American Gastrointestinal Endoscopic Surgeons
Paresh C. Shah, MD
Society of Critical Care Medicine
George A. Sample, MD, FCCP
Society of Nuclear Medicine
Kenneth A. McKusick, MD
Society of Thoracic Surgeons
Cameron D. Wright, MD
The Academy of Pharamaceutical Physicians and Investigators
Grant P. Bagley, MD
The Endocrine Society
Richard A. Guthrie, MD
The Society of Interventional Radiology
Katharine L. Krol, MD
The Triological Society
James H. Kelly, MD
United States and Canadian Academy of Pathology
David S. Wilkinson, MD, PhD

AMA Health Care Professionals Advisory Committee (HCPAC)

Tracy R. Gordy, MD, Co-Chair
AMA CPT Editorial Panel
Helene Fearon, PT, Co-Chair
AMA CPT Editorial Panel
American Academy of Physician Assistants
Terry E. Carlisle, PA-C, MPAS
American Association of Naturopathic Physicians
Wendell B. Milliman, ND
American Association for Respiratory Care
Susan Rinaldo-Gallo, Med, RRT
American Chiropractic Association
Craig S. Little, DC, FACO
American Dietetic Association
Keith Thomas-Ayoob, EdD, RD, FADA, CSP
American Massage Therapy Association
Whitney W. Lowe
Susan B. Rosen‡
American Nurses Association
David Keepnews, PhD, JD, RN
American Occupational Therapy Association
Leslie F. Davidson, MS, Ed, OTR/L
American Optometric Association
Douglas C. Morrow, OD
Pharmacist Services Technical Advisory Coalition
Daniel E. Buffington, PharmD, MBA
American Physical Therapy Association
Paul A. Rockar, Jr, PT, MS
American Podiatric Medical Association
Michael J. King, DPM
American Psychological Association
Antonio E. Puente, PhD
American Speech-Language Hearing Association
R. Wayne Holland, EdD
National Athletic Trainers' Association
J. David Jones, MSHA, MS, ATC‡
National Association of Social Workers
Nelda Spyres, ACSW, LCSW
National Society of Genetic Counselors
Debra L. Doyle, MS, CGC

Stedman's CPT® Dictionary

Understanding medical definitions can be one of the biggest struggles a coding or reimbursement professional can face. Confusion often surrounds the process of reconciling differences between physician's notes and terminology used in CPT® code descriptions. Now, you can end the guesswork of code assignment by truly understanding CPT code descriptions. In conjunction with the best-selling *Stedman's Medical Dictionary*, the AMA's CPT® experts have developed a reference aimed at reducing this frustration – *Stedman's CPT® Dictionary*.

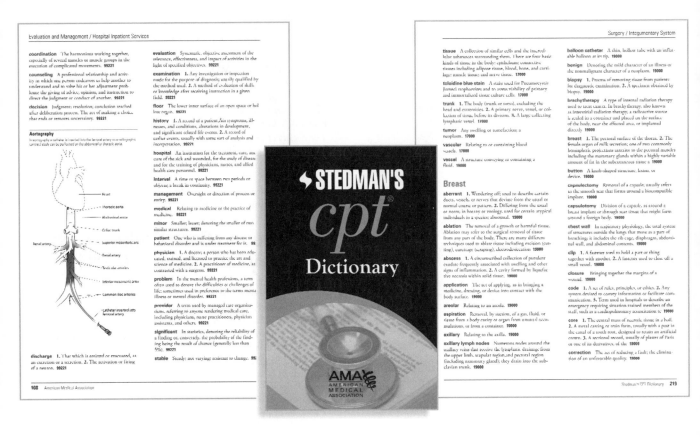

This new reference contains definitions of medical terms found within the CPT codebook descriptions. Definitions are organized by CPT section, giving the user the context to further understand the meaning behind these descriptions. This reference was designed for side-by-side usage with the AMA CPT codebook in an effort to clear confusion surrounding complicated medical terms.

Stedman's CPT® Dictionary also contains other information critical for medical understanding, including eponym, abbreviation, and medical terminology appendixes. Illustrations from *Stedman's Medical Dictionary* are also included to supplement definitions and further understanding.

Available December 2007
Order #: OP300607
Price: $124.95

ISBN: 978-1-57947-882-7
AMA member price: $94.95

To order, call **(800) 621-8335** or go to *www.amabookstore.com*

AMA
AMERICAN
MEDICAL
ASSOCIATION

Contents

Contents

Introduction

Current Procedural Terminology (CPT®), Fourth Edition, is a set of codes, descriptions, and guidelines intended to describe procedures and services performed by physicians and other health care providers. Each procedure or service is identified with a five-digit code. The use of CPT codes simplifies the reporting of services.

Inclusion of a descriptor and its associated five-digit code number in the CPT codebook is based on whether the procedure is consistent with contemporary medical practice and is performed by many practitioners in clinical practice in multiple locations. Inclusion in the CPT codebook does not represent endorsement by the American Medical Association (AMA) of any particular diagnostic or therapeutic procedure. Inclusion or exclusion of a procedure does not imply any health insurance coverage or reimbursement policy.

The CPT code set is published annually in the late summer or early fall as both electronic data files and books. The release of CPT data files on the Internet typically precedes the book by several weeks. In any case, January 1 is the effective date for use of the update of the CPT code set. The interval between the release of the update and the effective date is considered the implementation period and is intended to allow physicians and other providers, payers, and vendors to incorporate CPT changes into their systems. The exceptions to this schedule of release and effective dates are CPT Category III and vaccine product codes, which are released twice a year on January 1 or July 1 with effective dates for use six months later, and CPT Category II codes.

The main body of the material is listed in six sections. Each section is divided into subsections with anatomic, procedural, condition, or descriptor subheadings. The procedures and services with their identifying codes are presented in numeric order with one exception—the entire **Evaluation and Management** section (99201-99499) appears at the beginning of the listed procedures. These items are used by most physicians in reporting a significant portion of their services.

Section Numbers and Their Sequences

Category I

Evaluation and Management 99201-99499
Anesthesiology 00100-01999, 99100-99140
Surgery 10021-69990
Radiology (Including Nuclear Medicine and Diagnostic Ultrasound) .70010-79999
Pathology and Laboratory 80048-89356
Medicine
   (except Anesthesiology) . . 90281-99199, 99500-99602

Category II 0001F-6020F
Category III 0016T-0183T

The first and last code numbers and the subsection name of the items appear at the top margin of most pages (eg, "11010-11306 Surgery/Integumentary System"). The continuous pagination of the CPT codebook is found on the lower margin of each page along with explanation of any code symbols that are found on that page.

Instructions for Use of the CPT Codebook

Select the name of the procedure or service that accurately identifies the service performed. Do not select a CPT code that merely approximates the service provided. If no such specific code exists, then report the service using the appropriate unlisted procedure or service code. In surgery, it may be an operation; in medicine, a diagnostic or therapeutic procedure; in radiology, a radiograph. Other additional procedures performed or pertinent special services are also listed. When necessary, any modifying or extenuating circumstances are added. Any service or procedure should be adequately documented in the medical record.

It is important to recognize that the listing of a service or procedure and its code number in a specific section of this book does not restrict its use to a specific specialty group. Any procedure or service in any section of this book may be used to designate the services rendered by any qualified physician or other qualified health care professional.

Instructions, typically included as parenthetical notes with selected codes, indicate that a code should not be reported with another code or codes. These instructions are intended to prevent errors of significant probability and are not all inclusive. For example, the code with such instructions may be a component of another code and therefore it would be incorrect to report both codes even when the component service is performed. These instructions are not intended as a listing of all possible code combinations that should not be reported, nor to indicate all possible code combinations that are appropriately reported. When reporting codes for services provided, it is important to assure the accuracy and quality of coding through verification of the intent of the code by use of the related guidelines, parenthetical instructions, and coding resources, including *CPT Assistant* and other publications resulting from collaborative efforts of the American Medical Association with the medical specialty societies (ie, *Clinical Examples in Radiology*).

Format of the Terminology

The CPT code set has been developed as stand-alone descriptions of medical procedures. However, some of the procedures in the CPT codebook are not printed in their entirety but refer back to a common portion of the procedure listed in a preceding entry. This is evident when an entry is followed by one or more indentations. This is done in an effort to conserve space.

Example

25100	Arthrotomy, wrist joint; with biopsy
25105	with synovectomy

Note that the common part of code 25100 (the part before the semicolon) should be considered part of code 25105. Therefore, the full procedure represented by code 25105 should read:

25105	Arthrotomy, wrist joint; with synovectomy

Requests to Update the CPT Nomenclature

The effectiveness of the CPT nomenclature depends on constant updating to reflect changes in medical practice. This can only be accomplished through the interest and timely suggestions of practicing physicians, medical specialty societies, state medical associations, and other organizations and agencies. Accordingly, the AMA welcomes correspondence, inquiries, and suggestions concerning old and new procedures, as well as other matters such as codes and indices.

To submit a suggestion to add, delete, or revise procedures contained in the CPT codebook, please contact:

CPT Editorial Research & Development
American Medical Association
515 North State Street
Chicago, Illinois 60610

Coding change request forms are available at the AMA's CPT Web site: www.ama-assn.org/ama/pub/category/3866.html.

All proposed changes of the CPT codebook will be considered by the CPT Editorial Panel with consultation of appropriate medical specialty societies.

Guidelines

Specific guidelines are presented at the beginning of each of the six sections. These guidelines define items that are necessary to appropriately interpret and report the procedures and services contained in that section. For example, in the **Medicine** section, specific instructions are provided for handling unlisted services or procedures, special reports, and supplies and materials provided. Guidelines also provide explanations regarding terms that apply only to a particular section. For instance, **Radiology Guidelines** provide a definition of the unique term, "radiological supervision and interpretation." While in **Anesthesia,** a discussion of reporting time is included.

Add-on Codes

Some of the listed procedures are commonly carried out in addition to the primary procedure performed. These additional or supplemental procedures are designated as add-on codes with the symbol ✚ and they are listed in **Appendix D** of the CPT codebook. Add-on codes in *CPT 2008* can be readily identified by specific descriptor nomenclature that includes phrases such as "each additional" or "(List separately in addition to primary procedure)."

The add-on code concept in *CPT 2008* applies only to add-on procedures or services performed by the same physician. Add-on codes describe additional intra-service work associated with the primary procedure, eg, additional digit(s), lesion(s), neurorrhaphy(s), vertebral segment(s), tendon(s), joint(s).

Add-on codes are always performed in addition to the primary service or procedure and must never be reported as a stand-alone code. All add-on codes found in the CPT codebook are exempt from the multiple procedure concept (see the modifier 51 definition in **Appendix A**).

Modifiers

A modifier provides the means to report or indicate that a service or procedure that has been performed has been altered by some specific circumstance but not changed in its definition or code. Modifiers also enable health care professionals to effectively respond to payment policy requirements established by other entities. The judicious application of modifiers obviates the necessity for separate procedure listings that may describe the modifying circumstance. Modifiers may be used to indicate to the recipient of a report that:

- A service or procedure had both a professional and technical component.
- A service or procedure was performed by more than one physician and/or in more than one location.
- A service or procedure was increased or reduced.
- Only part of a service was performed.
- An adjunctive service was performed.
- A bilateral procedure was performed.
- A service or procedure was provided more than once.
- Unusual events occurred.

Example

A physician providing diagnostic or therapeutic radiology services, ultrasound, or nuclear medicine services in a hospital would add modifier 26 to report the professional component.

73090 with modifier 26 = Professional component only for an X ray of the forearm

Example

Two surgeons may be required to manage a specific surgical problem. When two surgeons work together as primary surgeons performing distinct part(s) of a procedure, each surgeon should report his/her distinct operative work by adding modifier 62 to the procedure code and any associated code(s) for that procedure as long as both surgeons continue to work together as primary surgeons. Each surgeon should report the co-surgery once using the same procedure code. Modifier 62 would be applicable. For instance, a neurological surgeon and an otolaryngologist are working as co-surgeons in performing transphenoidal excision of a pituitary neoplasm.

The first surgeon would report:

61548 62 = Hypophysectomy or excision of pituitary tumor, transnasal or transseptal approach, nonstereotactic + two surgeons modifier

AND the second surgeon would report:

61548 62 = Hypophysectomy or excision of pituitary tumor, transnasal or transseptal approach, nonstereotactic + two surgeons modifier

If additional procedure(s) (including add-on procedure[s]) are performed during the same surgical session, separate code(s) may also be reported with modifier 62 added. It should be noted that if a co-surgeon acts as an assistant in the performance of additional procedure(s) during the same surgical session, those services may be reported using separate procedure code(s) with modifier 80 or modifier 82 added, as appropriate. A complete listing of modifiers is found in **Appendix A**.

Place of Service and Facility Reporting

Some codes have specified places of service (eg, evaluation and management codes are specific to a setting). Other services and procedures may have instructions specific to the place of service (eg, therapeutic, prophylactic, and diagnostic injections and infusions). The CPT code set is designated for reporting physician and qualified health care professional services. It is also the designated code set for reporting services by organizational or facility providers (eg, hospitals) in specific circumstances. Facilities are entities that may report services in addition to the physician or qualified health care professional for the same service. For example, a physician may report a procedure performed in the outpatient department of the hospital and the hospital may report the same procedure. The CPT codebook uses the term *facility* to describe such providers and the term *nonfacility* to describe services where no facility reporting may occur. Services provided in the home by an agency are facility services. Services provided in the home by a physician or qualified health care professional who is not a representative of the agency are nonfacility services.

Unlisted Procedure or Service

It is recognized that there may be services or procedures performed by physicians that are not found in the CPT codebook. Therefore, a number of specific code numbers have been designated for reporting unlisted procedures. When an unlisted procedure number is used, the service or procedure should be described. Each of these unlisted procedural code numbers (with the appropriate accompanying topical entry) relates to a specific section of the book and is presented in the guidelines of that section.

Results, Testing, Interpretation, and Report

Results are the technical component of a service. Testing leads to results; results lead to interpretation. Reports are the work product of the interpretation of test results. Certain procedures or services described in the CPT codebook involve a technical component (eg, tests), which produce results (eg, data, images, slides). For clinical use, some of these results require interpretation. Some CPT descriptors specifically require interpretation and reporting to report that code.

Special Report

A service that is rarely provided, unusual, variable, or new may require a special report in determining medical appropriateness of the service. Pertinent information should include an adequate definition or description of the nature, extent, and need for the procedure and the time, effort, and equipment necessary to provide the service. Additional items may include complexity of symptoms, final diagnosis, pertinent physical findings, diagnostic and therapeutic procedures, concurrent problems, and follow-up care.

Code Symbols

A summary listing of additions, deletions, and revisions applicable to the CPT codebook is found in **Appendix B**. New procedure numbers added to the CPT codebook are identified throughout the text with the symbol ● placed before the code number. In instances where a code revision has resulted in a substantially altered procedure descriptor, the symbol ▲ is placed before the code number. The symbols ► ◄ are used to indicate new and revised text other than the procedure descriptors. These symbols indicate CPT Editorial Panel actions. The AMA reserves the right to correct typographical errors and make stylistic improvements. CPT add-on codes are annotated by the symbol ✚ and are listed in **Appendix D**. The symbol ⊘ is used to identify codes that are exempt from the use of modifier 51 but have not been designated as CPT add-on procedures or services. A list of codes exempt from modifier 51 usage is included in **Appendix E**. The symbol ⊙ is used to identify codes that include moderate sedation (see **Appendix G**). The symbol ∕ is used to identify codes for vaccines that are pending FDA approval (see **Appendix K**).

Alphabetical Reference Index

This codebook features an expanded alphabetical index that includes listings by procedure and anatomic site. Procedures and services commonly known by their eponyms or other designations are also included.

CPT 2008 in Electronic Formats

CPT 2008 procedure codes and descriptions are available on CD-ROM as data files and electronic software. Data files are available in ASCII and EBCDIC formats and can be imported into any billing and claims reporting software that accepts a text (TXT) file format. *CPT 2008 Electronic Professional* software, now with *Netter's Atlas of Human Anatomy for CPT Coding*, provides access to the entire *CPT 2008 Professional Edition* codebook on your desktop. Easy-to-use and fully searchable, this invaluable software contains all of the favorite *CPT Professional* features plus CPT codes and quick linking access between CPT codes, guidelines, modifiers, appendixes, index, and more. For more information call (800) 621-8335 or visit *www.amabookstore.com*.

References to AMA Resources

The symbols ⮞ and ⮞ appear after many codes throughout this codebook and indicate that the AMA has published reference material regarding that particular code.

The symbol ⮞ refers to the *CPT Assistant* monthly newsletter and *CPT Changes: An Insider's View*, an annual book with all of the coding changes for the current year. The symbol ⮞ refers to the quarterly newsletter *Clinical Examples in Radiology*.

Example

36569   age 5 years or older

> ⮞ *CPT Assistant* Oct 04:4, Dec 04:8; *CPT Changes: An Insider's View* 2004

> ⮞ *Clinical Examples in Radiology* Inaugural 04:1-2

(For placement of centrally inserted non-tunneled central venous catheter, without subcutaneous port or pump, age 5 years or older, use 36556)

In this example, the green reference sysmbol indicates that in two issues of *CPT Assistant* (October 2004, page 4, and December 2004, page 8) and in the 2004 edition of *CPT Changes: An Insider's View* material is available that may assist in understanding the application of the code. The red reference symbol indicates that the 2004 Inaugural issue of *Clinical Examples in Radiology* (pages 1-2) should be consulted.

Subscriptions to *CPT Assistant* and *Clinical Examples in Radiology* can be purchased by calling the AMA's Unified Service Center at (800) 621-8335. Individual back issues are available for purchase and immediate download at *www.amabookstore.com*.

An archive software product with every issue of *CPT Assistant* is also available. *CPT Assistant Archives 1990-2007* (available February 2007) provides convenient access to 18 years of *CPT Assistant* newsletter articles on your desktop. Search past issues of the AMA's authoritative coding newsletter by keyword, phrase, CPT code number, newsletter issue, article index, or codebook table of contents. This product offers simple search capabilities and a complete historical CPT code list from 1990-2007 that references when a code was added, deleted, and/or revised. Call (800) 621-8335 or visit *www.amabookstore.com* for more information.

Current and past editions of *CPT Changes: An Insider's View* can be purchased by calling the AMA's Unified Service Center at (800) 621-8335 or visiting *www.amabookstore.com*.

Additionally, an archives software product with all content from past and present editions of *CPT Changes: An Insider's View* is available. *CPT Changes Archives 2000-2008* provides access to current and historical CPT code and guideline changes on your computer desktop. Search by keyword, phrase, CPT code number, edition, and CPT codebook table of contents. For more information, call (800) 621-8335 or visit *www.amabookstore.com*.

Illustrated Anatomical and Procedural Review

It is essential that coders have a thorough understanding of medical terminology and anatomy to code accurately. The following section reviewing the basics of vocabulary and anatomy can be used as a quick reference to help you with your coding. It is not intended as a replacement for up-to-date medical dictionaries and anatomy texts, which are essential tools for accurate coding.

Prefixes, Suffixes, and Roots

Although medical terminology may seem complex, many medical terms can be broken into component parts, which makes them easier to understand. Many of these terms are derived from Latin or Greek words, but some include the names of physicians.

Prefixes are word parts that appear at the beginning of a word and modify its meaning; suffixes are found at the end of words. By learning what various prefixes and suffixes mean, it is possible to decipher the meaning of a word quickly. The following lists are a quick reference for some common prefixes and suffixes.

Numbers

Prefix	Meaning	Example
mono-, uni-	one	monocyte, unilateral
bi-	two	bilateral
tri-	three	triad
quadr-	four	quadriplegia
hex-, sex-	six	hexose
diplo-	double	diplopia

Surgical Procedures

Suffix	Meaning	Example
-centesis	puncture a cavity to remove fluid	amniocentesis
-ectomy	surgical removal (excision)	appendectomy
-ostomy	a new permanent opening	colostomy
-otomy	cutting into (incision)	tracheotomy
-orrhaphy	surgical repair/suture	herniorrhaphy
-opexy	surgical fixation	nephropexy
-oplasty	surgical repair	rhinoplasty
-otripsy	crushing, destroying	lithotripsy

Conditions

Prefix	Meaning	Example
ambi-	both	ambidextrous
aniso-	unequal	anisocoria
dys-	bad, painful, difficult	dysphoria
eu-	good, normal	euthanasia
hetero-	different	heterogeneous
homo-	same	homogeneous
hyper-	excessive, above	hypergastric
hypo-	deficient, below	hypogastric
iso-	equal, same	isotonic
mal-	bad, poor	malaise
megalo-	large	megalocardia

Conditions (continued)

Suffix	Meaning	Example
-algia	pain	neuralgia
-asthenia	weakness	myasthenia
-emia	blood	anemia
-iasis	condition of	amebiasis
-itis	inflammation	appendicitis
-lysis	destruction, break down	hemolysis
-lytic	destroy, break down	hemolytic
-oid	like	lipoid
-oma	tumor	carcinoma
-opathy	disease of	arthropathy
-orrhagia	hemorrhage	menorrhagia
-orrhea	flow or discharge	amenorrhea
-osis	abnormal condition of	tuberculosis
-paresis	weakness	hemiparesis
-plasia	growth	hyperplasia
-plegia	paralysis	paraplegia
-pnea	breathing	apnea

Directions and Positions

Prefix	Meaning	Example
ab-	away from	abduction
ad-	toward	adduction
ecto, exo-	outside	ectopic, exocrine
endo-	within	endoscope
epi-	upon	epigastric
infra-	below, under	infrastructure
ipsi-	same	ipsilateral
meso-	middle	mesopexy
meta-	after, beyond, transformation	metastasis
peri-	surrounding	pericardium
retro-	behind, back	retroversion
trans-	across, through	transvaginal

Word	Meaning
anterior or ventral	at or near the front surface of the body
posterior or dorsal	at or near the back surface of the body
superior	above
inferior	below
lateral	side

Directions and Positions (continued)

Word	Meaning
distal	farthest from center
proximal	nearest to center
medial	middle
supine	face up or palm up
prone	face down or palm down
sagittal	vertical body plane, divides the body into equal right and left sides
transverse	horizontal body plane, divides the body into top and bottom sections
coronal	vertical body plane, divides the body into front and back sections

Additional References

For best coding results, you will need to use other reference materials in addition to your coding books. These references include a medical dictionary and one or more anatomy books that can be purchased from the American Medical Association by calling 800 621-8335.

Medical Dictionaries

Stedman's CPT® Dictionary
Chicago, IL: American Medical Association, 2007.
OP300607

Merriam-Webster's Medical Desk Dictionary.
Springfield, Mass: Merriam Webster.
OP941493

Stedman's Medical Dictionary. 27th ed.
Baltimore, Md: Williams & Wilkins; 2000.
OP982900

Anatomy References

Kirschner, CG. *Netter's Atlas of Anatomy for CPT® and ICD-9-CM Coding Series: Musculoskeletal.*
Chicago, Ill: American Medical Association; *Coming Soon.*
OP492206

Kirschner, CG. *Netter's Atlas of Human Anatomy for CPT® Coding.*
Chicago, Ill: American Medical Association; 2005.
OP490605

Netter, FH. *Atlas of Human Anatomy.* 3rd ed.
East Hanover, NJ: Novartis; 2003.
OP936798

Lists of Illustrations

To further aid coders in properly assigning CPT codes, the codebook contains a number of anatomical and procedural illustrations.

Anatomical Illustrations

Pages xxiii-xl provide the following 29 anatomical illustrations.

Procedural Illustrations

Procedural illustrations are placed throughout the codebook and are associated with the following specific CPT codes.

CPT Code(s)	Illustration Title
69930	Cochlear Device Implantation
69990	Operating Microscope
72275	Epidurography
75600-75630	Aortography
75660-75680	Angiography, Carotid Artery
75820-75822	Venography
77057	Screening Mammography
91034	Esophageal Acid Reflux Test
91105	Gastric Intubation
92225, 92226	Extended Ophthalmoscopy
92235	Fluoroscein Angiography
92601-92604	A View of the Outer Cochlear Implant
92978	Intravascular Ultrasound (Coronary Vessel or Graft)
92982	Percutaneous Transluminal Coronary Angioplasty (PTCA)
93312-93318	Transesophageal Echocardiography (TEE)
93501	Right Heart Catheterization
93508	Coronary Angiography Without Concomitant Left Heart Catheterization
93510	Left Heart Catheterization
93571	Intravascular Distal Blood Flow Velocity
95951	Electroencephalographic (EEG) Monitoring and Video Recording
97810-97811	Acupuncture, Needle

Figure 1A
Body Planes — 3/4 View

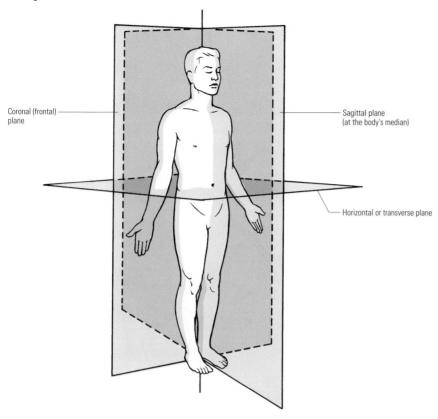

Coronal (frontal) plane

Sagittal plane (at the body's median)

Horizontal or transverse plane

Figure 1B
Body Aspects — Side View

Superior (cranial) aspect

Posterior aspect

Anterior aspect

Dorsal surface of hand

Palmar surface of hand

Dorsal surface of foot

Plantar surface of foot

Inferior aspect

Figure 1C
Body Planes — Front View

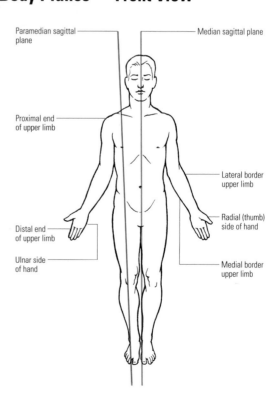

Paramedian sagittal plane

Median sagittal plane

Proximal end of upper limb

Lateral border upper limb

Radial (thumb) side of hand

Distal end of upper limb

Ulnar side of hand

Medial border upper limb

Figure 2
Structure of Skin

Epidermis

Dermis

Subcutaneous
tissue

Hair shaft

Hair root

Sebaceous
gland

Nerve endings

Hair bulb

Sweat gland

Cutaneous
nerve

Blood
vessels

Figure 3
Skeletal System

Skull

Maxilla

Mandible

Cervical vertebra

First rib

Clavicle

Scapula

Sternum

Humerus

Lumbar vertebra

Ilium

Radius

Sacrum

Ulna

Pubis

Ischium

Carpals

Metacarpals

Phalanges

Femur

Patella

Tibia

Fibula

Tarsals

Metatarsals

Phalanges

Figure 4A
Muscular System — Front

Sternocleidomastoid m.
Omohyoid m.
Sternohyoid m.
Trapezius m.
Deltoid m.
Pectoralis major m.
Latissimus dorsi m.
Serratas anterior m.
Oblique external m.
Rectus abdominus m.

Biceps m.
Brachialus m.
Brachioradialus m.
Pronator teres m.
Flexor carpi radialus m.
Palmaris longus m.
Flexor digitorum superficialus m.
Flexor carpi ulnaris m.

Pectineus m.
Adductor longus m.
Adductor magnus m.
Gracilis m.
Sartorius m.
Rectus femoris m.
Vastus medialis m.
Vastus lateralis m.
} Quadriceps

Peroneus longus m.
Tibialis anterior m.
Gastrocnemius m.
Extensor digitorum longus m.
Soleus m.

Figure 4B
Muscular System — Back

Trapezius m.
Deltoid m.
Infraspinatus m.
Teres minor m.
Teres major m.
Triceps m.
Latissimus dorsi m.
Anconeus m.
Extensor carpi radialis longus m.
Flexor carpi ulnaris m.
Extensor carpi radialis brevis m.
Extensor digitorum m.
Extensor carpi ulnaris m.
Abductor pollicis longus m.
Extensor pollicis brevis m.

Gluteus medius m.
Gluteus maximus m.
Adductor magnus m.
Biceps femoris m.
Semitendinosus m.
Gracilis m.
Semimembranosus m.
Vastus lateralis m.
Sartorius m.
Gastrocnemius m.
Peroneus longus m.
Flexor hallicis longus m.

Figure 5
Respiratory System

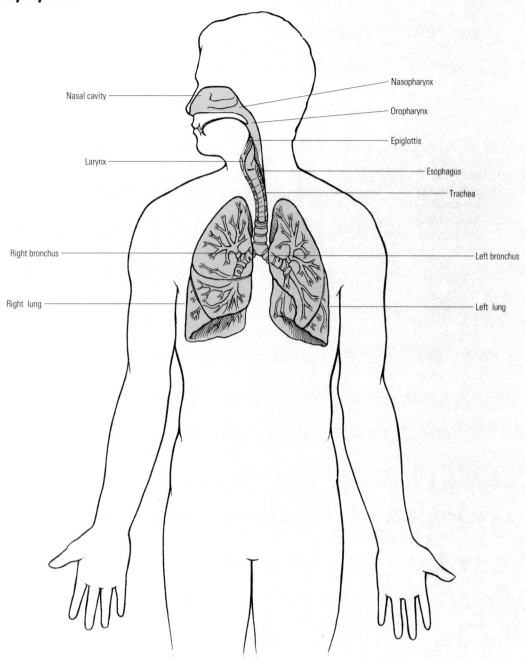

Nasal cavity

Larynx

Right bronchus

Right lung

Nasopharynx

Oropharynx

Epiglottis

Esophagus

Trachea

Left bronchus

Left lung

Figure 6A
Circulatory System — Arteries

Superficial temporal a.
Posterior auricular a.
External carotid a.
Internal carotid a.
Common carotid a.
Vertebral a.
Subclavian a.
Aorta and arch
Brachiocephalic trunk
Pulmonary a.
Axillary a.
Cardiac a.
Deep brachial a.
Thoracic aorta
Brachial a.
Celiac trunk
Aorta
Superior mesenteric a.
Radial a.
Renal a.
Interosseous a.
Gonadal a.
Ulnar a.
Inferior mesenteric a.
Common iliac a.
Deep palmar arch
External iliac a.
Superficial palmar arch
Internal iliac a.
Deep femoral a.
Femoral a.
Descending genicular a.
Popliteal a.
Anterior tibial a.
Peroneal a.
Posterior tibial a.

Figure 6B
Circulatory System — Veins

Superficial temporal v.
Facial v.
External jugular v.
Internal jugular v.
Subclavian v.
Brachiocephalic v.
Axillary v.
Superior vena cava
Brachial v.
Cephalic v.
Basilic v.
Hepatic v.
Median cubital v.
Renal v.
Gonadal v.
Inferior vena cava
Medial antebrachial v.
Common iliac v.
Internal iliac v.
External iliac v.
Superficial venous palmar arch
Deep femoral v.
Femoral v.
Great saphenous v.
Popliteal v.
Small saphenous v.
Anterior tibial v.
Posterior tibial v.
Dorsal venous arch

Figure 7
Lymphatic System

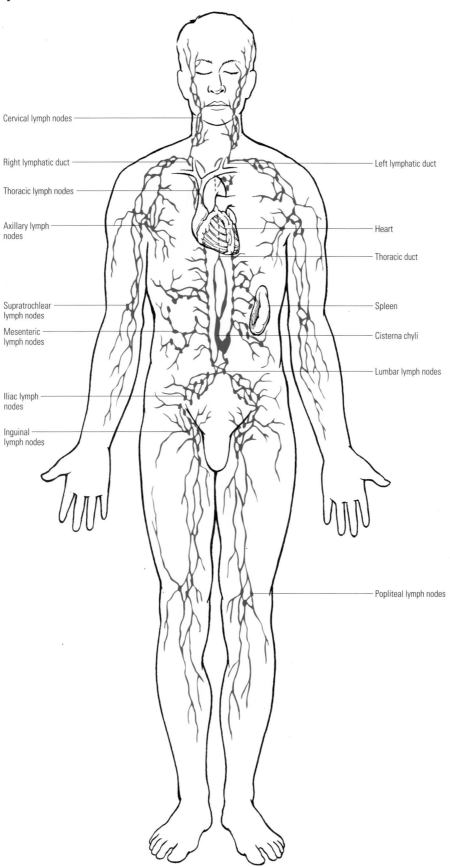

Cervical lymph nodes

Right lymphatic duct

Thoracic lymph nodes

Axillary lymph nodes

Supratrochlear lymph nodes

Mesenteric lymph nodes

Iliac lymph nodes

Inguinal lymph nodes

Left lymphatic duct

Heart

Thoracic duct

Spleen

Cisterna chyli

Lumbar lymph nodes

Popliteal lymph nodes

Figure 8
Digestive System

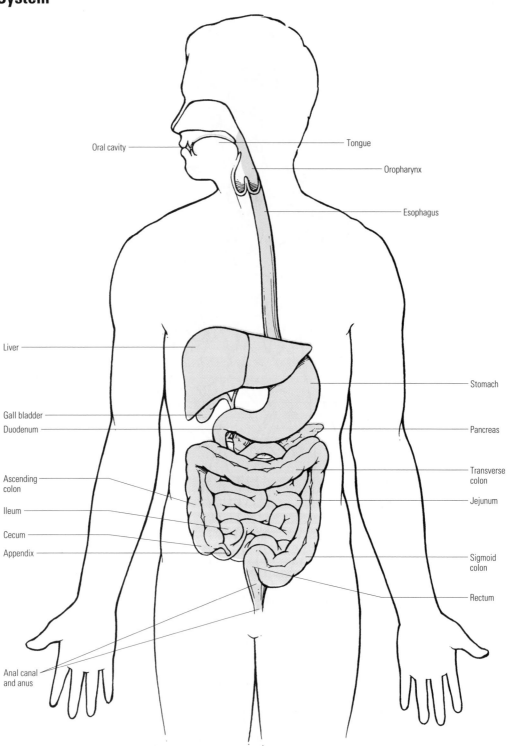

Oral cavity

Tongue

Oropharynx

Esophagus

Liver

Stomach

Gall bladder

Duodenum

Pancreas

Ascending colon

Transverse colon

Ileum

Jejunum

Cecum

Appendix

Sigmoid colon

Rectum

Anal canal and anus

Figure 9
Urinary System

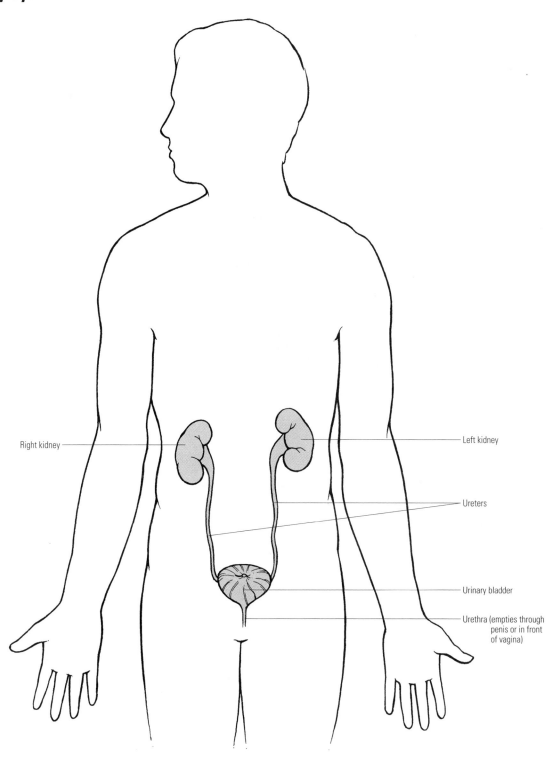

Right kidney

Left kidney

Ureters

Urinary bladder

Urethra (empties through penis or in front of vagina)

Figure 10
Male Genital System

Deferent duct

Urinary bladder and cavity

Corpus cavernosa

Corpus spongiosum

Penis

Glans penis

Prepuce

Seminal vesicle

Ejaculatory duct

Prostate gland

Spermatic cord and deferent duct

Epididymus

Testes

Scrotum

Figure 11
Female Genital System

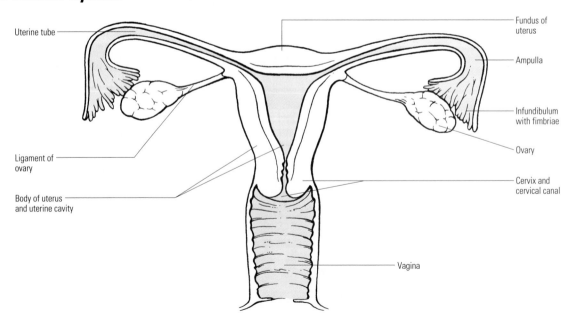

Uterine tube

Ligament of ovary

Body of uterus and uterine cavity

Fundus of uterus

Ampulla

Infundibulum with fimbriae

Ovary

Cervix and cervical canal

Vagina

Figure 12
Endocrine System

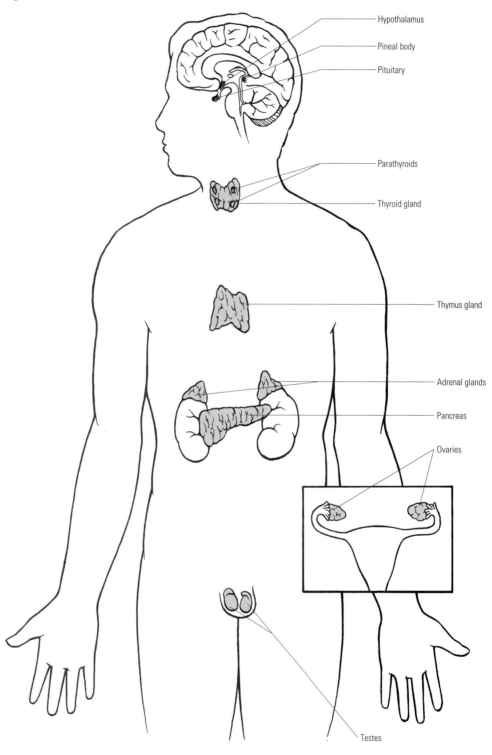

Hypothalamus

Pineal body

Pituitary

Parathyroids

Thyroid gland

Thymus gland

Adrenal glands

Pancreas

Ovaries

Testes

Figure 13
Nervous System

Brain

Cerebellum

Spinal cord

Brachial plexus

Musculocutaneous n.

Radial n.

Intercostal nerves
(with ribs)

Subcostal nerve
(12th thoracic)

Lumbar plexus

Median n.

Iliohypogastric n.

Ilioinguinal n.

Deep branch of radial n.

Lat. femoral cutaneous n.

Genitofemoral n.

Superficial branch of radial n.

Obturator n.

Sacral plexus

Femoral n.

Pudendal n.

Ulnar n.

Sciatic n.

Muscular branches
of femoral n.

Saphenous n.

Common peroneal n.

Tibial n.

Deep peroneal n.

Superficial peroneal n.

Figure 14
Skull

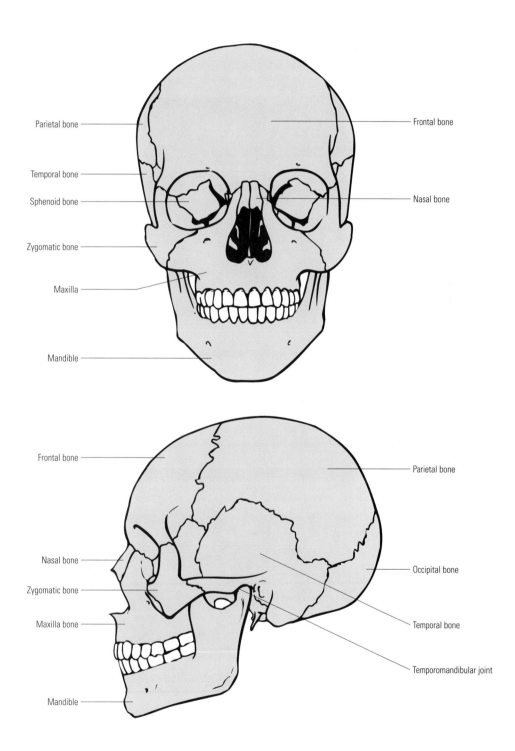

Figure 15
Bones, Muscles, and Tendons of Hand

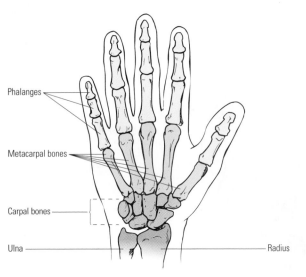

Phalanges

Metacarpal bones

Carpal bones

Ulna

Radius

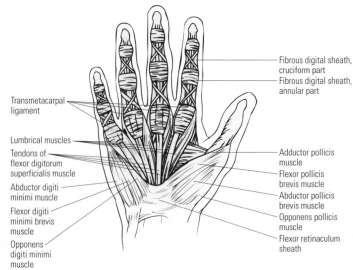

Transmetacarpal ligament

Lumbrical muscles

Tendons of flexor digitorum superficialis muscle

Abductor digiti minimi muscle

Flexor digiti minimi brevis muscle

Opponens digiti minimi muscle

Fibrous digital sheath, cruciform part

Fibrous digital sheath, annular part

Adductor pollicis muscle

Flexor pollicis brevis muscle

Abductor pollicis brevis muscle

Opponens pollicis muscle

Flexor retinaculum sheath

Figure 16
Bones and Muscles of Foot

Phalanges

Metatarsal bones

Tarsal bones

Talus

Calcaneus

Tendon of flexor hallucis longus muscle

Flexor hallucis brevis muscle

Abductor hallucis muscle

Lumbrical muscles

Flexor digitorum brevis muscle

Flexor digiti minimi brevis muscle

Abductor digiti minimi muscle

Figure 17A
Thoracic Vertebra—Superior View

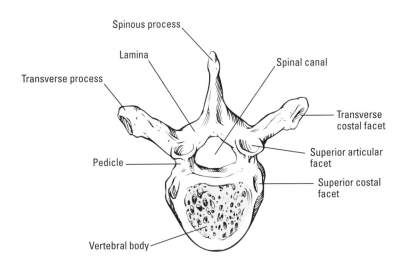

Spinous process

Lamina

Transverse process

Spinal canal

Transverse costal facet

Superior articular facet

Pedicle

Superior costal facet

Vertebral body

Figure 17B
Lumbar Vertebra—Superior View

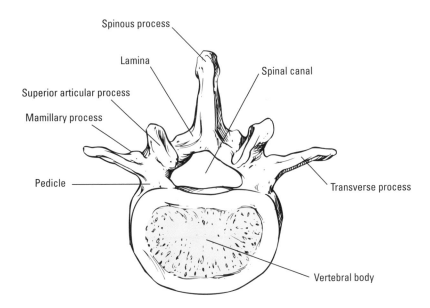

Spinous process

Lamina

Superior articular process

Spinal canal

Mamillary process

Pedicle

Transverse process

Vertebral body

Figure 17C
Lumbar Vertebrae—Lateral View

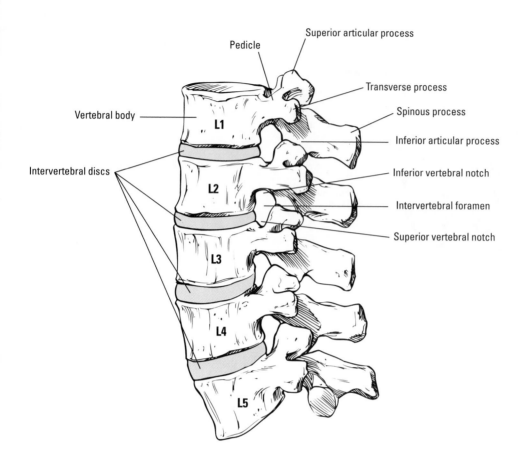

Pedicle

Superior articular process

Transverse process

Spinous process

Vertebral body

Inferior articular process

L1

Inferior vertebral notch

Intervertebral discs

Intervertebral foramen

L2

Superior vertebral notch

L3

L4

L5

Figure 18A
Brain Anatomy

Figure 18B
Sagittal Section of Brain and Brain Stem

Figure 19
Eyeball

Transverse (horizontal) section of eyeball

Figure 20
Ear

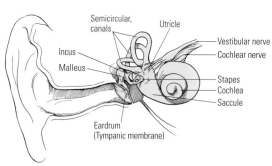

Figure 21
Paranasal Sinuses

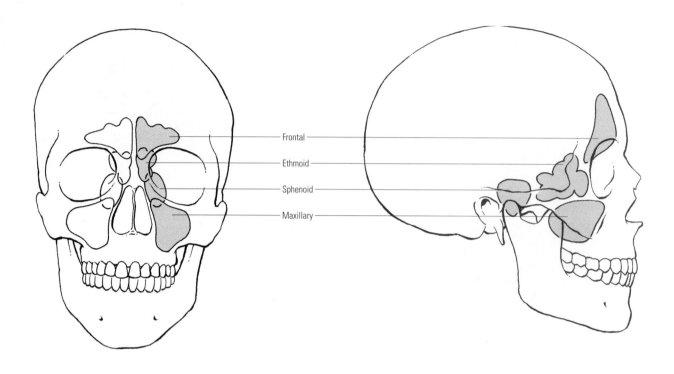

Frontal
Ethmoid
Sphenoid
Maxillary

Figure 22
Cardiac Anatomy

Superior vena cava
Right pulmonary artery
Pulmonary valve
Location of sinoatrial node
Location of atrioventricular node
Right atrium
Tricuspid valve
Right ventricle
Inferior vena cava

Aorta
Pulmonary artery
Left atrium
Aortic valve
Mitral valve
Left ventricle
Ventricular septum
Descending thoracic aorta

Evaluation and Management (E/M) Services Guidelines

In addition to the information presented in the Introduction, several other items unique to this section are defined or identified here.

Classification of Evaluation and Management (E/M) Services

The E/M section is divided into broad categories such as office visits, hospital visits, and consultations. Most of the categories are further divided into two or more subcategories of E/M services. For example, there are two subcategories of office visits (new patient and established patient) and there are two subcategories of hospital visits (initial and subsequent). The subcategories of E/M services are further classified into levels of E/M services that are identified by specific codes. This classification is important because the nature of physician work varies by type of service, place of service, and the patient's status.

The basic format of the levels of E/M services is the same for most categories. First, a unique code number is listed. Second, the place and/or type of service is specified, eg, office consultation. Third, the content of the service is defined, eg, comprehensive history and comprehensive examination. (See "Levels of E/M Services," page 3, for details on the content of E/M services.) Fourth, the nature of the presenting problem(s) usually associated with a given level is described. Fifth, the time typically required to provide the service is specified. (A detailed discussion of time is provided on page 4.)

Definitions of Commonly Used Terms

Certain key words and phrases are used throughout the E/M section. The following definitions are intended to reduce the potential for differing interpretations and to increase the consistency of reporting by physicians in differing specialties.

New and Established Patient

Solely for the purposes of distinguishing between new and established patients, **professional services** are those face-to-face services rendered by a physician and reported by a specific CPT code(s). A new patient is one who has not received any professional services from the physician or another physician of the same specialty who belongs to the same group practice, within the past three years.

An established patient is one who has received professional services from the physician or another physician of the same specialty who belongs to the same group practice, within the past three years.

In the instance where a physician is on call for or covering for another physician, the patient's encounter will be classified as it would have been by the physician who is not available.

No distinction is made between new and established patients in the emergency department. E/M services in the emergency department category may be reported for any new or established patient who presents for treatment in the emergency department.

The decision tree on page 2 is provided to aid in determining whether to report the E/M service provided as a new or an established patient encounter.

Chief Complaint

A chief complaint is a concise statement describing the symptom, problem, condition, diagnosis, or other factor that is the reason for the encounter, usually stated in the patient's words.

Concurrent Care

Concurrent care is the provision of similar services, eg, hospital visits, to the same patient by more than one physician on the same day. When concurrent care is provided, no special reporting is required. Modifier 75 has been deleted.

Counseling

Counseling is a discussion with a patient and/or family concerning one or more of the following areas:

- Diagnostic results, impressions, and/or recommended diagnostic studies
- Prognosis
- Risks and benefits of management (treatment) options
- Instructions for management (treatment) and/or follow-up
- Importance of compliance with chosen management (treatment) options
- Risk factor reduction
- Patient and family education

(For psychotherapy, see 90804-90857)

Decision Tree for New vs Established Patients

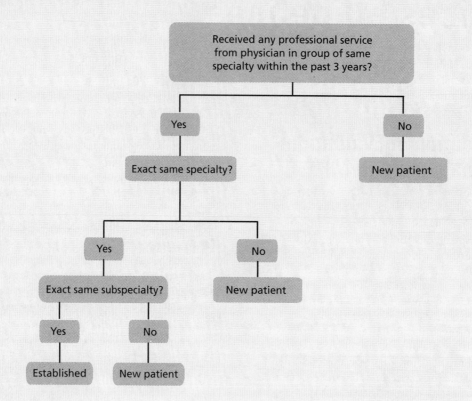

Family History

A review of medical events in the patient's family that includes significant information about:

- The health status or cause of death of parents, siblings, and children

- Specific diseases related to problems identified in the Chief Complaint or History of the Present Illness, and/or System Review

- Diseases of family members that may be hereditary or place the patient at risk

History of Present Illness

A chronological description of the development of the patient's present illness from the first sign and/or symptom to the present. This includes a description of location, quality, severity, timing, context, modifying factors, and associated signs and symptoms significantly related to the presenting problem(s).

Levels of E/M Services

Within each category or subcategory of E/M service, there are three to five levels of E/M services available for reporting purposes. Levels of E/M services are **not** interchangeable among the different categories or subcategories of service. For example, the first level of E/M services in the subcategory of office visit, new patient, does not have the same definition as the first level of E/M services in the subcategory of office visit, established patient.

The levels of E/M services include examinations, evaluations, treatments, conferences with or concerning patients, preventive pediatric and adult health supervision, and similar medical services, such as the determination of the need and/or location for appropriate care. Medical screening includes the history, examination, and medical decision-making required to determine the need and/or location for appropriate care and treatment of the patient (eg, office and other outpatient setting, emergency department, nursing facility). The levels of E/M services encompass the wide variations in skill, effort, time, responsibility, and medical knowledge required for the prevention or diagnosis and treatment of illness or injury and the promotion of optimal health. Each level of E/M services may be used by all physicians.

The descriptors for the levels of E/M services recognize seven components, six of which are used in defining the levels of E/M services. These components are:

- History
- Examination
- Medical decision making
- Counseling
- Coordination of care
- Nature of presenting problem
- Time

The first three of these components (history, examination, and medical decision making) are considered the **key** components in selecting a level of E/M services. (See "Determine the Extent of History Obtained," page 6.)

The next three components (counseling, coordination of care, and the nature of the presenting problem) are considered **contributory** factors in the majority of encounters. Although the first two of these contributory factors are important E/M services, it is not required that these services be provided at every patient encounter.

Coordination of care with other providers or agencies without a patient encounter on that day is reported using the case management codes.

The final component, time, is discussed in detail (see page 4).

Any specifically identifiable procedure (ie, identified with a specific CPT code) performed on or subsequent to the date of initial or subsequent E/M services should be reported separately.

The actual performance and/or interpretation of diagnostic tests/studies ordered during a patient encounter are not included in the levels of E/M services. Physician performance of diagnostic tests/studies for which specific CPT codes are available may be reported separately, in addition to the appropriate E/M code. The physician's interpretation of the results of diagnostic tests/studies (ie, professional component) with preparation of a separate distinctly identifiable signed written report may also be reported separately, using the appropriate CPT code with modifier 26 appended.

The physician may need to indicate that on the day a procedure or service identified by a CPT code was performed, the patient's condition required a significant separately identifiable E/M service above and beyond other services provided or beyond the usual preservice and postservice care associated with the procedure that was performed. The E/M service may be caused or prompted by the symptoms or condition for which the procedure and/or service was provided. This circumstance may be reported by adding modifier 25 to the appropriate level of E/M service. As such, different diagnoses are not required for reporting of the procedure and the E/M services on the same date.

Nature of Presenting Problem

A presenting problem is a disease, condition, illness, injury, symptom, sign, finding, complaint, or other reason for encounter, with or without a diagnosis being established at the time of the encounter. The E/M codes recognize five types of presenting problems that are defined as follows:

Minimal: A problem that may not require the presence of the physician, but service is provided under the physician's supervision.

Self-limited or minor: A problem that runs a definite and prescribed course, is transient in nature, and is not likely to permanently alter health status OR has a good prognosis with management/compliance.

Low severity: A problem where the risk of morbidity without treatment is low; there is little to no risk of mortality without treatment; full recovery without functional impairment is expected.

Moderate severity: A problem where the risk of morbidity without treatment is moderate; there is moderate risk of mortality without treatment; uncertain prognosis OR increased probability of prolonged functional impairment.

High severity: A problem where the risk of morbidity without treatment is high to extreme; there is a moderate to high risk of mortality without treatment OR high probability of severe, prolonged functional impairment.

Past History

A review of the patient's past experiences with illnesses, injuries, and treatments that includes significant information about:

- Prior major illnesses and injuries
- Prior operations
- Prior hospitalizations
- Current medications
- Allergies (eg, drug, food)
- Age appropriate immunization status
- Age appropriate feeding/dietary status

Social History

An age appropriate review of past and current activities that includes significant information about:

- Marital status and/or living arrangements
- Current employment
- Occupational history
- Use of drugs, alcohol, and tobacco
- Level of education
- Sexual history
- Other relevant social factors

System Review (Review of Systems)

An inventory of body systems obtained through a series of questions seeking to identify signs and/or symptoms that the patient may be experiencing or has experienced. For the purposes of the CPT codebook the following elements of a system review have been identified:

- Constitutional symptoms (fever, weight loss, etc)
- Eyes
- Ears, nose, mouth, throat
- Cardiovascular
- Respiratory
- Gastrointestinal
- Genitourinary
- Musculoskeletal
- Integumentary (skin and/or breast)
- Neurological
- Psychiatric
- Endocrine
- Hematologic/lymphatic
- Allergic/immunologic

The review of systems helps define the problem, clarify the differential diagnosis, identify needed testing, or serves as baseline data on other systems that might be affected by any possible management options.

Time

The inclusion of time in the definitions of levels of E/M services has been implicit in prior editions of the CPT codebook. The inclusion of time as an explicit factor beginning in *CPT 1992* is done to assist physicians in selecting the most appropriate level of E/M services. It should be recognized that the specific times expressed in the visit code descriptors are averages and, therefore, represent a range of times that may be higher or lower depending on actual clinical circumstances.

Time is **not** a descriptive component for the emergency department levels of E/M services because emergency department services are typically provided on a variable intensity basis, often involving multiple encounters with several patients over an extended period of time. Therefore, it is often difficult for physicians to provide accurate estimates of the time spent face-to-face with the patient.

Studies to establish levels of E/M services employed surveys of practicing physicians to obtain data on the amount of time and work associated with typical E/M services. Since "work" is not easily quantifiable, the codes must rely on other objective, verifiable measures that correlate with physicians' estimates of their "work." It has been demonstrated that physicians' estimations of **intraservice** time (as explained on the next page), both within and across specialties, is a variable that is predictive of the "work" of E/M services. This same research has shown there is a strong relationship between intraservice time and total time for E/M services. Intraservice time, rather than total time, was chosen for inclusion with the codes because of its relative ease of measurement and because of its direct correlation with measurements of the total amount of time and work associated with typical E/M services.

Intraservice times are defined as **face-to-face** time for office and other outpatient visits and as **unit/floor** time for hospital and other inpatient visits. This distinction is necessary because most of the work of typical office visits takes place during the face-to-face time with the patient, while most of the work of typical hospital visits takes place during the time spent on the patient's floor or unit.

Face-to-face time (office and other outpatient visits and office consultations): For coding purposes, face-to-face time for these services is defined as only that time that the physician spends face-to-face with the patient and/or family. This includes the time in which the physician performs such tasks as obtaining a history, performing an examination, and counseling the patient.

Physicians also spend time doing work before or after the face-to-face time with the patient, performing such tasks as reviewing records and tests, arranging for further services, and communicating further with other professionals and the patient through written reports and telephone contact.

This **non-face-to-face** time for office services—also called pre- and postencounter time—is not included in the time component described in the E/M codes. However, the pre- and post-face-to-face work associated with an encounter was included in calculating the total work of typical services in physician surveys.

Thus, the face-to-face time associated with the services described by any E/M code is a valid proxy for the total work done before, during, and after the visit.

Unit/floor time (hospital observation services, inpatient hospital care, initial and follow-up hospital consultations, nursing facility): For reporting purposes, intraservice time for these services is defined as unit/floor time, which includes the time that the physician is present on the patient's hospital unit and at the bedside rendering services for that patient. This includes the time in which the physician establishes and/or reviews the patient's chart, examines the patient, writes notes, and communicates with other professionals and the patient's family.

In the hospital, pre- and post-time includes time spent off the patient's floor performing such tasks as reviewing pathology and radiology findings in another part of the hospital.

This pre- and postvisit time is not included in the time component described in these codes. However, the pre- and postwork performed during the time spent off the floor or unit was included in calculating the total work of typical services in physician surveys.

Thus, the unit/floor time associated with the services described by any code is a valid proxy for the total work done before, during, and after the visit.

Unlisted Service

An E/M service may be provided that is not listed in this section of the CPT codebook. When reporting such a service, the appropriate "Unlisted" code may be used to indicate the service, identifying it by "Special Report," as discussed in the following paragraph. The "Unlisted Services" and accompanying codes for the E/M section are as follows:

99429   **Unlisted preventive** medicine service

99499   **Unlisted evaluation and management** service

Special Report

An unlisted service or one that is unusual, variable, or new may require a special report demonstrating the medical appropriateness of the service. Pertinent information should include an adequate definition or description of the nature, extent, and need for the procedure and the time, effort, and equipment necessary to provide the service. Additional items that may be included are complexity of symptoms, final diagnosis, pertinent physical findings, diagnostic and therapeutic procedures, concurrent problems, and follow-up care.

Clinical Examples

Clinical examples of the codes for E/M services are provided to assist physicians in understanding the meaning of the descriptors and selecting the correct code. The clinical examples are listed in Appendix C. Each example was developed by physicians in the specialties shown.

The same problem, when seen by physicians in different specialties, may involve different amounts of work. Therefore, the appropriate level of encounter should be reported using the descriptors rather than the examples.

The examples have been tested for validity and approved by the CPT Editorial Panel. Physicians were given the examples and asked to assign a code or assess the amount of time and work involved. Only examples that were rated consistently have been included in Appendix C.

Instructions for Selecting a Level of E/M Service

Identify the Category and Subcategory of Service

The categories and subcategories of codes available for reporting E/M services are shown in Table 1.

Table 1
Categories and Subcategories of Service

Category/Subcategory	Code Numbers	Category/Subcategory	Code Numbers
Office or Other Outpatient Services		Domiciliary, Rest Home or	
New Patient	99201-99205	Custodial Care Services	
Established Patient	99211-99215	New Patient	99324-99328
Hospital Observation Services		Established Patient	99334-99337
Hospital Observation Discharge Services	99217	Domiciliary, Rest Home (eg, Assisted	
Initial Hospital Observation Services	99218-99220	Living Facility), or Home Care Plan	
Hospital Observation or Inpatient Care		Oversight Services	99339-99340
Services (Including Admission and		Home Services	
Discharge Services)	99234-99236	New Patient	99341-99345
Hospital Inpatient Services		Established Patient	99347-99350
Initial Hospital Care	99221-99223	Prolonged Services	
Subsequent Hospital Care	99231-99233	With Direct Patient Contact	99354-99357
Hospital Discharge Services	99238-99239	Without Direct Patient Contact	99358-99359
Consultations		Standby Services	99360
Office Consultations	99241-99245	Case Management Services	
Inpatient Consultations	99251-99255	▶ Anticoagulant Management	99363-99364◀
Emergency Department Services	99281-99288	▶ Medical Team Conferences	99366-99368◀
Pediatric Patient Transport	99289-99290	Care Plan Oversight Services	99374-99380
Critical Care Services		Preventive Medicine Services	
Adult (over 24 months of age)	99291-99292	New Patient	99381-99387
Pediatric	99293-99294	Established Patient	99391-99397
Neonatal	99295-99296	Individual Counseling	99401-99404
Continuing Intensive Care Services	99298-99300	Group Counseling	99411-99412
Nursing Facility Services		Other	99420-99429
Initial Nursing Facility Care	99304-99306	Newborn Care	99431-99440
Subsequent Nursing Facility Care	99307-99310	▶Non-Face-to-Face Physician Services◀	
▶ Nursing Facility Discharge Services	99315-99316◀	▶ Telephone Services	99441-99443◀
Other Nursing Facility Services	99318	▶ Online Medical Evaluation	99444◀
		Special E/M Services	99450-99456
		▶Other E/M Services	99477-99499◀

Review the Reporting Instructions for the Selected Category or Subcategory

Most of the categories and many of the subcategories of service have special guidelines or instructions unique to that category or subcategory. Where these are indicated, eg, "Inpatient Hospital Care," special instructions will be presented preceding the levels of E/M services.

Review the Level of E/M Service Descriptors and Examples in the Selected Category or Subcategory

The descriptors for the levels of E/M services recognize seven components, six of which are used in defining the levels of E/M services. These components are:

- History
- Examination
- Medical decision making
- Counseling
- Coordination of care
- Nature of presenting problem
- Time

The first three of these components (ie, history, examination, and medical decision making) should be considered the **key** components in selecting the level of E/M services. An exception to this rule is in the case of visits that consist predominantly of counseling or coordination of care (see numbered paragraph 3, page 8).

The nature of the presenting problem and time are provided in some levels to assist the physician in determining the appropriate level of E/M service.

Determine the Extent of History Obtained

The extent of the history is dependent upon clinical judgment and on the nature of the presenting problems(s). The levels of E/M services recognize four types of history that are defined as follows:

Problem focused: Chief complaint; brief history of present illness or problem.

Expanded problem focused: Chief complaint; brief history of present illness; problem pertinent system review.

Detailed: Chief complaint; extended history of present illness; problem pertinent system review extended to include a review of a limited number of additional systems; **pertinent** past, family, and/or social history **directly related to the patient's problems.**

Comprehensive: Chief complaint; extended history of present illness; review of systems that is directly related to the problem(s) identified in the history of the present illness plus a review of all additional body systems; **complete** past, family, and social history.

The comprehensive history obtained as part of the preventive medicine E/M service is not problem-oriented and does not involve a chief complaint or present illness. It does, however, include a comprehensive system review and comprehensive or interval past, family, and social history as well as a comprehensive assessment/history of pertinent risk factors.

Determine the Extent of Examination Performed

The extent of the examination performed is dependent on clinical judgment and on the nature of the presenting problem(s). The levels of E/M services recognize four types of examination that are defined as follows:

Problem focused: A limited examination of the affected body area or organ system.

Expanded problem focused: A limited examination of the affected body area or organ system and other symptomatic or related organ system(s).

Detailed: An extended examination of the affected body area(s) and other symptomatic or related organ system(s).

Comprehensive: A general multisystem examination or a complete examination of a single organ system. **Note:** The comprehensive examination performed as part of the preventive medicine E/M service is multisystem, but its extent is based on age and risk factors identified.

For the purposes of these CPT definitions, the following body areas are recognized:

- Head, including the face
- Neck
- Chest, including breasts and axilla
- Abdomen
- Genitalia, groin, buttocks
- Back
- Each extremity

For the purposes of these CPT definitions, the following organ systems are recognized:

- Eyes
- Ears, nose, mouth, and throat
- Cardiovascular
- Respiratory

- Gastrointestinal
- Genitourinary
- Musculoskeletal
- Skin
- Neurologic
- Psychiatric
- Hematologic/lymphatic/immunologic

Determine the Complexity of Medical Decision Making

Medical decision making refers to the complexity of establishing a diagnosis and/or selecting a management option as measured by:

- The number of possible diagnoses and/or the number of management options that must be considered
- The amount and/or complexity of medical records, diagnostic tests, and/or other information that must be obtained, reviewed, and analyzed
- The risk of significant complications, morbidity, and/or mortality, as well as comorbidities, associated with the patient's presenting problems(s), the diagnostic procedure(s), and/or the possible management options

Four types of medical decision making are recognized: straightforward, low complexity, moderate complexity, and high complexity. To qualify for a given type of decision making, two of the three elements in Table 2 must be met or exceeded.

Comorbidities/underlying diseases, in and of themselves, are not considered in selecting a level of E/M services *unless* their presence significantly increases the complexity of the medical decision making.

Select the Appropriate Level of E/M Services Based on the Following

1. For the following categories/subcategories, **all of the key components,** ie, history, examination, and medical decision making, must meet or exceed the stated requirements to qualify for a particular level of E/M service: office, new patient; hospital observation services; initial hospital care; office consultations; initial inpatient consultations; emergency department services; initial nursing facility care; domiciliary care, new patient; and home, new patient.

2. For the following categories/subcategories, **two of the three key components** (ie, history, examination, and medical decision making) must meet or exceed the stated requirements to qualify for a particular level of E/M services: office, established patient; subsequent hospital care; subsequent nursing facility care; domiciliary care, established patient; and home, established patient.

Table 2

Complexity of Medical Decision Making

Number of Diagnoses or Management Options	Amount and/or Complexity of Data to be Reviewed	Risk of Complications and/or Morbidity or Mortality	Type of Decision Making
minimal	minimal or none	minimal	**straightforward**
limited	limited	low	**low complexity**
multiple	moderate	moderate	**moderate complexity**
extensive	extensive	high	**high complexity**

3. When counseling and/or coordination of care dominates (more than 50%) the physician/patient and/or family encounter (face-to-face time in the office or other outpatient setting or floor/unit time in the hospital or nursing facility), then **time** may be considered the key or controlling factor to qualify for a particular level of E/M services. This includes time spent with parties who have assumed responsibility for the care of the patient or decision making whether or not they are family members (eg, foster parents, person acting in loco parentis, legal guardian). The extent of counseling and/or coordination of care must be documented in the medical record.

Evaluation and Management

Office or Other Outpatient Services

The following codes are used to report evaluation and management services provided in the physician's office or in an outpatient or other ambulatory facility. A patient is considered an outpatient until inpatient admission to a health care facility occurs.

To report services provided to a patient who is admitted to a hospital or nursing facility in the course of an encounter in the office or other ambulatory facility, see the notes for initial hospital inpatient care (page 12) or initial nursing facility care (page 22).

For services provided by physicians in the emergency department, see 99281-99285.

For observation care, see 99217-99220.

For observation or inpatient care services (including admission and discharge services), see 99234-99236.

New Patient

99201   **Office or other outpatient visit** for the evaluation and management of a new patient, which requires these 3 key components:

- **A problem focused history;**
- **A problem focused examination;**
- **Straightforward medical decision making.**

Counseling and/or coordination of care with other providers or agencies are provided consistent with the nature of the problem(s) and the patient's and/or family's needs.

Usually, the presenting problem(s) are self limited or minor. Physicians typically spend 10 minutes face-to-face with the patient and/or family.

➲ *CPT Assistant* Winter 91:11, Spring 92:13, 24, Summer 92:1, 24, Spring 93:34, Summer 93:2, Fall 93:9, Spring 95:1, Summer 95:4, Fall 95:9, Jul 98:9, Sep 98:5, Jun 99:8, Feb 00:3, 9, 11, Aug 01:2, Oct 04:11, Mar 05:11, Apr 05:1, May 05:1, Jun 05:11, Dec 05:10, Feb 06:14, May 06:1, Jun 06:1, Aug 06:12, Oct 06:15, Apr 07:11

99202   **Office or other outpatient visit** for the evaluation and management of a new patient, which requires these 3 key components:

- **An expanded problem focused history;**
- **An expanded problem focused examination;**
- **Straightforward medical decision making.**

Counseling and/or coordination of care with other providers or agencies are provided consistent with the nature of the problem(s) and the patient's and/or family's needs.

Usually, the presenting problem(s) are of low to moderate severity. Physicians typically spend 20 minutes face-to-face with the patient and/or family.

➲ *CPT Assistant* Winter 91:11, Spring 92:13, 24, Summer 92:1, 24, Spring 93:34, Summer 93:2, Fall 93:9, Spring 95:1, Summer 95:4, Fall 95:9, Jul 98:9, Sep 98:5, Feb 00:11, Aug 01:2, Apr 02:14, Oct 04:10, Apr 05:1, 3, Jun 05:11, Dec 05:10, May 06:1, Jun 06:1, Oct 06:15, Apr 07:11

99203   **Office or other outpatient visit** for the evaluation and management of a new patient, which requires these 3 key components:

- **A detailed history;**
- **A detailed examination;**
- **Medical decision making of low complexity.**

Counseling and/or coordination of care with other providers or agencies are provided consistent with the nature of the problem(s) and the patient's and/or family's needs.

Usually, the presenting problem(s) are of moderate severity. Physicians typically spend 30 minutes face-to-face with the patient and/or family.

➲ *CPT Assistant* Winter 91:11, Spring 92:14, 24, Summer 92:1, 24, Spring 93:34, Summer 93:2, Fall 93:9, Spring 95:1, Summer 95:4, Fall 95:9, Jul 98:9, Sep 98:5, Feb 00:11, Aug 01:2, Apr 02:14, Oct 04:10, Feb 05:9, Apr 05:1, 3, Jun 05:11, Dec 05:10, May 06:1, Jun 06:1, Oct 06:15, Apr 07:11

99204   **Office or other outpatient visit** for the evaluation and management of a new patient, which requires these 3 key components:

- **A comprehensive history;**
- **A comprehensive examination;**
- **Medical decision making of moderate complexity.**

Counseling and/or coordination of care with other providers or agencies are provided consistent with the nature of the problem(s) and the patient's and/or family's needs.

Usually, the presenting problem(s) are of moderate to high severity. Physicians typically spend 45 minutes face-to-face with the patient and/or family.

➲ *CPT Assistant* Winter 91:11, Spring 92:14, 24, Summer 92:1, 24, Spring 93:34, Summer 93:2, Fall 93:9, Spring 95:1, Summer 95:4, Fall 95:9, Jul 98:9, Sep 98:5, Feb 00:11, Aug 01:2, Apr 02:14, May 02:1, Oct 04:10, Apr 05:1, 3, Jun 05:11, Dec 05:10, May 06:1, Jun 06:1, Oct 06:15, Apr 07:11

99205   **Office or other outpatient visit** for the evaluation and management of a new patient, which requires these 3 key components:

- **A comprehensive history;**
- **A comprehensive examination;**
- **Medical decision making of high complexity.**

Counseling and/or coordination of care with other providers or agencies are provided consistent with the nature of the problem(s) and the patient's and/or family's needs.

Usually, the presenting problem(s) are of moderate to high severity. Physicians typically spend 60 minutes face-to-face with the patient and/or family.

➔ *CPT Assistant* Winter 91:11, Spring 92:14, 24, Summer 92:1, 24, Spring 93:34, Summer 93:2, Fall 93:9, Spring 95:1, Summer 95:4, Fall 95:9, Jul 98:9, Sep 98:5, Feb 00:11, Aug 01:2, Apr 02:2, May 02:1, Oct 04:10, Apr 05:1, 3, Jun 05:11, Dec 05:10, May 06:1, Jun 06:1, Oct 06:15, Apr 07:11

Established Patient

99211   **Office or other outpatient visit** for the evaluation and management of an established patient, that may not require the presence of a physician. Usually, the presenting problem(s) are minimal. Typically, 5 minutes are spent performing or supervising these services.

➔ *CPT Assistant* Winter 91:11, Spring 92:14, 24, Summer 92:1, 24, Spring 93:34, Summer 93:2, Fall 93:9, Spring 95:1, Summer 95:4, Fall 95:9, Oct 96:10, Feb 97:9, May 97:4, Jul 98:9, Sep 98:5, Oct 99:9, Feb 00:11, Aug 01:2, Jan 02:2, Oct 04:10, Feb 05:15, Mar 05:11, Apr 05:1, 3, May 05:1, Jun 05:11, Nov 05:1, Dec 05:10, Feb 06:14, May 06:1, Jun 06:1, Jul 06:19, Oct 06:15, Nov 06:21, Apr 07:11

99212   **Office or other outpatient visit** for the evaluation and management of an established patient, which requires at least 2 of these 3 key components:

- **A problem focused history;**
- **A problem focused examination;**
- **Straightforward medical decision making.**

Counseling and/or coordination of care with other providers or agencies are provided consistent with the nature of the problem(s) and the patient's and/or family's needs.

Usually, the presenting problem(s) are self limited or minor. Physicians typically spend 10 minutes face-to-face with the patient and/or family.

➔ *CPT Assistant* Winter 91:11, Spring 92:14, 24, Summer 92:1, 24, Spring 93:34, Summer 93:2, Fall 93:9, Spring 95:1, Summer 95:4, Fall 95:9, Jul 98:9, Sep 98:5, Feb 00:11, Jun 00:11, Aug 01:2, Jan 02:2, May 02:3, Apr 04:14, Oct 04:10, Apr 05:1, 3 Jun 05:11, Dec 05:10, May 06:1, Jun 06:1, 11, Sep 06:8, Oct 06:15, Apr 07:11

99213   **Office or other outpatient visit** for the evaluation and management of an established patient, which requires at least 2 of these 3 key components:

- **An expanded problem focused history;**
- **An expanded problem focused examination;**
- **Medical decision making of low complexity.**

Counseling and coordination of care with other providers or agencies are provided consistent with the nature of the problem(s) and the patient's and/or family's needs.

Usually, the presenting problem(s) are of low to moderate severity. Physicians typically spend 15 minutes face-to-face with the patient and/or family.

➔ *CPT Assistant* Winter 91:11, Spring 92:14, 24, Summer 92:1, 24, Spring 93:34, Summer 93:2, Fall 93:9, Spring 95:1, Summer 95:4, Fall 95:9, Jan 97:10, Jul 98:9, Sep 98:5, Aug 01:2, May 02:3, Oct 03:5, Apr 04:14, Oct 04:10, Mar 05:11, Apr 05:1, 3, Jun 05:11, Dec 05:10, May 06:1, Jun 06:1, 11, Sep 06:8, Oct 06:15, Apr 07:11

99214   **Office or other outpatient visit** for the evaluation and management of an established patient, which requires at least 2 of these 3 key components:

- **A detailed history;**
- **A detailed examination;**
- **Medical decision making of moderate complexity.**

Counseling and/or coordination of care with other providers or agencies are provided consistent with the nature of the problem(s) and the patient's and/or family's needs.

Usually, the presenting problem(s) are of moderate to high severity. Physicians typically spend 25 minutes face-to-face with the patient and/or family.

➔ *CPT Assistant* Winter 91:11, Spring 92:15, 24, Summer 92:1, 24, Spring 93:34, Summer 93:2, Fall 93:9, Spring 95:1, Summer 95:4, Fall 95:9, May 97:4, Jul 98:9, Sep 98:5, Aug 01:2, Jan 02:2, May 02:1-2, Oct 03:5, Apr 04:14, Oct 04:10, Apr 05:1, 3, Jun 05:11, Dec 05:10, May 06:1, Jun 06:1, 11, Sep 06:8, Oct 06:15, Apr 07:11

99215   **Office or other outpatient visit** for the evaluation and management of an established patient, which requires at least 2 of these 3 key components:

- **A comprehensive history;**
- **A comprehensive examination;**
- **Medical decision making of high complexity.**

Counseling and/or coordination of care with other providers or agencies are provided consistent with the nature of the problem(s) and the patient's and/or family's needs.

Usually, the presenting problem(s) are of moderate to high severity. Physicians typically spend 40 minutes face-to-face with the patient and/or family.

➔ *CPT Assistant* Winter 91:11, Spring 92:15, 24, Summer 92:1, 24, Spring 93:34, Summer 93:2, Fall 93:9, Spring 95:1, Summer 95:4, Fall 95:9, Jan 97:10, Jul 98:9, Sep 98:5, Aug 01:2, Jan 02:2, May 02:1, 3, Apr 04:14, Oct 04:10, Mar 05:11, Apr 05:1, 3, Jun 05:11, Dec 05:10, May 06:1, Jun 06:1, 11, Sep 06:8, Oct 06:15, Apr 07:11

Hospital Observation Services

The following codes are used to report evaluation and management services provided to patients designated/admitted as "observation status" in a hospital. It is not necessary that the patient be located in an observation area designated by the hospital.

If such an area does exist in a hospital (as a separate unit in the hospital, in the emergency department, etc), these codes are to be utilized if the patient is placed in such an area.

For definitions of key components and commonly used terms, please see **Evaluation and Management Services Guidelines.**

Typical times have not yet been established for this category of services.

Observation Care Discharge Services

Observation care discharge of a patient from "observation status" includes final examination of the patient, discussion of the hospital stay, instructions for continuing care, and preparation of discharge records. For observation or inpatient hospital care including the admission and discharge of the patient on the same date, see codes 99234-99236 as appropriate.

99217 **Observation care discharge** day management (This code is to be utilized by the physician to report all services provided to a patient on discharge from "observation status" if the discharge is on other than the initial date of "observation status." To report services to a patient designated as "observation status" or "inpatient status" and discharged on the same date, use the codes for Observation or Inpatient Care Services [including Admission and Discharge Services, 99234-99236 as appropriate.])

> ➔ *CPT Assistant* Nov 97:2, Mar 98:1, May 98:3, Sep 98:5, Sep 00:3, May 05:1, Nov 05:10, Sep 06:8, Dec 06:14

Initial Observation Care

New or Established Patient

The following codes are used to report the encounter(s) by the supervising physician with the patient when designated as "observation status." This refers to the initiation of observation status, supervision of the care plan for observation and performance of periodic reassessments. For observation encounters by other physicians, see Office or Other Outpatient Consultation codes (99241-99245).

To report services provided to a patient who is admitted to the hospital after receiving hospital observation care services on the same date, see the notes for initial hospital inpatient care (page 12). For a patient admitted to the hospital on a date subsequent to the date of observation status, the hospital admission would be reported with the appropriate Initial Hospital Care code (99221-99223). For a patient admitted and discharged from observation or inpatient status on the same date, the services should be reported with codes 99234-99236 as appropriate. Do not report observation discharge (99217) in conjunction with a hospital admission.

When "observation status" is initiated in the course of an encounter in another site of service (eg, hospital emergency department, physician's office, nursing facility) all evaluation and management services provided by the supervising physician in conjunction with initiating "observation status" are considered part of the initial observation care when performed on the same date. The observation care level of service reported by the supervising physician should include the services related to initiating "observation status" provided in the other sites of service as well as in the observation setting.

Evaluation and management services on the same date provided in sites that are related to initiating "observation status" should NOT be reported separately.

These codes may not be utilized for post-operative recovery if the procedure is considered part of the surgical "package." These codes apply to all evaluation and management services that are provided on the same date of initiating "observation status."

99218 **Initial observation care,** per day, for the evaluation and management of a patient which requires these 3 key components:

- **A detailed or comprehensive history;**
- **A detailed or comprehensive examination; and**
- **Medical decision making that is straightforward or of low complexity.**

Counseling and/or coordination of care with other providers or agencies are provided consistent with the nature of the problem(s) and the patient's and/or family's needs.

Usually, the problem(s) requiring admission to "observation status" are of low severity.

> ➔ *CPT Assistant* Spring 93:34, Fall 95:9, Nov 97:2, Mar 98:1, Sep 98:5, Sep 00:3, Jan 03:10, Aug 04:11, May 05:1, Nov 05:10, Sep 06:8, Dec 06:14

99219 **Initial observation care,** per day, for the evaluation and management of a patient, which requires these 3 key components:

- **A comprehensive history;**
- **A comprehensive examination; and**
- **Medical decision making of moderate complexity.**

Counseling and/or coordination of care with other providers or agencies are provided consistent with the nature of the problem(s) and the patient's and/or family's needs.

Usually, the problem(s) requiring admission to "observation status" are of moderate severity.

➔ *CPT Assistant* Spring 93:34, Fall 95:16, Nov 97:2, Mar 98:1, Sep 98:5, Sep 00:3, Jan 03:10, Aug 04:11, Nov 05:10, Sep 06:8, Dec 06:14

99220 **Initial observation care,** per day, for the evaluation and management of a patient, which requires these 3 key components:

- **A comprehensive history;**
- **A comprehensive examination; and**
- **Medical decision making of high complexity.**

Counseling and/or coordination of care with other providers or agencies are provided consistent with the nature of the problem(s) and the patient's and/or family's needs.

Usually, the problem(s) requiring admission to "observation status" are of high severity.

➔ *CPT Assistant* Spring 93:34, Fall 95:16, Nov 97:2, Mar 98:1, Sep 98:5, Sep 00:3, Jan 03:10, Aug 04:11, Nov 05:10, Sep 06:8, Dec 06:14

Hospital Inpatient Services

The following codes are used to report evaluation and management services provided to hospital inpatients. Hospital inpatient services include those services provided to patients in a "partial hospital" setting. These codes are to be used to report these partial hospitalization services. See also psychiatry notes in the full text of CPT codebook.

For definitions of key components and commonly used terms, please see **Evaluation and Management Services Guidelines.** For Hospital Observation Services, see 99218-99220. For a patient admitted and discharged from observation or inpatient status on the same date, the services should be reported with codes 99234-99236 as appropriate.

Initial Hospital Care

New or Established Patient

The following codes are used to report the first hospital inpatient encounter with the patient by the admitting physician.

For initial inpatient encounters by physicians other than the admitting physician, see initial inpatient consultation codes (99251-99255) or subsequent hospital care codes (99231-99233) as appropriate.

▶For admission services for the neonate (28 days of age or less) requiring intensive observation, frequent interventions, and other intensive care services, see 99477.◀

When the patient is admitted to the hospital as an inpatient in the course of an encounter in another site of service (eg, hospital emergency department, observation status in a hospital, physician's office, nursing facility) all evaluation and management services provided by that physician in conjunction with that admission are considered part of the initial hospital care when performed on the same date as the admission. The inpatient care level of service reported by the admitting physician should include the services related to the admission he/she provided in the other sites of service as well as in the inpatient setting.

Evaluation and management services on the same date provided in sites that are related to the admission "observation status" should NOT be reported separately. For a patient admitted and discharged from observation or inpatient status on the same date, the services should be reported with codes 99234-99236 as appropriate.

99221 **Initial hospital care,** per day, for the evaluation and management of a patient, which requires these 3 key components:

- **A detailed or comprehensive history;**
- **A detailed or comprehensive examination; and**
- **Medical decision making that is straightforward or of low complexity.**

Counseling and/or coordination of care with other providers or agencies are provided consistent with the nature of the problem(s) and the patient's and/or family's needs.

Usually, the problem(s) requiring admission are of low severity. Physicians typically spend 30 minutes at the bedside and on the patient's hospital floor or unit.

➔ *CPT Assistant* Winter 91:11, Spring 92:14, 24, Summer 92:10, 24, Fall 92:1, Spring 93:34, Spring 95:1, Fall 95:9, Jul 96:11, Sep 96:10, Nov 97:2, Mar 98:1, Sep 98:5, Jan 02:2-3, Apr 03:26, Apr 04:14, Aug 04:11, May 05:1, Sep 06:8

99222 **Initial hospital care,** per day, for the evaluation and management of a patient, which requires these 3 key components:

- **A comprehensive history;**
- **A comprehensive examination; and**
- **Medical decision making of moderate complexity.**

Counseling and/or coordination of care with other providers or agencies are provided consistent with the nature of the problem(s) and the patient's and/or family's needs.

Usually, the problem(s) requiring admission are of moderate severity. Physicians typically spend 50 minutes at the bedside and on the patient's hospital floor or unit.

➔ *CPT Assistant* Winter 91:11, Spring 92:14, 24, Summer 92:10, 24, Fall 92:1, Spring 93:34, Spring 95:1, Fall 95:9, Jul 96:11, Sep 96:10, Nov 97:2, Mar 98:1, Sep 98:5, Jan 02:2-3, Apr 03:26, Apr 04:14, Aug 04:11, Sep 06:8

99223   **Initial hospital care,** per day, for the evaluation and management of a patient, which requires these 3 key components:

- **A comprehensive history;**
- **A comprehensive examination; and**
- **Medical decision making of high complexity.**

Counseling and/or coordination of care with other providers or agencies are provided consistent with the nature of the problem(s) and the patient's and/or family's needs.

Usually, the problem(s) requiring admission are of high severity. Physicians typically spend 70 minutes at the bedside and on the patient's hospital floor or unit.

➔ *CPT Assistant* Winter 91:11, Spring 92:14, 24, Summer 92:10, 24, Fall 92:1, Spring 93:34, Spring 95:1, Fall 95:9, Jul 96:11, Sep 96:10, Nov 97:2, Mar 98:1, Sep 98:5, Jan 02:2-3, Apr 03:26, Apr 04:14, Aug 04:11, Sep 06:8

Subsequent Hospital Care

All levels of subsequent hospital care include reviewing the medical record and reviewing the results of diagnostic studies and changes in the patient's status (ie, changes in history, physical condition and response to management) since the last assessment by the physician.

99231   **Subsequent hospital care,** per day, for the evaluation and management of a patient, which requires at least 2 of these 3 key components:

- **A problem focused interval history;**
- **A problem focused examination;**
- **Medical decision making that is straightforward or of low complexity.**

Counseling and/or coordination of care with other providers or agencies are provided consistent with the nature of the problem(s) and the patient's and/or family's needs.

Usually, the patient is stable, recovering or improving. Physicians typically spend 15 minutes at the bedside and on the patient's hospital floor or unit.

➔ *CPT Assistant* Winter 91:11, Spring 92:14, 24, Summer 92:10, 24, Fall 92:1, Spring 93:34, Spring 95:1, Fall 95:16, Nov 97:2, Sep 98:5, Jan 99:10, Nov 99:5, Aug 01:2, Jan 02:2-3, Apr 04:14, Aug 04:11, Mar 05:11, May 05:1, May 06:1, 16, Jul 06:4, Mar 07:9

99232   **Subsequent hospital care,** per day, for the evaluation and management of a patient, which requires at least 2 of these 3 key components:

- **An expanded problem focused interval history;**
- **An expanded problem focused examination;**
- **Medical decision making of moderate complexity.**

Counseling and/or coordination of care with other providers or agencies are provided consistent with the nature of the problem(s) and the patient's and/or family's needs.

Usually, the patient is responding inadequately to therapy or has developed a minor complication. Physicians typically spend 25 minutes at the bedside and on the patient's hospital floor or unit.

➔ *CPT Assistant* Winter 91:11, Spring 92:14, 24, Summer 92:10, 24, Fall 92:1, Spring 93:34, Spring 95:1, Fall 95:16, Nov 97:2, Sep 98:5, Jan 99:10, Nov 99:5, Jan 00:11, Aug 01:2, Apr 04:14, Aug 04:11, May 06:1, 16, Jul 06:4, Mar 07:9

99233   **Subsequent hospital care,** per day, for the evaluation and management of a patient, which requires at least 2 of these 3 key components:

- **A detailed interval history;**
- **A detailed examination;**
- **Medical decision making of high complexity.**

Counseling and/or coordination of care with other providers or agencies are provided consistent with the nature of the problem(s) and the patient's and/or family's needs.

Usually, the patient is unstable or has developed a significant complication or a significant new problem. Physicians typically spend 35 minutes at the bedside and on the patient's hospital floor or unit.

➔ *CPT Assistant* Winter 91:11, Spring 92:14, 24, Summer 92:10, 24, Fall 92:1, Spring 93:34, Spring 95:1, Fall 95:16, Nov 97:2, Sep 98:5, Jan 99:10, Nov 99:5, Aug 01:2, Apr 04:14, Aug 04:11, May 06:1, 16, Jul 06:4, Mar 07:9

Observation or Inpatient Care Services (Including Admission and Discharge Services)

The following codes are used to report observation or inpatient hospital care services provided to patients admitted and discharged on the same date of service. When a patient is admitted to the hospital from observation status on the same date, the physician should report only the initial hospital care code. The initial hospital care code reported by the admitting physician should include the services related to the observation status services he/she provided on the same date of inpatient admission.

When "observation status" is initiated in the course of an encounter in another site of service (eg, hospital emergency department, physician's office, nursing facility) all evaluation and management services provided by the supervising physician in conjunction with initiating "observation status" are considered part of the initial observation care when performed on the same date. The observation care level of service should include the services related to initiating "observation status" provided in the other sites of service as well as in the observation setting when provided by the same physician.

For patients admitted to observation or inpatient care and discharged on a different date, see codes 99218-99220 and 99217, or 99221-99223 and 99238, 99239.

99234   **Observation or inpatient hospital care,** for the evaluation and management of a patient including admission and discharge on the same date, which requires these 3 key components:

- **A detailed or comprehensive history;**
- **A detailed or comprehensive examination; and**
- **Medical decision making that is straightforward or of low complexity.**

Counseling and/or coordination of care with other providers or agencies are provided consistent with the nature of the problem(s) and the patient's and/or family's needs.

Usually the presenting problem(s) requiring admission are of low severity.

➲ *CPT Assistant* Nov 97:2, Mar 98:2, May 98:1, Sep 98:5, Jan 00:11, Sep 00:3, Jan 02:2, Jun 02:10, Jan 03:10, May 05:1, Nov 05:10, Sep 06:8, Dec 06:14

99235   **Observation or inpatient hospital care,** for the evaluation and management of a patient including admission and discharge on the same date, which requires these 3 key components:

- **A comprehensive history;**
- **A comprehensive examination; and**
- **Medical decision making of moderate complexity.**

Counseling and/or coordination of care with other providers or agencies are provided consistent with the nature of the problem(s) and the patient's and/or family's needs.

Usually the presenting problem(s) requiring admission are of moderate severity.

➲ *CPT Assistant* Nov 97:2, Mar 98:2, May 98:1, Sep 98:5, Jan 00:11, Sep 00:3, Jan 02:2, Jun 02:10, Jan 03:10, Nov 05:10, Sep 06:8, Dec 06:14

99236   **Observation or inpatient hospital care,** for the evaluation and management of a patient including admission and discharge on the same date, which requires these 3 key components:

- **A comprehensive history;**
- **A comprehensive examination; and**
- **Medical decision making of high complexity.**

Counseling and/or coordination of care with other providers or agencies are provided consistent with the nature of the problem(s) and the patient's and/or family's needs.

Usually the presenting problem(s) requiring admission are of high severity.

➲ *CPT Assistant* Nov 97:2, Mar 98:2, May 98:1, Sep 98:5, Jan 00:11, Sep 00:3, Jan 02:2, Jun 02:10, Jan 03:10, Nov 05:10, Sep 06:8, Dec 06:14

Hospital Discharge Services

The hospital discharge day management codes are to be used to report the total duration of time spent by a physician for final hospital discharge of a patient. The codes include, as appropriate, final examination of the patient, discussion of the hospital stay, even if the time spent by the physician on that date is not continuous, instructions for continuing care to all relevant caregivers, and preparation of discharge records, prescriptions and referral forms. For a patient admitted and discharged from observation or inpatient status on the same date, the services should be reported with codes 99234-99236 as appropriate.

99238   **Hospital discharge day management;** 30 minutes or less

➲ *CPT Assistant* Fall 92:1, Spring 93:4, Nov 97:4, Mar 98:3, 11, May 98:2, Jan 99:10, Jan 02:2, Aug 04:11, May 05:1, Sep 06:8

99239   more than 30 minutes

➲ *CPT Assistant* Nov 97:4, Mar 98:3, 11, May 98:2, Jan 99:10, Jan 02:2, Aug 04:11, Sep 06:8

(These codes are to be utilized by the physician to report all services provided to a patient on the date of discharge, if other than the initial date of inpatient status. To report services to a patient who is admitted as an inpatient and discharged on the same date, see codes 99234-99236 for observation or inpatient hospital care including the admission and discharge of the patient on the same date. To report concurrent care services provided by a physician[s] other than the attending physician, use subsequent hospital care codes [99231-99233] on the day of discharge.)

(For Observation Care Discharge, use 99217)

(For observation or inpatient hospital care including the admission and discharge of the patient on the same date, see 99234-99236)

(For Nursing Facility Care Discharge, see 99315, 99316)

(For discharge services provided to newborns admitted and discharged on the same date, use 99435)

Consultations

A consultation is a type of service provided by a physician whose opinion or advice regarding evaluation and/or management of a specific problem is requested by another physician or other appropriate source.

A physician consultant may initiate diagnostic and/or therapeutic services at the same or subsequent visit.

The written or verbal request for a consult may be made by a physician or other appropriate source and documented in the patient's medical record. The consultant's opinion and any services that were ordered or performed must also be documented in the patient's medical record and communicated by written report to the requesting physician or other appropriate source.

A "consultation" initiated by a patient and/or family, and not requested by a physician or other appropriate source (eg, physician assistant, nurse practitioner, doctor of chiropractic, physical therapist, occupational therapist, speech-language pathologist, psychologist, social worker, lawyer, or insurance company), is not reported using the consultation codes but may be reported using the office visit, home service, or domiciliary/rest home care codes.

If a consultation is mandated, eg, by a third-party payer, modifier 32 should also be reported.

Any specifically identifiable procedure (ie, identified with a specific CPT code) performed on or subsequent to the date of the initial consultation should be reported separately.

If subsequent to the completion of a consultation the consultant assumes responsibility for management of a portion or all of the patient's condition(s), the appropriate **Evaluation and Management** services code for the site of service should be reported. In the hospital or nursing facility setting, the consulting physician should use the appropriate inpatient consultation code for the initial encounter and then subsequent hospital or nursing facility care codes. In the office setting, the physician should use the appropriate office or other outpatient consultation codes and then the established patient office or other outpatient services codes.

For definitions of key components and commonly used terms, please see **Evaluation and Management Services Guidelines.**

Office or Other Outpatient Consultations

New or Established Patient

The following codes are used to report consultations provided in the physician's office or in an outpatient or other ambulatory facility, including hospital observation services, home services, domiciliary, rest home, or emergency department (see the preceding consultation definition above). Follow-up visits in the consultant's office or other outpatient facility that are initiated by the physician consultant or patient are reported using the appropriate codes for established patients, office visits (99211-99215), domiciliary, rest home (99334-99337), or home (99347-99350). If an additional request for an opinion or advice regarding the same or a new problem is received from another physician or other appropriate source and documented in the medical record, the office consultation codes may be used again.

99241   **Office consultation** for a new or established patient, which requires these 3 key components:

- **A problem focused history;**
- **A problem focused examination; and**
- **Straightforward medical decision making.**

Counseling and/or coordination of care with other providers or agencies are provided consistent with the nature of the problem(s) and the patient's and/or family's needs.

Usually, the presenting problem(s) are self limited or minor. Physicians typically spend 15 minutes face-to-face with the patient and/or family.

➔ *CPT Assistant* Winter 91:11, Spring 92:4, 23-24, Summer 92:12, Spring 93:4, Spring 95:1, Oct 97:1, Sep 98:5, Jun 99:10, Apr 00:10, Aug 01:3, Jan 02:2, Jul 02:2, Sep 02:11, May 05:1, Dec 05:10, Jan 06:46, May 06:1, 16, Jun 06:1, Sep 06:8, Jan 07:28, Apr 07:11

99242   **Office consultation** for a new or established patient, which requires these 3 key components:

- **An expanded problem focused history;**
- **An expanded problem focused examination; and**
- **Straightforward medical decision making.**

Counseling and/or coordination of care with other providers or agencies are provided consistent with the nature of the problem(s) and the patient's and/or family's needs.

Usually, the presenting problem(s) are of low severity. Physicians typically spend 30 minutes face-to-face with the patient and/or family.

➔ *CPT Assistant* Winter 91:11, Spring 92:4, 23-24, Summer 92:12, Spring 93:2, 34, Spring 95:1, Oct 97:1, Sep 98:5, Aug 01:3, Jan 02:2, Jul 02:2, Sep 02:11, Dec 05:10, May 06:1, 16, Jun 06:1, Sep 06:8, Apr 07:11; *CPT Changes: An Insider's View* 2000

99243   **Office consultation** for a new or established patient, which requires these 3 key components:

- **A detailed history;**
- **A detailed examination; and**
- **Medical decision making of low complexity.**

Counseling and/or coordination of care with other providers or agencies are provided consistent with the nature of the problem(s) and the patient's and/or family's needs.

Usually, the presenting problem(s) are of moderate severity. Physicians typically spend 40 minutes face-to-face with the patient and/or family.

➔ *CPT Assistant* Winter 91:11, Spring 92:4, 23-24, Summer 92:12, Spring 93:2, 34, Spring 95:1, Oct 97:1, Sep 98:5, Aug 01:3, Jan 02:2, Jul 02:2, Sep 02:11, Oct 03:5, Dec 05:10, May 06:1, 16, Jun 06:1, Sep 06:8, Apr 07:11

99244   **Office consultation** for a new or established patient, which requires these 3 key components:

- **A comprehensive history;**
- **A comprehensive examination; and**
- **Medical decision making of moderate complexity.**

Counseling and/or coordination of care with other providers or agencies are provided consistent with the nature of the problem(s) and the patient's and/or family's needs.

Usually, the presenting problem(s) are of moderate to high severity. Physicians typically spend 60 minutes face-to-face with the patient and/or family.

➔ *CPT Assistant* Winter 91:11, Spring 92:3, 23-24, Summer 92:12, Spring 93:2, 34, Spring 95:1, Oct 97:1, Sep 98:5, Aug 01:3, Jan 02:2, Jul 02:2, Sep 02:11, Oct 03:5, Dec 05:10, May 06:1, 16, Jun 06:1, Sep 06:8, Apr 07:11

99245   **Office consultation** for a new or established patient, which requires these 3 key components:

- **A comprehensive history;**

- **A comprehensive examination; and**

- **Medical decision making of high complexity.**

Counseling and/or coordination of care with other providers or agencies are provided consistent with the nature of the problem(s) and the patient's and/or family's needs.

Usually, the presenting problem(s) are of moderate to high severity. Physicians typically spend 80 minutes face-to-face with the patient and/or family.

> *CPT Assistant* Winter 91:11, Spring 92:4, 23-24, Summer 92:12, Spring 93:2, 34, Spring 95:1, Oct 97:1, Sep 98:5, Aug 01:2, Jan 02:2, Jul 02:2, Sep 02:11, Dec 05:10, May 06:1, 16, Jun 06:1, Sep 06:8, Apr 07:11

Inpatient Consultations

New or Established Patient

The following codes are used to report physician consultations provided to hospital inpatients, residents of nursing facilities, or patients in a partial hospital setting. Only one consultation should be reported by a consultant per admission. Subsequent services during the same admission are reported using Subsequent Hospital Care codes (99231-99233) or Subsequent Nursing Facility Care codes (99307-99310), including services to complete the initial consultation, monitor progress, revise recommendations, or address a new problem.

99251   **Inpatient consultation** for a new or established patient, which requires these 3 key components:

- **A problem focused history;**

- **A problem focused examination; and**

- **Straightforward medical decision making.**

Counseling and/or coordination of care with other providers or agencies are provided consistent with the nature of the problem(s) and the patient's and/or family's needs.

Usually, the presenting problem(s) are self limited or minor. Physicians typically spend 20 minutes at the bedside and on the patient's hospital floor or unit.

> *CPT Assistant* Winter 91:11, Spring 92:16, 23-24, Summer 92:12, Spring 93:34, Spring 95:1, Oct 97:1, Sep 98:5, Aug 01:3, Sep 02:11, May 05:1, May 06:1, 16, Jun 06:1, Jul 06:19; *CPT Changes: An Insider's View* 2007

99252   **Inpatient consultation** for a new or established patient, which requires these 3 key components:

- **An expanded problem focused history;**

- **An expanded problem focused examination; and**

- **Straightforward medical decision making.**

Counseling and/or coordination of care with other providers or agencies are provided consistent with the nature of the problem(s) and the patient's and/or family's needs.

Usually, the presenting problem(s) are of low severity. Physicians typically spend 40 minutes at the bedside and on the patient's hospital floor or unit.

> *CPT Assistant* Winter 91:11, Spring 92:16, 23-24, Summer 92:12, Summer 93:34, Spring 95:1, Oct 97:1, Sep 98:5, Aug 01:4, Sep 02:11, May 06:1, 16, Jun 06:1, Jul 06:19; *CPT Changes: An Insider's View* 2007

99253   **Inpatient consultation** for a new or established patient, which requires these 3 key components:

- **A detailed history;**

- **A detailed examination; and**

- **Medical decision making of low complexity.**

Counseling and/or coordination of care with other providers or agencies are provided consistent with the nature of the problem(s) and the patient's and/or family's needs.

Usually, the presenting problem(s) are of moderate severity. Physicians typically spend 55 minutes at the bedside and on the patient's hospital floor or unit.

> *CPT Assistant* Winter 91:11, Spring 92:16, 23-24, Summer 92:12, Summer 93:34, Spring 95:1, Oct 97:1, Oct 97:1, Sep 98:5, Aug 01:4, Sep 02:11, May 06:1, 16, Jun 06:1, Jul 06:19; *CPT Changes: An Insider's View* 2007

99254   **Inpatient consultation** for a new or established patient, which requires these 3 key components:

- **A comprehensive history;**

- **A comprehensive examination; and**

- **Medical decision making of moderate complexity.**

Counseling and/or coordination of care with other providers or agencies are provided consistent with the nature of the problem(s) and the patient's and/or family's needs.

Usually, the presenting problem(s) are of moderate to high severity. Physicians typically spend 80 minutes at the bedside and on the patient's hospital floor or unit.

> *CPT Assistant* Winter 91:11, Spring 92:16, 23-24, Summer 92:12, Summer 93:34, Spring 95:1, Oct 97:1, Sep 98:5, Aug 01:4, Sep 02:11, May 06:1, 16, Jun 06:1, Jul 06:19; *CPT Changes: An Insider's View* 2007

99255   **Inpatient consultation** for a new or established patient, which requires these 3 key components:

- **A comprehensive history;**

- **A comprehensive examination; and**

- **Medical decision making of high complexity.**

Counseling and/or coordination of care with other providers or agencies are provided consistent with the nature of the problem(s) and the patient's and/or family's needs.

Usually, the presenting problem(s) are of moderate to high severity. Physicians typically spend 110 minutes at the bedside and on the patient's hospital floor or unit.

> *CPT Assistant* Winter 91:11, Spring 92:16, 23-24, Summer 92:12, Summer 93:34, Spring 95:1, Oct 97:1, Sep 98:5, Aug 01:4, Sep 02:11, May 06:1, 16, Jun 06:1, Jul 06:19; *CPT Changes: An Insider's View* 2007

Emergency Department Services

New or Established Patient

The following codes are used to report evaluation and management services provided in the emergency department. No distinction is made between new and established patients in the emergency department.

An emergency department is defined as an organized hospital-based facility for the provision of unscheduled episodic services to patients who present for immediate medical attention. The facility must be available 24 hours a day.

For critical care services provided in the emergency department, see Critical Care notes and 99291, 99292.

For evaluation and management services provided to a patient in an observation area of a hospital, see 99217-99220.

For observation or inpatient care services (including admission and discharge services), see 99234-99236.

99281   **Emergency department visit** for the evaluation and management of a patient, which requires these 3 key components:

- **A problem focused history;**
- **A problem focused examination; and**
- **Straightforward medical decision making.**

Counseling and/or coordination of care with other providers or agencies are provided consistent with the nature of the problem(s) and the patient's and/or family's needs.

Usually, the presenting problem(s) are self limited or minor.

➔ *CPT Assistant* Winter 91:11, Spring 92:24, Summer 92:18, Spring 93:34, Spring 95:1, Feb 96:3, Sep 98:5, Jan 00:11, Feb 00:11, Sep 00:3, Apr 02:14, Jul 02:2, May 05:1, Nov 05:10, Feb 06:14, Dec 06:14

99282   **Emergency department visit** for the evaluation and management of a patient, which requires these 3 key components:

- **An expanded problem focused history;**
- **An expanded problem focused examination; and**
- **Medical decision making of low complexity.**

Counseling and/or coordination of care with other providers or agencies are provided consistent with the nature of the problem(s) and the patient's and/or family's needs.

Usually, the presenting problem(s) are of low to moderate severity.

➔ *CPT Assistant* Winter 91:11, Spring 92:24, Summer 92:18, Spring 93:34, Spring 95:1, Summer 95:1, Feb 96:3, Sep 98:5, Jan 00:11, Feb 00:11, Sep 00:3, Apr 02:14, Jul 02:2, Nov 05:10, Feb 06:14, Dec 06:14

99283   **Emergency department visit** for the evaluation and management of a patient, which requires these 3 key components:

- **An expanded problem focused history;**
- **An expanded problem focused examination; and**
- **Medical decision making of moderate complexity.**

Counseling and/or coordination of care with other providers or agencies are provided consistent with the nature of the problem(s) and the patient's and/or family's needs.

Usually, the presenting problem(s) are of moderate severity.

➔ *CPT Assistant* Winter 91:11, Spring 92:24, Summer 92:18, Spring 93:34, Spring 95:1, Summer 95:1, Feb 96:3, Sep 98:5, Jan 00:11, Feb 00:11, Sep 00:3, Apr 02:14, Jul 02:2, Nov 05:10, Feb 06:14, Dec 06:14

99284   **Emergency department visit** for the evaluation and management of a patient, which requires these 3 key components:

- **A detailed history;**
- **A detailed examination; and**
- **Medical decision making of moderate complexity.**

Counseling and/or coordination of care with other providers or agencies are provided consistent with the nature of the problem(s) and the patient's and/or family's needs.

Usually, the presenting problem(s) are of high severity, and require urgent evaluation by the physician but do not pose an immediate significant threat to life or physiologic function.

➔ *CPT Assistant* Winter 91:11, Spring 92:24, Summer 92:18, Spring 93:34, Spring 95:1, Summer 95:1, Feb 96:3, Sep 98:5, Jan 00:11, Feb 00:11, Sep 00:3, Apr 02:14, Jul 02:2, Nov 05:10, Feb 06:14, Dec 06:14

99285   **Emergency department visit** for the evaluation and management of a patient, which requires these 3 key components within the constraints imposed by the urgency of the patient's clinical condition and/or mental status:

- **A comprehensive history;**
- **A comprehensive examination; and**
- **Medical decision making of high complexity.**

Counseling and/or coordination of care with other providers or agencies are provided consistent with the nature of the problem(s) and the patient's and/or family's needs.

Usually, the presenting problem(s) are of high severity and pose an immediate significant threat to life or physiologic function.

➔ *CPT Assistant* Winter 91:11, Spring 92:24, Summer 92:18, Spring 93:34, Spring 95:1, Summer 95:1, Feb 96:3, Aug 98:8, Sep 98:5, Nov 99:23, Jan 00:11, Feb 00:11, Sep 00:3, Apr 02:14, Jul 02:2, Sep 02:11, Mar 05:11, Nov 05:10, Feb 06:14, Dec 06:14; *CPT Changes: An Insider's View* 2000

Other Emergency Services

In physician directed emergency care, advanced life support, the physician is located in a hospital emergency or critical care department, and is in two-way voice communication with ambulance or rescue personnel outside the hospital. The physician directs the performance of necessary medical procedures, including but not limited to: telemetry of cardiac rhythm; cardiac and/or pulmonary resuscitation; endotracheal or esophageal obturator airway intubation; administration of intravenous fluids and/or administration of intramuscular, intratracheal or subcutaneous drugs; and/or electrical conversion of arrhythmia.

99288   **Physician direction of** emergency medical systems (EMS) emergency care, advanced life support

> *CPT Assistant* Summer 92:18, May 05:1

Pediatric Critical Care Patient Transport

The following codes 99289 and 99290 are used to report the physical attendance and direct face-to-face care by a physician during the interfacility transport of a critically ill or critically injured pediatric patient. For the purpose of reporting codes 99289 and 99290, face-to-face care begins when the physician assumes primary responsibility of the pediatric patient at the referring hospital/facility, and ends when the receiving hospital/facility accepts responsibility for the pediatric patient's care. Only the time the physician spends in direct face-to-face contact with the patient during the transport should be reported. Pediatric patient transport services involving less than 30 minutes of face-to-face physician care should not be reported using codes 99289, 99290. Procedure(s) or service(s) performed by other members of the transporting team may not be reported by the supervising physician.

▶The following services are included when performed during the pediatric patient transport by the physician providing critical care and may not be reported separately: routine monitoring evaluations (eg, heart rate, respiratory rate, blood pressure, and pulse oximetry), the interpretation of cardiac output measurements (93561, 93562), chest X rays (71010, 71015, 71020), pulse oximetry (94760, 94761, 94762), blood gases and information data stored in computers (eg, ECGs, blood pressures, hematologic data) (99090), gastric intubation (43752, 91105), temporary transcutaneous pacing (92953), ventilatory management (94002-94004, 94660, 94662) and vascular access procedures (36000, 36400, 36405, 36406, 36410, 36415, 36591, 36600). Any services performed that are not listed above should be reported separately.◀

Critical care is the direct delivery by a physician(s) of medical care for a critically ill or critically injured patient. A critical illness or injury acutely impairs one or more vital organ systems such that there is a high probability of imminent or life threatening deterioration in the patient's condition. Critical care involves high complexity decision making to assess, manipulate, and support vital system function(s) to treat single or multiple vital organ system failure and/or to prevent further life threatening deterioration of the patient's condition. Examples of vital organ system failure include, but are not limited to: central nervous system failure, circulatory failure, shock, renal, hepatic, metabolic, and/or respiratory failure.

Providing medical care to a critically ill, injured, or post-operative patient qualifies as a critical care service only if both the illness or injury and the treatment being provided meet the above requirements.

The direction of emergency care to transporting staff by a physician located in a hospital or other facility by two-way communication is not considered direct face-to-face care and should not be reported with codes 99289, 99290. Physician directed emergency care through outside voice communication to transporting staff personnel is reported with code 99288.

The emergency department services codes (99281-99285), initial hospital care codes (99221-99223), hourly critical care codes (99291, 99292), or initial date neonatal intensive care code (99295) are only reported after the patient has been admitted to the emergency department, the inpatient floor or the critical care unit of the receiving facility.

Code 99289 is used to report the first 30-74 minutes of direct face-to-face time with the transport pediatric patient and should be reported only once on a given date. Code 99290 is used to report each additional 30 minutes provided on a given date. Face-to-face services less than 30 minutes should not be reported with these codes.

99289   Critical care services delivered by a physician, face-to-face, during an interfacility transport of critically ill or critically injured pediatric patient, 24 months of age or less; first 30-74 minutes of hands on care during transport

> *CPT Assistant* May 05:1, Jul 06:4; *CPT Changes: An Insider's View* 2002, 2003

+ 99290   each additional 30 minutes (List separately in addition to code for primary service)

> *CPT Changes: An Insider's View* 2002

(Use 99290 in conjunction with 99289)

(Critical care of less than 30 minutes total duration should be reported with the appropriate E/M code)

Critical Care Services

Critical care is the direct delivery by a physician(s) of medical care for a critically ill or critically injured patient. A critical illness or injury acutely impairs one or more vital organ systems such that there is a high probability of imminent or life threatening deterioration in the patient's condition. Critical care involves high complexity decision making to assess, manipulate, and support vital system function(s) to treat single or multiple vital organ system failure and/or to prevent further life threatening deterioration of the patient's condition. Examples of vital organ system failure include, but are not limited to: central nervous system failure, circulatory failure, shock, renal, hepatic, metabolic, and/or respiratory failure. Although critical care typically requires interpretation of multiple physiologic parameters and/or application of advanced technology(s), critical care may be provided in life threatening situations when these elements are not present. Critical care may be provided on multiple days, even if no changes are made in the treatment rendered to the patient, provided that the patient's condition continues to require the level of physician attention described above.

Providing medical care to a critically ill, injured, or post-operative patient qualifies as a critical care service only if both the illness or injury and the treatment being provided meet the above requirements. Critical care is usually, but not always, given in a critical care area, such as the coronary care unit, intensive care unit, pediatric intensive care unit, respiratory care unit, or the emergency care facility.

Inpatient critical care services provided to infants 29 days through 24 months of age are reported with pediatric critical care codes 99293 and 99294. The pediatric critical care codes are reported as long as the infant/young child qualifies for critical care services during the hospital stay through 24 months of age. Inpatient critical care services provided to neonates (28 days of age or less) are reported with the neonatal critical care codes 99295 and 99296. The neonatal critical care codes are reported as long as the neonate qualifies for critical care services during the hospital stay through the 28th postnatal day. The reporting of the pediatric and neonatal critical care services is not based on time or the type of unit (eg, pediatric or neonatal critical care unit) and it is not dependent upon the type of provider delivering the care. To report critical care services provided in the outpatient setting (eg, emergency department or office), for neonates and pediatric patients up through 24 months of age, see the hourly Critical Care codes 99291, 99292. If the same physician provides critical care services for a neonatal or pediatric patient in both the outpatient and inpatient settings on the same day, report only the appropriate Neonatal or Pediatric Critical Care code (99293-99296) for all critical care services provided on that day. For

additional instructions on reporting these services, see the Neonatal and Pediatric Critical Care section and codes 99293-99296.

Services for a patient who is not critically ill but happens to be in a critical care unit are reported using other appropriate E/M codes.

Critical care and other E/M services may be provided to the same patient on the same date by the same physician.

▶The following services are included in reporting critical care when performed during the critical period by the physician(s) providing critical care: the interpretation of cardiac output measurements (93561, 93562), chest X rays (71010, 71015, 71020), pulse oximetry (94760, 94761, 94762), blood gases, and information data stored in computers (eg, ECGs, blood pressures, hematologic data [99090]); gastric intubation (43752, 91105); temporary transcutaneous pacing (92953); ventilatory management (94002-94004, 94660, 94662); and vascular access procedures (36000, 36410, 36415, 36591, 36600). Any services performed that are not listed above should be reported separately.◀

Codes 99291, 99292 should be reported for the physician's attendance during the transport of critically ill or critically injured patients over 24 months of age to or from a facility or hospital. For physician transport services of critically ill or critically injured pediatric patients 24 months of age or less see 99289, 99290.

The critical care codes 99291 and 99292 are used to report the total duration of time spent by a physician providing critical care services to a critically ill or critically injured patient, even if the time spent by the physician on that date is not continuous. For any given period of time spent providing critical care services, the physician must devote his or her full attention to the patient and, therefore, cannot provide services to any other patient during the same period of time.

Time spent with the individual patient should be recorded in the patient's record. The time that can be reported as critical care is the time spent engaged in work directly related to the individual patient's care whether that time was spent at the immediate bedside or elsewhere on the floor or unit. For example, time spent on the unit or at the nursing station on the floor reviewing test results or imaging studies, discussing the critically ill patient's care with other medical staff or documenting critical care services in the medical record would be reported as critical care, even though it does not occur at the bedside. Also, when the patient is unable or clinically incompetent to participate in discussions, time spent on the floor or unit with family members or surrogate decision makers obtaining a medical history, reviewing the patient's condition or prognosis, or discussing treatment or limitation(s) of treatment may be reported as critical care, provided that the conversation bears directly on the management of the patient.

Time spent in activities that occur outside of the unit or off the floor (eg, telephone calls, whether taken at home, in the office, or elsewhere in the hospital) may not be reported as critical care since the physician is not immediately available to the patient. Time spent in activities that do not directly contribute to the treatment of the patient may not be reported as critical care, even if they are performed in the critical care unit (eg, participation in administrative meetings or telephone calls to discuss other patients). Time spent performing separately reportable procedures or services should not be included in the time reported as critical care time.

Code 99291 is used to report the first 30-74 minutes of critical care on a given date. It should be used only once per date even if the time spent by the physician is not continuous on that date. Critical care of less than 30 minutes total duration on a given date should be reported with the appropriate E/M code.

Code 99292 is used to report additional block(s) of time, of up to 30 minutes each beyond the first 74 minutes. (See table below.)

The following examples illustrate the correct reporting of critical care services:

Total Duration of Critical Care	Codes
less than 30 minutes (less than 30 minutes)	appropriate E/M codes
30-74 minutes (30 minutes - 1 hr. 14 min.)	99291 X 1
75-104 minutes (1 hr. 15 min. - 1 hr. 44 min.)	99291 X 1 AND 99292 X 1
105-134 minutes (1 hr. 45 min. - 2 hr. 14 min.)	99291 X 1 AND 99292 X 2
135 - 164 minutes (2 hr. 15 min. - 2 hr. 44 min.)	99291 X 1 AND 99292 X 3
165 - 194 minutes (2 hr. 45 min. - 3 hr. 14 min.)	99291 X 1 AND 99292 X 4
194 minutes or longer (3 hr. 14 min. - etc.)	99291 and 99292 as appropriate (see illustrated reporting examples above)

99291 **Critical care, evaluation and management** of the critically ill or critically injured patient; first 30-74 minutes

➔ *CPT Assistant* Summer 92:18, Summer 93:1, Summer 95:1, Jan 96:7, Apr 97:3, Dec 98:6, Nov 99:3, Apr 00:6, Sep 00:1, Dec 00:15, Jul 02:2, Feb 03:15, Oct 03:2, Aug 04:7, 10, Oct 04:14, May 05:1, Jul 05:15, Nov 05:10, Jul 06:4, Dec 06:13

+ 99292 each additional 30 minutes (List separately in addition to code for primary service)

➔ *CPT Assistant* Summer 92:18, Summer 93:1, Summer 95:1, Jan 96:7, Apr 97:3, Dec 98:6, Nov 99:3, Apr 00:6, Sep 00:1, Dec 00:15, Feb 03:15, Oct 03:2, Aug 04:10, Oct 04:14, Jul 05:15, Nov 05:10, Jul 06:4, Dec 06:13

(Use 99292 in conjunction with 99291)

▶Inpatient Neonatal and Pediatric Critical Care and Intensive Services◀

The following codes (99293-99296) are used to report services provided by a physician directing the inpatient care of a critically ill neonate/infant. The same definitions for critical care services apply for the adult, child, and neonate.

The initial day neonatal critical care code (99295) can be used in addition to codes 99360, 99436 or 99440 as appropriate, when the physician is present for the delivery (99360 or 99436) and newborn resuscitation (99440) is required. Other procedures performed as a necessary part of the resuscitation (eg, endotracheal intubation (31500)) are also reported separately when performed as part of the pre-admission delivery room care. In order to report these procedures separately, they must be performed as a necessary component of the resuscitation and not simply as a convenience before admission to the neonatal intensive care unit.

Codes 99295, 99296 are used to report services provided by a physician directing the inpatient care of a critically ill neonate through the first 28 days of life. They represent care starting with the date of admission (99295) and subsequent day(s) (99296) and may be reported only once per day, per patient.

Codes 99293, 99294 are used to report services provided by a physician directing the inpatient care of a critically ill infant or young child from 29 days of postnatal age through 24 months of age. They represent care starting with the date of admission (99293) and subsequent day(s) (99294) and may be reported by a single physician only once per day, per patient in a given setting. The critically ill or critically injured child older than 24 months of age would be reported with hourly critical care service codes (99291, 99292).

▶When a neonate or infant is not critically ill, but requires intensive observation, frequent interventions and other intensive care services, the Continuing Intensive Care Services codes (99298, 99299, 99300) should be used to report services for those neonates/infants with present body weight of 5000 grams or less. When the present body weight of those neonates/infants exceeds 5000 grams, the Subsequent Hospital Care Services codes (99231-99233) should be used. To report initial services for the neonate requiring intensive observation, frequent interventions and other intensive care services, use 99477.◄

To report critical care services provided in the outpatient setting (eg, emergency department or office) for neonates and pediatric patients up through 24 months of age, see the hourly Critical Care codes 99291, 99292. If the same physician provides critical care services for a neonatal or pediatric patient in both the outpatient and inpatient settings on the same day, report only the appropriate Neonatal or Pediatric Critical Care code (99293-99296) for all critical care services provided on that day.

Care rendered under 99293-99296 includes management, monitoring, and treatment of the patient including respiratory, pharmacologic control of the circulatory system, enteral and parenteral nutrition, metabolic and hematologic maintenance, parent/family counseling, case management services, and personal direct supervision of the health care team in the performance of cognitive and procedural activities.

►The pediatric and neonatal critical care codes include those procedures listed above for the hourly critical care codes (99291, 99292). In addition, the following procedures are also included in the bundled (global) pediatric and neonatal critical care service codes (99293-99296), and the initial and continuing intensive care codes (99298-99300, 99477), umbilical venous (36510) and umbilical arterial catheters (36660), other arterial catheters (36140, 36620), central (36555) or peripheral vessel catheterization (36000), vascular access procedures (36400, 36405, 36406), vascular punctures (36420, 36600), oral or nasogastric tube placement (43752), endotracheal intubation (31500), lumbar puncture (62270), suprapubic bladder aspiration (51100), bladder catheterization (51701, 51702), ventilatory management (94002-94004), continuous positive airway pressure (CPAP) (94660), surfactant administration (94610), transfusion of blood components (36430, 36440), invasive or noninvasive electronic monitoring of vital signs, bedside pulmonary function testing (94375), and/or monitoring or interpretation of blood gases or oxygen saturation (94760-94762). Any services performed that are not listed above should be reported separately.◄

For additional instructions, see descriptions listed for 99293-99296

Inpatient Pediatric Critical Care

99293 **Initial inpatient pediatric critical care,** per day, for the evaluation and management of a critically ill infant or young child, 29 days through 24 months of age

➔ *CPT Assistant* Feb 03:15, Oct 03:2, Aug 04:7, 10, May 05:1, Nov 05:10, Jul 06:4, Apr 07:3; *CPT Changes: An Insider's View* 2003, 2004, 2005

99294 **Subsequent inpatient pediatric critical care,** per day, for the evaluation and management of a critically ill infant or young child, 29 days through 24 months of age

➔ *CPT Assistant* Feb 03:15, Oct 03:2, Aug 04:7, Nov 05:10, Jul 06:4, Apr 07:3; *CPT Changes: An Insider's View* 2003, 2004, 2005

Inpatient Neonatal Critical Care

99295 **Initial inpatient neonatal critical care,** per day, for the evaluation and management of a critically ill neonate, 28 days of age or less

This code is reserved for the date of admission for neonates who are critically ill. Critically ill neonates require cardiac and/or respiratory support (including ventilator or nasal CPAP when indicated), continuous or frequent vital sign monitoring, laboratory and blood gas interpretations, follow-up physician reevaluations, and constant observation by the health care team under direct physician supervision. Immediate preoperative evaluation and stabilization of neonates with life threatening surgical or cardiac conditions are included under this code. Neonates with life threatening surgical or cardiac conditions are included under this code.

Care for neonates who require an intensive care setting but who are not critically ill is reported using the initial hospital care codes (99221-99223).

➔ *CPT Assistant* Summer 93:1, Nov 97:4-5, Mar 98:11, Nov 99:5-6, Dec 00:14, Feb 03:15, Oct 03:1, May 05:1, Nov 05:10; *CPT Changes: An Insider's View* 2000, 2003, 2004, 2005

▲ **99296** **Subsequent inpatient neonatal critical care,** per day, for the evaluation and management of a critically ill neonate, 28 days of age or less

➔ *CPT Changes: An Insider's View* 2008

A critically ill neonate will require cardiac and/or respiratory support (including ventilator or nasal CPAP when indicated), continuous or frequent vital sign monitoring, laboratory and blood gas interpretations, follow-up physician re-evaluations throughout a 24-hour period, and constant observation by the health care team under direct physician supervision.

►(Subsequent care for neonates who require an intensive setting but who are not critically ill is reported using either the intensive low birth weight services codes [99298, 99299 for those 5000 grams or less] or the subsequent hospital care codes [99231-99233 for those greater than 5000 grams])◄

➔ *CPT Assistant* Summer 93:1, Nov 97:4-5, Mar 98:11, Nov 99:5-6, Dec 00: 14, Feb 03:15, Oct 03:1, Nov 05:10; *CPT Changes: An Insider's View* 2000, 2003, 2004, 2005, 2008

Continuing Intensive Care Services

Codes 99298, 99299, 99300 are used to report services subsequent to the day of admission provided by a physician directing the continuing intensive care of the low birth weight (LBW, 1500-2500 grams present body weight) infant, very low birth weight (VLBW, less than 1500 grams present body weight) infant, or normal weight (2501-5000 grams present body weight) newborn who do not meet the definition of critically ill but continue to require intensive observation, frequent interventions, and other intensive services. Codes 99298, 99299, 99300 represent subsequent day(s) of care and may be reported only once per calendar day, per patient and are global codes with the same services bundled as outlined under codes 99293-99296.

For additional instructions, see descriptions listed for 99298, 99299, 99300.

99298 **Subsequent intensive care,** per day, for the evaluation and management of the recovering very low birth weight infant (present body weight less than 1500 g)

Infants with present body weight less than 1500 grams who are not critically ill but continue to require intensive cardiac and respiratory monitoring, continuous and/or frequent vital sign monitoring, heat maintenance, enteral and/or parenteral nutritional adjustments, laboratory and oxygen monitoring and constant observation by the health care team under direct physician supervision.

➔ *CPT Assistant* Nov 98:2-3, Nov 99:5-6, Aug 00:4, Dec 00:15, Oct 03:2, May 05:1, Nov 05:10; *CPT Changes: An Insider's View* 2000, 2003

99299 **Subsequent intensive care,** per day, for the evaluation and management of the recovering low birth weight infant (present body weight of 1500-2500 g)

Infants with present body weight of 1500-2500 grams who are not critically ill but continue to require intensive cardiac and respiratory monitoring, continuous and/or frequent vital sign monitoring, heat maintenance, enteral and/or parenteral nutritional adjustments, laboratory and oxygen monitoring, and constant observation by the health care team under direct physician supervision.

➔ *CPT Assistant* Oct 03:2, Nov 05:10; *CPT Changes: An Insider's View* 2003

99300 **Subsequent intensive care,** per day, for the evaluation and management of the recovering infant (present body weight of 2501-5000 g)

Infants with present body weight of 2501-5000 grams who are not critically ill but continue to require intensive cardiac and respiratory monitoring, continuous and/or frequent vital sign monitoring, heat maintenance, enteral and/or parenteral nutritional adjustments, laboratory and oxygen monitoring and constant observation by the health care team under direct physician supervision.

➔ *CPT Changes: An Insider's View* 2006

Nursing Facility Services

The following codes are used to report evaluation and management services to patients in nursing facilities (formerly called skilled nursing facilities [SNFs], intermediate care facilities [ICFs], or long-term care facilities [LTCFs]).

These codes should also be used to report evaluation and management services provided to a patient in a psychiatric residential treatment center (a facility or a distinct part of a facility for psychiatric care, which provides a 24-hour therapeutically planned and professionally staffed group living and learning environment). If procedures such as medical psychotherapy are provided in addition to evaluation and management services, these should be reported in addition to the evaluation and management services provided.

Nursing facilities that provide convalescent, rehabilitative, or long term care are required to conduct comprehensive, accurate, standardized, and reproducible assessments of each resident's functional capacity using a Resident Assessment Instrument (RAI). All RAIs include the Minimum Data Set (MDS), Resident Assessment Protocols (RAPs), and utilization guidelines. The MDS is the primary screening and assessment tool; the RAPs trigger the identification of potential problems and provide guidelines for follow-up assessments.

Physicians have a central role in assuring that all residents receive thorough assessments and that medical plans of care are instituted or revised to enhance or maintain the residents' physical and psychosocial functioning. This role includes providing input in the development of the MDS and a multi-disciplinary plan of care, as required by regulations pertaining to the care of nursing facility residents.

Two major subcategories of nursing facility services are recognized: Initial Nursing Facility Care and Subsequent Nursing Facility Care. Both subcategories apply to new or established patients.

For definitions of key components and commonly used terms, please see **Evaluation and Management Services Guidelines.**

(For care plan oversight services provided to nursing facility residents, see 99379-99380)

Initial Nursing Facility Care

New or Established Patient

When the patient is admitted to the nursing facility in the course of an encounter in another site of service (eg, hospital emergency department, physician's office), all evaluation and management services provided by that physician in conjunction with that admission are considered part of the initial nursing facility care when performed on the same date as the admission or readmission. The nursing facility care level of service reported by the admitting physician should include the services related to the admission he/she provided in the other sites of service as well as in the nursing facility setting.

Hospital discharge or observation discharge services performed on the same date of nursing facility admission or readmission may be reported separately. For a patient discharged from inpatient status on the same date of nursing facility admission or readmission, the hospital discharge services should be reported with codes 99238, 99239 as appropriate. For a patient discharged from observation status on the same date of nursing facility admission or readmission, the observation care discharge services should be reported with code 99217. For a patient admitted and discharged from observation or inpatient status on the same date, see codes 99234-99236.

(For nursing facility care discharge, see 99315, 99316)

(99301-99303 have been deleted)

▲ **99304**   Initial nursing facility care, per day, for the evaluation and management of a patient, which requires these 3 key components:

- **A detailed or comprehensive history;**
- **A detailed or comprehensive examination; and**
- **Medical decision making that is straightforward or of low complexity.**

Counseling and/or coordination of care with other providers or agencies are provided consistent with the nature of the problem(s) and the patient's and/or family's needs.

Usually, the problem(s) requiring admission are of low severity. Physicians typically spend 25 minutes with the patient and/or family or caregiver.

➔ *CPT Changes: An Insider's View* 2006, 2008

▲ **99305**   Initial nursing facility care, per day, for the evaluation and management of a patient, which requires these 3 key components:

- **A comprehensive history;**
- **A comprehensive examination; and**
- **Medical decision making of moderate complexity.**

Counseling and/or coordination of care with other providers or agencies are provided consistent with the nature of the problem(s) and the patient's and/or family's needs.

Usually, the problem(s) requiring admission are of moderate severity. Physicians typically spend 35 minutes with the patient and/or family or caregiver.

➔ *CPT Changes: An Insider's View* 2006, 2008

▲ **99306**   Initial nursing facility care, per day, for the evaluation and management of a patient, which requires these 3 key components:

- **A comprehensive history;**
- **A comprehensive examination; and**
- **Medical decision making of high complexity.**

Counseling and/or coordination of care with other providers or agencies are provided consistent with the nature of the problem(s) and the patient's and/or family's needs.

Usually, the problem(s) requiring admission are of high severity. Physicians typically spend 45 minutes with the patient and/or family or caregiver.

➔ *CPT Changes: An Insider's View* 2006, 2008

Subsequent Nursing Facility Care

All levels of subsequent nursing facility care include reviewing the medical record and reviewing the results of diagnostic studies and changes in the patient's status (ie, changes in history, physical condition, and response to management) since the last assessment by the physician.

▲ **99307**   Subsequent nursing facility care, per day, for the evaluation and management of a patient, which requires at least 2 of these 3 key components:

- **A problem focused interval history;**
- **A problem focused examination;**
- **Straightforward medical decision making.**

Counseling and/or coordination of care with other providers or agencies are provided consistent with the nature of the problem(s) and the patient's and/or family's needs.

Usually, the patient is stable, recovering, or improving. Physicians typically spend 10 minutes with the patient and/or family or caregiver.

➔ *CPT Changes: An Insider's View* 2006, 2008

▲ **99308**   Subsequent nursing facility care, per day, for the evaluation and management of a patient, which requires at least 2 of these 3 key components:

- **An expanded problem focused interval history;**
- **An expanded problem focused examination;**
- **Medical decision making of low complexity.**

Counseling and/or coordination of care with other providers or agencies are provided consistent with the nature of the problem(s) and the patient's and/or family's needs.

Usually, the patient is responding inadequately to therapy or has developed a minor complication. Physicians typically spend 15 minutes with the patient and/or family or caregiver.

➔ *CPT Changes: An Insider's View* 2006, 2008

▲ **99309**   Subsequent nursing facility care, per day, for the evaluation and management of a patient, which requires at least 2 of these 3 key components:

- **A detailed interval history;**
- **A detailed examination;**
- **Medical decision making of moderate complexity.**

Counseling and/or coordination of care with other providers or agencies are provided consistent with the nature of the problem(s) and the patient's and/or family's needs.

Usually, the patient has developed a significant complication or a significant new problem. Physicians typically spend 25 minutes with the patient and/or family or caregiver.

➔ *CPT Changes: An Insider's View* 2006, 2008

▲ **99310**   Subsequent nursing facility care, per day, for the evaluation and management of a patient, which requires at least 2 of these 3 key components:

- **A comprehensive interval history;**
- **A comprehensive examination;**
- **Medical decision making of high complexity.**

Counseling and/or coordination of care with other providers or agencies are provided consistent with the nature of the problem(s) and the patient's and/or family's needs.

The patient may be unstable or may have developed a significant new problem requiring immediate physician attention. Physicians typically spend 35 minutes with the patient and/or family or caregiver.

➔ *CPT Changes: An Insider's View* 2006, 2008

(99311-99313 have been deleted)

Nursing Facility Discharge Services

The nursing facility discharge day management codes are to be used to report the total duration of time spent by a physician for the final nursing facility discharge of a patient. The codes include, as appropriate, final examination of the patient, discussion of the nursing facility stay, even if the time spent by the physician on that date is not continuous. Instructions are given for continuing care to all relevant caregivers, and preparation of discharge records, prescriptions and referral forms.

99315   Nursing facility discharge day management; 30 minutes or less

➔ *CPT Assistant* Nov 97:5-6, Sep 98:5, May 02:19, Nov 02:11, May 05:1

99316   more than 30 minutes

➔ *CPT Assistant* Nov 97:5-6, Sep 98:5, May 02:19, Nov 02:11

Other Nursing Facility Services

▲ **99318**   Evaluation and management of a patient involving an annual nursing facility assessment, which requires these 3 key components:

- **A detailed interval history;**
- **A comprehensive examination; and**
- **Medical decision making that is of low to moderate complexity.**

Counseling and/or coordination of care with other providers or agencies are provided consistent with the nature of the problem(s) and the patient's and/or family's needs.

Usually, the patient is stable, recovering, or improving. Physicians typically spend 30 minutes with the patient and/or family or caregiver.

➔ *CPT Changes: An Insider's View* 2006, 2008

(Do not report 99318 on the same date of service as nursing facility services codes 99304-99316)

Domiciliary, Rest Home (eg, Boarding Home), or Custodial Care Services

The following codes are used to report evaluation and management services in a facility which provides room, board and other personal assistance services, generally on a long-term basis. They also are used to report evaluation and management services in an assisted living facility.

The facility's services do not include a medical component.

For definitions of key components and commonly used terms, please see **Evaluation and Management Services Guidelines.**

(For care plan oversight services provided to a patient in a domiciliary facility under the care of a home health agency, see 99374-99375)

(For care plan oversight services provided to a patient in a domiciliary facility under the individual supervision of a physician, see 99339, 99340)

New Patient

(99321-99323 have been deleted)

99324   Domiciliary or rest home visit for the evaluation and management of a new patient, which requires these 3 key components:

- **A problem focused history;**
- **A problem focused examination; and**
- **Straightforward medical decision making.**

Counseling and/or coordination of care with other providers or agencies are provided consistent with the nature of the problem(s) and the patient's and/or family's needs.

Usually, the presenting problem(s) are of low severity. Physicians typically spend 20 minutes with the patient and/or family or caregiver.

➔ *CPT Assistant* Jan 06:1, Jun 06:1; *CPT Changes: An Insider's View* 2006

99325   Domiciliary or rest home visit for the evaluation and management of a new patient, which requires these 3 key components:

- **An expanded problem focused history;**
- **An expanded problem focused examination; and**
- **Medical decision making of low complexity.**

Counseling and/or coordination of care with other providers or agencies are provided consistent with the nature of the problem(s) and the patient's and/or family's needs.

Usually, the presenting problem(s) are of moderate severity. Physicians typically spend 30 minutes with the patient and/or family or caregiver.

➔ *CPT Assistant* Jan 06:1, Jun 06:1; *CPT Changes: An Insider's View* 2006

99326   Domiciliary or rest home visit for the evaluation and management of a new patient, which requires these 3 key components:

- **A detailed history;**
- **A detailed examination; and**
- **Medical decision making of moderate complexity.**

Counseling and/or coordination of care with other providers or agencies are provided consistent with the nature of the problem(s) and the patient's and/or family's needs.

Usually, the presenting problem(s) are of moderate to high severity. Physicians typically spend 45 minutes with the patient and/or family or caregiver.

➔ *CPT Assistant* Jan 06:1, Jun 06:1; *CPT Changes: An Insider's View* 2006

99327   Domiciliary or rest home visit for the evaluation and management of a new patient, which requires these 3 key components:

- **A comprehensive history;**
- **A comprehensive examination; and**
- **Medical decision making of moderate complexity.**

Counseling and/or coordination of care with other providers or agencies are provided consistent with the nature of the problem(s) and the patient's and/or family's needs.

Usually, the presenting problem(s) are of high severity. Physicians typically spend 60 minutes with the patient and/or family or caregiver.

➔ *CPT Assistant* Jan 06:1, Jun 06:1; *CPT Changes: An Insider's View* 2006

99328   Domiciliary or rest home visit for the evaluation and management of a new patient, which requires these 3 key components:

- **A comprehensive history;**
- **A comprehensive examination; and**
- **Medical decision making of high complexity.**

Counseling and/or coordination of care with other providers or agencies are provided consistent with the nature of the problem(s) and the patient's and/or family's needs.

Usually, the patient is unstable or has developed a significant new problem requiring immediate physician attention. Physicians typically spend 75 minutes with the patient and/or family or caregiver.

➔ *CPT Assistant* Jan 06:1, Jun 06:1; *CPT Changes: An Insider's View* 2006

Established Patient

(99331-99333 have been deleted)

99334   Domiciliary or rest home visit for the evaluation and management of an established patient, which requires at least 2 of these 3 key components:

- **A problem focused interval history;**
- **A problem focused examination;**
- **Straightforward medical decision making.**

Counseling and/or coordination of care with other providers or agencies are provided consistent with the nature of the problem(s) and the patient's and/or family's needs.

Usually, the presenting problem(s) are self-limited or minor. Physicians typically spend 15 minutes with the patient and/or family or caregiver.

➔ *CPT Assistant* Jan 06:1, Jun 06:1; *CPT Changes: An Insider's View* 2006

99335   Domiciliary or rest home visit for the evaluation and management of an established patient, which requires at least 2 of these 3 key components:

- **An expanded problem focused interval history;**
- **An expanded problem focused examination;**
- **Medical decision making of low complexity.**

Counseling and/or coordination of care with other providers or agencies are provided consistent with the nature of the problem(s) and the patient's and/or family's needs.

Usually, the presenting problem(s) are of low to moderate severity. Physicians typically spend 25 minutes with the patient and/or family or caregiver.

➔ *CPT Assistant* Jan 06:1, Jun 06:1; *CPT Changes: An Insider's View* 2006

99336 Domiciliary or rest home visit for the evaluation and management of an established patient, which requires at least 2 of these 3 key components:

- **A detailed interval history;**
- **A detailed examination;**
- **Medical decision making of moderate complexity.**

Counseling and/or coordination of care with other providers or agencies are provided consistent with the nature of the problem(s) and the patient's and/or family's needs.

Usually, the presenting problem(s) are of moderate to high severity. Physicians typically spend 40 minutes with the patient and/or family or caregiver.

➔ *CPT Assistant* Jan 06:1, Jun 06:1; *CPT Changes: An Insider's View* 2006

99337 Domiciliary or rest home visit for the evaluation and management of an established patient, which requires at least 2 of these 3 key components:

- **A comprehensive interval history;**
- **A comprehensive examination;**
- **Medical decision making of moderate to high complexity.**

Counseling and/or coordination of care with other providers or agencies are provided consistent with the nature of the problem(s) and the patient's and/or family's needs.

Usually, the presenting problem(s) are of moderate to high severity. The patient may be unstable or may have developed a significant new problem requiring immediate physician attention. Physicians typically spend 60 minutes with the patient and/or family or caregiver.

➔ *CPT Assistant* Jan 06:1, Jun 06:1; *CPT Changes: An Insider's View* 2006

Domiciliary, Rest Home (eg, Assisted Living Facility), or Home Care Plan Oversight Services

(For instructions on the use of 99339, 99340, see introductory notes for 99374-99380)

(For care plan oversight services for patients under the care of a home health agency, hospice, or nursing facility, see 99374-99380)

▶(Do not report 99339, 99340 for time reported with 98966-98969, 99441-99444)◀

99339 Individual physician supervision of a patient (patient not present) in home, domiciliary or rest home (eg, assisted living facility) requiring complex and multidisciplinary care modalities involving regular physician development and/or revision of care plans, review of subsequent reports of patient status, review of related laboratory and other studies, communication (including telephone calls) for purposes of assessment or care decisions with health care professional(s), family member(s), surrogate decision maker(s) (eg, legal guardian) and/or key caregiver(s) involved in patient's care, integration of new information into the medical treatment plan and/or adjustment of medical therapy, within a calendar month; 15-29 minutes

➔ *CPT Assistant* Jan 06:1, Dec 06:4, Mar 07:11; *CPT Changes: An Insider's View* 2006

99340 30 minutes or more

➔ *CPT Assistant* Jan 06:1, Dec 06:4, Mar 07:11; *CPT Changes: An Insider's View* 2006

(Do not report 99339, 99340 for patients under the care of a home health agency, enrolled in a hospice program, or for nursing facility residents)

Home Services

The following codes are used to report evaluation and management services provided in a private residence.

For definitions of key components and commonly used terms, please see **Evaluation and Management Services Guidelines.**

(For care plan oversight services provided to a patient in the home under the care of a home health agency, see 99374-99375)

(For care plan oversight services provided to a patient in the home under the individual supervision of a physician, see 99339, 99340)

New Patient

99341 **Home visit** for the evaluation and management of a new patient, which requires these 3 key components:

- **A problem focused history;**
- **A problem focused examination; and**
- **Straightforward medical decision making.**

Counseling and/or coordination of care with other providers or agencies are provided consistent with the nature of the problem(s) and the patient's and/or family's needs.

Usually, the presenting problem(s) are of low severity. Physicians typically spend 20 minutes face-to-face with the patient and/or family.

➔ *CPT Assistant* Winter 91:11, Spring 92:24, Summer 92:12, Spring 93:34, Spring 95:1, Jun 97:6, Nov 97:6-8, Oct 98:6, Oct 03:7, May 05:1, Jan 06:1

99342   **Home visit** for the evaluation and management of a new patient, which requires these 3 key components:

- **An expanded problem focused history;**
- **An expanded problem focused examination; and**
- **Medical decision making of low complexity.**

Counseling and/or coordination of care with other providers or agencies are provided consistent with the nature of the problem(s) and the patient's and/or family's needs.

Usually, the presenting problem(s) are of moderate severity. Physicians typically spend 30 minutes face-to-face with the patient and/or family.

➔ *CPT Assistant* Winter 91:11, Spring 92:24, Summer 92:12, Spring 93:34, Spring 95:1, Jun 97:6, Nov 97:6-8, Oct 98:6, Jan 06:1

99343   **Home visit** for the evaluation and management of a new patient, which requires these 3 key components:

- **A detailed history;**
- **A detailed examination; and**
- **Medical decision making of moderate complexity.**

Counseling and/or coordination of care with other providers or agencies are provided consistent with the nature of the problem(s) and the patient's and/or family's needs.

Usually, the presenting problem(s) are of moderate to high severity. Physicians typically spend 45 minutes face-to-face with the patient and/or family.

➔ *CPT Assistant* Winter 91:11, Spring 92:24, Summer 92:12, Spring 93:34, Spring 95:1, Jun 97:6, Nov 97:6-8, Oct 98:6, Jan 06:1

99344   **Home visit** for the evaluation and management of a new patient, which requires these 3 key components:

- **A comprehensive history;**
- **A comprehensive examination; and**
- **Medical decision making of moderate complexity.**

Counseling and/or coordination of care with other providers or agencies are provided consistent with the nature of the problem(s) and the patient's and/or family's needs.

Usually, the presenting problem(s) are of high severity. Physicians typically spend 60 minutes face-to-face with the patient and/or family.

➔ *CPT Assistant* Nov 97:6-8, Oct 98:6, Jan 06:1

99345   **Home visit** for the evaluation and management of a new patient, which requires these 3 key components:

- **A comprehensive history;**
- **A comprehensive examination; and**
- **Medical decision making of high complexity.**

Counseling and/or coordination of care with other providers or agencies are provided consistent with the nature of the problem(s) and the patient's and/or family's needs.

Usually, the patient is unstable or has developed a significant new problem requiring immediate physician attention. Physicians typically spend 75 minutes face-to-face with the patient and/or family.

➔ *CPT Assistant* Nov 97:6-8, Oct 98:6, Jan 06:1

Established Patient

99347   **Home visit** for the evaluation and management of an established patient, which requires at least 2 of these 3 key components:

- **A problem focused interval history;**
- **A problem focused examination;**
- **Straightforward medical decision making.**

Counseling and/or coordination of care with other providers or agencies are provided consistent with the nature of the problem(s) and the patient's and/or family's needs.

Usually, the presenting problem(s) are self limited or minor. Physicians typically spend 15 minutes face-to-face with the patient and/or family.

➔ *CPT Assistant* Nov 97:6-8, Oct 98:6, May 05:1, Jan 06:1

99348   **Home visit** for the evaluation and management of an established patient, which requires at least 2 of these 3 key components:

- **An expanded problem focused interval history;**
- **An expanded problem focused examination;**
- **Medical decision making of low complexity.**

Counseling and/or coordination of care with other providers or agencies are provided consistent with the nature of the problem(s) and the patient's and/or family's needs.

Usually, the presenting problem(s) are of low to moderate severity. Physicians typically spend 25 minutes face-to-face with the patient and/or family.

➔ *CPT Assistant* Nov 97:6-8, Oct 98:6, Jan 06:1

99349   **Home visit** for the evaluation and management of an established patient, which requires at least 2 of these 3 key components:

- **A detailed interval history;**
- **A detailed examination;**
- **Medical decision making of moderate complexity.**

Counseling and/or coordination of care with other providers or agencies are provided consistent with the nature of the problem(s) and the patient's and/or family's needs.

Usually, the presenting problem(s) are moderate to high severity. Physicians typically spend 40 minutes face-to-face with the patient and/or family.

➔ *CPT Assistant* Nov 97:6-8, Oct 98:6, Jan 06:1

99350 **Home visit** for the evaluation and management of an established patient, which requires at least 2 of these 3 key components:

- **A comprehensive interval history;**

- **A comprehensive examination;**

- **Medical decision making of moderate to high complexity.**

Counseling and/or coordination of care with other providers or agencies are provided consistent with the nature of the problem(s) and the patient's and/or family's needs.

Usually, the presenting problem(s) are of moderate to high severity. The patient may be unstable or may have developed a significant new problem requiring immediate physician attention. Physicians typically spend 60 minutes face-to-face with the patient and/or family.

➔ *CPT Assistant* Nov 97:6-8, Oct 98:6, Oct 03:7, Jan 06:1

Prolonged Services

Prolonged Physician Service With Direct (Face-To-Face) Patient Contact

Codes 99354-99357 are used when a physician provides prolonged service involving direct (face-to-face) patient contact that is beyond the usual service in either the inpatient or outpatient setting. This service is reported in addition to other physician services, including evaluation and management services at any level. Appropriate codes should be selected for supplies provided or procedures performed in the care of the patient during this period.

Codes 99354-99357 are used to report the total duration of face-to-face time spent by a physician on a given date providing prolonged service, even if the time spent by the physician on that date is not continuous.

Code 99354 or 99356 is used to report the first hour of prolonged service on a given date, depending on the place of service.

Either code also may be used to report a total duration of prolonged service of 30-60 minutes on a given date. Either code should be used only once per date, even if the

time spent by the physician is not continuous on that date. Prolonged service of less than 30 minutes total duration on a given date is not separately reported because the work involved is included in the total work of the evaluation and management codes.

Code 99355 or 99357 is used to report each additional 30 minutes beyond the first hour, depending on the place of service. Either code may also be used to report the final 15-30 minutes of prolonged service on a given date. Prolonged service of less than 15 minutes beyond the first hour or less than 15 minutes beyond the final 30 minutes is not reported separately.

The following examples illustrate the correct reporting of prolonged physician service with direct patient contact in the office setting:

Total Duration of Prolonged Services	Code(s)
less than 30 minutes (less than 30 minutes)	Not reported separately
30-74 minutes (30 minutes - 1 hr. 14 min.)	99354 X 1
75-104 minutes (1 hr. 15 min. - 1 hr. 44 min.)	99354 X 1 AND 99355 X 1
105-134 minutes (1 hr. 45 min. - 2 hr. 14 min.)	99354 X 1 AND 99355 X 2
135-164 minutes (2 hr. 15 min. - 2 hr. 44 min.)	99354 X 1 AND 99355 X 3
165-194 minutes (2 hr. 45 min. - 3 hr. 14 min.)	99354 X 1 AND 99355 X 4

+ 99354 Prolonged physician service in the office or other outpatient setting requiring direct (face-to-face) patient contact beyond the usual service (eg, prolonged care and treatment of an acute asthmatic patient in an outpatient setting); first hour (List separately in addition to code for office or other outpatient **Evaluation and Management** service)

➔ *CPT Assistant* Spring 94:30, 32, May 97:3, Sep 98:5, Sep 00:2, Jul 01:2, May 05:1, Nov 05:10

(Use 99354 in conjunction with 99201-99215, 99241-99245, 99304-99350)

+ 99355 each additional 30 minutes (List separately in addition to code for prolonged physician service)

➔ *CPT Assistant* Spring 94:30, 32, May 97:3, Sep 98:5, Sep 00:2, Jul 01:2, Nov 05:10

(Use 99355 in conjunction with 99354)

+ 99356   Prolonged physician service in the inpatient setting, requiring direct (face-to-face) patient contact beyond the usual service (eg, maternal fetal monitoring for high risk delivery or other physiological monitoring, prolonged care of an acutely ill inpatient); first hour (List separately in addition to code for inpatient Evaluation and Management service)

➜ *CPT Assistant* Spring 94:30, 32, Apr 97:3, May 97:3, Sep 98:5, Sep 00:2, Jul 01:2, Nov 05:10

(Use 99356 in conjunction with 99221-99233, 99251-99255)

+ 99357   each additional 30 minutes (List separately in addition to code for prolonged physician service)

➜ *CPT Assistant* Spring 94:34, Apr 97:3, May 97:3, Sep 98:5, Sep 00:2, Jul 01:2, Nov 05:10

(Use 99357 in conjunction with 99356)

Prolonged Physician Service Without Direct (Face-To-Face) Patient Contact

Codes 99358 and 99359 are used when a physician provides prolonged service not involving direct (face-to-face) care that is beyond the usual service in either the inpatient or outpatient setting.

This service is to be reported in addition to other physician service, including evaluation and management services at any level.

Codes 99358 and 99359 are used to report the total duration of non-face-to-face time spent by a physician on a given date providing prolonged service, even if the time spent by the physician on that date is not continuous. Code 99358 is used to report the first hour of prolonged service on a given date regardless of the place of service.

It may also be used to report a total duration of prolonged service of 30-60 minutes on a given date. It should be used only once per date even if the time spent by the physician is not continuous on that date.

Prolonged service of less than 30 minutes total duration on a given date is not separately reported.

Code 99359 is used to report each additional 30 minutes beyond the first hour regardless of the place of service. It may also be used to report the final 15-30 minutes of prolonged service on a given date.

Prolonged service of less than 15 minutes beyond the first hour or less than 15 minutes beyond the final 30 minutes is not reported separately.

+ 99358   **Prolonged evaluation and management service** before and/or after direct (face-to-face) patient care (eg, review of extensive records and tests, communication with other professionals and/or the patient/family); first hour (List separately in addition to code(s) for other physician service(s) and/or inpatient or outpatient Evaluation and Management service)

➜ *CPT Assistant* Spring 94:34, Nov 98:3, Sep 00:3, May 05:1, Nov 05:10

+ 99359   each additional 30 minutes (List separately in addition to code for prolonged physician service)

➜ *CPT Assistant* Spring 94:34, Sep 00:3, Nov 05:10

(Use 99359 in conjunction with 99358)

▶(To report telephone evaluation and management services, see 99441-99443)◀

Physician Standby Services

Code 99360 is used to report physician standby service that is requested by another physician and that involves prolonged physician attendance without direct (face-to-face) patient contact. The physician may not be providing care or services to other patients during this period. This code is not used to report time spent proctoring another physician. It is also not used if the period of standby ends with the performance of a procedure subject to a "surgical" package by the physician who was on standby.

Code 99360 is used to report the total duration of time spent by a physician on a given date on standby. Standby service of less than 30 minutes total duration on a given date is not reported separately.

Second and subsequent periods of standby beyond the first 30 minutes may be reported only if a full 30 minutes of standby was provided for each unit of service reported.

99360   **Physician standby service,** requiring prolonged physician attendance, each 30 minutes (eg, operative standby, standby for frozen section, for cesarean/high risk delivery, for monitoring EEG)

➜ *CPT Assistant* Spring 94:32, Apr 97:10, Aug 97:18, Nov 97:8, Nov 99:5-6, Aug 00:3, Sep 00:3, May 05:1, Nov 05:10, Nov 06:23

(For hospital mandated on call services, see 99026, 99027)

(99360 may be reported in addition to 99431, 99440 as appropriate)

(Do not report 99360 in conjunction with 99436)

Case Management Services

▶Case management is a process in which a physician or another qualified health care professional is responsible for direct care of a patient and, additionally, for coordinating, managing access to, initiating, and/or supervising other health care services needed by the patient.◀

▶(99361, 99362 have been deleted. To report, see 99366-99368)◀

Anticoagulant Management

Anticoagulant services are intended to describe the outpatient management of warfarin therapy, including ordering, review, and interpretation of International Normalized Ratio (INR) testing, communication with patient, and dosage adjustments as appropriate.

▶When reporting these services, the work of anticoagulant management may not be used as a basis for reporting an evaluation and management (E/M) service or care plan oversight time during the reporting period. Do not report these services with 98966-98969, 99441-99444 when telephone or on-line services address anticoagulation with warfarin management. If a significant, separately identifiable E/M service is performed, report the appropriate E/M service code using modifier 25.◀

These services are outpatient services only. When anticoagulation therapy is initiated or continued in the inpatient or observation setting, a new period begins after discharge and is reported with 99364. Do not report 99363-99364 with 99217-99239, 99291-99300, 99304-99318 or other code(s) for physician review, interpretation, and patient management of home INR testing for a patient with mechanical heart valve(s).

Any period less than 60 continuous outpatient days is not reported. If less than the specified minimum number of services per period are performed, do not report the anticoagulant management services (99363-99364).

99363 Anticoagulant management for an outpatient taking warfarin, physician review and interpretation of International Normalized Ratio (INR) testing, patient instructions, dosage adjustment (as needed), and ordering of additional tests; initial 90 days of therapy (must include a minimum of 8 INR measurements)
➔ *CPT Changes: An Insider's View* 2007

99364 each subsequent 90 days of therapy (must include a minimum of 3 INR measurements)
➔ *CPT Changes: An Insider's View* 2007

▶Medical Team Conferences◀

▶Medical team conferences include face-to-face participation by a minimum of three qualified health care professionals from different specialties or disciplines (each of whom provide direct care to the patient), with or without the presence of the patient, family member(s), community agencies, surrogate decision maker(s) (eg, legal guardian), and/or caregiver(s). The participants are actively involved in the development, revision, coordination, and implementation of health care services needed by the patient. Reporting participants shall have performed face-to-face evaluations or treatments of the patient, independent of any team conference, within the previous 60 days.

Physicians may report their time spent in a team conference with the patient and/or family present using evaluation and management (E/M) codes (and time as the key controlling factor for code selection when counseling and/or coordination of care dominates the service). These introductory guidelines do not apply to services reported using E/M codes (see E/M services guidelines). However, the physician must be directly involved with the patient, providing face-to-face services outside of the conference visit with other providers or agencies.

Reporting participants shall document their participation in the team conference as well as their contributed information and subsequent treatment recommendations.

No more than one individual from the same specialty may report 99366-99368 at the same encounter.

Individuals should not report 99366-99368 when their participation in the medical team conference is part of a facility or organizational service contractually provided by the organizational or facility provider.

The team conference starts at the beginning of the review of an individual patient and ends at the conclusion of the review. Time related to record keeping and report generation is not reported. The reporting participant shall be present for all time reported. The time reported is not limited to the time that the participant is communicating to the other team members or patient and/or family. Time reported for medical team conferences may not be used in the determination of time for other services such as care plan oversight (99374-99380), home, domiciliary, or rest home care plan oversight (99339-99340), prolonged services (99354-99359), psychotherapy, or any E/M service. For team conferences where the patient is present for any part of the duration of the conference, nonphysician qualified health care professionals report the team conference face-to-face code 99366.◀

▶Medical Team Conference, Direct (Face-to-Face) Contact With Patient and/or Family◀

● **99366** **Medical team conference** with interdisciplinary team of health care professionals, face-to-face with patient and/or family, 30 minutes or more, participation by nonphysician qualified health care professional
➔ *CPT Changes: An Insider's View* 2008

▶(Team conference services of less than 30 minutes duration are not reported separately)◀

▶(For team conference services by a physician with patient and/or family present, see Evaluation and Management services)◀

▶Medical Team Conference, Without Direct (Face-to-Face) Contact With Patient and/or Family◀

● **99367** **Medical team conference** with interdisciplinary team of health care professionals, patient and/or family not present, 30 minutes or more; participation by physician
➔ *CPT Changes: An Insider's View* 2008

● **99368**   participation by nonphysician qualified health care professional

⮕ *CPT Changes: An Insider's View* 2008

►(Team conference services of less than 30 minutes duration are not reported separately)◄

►(99371-99373 have been deleted. To report telephone evaluation and management services, see 99441-99443)◄

Care Plan Oversight Services

►Care plan oversight services are reported separately from codes for office/outpatient, hospital, home, nursing facility or domiciliary, or non-face-to-face services. The complexity and approximate physician time of the care plan oversight services provided within a 30-day period determine code selection. Only one physician may report services for a given period of time, to reflect that physician's sole or predominant supervisory role with a particular patient. These codes should not be reported for supervision of patients in nursing facilities or under the care of home health agencies unless they require recurrent supervision of therapy.◄

The work involved in providing very low intensity or infrequent supervision services is included in the pre- and post-encounter work for home, office/outpatient and nursing facility or domiciliary visit codes.

(For care plan oversight services of patients in the home, domiciliary, or rest home (eg, assisted living facility) under the individual supervision of a physician, see 99339, 99340)

►(Do not report 99374-99380 for time reported with 98966-98969, 99441-99444)◄

99374   **Physician supervision** of a patient under care of home health agency (patient not present) in home, domiciliary or equivalent environment (eg, Alzheimer's facility) requiring complex and multidisciplinary care modalities involving regular physician development and/or revision of care plans, review of subsequent reports of patient status, review of related laboratory and other studies, communication (including telephone calls) for purposes of assessment or care decisions with health care professional(s), family member(s), surrogate decision maker(s) (eg, legal guardian) and/or key caregiver(s) involved in patient's care, integration of new information into the medical treatment plan and/or adjustment of medical therapy, within a calendar month; 15-29 minutes

⮕ *CPT Assistant* Summer 94:9, Nov 97:8-9, May 05:1, Dec 06:4, Mar 07:11; *CPT Changes: An Insider's View* 2002

99375   30 minutes or more

⮕ *CPT Assistant* Summer 94:9, Nov 97:8-9, Dec 06:4, Mar 07:11

99377   **Physician supervision** of a hospice patient (patient not present) requiring complex and multidisciplinary care modalities involving regular physician development and/or revision of care plans, review of subsequent reports of patient status, review of related laboratory and other studies, communication (including telephone calls) for purposes of assessment or care decisions with health care professional(s), family member(s), surrogate decision maker(s) (eg, legal guardian) and/or key caregiver(s) involved in patient's care, integration of new information into the medical treatment plan and/or adjustment of medical therapy, within a calendar month; 15-29 minutes

⮕ *CPT Assistant* Nov 97:8-9, Dec 06:4, Mar 07:11; *CPT Changes: An Insider's View* 2001, 2002

99378   30 minutes or more

⮕ *CPT Assistant* Nov 97:8-9, Dec 06:4, Mar 07:11

99379   **Physician supervision** of a nursing facility patient (patient not present) requiring complex and multidisciplinary care modalities involving regular physician development and/or revision of care plans, review of subsequent reports of patient status, review of related laboratory and other studies, communication (including telephone calls) for purposes of assessment or care decisions with health care professional(s), family member(s), surrogate decision maker(s) (eg, legal guardian) and/or key caregiver(s) involved in patient's care, integration of new information into the medical treatment plan and/or adjustment of medical therapy, within a calendar month; 15-29 minutes

⮕ *CPT Changes: An Insider's View* 2002

99380   30 minutes or more

⮕ *CPT Assistant* Nov 97:8-9, Dec 06:4

Preventive Medicine Services

The following codes are used to report the preventive medicine evaluation and management of infants, children, adolescents and adults.

The extent and focus of the services will largely depend on the age of the patient.

If an abnormality/ies is encountered or a preexisting problem is addressed in the process of performing this preventive medicine evaluation and management service, and if the problem/abnormality is significant enough to require additional work to perform the key components of a problem-oriented E/M service, then the appropriate Office/Outpatient code 99201-99215 should also be reported. Modifier 25 should be added to the Office/Outpatient code to indicate that a significant, separately identifiable Evaluation and Management service was provided by the same physician on the same day as the preventive medicine service. The appropriate preventive medicine service is additionally reported.

An insignificant or trivial problem/abnormality that is encountered in the process of performing the preventive medicine evaluation and management service and which does not require additional work and the performance of the key components of a problem-oriented E/M service should not be reported.

The "comprehensive" nature of the Preventive Medicine Services codes 99381-99397 reflects an age and gender appropriate history/exam and is NOT synonymous with the "comprehensive" examination required in Evaluation and Management codes 99201-99350.

Codes 99381-99397 include counseling/anticipatory guidance/risk factor reduction interventions which are provided at the time of the initial or periodic comprehensive preventive medicine examination. (Refer to codes 99401-99412 for reporting those counseling/anticipatory guidance/risk factor reduction interventions that are provided at an encounter separate from the preventive medicine examination.)

Immunizations and ancillary studies involving laboratory, radiology, other procedures, or screening tests identified with a specific CPT code are reported separately. For immunizations, see 90465-90474 and 90476-90749.

New Patient

99381   **Initial comprehensive preventive medicine** evaluation and management of an individual including an age and gender appropriate history, examination, counseling/anticipatory guidance/risk factor reduction interventions, and the ordering of appropriate immunization(s), laboratory/diagnostic procedures, new patient; infant (age younger than 1 year)
➔ *CPT Assistant* Winter 91:11, Spring 93:14, 34, Spring 95:1, Aug 97:1, Jul 98:9, Sep 98:5, Nov 98:3-4, May 02:1, May 05:1, Aug 05:15, Oct 06:15; *CPT Changes: An Insider's View* 2002

99382   early childhood (age 1 through 4 years)
➔ *CPT Assistant* Winter 91:11, Spring 93:14, 34, Spring 95:1, Aug 97:1, Jul 98:9, Sep 98:5, Nov 98:3-4, May 02:1, Aug 05:15, Oct 06:15

99383   late childhood (age 5 through 11 years)
➔ *CPT Assistant* Winter 91:11, Spring 93:14, 34, Spring 95:1, Aug 97:1, Jul 98:9, Sep 98:5, Nov 98:3-4, May 02:1, Aug 05:15, Oct 06:15

99384   adolescent (age 12 through 17 years)
➔ *CPT Assistant* Winter 91:11, Spring 93:14, 34, Spring 95:1, Aug 97:1, Jul 98:9, Sep 98:5, Nov 98:3-4, May 02:1, Aug 05:15, Oct 06:15

99385   18-39 years
➔ *CPT Assistant* Winter 91:11, Spring 93:14, 34, Spring 95:1, Aug 97:1, Jul 98:9, Sep 98:5, Nov 98:3-4, May 02:1, Aug 05:15, Oct 06:15

99386   40-64 years
➔ *CPT Assistant* Winter 91:11, Spring 93:14, 34, Spring 95:1, Aug 97:1, Jul 98:9, Sep 98:5, Nov 98:3-4, May 02:1, Aug 05:15, Oct 06:15

99387   65 years and older
➔ *CPT Assistant* Winter 91:11, Spring 93:14, 34, Spring 95:1, Aug 97:1, Jul 98:9, Sep 98:5, Nov 98:3-4, May 02:1, Aug 05:15, Oct 06:15

Established Patient

99391   **Periodic comprehensive preventive medicine** reevaluation and management of an individual including an age and gender appropriate history, examination, counseling/anticipatory guidance/risk factor reduction interventions, and the ordering of appropriate immunization(s), laboratory/diagnostic procedures, established patient; infant (age younger than 1 year)
➔ *CPT Assistant* Winter 91:11, Spring 93:14, 34, Spring 95:1, Aug 97:1, Jul 98:9, Sep 98:5, Nov 98:3-4, May 02:1, May 05:1, Aug 05:15, Oct 06:15; *CPT Changes: An Insider's View* 2002

99392   early childhood (age 1 through 4 years)
➔ *CPT Assistant* Winter 91:11, Spring 93:14, 34, Spring 95:1, Aug 97:1, Jul 98:9, Sep 98:5, Nov 98:3-4, May 02:1, Aug 05:15, Oct 06:15

99393   late childhood (age 5 through 11 years)
➔ *CPT Assistant* Winter 91:11, Spring 93:14, 34, Spring 95:1, Aug 97:1, Jul 98:9, Sep 98:5, Nov 98:3-4, May 02:1, Aug 05:15, Oct 06:15

99394   adolescent (age 12 through 17 years)
➔ *CPT Assistant* Winter 91:11, Spring 93:14, 34, Spring 95:1, Aug 97:1, Jul 98:9, Sep 98:5, Nov 98:3-4, May 02:1, Aug 05:15, Oct 06:15

99395   18-39 years
➔ *CPT Assistant* Winter 91:11, Spring 93:14, 34, Spring 95:1, Aug 97:1, Jul 98:9, Sep 98:5, Nov 98:3-4, May 02:1, Aug 05:15, Oct 06:15

99396   40-64 years
➔ *CPT Assistant* Winter 91:11, Spring 93:14, 34, Spring 95:1, Aug 97:1, Jul 98:9, Sep 98:5, Nov 98:3-4, May 02:1, Aug 05:15, Oct 06:15

99397   65 years and older
➔ *CPT Assistant* Winter 91:11, Spring 93:14, 34, Spring 95:1, Aug 97:1, Jul 98:9, Sep 98:5, Nov 98:3-4, May 02:1, Aug 05:15, Oct 06:15

▶Counseling Risk Factor Reduction and Behavior Change Intervention◀

New or Established Patient

▶These codes are used to report services provided face-to-face by a physician or other qualified health care professional for the purpose of promoting health and preventing illness or injury. They are distinct from evaluation and management (E/M) services that may be reported separately when performed. Risk factor reduction services are used for persons without a specific illness for which the counseling might otherwise be used as part of treatment.

Preventive medicine counseling and risk factor reduction interventions will vary with age and should address such issues as family problems, diet and exercise, substance use, sexual practices, injury prevention, dental health, and diagnostic and laboratory test results available at the time of the encounter.

Behavior change interventions are for persons who have a behavior that is often considered an illness itself, such as tobacco use and addiction, substance abuse/misuse, or obesity. Behavior change services may be reported when performed as part of the treatment of condition(s) related to or potentially exacerbated by the behavior or when performed to change the harmful behavior that has not yet resulted in illness. Any E/M services reported on the same day must be distinct, and time spent providing these services may not be used as a basis for the E/M code selection. Behavior change services involve specific validated interventions of assessing readiness for change and barriers to change, advising a change in behavior, assisting by providing specific suggested actions and motivational counseling, and arranging for services and follow-up.

For counseling groups of patients with symptoms or established illness, use 99078.◄

Preventive Medicine, Individual Counseling

99401   **Preventive medicine counseling** and/or risk factor reduction intervention(s) provided to an individual (separate procedure); approximately 15 minutes
➔ *CPT Assistant* Aug 97:1, Jan 98:12, May 05:1

99402   approximately 30 minutes
➔ *CPT Assistant* Aug 97:1, Jan 98:12, May 05:1

99403   approximately 45 minutes
➔ *CPT Assistant* Aug 97:1, Jan 98:12, May 05:1

99404   approximately 60 minutes
➔ *CPT Assistant* Aug 97:1, Jan 98:12, May 05:1

►Behavior Change Interventions, Individual◄

● **99406**   Smoking and tobacco use cessation counseling visit; intermediate, greater than 3 minutes up to 10 minutes
➔ *CPT Changes: An Insider's View* 2008

● **99407**   intensive, greater than 10 minutes
➔ *CPT Changes: An Insider's View* 2008

►(Do not report 99407 in conjunction with 99406)◄

● **99408**   Alcohol and/or substance (other than tobacco) abuse structured screening (eg, AUDIT, DAST), and brief intervention (SBI) services; 15 to 30 minutes
➔ *CPT Changes: An Insider's View* 2008

►(Do not report services of less than 15 minutes with 99408)◄

● **99409**   greater than 30 minutes
➔ *CPT Changes: An Insider's View* 2008

►(Do not report 99409 in conjunction with 99408)◄

►(Do not report 99408, 99409 in conjunction with 99420)◄

►(Use 99408, 99409 only for initial screening and brief intervention)◄

Preventive Medicine, Group Counseling

99411   **Preventive medicine counseling** and/or risk factor reduction intervention(s) provided to individuals in a group setting (separate procedure); approximately 30 minutes
➔ *CPT Assistant* Aug 97:1, Jan 98:12, Sep 98:5, May 05:1

99412   approximately 60 minutes
➔ *CPT Assistant* Aug 97:1, Jan 98:12, Sep 98:5, May 05:1

Other Preventive Medicine Services

99420   **Administration and interpretation** of health risk assessment instrument (eg, health hazard appraisal)
➔ *CPT Assistant* May 05:1

99429   **Unlisted preventive** medicine service
➔ *CPT Assistant* Sep 98:5, May 05:1

Newborn Care

The following codes are used to report the services provided to newborns in several different settings.

For newborn hospital discharge services provided on a date subsequent to the admission date of the newborn, use 99238.

For discharge services provided to newborns admitted and discharged on the same date, use 99435.

99431   **History and examination** of the normal newborn infant, initiation of diagnostic and treatment programs and preparation of hospital records. (This code should also be used for birthing room deliveries.)
➔ *CPT Assistant* Apr 97:10, Nov 97:9, Sep 98:5, Apr 04:14, May 05:1

99432   **Normal newborn care** in other than hospital or birthing room setting, including physical examination of baby and conference(s) with parent(s)
➔ *CPT Assistant* Sep 98:5, May 99:11, Apr 04:14

99433   **Subsequent hospital care,** for the evaluation and management of a normal newborn, per day
➔ *CPT Assistant* Sep 98:5, Apr 03:27

99435   **History and examination** of the normal newborn infant, including the preparation of medical records. (This code should only be used for newborns assessed and discharged from the hospital or birthing room on the same date.)
➔ *CPT Assistant* Sep 98:5, Apr 04:14

99436   **Attendance** at delivery (when requested by delivering physician) and initial stabilization of newborn

→ *CPT Assistant* Nov 97:9-10, Sep 98:5, Nov 99:5-6, Aug 00:3, Aug 04:9, Nov 05:15

(99436 may be reported in addition to 99431)

(Do not report 99436 in conjunction with 99440)

99440   **Newborn resuscitation**: provision of positive pressure ventilation and/or chest compressions in the presence of acute inadequate ventilation and/or cardiac output

→ *CPT Assistant* Summer 93:3, Mar 96:10, Nov 97:9, Sep 98:5, Nov 99:5-6, Aug 00:3, Oct 03:3, Aug 04:9, Apr 07:3

▶Non-Face-to-Face Physician Services◀

▶Telephone Services◀

▶Telephone services are non-face-to-face evaluation and management (E/M) services provided by a physician to a patient using the telephone. These codes are used to report episodes of care by the physician initiated by an established patient or guardian of an established patient. If the telephone service ends with a decision to see the patient within 24 hours or next available urgent visit appointment, the code is not reported; rather the encounter is considered part of the preservice work of the subsequent E/M service, procedure, and visit. Likewise if the telephone call refers to an E/M service performed and reported by the physician within the previous seven days (either physician requested or unsolicited patient follow-up) or within the postoperative period of the previously completed procedure, then the service(s) are considered part of that previous E/M service or procedure. (Do not report 99441-99443 if reporting 99441-99444 performed in the previous seven days.)◀

▶(For telephone services provided by a qualified nonphysician health care professional, see 98966-98968)◀

● **99441**   Telephone evaluation and management service provided by a physician to an established patient, parent, or guardian not originating from a related E/M service provided within the previous 7 days nor leading to an E/M service or procedure within the next 24 hours or soonest available appointment; 5-10 minutes of medical discussion

→ *CPT Changes: An Insider's View* 2008

● **99442**   11-20 minutes of medical discussion

→ *CPT Changes: An Insider's View* 2008

● **99443**   21-30 minutes of medical discussion

→ *CPT Changes: An Insider's View* 2008

▶(Do not report 99441-99443 when using 99339-99340, 99374-99380 for the same call[s])◀

▶(Do not report 99441-99443 for anticoagulation management when reporting 99363-99364)◀

▶On-Line Medical Evaluation◀

▶An on-line electronic medical evaluation is a non-face-to-face evaluation and management (E/M) service by a physician to a patient using Internet resources in response to a patient's on-line inquiry. Reportable services involve the physician's personal timely response to the patient's inquiry and must involve permanent storage (electronic or hard copy) of the encounter. This service is reported only once for the same episode of care during a seven-day period, although multiple physicians could report their exchange with the same patient. If the on-line medical evaluation refers to an E/M service previously performed and reported by the physician within the previous seven days (either physician requested or unsolicited patient follow-up) or within the postoperative period of the previously completed procedure, then the service(s) are considered covered by the previous E/M service or procedure. A reportable service encompasses the sum of communication (eg, related telephone calls, prescription provision, laboratory orders) pertaining to the on-line patient encounter.◀

▶(For an on-line medical evaluation provided by a qualified nonphysician health care professional, use 98969)◀

● **99444**   Online evaluation and management service provided by a physician to an established patient, guardian, or health care provider not originating from a related E/M service provided within the previous 7 days, using the Internet or similar electronic communications network

→ *CPT Changes: An Insider's View* 2008

▶(Do not report 99444 when using 99339-99340, 99374-99380 for the same communication[s])◀

▶(Do not report 99444 for anticoagulation management when reporting 99363, 99364)◀

Special Evaluation and Management Services

The following codes are used to report evaluations performed to establish baseline information prior to life or disability insurance certificates being issued. This service is performed in the office or other setting, and applies to both new and established patients. When using these codes, no active management of the problem(s) is undertaken during the encounter.

If other evaluation and management services and/or procedures are performed on the same date, the appropriate E/M or procedure code(s) should be reported in addition to these codes.

Basic Life and/or Disability Evaluation Services

99450   **Basic life** and/or disability examination that includes:

- **Measurement of height, weight, and blood pressure;**
- **Completion of a medical history following a life insurance pro forma;**
- **Collection of blood sample and/or urinalysis complying with "chain of custody" protocols; and**
- **Completion of necessary documentation/certificates.**

➔ *CPT Assistant* Summer 95:14, Sep 98:5, May 05:1

Work Related or Medical Disability Evaluation Services

99455   **Work related** or medical disability examination by the treating physician that includes:

- **Completion of a medical history commensurate with the patient's condition;**
- **Performance of an examination commensurate with the patient's condition;**
- **Formulation of a diagnosis, assessment of capabilities and stability, and calculation of impairment;**
- **Development of future medical treatment plan; and**
- **Completion of necessary documentation/certificates and report.**

➔ *CPT Assistant* Summer 95:14, Sep 98:5, May 05:1

99456   **Work related** or medical disability examination by other than the treating physician that includes:

- **Completion of a medical history commensurate with the patient's condition;**
- **Performance of an examination commensurate with the patient's condition;**
- **Formulation of a diagnosis, assessment of capabilities and stability, and calculation of impairment;**
- **Development of future medical treatment plan; and**
- **Completion of necessary documentation/certificates and report.**

➔ *CPT Assistant* Summer 95:14, Sep 98:5

(Do not report 99455, 99456 in conjunction with 99080 for the completion of Workman's Compensation forms)

Other Evaluation and Management Services

● **99477**   Initial hospital care, per day, for the evaluation and management of the neonate, 28 days of age or less, who requires intensive observation, frequent interventions, and other intensive care services

➔ *CPT Changes: An Insider's View* 2008

►(For the initiation of inpatient care of the normal newborn, report 99431)◄

►(For the initiation of care of the critically ill neonate, use 99295)◄

►(For initiation of inpatient hospital care of the neonate not requiring intensive observation, frequent interventions, and other intensive care services, see 99221-99223)◄

99499   **Unlisted evaluation and management** service

➔ *CPT Assistant* Apr 96:11, Mar 05:11, May 05:1, Jan 06:46, Sep 06:8, Jan 07:30

Notes

⊙=Moderate sedation   ✚=Add-on code   ✗=FDA approval pending   ➔➔=See p xvii for details

Anesthesia Guidelines

Services involving administration of anesthesia are reported by the use of the anesthesia five-digit procedure code (00100-01999) plus modifier codes (defined under "Anesthesia Modifiers" later in these Guidelines).

The reporting of anesthesia services is appropriate by or under the responsible supervision of a physician. These services may include but are not limited to general, regional, supplementation of local anesthesia, or other supportive services in order to afford the patient the anesthesia care deemed optimal by the anesthesiologist during any procedure. These services include the usual preoperative and postoperative visits, the anesthesia care during the procedure, the administration of fluids and/or blood and the usual monitoring services (eg, ECG, temperature, blood pressure, oximetry, capnography, and mass spectrometry). Unusual forms of monitoring (eg, intra-arterial, central venous, and Swan-Ganz) are not included.

Items used by all physicians in reporting their services are presented in the **Introduction.** Some of the commonalities are repeated in this section for the convenience of those physicians referring to this section on **Anesthesia.** Other definitions and items unique to anesthesia are also listed.

To report moderate (conscious) sedation provided by a physician also performing the service for which conscious sedation is being provided, see codes 99143-99145.

For the procedures listed in Appendix G, when a second physician other than the health care professional performing the diagnostic or therapeutic services provides moderate (conscious) sedation in the facility setting (eg, hospital, outpatient hospital/ambulatory surgery center, skilled nursing facility), the second physician reports the associated moderate sedation procedure/service 99148-99150; when these services are performed by the second physician in the nonfacility setting (eg, physician office, freestanding imaging center), codes 99148-99150 would not be reported. Moderate sedation does not include minimal sedation (anxiolysis), deep sedation, or monitored anesthesia care (00100-01999).

To report regional or general anesthesia provided by a physician also performing the services for which the anesthesia is being provided, see modifier 47 in Appendix A.

Time Reporting

Time for anesthesia procedures may be reported as is customary in the local area. Anesthesia time begins when the anesthesiologist begins to prepare the patient for the induction of anesthesia in the operating room or in an equivalent area and ends when the anesthesiologist is no longer in personal attendance, that is, when the patient may be safely placed under postoperative supervision.

Physician's Services

Physician's services rendered in the office, home, or hospital; consultation; and other medical services are listed in the section titled **Evaluation and Management Services** (99201-99499 series) found on page 1. "Special Services and Reporting" (99000-99091 series) are listed in the **Medicine** section.

Materials Supplied by Physician

Supplies and materials provided by the physician (eg, sterile trays, drugs) over and above those usually included with the office visit or other services rendered may be listed separately. Drugs, tray supplies, and materials provided should be listed and identified with 99070 or the appropriate supply code.

Separate or Multiple Procedures

When multiple surgical procedures are performed during a single anesthetic administration, the anesthesia code representing the most complex procedure is reported. The time reported is the combined total for all procedures.

Special Report

A service that is rarely provided, unusual, variable, or new may require a special report in determining medical appropriateness of the service. Pertinent information should include an adequate definition or description of the nature, extent, and need for the procedure and the time, effort, and equipment necessary to provide the service. Additional items may include:

- Complexity of symptoms
- Final diagnosis
- Pertinent physical findings
- Diagnostic and therapeutic procedures
- Concurrent problems
- Follow-up care

Anesthesia Modifiers

All anesthesia services are reported by use of the anesthesia five-digit procedure code (00100-01999) plus the addition of a physical status modifier. The use of other optional modifiers may be appropriate.

Physical Status Modifiers

Physical Status modifiers are represented by the initial letter 'P' followed by a single digit from 1 to 6 as defined in the following list.

P1: A normal healthy patient

P2: A patient with mild systemic disease

P3: A patient with severe systemic disease

P4: A patient with severe systemic disease that is a constant threat to life

P5: A moribund patient who is not expected to survive without the operation

P6: A declared brain-dead patient whose organs are being removed for donor purposes

These six levels are consistent with the American Society of Anesthesiologists (ASA) ranking of patient physical status. Physical status is included in the CPT codebook to distinguish among various levels of complexity of the anesthesia service provided.

Example: 00100-P1

Qualifying Circumstances

More than one qualifying circumstance may be selected.

Many anesthesia services are provided under particularly difficult circumstances, depending on factors such as extraordinary condition of patient, notable operative conditions, and/or unusual risk factors. This section includes a list of important qualifying circumstances that significantly affect the character of the anesthesia service provided. These procedures would not be reported alone but would be reported as additional procedure numbers qualifying an anesthesia procedure or service.

+ **99100** Anesthesia for patient of extreme age, younger than 1 year and older than 70 (List separately in addition to code for primary anesthesia procedure)

(For procedure performed on infants younger than 1 year of age at time of surgery, see 00326, 00561, 00834, 00836)

+ **99116** Anesthesia complicated by utilization of total body hypothermia (List separately in addition to code for primary anesthesia procedure)

+ **99135** Anesthesia complicated by utilization of controlled hypotension (List separately in addition to code for primary anesthesia procedure)

+ **99140** Anesthesia complicated by emergency conditions (specify) (List separately in addition to code for primary anesthesia procedure)

(An emergency is defined as existing when delay in treatment of the patient would lead to a significant increase in the threat to life or body part.)

Anesthesia

Head

00100   Anesthesia for procedures on salivary glands, including biopsy

> *CPT Assistant* Feb 97:4, Nov 99:6, Feb 06:9, Mar 06:15

00102   Anesthesia for procedures involving plastic repair of cleft lip

> *CPT Assistant* Nov 99:6; *CPT Changes: An Insider's View* 2000

00103   Anesthesia for reconstructive procedures of eyelid (eg, blepharoplasty, ptosis surgery)

> *CPT Assistant* Nov 99:6; *CPT Changes: An Insider's View* 2000

00104   Anesthesia for electroconvulsive therapy

00120   Anesthesia for procedures on external, middle, and inner ear including biopsy; not otherwise specified

00124   otoscopy

> *CPT Assistant* Nov 99:7

00126   tympanotomy

00140   Anesthesia for procedures on eye; not otherwise specified

00142   lens surgery

00144   corneal transplant

00145   vitreoretinal surgery

> *CPT Changes: An Insider's View* 2001

00147   iridectomy

00148   ophthalmoscopy

00160   Anesthesia for procedures on nose and accessory sinuses; not otherwise specified

00162   radical surgery

00164   biopsy, soft tissue

00170   Anesthesia for intraoral procedures, including biopsy; not otherwise specified

00172   repair of cleft palate

00174   excision of retropharyngeal tumor

00176   radical surgery

00190   Anesthesia for procedures on facial bones or skull; not otherwise specified

> *CPT Changes: An Insider's View* 2001

00192   radical surgery (including prognathism)

00210   Anesthesia for intracranial procedures; not otherwise specified

00212   subdural taps

00214   burr holes, including ventriculography

> *CPT Assistant* Nov 99:7; *CPT Changes: An Insider's View* 2000

00215   cranioplasty or elevation of depressed skull fracture, extradural (simple or compound)

> *CPT Changes: An Insider's View* 2001

00216   vascular procedures

00218   procedures in sitting position

00220   cerebrospinal fluid shunting procedures

00222   electrocoagulation of intracranial nerve

Neck

00300   Anesthesia for all procedures on the integumentary system, muscles and nerves of head, neck, and posterior trunk, not otherwise specified

> *CPT Assistant* Nov 99:7, Mar 06:15

00320   Anesthesia for all procedures on esophagus, thyroid, larynx, trachea and lymphatic system of neck; not otherwise specified, age 1 year or older

> *CPT Changes: An Insider's View* 2003

00322   needle biopsy of thyroid

(For procedures on cervical spine and cord, see 00600, 00604, 00670)

00326   Anesthesia for all procedures on the larynx and trachea in children younger than 1 year of age

> *CPT Changes: An Insider's View* 2003

(Do not report 00326 in conjunction with 99100)

00350   Anesthesia for procedures on major vessels of neck; not otherwise specified

00352   simple ligation

(For arteriography, use 01916)

Thorax (Chest Wall and Shoulder Girdle)

00400   Anesthesia for procedures on the integumentary system on the extremities, anterior trunk and perineum; not otherwise specified

> *CPT Assistant* Mar 06:15

00402   reconstructive procedures on breast (eg, reduction or augmentation mammoplasty, muscle flaps)

00404   radical or modified radical procedures on breast

00406	radical or modified radical procedures on breast with internal mammary node dissection
00410	electrical conversion of arrhythmias
00450	Anesthesia for procedures on clavicle and scapula; not otherwise specified
00452	radical surgery
00454	biopsy of clavicle
00470	Anesthesia for partial rib resection; not otherwise specified
00472	thoracoplasty (any type)
00474	radical procedures (eg, pectus excavatum)

Intrathoracic

00500	Anesthesia for all procedures on esophagus
➔ *CPT Assistant* Mar 06:15
00520	Anesthesia for closed chest procedures; (including bronchoscopy) not otherwise specified
➔ *CPT Assistant* Nov 99:7; *CPT Changes: An Insider's View* 2000
00522	needle biopsy of pleura
00524	pneumocentesis
00528	mediastinoscopy and diagnostic thoracoscopy not utilizing one lung ventilation
➔ *CPT Assistant* Nov 99:7; *CPT Changes: An Insider's View* 2000, 2003, 2004

(For tracheobronchial reconstruction, use 00539)

00529	mediastinoscopy and diagnostic thoracoscopy utilizing one lung ventilation
➔ *CPT Assistant* Jun 04:3; *CPT Changes: An Insider's View* 2004
00530	Anesthesia for permanent transvenous pacemaker insertion
➔ *CPT Changes: An Insider's View* 2001
00532	Anesthesia for access to central venous circulation
00534	Anesthesia for transvenous insertion or replacement of pacing cardioverter-defibrillator
➔ *CPT Changes: An Insider's View* 2001

(For transthoracic approach, use 00560)

00537	Anesthesia for cardiac electrophysiologic procedures including radiofrequency ablation
➔ *CPT Changes: An Insider's View* 2001
00539	Anesthesia for tracheobronchial reconstruction
➔ *CPT Changes: An Insider's View* 2003
00540	Anesthesia for thoracotomy procedures involving lungs, pleura, diaphragm, and mediastinum (including surgical thoracoscopy); not otherwise specified
00541	utilizing one lung ventilation
➔ *CPT Changes: An Insider's View* 2003

(For thoracic spine and cord anesthesia procedures via an anterior transthoracic approach, see 00625-00626)

00542	decortication
00546	pulmonary resection with thoracoplasty
00548	intrathoracic procedures on the trachea and bronchi
➔ *CPT Assistant* Nov 97:10
00550	Anesthesia for sternal debridement
➔ *CPT Changes: An Insider's View* 2001
00560	Anesthesia for procedures on heart, pericardial sac, and great vessels of chest; without pump oxygenator
➔ *CPT Changes: An Insider's View* 2002
00561	with pump oxygenator, younger than one year of age
➔ *CPT Changes: An Insider's View* 2005

(Do not report 00561 in conjunction with 99100, 99116, and 99135)

00562	with pump oxygenator
00563	with pump oxygenator with hypothermic circulatory arrest
➔ *CPT Changes: An Insider's View* 2001
00566	Anesthesia for direct coronary artery bypass grafting without pump oxygenator
➔ *CPT Changes: An Insider's View* 2001
00580	Anesthesia for heart transplant or heart/lung transplant

Spine and Spinal Cord

00600	Anesthesia for procedures on cervical spine and cord; not otherwise specified
➔ *CPT Assistant* Mar 06:15

►(For percutaneous image-guided spine and spinal cord anesthesia procedures, see 01935, 01936)◄

00604	procedures with patient in the sitting position
➔ *CPT Changes: An Insider's View* 2001
00620	Anesthesia for procedures on thoracic spine and cord; not otherwise specified
00622	thoracolumbar sympathectomy
00625	Anesthesia for procedures on the thoracic spine and cord, via an anterior transthoracic approach; not utilizing one lung ventilation
➔ *CPT Changes: An Insider's View* 2007
00626	utilizing one lung ventilation
➔ *CPT Changes: An Insider's View* 2007

(For anesthesia for thoracotomy procedures other than spinal, see 00540-00541)

00630	Anesthesia for procedures in lumbar region; not otherwise specified
00632	lumbar sympathectomy

00634	chemonucleolysis
00635	diagnostic or therapeutic lumbar puncture
	➔ *CPT Changes: An Insider's View* 2001
00640	Anesthesia for manipulation of the spine or for closed procedures on the cervical, thoracic or lumbar spine
	➔ *CPT Changes: An Insider's View* 2003
00670	Anesthesia for extensive spine and spinal cord procedures (eg, spinal instrumentation or vascular procedures)
	➔ *CPT Changes: An Insider's View* 2001

Upper Abdomen

00700	Anesthesia for procedures on upper anterior abdominal wall; not otherwise specified
	➔ *CPT Assistant* Mar 06:15
00702	percutaneous liver biopsy
00730	Anesthesia for procedures on upper posterior abdominal wall
00740	Anesthesia for upper gastrointestinal endoscopic procedures, endoscope introduced proximal to duodenum
	➔ *CPT Assistant* Nov 99:7; *CPT Changes: An Insider's View* 2000
00750	Anesthesia for hernia repairs in upper abdomen; not otherwise specified
00752	lumbar and ventral (incisional) hernias and/or wound dehiscence
00754	omphalocele
00756	transabdominal repair of diaphragmatic hernia
00770	Anesthesia for all procedures on major abdominal blood vessels
00790	Anesthesia for intraperitoneal procedures in upper abdomen including laparoscopy; not otherwise specified
00792	partial hepatectomy or management of liver hemorrhage (excluding liver biopsy)
	➔ *CPT Changes: An Insider's View* 2001
00794	pancreatectomy, partial or total (eg, Whipple procedure)
00796	liver transplant (recipient)
	(For harvesting of liver, use 01990)
00797	gastric restrictive procedure for morbid obesity
	➔ *CPT Changes: An Insider's View* 2002

Lower Abdomen

00800	Anesthesia for procedures on lower anterior abdominal wall; not otherwise specified
	➔ *CPT Assistant* Mar 06:15
00802	panniculectomy

00810	Anesthesia for lower intestinal endoscopic procedures, endoscope introduced distal to duodenum
	➔ *CPT Assistant* Nov 99:7; *CPT Changes: An Insider's View* 2000
00820	Anesthesia for procedures on lower posterior abdominal wall
00830	Anesthesia for hernia repairs in lower abdomen; not otherwise specified
00832	ventral and incisional hernias
	(For hernia repairs in the infant 1 year of age or younger, see 00834, 00836)
00834	Anesthesia for hernia repairs in the lower abdomen not otherwise specified, younger than 1 year of age
	➔ *CPT Changes: An Insider's View* 2003
	(Do not report 00834 in conjunction with 99100)
00836	Anesthesia for hernia repairs in the lower abdomen not otherwise specified, infants younger than 37 weeks gestational age at birth and younger than 50 weeks gestational age at time of surgery
	➔ *CPT Changes: An Insider's View* 2003
	(Do not report 00836 in conjunction with 99100)
00840	Anesthesia for intraperitoneal procedures in lower abdomen including laparoscopy; not otherwise specified
00842	amniocentesis
00844	abdominoperineal resection
00846	radical hysterectomy
00848	pelvic exenteration
00851	tubal ligation/transection
	➔ *CPT Changes: An Insider's View* 2002
00860	Anesthesia for extraperitoneal procedures in lower abdomen, including urinary tract; not otherwise specified
00862	renal procedures, including upper one-third of ureter, or donor nephrectomy
00864	total cystectomy
00865	radical prostatectomy (suprapubic, retropubic)
00866	adrenalectomy
00868	renal transplant (recipient)
	(For donor nephrectomy, use 00862)
	(For harvesting kidney from brain-dead patient, use 01990)
00870	cystolithotomy
00872	Anesthesia for lithotripsy, extracorporeal shock wave; with water bath
00873	without water bath
00880	Anesthesia for procedures on major lower abdominal vessels; not otherwise specified
00882	inferior vena cava ligation

Perineum

(For perineal procedures on integumentary system, muscles and nerves, see 00300, 00400)

00902 Anesthesia for; anorectal procedure
➔ *CPT Assistant* Mar 06:15; *CPT Changes: An Insider's View* 2001

00904 radical perineal procedure

00906 vulvectomy

00908 perineal prostatectomy

00910 Anesthesia for transurethral procedures (including urethrocystoscopy); not otherwise specified

00912 transurethral resection of bladder tumor(s)

00914 transurethral resection of prostate

00916 post-transurethral resection bleeding

00918 with fragmentation, manipulation and/or removal of ureteral calculus
➔ *CPT Assistant* Nov 99:8; *CPT Changes: An Insider's View* 2000

00920 Anesthesia for procedures on male genitalia (including open urethral procedures); not otherwise specified
➔ *CPT Changes: An Insider's View* 2001

00921 vasectomy, unilateral or bilateral
➔ *CPT Changes: An Insider's View* 2003

00922 seminal vesicles

00924 undescended testis, unilateral or bilateral

00926 radical orchiectomy, inguinal

00928 radical orchiectomy, abdominal

00930 orchiopexy, unilateral or bilateral

00932 complete amputation of penis

00934 radical amputation of penis with bilateral inguinal lymphadenectomy

00936 radical amputation of penis with bilateral inguinal and iliac lymphadenectomy

00938 insertion of penile prosthesis (perineal approach)

00940 Anesthesia for vaginal procedures (including biopsy of labia, vagina, cervix or endometrium); not otherwise specified

00942 colpotomy, vaginectomy, colporrhaphy, and open urethral procedures
➔ *CPT Changes: An Insider's View* 2001, 2002

00944 vaginal hysterectomy

00948 cervical cerclage

00950 culdoscopy

00952 hysteroscopy and/or hysterosalpingography
➔ *CPT Assistant* Nov 99:8; *CPT Changes: An Insider's View* 2000

Pelvis (Except Hip)

01112 Anesthesia for bone marrow aspiration and/or biopsy, anterior or posterior iliac crest
➔ *CPT Assistant* Mar 06:15; *CPT Changes: An Insider's View* 2001

01120 Anesthesia for procedures on bony pelvis

01130 Anesthesia for body cast application or revision

01140 Anesthesia for interpelviabdominal (hindquarter) amputation

01150 Anesthesia for radical procedures for tumor of pelvis, except hindquarter amputation

01160 Anesthesia for closed procedures involving symphysis pubis or sacroiliac joint

01170 Anesthesia for open procedures involving symphysis pubis or sacroiliac joint

01173 Anesthesia for open repair of fracture disruption of pelvis or column fracture involving acetabulum
➔ *CPT Assistant* Jun 04:3-4; *CPT Changes: An Insider's View* 2004

01180 Anesthesia for obturator neurectomy; extrapelvic

01190 intrapelvic

Upper Leg (Except Knee)

01200 Anesthesia for all closed procedures involving hip joint
➔ *CPT Assistant* Mar 06:15

01202 Anesthesia for arthroscopic procedures of hip joint

01210 Anesthesia for open procedures involving hip joint; not otherwise specified

01212 hip disarticulation

01214 total hip arthroplasty
➔ *CPT Changes: An Insider's View* 2001, 2002

01215 revision of total hip arthroplasty
➔ *CPT Changes: An Insider's View* 2001, 2002

01220 Anesthesia for all closed procedures involving upper two-thirds of femur

01230 Anesthesia for open procedures involving upper two-thirds of femur; not otherwise specified

01232 amputation

01234 radical resection

01250 Anesthesia for all procedures on nerves, muscles, tendons, fascia, and bursae of upper leg

01260 Anesthesia for all procedures involving veins of upper leg, including exploration

01270 Anesthesia for procedures involving arteries of upper leg, including bypass graft; not otherwise specified

01272   femoral artery ligation

01274   femoral artery embolectomy

Knee and Popliteal Area

01320 Anesthesia for all procedures on nerves, muscles, tendons, fascia, and bursae of knee and/or popliteal area
➔ *CPT Assistant* Mar 06:15

01340 Anesthesia for all closed procedures on lower one-third of femur

01360 Anesthesia for all open procedures on lower one-third of femur

01380 Anesthesia for all closed procedures on knee joint

01382 Anesthesia for diagnostic arthroscopic procedures of knee joint
➔ *CPT Changes: An Insider's View* 2003

01390 Anesthesia for all closed procedures on upper ends of tibia, fibula, and/or patella

01392 Anesthesia for all open procedures on upper ends of tibia, fibula, and/or patella

01400 Anesthesia for open or surgical arthroscopic procedures on knee joint; not otherwise specified
➔ *CPT Changes: An Insider's View* 2003

01402   total knee arthroplasty
➔ *CPT Changes: An Insider's View* 2002

01404   disarticulation at knee

01420 Anesthesia for all cast applications, removal, or repair involving knee joint

01430 Anesthesia for procedures on veins of knee and popliteal area; not otherwise specified

01432   arteriovenous fistula

01440 Anesthesia for procedures on arteries of knee and popliteal area; not otherwise specified

01442   popliteal thromboendarterectomy, with or without patch graft

01444   popliteal excision and graft or repair for occlusion or aneurysm

Lower Leg (Below Knee, Includes Ankle and Foot)

01462 Anesthesia for all closed procedures on lower leg, ankle, and foot
➔ *CPT Assistant* Mar 06:15

01464 Anesthesia for arthroscopic procedures of ankle and/or foot
➔ *CPT Changes: An Insider's View* 2003

01470 Anesthesia for procedures on nerves, muscles, tendons, and fascia of lower leg, ankle, and foot; not otherwise specified

01472   repair of ruptured Achilles tendon, with or without graft

01474   gastrocnemius recession (eg, Strayer procedure)

01480 Anesthesia for open procedures on bones of lower leg, ankle, and foot; not otherwise specified

01482   radical resection (including below knee amputation)
➔ *CPT Changes: An Insider's View* 2001

01484   osteotomy or osteoplasty of tibia and/or fibula

01486   total ankle replacement

01490 Anesthesia for lower leg cast application, removal, or repair

01500 Anesthesia for procedures on arteries of lower leg, including bypass graft; not otherwise specified

01502   embolectomy, direct or with catheter

01520 Anesthesia for procedures on veins of lower leg; not otherwise specified

01522   venous thrombectomy, direct or with catheter

Shoulder and Axilla

Includes humeral head and neck, sternoclavicular joint, acromioclavicular joint, and shoulder joint.

01610 Anesthesia for all procedures on nerves, muscles, tendons, fascia, and bursae of shoulder and axilla
➔ *CPT Assistant* Mar 06:15

01620 Anesthesia for all closed procedures on humeral head and neck, sternoclavicular joint, acromioclavicular joint, and shoulder joint

01622 Anesthesia for diagnostic arthroscopic procedures of shoulder joint
➔ *CPT Changes: An Insider's View* 2003

01630 Anesthesia for open or surgical arthroscopic procedures on humeral head and neck, sternoclavicular joint, acromioclavicular joint, and shoulder joint; not otherwise specified

➔ *CPT Changes: An Insider's View* 2003

01632   radical resection

01634   shoulder disarticulation

01636   interthoracoscapular (forequarter) amputation

01638   total shoulder replacement

01650 Anesthesia for procedures on arteries of shoulder and axilla; not otherwise specified

01652   axillary-brachial aneurysm

01654   bypass graft

01656   axillary-femoral bypass graft

01670 Anesthesia for all procedures on veins of shoulder and axilla

01680 Anesthesia for shoulder cast application, removal or repair; not otherwise specified

01682   shoulder spica

Upper Arm and Elbow

01710 Anesthesia for procedures on nerves, muscles, tendons, fascia, and bursae of upper arm and elbow; not otherwise specified

➔ *CPT Assistant* Mar 06:15

01712   tenotomy, elbow to shoulder, open

01714   tenoplasty, elbow to shoulder

01716   tenodesis, rupture of long tendon of biceps

01730 Anesthesia for all closed procedures on humerus and elbow

01732 Anesthesia for diagnostic arthroscopic procedures of elbow joint

➔ *CPT Changes: An Insider's View* 2003

01740 Anesthesia for open or surgical arthroscopic procedures of the elbow; not otherwise specified

➔ *CPT Changes: An Insider's View* 2003

01742   osteotomy of humerus

01744   repair of nonunion or malunion of humerus

01756   radical procedures

01758   excision of cyst or tumor of humerus

01760   total elbow replacement

01770 Anesthesia for procedures on arteries of upper arm and elbow; not otherwise specified

01772   embolectomy

01780 Anesthesia for procedures on veins of upper arm and elbow; not otherwise specified

01782   phleborrhaphy

Forearm, Wrist, and Hand

01810 Anesthesia for all procedures on nerves, muscles, tendons, fascia, and bursae of forearm, wrist, and hand

➔ *CPT Assistant* Mar 06:15

01820 Anesthesia for all closed procedures on radius, ulna, wrist, or hand bones

01829 Anesthesia for diagnostic arthroscopic procedures on the wrist

➔ *CPT Changes: An Insider's View* 2003

01830 Anesthesia for open or surgical arthroscopic/endoscopic procedures on distal radius, distal ulna, wrist, or hand joints; not otherwise specified

➔ *CPT Changes: An Insider's View* 2003

01832   total wrist replacement

01840 Anesthesia for procedures on arteries of forearm, wrist, and hand; not otherwise specified

01842   embolectomy

01844 Anesthesia for vascular shunt, or shunt revision, any type (eg, dialysis)

01850 Anesthesia for procedures on veins of forearm, wrist, and hand; not otherwise specified

01852   phleborrhaphy

01860 Anesthesia for forearm, wrist, or hand cast application, removal, or repair

Radiological Procedures

▶(01905 has been deleted. To report, see 01935, 01936)◀

01916 Anesthesia for diagnostic arteriography/venography

➔ *CPT Changes: An Insider's View* 2002

(Do not report 01916 in conjunction with therapeutic codes 01924-01926, 01930-01933)

01920 Anesthesia for cardiac catheterization including coronary angiography and ventriculography (not to include Swan-Ganz catheter)

01922 Anesthesia for non-invasive imaging or radiation therapy

01924 Anesthesia for therapeutic interventional radiological procedures involving the arterial system; not otherwise specified

➜ *CPT Changes: An Insider's View* 2002

01925 carotid or coronary

➜ *CPT Changes: An Insider's View* 2002

01926 intracranial, intracardiac, or aortic

➜ *CPT Changes: An Insider's View* 2002

01930 Anesthesia for therapeutic interventional radiological procedures involving the venous/lymphatic system (not to include access to the central circulation); not otherwise specified

➜ *CPT Changes: An Insider's View* 2002

▲ **01931** intrahepatic or portal circulation (eg, transvenous intrahepatic portosystemic shunt[s] [TIPS])

➜ *CPT Changes: An Insider's View* 2002, 2008

01932 intrathoracic or jugular

➜ *CPT Changes: An Insider's View* 2002

01933 intracranial

➜ *CPT Changes: An Insider's View* 2002

● **01935** Anesthesia for percutaneous image guided procedures on the spine and spinal cord; diagnostic

➜ *CPT Changes: An Insider's View* 2008

● **01936** therapeutic

➜ *CPT Changes: An Insider's View* 2008

Burn Excisions or Debridement

01951 Anesthesia for second- and third-degree burn excision or debridement with or without skin grafting, any site, for total body surface area (TBSA) treated during anesthesia and surgery; less than 4% total body surface area

➜ *CPT Assistant* Mar 06:15; *CPT Changes: An Insider's View* 2001, 2002

01952 between 4% and 9% of total body surface area

➜ *CPT Changes: An Insider's View* 2001, 2002

+ **01953** each additional 9% total body surface area or part thereof (List separately in addition to code for primary procedure)

➜ *CPT Changes: An Insider's View* 2001

(Use 01953 in conjunction with 01952)

Obstetric

01958 Anesthesia for external cephalic version procedure

➜ *CPT Assistant* Jun 04:5-6; *CPT Changes: An Insider's View* 2004

01960 Anesthesia for vaginal delivery only

➜ *CPT Assistant* Dec 01:3; *CPT Changes: An Insider's View* 2002

01961 Anesthesia for cesarean delivery only

➜ *CPT Changes: An Insider's View* 2002, 2003

01962 Anesthesia for urgent hysterectomy following delivery

➜ *CPT Changes: An Insider's View* 2002, 2003

01963 Anesthesia for cesarean hysterectomy without any labor analgesia/anesthesia care

➜ *CPT Changes: An Insider's View* 2002, 2003

(01964 has been deleted. To report, see 01965, 01966)

01965 Anesthesia for incomplete or missed abortion procedures

➜ *CPT Changes: An Insider's View* 2006

01966 Anesthesia for induced abortion procedures

➜ *CPT Changes: An Insider's View* 2006

01967 Neuraxial labor analgesia/anesthesia for planned vaginal delivery (this includes any repeat subarachnoid needle placement and drug injection and/or any necessary replacement of an epidural catheter during labor)

➜ *CPT Assistant* Dec 01:3; *CPT Changes: An Insider's View* 2002

+ **01968** Anesthesia for cesarean delivery following neuraxial labor analgesia/anesthesia (List separately in addition to code for primary procedure performed)

➜ *CPT Assistant* Dec 01:3; *CPT Changes: An Insider's View* 2002, 2003

(Use 01968 in conjunction with 01967)

+ **01969** Anesthesia for cesarean hysterectomy following neuraxial labor analgesia/anesthesia (List separately in addition to code for primary procedure performed)

➜ *CPT Assistant* Dec 01:3; *CPT Changes: An Insider's View* 2002, 2003

(Use 01969 in conjunction with 01967)

Other Procedures

01990 Physiological support for harvesting of organ(s) from brain-dead patient

➜ *CPT Assistant* Mar 06:15

01991 Anesthesia for diagnostic or therapeutic nerve blocks and injections (when block or injection is performed by a different provider); other than the prone position

➔ *CPT Changes: An Insider's View* 2003

01992 prone position

➔ *CPT Changes: An Insider's View* 2003

(Do not report 01991 or 01992 in conjunction with 99143-99150)

(When regional intravenous administration of local anesthetic agent or other medication in the upper or lower extremity is used as the anesthetic for a surgical procedure, report the appropriate anesthesia code. To report a Bier block for pain management, use 64999. For intra-arterial or intravenous injections, see 90773, 90774)

(For intra-arterial or intravenous therapy for pain management, see 90773, 90774)

(01995 has been deleted)

01996 Daily hospital management of epidural or subarachnoid continuous drug administration

➔ *CPT Assistant* Feb 97:5, Nov 97:10, May 99:6; *CPT Changes: An Insider's View* 2003

(Report code 01996 for daily hospital management of continuous epidural or subarachnoid drug administration performed after insertion of an epidural or subarachnoid catheter)

01999 Unlisted anesthesia procedure(s)

➔ *CPT Assistant* Feb 97:4, Feb 06:9, Mar 06:15, Jan 07:30

Surgery Guidelines

Items used by all physicians in reporting their services are presented in the **Introduction.** Some of the commonalities are repeated here for the convenience of those physicians referring to this section on **Surgery.** Other definitions and items unique to Surgery are also listed.

Physicians' Services

Physicians' services rendered in the office, home, or hospital, consultations, and other medical services are listed in the section entitled **Evaluation and Management Services** (99201-99499) found in the front of the book, beginning on page 9. "Special Services and Reports" (99000 series) is presented in the **Medicine** section.

CPT Surgical Package Definition

The services provided by the physician to any patient by their very nature are variable. The CPT codes that represent a readily identifiable surgical procedure thereby include, on a procedure-by-procedure basis, a variety of services. In defining the specific services "included" in a given CPT surgical code, the following services are always included in addition to the operation per se:

- Local infiltration, metacarpal/metatarsal/digital block or topical anesthesia
- Subsequent to the decision for surgery, one related E/M encounter on the date immediately prior to or on the date of procedure (including history and physical)
- Immediate postoperative care, including dictating operative notes, talking with the family and other physicians
- Writing orders
- Evaluating the patient in the postanesthesia recovery area
- Typical postoperative follow-up care

Follow-Up Care for Diagnostic Procedures

Follow-up care for diagnostic procedures (eg, endoscopy, arthroscopy, injection procedures for radiography) includes only that care related to recovery from the diagnostic procedure itself. Care of the condition for which the diagnostic procedure was performed or of other concomitant conditions is not included and may be listed separately.

Follow-Up Care for Therapeutic Surgical Procedures

Follow-up care for therapeutic surgical procedures includes only that care which is usually a part of the surgical service. Complications, exacerbations, recurrence, or the presence of other diseases or injuries requiring additional services should be separately reported.

Materials Supplied by Physician

Supplies and materials provided by the physician (eg, sterile trays/drugs), over and above those usually included with the procedure(s) rendered are reported separately. List drugs, trays, supplies, and materials provided. Identify as 99070 or specific supply code.

Reporting More Than One Procedure/Service

When a physician performs more than one procedure/service on the same date, same session or during a post-operative period (subject to the "surgical package" concept), several CPT modifiers may apply (see Appendix A for definition).

Separate Procedure

Some of the procedures or services listed in the CPT codebook that are commonly carried out as an integral component of a total service or procedure have been identified by the inclusion of the term "separate procedure." The codes designated as "separate procedure" should not be reported in addition to the code for the total procedure or service of which it is considered an integral component.

However, when a procedure or service that is designated as a "separate procedure" is carried out independently or considered to be unrelated or distinct from other procedures/services provided at that time, it may be reported by itself, or in addition to other procedures/services by appending modifier 59 to the specific "separate procedure" code to indicate that the procedure is not considered to be a component of another procedure, but is a distinct, independent procedure. This may represent a different session, different procedure or surgery, different site or organ system, separate incision/excision, separate lesion, or separate injury (or area of injury in extensive injuries).

Subsection Information

Several of the subheadings or subsections have special needs or instructions unique to that section. Where these are indicated (eg, "Maternity Care and Delivery"), special **"Notes"** will be presented preceding those procedural terminology listings, referring to that subsection specifically. If there is an "Unlisted Procedure" code number (see below) for the individual subsection, it will also be shown. Those subsections within the **Surgery** section that have **"Notes"** are as follows:

Digestive:
Endoscopy/Laparoscopy.......... 43200-43272,
      43280-43289, 43651-43659, 43770-43774,
      44180-44238, 44360-44397, 44970-44979,
      45300-45387, 45395-45397, 45400-45402,
      46600-46615, 47370-47379, 47550-47556,
          47560-47562, 49320-49329,
                   49650-49659

Pancreas Transplantation.......... 48550-48556

Herniotomy..................... 49491-49611

Renal Transplantation 50300-50380

Urodynamics 51725-51798

Endoscopy/Laparoscopy

    Urinary.......... 50541-50545, 50945-50980,
                   51990-52648

    Male Genital   54690-54699, 55550-55559, 55866

    Female Genital 58541-58579, 58660-58679

    Endocrine 60650-60659

Maternity Care and Delivery 59000-59899

Nervous System:
Surgery of Skull Base............. 61580-61619

Neurostimulators (Intracranial) 61850-61888,
                   62160-62319

Neurostimulators (Spinal) 63650-63688

Neurostimulators (Peripheral Nerve). 64553-64595

Secondary Implants(s) 65125-65175

Removal Cataract................ 66830-66999

Prophylaxis 67141-67229

Eyelid:
    Excision, Destruction........... 67800-67840

    Reconstruction................ 67930-67975

Operating Microscope 69990

Unlisted Service or Procedure

A service or procedure may be provided that is not listed
in this edition of the CPT codebook. When reporting
such a service, the appropriate "Unlisted Procedure" code
may be used to indicate the service, identifying it by
"Special Report" as discussed in the section below. The
"Unlisted Procedures" and accompanying codes for
Surgery are as follows:

15999   Unlisted procedure, excision pressure ulcer

17999   Unlisted procedure, skin, mucous membrane and
         subcutaneous tissue

19499   Unlisted procedure, breast

20999   Unlisted procedure, musculoskeletal system, general

21089   Unlisted maxillofacial prosthetic procedure

21299	Unlisted craniofacial and maxillofacial procedure
21499	Unlisted musculoskeletal procedure, head
21899	Unlisted procedure, neck or thorax
22899	Unlisted procedure, spine
22999	Unlisted procedure, abdomen, musculoskeletal system
23929	Unlisted procedure, shoulder
24999	Unlisted procedure, humerus or elbow
25999	Unlisted procedure, forearm or wrist
26989	Unlisted procedure, hands or fingers
27299	Unlisted procedure, pelvis or hip joint
27599	Unlisted procedure, femur or knee
27899	Unlisted procedure, leg or ankle
28899	Unlisted procedure, foot or toes
29799	Unlisted procedure, casting or strapping
29999	Unlisted procedure, arthroscopy
30999	Unlisted procedure, nose
31299	Unlisted procedure, accessory sinuses
31599	Unlisted procedure, larynx
31899	Unlisted procedure, trachea, bronchi
32999	Unlisted procedure, lungs and pleura
33999	Unlisted procedure, cardiac surgery
36299	Unlisted procedure, vascular injection
37501	Unlisted vascular endoscopy procedure
37799	Unlisted procedure, vascular surgery
38129	Unlisted laparoscopy procedure, spleen
38589	Unlisted laparoscopy procedure, lymphatic system
38999	Unlisted procedure, hemic or lymphatic system
39499	Unlisted procedure, mediastinum
39599	Unlisted procedure, diaphragm
40799	Unlisted procedure, lips
40899	Unlisted procedure, vestibule of mouth
41599	Unlisted procedure, tongue, floor of mouth
41899	Unlisted procedure, dentoalveolar structures
42299	Unlisted procedure, palate, uvula
42699	Unlisted procedure, salivary glands or ducts
42999	Unlisted procedure, pharynx, adenoids, or tonsils
43289	Unlisted laparoscopy procedure, esophagus
43499	Unlisted procedure, esophagus
43659	Unlisted laparoscopy procedure, stomach
43999	Unlisted procedure, stomach
44238	Unlisted laparoscopy procedure, intestine (except rectum)

44799	Unlisted procedure, intestine
44899	Unlisted procedure, Meckel's diverticulum and the mesentery
44979	Unlisted laparoscopy procedure, appendix
45499	Unlisted laparoscopy procedure, rectum
45999	Unlisted procedure, rectum
46999	Unlisted procedure, anus
47379	Unlisted laparoscopic procedure, liver
47399	Unlisted procedure, liver
47579	Unlisted laparoscopy procedure, biliary tract
47999	Unlisted procedure, biliary tract
48999	Unlisted procedure, pancreas
49329	Unlisted laparoscopy procedure, abdomen, peritoneum and omentum
49659	Unlisted laparoscopy procedure, hernioplasty, herniorrhaphy, herniotomy
49999	Unlisted procedure, abdomen, peritoneum and omentum
50549	Unlisted laparoscopy procedure, renal
50949	Unlisted laparoscopy procedure, ureter
51999	Unlisted laparoscopy procedure, bladder
53899	Unlisted procedure, urinary system
54699	Unlisted laparoscopy procedure, testis
55559	Unlisted laparoscopy procedure, spermatic cord
55899	Unlisted procedure, male genital system
58578	Unlisted laparoscopy procedure, uterus
58579	Unlisted hysteroscopy procedure, uterus
58679	Unlisted laparoscopy procedure, oviduct, ovary
58999	Unlisted procedure, female genital system (nonobstetrical)
59897	Unlisted fetal invasive procedure, including ultrasound guidance
59898	Unlisted laparoscopy procedure, maternity care and delivery
59899	Unlisted procedure, maternity care and delivery
60659	Unlisted laparoscopy procedure, endocrine system
60699	Unlisted procedure, endocrine system
64999	Unlisted procedure, nervous system
66999	Unlisted procedure, anterior segment of eye
67299	Unlisted procedure, posterior segment
67399	Unlisted procedure, ocular muscle
67599	Unlisted procedure, orbit
67999	Unlisted procedure, eyelids

68399	Unlisted procedure, conjunctiva
68899	Unlisted procedure, lacrimal system
69399	Unlisted procedure, external ear
69799	Unlisted procedure, middle ear
69949	Unlisted procedure, inner ear
69979	Unlisted procedure, temporal bone, middle fossa approach

Special Report

A service that is rarely provided, unusual, variable, or new may require a special report in determining medical appropriateness of the service. Pertinent information should include an adequate definition or description of the nature, extent, and need for the procedure, and the time, effort, and equipment necessary to provide the service. Additional items which may be included are:

- Complexity of symptoms
- Final diagnosis
- Pertinent physical findings (such as size, locations, and number of lesion(s), if appropriate)
- Diagnostic and therapeutic procedures (including major and supplementary surgical procedures, if appropriate)
- Concurrent problems
- Follow-up care

Surgical Destruction

Surgical destruction is a part of a surgical procedure and different methods of destruction are not ordinarily listed separately unless the technique substantially alters the standard management of a problem or condition. Exceptions under special circumstances are provided for by separate code numbers.

Surgery

General

10021   Fine needle aspiration; without imaging guidance
> *CPT Assistant* Aug 02:10, Mar 05:11; *CPT Changes: An Insider's View* 2002

10022   with imaging guidance
> *CPT Changes: An Insider's View* 2002
> *Clinical Examples in Radiology* Summer 05:1, 6

(For radiological supervision and interpretation, see 76942, 77002, 77012, 77021)

(For percutaneous needle biopsy other than fine needle aspiration, see 20206 for muscle, 32400 for pleura, 32405 for lung or mediastinum, 42400 for salivary gland, 47000, 47001 for liver, 48102 for pancreas, 49180 for abdominal or retroperitoneal mass, 60100 for thyroid, 62269 for spinal cord)

(For evaluation of fine needle aspirate, see 88172, 88173)

Integumentary System

Skin, Subcutaneous and Accessory Structures

Incision and Drainage

(For excision, see 11400, et seq)

10040   Acne surgery (eg, marsupialization, opening or removal of multiple milia, comedones, cysts, pustules)

10060   Incision and drainage of abscess (eg, carbuncle, suppurative hidradenitis, cutaneous or subcutaneous abscess, cyst, furuncle, or paronychia); simple or single

10061   complicated or multiple

10080   Incision and drainage of pilonidal cyst; simple
> *CPT Assistant* Fall 92:13, Dec 06:15

10081   complicated
> *CPT Assistant* Fall 92:13, Dec 06:15

(For excision of pilonidal cyst, see 11770-11772)

10120   Incision and removal of foreign body, subcutaneous tissues; simple

10121   complicated
> *CPT Assistant* Spring 91:7, Dec 06:15

(To report wound exploration due to penetrating trauma without laparotomy or thoracotomy, see 20100-20103, as appropriate)

(To report debridement associated with open fracture(s) and/or dislocation(s), use 11010-11012, as appropriate)

10140   Incision and drainage of hematoma, seroma or fluid collection
> *CPT Changes: An Insider's View* 2002

(If imaging guidance is performed, see 76942, 77012, 77021)

10160   Puncture aspiration of abscess, hematoma, bulla, or cyst
> *CPT Changes: An Insider's View* 2002

(If imaging guidance is performed, see 76942, 77012, 77021)

10180   Incision and drainage, complex, postoperative wound infection

(For secondary closure of surgical wound, see 12020, 12021, 13160)

Excision—Debridement

(For dermabrasions, see 15780-15783)

(For nail debridement, see 11720-11721)

(For burn(s), see 16000-16035)

11000   Debridement of extensive eczematous or infected skin; up to 10% of body surface
> *CPT Assistant* May 99:10

(For abdominal wall or genitalia debridement for necrotizing soft tissue infection, see 11004-11006)

+ 11001   each additional 10% of the body surface (List separately in addition to code for primary procedure)
> *CPT Assistant* May 99:10

(Use 11001 in conjunction with 11000)

11004   Debridement of skin, subcutaneous tissue, muscle and fascia for necrotizing soft tissue infection; external genitalia and perineum
> *CPT Changes: An Insider's View* 2005

11005   abdominal wall, with or without fascial closure

→ *CPT Changes: An Insider's View* 2005

Debridement of Abdominal Wall
11005

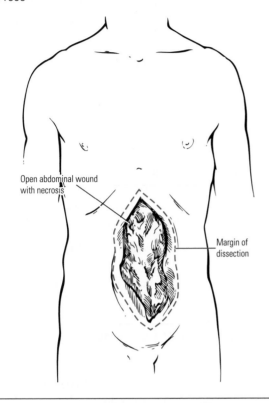

Open abdominal wound with necrosis

Margin of dissection

11006   external genitalia, perineum and abdominal wall, with or without fascial closure

→ *CPT Changes: An Insider's View* 2005

+▲ 11008   Removal of prosthetic material or mesh, abdominal wall for infection (eg, for chronic or recurrent mesh infection or necrotizing soft tissue infection) (List separately in addition to code for primary procedure)

→ *CPT Changes: An Insider's View* 2005, 2008

▶(Use 11008 in conjunction with 10180, 11004-11006)◀

(Do not report 11008 in conjunction with 11000-11001, 11010-11044)

(Report skin grafts or flaps separately when performed for closure at the same session as 11004-11008)

(When insertion of mesh is used for closure, use 49568)

(If orchiectomy is performed, use 54520)

(If testicular transplantation is performed, use 54680)

11010   Debridement including removal of foreign material associated with open fracture(s) and/or dislocation(s); skin and subcutaneous tissues

→ *CPT Assistant* Mar 97:2, Apr 97:10, Aug 97:6, Oct 03:10

11011   skin, subcutaneous tissue, muscle fascia, and muscle

→ *CPT Assistant* Mar 97:2, Apr 97:10, Aug 97:6

11012   skin, subcutaneous tissue, muscle fascia, muscle, and bone

→ *CPT Assistant* Mar 97:2, Apr 97:10, Aug 97:6, Oct 03:10

11040   Debridement; skin, partial thickness

→ *CPT Assistant* Fall 93:21, May 96:6, Feb 97:7, Aug 97:6

11041   skin, full thickness

→ *CPT Assistant* Fall 93:21, May 96:6, Feb 97:7, Aug 97:6, Jun 05:1, 0

11042   skin, and subcutaneous tissue

→ *CPT Assistant* Winter 92:10, May 96:6, Feb 97:7, Aug 97:6

11043   skin, subcutaneous tissue, and muscle

→ *CPT Assistant* May 96:6, Feb 97:7, Apr 97:11, Aug 97:6, Dec 99:10

11044   skin, subcutaneous tissue, muscle, and bone

→ *CPT Assistant* Fall 93:21, Mar 96:10, May 96:6, Feb 97:7, Apr 97:11, Aug 97:6

(Do not report 11040-11044 in conjunction with 97597-97602)

Paring or Cutting

(To report destruction, see 17000-17004)

11055   Paring or cutting of benign hyperkeratotic lesion (eg, corn or callus); single lesion

→ *CPT Assistant* Nov 97:11, Jan 99:11

11056   2 to 4 lesions

→ *CPT Assistant* Nov 97:11, Jan 99:11

11057   more than 4 lesions

→ *CPT Assistant* Nov 97:11, Jan 99:11, May 99:10

Biopsy

During certain surgical procedures in the integumentary system, such as excision, destruction, or shave removals, the removed tissue is often submitted for pathologic examination. The obtaining of tissue for pathology during the course of these procedures is a routine component of such procedures. This obtaining of tissue is not considered a separate biopsy procedure and is not separately reported. The use of a biopsy procedure code (eg, 11100, 11101) indicates that the procedure to obtain tissue for pathologic examination was performed independently, or was unrelated or distinct from other procedures/services provided at that time. Such biopsies are not considered components of other procedures when performed on different lesions or different sites on the same date, and are to be reported separately.

(For biopsy of conjunctiva, use 68100; eyelid, use 67810)

11100   Biopsy of skin, subcutaneous tissue and/or mucous membrane (including simple closure), unless otherwise listed; single lesion

→ *CPT Assistant* Fall 94:20, Mar 97:12, Jun 97:12, Apr 00:7, Nov 02:6, Jul 04:5, Oct 04:4, Nov 06:1; *CPT Changes: An Insider's View* 2004

+ 11101   each separate/additional lesion (List separately in addition to code for primary procedure)

> *CPT Assistant* Fall 94:20, Apr 00:6, Apr 00:7, Nov 02:6, Jul 04:5, Oct 04:4, Nov 06:1

(Use 11101 in conjunction with 11100)

Removal of Skin Tags

▶Removal by scissoring or any sharp method, ligature strangulation, electrosurgical destruction or combination of treatment modalities, including chemical destruction or electrocauterization of wound, with or without local anesthesia.◀

11200   Removal of skin tags, multiple fibrocutaneous tags, any area; up to and including 15 lesions

> *CPT Assistant* Winter 90:3, Nov 97:11-12, Nov 02:11

+ 11201   each additional 10 lesions (List separately in addition to code for primary procedure)

> *CPT Assistant* Winter 90:3, Nov 97:11-12, Nov 02:11

(Use 11201 in conjunction with 11200)

Removal of Skin Tags
11200, 11201

Skin tags

Scissor excision of skin tag

Shaving of Epidermal or Dermal Lesions

Shaving is the sharp removal by transverse incision or horizontal slicing to remove epidermal and dermal lesions without a full-thickness dermal excision. This includes local anesthesia, chemical or electrocauterization of the wound. The wound does not require suture closure.

11300   Shaving of epidermal or dermal lesion, single lesion, trunk, arms or legs; lesion diameter 0.5 cm or less

> *CPT Assistant* Feb 00:11, Nov 02:11

11301   lesion diameter 0.6 to 1.0 cm

> *CPT Assistant* Feb 00:11

11302   lesion diameter 1.1 to 2.0 cm

> *CPT Assistant* Feb 00:11

11303   lesion diameter over 2.0 cm

> *CPT Assistant* Feb 00:11

11305   Shaving of epidermal or dermal lesion, single lesion, scalp, neck, hands, feet, genitalia; lesion diameter 0.5 cm or less

> *CPT Assistant* Feb 00:11

11306   lesion diameter 0.6 to 1.0 cm

> *CPT Assistant* Feb 00:11

11307   lesion diameter 1.1 to 2.0 cm

> *CPT Assistant* Feb 00:11

11308   lesion diameter over 2.0 cm

> *CPT Assistant* Feb 00:11

11310   Shaving of epidermal or dermal lesion, single lesion, face, ears, eyelids, nose, lips, mucous membrane; lesion diameter 0.5 cm or less

> *CPT Assistant* Feb 00:11

11311   lesion diameter 0.6 to 1.0 cm

> *CPT Assistant* Feb 00:11

11312   lesion diameter 1.1 to 2.0 cm

> *CPT Assistant* Feb 00:11

11313   lesion diameter over 2.0 cm

> *CPT Assistant* Feb 00:11

Measuring and Coding the Removal of a Lesion

Measuring lesion removal.
A. Example: excision, malignant lesion of the back, 1.0 cm. Code 11606.

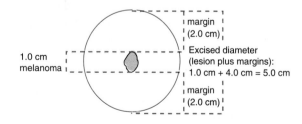

1.0 cm melanoma

margin (2.0 cm)

Excised diameter (lesion plus margins): 1.0 cm + 4.0 cm = 5.0 cm

margin (2.0 cm)

B. Example: Excision of benign lesion of the neck, 1.0 cm by 2.0 cm. Code 11423.

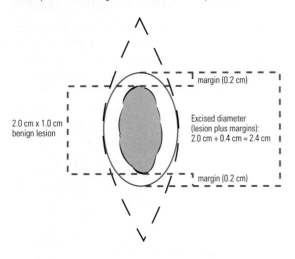

C. Example: Excision, malignant lesion of the nose, 0.9 cm. Code 11642.

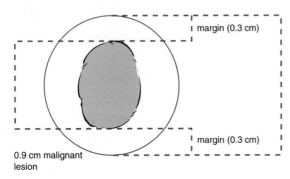

Excision—Benign Lesions

Excision (including simple closure) of benign lesions of skin (eg, neoplasm, cicatricial, fibrous, inflammatory, congenital, cystic lesions), includes local anesthesia. See appropriate size and area below. For shave removal, see 11300 et seq., and for electrosurgical and other methods see 17000 et seq.

Excision is defined as full-thickness (through the dermis) removal of a lesion, including margins, and includes simple (non-layered) closure when performed. Report separately each benign lesion excised. Code selection is determined by measuring the greatest clinical diameter of the apparent lesion plus that margin required for complete excision (lesion diameter plus the most narrow margins required equals the excised diameter). The margins refer to the most narrow margin required to

adequately excise the lesion, based on the physician's judgment. The measurement of lesion plus margin is made prior to excision. The excised diameter is the same whether the surgical defect is repaired in a linear fashion, or reconstructed (eg, with a skin graft).

▶The closure of defects created by incision, excision, or trauma may require intermediate or complex closure. Repair by intermediate or complex closure should be reported separately. For excision of benign lesions requiring more than simple closure, ie, requiring intermediate or complex closure, report 11400-11446 in addition to appropriate intermediate (12031-12057) or complex closure (13100-13153) codes. For reconstructive closure, see 15002-15261, 15570-15770. For excision performed in conjunction with adjacent tissue transfer, report only the adjacent tissue transfer code (14000-14300). Excision of lesion (11400–11446) is not separately reportable with adjacent tissue transfer. See page 58 for the definition of *intermediate* or *complex* closure.◀

11400 Excision, benign lesion including margins, except skin tag (unless listed elsewhere), trunk, arms or legs; excised diameter 0.5 cm or less
➔ *CPT Assistant* Summer 92:22, Fall 93:7, Fall 95:3, May 96:11, Aug 00:5, Nov 02:5, 7, Aug 06:10; *CPT Changes: An Insider's View* 2003

11401 excised diameter 0.6 to 1.0 cm
➔ *CPT Assistant* Summer 92:22, Fall 93:7, Fall 95:3, May 96:11, Nov 02:5, 7; *CPT Changes: An Insider's View* 2003

11402 excised diameter 1.1 to 2.0 cm
➔ *CPT Assistant* Summer 92:22, Fall 93:7, Fall 95:3, May 96:11, Nov 02:5, 7; *CPT Changes: An Insider's View* 2003

11403 excised diameter 2.1 to 3.0 cm
➔ *CPT Assistant* Summer 92:22, Fall 93:7, Fall 95:3, May 96:11, Nov 02:5, 7; *CPT Changes: An Insider's View* 2003

11404 excised diameter 3.1 to 4.0 cm
➔ *CPT Assistant* Summer 92:22, Fall 93:7, Fall 95:3, May 96:11, Nov 02:5, 7; *CPT Changes: An Insider's View* 2003

11406 excised diameter over 4.0 cm
➔ *CPT Assistant* Summer 92:22, Fall 93:7, Fall 95:3, May 96:11, Nov 02:5, 7; *CPT Changes: An Insider's View* 2003

(For unusual or complicated excision, add modifier 22)

11420 Excision, benign lesion including margins, except skin tag (unless listed elsewhere), scalp, neck, hands, feet, genitalia; excised diameter 0.5 cm or less
➔ *CPT Assistant* Summer 92:22, Fall 95:3; *CPT Changes: An Insider's View* 2003

11421 excised diameter 0.6 to 1.0 cm
➔ *CPT Assistant* Summer 92:22, Fall 95:3, May 96:11; *CPT Changes: An Insider's View* 2003

11422 excised diameter 1.1 to 2.0 cm
➔ *CPT Assistant* Summer 92:22, Fall 95:3, May 96:11, Aug 00:5; *CPT Changes: An Insider's View* 2003

11423   excised diameter 2.1 to 3.0 cm
➔ *CPT Assistant* Summer 92:22, Fall 95:3, May 96:11;
CPT Changes: An Insider's View 2003

11424   excised diameter 3.1 to 4.0 cm
➔ *CPT Assistant* Summer 92:22, Fall 95:3, May 96:11;
CPT Changes: An Insider's View 2003

11426   excised diameter over 4.0 cm
➔ *CPT Assistant* Summer 92:22, Fall 95:3, May 96:11;
CPT Changes: An Insider's View 2003

(For unusual or complicated excision, add modifier 22)

11440   Excision, other benign lesion including margins, except
skin tag (unless listed elsewhere), face, ears, eyelids,
nose, lips, mucous membrane; excised diameter 0.5 cm
or less
➔ *CPT Assistant* Summer 92:22, Fall 95:3, May 96:11;
CPT Changes: An Insider's View 2003

11441   excised diameter 0.6 to 1.0 cm
➔ *CPT Assistant* Summer 92:22, Fall 95:3, May 96:11;
CPT Changes: An Insider's View 2003

11442   excised diameter 1.1 to 2.0 cm
➔ *CPT Assistant* Summer 92:22, Fall 95:3, May 96:11,
Aug 00:5; *CPT Changes: An Insider's View* 2003

11443   excised diameter 2.1 to 3.0 cm
➔ *CPT Assistant* Summer 92:22, Fall 95:3, May 96:11;
CPT Changes: An Insider's View 2003

11444   excised diameter 3.1 to 4.0 cm
➔ *CPT Assistant* Summer 92:22, Fall 95:3, May 96:11;
CPT Changes: An Insider's View 2003

11446   excised diameter over 4.0 cm
➔ *CPT Assistant* Summer 92:22, Fall 95:3, May 96:11,
Aug 06:10; *CPT Changes: An Insider's View* 2003

(For unusual or complicated excision, add modifier 22)

(For eyelids involving more than skin, see also 67800 et
seq)

11450   Excision of skin and subcutaneous tissue for hidradenitis,
axillary; with simple or intermediate repair

11451   with complex repair

11462   Excision of skin and subcutaneous tissue for hidradenitis,
inguinal; with simple or intermediate repair

11463   with complex repair

11470   Excision of skin and subcutaneous tissue for hidradenitis,
perianal, perineal, or umbilical; with simple or
intermediate repair

11471   with complex repair

(When skin graft or flap is used for closure, use
appropriate procedure code in addition)

(For bilateral procedure, add modifier 50)

Excision—Malignant Lesions

Excision (including simple closure) of malignant lesions
of skin (eg, basal cell carcinoma, squamous cell
carcinoma, melanoma) includes local anesthesia. (See
appropriate size and body area below.) For destruction of
malignant lesions of skin, see destruction codes 17260-
17286.

Excision is defined as full-thickness (through the dermis)
removal of a lesion including margins, and includes
simple (non-layered) closure when performed. Report
separately each malignant lesion excised. Code selection is
determined by measuring the greatest clinical diameter of
the apparent lesion plus that margin required for
complete excision (lesion diameter plus the most narrow
margins required equals the excised diameter). The
margins refer to the most narrow margin required to
adequately excise the lesion, based on the physician's
judgment. The measurement of lesion plus margin is
made prior to excision. The excised diameter is the same
whether the surgical defect is repaired in a linear fashion,
or reconstructed (eg, with a skin graft).

▶The closure of defects created by incision, excision, or
trauma may require intermediate or complex closure.
Repair by intermediate or complex closure should be
reported separately. For excision of malignant lesions
requiring more than simple closure, ie, requiring
intermediate or complex closure, report 11600-11646 in
addition to appropriate intermediate (12031-12057) or
complex closure (13100-13153) codes. For reconstructive
closure, see 15002-15261, 15570-15770. For excision
performed in conjunction with adjacent tissue transfer,
report only the adjacent tissue transfer code (14000-
14300). Excision of lesion (11600–11646) is not
separately reportable with adjacent tissue transfer. See
page 58 for the definition of *intermediate* or *complex*
closure.◀

When frozen section pathology shows the margins of
excision were not adequate, an additional excision may be
necessary for complete tumor removal. Use only one code
to report the additional excision and re-excision(s) based
on the final widest excised diameter required for complete
tumor removal at the same operative session. To report a
re-excision procedure performed to widen margins at a
subsequent operative session, see codes 11600-11646, as
appropriate. Append modifier 58 if the re-excision
procedure is performed during the postoperative period
of the primary excision procedure.

11600 Excision, malignant lesion including margins, trunk, arms, or legs; excised diameter 0.5 cm or less

 CPT Assistant Fall 95:3, May 96:11, Nov 02:5; *CPT Changes: An Insider's View* 2003

Measuring and Coding the Removal of a Lesion
11600

Example: Excision, malignant lesion, 0.4 cm. Code 11600.

0.2 cm lesion

margin (0.1 cm)   margin (0.1 cm)

Excised diameter
(lesion plus margins):
0.2 cm + 0.2 cm = 0.4 cm

11601 excised diameter 0.6 to 1.0 cm

 CPT Assistant Fall 95:3, May 96:11, Nov 02:5; *CPT Changes: An Insider's View* 2003

11602 excised diameter 1.1 to 2.0 cm

 CPT Assistant Fall 95:3, May 96:11, Nov 02:5; *CPT Changes: An Insider's View* 2003

11603 excised diameter 2.1 to 3.0 cm

 CPT Assistant Fall 95:3, May 96:11, Nov 02:5; *CPT Changes: An Insider's View* 2003

11604 excised diameter 3.1 to 4.0 cm

 CPT Assistant Fall 95:3, May 96:11, Nov 02:5; *CPT Changes: An Insider's View* 2003

11606 excised diameter over 4.0 cm

 CPT Assistant Fall 91:6, Fall 95:3, May 96:11, Nov 02:5; *CPT Changes: An Insider's View* 2003

11620 Excision, malignant lesion including margins, scalp, neck, hands, feet, genitalia; excised diameter 0.5 cm or less

 CPT Assistant Fall 95:3, Nov 02:5; *CPT Changes: An Insider's View* 2003

11621 excised diameter 0.6 to 1.0 cm

 CPT Assistant Fall 95:3, May 96:11, Nov 02:5; *CPT Changes: An Insider's View* 2003

11622 excised diameter 1.1 to 2.0 cm

 CPT Assistant Fall 95:3, May 96:11, Nov 02:5; *CPT Changes: An Insider's View* 2003

11623 excised diameter 2.1 to 3.0 cm

 CPT Assistant Fall 95:3, May 96:11, Nov 02:5; *CPT Changes: An Insider's View* 2003

11624 excised diameter 3.1 to 4.0 cm

 CPT Assistant Fall 95:3, May 96:11, Nov 02:5; *CPT Changes: An Insider's View* 2003

11626 excised diameter over 4.0 cm

 CPT Assistant Fall 95:3, May 96:11, Nov 02:5; *CPT Changes: An Insider's View* 2003

11640 Excision, malignant lesion including margins, face, ears, eyelids, nose, lips; excised diameter 0.5 cm or less

 CPT Assistant Fall 95:3, May 96:11, Nov 02:5; *CPT Changes: An Insider's View* 2003

11641 excised diameter 0.6 to 1.0 cm

 CPT Assistant Fall 95:3, May 96:11; *CPT Changes: An Insider's View* 2003

11642 excised diameter 1.1 to 2.0 cm

 CPT Assistant Fall 95:3, May 96:11; *CPT Changes: An Insider's View* 2003

11643 excised diameter 2.1 to 3.0 cm

 CPT Assistant Fall 95:3, May 96:11; *CPT Changes: An Insider's View* 2003

11644 excised diameter 3.1 to 4.0 cm

 CPT Assistant Fall 95:3, May 96:11; *CPT Changes: An Insider's View* 2003

11646 excised diameter over 4.0 cm

 CPT Assistant Fall 95:3, May 96:11; *CPT Changes: An Insider's View* 2003

(For eyelids involving more than skin, see also 67800 et seq)

Nails

(For drainage of paronychia or onychia, see 10060, 10061)

11719 Trimming of nondystrophic nails, any number

 CPT Assistant Nov 97:12, Dec 02:4

Lateral Nail View
11719-11765

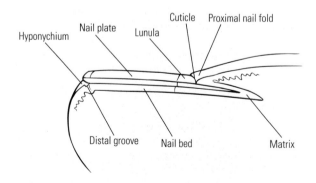

Cuticle   Proximal nail fold

Nail plate   Lunula

Hyponychium

Distal groove   Nail bed   Matrix

11720 Debridement of nail(s) by any method(s); one to five
➔ *CPT Assistant* Nov 96:3, Dec 02:4

11721 six or more
➔ *CPT Assistant* Nov 96:3, Dec 02:4

11730 Avulsion of nail plate, partial or complete, simple; single
➔ *CPT Assistant* Mar 96:10, Dec 02:4, Dec 03:11

+ 11732 each additional nail plate (List separately in addition to code for primary procedure)
➔ *CPT Assistant* Dec 02:4

(Use 11732 in conjunction with 11730)

11740 Evacuation of subungual hematoma
➔ *CPT Assistant* Dec 02:4

11750 Excision of nail and nail matrix, partial or complete (eg, ingrown or deformed nail), for permanent removal;
➔ *CPT Assistant* Dec 02:4

11752 with amputation of tuft of distal phalanx
➔ *CPT Assistant* Dec 02:4

(For skin graft, if used, use 15050)

11755 Biopsy of nail unit (eg, plate, bed, matrix, hyponychium, proximal and lateral nail folds) (separate procedure)
➔ *CPT Assistant* Mar 96:11, Dec 02:4, Oct 04:14; *CPT Changes: An Insider's View* 2002

11760 Repair of nail bed
➔ *CPT Assistant* Dec 02:4

11762 Reconstruction of nail bed with graft
➔ *CPT Assistant* Dec 02:4

11765 Wedge excision of skin of nail fold (eg, for ingrown toenail)
➔ *CPT Assistant* Dec 02:4

Dorsal Nail View
11719-11765

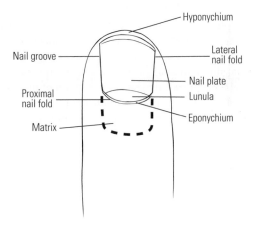

Hyponychium

Lateral nail fold

Nail groove

Nail plate

Proximal nail fold

Lunula

Matrix

Eponychium

Pilonidal Cyst

11770 Excision of pilonidal cyst or sinus; simple

11771 extensive

11772 complicated

(For incision of pilonidal cyst, see 10080, 10081)

Introduction

11900 Injection, intralesional; up to and including 7 lesions
➔ *CPT Assistant* Sep 96:5, May 98:10, Nov 99:8, Feb 00:11, Sep 04:12

11901 more than 7 lesions
➔ *CPT Assistant* Sep 96:5, May 98:10, Nov 99:8, Feb 00:11, Sep 04:12

(11900, 11901 are not to be used for preoperative local anesthetic injection)

(For veins, see 36470, 36471)

(For intralesional chemotherapy administration, see 96405, 96406)

11920 Tattooing, intradermal introduction of insoluble opaque pigments to correct color defects of skin, including micropigmentation; 6.0 sq cm or less

11921 6.1 to 20.0 sq cm

+ 11922 each additional 20.0 sq cm (List separately in addition to code for primary procedure)

(Use 11922 in conjunction with 11921)

11950 Subcutaneous injection of filling material (eg, collagen); 1 cc or less

11951 1.1 to 5.0 cc

11952 5.1 to 10.0 cc

11954 over 10.0 cc

11960 Insertion of tissue expander(s) for other than breast, including subsequent expansion
➔ *CPT Assistant* Winter 91:2

(For breast reconstruction with tissue expander(s), use 19357)

11970 Replacement of tissue expander with permanent prosthesis
➔ *CPT Assistant* Aug 05:1

11971 Removal of tissue expander(s) without insertion of prosthesis
➔ *CPT Assistant* Jun 05:11

11975 Insertion, implantable contraceptive capsules

11976 Removal, implantable contraceptive capsules

11977 Removal with reinsertion, implantable contraceptive capsules

11980 Subcutaneous hormone pellet implantation (implantation of estradiol and/or testosterone pellets beneath the skin)
➔ *CPT Assistant* Nov 99:8; *CPT Changes: An Insider's View* 2000

11981 Insertion, non-biodegradable drug delivery implant
➔ *CPT Changes: An Insider's View* 2002

11982 Removal, non-biodegradable drug delivery implant
➔ *CPT Changes: An Insider's View* 2002

11983 Removal with reinsertion, non-biodegradable drug delivery implant
➔ *CPT Changes: An Insider's View* 2002

Repair (Closure)

Use the codes in this section to designate wound closure utilizing sutures, staples, or tissue adhesives (eg, 2-cyanoacrylate), either singly or in combination with each other, or in combination with adhesive strips. Wound closure utilizing adhesive strips as the sole repair material should be coded using the appropriate E/M code.

Definitions

The repair of wounds may be classified as Simple, Intermediate, or Complex.

Simple repair is used when the wound is superficial; eg, involving primarily epidermis or dermis, or subcutaneous tissues without significant involvement of deeper structures, and requires simple one layer closure. This includes local anesthesia and chemical or electrocauterization of wounds not closed.

Intermediate repair includes the repair of wounds that, in addition to the above, require layered closure of one or more of the deeper layers of subcutaneous tissue and superficial (non-muscle) fascia, in addition to the skin (epidermal and dermal) closure. Single-layer closure of heavily contaminated wounds that have required extensive cleaning or removal of particulate matter also constitutes intermediate repair.

Complex repair includes the repair of wounds requiring more than layered closure, viz., scar revision, debridement (eg, traumatic lacerations or avulsions), extensive undermining, stents or retention sutures. Necessary preparation includes creation of a defect for repairs (eg, excision of a scar requiring a complex repair) or the debridement of complicated lacerations or avulsions. Complex repair does not include excision of benign (11400-11446) or malignant (11600-11646) lesions.

Instructions for listing services at time of wound repair:

1. The repaired wound(s) should be measured and recorded in centimeters, whether curved, angular, or stellate.

2. When multiple wounds are repaired, add together the lengths of those in the same classification (see above) and from all anatomic sites that are grouped together into the same code descriptor. For example, add together the lengths of intermediate repairs to the trunk and extremities. Do not add lengths of repairs from different groupings of anatomic sites (eg, face and extremities). Also, do not add together lengths of different classifications (eg, intermediate and complex repairs).

When more than one classification of wounds is repaired, list the more complicated as the primary procedure and the less complicated as the secondary procedure, using modifier 51.

3. Decontamination and/or debridement: Debridement is considered a separate procedure only when gross contamination requires prolonged cleansing, when appreciable amounts of devitalized or contaminated tissue are removed, or when debridement is carried out separately without immediate primary closure. (For extensive debridement of soft tissue and/or bone, see 11040-11044.)

(For extensive debridement of soft tissue and/or bone, not associated with open fracture(s) and/or dislocation(s) resulting from penetrating and/or blunt trauma, see 11040-11044.)

(For extensive debridement of subcutaneous tissue, muscle fascia, muscle, and/or bone associated with open fracture(s) and/or dislocation(s), see 11010-11012.)

4. Involvement of nerves, blood vessels and tendons: Report under appropriate system (Nervous, Cardiovascular, Musculoskeletal) for repair of these structures. The repair of these associated wounds is included in the primary procedure unless it qualifies as a complex wound, in which case modifier 51 applies.

Simple ligation of vessels in an open wound is considered as part of any wound closure.

Simple "exploration" of nerves, blood vessels or tendons exposed in an open wound is also considered part of the essential treatment of the wound and is not a separate procedure unless appreciable dissection is required. If the wound requires enlargement, extension of dissection (to determine penetration), debridement, removal of foreign body(s), ligation or coagulation of minor subcutaneous and/or muscular blood vessel(s) of the subcutaneous tissue, muscle fascia, and/or muscle, not requiring thoracotomy or laparotomy, use codes 20100-20103, as appropriate.

Repair—Simple

Sum of lengths of repairs for each group of anatomic sites.

12001   Simple repair of superficial wounds of scalp, neck, axillae, external genitalia, trunk and/or extremities (including hands and feet); 2.5 cm or less
➡ *CPT Assistant* Jun 96:7, Feb 98:11, Jan 00:11, Feb 00:10, Apr 00:8, Jul 00:10, Jan 02:10, Feb 07:10

12002   2.6 cm to 7.5 cm
➡ *CPT Assistant* Feb 00:10, Jan 02:10

12004   7.6 cm to 12.5 cm
➡ *CPT Assistant* Feb 00:10, Jan 02:10

12005   12.6 cm to 20.0 cm
➡ *CPT Assistant* Feb 00:10, Jan 02:10

12006   20.1 cm to 30.0 cm
➡ *CPT Assistant* Feb 98:11, Feb 00:10, Jan 02:10

12007   over 30.0 cm
➡ *CPT Assistant* Feb 00:10, Jan 02:10

12011   Simple repair of superficial wounds of face, ears, eyelids, nose, lips and/or mucous membranes; 2.5 cm or less
➡ *CPT Assistant* Feb 00:10, May 00:8, Jan 02:10

12013   2.6 cm to 5.0 cm
➡ *CPT Assistant* Feb 00:10, Jan 02:10

12014   5.1 cm to 7.5 cm
➡ *CPT Assistant* Feb 00:10, Jan 02:10

12015   7.6 cm to 12.5 cm
➡ *CPT Assistant* Feb 00:10, Jan 02:10

12016   12.6 cm to 20.0 cm
➡ *CPT Assistant* Feb 00:10, Jan 02:10

12017   20.1 cm to 30.0 cm
➡ *CPT Assistant* Feb 00:10, Jan 02:10

12018   over 30.0 cm
➡ *CPT Assistant* Feb 00:10, Jan 02:10, Feb 07:10

12020   Treatment of superficial wound dehiscence; simple closure
➡ *CPT Assistant* Feb 00:10, Jan 02:10

12021   with packing
➡ *CPT Assistant* Feb 00:10, Jan 02:10

(For extensive or complicated secondary wound closure, use 13160)

Repair—Intermediate

Sum of lengths of repairs for each group of anatomic sites.

12031   Layer closure of wounds of scalp, axillae, trunk and/or extremities (excluding hands and feet); 2.5 cm or less
➡ *CPT Assistant* Sep 97:11, Feb 00:10, Apr 00:8, Jan 02:10, Aug 06:1, Feb 07:10

12032   2.6 cm to 7.5 cm
➡ *CPT Assistant* May 96:6, Jun 96:8, Feb 00:10, Jan 02:10, Feb 07:10

12034   7.6 cm to 12.5 cm
➡ *CPT Assistant* Fall 91:6, Feb 00:10, Jan 02:10, Feb 07:10

12035   12.6 cm to 20.0 cm
➡ *CPT Assistant* Feb 00:10, Jan 02:10, Feb 07:10

12036   20.1 cm to 30.0 cm
➡ *CPT Assistant* Feb 00:10, Jan 02:10, Feb 07:10

12037   over 30.0 cm
➡ *CPT Assistant* Feb 00:10, Jan 02:10, Feb 07:10

12041   Layer closure of wounds of neck, hands, feet and/or external genitalia; 2.5 cm or less
➡ *CPT Assistant* Sep 97:11, Feb 00:10, Apr 00:8, Jan 02:10, Feb 07:10

12042   2.6 cm to 7.5 cm
➡ *CPT Assistant* Feb 00:10, Apr 00:9, Jan 02:10, Feb 07:10

12044   7.6 cm to 12.5 cm
➡ *CPT Assistant* Feb 00:10, Jan 02:10, Feb 07:10

12045   12.6 cm to 20.0 cm
➡ *CPT Assistant* Feb 00:10, Jan 02:10, Feb 07:10

12046   20.1 cm to 30.0 cm
➡ *CPT Assistant* Feb 00:10, Jan 02:10, Feb 07:10

12047   over 30.0 cm
➡ *CPT Assistant* Feb 00:10, Jan 02:10, Feb 07:10

12051   Layer closure of wounds of face, ears, eyelids, nose, lips and/or mucous membranes; 2.5 cm or less
➡ *CPT Assistant* Sep 97:11, Feb 00:10, Apr 00:8, Jan 02:10, Feb 07:10

12052   2.6 cm to 5.0 cm
➡ *CPT Assistant* Feb 00:10, Aug 00:9, Jan 02:10, Feb 07:10

12053   5.1 cm to 7.5 cm
➡ *CPT Assistant* Feb 00:10, Jan 02:10, Feb 07:10

12054   7.6 cm to 12.5 cm
➡ *CPT Assistant* Feb 00:10, Jan 02:10, Feb 07:10

12055   12.6 cm to 20.0 cm
➡ *CPT Assistant* Feb 00:10, Jan 02:10, Feb 07:10

12056   20.1 cm to 30.0 cm
➡ *CPT Assistant* Feb 00:10, Jan 02:10, Feb 07:10

12057   over 30.0 cm
➡ *CPT Assistant* Feb 00:10, Jan 02:10, Feb 07:10

Repair—Complex

Reconstructive procedures, complicated wound closure.

Sum of lengths of repairs for each group of anatomic sites.

(For full thickness repair of lip or eyelid, see respective anatomical subsections)

13100   Repair, complex, trunk; 1.1 cm to 2.5 cm
➡ *CPT Assistant* Sep 97:11, Dec 98:5, Nov 99:9-10, Feb 00:10, Apr 00:8

(For 1.0 cm or less, see simple or intermediate repairs)

13101   2.6 cm to 7.5 cm
➡ *CPT Assistant* Dec 98:5, Nov 99:9-10, Feb 00:10, Apr 00:9

+ 13102   each additional 5 cm or less (List separately in addition to code for primary procedure)
➡ *CPT Assistant* Nov 99:9-10, Feb 00:10, Apr 00:9; *CPT Changes: An Insider's View* 2000

(Use 13102 in conjunction with 13101)

13120   Repair, complex, scalp, arms, and/or legs; 1.1 cm to 2.5 cm
➡ *CPT Assistant* Sep 97:11, Apr 99:11, Nov 99:9-10, Feb 00:10, Apr 00:8

(For 1.0 cm or less, see simple or intermediate repairs)

13121   2.6 cm to 7.5 cm
➡ *CPT Assistant* Dec 98:5, Nov 99:9-10, Feb 00:10

+ 13122   each additional 5 cm or less (List separately in addition to code for primary procedure)
➡ *CPT Assistant* Nov 99:10; *CPT Changes: An Insider's View* 2000

(Use 13122 in conjunction with 13121)

13131   Repair, complex, forehead, cheeks, chin, mouth, neck, axillae, genitalia, hands and/or feet; 1.1 cm to 2.5 cm
➡ *CPT Assistant* Fall 93:7, Sep 97:11, Dec 98:5, Nov 99:10, Feb 00:10, Apr 00:8

(For 1.0 cm or less, see simple or intermediate repairs)

13132   2.6 cm to 7.5 cm
➡ *CPT Assistant* Fall 93:7, Dec 98:5, Nov 99:10, Dec 99:10, Feb 00:10, Apr 00:9, Aug 00:9

+ 13133   each additional 5 cm or less (List separately in addition to code for primary procedure)
➡ *CPT Assistant* Fall 93:7, Feb 00:10, Apr 00:9; *CPT Changes: An Insider's View* 2000

(Use 13133 in conjunction with 13132)

13150   Repair, complex, eyelids, nose, ears and/or lips; 1.0 cm or less
➡ *CPT Assistant* Sep 97:11, Dec 98:5, Nov 99:10, Feb 00:10, Apr 00:8

(See also 40650-40654, 67961-67975)

13151   1.1 cm to 2.5 cm
➡ *CPT Assistant* Dec 98:5, Nov 99:10, Feb 00:10

13152   2.6 cm to 7.5 cm
➡ *CPT Assistant* Dec 98:5, Nov 99:10, Feb 00:10

+ 13153   each additional 5 cm or less (List separately in addition to code for primary procedure)
➡ *CPT Assistant* Nov 99:10, Feb 00:10; *CPT Changes: An Insider's View* 2000

(Use 13153 in conjunction with 13152)

13160   Secondary closure of surgical wound or dehiscence, extensive or complicated
➡ *CPT Assistant* Sep 97:11, Dec 98:5, Apr 00:8

(For packing or simple secondary wound closure, see 12020, 12021)

Adjacent Tissue Transfer or Rearrangement

For full thickness repair of lip or eyelid, see respective anatomical subsections.

▶Codes 14000-14300 are used for excision (including lesion) and/or repair by adjacent tissue transfer or rearrangement (eg, Z-plasty, W-plasty, V-Y plasty, rotation flap, advancement flap, double pedicle flap). When applied in repairing lacerations, the procedures listed must be performed by the surgeon to accomplish the repair. They do not apply to direct closure or rearrangement of traumatic wounds incidentally resulting in these configurations. The excision of a benign lesion (11400-11446) or a malignant lesion (11600-11646) is not separately reportable with codes 14000-14300.◀

Skin graft necessary to close secondary defect is considered an additional procedure. For purposes of code selection, the term "defect" includes the primary and secondary defects. The primary defect resulting from the excision and the secondary defect resulting from flap design to perform the reconstruction are measured together to determine the code.

14000   Adjacent tissue transfer or rearrangement, trunk; defect 10 sq cm or less
➡ *CPT Assistant* Sep 96:11, Jul 99:3, Jul 00:10, Jan 06:47, Dec 06:15

14001   defect 10.1 sq cm to 30.0 sq cm
➡ *CPT Assistant* Aug 96:8, Jul 99:3, Jan 06:47, Dec 06:15

14020   Adjacent tissue transfer or rearrangement, scalp, arms and/or legs; defect 10 sq cm or less
➡ *CPT Assistant* Jul 99:3, Jan 06:47, Dec 06:15

14021   defect 10.1 sq cm to 30.0 sq cm
➡ *CPT Assistant* Jul 99:3, Jan 06:47, Dec 06:15

14040   Adjacent tissue transfer or rearrangement, forehead, cheeks, chin, mouth, neck, axillae, genitalia, hands and/or feet; defect 10 sq cm or less
➡ *CPT Assistant* Jul 99:3, Jul 00:10, Jan 06:47, Dec 06:15

14041   defect 10.1 sq cm to 30.0 sq cm
➡ *CPT Assistant* Jul 99:3, Jan 06:47, Dec 06:15

14060   Adjacent tissue transfer or rearrangement, eyelids, nose, ears and/or lips; defect 10 sq cm or less
> *CPT Assistant* Fall 93:7, Jul 99:3, Dec 99:10, Jan 06:47, Dec 06:15

14061   defect 10.1 sq cm to 30.0 sq cm
> *CPT Assistant* Jul 99:3, Jan 06:47, Dec 06:15

(For eyelid, full thickness, see 67961 et seq)

Adjacent Tissue Repairs
14000-14061

Repair of primary and secondary defects requires assignment of a code based upon the repair location and the approximate description (as demonstrated below) of the area repaired.

A. Advancement Flap

Area 1: 1.0 cm x 1.0 cm = 1.0 sq cm
Area 2: 1.0 cm x 2.0 cm = 2.0 sq cm
(Area 1) + (Area 2) = 1.0 sq cm + 2.0 sq cm = 3.0 sq cm

B. Rotation Flap

Area 1: 1.0 cm x 1.0 cm = 1.0 sq cm
Area 2: 2.5 cm x 1.2 cm = 3.0 sq cm
(Area 1) + (Area 2) = 1.0 sq cm + 3.0 sq cm = 4.0 sq cm

14300   Adjacent tissue transfer or rearrangement, more than 30 sq cm, unusual or complicated, any area
> *CPT Assistant* Aug 96:8, Sep 96:11, Jul 99:3, Jan 06:47, Dec 06:15

14350   Filleted finger or toe flap, including preparation of recipient site
> *CPT Assistant* Jan 06:47

Skin Replacement Surgery and Skin Substitutes

Identify by size and location of the defect (recipient area) and the type of graft or skin substitute; includes simple debridement of granulation tissue or recent avulsion.

When a primary procedure such as orbitectomy, radical mastectomy, or deep tumor removal requires skin graft for definitive closure, see appropriate anatomical subsection for primary procedure and this section for skin graft or skin substitute.

Use 15002-15005 for initial wound recipient site preparation.

Use 15100-15261 for autologous skin grafts. For autologous tissue-cultured epidermal grafts, use 15150-15157. For harvesting of autologous keratinocytes and dermal tissue for tissue-cultured skin grafts, use 15040. Procedures are coded by recipient site. Use 15170-15176 for acellular dermal replacement. Use modifier 58 for staged application procedure(s).

Repair of donor site requiring skin graft or local flaps is to be added as an additional procedure.

Codes 15002-15005 describe burn and wound preparation or incisional or excisional release of scar contracture resulting in an open wound requiring a skin graft. Codes 15100-15431 describe the application of skin replacements and skin substitutes. The following definition should be applied to those codes that reference "100 sq cm or 1% of body area of infants and children" when determining the involvement of body size: The measurement of 100 sq cm is applicable to adults and children age 10 and older; percentages of body surface area apply to infants and children younger than the age of 10.

These codes are not intended to be reported for simple graft application alone or application stabilized with dressings (eg, by simple gauze wrap). The skin substitute/graft is anchored using the surgeon's choice of fixation. When services are performed in the office, the supply of the skin substitute/graft should be reported separately. Routine dressing supplies are not reported separately.

(For microvascular flaps, see 15756-15758)

Surgical Preparation

(15000, 15001 have been deleted. To report, see 15002-15005)

15002 Surgical preparation or creation of recipient site by excision of open wounds, burn eschar, or scar (including subcutaneous tissues), or incisional release of scar contracture, trunk, arms, legs; first 100 sq cm or 1% of body area of infants and children
➲ *CPT Changes: An Insider's View* 2007

+ 15003 each additional 100 sq cm or each additional 1% of body area of infants and children (List separately in addition to code for primary procedure)
➲ *CPT Changes: An Insider's View* 2007

(Use 15003 in conjunction with 15002)

15004 Surgical preparation or creation of recipient site by excision of open wounds, burn eschar, or scar (including subcutaneous tissues), or incisional release of scar contracture, face, scalp, eyelids, mouth, neck, ears, orbits, genitalia, hands, feet and/or multiple digits; first 100 sq cm or 1% of body area of infants and children
➲ *CPT Changes: An Insider's View* 2007

+ 15005 each additional 100 sq cm or each additional 1% of body area of infants and children (List separately in addition to code for primary procedure)
➲ *CPT Changes: An Insider's View* 2007

(Use 15005 in conjunction with 15004)

(Report 15002-15005 in conjunction with code for appropriate skin grafts or replacements [15050-15261, 15330-15336]. List the graft or replacement separately by its procedure number when the graft, immediate or delayed, is applied)

(For excision of benign lesions, see 11400-11471)

(For excision of malignant lesions, see 11600-11646)

(For excision to prepare or create recipient site with dressings or materials not listed in 15040-15431, use 15002-15005 only)

(For excision with immediate skin grafting, use 15002-15005 in conjunction with 15050-15261)

(For excision with immediate allograft skin placement, use 15002-15005 in conjunction with 15300-15336 and 15360-15366)

(For excision with immediate xenogeneic dermis placement, use 15002-15005 in conjunction with 15400-15421)

Grafts

Autograft/Tissue Cultured Autograft

15040 Harvest of skin for tissue cultured skin autograft, 100 sq cm or less
➲ *CPT Changes: An Insider's View* 2006

15050 Pinch graft, single or multiple, to cover small ulcer, tip of digit, or other minimal open area (except on face), up to defect size 2 cm diameter
➲ *CPT Assistant* Apr 97:4, Sep 97:2, Nov 98:6

15100 Split-thickness autograft, trunk, arms, legs; first 100 sq cm or less, or 1% of body area of infants and children (except 15050)
➲ *CPT Assistant* Fall 93:7, Apr 97:4, Aug 97:6, Sep 97:3, Nov 98:6, Sep 02:3, Oct 06:1; *CPT Changes: An Insider's View* 2002, 2006

+ 15101 each additional 100 sq cm, or each additional 1% of body area of infants and children, or part thereof (List separately in addition to code for primary procedure)
➲ *CPT Assistant* Apr 97:4, Nov 98:6, Sep 02:3; *CPT Changes: An Insider's View* 2002

(Use 15101 in conjunction with 15100)

15110 Epidermal autograft, trunk, arms, legs; first 100 sq cm or less, or 1% of body area of infants and children
➲ *CPT Changes: An Insider's View* 2006

+ 15111 each additional 100 sq cm, or each additional 1% of body area of infants and children, or part thereof (List separately in addition to code for primary procedure)
➲ *CPT Changes: An Insider's View* 2006

(Use 15111 in conjunction with 15110)

15115 Epidermal autograft, face, scalp, eyelids, mouth, neck, ears, orbits, genitalia, hands, feet, and/or multiple digits; first 100 sq cm or less, or 1% of body area of infants and children
➲ *CPT Changes: An Insider's View* 2006

+ 15116 each additional 100 sq cm, or each additional 1% of body area of infants and children, or part thereof (List separately in addition to code for primary procedure)
➲ *CPT Changes: An Insider's View* 2006

(Use 15116 in conjunction with 15115)

15120 Split-thickness autograft, face, scalp, eyelids, mouth, neck, ears, orbits, genitalia, hands, feet, and/or multiple digits; first 100 sq cm or less, or 1% of body area of infants and children (except 15050)
➲ *CPT Assistant* Apr 97:4, Aug 97:6, Sep 97:3, Nov 98:6, Jan 99:4, Sep 02:3; *CPT Changes: An Insider's View* 2002, 2006

+ 15121 each additional 100 sq cm, or each additional 1% of body area of infants and children, or part thereof (List separately in addition to code for primary procedure)
➲ *CPT Assistant* Apr 97:4, Aug 97:6, Sep 97:3, Nov 98:6, Jan 99:4, Sep 02:3; *CPT Changes: An Insider's View* 2002

(Use 15121 in conjunction with 15120)

(For eyelids, see also 67961 et seq)

15130 Dermal autograft, trunk, arms, legs; first 100 sq cm or less, or 1% of body area of infants and children
➲ *CPT Changes: An Insider's View* 2006

+ 15131 each additional 100 sq cm, or each additional 1% of body area of infants and children, or part thereof (List separately in addition to code for primary procedure)
➲ *CPT Changes: An Insider's View* 2006

(Use 15131 in conjunction with 15130)

15135   Dermal autograft, face, scalp, eyelids, mouth, neck, ears, orbits, genitalia, hands, feet, and/or multiple digits; first 100 sq cm or less, or 1% of body area of infants and children
➔ *CPT Changes: An Insider's View* 2006

+ 15136   each additional 100 sq cm, or each additional 1% of body area of infants and children, or part thereof (List separately in addition to code for primary procedure)
➔ *CPT Changes: An Insider's View* 2006

(Use 15136 in conjunction with 15135)

15150   Tissue cultured epidermal autograft, trunk, arms, legs; first 25 sq cm or less
➔ *CPT Changes: An Insider's View* 2006

+ 15151   additional 1 sq cm to 75 sq cm (List separately in addition to code for primary procedure)
➔ *CPT Changes: An Insider's View* 2006

(Do not report 15151 more than once per session)

(Use 15151 in conjunction with 15150)

+ 15152   each additional 100 sq cm, or each additional 1% of body area of infants and children, or part thereof (List separately in addition to code for primary procedure)
➔ *CPT Changes: An Insider's View* 2006

(Use 15152 in conjunction with 15151)

15155   Tissue cultured epidermal autograft, face, scalp, eyelids, mouth, neck, ears, orbits, genitalia, hands, feet, and/or multiple digits; first 25 sq cm or less
➔ *CPT Changes: An Insider's View* 2006

+ 15156   additional 1 sq cm to 75 sq cm (List separately in addition to code for primary procedure)
➔ *CPT Changes: An Insider's View* 2006

(Do not report 15156 more than once per session)

(Use 15156 in conjunction with 15155)

+ 15157   each additional 100 sq cm, or each additional 1% of body area of infants and children, or part thereof (List separately in addition to code for primary procedure)
➔ *CPT Changes: An Insider's View* 2006

(Use 15157 in conjunction with 15156)

Acellular Dermal Replacement

15170   Acellular dermal replacement, trunk, arms, legs; first 100 sq cm or less, or 1% of body area of infants and children
➔ *CPT Changes: An Insider's View* 2006

+ 15171   each additional 100 sq cm, or each additional 1% of body area of infants and children, or part thereof (List separately in addition to code for primary procedure)
➔ *CPT Changes: An Insider's View* 2006

(Use 15171 in conjunction with 15170)

15175   Acellular dermal replacement, face, scalp, eyelids, mouth, neck, ears, orbits, genitalia, hands, feet, and/or multiple digits; first 100 sq cm or less, or 1% of body area of infants and children
➔ *CPT Changes: An Insider's View* 2006

+ 15176   each additional 100 sq cm, or each additional 1% of body area of infants and children, or part thereof (List separately in addition to code for primary procedure)
➔ *CPT Changes: An Insider's View* 2006

(Use 15176 in conjunction with 15175)

15200   Full thickness graft, free, including direct closure of donor site, trunk; 20 sq cm or less
➔ *CPT Assistant* Aug 96:11, Aug 97:6, Sep 97:3; *CPT Changes: An Insider's View* 2002

+ 15201   each additional 20 sq cm (List separately in addition to code for primary procedure)
➔ *CPT Assistant* Apr 97:4, Aug 97:6, Sep 97:3; *CPT Changes: An Insider's View* 2002

(Use 15201 in conjunction with 15200)

15220   Full thickness graft, free, including direct closure of donor site, scalp, arms, and/or legs; 20 sq cm or less
➔ *CPT Assistant* Apr 97:4, Aug 97:6, Sep 97:3, Aug 98:9; *CPT Changes: An Insider's View* 2002

+ 15221   each additional 20 sq cm (List separately in addition to code for primary procedure)
➔ *CPT Assistant* Apr 97:4, Aug 97:6, Sep 97:3, Aug 98:9; *CPT Changes: An Insider's View* 2002

(Use 15221 in conjunction with 15220)

15240   Full thickness graft, free, including direct closure of donor site, forehead, cheeks, chin, mouth, neck, axillae, genitalia, hands, and/or feet; 20 sq cm or less
➔ *CPT Assistant* Apr 97:4, Aug 97:6, Sep 97:3, Nov 00:10; *CPT Changes: An Insider's View* 2002

(For finger tip graft, use 15050)

(For repair of syndactyly, fingers, see 26560-26562)

+ 15241   each additional 20 sq cm (List separately in addition to code for primary procedure)
➔ *CPT Assistant* Apr 97:4, Aug 97:6, Sep 97:3; *CPT Changes: An Insider's View* 2002

(Use 15241 in conjunction with 15240)

15260   Full thickness graft, free, including direct closure of donor site, nose, ears, eyelids, and/or lips; 20 sq cm or less
➔ *CPT Assistant* Fall 91:7, Fall 93:7, Apr 97:4, Aug 97:6, Sep 97:3, Jul 99:3; *CPT Changes: An Insider's View* 2002

+ 15261   each additional 20 sq cm (List separately in addition to code for primary procedure)
➔ *CPT Assistant* Fall 91:7, Apr 97:4, Aug 97:6, Sep 97:3; *CPT Changes: An Insider's View* 2002

(Use 15261 in conjunction with 15260)

(For eyelids, see also 67961 et seq)

(Repair of donor site requiring skin graft or local flaps, to be added as additional separate procedure)

Allograft/Tissue Cultured Allogeneic Skin Substitute

Application of a non-autologous human skin graft (ie, homograft) from a donor to a part of the recipient's body to resurface an area damaged by burns, traumatic injury, soft tissue infection and/or tissue necrosis or surgery.

15300 Allograft skin for temporary wound closure, trunk, arms, legs; first 100 sq cm or less, or 1% of body area of infants and children

→ *CPT Changes: An Insider's View* 2006

+ 15301 each additional 100 sq cm, or each additional 1% of body area of infants and children, or part thereof (List separately in addition to code for primary procedure)

→ *CPT Changes: An Insider's View* 2006

(Use 15301 in conjunction with 15300)

15320 Allograft skin for temporary wound closure, face, scalp, eyelids, mouth, neck, ears, orbits, genitalia, hands, feet, and/or multiple digits; first 100 sq cm or less, or 1% of body area of infants and children

→ *CPT Changes: An Insider's View* 2006

+ 15321 each additional 100 sq cm, or each additional 1% of body area of infants and children, or part thereof (List separately in addition to code for primary procedure)

→ *CPT Changes: An Insider's View* 2006

(Use 15321 in conjunction with 15320)

Allograft, Skin
15300-15321

Application of allograft skin (homograft) from a healthy cadaveric donor is applied to a part of the patient's body to resurface an area damaged by burns, traumatic injury, or surgery.

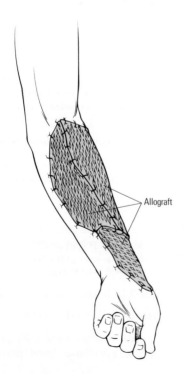

Allograft

15330 Acellular dermal allograft, trunk, arms, legs; first 100 sq cm or less, or 1% of body area of infants and children

→ *CPT Changes: An Insider's View* 2006

+ 15331 each additional 100 sq cm, or each additional 1% of body area of infants and children, or part thereof (List separately in addition to code for primary procedure)

→ *CPT Changes: An Insider's View* 2006

(Use 15331 in conjunction with 15330)

15335 Acellular dermal allograft, face, scalp, eyelids, mouth, neck, ears, orbits, genitalia, hands, feet, and/or multiple digits; first 100 sq cm or less, or 1% of body area of infants and children

→ *CPT Changes: An Insider's View* 2006

+ 15336 each additional 100 sq cm, or each additional 1% of body area of infants and children, or part thereof (List separately in addition to code for primary procedure)

→ *CPT Changes: An Insider's View* 2006, 2007

(Use 15336 in conjunction with 15335)

15340 Tissue cultured allogeneic skin substitute; first 25 sq cm or less

→ *CPT Changes: An Insider's View* 2006

+ 15341 each additional 25 sq cm

→ *CPT Changes: An Insider's View* 2006

(Use 15341 in conjunction with 15340)

(Do not report 15340, 15341 in conjunction with 11040-11042, 15002-15005)

(15342 has been deleted. To report, see 15170, 15175, 15340, 15360, 15365)

(15343 has been deleted. To report, see 15171, 15176, 15341, 15361, 15366)

(15350 has been deleted. To report, see 15300, 15320, 15330, 15335)

(15351 has been deleted. To report, see 15301, 15321, 15331, 15336)

15360 Tissue cultured allogeneic dermal substitute, trunk, arms, legs; first 100 sq cm or less, or 1% of body area of infants and children

→ *CPT Changes: An Insider's View* 2006

+ 15361 each additional 100 sq cm, or each additional 1% of body area of infants and children, or part thereof (List separately in addition to code for primary procedure)

→ *CPT Changes: An Insider's View* 2006

(Use 15361 in conjunction with 15360)

15365   Tissue cultured allogeneic dermal substitute, face, scalp, eyelids, mouth, neck, ears, orbits, genitalia, hands, feet, and/or multiple digits; first 100 sq cm or less, or 1% of body area of infants and children
➜ *CPT Changes: An Insider's View* 2006

+ 15366   each additional 100 sq cm, or each additional 1% of body area of infants and children, or part thereof (List separately in addition to code for primary procedure)
➜ *CPT Changes: An Insider's View* 2006, 2007

(Use 15366 in conjunction with 15365)

Xenograft

Application of a non-human skin graft or biologic wound dressing (eg, porcine tissue or pigskin) to a part of the recipient's body following debridement of the burn wound or area of traumatic injury, soft tissue infection and/or tissue necrosis, or surgery.

15400   Xenograft, skin (dermal), for temporary wound closure, trunk, arms, legs; first 100 sq cm or less, or 1% of body area of infants and children
➜ *CPT Assistant* Apr 97:4, Sep 97:3, Nov 98:6, Jan 99:4, Apr 01:10, Nov 03:15, Jan 06:1, Aug 06:10, Oct 06:1; *CPT Changes: An Insider's View* 2006

Xenograft, Skin
15400-15401

Application of porcine skin graft following excision of the burn wound and/or surgical preparation of the site

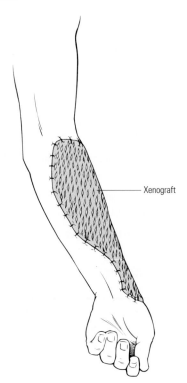

Xenograft

+ 15401   each additional 100 sq cm, or each additional 1% of body area of infants and children, or part thereof (List separately in addition to code for primary procedure)
➜ *CPT Assistant* Nov 98:6, Jan 99:4, Jan 06:1; *CPT Changes: An Insider's View* 2006

(Use 15401 in conjunction with 15400)

15420   Xenograft skin (dermal), for temporary wound closure, face, scalp, eyelids, mouth, neck, ears, orbits, genitalia, hands, feet, and/or multiple digits; first 100 sq cm or less, or 1% of body area of infants and children
➜ *CPT Changes: An Insider's View* 2006

+ 15421   each additional 100 sq cm, or each additional 1% of body area of infants and children, or part thereof (List separately in addition to code for primary procedure)
➜ *CPT Changes: An Insider's View* 2006

(Use 15421 in conjunction with 15420)

15430   Acellular xenograft implant; first 100 sq cm or less, or 1% of body area of infants and children
➜ *CPT Changes: An Insider's View* 2006

+ 15431   each additional 100 sq cm, or each additional 1% of body area of infants and children, or part thereof (List separately in addition to code for primary procedure)
➜ *CPT Changes: An Insider's View* 2006

(Use 15431 in conjunction with 15430)

(Do not report 15430, 15431 in conjunction with 11040-11042, 15002-15005, 0170T)

Flaps (Skin and/or Deep Tissues)

The regions listed refer to the recipient area (not the donor site) when a flap is being attached in a transfer or to a final site.

The regions listed refer to a donor site when a tube is formed for later or when a "delay" of flap is prior to the transfer.

Procedures 15570-15738 do not include extensive immobilization (eg, large plaster casts and other immobilizing devices are considered additional separate procedures).

A repair of a donor site requiring a skin graft or local flaps is considered an additional separate procedure.

(For microvascular flaps, see 15756-15758)

(For flaps without inclusion of a vascular pedicle, see 15570-15576)

(For adjacent tissue transfer flaps, see 14000-14300)

15570   Formation of direct or tubed pedicle, with or without transfer; trunk
➜ *CPT Assistant* Nov 02:7

15572   scalp, arms, or legs

15574 forehead, cheeks, chin, mouth, neck, axillae, genitalia, hands or feet

15576 eyelids, nose, ears, lips, or intraoral

15600 Delay of flap or sectioning of flap (division and inset); at trunk

➔ *CPT Assistant* Nov 99:10

15610 at scalp, arms, or legs

15620 at forehead, cheeks, chin, neck, axillae, genitalia, hands, or feet

15630 at eyelids, nose, ears, or lips

15650 Transfer, intermediate, of any pedicle flap (eg, abdomen to wrist, Walking tube), any location

(For eyelids, nose, ears, or lips, see also anatomical area)

(For revision, defatting or rearranging of transferred pedicle flap or skin graft, see 13100-14300)

(Procedures 15732-15738 are described by donor site of the muscle, myocutaneous, or fasciocutaneous flap)

15731 Forehead flap with preservation of vascular pedicle (eg, axial pattern flap, paramedian forehead flap)

➔ *CPT Changes: An Insider's View* 2007

(For muscle, myocutaneous, or fasciocutaneous flap of the head or neck, use 15732)

Axial Pattern Forehead Flap
15731

Reconstruction of a nasal defect with a forehead flap based on the left supratrochlear vessels

Donor defect

Forehead flap

15732 Muscle, myocutaneous, or fasciocutaneous flap; head and neck (eg, temporalis, masseter muscle, sternocleidomastoid, levator scapulae)

➔ *CPT Changes: An Insider's View* 2002

(For forehead flap with preservation of vascular pedicle, use 15731)

15734 trunk

15736 upper extremity

15738 lower extremity

➔ *CPT Assistant* Sep 03:15

Other Flaps and Grafts

Repair of donor site requiring skin graft or local flaps should be reported as an additional procedure.

15740 Flap; island pedicle

➔ *CPT Assistant* Mar 04:11, Sep 04:12, Oct 04:15

15750 neurovascular pedicle

15756 Free muscle or myocutaneous flap with microvascular anastomosis

➔ *CPT Assistant* Apr 97:5, Nov 97:12, Nov 98:6; *CPT Changes: An Insider's View* 2003

(Do not report code 69990 in addition to code 15756)

15757 Free skin flap with microvascular anastomosis

➔ *CPT Assistant* Apr 97:5, Nov 98:6

(Do not report code 69990 in addition to code 15757)

15758 Free fascial flap with microvascular anastomosis

➔ *CPT Assistant* Apr 97:5, Nov 98:6

(Do not report code 69990 in addition to code 15758)

15760 Graft; composite (eg, full thickness of external ear or nasal ala), including primary closure, donor area

➔ *CPT Assistant* Sep 97:3

15770 derma-fat-fascia

➔ *CPT Assistant* Sep 97:3

15775 Punch graft for hair transplant; 1 to 15 punch grafts

➔ *CPT Assistant* Sep 97:3

15776 more than 15 punch grafts

➔ *CPT Assistant* Sep 97:3

(For strip transplant, use 15220)

Other Procedures

15780 Dermabrasion; total face (eg, for acne scarring, fine wrinkling, rhytids, general keratosis)

➔ *CPT Assistant* Apr 03:27

15781 segmental, face

15782 regional, other than face

15783 superficial, any site (eg, tattoo removal)

➔ *CPT Assistant* Apr 03:27

15786	Abrasion; single lesion (eg, keratosis, scar)
+ 15787	each additional four lesions or less (List separately in addition to code for primary procedure)
	(Use 15787 in conjunction with 15786)
15788	Chemical peel, facial; epidermal
15789	dermal
15792	Chemical peel, nonfacial; epidermal
15793	dermal
	(15810, 15811 have been deleted)
15819	Cervicoplasty
15820	Blepharoplasty, lower eyelid;
	➔ *CPT Assistant* Feb 04:11, May 04:12, Feb 05:16
15821	with extensive herniated fat pad
	➔ *CPT Assistant* Feb 04:11, May 04:12, Feb 05:16
15822	Blepharoplasty, upper eyelid;
	➔ *CPT Assistant* Feb 04:11, May 04:12, Feb 05:16
15823	with excessive skin weighting down lid
	➔ *CPT Assistant* Sep 00:7, Feb 04:11, May 04:12, Feb 05:16
	(For bilateral blepharoplasty, add modifier 50)
15824	Rhytidectomy; forehead
	(For repair of brow ptosis, use 67900)
15825	neck with platysmal tightening (platysmal flap, P-flap)
15826	glabellar frown lines
15828	cheek, chin, and neck
15829	superficial musculoaponeurotic system (SMAS) flap
	(For bilateral rhytidectomy, add modifier 50)
15830	Excision, excessive skin and subcutaneous tissue (includes lipectomy); abdomen, infraumbilical panniculectomy
	➔ *CPT Changes: An Insider's View* 2007
	(Do not report 15830 in conjunction with 12031, 12032, 12034, 12035, 12036, 12037, 13100, 13101, 13102, 14000-14001, 14300)
	(15831 has been deleted. To report abdominoplasty with panniculectomy, use 15830 in conjunction with 15847. To report other abdominoplasty, use 17999)
15832	thigh
15833	leg
15834	hip
15835	buttock
15836	arm
15837	forearm or hand
15838	submental fat pad
15839	other area
	(For bilateral procedure, add modifier 50)

15840	Graft for facial nerve paralysis; free fascia graft (including obtaining fascia)
	(For bilateral procedure, add modifier 50)
15841	free muscle graft (including obtaining graft)
15842	free muscle flap by microsurgical technique
	➔ *CPT Changes: An Insider's View* 2001
	(Do not report code 69990 in addition to code 15842)
15845	regional muscle transfer
	(For intravenous fluorescein examination of blood flow in graft or flap, use 15860)
	(For nerve transfers, decompression, or repair, see 64831-64876, 64905, 64907, 69720, 69725, 69740, 69745, 69955)
+ 15847	Excision, excessive skin and subcutaneous tissue (includes lipectomy), abdomen (eg, abdominoplasty) (includes umbilical transposition and fascial plication) (List separately in addition to code for primary procedure)
	➔ *CPT Changes: An Insider's View* 2007
	(Use 15847 in conjunction with 15830)
	(For abdominal wall hernia repair, see 49491-49587)
	(To report other abdominoplasty, use 17999)
15850	Removal of sutures under anesthesia (other than local), same surgeon
	➔ *CPT Assistant* Spring 93:34, Nov 97:22
15851	Removal of sutures under anesthesia (other than local), other surgeon
	➔ *CPT Assistant* Spring 93:34, Nov 97:22
15852	Dressing change (for other than burns) under anesthesia (other than local)
15860	Intravenous injection of agent (eg, fluorescein) to test vascular flow in flap or graft
	➔ *CPT Changes: An Insider's View* 2002
15876	Suction assisted lipectomy; head and neck
15877	trunk
	➔ *CPT Assistant* Oct 99:10, Feb 05:14
15878	upper extremity
15879	lower extremity

Pressure Ulcers (Decubitus Ulcers)

15920	Excision, coccygeal pressure ulcer, with coccygectomy; with primary suture
15922	with flap closure
15931	Excision, sacral pressure ulcer, with primary suture;
15933	with ostectomy
15934	Excision, sacral pressure ulcer, with skin flap closure;
15935	with ostectomy

15936 Excision, sacral pressure ulcer, in preparation for muscle or myocutaneous flap or skin graft closure;

➡ *CPT Assistant* Nov 98:6-7

15937 with ostectomy

(For repair of defect using muscle or myocutaneous flap, use code(s) 15734 and/or 15738 in addition to 15936, 15937. For repair of defect using split skin graft, use codes 15100 and/or 15101 in addition to 15936, 15937)

15940 Excision, ischial pressure ulcer, with primary suture;

15941 with ostectomy (ischiectomy)

15944 Excision, ischial pressure ulcer, with skin flap closure;

15945 with ostectomy

15946 Excision, ischial pressure ulcer, with ostectomy, in preparation for muscle or myocutaneous flap or skin graft closure

➡ *CPT Assistant* Nov 98:6-7, Jun 02:10, Jan 03:23

(For repair of defect using muscle or myocutaneous flap, use code(s) 15734 and/or 15738 in addition to 15946. For repair of defect using split skin graft, use codes 15100 and/or 15101 in addition to 15946)

15950 Excision, trochanteric pressure ulcer, with primary suture;

15951 with ostectomy

15952 Excision, trochanteric pressure ulcer, with skin flap closure;

15953 with ostectomy

15956 Excision, trochanteric pressure ulcer, in preparation for muscle or myocutaneous flap or skin graft closure;

➡ *CPT Assistant* Nov 98:6-7

15958 with ostectomy

➡ *CPT Assistant* Nov 98:6-7

(For repair of defect using muscle or myocutaneous flap, use code(s) 15734 and/or 15738 in addition to 15956, 15958. For repair of defect using split skin graft, use codes 15100 and/or 15101 in addition to 15956, 15958)

15999 Unlisted procedure, excision pressure ulcer

(For free skin graft to close ulcer or donor site, see 15002 et seq)

Burns, Local Treatment

Procedures 16000-16036 refer to local treatment of burned surface only. Codes 16020-16030 include the application of materials (eg, dressings) not described in 15100-15431.

List percentage of body surface involved and depth of burn.

For necessary related medical services (eg, hospital visits, detention) in management of burned patients, see appropriate services in **Evaluation and Management** and **Medicine** sections.

For the application of skin grafts or skin substitutes, see 15100-15650.

16000 Initial treatment, first degree burn, when no more than local treatment is required

➡ *CPT Assistant* Aug 97:6

Calculation of Total Body Surface Area (TBSA) Burn
16000

Calculation of the percentage of a body burned is achieved by dividing the total body surface area into 9% or multiples of 9% segments. In the infant or child, the "rule" deviates because of the large surface area of the child's head.

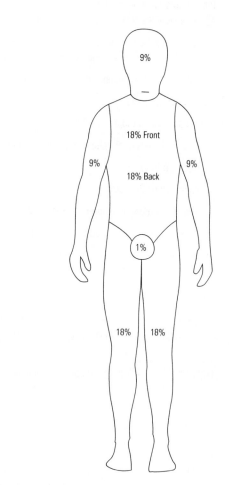

(16010, 16015 have been deleted. To report, see 16020-16030)

16020 Dressings and/or debridement of partial-thickness burns, initial or subsequent; small (less than 5% total body surface area)

➡ *CPT Assistant* Aug 97:6; *CPT Changes: An Insider's View* 2006

16025   medium (eg, whole face or whole extremity, or 5% to
                 10% total body surface area)
                 ➔ *CPT Assistant* Aug 97:6; *CPT Changes: An Insider's View*
                 2006

16030   large (eg, more than one extremity, or greater than
                 10% total body surface area)
                 ➔ *CPT Assistant* Aug 97:6; *CPT Changes: An Insider's View*
                 2006

16035   Escharotomy; initial incision
                 ➔ *CPT Assistant* Aug 97:6; *CPT Changes: An Insider's View* 2001

+ 16036   each additional incision (List separately in addition to
                 code for primary procedure)
                 ➔ *CPT Changes: An Insider's View* 2001

                 (Use 16036 in conjunction with 16035)

                 (For debridement, curettement of burn wound, see 16020-
                 16030)

Destruction

Destruction means the ablation of benign, premalignant
or malignant tissues by any method, with or without
curettage, including local anesthesia, and not usually
requiring closure.

Any method includes electrosurgery, cryosurgery, laser
and chemical treatment. Lesions include condylomata,
papillomata, molluscum contagiosum, herpetic lesions,
warts (ie, common, plantar, flat), milia, or other benign,
premalignant (eg, actinic keratoses), or malignant lesions.

          (For destruction of lesion(s) in specific anatomic sites,
          see 40820, 46900-46917, 46924, 54050-54057, 54065,
          56501, 56515, 57061, 57065, 67850, 68135)

          (For paring or cutting of benign hyperkeratotic lesions (eg,
          corns or calluses), see 11055-11057)

          (For sharp removal or electrosurgical destruction of skin
          tags and fibrocutaneous tags, see 11200, 11201)

          (For cryotherapy of acne, use 17340)

          (For initiation or follow-up care of topical chemotherapy
          (eg, 5-FU or similar agents), see appropriate office visits)

          (For shaving of epidermal or dermal lesions, see 11300-
          11313)

Destruction, Benign or Premalignant Lesions

17000   Destruction (eg, laser surgery, electrosurgery,
                 cryosurgery, chemosurgery, surgical curettement),
                 premalignant lesions (eg, actinic keratoses); first lesion
                 ➔ *CPT Assistant* Winter 90:3, Nov 97:12, Jun 99:10, May 06:19,
                 Feb 07:10; *CPT Changes: An Insider's View* 2002, 2007

+ 17003   second through 14 lesions, each (List separately in
                 addition to code for first lesion)
                 ➔ *CPT Assistant* Nov 97:12, Jun 99:10, May 06:19, Feb 07:10

          (Use 17003 in conjunction with 17000)

          (For destruction of common or plantar warts, see 17110,
          17111)

⊘ 17004   Destruction (eg, laser surgery, electrosurgery,
                 cryosurgery, chemosurgery, surgical curettement),
                 premalignant lesions (eg, actinic keratoses), 15 or more
                 lesions
                 ➔ *CPT Assistant* Nov 97:12, Nov 98:7, Jun 99:10, Mar 03:21,
                 Feb 07:10; *CPT Changes: An Insider's View* 2002, 2007

          (Do not report 17004 in conjunction with 17000-17003)

Destruction, Benign or Premalignant Lesions
17004

The lesions, seen as rough scaling patches
scattered over the face, scalp, and ears, are
destroyed by cryosurgery or other surgical means.

Ice field

Cryo probe
(spray nozzle)

17106 Destruction of cutaneous vascular proliferative lesions (eg, laser technique); less than 10 sq cm
→ *CPT Assistant* Winter 90:3, Apr 07:11

17107 10.0 to 50.0 sq cm
→ *CPT Assistant* Winter 90:3, Apr 07:11

17108 over 50.0 sq cm
→ *CPT Assistant* Winter 90:3, Apr 07:11

▲ **17110** Destruction (eg, laser surgery, electrosurgery, cryosurgery, chemosurgery, surgical curettement), of benign lesions other than skin tags or cutaneous vascular proliferative lesions; up to 14 lesions
→ *CPT Assistant* Nov 97:13, Feb 07:10, Apr 07:11; *CPT Changes: An Insider's View* 2002, 2007, 2008

17111 15 or more lesions
→ *CPT Assistant* Nov 97:13, Feb 07:10, Apr 07:11

17250 Chemical cauterization of granulation tissue (proud flesh, sinus or fistula)

(17250 is not to be used with removal or excision codes for the same lesion)

Destruction, Malignant Lesions, Any Method

17260 Destruction, malignant lesion (eg, laser surgery, electrosurgery, cryosurgery, chemosurgery, surgical curettement), trunk, arms or legs; lesion diameter 0.5 cm or less
→ *CPT Changes: An Insider's View* 2002

17261 lesion diameter 0.6 to 1.0 cm

17262 lesion diameter 1.1 to 2.0 cm

17263 lesion diameter 2.1 to 3.0 cm

17264 lesion diameter 3.1 to 4.0 cm

17266 lesion diameter over 4.0 cm

17270 Destruction, malignant lesion (eg, laser surgery, electrosurgery, cryosurgery, chemosurgery, surgical curettement), scalp, neck, hands, feet, genitalia; lesion diameter 0.5 cm or less
→ *CPT Changes: An Insider's View* 2002

17271 lesion diameter 0.6 to 1.0 cm

17272 lesion diameter 1.1 to 2.0 cm

17273 lesion diameter 2.1 to 3.0 cm

17274 lesion diameter 3.1 to 4.0 cm

17276 lesion diameter over 4.0 cm

17280 Destruction, malignant lesion (eg, laser surgery, electrosurgery, cryosurgery, chemosurgery, surgical curettement), face, ears, eyelids, nose, lips, mucous membrane; lesion diameter 0.5 cm or less
→ *CPT Changes: An Insider's View* 2002

17281 lesion diameter 0.6 to 1.0 cm

17282 lesion diameter 1.1 to 2.0 cm

17283 lesion diameter 2.1 to 3.0 cm

17284 lesion diameter 3.1 to 4.0 cm

17286 lesion diameter over 4.0 cm

Mohs Micrographic Surgery

Mohs micrographic surgery is a technique for the removal of complex or ill-defined skin cancer with histologic examination of 100% of the surgical margins. It requires a single physician to act in two integrated but separate and distinct capacities: surgeon and pathologist. If either of these responsibilities is delegated to another physician who reports the services separately, these codes should not be reported. The Mohs surgeon removes the tumor tissue and maps and divides the tumor specimen into pieces, and each piece is embedded into an individual tissue block for histopathologic examination. Thus a tissue block in Mohs surgery is defined as an individual tissue piece embedded in a mounting medium for sectioning.

If repair is performed, use separate repair, flap, or graft codes. If a biopsy of a suspected skin cancer is performed on the same day as Mohs surgery because there was no prior pathology confirmation of a diagnosis, then report diagnostic skin biopsy (11100, 11101) and frozen section pathology (88331) with modifier 59 to distinguish from the subsequent definitive surgical procedure of Mohs surgery.

(17304-17310 have been deleted. To report, see 17311-17315)

(If additional special pathology procedures, stains or immunostains are required, use 88311-88314, 88342)

(Do not report 88314 in conjunction with 17311-17315 for routine frozen section stain (eg, hematoxylin and eosin, toluidine blue) performed during Mohs surgery. When a nonroutine histochemical stain on frozen tissue is utilized, report 88314 with modifier 59)

(Do not report 88302-88309 on the same specimen as part of the Mohs surgery)

17311 Mohs micrographic technique, including removal of all gross tumor, surgical excision of tissue specimens, mapping, color coding of specimens, microscopic examination of specimens by the surgeon, and histopathologic preparation including routine stain(s) (eg, hematoxylin and eosin, toluidine blue), head, neck, hands, feet, genitalia, or any location with surgery directly involving muscle, cartilage, bone, tendon, major nerves, or vessels; first stage, up to 5 tissue blocks
→ *CPT Changes: An Insider's View* 2007

+ **17312** each additional stage after the first stage, up to 5 tissue blocks (List separately in addition to code for primary procedure)
→ *CPT Changes: An Insider's View* 2007

(Use 17312 in conjunction with 17311)

17313 Mohs micrographic technique, including removal of all gross tumor, surgical excision of tissue specimens, mapping, color coding of specimens, microscopic examination of specimens by the surgeon, and histopathologic preparation including routine stain(s) (eg, hematoxylin and eosin, toluidine blue), of the trunk, arms, or legs; first stage, up to 5 tissue blocks
→ *CPT Changes: An Insider's View* 2007

+ 17314 each additional stage after the first stage, up to 5 tissue blocks (List separately in addition to code for primary procedure)
→ *CPT Changes: An Insider's View* 2007

(Use 17314 in conjunction with 17313)

+ 17315 Mohs micrographic technique, including removal of all gross tumor, surgical excision of tissue specimens, mapping, color coding of specimens, microscopic examination of specimens by the surgeon, and histopathologic preparation including routine stain(s) (eg, hematoxylin and eosin, toluidine blue), each additional block after the first 5 tissue blocks, any stage (List separately in addition to code for primary procedure)
→ *CPT Changes: An Insider's View* 2007

(Use 17315 in conjunction with 17311-17314)

Other Procedures

17340 Cryotherapy (CO_2 slush, liquid N_2) for acne

17360 Chemical exfoliation for acne (eg, acne paste, acid)

17380 Electrolysis epilation, each 30 minutes

(For actinotherapy, use 96900)

17999 Unlisted procedure, skin, mucous membrane and subcutaneous tissue
→ *CPT Assistant* Dec 98:9, May 99:11, Jun 05:11

Breast

Incision

19000 Puncture aspiration of cyst of breast;
→ *CPT Assistant* Fall 94:18, Apr 05:6

+ 19001 each additional cyst (List separately in addition to code for primary procedure)
→ *CPT Assistant* Fall 94:18, Apr 05:6

(Use 19001 in conjunction with 19000)

(If imaging guidance is performed, see 76942, 77021, 77031, 77032)

19020 Mastotomy with exploration or drainage of abscess, deep
→ *CPT Assistant* Apr 05:6

19030 Injection procedure only for mammary ductogram or galactogram
→ *CPT Assistant* Jul 04:8, Apr 05:6

(For radiological supervision and interpretation, see 77053, 77054)

(For catheter lavage of mammary ducts for collection of cytology specimens, use Category III codes 0046T, 0047T)

Excision

Excisional breast surgery includes certain biopsy procedures, the removal of cysts or other benign or malignant tumors or lesions, and the surgical treatment of breast and chest wall malignancies. Biopsy procedures may be percutaneous or open, and they involve the removal of differing amounts of tissue for diagnosis.

Breast biopsies are reported using codes 19100-19103. The open excision of breast lesions (eg, lesions of the breast ducts, cysts, benign or malignant tumors), without specific attention to adequate surgical margins, with or without the preoperative placement of radiological markers, is reported using codes 19110-19126. Partial mastectomy procedures (eg, lumpectomy, tylectomy, quadrantectomy, or segmentectomy) describe open excisions of breast tissue with specific attention to adequate surgical margins.

Partial mastectomy procedures are reported using codes 19301 or 19302 as appropriate. Documentation for partial mastectomy procedures includes attention to the removal of adequate surgical margins surrounding the breast mass or lesion.

Total mastectomy procedures include simple mastectomy, complete mastectomy, subcutaneous mastectomy, modified radical mastectomy, radical mastectomy, and more extended procedures (eg, Urban type operation). Total mastectomy procedures are reported using codes 19303-19307 as appropriate.

Excisions or resections of chest wall tumors including ribs, with or without reconstruction, with or without mediastinal lymphadenectomy, are reported using codes 19260, 19271, or 19272. Codes 19260-19272 are not restricted to breast tumors and are used to report resections of chest wall tumors originating from any chest wall component. (For excision of lung or pleura, see 32310 et seq.)

(To report bilateral procedures, report modifier 50 with the procedure code)

19100 Biopsy of breast; percutaneous, needle core, not using imaging guidance (separate procedure)
→ *CPT Assistant* Spring 93:35, Fall 94:18, Apr 96:8, Mar 97:4, Nov 97:24, Nov 98:7, Jan 01:10, May 02:18, Apr 05:6, Dec 06:10; *CPT Changes: An Insider's View* 2001

(For fine needle aspiration, use 10021)

(For image guided breast biopsy, see 19102, 19103, 10022)

19101   open, incisional
> *CPT Assistant* Spring 93:35, Fall 94:19, Nov 97:24, Jan 01:8, May 02:18, Apr 05:6; *CPT Changes: An Insider's View* 2001

19102   percutaneous, needle core, using imaging guidance
> *CPT Assistant* Jan 01:10, May 02:18, Apr 05:6; *CPT Changes: An Insider's View* 2001
> *Clinical Examples in Radiology* Summer 05:1, 2

(For placement of percutaneous localization clip, use 19295)

19103   percutaneous, automated vacuum assisted or rotating biopsy device, using imaging guidance
> *CPT Assistant* Jan 01:10, May 02:18, Apr 03:7, Apr 05:6; *CPT Changes: An Insider's View* 2001

(For imaging guidance performed in conjunction with 19102, 19103, see 76942, 77012, 77021, 77031, 77032)

(For placement of percutaneous localization clip, use 19295)

19105   Ablation, cryosurgical, of fibroadenoma, including ultrasound guidance, each fibroadenoma
> *CPT Changes: An Insider's View* 2007

(Do not report 19105 in conjunction with 76940, 76942)

(For adjacent lesions treated with one cryoprobe insertion, report once)

19110   Nipple exploration, with or without excision of a solitary lactiferous duct or a papilloma lactiferous duct
> *CPT Assistant* Apr 05:6

19112   Excision of lactiferous duct fistula
> *CPT Assistant* Apr 05:6

19120   Excision of cyst, fibroadenoma, or other benign or malignant tumor, aberrant breast tissue, duct lesion, nipple or areolar lesion (except 19300), open, male or female, one or more lesions
> *CPT Assistant* Feb 96:9, Nov 97:14, Jan 01:8, May 01:10, Apr 05:6, 13; *CPT Changes: An Insider's View* 2001, 2007

19125   Excision of breast lesion identified by preoperative placement of radiological marker, open; single lesion
> *CPT Assistant* Fall 94:18, Mar 98:10, Jan 01:8, Apr 05:6; *CPT Changes: An Insider's View* 2001

+ 19126   each additional lesion separately identified by a preoperative radiological marker (List separately in addition to code for primary procedure)
> *CPT Assistant* Fall 94:18, Mar 98:10, Jan 01:8, Apr 05:6; *CPT Changes: An Insider's View* 2001

(Use 19126 in conjunction with 19125)

(19140-19240 have been deleted. To report, see 19300-19307)

19260   Excision of chest wall tumor including ribs
> *CPT Assistant* Apr 05:6, 7

19271   Excision of chest wall tumor involving ribs, with plastic reconstruction; without mediastinal lymphadenectomy
> *CPT Assistant* Apr 05:6, 7

19272   with mediastinal lymphadenectomy
> *CPT Assistant* Apr 05:6, 7

▶(Do not report 19260, 19271, 19272 in conjunction with 32100, 32422, 32503, 32504, 32551)◀

Introduction

19290   Preoperative placement of needle localization wire, breast;
> *CPT Assistant* Fall 94:19, Apr 05:6
> *Clinical Examples in Radiology* Fall 05:01

+ 19291   each additional lesion (List separately in addition to code for primary procedure)
> *CPT Assistant* Fall 94:19, Apr 05:6

(Use 19291 in conjunction with 19290)

(For radiological supervision and interpretation, see 76942, 77031, 77032)

+ 19295   Image guided placement, metallic localization clip, percutaneous, during breast biopsy (List separately in addition to code for primary procedure)
> *CPT Assistant* Jan 01:10, Apr 05:6; *CPT Changes: An Insider's View* 2001

(Use 19295 in conjunction with 19102, 19103)

19296   Placement of radiotherapy afterloading balloon catheter into the breast for interstitial radioelement application following partial mastectomy, includes imaging guidance; on date separate from partial mastectomy
> *CPT Assistant* Apr 05:6-8, Nov 05:15; *CPT Changes: An Insider's View* 2005

+ 19297   concurrent with partial mastectomy (List separately in addition to code for primary procedure)
> *CPT Assistant* Apr 05:6-8, Nov 05:15; *CPT Changes: An Insider's View* 2005

(Use 19297 in conjunction with 19301 or 19302)

⊙ 19298   Placement of radiotherapy afterloading brachytherapy catheters (multiple tube and button type) into the breast for interstitial radioelement application following (at the time of or subsequent to) partial mastectomy, includes imaging guidance
> *CPT Assistant* Apr 05:6-7, 9, 16, Nov 05:15; *CPT Changes: An Insider's View* 2005

Mastectomy Procedures

19300   Mastectomy for gynecomastia
→ *CPT Changes: An Insider's View* 2007

19301   Mastectomy, partial (eg, lumpectomy, tylectomy, quadrantectomy, segmentectomy);
→ *CPT Changes: An Insider's View* 2007

19302   with axillary lymphadenectomy
→ *CPT Changes: An Insider's View* 2007

(For placement of radiotherapy afterloading balloon/brachytherapy catheters, see 19296-19298)

19303   Mastectomy, simple, complete
→ *CPT Changes: An Insider's View* 2007

(For immediate or delayed insertion of implant, see 19340, 19342)

(For gynecomastia, use 19300)

19304   Mastectomy, subcutaneous
→ *CPT Changes: An Insider's View* 2007

(For immediate or delayed insertion of implant, see 19340, 19342)

19305   Mastectomy, radical, including pectoral muscles, axillary lymph nodes
→ *CPT Changes: An Insider's View* 2007

(For immediate or delayed insertion of implant, see 19340, 19342)

19306   Mastectomy, radical, including pectoral muscles, axillary and internal mammary lymph nodes (Urban type operation)
→ *CPT Changes: An Insider's View* 2007

(For immediate or delayed insertion of implant, see 19340, 19342)

19307   Mastectomy, modified radical, including axillary lymph nodes, with or without pectoralis minor muscle, but excluding pectoralis major muscle
→ *CPT Changes: An Insider's View* 2007

(For immediate or delayed insertion of implant, see 19340, 19342)

Repair and/or Reconstruction

(To report bilateral procedures, report modifier 50 with the procedure code)

19316   Mastopexy
→ *CPT Assistant* Jan 03:7, Apr 05:6

19318   Reduction mammaplasty
→ *CPT Assistant* Jan 03:7, Apr 05:6

19324   Mammaplasty, augmentation; without prosthetic implant
→ *CPT Assistant* Apr 05:6

19325   with prosthetic implant
→ *CPT Assistant* Apr 05:6

(For flap or graft, use also appropriate number)

19328   Removal of intact mammary implant
→ *CPT Assistant* Apr 05:6

19330   Removal of mammary implant material
→ *CPT Assistant* Nov 01:11, Apr 05:6

19340   Immediate insertion of breast prosthesis following mastopexy, mastectomy or in reconstruction
→ *CPT Assistant* Aug 96:8, Apr 05:6, Aug 05:1

19342   Delayed insertion of breast prosthesis following mastopexy, mastectomy or in reconstruction
→ *CPT Assistant* Aug 96:8, Apr 05:6, Aug 05:1

(For supply of implant, use 99070)

(For preparation of custom breast implant, use 19396)

19350   Nipple/areola reconstruction
→ *CPT Assistant* Aug 96:11, Apr 05:6

19355   Correction of inverted nipples
→ *CPT Assistant* Apr 05:6

19357   Breast reconstruction, immediate or delayed, with tissue expander, including subsequent expansion
→ *CPT Assistant* Winter 91:2, Apr 05:6, Aug 05:1

19361   Breast reconstruction with latissimus dorsi flap, without prosthetic implant
→ *CPT Assistant* Apr 05:6, Aug 05:1; *CPT Changes: An Insider's View* 2007

(For insertion of prosthesis, use also 19340)

19364   Breast reconstruction with free flap
→ *CPT Assistant* Aug 96:8, Nov 98:7, Apr 05:6, Aug 05:1

(Do not report code 69990 in addition to code 19364)

(19364 includes harvesting of the flap, microvascular transfer, closure of the donor site, and inset shaping the flap into a breast)

19366   Breast reconstruction with other technique
→ *CPT Assistant* Aug 96:8, Nov 98:7, Apr 05:6

(For operating microscope, use 69990)

(For insertion of prosthesis, use also 19340 or 19342)

19367   Breast reconstruction with transverse rectus abdominis myocutaneous flap (TRAM), single pedicle, including closure of donor site;
→ *CPT Assistant* Nov 98:7, Apr 05:6, Aug 05:1

19368   with microvascular anastomosis (supercharging)
→ *CPT Assistant* Nov 98:7, Apr 05:6, Aug 05:1

(Do not report code 69990 in addition to code 19368)

19369   Breast reconstruction with transverse rectus abdominis
          myocutaneous flap (TRAM), double pedicle, including
          closure of donor site
          ➲ *CPT Assistant* Oct 00:3, Apr 05:6, Aug 05:1

19370   Open periprosthetic capsulotomy, breast
          ➲ *CPT Assistant* Aug 96:8, Apr 05:6

19371   Periprosthetic capsulectomy, breast
          ➲ *CPT Assistant* Aug 96:8, Nov 01:11, Apr 05:6

19380   Revision of reconstructed breast
          ➲ *CPT Assistant* Apr 05:6

19396   Preparation of moulage for custom breast implant
          ➲ *CPT Assistant* Jan 03:7, Apr 05:6

Other Procedures

(For microwave thermotherapy of the breast, use
Category III code 0061T)

19499   Unlisted procedure, breast
          ➲ *CPT Assistant* Apr 05:6

Musculoskeletal System

Cast and strapping procedures appear at the end of this section.

The services listed below include the application and removal of the first cast or traction device only. Subsequent replacement of cast and/or traction device may require an additional listing.

Definitions

The terms "closed treatment," "open treatment," and "percutaneous skeletal fixation" have been carefully chosen to accurately reflect current orthopaedic procedural treatments.

Closed treatment specifically means that the fracture site is not surgically opened (exposed to the external environment and directly visualized). This terminology is used to describe procedures that treat fractures by three methods: 1) without manipulation; 2) with manipulation; or 3) with or without traction.

Open treatment is used when the fractured bone is either: 1) surgically opened (exposed to the external environment) and the fracture (bone ends) visualized and internal fixation may be used; or 2) the fractured bone is opened remote from the fracture site in order to insert an intramedullary nail across the fracture site (the fracture site is not opened and visualized).

Percutaneous skeletal fixation describes fracture treatment which is neither open nor closed. In this procedure, the fracture fragments are not visualized, but fixation (eg, pins) is placed across the fracture site, usually under X-ray imaging.

The type of fracture (eg, open, compound, closed) does not have any coding correlation with the type of treatment (eg, closed, open, or percutaneous) provided.

The codes for treatment of fractures and joint injuries (dislocations) are categorized by the type of manipulation (reduction) and stabilization (fixation or immobilization). These codes can apply to either open (compound) or closed fractures or joint injuries.

Skeletal traction is the application of a force (distracting or traction force) to a limb segment through a wire, pin, screw, or clamp that is attached (eg, penetrates) to bone.

Skin traction is the application of a force (longitudinal) to a limb using felt or strapping applied directly to skin only.

External fixation is the usage of skeletal pins plus an attaching mechanism/device used for temporary or definitive treatment of acute or chronic bony deformity.

Codes for obtaining autogenous bone grafts, cartilage, tendon, fascia lata grafts or other tissues through separate incisions are to be used only when the graft is not already listed as part of the basic procedure.

Re-reduction of a fracture and/or dislocation performed by the primary physician may be identified by the addition of the modifier 76 to the usual procedure number to indicate "Repeat Procedure or Service by Same Physician." (See guidelines.)

Codes for external fixation are to be used only when external fixation is not already listed as part of the basic procedure.

All codes for suction irrigation have been deleted. To report, list only the primary surgical procedure performed (eg, sequestrectomy, deep incision).

Manipulation is used throughout the musculoskeletal fracture and dislocation subsections to specifically mean the attempted reduction or restoration of a fracture or joint dislocation to its normal anatomic alignment by the application of manually applied forces.

General

Incision

20000   Incision of soft tissue abscess (eg, secondary to osteomyelitis); superficial

20005   deep or complicated

Wound Exploration—Trauma (eg, Penetrating Gunshot, Stab Wound)

20100-20103 relate to wound(s) resulting from penetrating trauma. These codes describe surgical exploration and enlargement of the wound, extension of dissection (to determine penetration), debridement, removal of foreign body(s), ligation or coagulation of minor subcutaneous and/or muscular blood vessel(s), of the subcutaneous tissue, muscle fascia, and/or muscle, not requiring thoracotomy or laparotomy. If a repair is done to major structure(s) or major blood vessel(s) requiring thoracotomy or laparotomy, then those specific code(s) would supersede the use of codes 20100-20103. To report Simple, Intermediate, or Complex repair of wound(s) that do not require enlargement of the wound, extension of dissection, etc., as stated above, use specific Repair code(s) in the **Integumentary System** section.

20100   Exploration of penetrating wound (separate procedure); neck
> *CPT Assistant* Jun 96:7, Aug 96:10, Sep 06:13

20101   chest
> *CPT Assistant* Jun 96:7, Sep 06:13

20102   abdomen/flank/back
> *CPT Assistant* Jun 96:7, Sep 06:13

20103   extremity
> *CPT Assistant* Jun 96:7, Aug 96:10, Sep 06:13

Excision

20150   Excision of epiphyseal bar, with or without autogenous soft tissue graft obtained through same fascial incision

(For aspiration of bone marrow, use 38220)

20200   Biopsy, muscle; superficial

20205   deep

20206   Biopsy, muscle, percutaneous needle

(If imaging guidance is performed, see 76942, 77012, 77021)

(For fine needle aspiration, use 10021 or 10022)

(For evaulation of fine needle aspirate, see 88172-88173)

(For excision of muscle tumor, deep, see specific anatomic section)

20220   Biopsy, bone, trocar, or needle; superficial (eg, ilium, sternum, spinous process, ribs)
   CPT Assistant Winter 92:17, Jul 98:4

20225   deep (eg, vertebral body, femur)
   CPT Assistant Winter 92:17, Jul 98:4; CPT Changes: An Insider's View 2002

(For bone marrow biopsy, use 38221)

(For radiologic supervision and interpretation, see 77002, 77012, 77021)

20240   Biopsy, bone, open; superficial (eg, ilium, sternum, spinous process, ribs, trochanter of femur)
   CPT Assistant Winter 92:17, Jul 98:4, Aug 04:11, Aug 05:13; CPT Changes: An Insider's View 2004

20245   deep (eg, humerus, ischium, femur)
   CPT Assistant Winter 92:17, Jul 98:4

20250   Biopsy, vertebral body, open; thoracic
   CPT Assistant Winter 92:17, Jul 98:4

20251   lumbar or cervical
   CPT Assistant Winter 92:17, Jul 98:4

(For sequestrectomy, osteomyelitis or drainage of bone abscess, see anatomical area)

Introduction or Removal

(For injection procedure for arthrography, see anatomical area)

20500   Injection of sinus tract; therapeutic (separate procedure)

20501   diagnostic (sinogram)

(For radiological supervision and interpretation, use 76080)

▶(For contrast injection[s] and radiological assessment of gastrostomy, duodenostomy, jejunostomy, gastro-jejunostomy, or cecostomy [or other colonic] tube including fluoroscopic imaging guidance, use 49465)◀

20520   Removal of foreign body in muscle or tendon sheath; simple

20525   deep or complicated

20526   Injection, therapeutic (eg, local anesthetic, corticosteroid), carpal tunnel
   CPT Assistant Mar 02:7; CPT Changes: An Insider's View 2002

20550   Injection(s); single tendon sheath, or ligament, aponeurosis (eg, plantar "fascia")
   CPT Assistant Jan 96:7, Jun 98:10, Mar 02:7, Aug 03:14, Sep 03:13, Dec 03:11; CPT Changes: An Insider's View 2002, 2003, 2004

20551   single tendon origin/insertion
   CPT Assistant Mar 02:7, Sep 03:13; CPT Changes: An Insider's View 2002, 2004

20552   Injection(s); single or multiple trigger point(s), one or two muscle(s)
   CPT Assistant Mar 02:7, May 03:19, Sep 03:11; CPT Changes: An Insider's View 2002, 2003, 2004

20553   single or multiple trigger point(s), three or more muscle(s)
   CPT Assistant Mar 02:7, May 03:19, Sep 03:11; CPT Changes: An Insider's View 2002, 2003

(If imaging guidance is performed, see 76942, 77002, 77021)

Trigger Point Injection
20552, 20553

Insertion of needle into muscle trigger point for injection of therapeutic agent

Injection site

Cross section through the body wall at level of lumbar vertebra

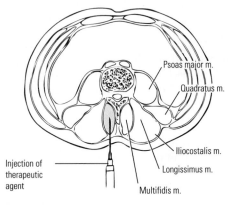

Psoas major m.

Quadratus m.

Injection of therapeutic agent

Iliocostalis m.

Longissimus m.

Multifidis m.

● **20555**   Placement of needles or catheters into muscle and/or soft tissue for subsequent interstitial radioelement application (at the time of or subsequent to the procedure)
→ *CPT Changes: An Insider's View* 2008

▶(For placement of devices into the breast for interstitial radioelement application, see 19296-19298)◀

▶(For placement of needles, catheters, or devices into muscle or soft tissue of the head and neck, for interstitial radioelement application, use 41019)◀

▶(For placement of needles or catheters for interstitial radioelement application into prostate, use 55875)◀

▶(For placement of needles or catheters into the pelvic organs or genitalia [except prostate] for interstitial radioelement application, use 55920)◀

▶(For interstitial radioelement application, see 77776-77784)◀

▶(For imaging guidance, see 76942, 77002, 77012, 77021)◀

20600   Arthrocentesis, aspiration and/or injection; small joint or bursa (eg, fingers, toes)
→ *CPT Changes: An Insider's View* 2003

20605   intermediate joint or bursa (eg, temporomandibular, acromioclavicular, wrist, elbow or ankle, olecranon bursa)
→ *CPT Changes: An Insider's View* 2003

20610   major joint or bursa (eg, shoulder, hip, knee joint, subacromial bursa)
→ *CPT Assistant* Spring 92:8, Mar 01:10, Apr 04:15, Jul 06:1

(If imaging guidance is performed, see 76942, 77002, 77012, 77021)

Arthrocentesis, Aspiration, or Injection of Major Joint or Bursa
20610

Insertion of needle into major joint or bursa for injection of therapeutic or diagnostic agent, aspiration, or arthrocentesis

Articular capsule of hip joint

20612   Aspiration and/or injection of ganglion cyst(s) any location
→ *CPT Changes: An Insider's View* 2003

(To report multiple ganglion cyst aspirations/injections, use 20612 and append modifier 59)

20615   Aspiration and injection for treatment of bone cyst

20650   Insertion of wire or pin with application of skeletal traction, including removal (separate procedure)

▲ **20660**   Application of cranial tongs, caliper, or stereotactic frame, including removal (separate procedure)
→ *CPT Assistant* Jun 96:10, Nov 97:14, Jan 06:46, Dec 06:10; *CPT Changes: An Insider's View* 2008

20661   Application of halo, including removal; cranial
→ *CPT Assistant* Nov 97:14

20662   pelvic

20663   femoral

20664   Application of halo, including removal, cranial, 6 or more pins placed, for thin skull osteology (eg, pediatric patients, hydrocephalus, osteogenesis imperfecta), requiring general anesthesia
→ *CPT Assistant* Nov 97:14

Halo Application for Thin Skull Osteology
20664

A cranial halo is placed on the head of a child whose skull is unusually thin due to congenital or developmental problems.

20665   Removal of tongs or halo applied by another physician

20670   Removal of implant; superficial (eg, buried wire, pin or rod) (separate procedure)

20680   deep (eg, buried wire, pin, screw, metal band, nail, rod or plate)

> → *CPT Assistant* Spring 92:11

▲ **20690**   Application of a uniplane (pins or wires in one plane), unilateral, external fixation system

> → *CPT Assistant* Winter 90:4, Winter 92:11, Fall 93:21, Oct 99:5, Jan 04:27, Jun 05:12; *CPT Changes: An Insider's View* 2008

Uniplane External Fixation System
20690

The following figures are examples of types of stabilization devices. Codes 20690 and 20692 describe the placement of types of external fixation devices. The method of stabilization depends upon fracture grade (degree of soft tissue injury/skin integrity disruption), type (eg, comminuted, spiral, impacted), and location (eg, extremity, pelvis).

External fixation system

Fracture

External fixation system

▲ **20692**   Application of a multiplane (pins or wires in more than one plane), unilateral, external fixation system (eg, Ilizarov, Monticelli type)

> → *CPT Assistant* Winter 90:4, Fall 93:21, Oct 99:5, Jul 00:11

Multiplane External Fixation System
20692

The following figure is an example of a type of multiplane stabilization device. Codes 20690 and 20692 describe the placement of types of external fixation devices. The method of stabilization depends upon fracture grade (degree of soft tissue injury/skin integrity disruption), type (eg, comminuted, spiral, impacted), and location (eg, extremity, pelvis).

Defect

External fixation system

20693   Adjustment or revision of external fixation system requiring anesthesia (eg, new pin(s) or wire(s) and/or new ring(s) or bar(s))

> → *CPT Assistant* Fall 93:21, Oct 99:5, Jul 00:11

20694   Removal, under anesthesia, of external fixation system

> → *CPT Assistant* Winter 92:10, Fall 93:21, Oct 99:5, Jul 00:11

Replantation

20802   Replantation, arm (includes surgical neck of humerus through elbow joint), complete amputation

(To report replantation of incomplete arm amputation, see specific code(s) for repair of bone(s), ligament(s), tendon(s), nerve(s), or blood vessel(s) with modifier 52)

20805   Replantation, forearm (includes radius and ulna to radial carpal joint), complete amputation

(To report replantation of incomplete forearm amputation, see specific code(s) for repair of bone(s), ligament(s), tendon(s), nerve(s), or blood vessel(s) with modifier 52)

20808   Replantation, hand (includes hand through metacarpophalangeal joints), complete amputation

(To report replantation of incomplete hand amputation, see specific code(s) for repair of bone(s), ligament(s), tendon(s), nerve(s), or blood vessel(s) with modifier 52)

20816   Replantation, digit, excluding thumb (includes metacarpophalangeal joint to insertion of flexor sublimis tendon), complete amputation
> *CPT Assistant* Oct 96:11

(To report replantation of incomplete digit amputation, excluding thumb, see specific code(s) for repair of bone(s), ligament(s), tendon(s), nerve(s), or blood vessel(s) with modifier 52)

20822   Replantation, digit, excluding thumb (includes distal tip to sublimis tendon insertion), complete amputation

(To report replantation of incomplete digit amputation, excluding thumb, see specific code(s) for repair of bone(s), ligament(s), tendon(s), nerve(s), or blood vessel(s) with modifier 52)

20824   Replantation, thumb (includes carpometacarpal joint to MP joint), complete amputation

(To report replantation of incomplete thumb amputation, see specific code(s) for repair of bone(s), ligament(s), tendon(s), nerve(s), or blood vessel(s) with modifier 52)

20827   Replantation, thumb (includes distal tip to MP joint), complete amputation

(To report replantation of incomplete thumb amputation, see specific code(s) for repair of bone(s), ligament(s), tendon(s), nerve(s), or blood vessel(s) with modifier 52)

(To report replantation of complete leg amputation, see specific code(s) for repair of bone(s), ligament(s), tendon(s), nerve(s), or blood vessel(s) with modifier 52)

(To report replantation of incomplete leg amputation, see specific code(s) for repair of bone(s), ligament(s), tendon(s), nerve(s), or blood vessel(s) with modifier 52)

20838   Replantation, foot, complete amputation

(To report replantation of incomplete foot amputation, see specific code(s) for repair of bone(s), ligament(s), tendon(s), nerve(s), or blood vessel(s) with modifier 52)

Grafts (or Implants)

Codes for obtaining autogenous bone, cartilage, tendon, fascia lata grafts, or other tissues through separate skin/fascial incisions should be reported separately unless the code descriptor references the harvesting of the graft or implant (eg, includes obtaining graft).

Do not append modifier 62 to bone graft codes 20900-20938.

(For spinal surgery bone graft(s) see codes 20930-20938)

▲ **20900**   Bone graft, any donor area; minor or small (eg, dowel or button)
> *CPT Assistant* Dec 00:15; *CPT Changes: An Insider's View* 2008

▲ **20902**   major or large
> *CPT Assistant* Dec 00:15; *CPT Changes: An Insider's View* 2008

▲ **20910**   Cartilage graft; costochondral
> *CPT Changes: An Insider's View* 2008

▲ **20912**   nasal septum
> *CPT Changes: An Insider's View* 2008

(For ear cartilage, use 21235)

▲ **20920**   Fascia lata graft; by stripper
> *CPT Assistant* Aug 99:5, Jan 05:8; *CPT Changes: An Insider's View* 2008

▲ **20922**   by incision and area exposure, complex or sheet
> *CPT Assistant* Jan 05:8; *CPT Changes: An Insider's View* 2008

▲ **20924**   Tendon graft, from a distance (eg, palmaris, toe extensor, plantaris)
> *CPT Changes: An Insider's View* 2008

▲ **20926**   Tissue grafts, other (eg, paratenon, fat, dermis)
> *CPT Assistant* Summer 91:12, Aug 99:5, Nov 99:10, May 06:16; *CPT Changes: An Insider's View* 2008

+▲ **20930**   Allograft for spine surgery only; morselized (List separately in addition to code for primary procedure)
> *CPT Assistant* Feb 96:6, Mar 96:4, Sep 97:8, Nov 99:10, Feb 02:6, Jan 04:27; *CPT Changes: An Insider's View* 2008

▶(Use 20930 in conjunction with 22319, 22532-22533, 22548-22558, 22590-22612, 22630, 22800-22812)◀

+▲ **20931**   structural (List separately in addition to code for primary procedure)
> *CPT Assistant* Feb 96:6, Feb 02:6, Feb 05:15; *CPT Changes: An Insider's View* 2008

▶(Use 20931 in conjunction with 22319, 22532-22533, 22548-22558, 22590-22612, 22630, 22800-22812)◀

+▲ **20936**   Autograft for spine surgery only (includes harvesting the graft); local (eg, ribs, spinous process, or laminar fragments) obtained from same incision (List separately in addition to code for primary procedure)
> *CPT Assistant* Feb 96:6, Sep 97:8, Feb 02:6; *CPT Changes: An Insider's View* 2008

▶(Use 20936 in conjunction with 22319, 22532-22533, 22548-22612, 22630, 22800-22812)◀

+▲ 20937 morselized (through separate skin or fascial incision) (List separately in addition to code for primary procedure)

→ *CPT Assistant* Feb 96:6, Sep 97:8, Dec 99:2, Feb 02:6; *CPT Changes: An Insider's View* 2008

▶(Use 20937 in conjunction with 22319, 22532-22533, 22548-22558, 22590-22612, 22630, 22800-22812)◀

+▲ 20938 structural, bicortical or tricortical (through separate skin or fascial incision) (List separately in addition to code for primary procedure)

→ *CPT Assistant* Feb 96:6, Mar 96:5, Sep 97:8, Feb 02:6; *CPT Changes: An Insider's View* 2008

▶(Use 20938 in conjunction with 22319, 22532-22533, 22548-22558, 22590-22612, 22630, 22800-22812)◀

(For needle aspiration of bone marrow for the purpose of bone grafting, use 38220)

Other Procedures

20950 Monitoring of interstitial fluid pressure (includes insertion of device, eg, wick catheter technique, needle manometer technique) in detection of muscle compartment syndrome

20955 Bone graft with microvascular anastomosis; fibula

→ *CPT Assistant* Apr 97:4

20956 iliac crest

→ *CPT Assistant* Apr 97:4

20957 metatarsal

→ *CPT Assistant* Apr 97:4

20962 other than fibula, iliac crest, or metatarsal

→ *CPT Assistant* Apr 97:4

(Do not report code 69990 in addition to codes 20955-20962)

20969 Free osteocutaneous flap with microvascular anastomosis; other than iliac crest, metatarsal, or great toe

→ *CPT Assistant* Apr 97:4

20970 iliac crest

→ *CPT Assistant* Apr 97:4

20972 metatarsal

→ *CPT Assistant* Apr 97:4

20973 great toe with web space

→ *CPT Assistant* Apr 97:4

(Do not report code 69990 in addition to codes 20969-20973)

(For great toe, wrap-around procedure, use 26551)

⊘ 20974 Electrical stimulation to aid bone healing; noninvasive (nonoperative)

→ *CPT Assistant* Sep 96:11, Nov 00:8

⊘ 20975 invasive (operative)

→ *CPT Assistant* Nov 00:8

20979 Low intensity ultrasound stimulation to aid bone healing, noninvasive (nonoperative)

→ *CPT Assistant* Nov 99:10, Nov 00:8; *CPT Changes: An Insider's View* 2000

⊙ 20982 Ablation, bone tumor(s) (eg, osteoid osteoma, metastasis) radiofrequency, percutaneous, including computed tomographic guidance

→ *CPT Changes: An Insider's View* 2004

(Do not report 20982 in conjunction with 77013)

+● 20985 Computer-assisted surgical navigational procedure for musculoskeletal procedures; image-less (List separately in addition to code for primary procedure)

→ *CPT Changes: An Insider's View* 2008

+● 20986 with image guidance based on intraoperatively obtained images (eg, fluoroscopy, ultrasound) (List separately in addition to code for primary procedure)

→ *CPT Changes: An Insider's View* 2008

▶(If multiple imaging modalities are used, report 20986 only once)◀

+● 20987 with image guidance based on preoperative images (List separately in addition to code for primary procedure)

→ *CPT Changes: An Insider's View* 2008

▶(If multiple imaging modalities are used, report 20987 only once)◀

▶(Do not report 20985-20987 in conjunction with 61795)◀

20999 Unlisted procedure, musculoskeletal system, general

→ *CPT Assistant* Sep 03:13

Head

Skull, facial bones, and temporomandibular joint.

Incision

(For drainage of superficial abscess and hematoma, use 20000)

(For removal of embedded foreign body from dentoalveolar structure, see 41805, 41806)

21010 Arthrotomy, temporomandibular joint

(To report bilateral procedures, report 21010 with modifier 50)

Excision

21015 Radical resection of tumor (eg, malignant neoplasm), soft tissue of face or scalp

(To report excision of skull tumor for osteomyelitis, use 61501)

21025 Excision of bone (eg, for osteomyelitis or bone abscess); mandible

21026 facial bone(s)

21029 Removal by contouring of benign tumor of facial bone (eg, fibrous dysplasia)

21030 Excision of benign tumor or cyst of maxilla or zygoma by enucleation and curettage
➔ *CPT Assistant* Nov 03:9; *CPT Changes: An Insider's View* 2003

21031 Excision of torus mandibularis

21032 Excision of maxillary torus palatinus

21034 Excision of malignant tumor of maxilla or zygoma
➔ *CPT Assistant* Nov 03:9; *CPT Changes: An Insider's View* 2003

21040 Excision of benign tumor or cyst of mandible, by enucleation and/or curettage
➔ *CPT Assistant* Nov 03:9; *CPT Changes: An Insider's View* 2003

(For enucleation and/or curettage of benign cysts or tumors of mandible not requiring osteotomy, use 21040)

(For excision of benign tumor or cyst of mandible requiring osteotomy, see 21046-21047)

21044 Excision of malignant tumor of mandible;

21045 radical resection

(For bone graft, use 21215)

21046 Excision of benign tumor or cyst of mandible; requiring intra-oral osteotomy (eg, locally aggressive or destructive lesion(s))
➔ *CPT Assistant* Nov 03:9; *CPT Changes: An Insider's View* 2003

21047 requiring extra-oral osteotomy and partial mandibulectomy (eg, locally aggressive or destructive lesion(s))
➔ *CPT Assistant* Nov 03:9; *CPT Changes: An Insider's View* 2003

21048 Excision of benign tumor or cyst of maxilla; requiring intra-oral osteotomy (eg, locally aggressive or destructive lesion(s))
➔ *CPT Assistant* Nov 03:9; *CPT Changes: An Insider's View* 2003

21049 requiring extra-oral osteotomy and partial maxillectomy (eg, locally aggressive or destructive lesion(s))
➔ *CPT Assistant* Nov 03:9; *CPT Changes: An Insider's View* 2003

21050 Condylectomy, temporomandibular joint (separate procedure)

(For bilateral procedures, report 21050 with modifier 50)

21060 Meniscectomy, partial or complete, temporomandibular joint (separate procedure)

(For bilateral procedures, report 21060 with modifier 50)

21070 Coronoidectomy (separate procedure)

(For bilateral procedures, report 21070 with modifier 50)

►Manipulation◄

● **21073** Manipulation of temporomandibular joint(s) (TMJ), therapeutic, requiring an anesthesia service (ie, general or monitored anesthesia care)
➔ *CPT Changes: An Insider's View* 2008

►(For TMJ manipulation without an anesthesia service [ie, general or monitored anesthesia care], see 97140, 98925-98929, 98943)◄

►(For closed treatment of temporomandibular dislocation, see 21480, 21485)◄

Head Prosthesis

Codes 21076-21089 describe professional services for the rehabilitation of patients with oral, facial, or other anatomical deficiencies by means of prostheses such as an artificial eye, ear, or nose or intraoral obturator to close a cleft. Codes 21076-21089 should only be used when the physician actually designs and prepares the prosthesis (ie, not prepared by an outside laboratory).

►(For application or removal of caliper or tongs, see 20660, 20665)◄

21076 Impression and custom preparation; surgical obturator prosthesis

21077 orbital prosthesis

21079 interim obturator prosthesis
➔ *CPT Assistant* Winter 90:5, Sep 06:13, Dec 06:10

21080 definitive obturator prosthesis
➔ *CPT Assistant* Winter 90:5, Sep 06:13, Dec 06:10

21081 mandibular resection prosthesis
➔ *CPT Assistant* Winter 90:5, Sep 06:13, Dec 06:10

21082 palatal augmentation prosthesis
➔ *CPT Assistant* Winter 90:5, Sep 06:13, Dec 06:10

21083 palatal lift prosthesis
➔ *CPT Assistant* Winter 90:5, Sep 06:13, Dec 06:10

21084 speech aid prosthesis
➔ *CPT Assistant* Winter 90:5, Sep 06:13, Dec 06:10

21085 oral surgical splint
➔ *CPT Assistant* Winter 90:5, Sep 06:13, Dec 06:10

21086 auricular prosthesis
➔ *CPT Assistant* Winter 90:5, Sep 06:13, Dec 06:10

21087 nasal prosthesis
➔ *CPT Assistant* Winter 90:5, Sep 06:13, Dec 06:10

21088 facial prosthesis
➔ *CPT Assistant* Winter 90:5, Sep 06:13, Dec 06:10

Other Procedures

21089 Unlisted maxillofacial prosthetic procedure
➔ *CPT Assistant* Winter 90:5, Sep 06:13, Dec 06:10

Introduction or Removal

21100 Application of halo type appliance for maxillofacial fixation, includes removal (separate procedure)

21110 Application of interdental fixation device for conditions other than fracture or dislocation, includes removal
➔ *CPT Assistant* Mar 97:10

(For removal of interdental fixation by another physician, see 20670-20680)

21116 Injection procedure for temporomandibular joint arthrography

(For radiological supervision and interpretation, use 70332. Do not report 77002 in conjunction with 70332)

Repair, Revision, and/or Reconstruction

(For cranioplasty, see 21179, 21180 and 62116, 62120, 62140-62147)

21120 Genioplasty; augmentation (autograft, allograft, prosthetic material)

21121 sliding osteotomy, single piece

21122 sliding osteotomies, two or more osteotomies (eg, wedge excision or bone wedge reversal for asymmetrical chin)

21123 sliding, augmentation with interpositional bone grafts (includes obtaining autografts)

21125 Augmentation, mandibular body or angle; prosthetic material

21127 with bone graft, onlay or interpositional (includes obtaining autograft)

21137 Reduction forehead; contouring only

21138 contouring and application of prosthetic material or bone graft (includes obtaining autograft)

21139 contouring and setback of anterior frontal sinus wall

21141 Reconstruction midface, LeFort I; single piece, segment movement in any direction (eg, for Long Face Syndrome), without bone graft

21142 two pieces, segment movement in any direction, without bone graft

21143 three or more pieces, segment movement in any direction, without bone graft

21145 single piece, segment movement in any direction, requiring bone grafts (includes obtaining autografts)

21146 two pieces, segment movement in any direction, requiring bone grafts (includes obtaining autografts) (eg, ungrafted unilateral alveolar cleft)

21147 three or more pieces, segment movement in any direction, requiring bone grafts (includes obtaining autografts) (eg, ungrafted bilateral alveolar cleft or multiple osteotomies)

21150 Reconstruction midface, LeFort II; anterior intrusion (eg, Treacher-Collins Syndrome)

21151 any direction, requiring bone grafts (includes obtaining autografts)

21154 Reconstruction midface, LeFort III (extracranial), any type, requiring bone grafts (includes obtaining autografts); without LeFort I

21155 with LeFort I

21159 Reconstruction midface, LeFort III (extra and intracranial) with forehead advancement (eg, mono bloc), requiring bone grafts (includes obtaining autografts); without LeFort I

21160 with LeFort I

21172 Reconstruction superior-lateral orbital rim and lower forehead, advancement or alteration, with or without grafts (includes obtaining autografts)

(For frontal or parietal craniotomy performed for craniosynostosis, use 61556)

21175 Reconstruction, bifrontal, superior-lateral orbital rims and lower forehead, advancement or alteration (eg, plagiocephaly, trigonocephaly, brachycephaly), with or without grafts (includes obtaining autografts)

(For bifrontal craniotomy performed for craniosynostosis, use 61557)

21179 Reconstruction, entire or majority of forehead and/or supraorbital rims; with grafts (allograft or prosthetic material)

21180 with autograft (includes obtaining grafts)

(For extensive craniectomy for multiple suture craniosynostosis, use only 61558 or 61559)

21181 Reconstruction by contouring of benign tumor of cranial bones (eg, fibrous dysplasia), extracranial

21182 Reconstruction of orbital walls, rims, forehead, nasoethmoid complex following intra- and extracranial excision of benign tumor of cranial bone (eg, fibrous dysplasia), with multiple autografts (includes obtaining grafts); total area of bone grafting less than 40 sq cm

21183 total area of bone grafting greater than 40 sq cm but less than 80 sq cm
➔ *CPT Changes: An Insider's View* 2002

21184 total area of bone grafting greater than 80 sq cm
➔ *CPT Changes: An Insider's View* 2002

(For excision of benign tumor of cranial bones, see 61563, 61564)

⊙ =Moderate sedation   ✚ =Add-on code   ⊮ =FDA approval pending   ➔➔ =See p xvii for details

21188 Reconstruction midface, osteotomies (other than LeFort type) and bone grafts (includes obtaining autografts)

21193 Reconstruction of mandibular rami, horizontal, vertical, C, or L osteotomy; without bone graft
➔ *CPT Assistant* Apr 96:11

21194 with bone graft (includes obtaining graft)
➔ *CPT Assistant* Apr 96:11

21195 Reconstruction of mandibular rami and/or body, sagittal split; without internal rigid fixation
➔ *CPT Assistant* Apr 96:11

21196 with internal rigid fixation
➔ *CPT Assistant* Apr 96:11, Mar 97:11

Reconstruction of Mandibular Rami
21196

The mandibular ramus is reconstructed to lengthen, set back, or rotate the mandible.

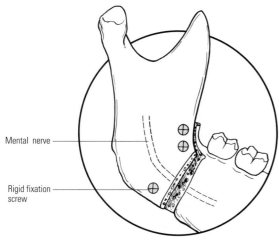

Mental nerve

Rigid fixation screw

21198 Osteotomy, mandible, segmental;
➔ *CPT Changes: An Insider's View* 2001

21199 with genioglossus advancement
➔ *CPT Changes: An Insider's View* 2001

(To report total osteotomy of the maxilla, see 21141-21160)

21206 Osteotomy, maxilla, segmental (eg, Wassmund or Schuchard)

21208 Osteoplasty, facial bones; augmentation (autograft, allograft, or prosthetic implant)

21209 reduction

21210 Graft, bone; nasal, maxillary or malar areas (includes obtaining graft)

(For cleft palate repair, see 42200-42225)

21215 mandible (includes obtaining graft)

21230 Graft; rib cartilage, autogenous, to face, chin, nose or ear (includes obtaining graft)

21235 ear cartilage, autogenous, to nose or ear (includes obtaining graft)

(To report graft augmentation of facial bones, use 21208)

21240 Arthroplasty, temporomandibular joint, with or without autograft (includes obtaining graft)

21242 Arthroplasty, temporomandibular joint, with allograft

21243 Arthroplasty, temporomandibular joint, with prosthetic joint replacement

21244 Reconstruction of mandible, extraoral, with transosteal bone plate (eg, mandibular staple bone plate)

21245 Reconstruction of mandible or maxilla, subperiosteal implant; partial

21246 complete

21247 Reconstruction of mandibular condyle with bone and cartilage autografts (includes obtaining grafts) (eg, for hemifacial microsomia)

21248 Reconstruction of mandible or maxilla, endosteal implant (eg, blade, cylinder); partial

21249 complete

(To report midface reconstruction, see 21141-21160)

21255 Reconstruction of zygomatic arch and glenoid fossa with bone and cartilage (includes obtaining autografts)

21256 Reconstruction of orbit with osteotomies (extracranial) and with bone grafts (includes obtaining autografts) (eg, micro-ophthalmia)

21260 Periorbital osteotomies for orbital hypertelorism, with bone grafts; extracranial approach

21261 combined intra- and extracranial approach

21263 with forehead advancement

21267 Orbital repositioning, periorbital osteotomies, unilateral, with bone grafts; extracranial approach

21268 combined intra- and extracranial approach

21270 Malar augmentation, prosthetic material

(For malar augmentation with bone graft, use 21210)

21275 Secondary revision of orbitocraniofacial reconstruction

21280 Medial canthopexy (separate procedure)

(For medial canthoplasty, use 67950)

21282 Lateral canthopexy

21295 Reduction of masseter muscle and bone (eg, for treatment of benign masseteric hypertrophy); extraoral approach

21296 intraoral approach

Other Procedures

21299 Unlisted craniofacial and maxillofacial procedure

Fracture and/or Dislocation

(For operative repair of skull fracture, see 62000-62010)

(21300 has been deleted)

(To report closed treatment of skull fracture, use the appropriate Evaluation and Management code)

21310 Closed treatment of nasal bone fracture without manipulation

21315 Closed treatment of nasal bone fracture; without stabilization

21320 with stabilization

21325 Open treatment of nasal fracture; uncomplicated

21330 complicated, with internal and/or external skeletal fixation

21335 with concomitant open treatment of fractured septum

21336 Open treatment of nasal septal fracture, with or without stabilization

21337 Closed treatment of nasal septal fracture, with or without stabilization

21338 Open treatment of nasoethmoid fracture; without external fixation

21339 with external fixation

21340 Percutaneous treatment of nasoethmoid complex fracture, with splint, wire or headcap fixation, including repair of canthal ligaments and/or the nasolacrimal apparatus

21343 Open treatment of depressed frontal sinus fracture

21344 Open treatment of complicated (eg, comminuted or involving posterior wall) frontal sinus fracture, via coronal or multiple approaches

21345 Closed treatment of nasomaxillary complex fracture (LeFort II type), with interdental wire fixation or fixation of denture or splint

21346 Open treatment of nasomaxillary complex fracture (LeFort II type); with wiring and/or local fixation

21347 requiring multiple open approaches

21348 with bone grafting (includes obtaining graft)

21355 Percutaneous treatment of fracture of malar area, including zygomatic arch and malar tripod, with manipulation

21356 Open treatment of depressed zygomatic arch fracture (eg, Gillies approach)

21360 Open treatment of depressed malar fracture, including zygomatic arch and malar tripod

21365 Open treatment of complicated (eg, comminuted or involving cranial nerve foramina) fracture(s) of malar area, including zygomatic arch and malar tripod; with internal fixation and multiple surgical approaches

21366 with bone grafting (includes obtaining graft)

21385 Open treatment of orbital floor blowout fracture; transantral approach (Caldwell-Luc type operation)

21386 periorbital approach

21387 combined approach

21390 periorbital approach, with alloplastic or other implant

21395 periorbital approach with bone graft (includes obtaining graft)

21400 Closed treatment of fracture of orbit, except blowout; without manipulation

21401 with manipulation

21406 Open treatment of fracture of orbit, except blowout; without implant

21407 with implant

21408 with bone grafting (includes obtaining graft)

21421 Closed treatment of palatal or maxillary fracture (LeFort I type), with interdental wire fixation or fixation of denture or splint

21422 Open treatment of palatal or maxillary fracture (LeFort I type);

21423 complicated (comminuted or involving cranial nerve foramina), multiple approaches

21431 Closed treatment of craniofacial separation (LeFort III type) using interdental wire fixation of denture or splint

21432 Open treatment of craniofacial separation (LeFort III type); with wiring and/or internal fixation

21433 complicated (eg, comminuted or involving cranial nerve foramina), multiple surgical approaches

21435 complicated, utilizing internal and/or external fixation techniques (eg, head cap, halo device, and/or intermaxillary fixation)

(For removal of internal or external fixation device, use 20670)

21436 complicated, multiple surgical approaches, internal fixation, with bone grafting (includes obtaining graft)

21440 Closed treatment of mandibular or maxillary alveolar ridge fracture (separate procedure)

21445 Open treatment of mandibular or maxillary alveolar ridge fracture (separate procedure)

21450 Closed treatment of mandibular fracture; without manipulation

21451 with manipulation

21452 Percutaneous treatment of mandibular fracture, with external fixation

21453 Closed treatment of mandibular fracture with interdental fixation

21454 Open treatment of mandibular fracture with external fixation

21461 Open treatment of mandibular fracture; without interdental fixation

21462 with interdental fixation

21465 Open treatment of mandibular condylar fracture

21470 Open treatment of complicated mandibular fracture by multiple surgical approaches including internal fixation, interdental fixation, and/or wiring of dentures or splints
➔ *CPT Assistant* Nov 02:10

21480 Closed treatment of temporomandibular dislocation; initial or subsequent

21485 complicated (eg, recurrent requiring intermaxillary fixation or splinting), initial or subsequent

21490 Open treatment of temporomandibular dislocation

(For interdental wire fixation, use 21497)

(21493 and 21494 have been deleted. To report, use the applicable Evaluation and Management codes)

21495 Open treatment of hyoid fracture

(For laryngoplasty with open reduction of fracture, use 31584)

(To report treatment of closed fracture of larynx, use the applicable Evaluation and Management codes)

21497 Interdental wiring, for condition other than fracture
➔ *CPT Assistant* Mar 97:10

Other Procedures

21499 Unlisted musculoskeletal procedure, head

(For unlisted craniofacial or maxillofacial procedure, use 21299)

Neck (Soft Tissues) and Thorax

(For cervical spine and back, see 21920 et seq)

(For injection of fracture site or trigger point, use 20550)

Incision

(For incision and drainage of abscess or hematoma, superficial, see 10060, 10140)

21501 Incision and drainage, deep abscess or hematoma, soft tissues of neck or thorax;

(For posterior spine subfascial incision and drainage, see 22010-22015)

21502 with partial rib ostectomy

21510 Incision, deep, with opening of bone cortex (eg, for osteomyelitis or bone abscess), thorax

Excision

(For bone biopsy, see 20220-20251)

21550 Biopsy, soft tissue of neck or thorax

(For needle biopsy of soft tissue, use 20206)

21555 Excision tumor, soft tissue of neck or thorax; subcutaneous
➔ *CPT Assistant* Oct 02:11

21556 deep, subfascial, intramuscular

21557 Radical resection of tumor (eg, malignant neoplasm), soft tissue of neck or thorax

21600 Excision of rib, partial

(For radical resection of chest wall and rib cage for tumor, use 19260)

(For radical debridement of chest wall and rib cage for injury, see 11040-11044)

21610 Costotransversectomy (separate procedure)

21615 Excision first and/or cervical rib;

21616 with sympathectomy

21620 Ostectomy of sternum, partial

21627 Sternal debridement

(For debridement and closure, use 21750)

21630 Radical resection of sternum;

21632 with mediastinal lymphadenectomy

Repair, Revision, and/or Reconstruction

(For superficial wound, see **Integumentary System** section under Repair—Simple)

21685 Hyoid myotomy and suspension
➔ *CPT Assistant* Aug 04:11; *CPT Changes: An Insider's View* 2004

21700 Division of scalenus anticus; without resection of cervical rib

21705 with resection of cervical rib

21720 Division of sternocleidomastoid for torticollis, open operation; without cast application

(For transection of spinal accessory and cervical nerves, see 63191, 64722)

21725 with cast application

21740 Reconstructive repair of pectus excavatum or carinatum; open
> *CPT Changes: An Insider's View* 2003

21742 minimally invasive approach (Nuss procedure), without thoracoscopy
> *CPT Changes: An Insider's View* 2003

21743 minimally invasive approach (Nuss procedure), with thoracoscopy
> *CPT Changes: An Insider's View* 2003

21750 Closure of median sternotomy separation with or without debridement (separate procedure)
> *CPT Changes: An Insider's View* 2002

Fracture and/or Dislocation

21800 Closed treatment of rib fracture, uncomplicated, each

21805 Open treatment of rib fracture without fixation, each

21810 Treatment of rib fracture requiring external fixation (flail chest)

21820 Closed treatment of sternum fracture

21825 Open treatment of sternum fracture with or without skeletal fixation

(For sternoclavicular dislocation, see 23520-23532)

Other Procedures

21899 Unlisted procedure, neck or thorax

Back and Flank

Excision

21920 Biopsy, soft tissue of back or flank; superficial

21925 deep

(For needle biopsy of soft tissue, use 20206)

21930 Excision, tumor, soft tissue of back or flank

21935 Radical resection of tumor (eg, malignant neoplasm), soft tissue of back or flank

Spine (Vertebral Column)

Cervical, thoracic, and lumbar spine.

Within the spine section, bone grafting procedures are reported separately and in addition to arthrodesis. For bone grafts in other Musculoskeletal sections, see specific code(s) descriptor(s) and/or accompanying guidelines.

▶To report bone grafts performed after arthrodesis, see 20930-20938. Do not append modifier 62 to bone graft codes 20900-20938.◀

Example:

Posterior arthrodesis of L5-S1 for degenerative disc disease utilizing morselized autogenous iliac bone graft harvested through a separate fascial incision.

Report as 22612 and 20937.

▶Within the spine section, instrumentation is reported separately and in addition to arthrodesis. To report instrumentation procedures performed with definitive vertebral procedure(s), see 22840-22855. Instrumentation procedure codes 22840-22848 and 22851 are reported in addition to the definitive procedure(s). Modifier 62 may not be appended to the definitive or add-on spinal instrumentation procedure code(s) 22840-22848 and 22850-22852.◀

Example:

Posterior arthrodesis of L4-S1, utilizing morselized autogenous iliac bone graft harvested through separate fascial incision, and pedicle screw fixation.

Report as 22612, 22614, 22842, and 20937.

Vertebral procedures are sometimes followed by arthrodesis and in addition may include bone grafts and instrumentation.

▶When arthrodesis is performed in addition to another procedure, the arthrodesis should be reported in addition to the original procedure with modifier 51 (multiple procedures). Examples are after osteotomy, fracture care, vertebral corpectomy, and laminectomy. Bone grafts and instrumentation are never performed without arthrodesis.◀

Example:

Treatment of a burst fracture of L2 by corpectomy followed by arthrodesis of L1-L3, utilizing anterior instrumentation L1-L3 and structural allograft.

Report as 63090, 22558-51, 22585, 22845, and 20931.

When two surgeons work together as primary surgeons performing distinct part(s) of a single reportable procedure, each surgeon should report his/her distinct operative work by appending modifier 62 to the single definitive procedure code. If additional procedure(s) (including add-on procedure(s)) are performed during the same surgical session, separate code(s) may be reported by each co-surgeon, with modifier 62 appended (see Appendix A).

Example:

A 42-year-old male with a history of posttraumatic degenerative disc disease at L3-4 and L4-5 (internal disc disruption) underwent surgical repair. Surgeon A performed an anterior exposure of the spine with mobilization of the great vessels. Surgeon B performed anterior (minimal) discectomy and fusion at L3-4 and L4-5 using anterior interbody technique.

Report surgeon A: 22558 append modifier 62, 22585 append modifier 62
Report surgeon B: 22558 append modifier 62, 22585 append modifier 62, 20931

> (Do not append modifier 62 to bone graft code 20931)

> (For injection procedure for myelography, use 62284)

> (For injection procedure for discography, see 62290, 62291)

> (For injection procedure, chemonucleolysis, single or multiple levels, use 62292)

> (For injection procedure for facet joints, see 64470-64476, 64622-64627)

> (For needle or trocar biopsy, see 20220-20225)

Incision

22010   Incision and drainage, open, of deep abscess (subfascial), posterior spine; cervical, thoracic, or cervicothoracic
> ➔ *CPT Changes: An Insider's View* 2006

22015   lumbar, sacral, or lumbosacral
> ➔ *CPT Changes: An Insider's View* 2006

> (Do not report 22015 in conjunction with 22010)

> (Do not report 22015 in conjunction with instrumentation removal, 10180, 22850, 22852)

> (For incision and drainage of abscess or hematoma, superficial, see 10060, 10140)

Excision

For the following codes, when two surgeons work together as primary surgeons performing distinct part(s) of partial vertebral body excision, each surgeon should report his/her distinct operative work by appending modifier 62 to the procedure code. In this situation, modifier 62 may be appended to the procedure code(s) 22100-22102, 22110-22114 and, as appropriate, to the associated additional vertebral segment add-on code(s) 22103, 22116 as long as both surgeons continue to work together as primary surgeons.

> (For bone biopsy, see 20220-20251)

> (To report soft tissue biopsy of back or flank, see 21920-21925)

> (For needle biopsy of soft tissue, use 20206)

> (To report excision of soft tissue tumor of back or flank, use 21930)

22100   Partial excision of posterior vertebral component (eg, spinous process, lamina or facet) for intrinsic bony lesion, single vertebral segment; cervical

22101   thoracic

22102   lumbar

> ▶(For insertion of posterior spinous process distraction devices, see 0171T, 0172T)◀

+ 22103   each additional segment (List separately in addition to code for primary procedure)
> ➔ *CPT Assistant* Feb 96:6

> (Use 22103 in conjunction with 22100, 22101, 22102)

22110   Partial excision of vertebral body, for intrinsic bony lesion, without decompression of spinal cord or nerve root(s), single vertebral segment; cervical

22112   thoracic

22114   lumbar

+ 22116   each additional vertebral segment (List separately in addition to code for primary procedure)
> ➔ *CPT Assistant* Feb 96:6

> (Use 22116 in conjunction with 22110, 22112, 22114)

> (For complete or near complete resection of vertebral body, see vertebral corpectomy, 63081-63091)

> (For spinal reconstruction with bone graft (autograft, allograft) and/or methylmethacrylate of cervical vertebral body, use 63081 and 22554 and 20931 or 20938)

> (For spinal reconstruction with bone graft (autograft, allograft) and/or methylmethacrylate of thoracic vertebral body, use 63085 or 63087 and 22556 and 20931 or 20938)

> (For spinal reconstruction with bone graft (autograft, allograft) and/or methylmethacrylate of lumbar vertebral body, use 63087 or 63090 and 22558 and 20931 or 20938)

> (For spinal reconstruction following vertebral body resection, use 63082 or 63086 or 63088 or 63091, and 22585)

> (For harvest of bone autograft for vertebral reconstruction, see 20931 or 20938)

> (For cervical spinal reconstruction with prosthetic replacement of resected vertebral bodies, see codes 63081 and 22554 and 20931 or 20938 and 22851)

> (For thoracic spinal reconstruction with prosthetic replacement of resected vertebral bodies, see codes 63085 or 63087 and 22556 and 20931 or 20938 and 22851)

> (For lumbar spinal reconstruction with prosthetic replacement of resected vertebral bodies, see codes 63087 or 63090 and 22558, and 20931 or 20938 and 22851)

> (For osteotomy of spine, see 22210-22226)

Osteotomy

To report arthrodesis, see codes 22590-22632. (Report in addition to code[s] for the definitive procedure with modifier 51.)

▶To report instrumentation procedures, see 22840-22855. (Report in addition to code[s] for the definitive procedure[s].) Do not append modifier 62 to spinal instrumentation codes 22840-22848 and 22850-22852.

To report bone graft procedures, see 20930-20938. (Report in addition to code[s] for the definitive procedure[s].) Do not append modifier 62 to bone graft codes 20900-20938.◀

For the following codes, when two surgeons work together as primary surgeons performing distinct part(s) of an anterior spine osteotomy, each surgeon should report his/her distinct operative work by appending modifier 62 to the procedure code. In this situation, modifier 62 may be appended to the procedure code(s) 22210-22214, 22220-22224 and, as appropriate, to associated additional segment add-on code(s) 22216, 22226 as long as both surgeons continue to work together as primary surgeons.

▶Spinal osteotomy procedures are reported when a portion(s) of the vertebral segment(s) is cut and removed in preparation for re-aligning the spine as part of a spinal deformity correction. For excision of an intrinsic lesion of the vertebra without deformity correction, see 22100-22116. For decompression of the spinal cord and/or nerve roots, see 63001-63308.

The three columns are defined as anterior (anterior two-thirds of the vertebral body), middle (posterior third of the vertebral body and the pedicle), and posterior (articular facets, lamina, and spinous process).◀

● **22206** Osteotomy of spine, posterior or posterolateral approach, three columns, one vertebral segment (eg, pedicle/vertebral body subtraction); thoracic
➔ *CPT Changes: An Insider's View* 2008

▶(Do not report 22206 in conjunction with 22207)◀

● **22207** lumbar
➔ *CPT Changes: An Insider's View* 2008

▶(Do not report 22207 in conjunction with 22206)◀

+ ● **22208** each additional vertebral segment (List separately in addition to code for primary procedure)
➔ *CPT Changes: An Insider's View* 2008

▶(Use 22208 in conjunction with 22206, 22207)◀

▶(Do not report 22206, 22207, 22208 in conjunction with 22210-22226, 22830, 63001-63048, 63055-63066, 63075-63091, 63101-63103, when performed at the same level)◀

22210 Osteotomy of spine, posterior or posterolateral approach, one vertebral segment; cervical

22212 thoracic

22214 lumbar

+ **22216** each additional vertebral segment (List separately in addition to primary procedure)

(Use 22216 in conjunction with 22210, 22212, 22214)

22220 Osteotomy of spine, including discectomy, anterior approach, single vertebral segment; cervical
➔ *CPT Assistant* Feb 02:4

22222 thoracic
➔ *CPT Assistant* Feb 02:4

22224 lumbar
➔ *CPT Assistant* Feb 02:4

+ **22226** each additional vertebral segment (List separately in addition to code for primary procedure)
➔ *CPT Assistant* Feb 96:6, Feb 02:4

(Use 22226 in conjunction with 22220, 22222, 22224)

(For vertebral corpectomy, see 63081-63091)

Fracture and/or Dislocation

To report arthrodesis, see codes 22590-22632. (Report in addition to code[s] for the definitive procedure with modifier 51.)

▶To report instrumentation procedures, see 22840-22855. (Report in addition to code[s] for the definitive procedure[s].) Do not append modifier 62 to spinal instrumentation codes 22840-22848 and 22850-22852.

To report bone graft procedures, see 20930-20938. (Report in addition to code[s] for the definitive procedure[s].) Do not append modifier 62 to bone graft codes 20900-20938.◀

For the following codes, when two surgeons work together as primary surgeons performing distinct part(s) of open fracture and/or dislocation procedure(s), each surgeon should report his/her distinct operative work by appending modifier 62 to the procedure code. In this situation, modifier 62 may be appended to the procedure code(s) 22318-22327 and, as appropriate, the associated additional fracture vertebrae or dislocated segment add-on code 22328 as long as both surgeons continue to work together as primary surgeons.

22305 Closed treatment of vertebral process fracture(s)

22310 Closed treatment of vertebral body fracture(s), without manipulation, requiring and including casting or bracing

22315 Closed treatment of vertebral fracture(s) and/or dislocation(s) requiring casting or bracing, with and including casting and/or bracing, with or without anesthesia, by manipulation or traction

(For spinal subluxation, use 97140)

22318 Open treatment and/or reduction of odontoid fracture(s) and or dislocation(s) (including os odontoideum), anterior approach, including placement of internal fixation; without grafting

➔ *CPT Assistant* Nov 99:11; *CPT Changes: An Insider's View* 2000

22319 with grafting

➔ *CPT Assistant* Nov 99:11; *CPT Changes: An Insider's View* 2000

22325 Open treatment and/or reduction of vertebral fracture(s) and/or dislocation(s), posterior approach, one fractured vertebra or dislocated segment; lumbar

➔ *CPT Assistant* Sep 97:8

22326 cervical

➔ *CPT Assistant* Sep 97:8

22327 thoracic

➔ *CPT Assistant* Sep 97:8

+ 22328 each additional fractured vertebra or dislocated segment (List separately in addition to code for primary procedure)

➔ *CPT Assistant* Feb 96:6

(Use 22328 in conjunction with 22325, 22326, 22327)

(For treatment of vertebral fracture by the anterior approach, see corpectomy 63081-63091, and appropriate arthrodesis, bone graft and instrument codes)

(For decompression of spine following fracture, see 63001-63091; for arthrodesis of spine following fracture, see 22548-22632)

Manipulation

(For spinal manipulation without anesthesia, use 97140)

22505 Manipulation of spine requiring anesthesia, any region

➔ *CPT Assistant* Mar 97:11, Jan 99:11

Vertebral Body, Embolization or Injection

22520 Percutaneous vertebroplasty, one vertebral body, unilateral or bilateral injection; thoracic

➔ *CPT Assistant* Mar 01:2, Oct 06:13; *CPT Changes: An Insider's View* 2001

22521 lumbar

➔ *CPT Assistant* Mar 01:2, Oct 06:13; *CPT Changes: An Insider's View* 2001

+ 22522 each additional thoracic or lumbar vertebral body (List separately in addition to code for primary procedure)

➔ *CPT Assistant* Mar 01:2, Oct 06:13; *CPT Changes: An Insider's View* 2001

(Use 22522 in conjunction with 22520, 22521 as appropriate)

(For radiological supervision and interpretation, see 72291, 72292)

Percutaneous Vertebroplasty
22520

Augmentation of a vertebral fracture is achieved by percutaneous injections of polymethylmethacrylate under fluoroscopic guidance.

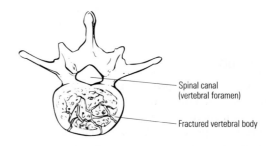

Spinal canal (vertebral foramen)

Fractured vertebral body

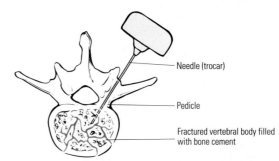

Needle (trocar)

Pedicle

Fractured vertebral body filled with bone cement

22523 Percutaneous vertebral augmentation, including cavity creation (fracture reduction and bone biopsy included when performed) using mechanical device, one vertebral body, unilateral or bilateral cannulation (eg, kyphoplasty); thoracic

➔ *CPT Changes: An Insider's View* 2006

➔ *Clinical Examples in Radiology* Winter 06:14

22524 lumbar

➔ *CPT Changes: An Insider's View* 2006

➔ *Clinical Examples in Radiology* Winter 06:14

+ 22525 each additional thoracic or lumbar vertebral body (List separately in addition to code for primary procedure)

➔ *CPT Changes: An Insider's View* 2006

➔ *Clinical Examples in Radiology* Winter 06:14

(Do not report 22525 in conjunction with 20225 when performed at the same level as 22523-22525)

(Use 22525 in conjunction with 22523, 22524)

(For radiological supervision and interpretation, see 72291, 72292)

⊙ **22526** Percutaneous intradiscal electrothermal annuloplasty, unilateral or bilateral including fluoroscopic guidance; single level

⮕ *CPT Changes: An Insider's View* 2007

⊙✛ **22527** one or more additional levels (List separately in addition to code for primary procedure)

⮕ *CPT Changes: An Insider's View* 2007

(Do not report codes 22526, 22527 in conjunction with 77002, 77003)

(For percutaneous intradiscal annuloplasty using method other than electrothermal, see 0062T, 0063T)

Arthrodesis

Arthrodesis may be performed in the absence of other procedures and therefore when it is combined with another definitive procedure (eg, osteotomy, fracture care, vertebral corpectomy or laminectomy), modifier 51 is appropriate. However, arthrodesis codes 22585, 22614, and 22632 are considered add-on procedure codes and should not be used with modifier 51.

▶To report instrumentation procedures, see 22840-22855. (Codes 22840-22848, 22851 are reported in conjunction with code[s] for the definitive procedure[s]. When instrumentation reinsertion or removal is reported in conjunction with other definitive procedures including arthrodesis, decompression, and exploration of fusion, append modifier 51 to 22849, 22850, 22852, and 22855.) To report exploration of fusion, use 22830. (When exploration is reported in conjunction with other definitive procedures, including arthrodesis and decompression, append modifier 51 to 22830.) Do not append modifier 62 to spinal instrumentation codes 22840-22848 and 22850-22852.

To report bone graft procedures, see 20930-20938. (Report in addition to code[s] for the definitive procedure[s].) Do not append modifier 62 to bone graft codes 20900-20938.◀

Lateral Extracavitary Approach Technique

22532 Arthrodesis, lateral extracavitary technique, including minimal discectomy to prepare interspace (other than for decompression); thoracic

⮕ *CPT Changes: An Insider's View* 2004

22533 lumbar

⮕ *CPT Changes: An Insider's View* 2004

✛ **22534** thoracic or lumbar, each additional vertebral segment (List separately in addition to code for primary procedure)

⮕ *CPT Changes: An Insider's View* 2004

(Use 22534 in conjunction with 22532 and 22533)

Anterior or Anterolateral Approach Technique

Procedure codes 22554-22558 are for SINGLE interspace; for additional interspaces, use 22585. A vertebral interspace is the non-bony compartment between two adjacent vertebral bodies, which contains the intervertebral disc, and includes the nucleus pulposus, annulus fibrosus, and two cartilagenous endplates.

For the following codes, when two surgeons work together as primary surgeons performing distinct part(s) of an anterior interbody arthrodesis, each surgeon should report his/her distinct operative work by appending modifier 62 to the procedure code. In this situation, modifier 62 may be appended to the procedure code(s) 22548-22558 and, as appropriate, to the associated additional interspace add-on code 22585 as long as both surgeons continue to work together as primary surgeons.

22548 Arthrodesis, anterior transoral or extraoral technique, clivus-C1-C2 (atlas-axis), with or without excision of odontoid process

⮕ *CPT Assistant* Spring 93:36, Feb 96:7, Sep 97:8, Sep 00:10, Feb 02:4

(For intervertebral disc excision by laminotomy or laminectomy, see 63020-63042)

Arthrodesis (Anterior Transoral Technique)
22548

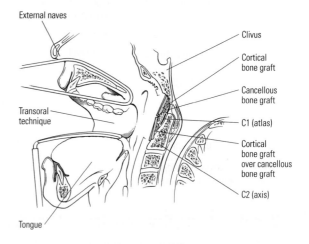

22554 Arthrodesis, anterior interbody technique, including minimal discectomy to prepare interspace (other than for decompression); cervical below C2

⮕ *CPT Assistant* Spring 93:36, Sep 97:8, Sep 00:10, Jan 01:12, Feb 02:4

22556 thoracic

⮕ *CPT Assistant* Spring 93:36, Jul 96:7, Sep 97:8, Sep 00:10, Feb 02:4

Anterior Approach for Cervical Fusion
22554

An example of an exposure technique used to reach anterior cervical vertebrae for spinal procedures (eg, discectomy, arthrodesis, spinal instrumentation)

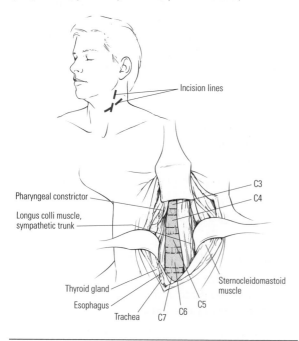

- Incision lines
- Pharyngeal constrictor
- Longus colli muscle, sympathetic trunk
- C3
- C4
- Thyroid gland
- Esophagus
- Sternocleidomastoid muscle
- Trachea
- C7
- C6
- C5

22558   lumbar

⊙ *CPT Assistant* Spring 93:36, Mar 96:6, Jul 96:7, Sep 97:8, Sep 00:10, Feb 02:4

Anterior Approach for Lumbar Fusion (Anterior Retroperitoneal Exposure)
22558

An example of an exposure technique used to reach anterior lumbar vertebrae for spinal procedures (eg, discectomy, arthrodesis, spinal instrumentation)

Incision line and approach to lumbar spine

- Body of vertebra
- Sympathetic trunk
- Psoas major muscle

+ 22585   each additional interspace (List separately in addition to code for primary procedure)

⊙ *CPT Assistant* Spring 93:36, Feb 96:6, Mar 96:6, Sep 97:8, Sep 00:10, Feb 02:4

(Use 22585 in conjunction with 22554, 22556, 22558)

Posterior, Posterolateral or Lateral Transverse Process Technique

►To report instrumentation procedures, see 22840-22855. (Report in addition to code[s] for the definitive procedure[s].) Do not append modifier 62 to spinal instrumentation codes 22840-22848 and 22850-22852.

To report bone graft procedures, see 20930-20938. (Report in addition to code[s] for the definitive procedure[s].) Do not append modifier 62 to bone graft codes 20900-20938.◄

A vertebral segment describes the basic constituent part into which the spine may be divided. It represents a single complete vertebral bone with its associated articular processes and laminae. A vertebral interspace is the non-bony compartment between two adjacent vertebral bodies which contains the intervertebral disc, and includes the nucleus pulposus, annulus fibrosus, and two cartilagenous endplates.

22590   Arthrodesis, posterior technique, craniocervical (occiput-C2)

⊙ *CPT Assistant* Spring 93:36, Sep 97:8

22595   Arthrodesis, posterior technique, atlas-axis (C1-C2)

⊙ *CPT Assistant* Spring 93:36, Sep 97:8

22600   Arthrodesis, posterior or posterolateral technique, single level; cervical below C2 segment

⊙ *CPT Assistant* Spring 93:36, Sep 97:8

22610   thoracic (with or without lateral transverse technique)

⊙ *CPT Assistant* Spring 93:36, Sep 97:8

22612   lumbar (with or without lateral transverse technique)

⊙ *CPT Assistant* Spring 93:36, Mar 96:7, Sep 97:8, 11

+ 22614   each additional vertebral segment (List separately in addition to code for primary procedure)

⊙ *CPT Assistant* Feb 96:6, Mar 96:7

(Use 22614 in conjunction with 22600, 22610, 22612)

22630   Arthrodesis, posterior interbody technique, including laminectomy and/or discectomy to prepare interspace (other than for decompression), single interspace; lumbar

⊙ *CPT Assistant* Spring 93:36, Sep 97:8, Nov 99:11, Dec 99:2, Jan 01:12; *CPT Changes: An Insider's View* 2000

+ 22632   each additional interspace (List separately in addition to code for primary procedure)

⊙ *CPT Assistant* Feb 96:6, Sep 97:8, Dec 99:2

(Use 22632 in conjunction with 22630)

Spine Deformity (eg, Scoliosis, Kyphosis)

▶To report instrumentation procedures, see 22840-22855. (Report in addition to code[s] for the definitive procedure[s].) Do not append modifier 62 to spinal instrumentation codes 22840-22848 and 22850-22852.

To report bone graft procedures, see 20930-20938. (Report in addition to code[s] for the definitive procedure[s].) Do not append modifier 62 to bone graft codes 20900-20938.◄

A vertebral segment describes the basic constituent part into which the spine may be divided. It represents a single complete vertebral bone with its associated articular processes and laminae.

For the following codes, when two surgeons work together as primary surgeons performing distinct part(s) of an arthrodesis for spinal deformity, each surgeon should report his/her distinct operative work by appending modifier 62 to the procedure code. In this situation, modifier 62 may be appended to procedure code(s) 22800-22819 as long as both surgeons continue to work together as primary surgeons.

22800 Arthrodesis, posterior, for spinal deformity, with or without cast; up to 6 vertebral segments

22802 7 to 12 vertebral segments
  ➲ CPT Assistant Mar 96:10

22804 13 or more vertebral segments

22808 Arthrodesis, anterior, for spinal deformity, with or without cast; 2 to 3 vertebral segments
  ➲ CPT Assistant Feb 02:4

22810 4 to 7 vertebral segments
  ➲ CPT Assistant Mar 96:10, Sep 97:8, Feb 02:4

22812 8 or more vertebral segments
  ➲ CPT Assistant Feb 02:4

22818 Kyphectomy, circumferential exposure of spine and resection of vertebral segment(s) (including body and posterior elements); single or 2 segments
  ➲ CPT Assistant Nov 97:14

22819 3 or more segments
  ➲ CPT Assistant Nov 97:14

(To report arthrodesis, see 22800-22804 and add modifier 51)

Exploration

▶To report instrumentation procedures, see 22840-22855. (Codes 22840-22848 and 22851 are reported in conjunction with code[s] for the definitive procedure[s]. When instrumentation reinsertion or removal is reported in conjunction with other definitive procedures including arthrodesis, decompression, and exploration of fusion, append modifier 51 to 22849, 22850, 22852 and 22855.) Code 22849 should not be reported with 22850, 22852, and 22855 at the same spinal levels. To report exploration of fusion, see 22830. (When exploration is reported in conjunction with other definitive procedures, including arthrodesis and decompression, append modifier 51 to 22830.)◄

(To report bone graft procedures, see 20930-20938)

22830 Exploration of spinal fusion
  ➲ CPT Assistant Sep 97:11

Spinal Instrumentation

Segmental instrumentation is defined as fixation at each end of the construct and at least one additional interposed bony attachment.

Non-segmental instrumentation is defined as fixation at each end of the construct and may span several vertebral segments without attachment to the intervening segments.

▶Insertion of spinal instrumentation is reported separately and in addition to arthrodesis. Instrumentation procedure codes 22840-22848 and 22851 are reported in addition to the definitive procedure(s). Do not append modifier 62 to spinal instrumentation codes 22840-22848 and 22850-22852.

To report bone graft procedures, see 20930-20938. (Report in addition to code[s] for definitive procedure[s].) Do not append modifier 62 to bone graft codes 20900-20938.◄

A vertebral segment describes the basic constituent part into which the spine may be divided. It represents a single complete vertebral bone with its associated articular processes and laminae. A vertebral interspace is the non-bony compartment between two adjacent vertebral bodies, which contains the intervertebral disc, and includes the nucleus pulposus, annulus fibrosus, and two cartilagenous endplates.

▶Codes 22849, 22850, 22852, and 22855 are subject to modifier 51 if reported with other definitive procedure(s), including arthrodesis, decompression, and exploration of fusion. Code 22849 should not be reported with 22850, 22852, and 22855 at the same spinal levels.◄

+▲ 22840 Posterior non-segmental instrumentation (eg, Harrington rod technique, pedicle fixation across one interspace, atlantoaxial transarticular screw fixation, sublaminar wiring at C1, facet screw fixation) (List separately in addition to code for primary procedure)

➲ *CPT Assistant* Feb 96:6, Jul 96:10, Sep 97:8, Nov 99:12, Feb 02:6; *CPT Changes: An Insider's View* 2000, 2008

▶(Use 22840 in conjunction with 22100-22102, 22110-22114, 22206-22208, 22210-22214, 22220-22224, 22305-22327, 22532-22533, 22548-22558, 22590-22612, 22630, 22800-22812, 63001-63030, 63040-63042, 63045-63047, 63050-63056, 63064, 63075, 63077, 63081, 63085, 63087, 63090, 63101-63102, 63170-63290, 63300-63307)◀

▶(For insertion of posterior spinous process distraction devices, see 0171T, 0172T)◀

Non-Segmental Spinal Instrumentation
22840

Fixation at each end of the construct

+▲ 22841 Internal spinal fixation by wiring of spinous processes (List separately in addition to code for primary procedure)

➲ *CPT Assistant* Feb 96:6, Sep 97:8, Feb 02:6; *CPT Changes: An Insider's View* 2008

▶(Use 22841 in conjunction with 22100-22102, 22110-22114, 22206-22208, 22210-22214, 22220-22224, 22305-22327, 22532-22533, 22548-22558, 22590-22612, 22630, 22800-22812, 63001-63030, 63040-63042, 63045-63047, 63050-63056, 63064, 63075, 63077, 63081, 63085, 63087, 63090, 63101-63102, 63170-63290, 63300-63307)◀

+▲ 22842 Posterior segmental instrumentation (eg, pedicle fixation, dual rods with multiple hooks and sublaminar wires); 3 to 6 vertebral segments (List separately in addition to code for primary procedure)

➲ *CPT Assistant* Feb 96:6, Mar 96:7, Sep 97:8, Feb 02:6; *CPT Changes: An Insider's View* 2008

▶(Use 22842 in conjunction with 22100-22102, 22110-22114, 22206-22208, 22210-22214, 22220-22224, 22305-22327, 22532-22533, 22548-22558, 22590-22612, 22630, 22800-22812, 63001-63030, 63040-63042, 63045-63047, 63050-63056, 63064, 63075, 63077, 63081, 63085, 63087, 63090, 63101-63102, 63170-63290, 63300-63307)◀

+▲ 22843 7 to 12 vertebral segments (List separately in addition to code for primary procedure)

➲ *CPT Assistant* Feb 96:6, Sep 97:8, Feb 02:6; *CPT Changes: An Insider's View* 2008

▶(Use 22843 in conjunction with 22100-22102, 22110-22114, 22206-22208, 22210-22214, 22220-22224, 22305-22327, 22532-22533, 22548-22558, 22590-22612, 22630, 22800-22812, 63001-63030, 63040-63042, 63045-63047, 63050-63056, 63064, 63075, 63077, 63081, 63085, 63087, 63090, 63101-63102, 63170-63290, 63300-63307)◀

+▲ 22844 13 or more vertebral segments (List separately in addition to code for primary procedure)

➲ *CPT Assistant* Feb 96:6, Sep 97:8, Feb 02:6; *CPT Changes: An Insider's View* 2008

▶(Use 22844 in conjunction with 22100-22102, 22110-22114, 22206-22208, 22210-22214, 22220-22224, 22305-22327, 22532-22533, 22548-22558, 22590-22612, 22630, 22800-22812, 63001-63030, 63040-63042, 63045-63047, 63050-63056, 63064, 63075, 63077, 63081, 63085, 63087, 63090, 63101-63102, 63170-63290, 63300-63307)◀

Segmental Spinal Instrumentation
22842-22844

Fixation at each end of the construct and at least one additional interposed bony attachment

---

▲ =Revised code   ● =New code   ▶ ◀ =Contains new or revised text   ⊘ =Modifier 51 exempt

+▲ 22845 Anterior instrumentation; 2 to 3 vertebral segments (List separately in addition to code for primary procedure)

➔ *CPT Assistant* Feb 96:6, Mar 96:10, Jul 96:7, 10, Sep 97:8, Feb 02:6; *CPT Changes: An Insider's View* 2008

▶(Use 22845 in conjunction with 22100-22102, 22110-22114, 22206-22208, 22210-22214, 22220-22224, 22305-22327, 22532-22533, 22548-22558, 22590-22612, 22630, 22800-22812, 63001-63030, 63040-63042, 63045-63047, 63050-63056, 63064, 63075, 63077, 63081, 63085, 63087, 63090, 63101-63102, 63170-63290, 63300-63307)◀

+▲ 22846 4 to 7 vertebral segments (List separately in addition to code for primary procedure)

➔ *CPT Assistant* Feb 96:6, Sep 97:8, Feb 02:6; *CPT Changes: An Insider's View* 2008

▶(Use 22846 in conjunction with 22100-22102, 22110-22114, 22206-22208, 22210-22214, 22220-22224, 22305-22327, 22532-22533, 22548-22558, 22590-22612, 22630, 22800-22812, 63001-63030, 63040-63042, 63045-63047, 63050-63056, 63064, 63075, 63077, 63081, 63085, 63087, 63090, 63101-63102, 63170-63290, 63300-63307)◀

+▲ 22847 8 or more vertebral segments (List separately in addition to code for primary procedure)

➔ *CPT Assistant* Feb 96:6, Sep 97:8, Feb 02:6; *CPT Changes: An Insider's View* 2008

▶(Use 22847 in conjunction with 22100-22102, 22110-22114, 22206-22208, 22210-22214, 22220-22224, 22305-22327, 22532-22533, 22548-22558, 22590-22612, 22630, 22800-22812, 63001-63030, 63040-63042, 63045-63047, 63050-63056, 63064, 63075, 63077, 63081, 63085, 63087, 63090, 63101-63102, 63170-63290, 63300-63307)◀

+▲ 22848 Pelvic fixation (attachment of caudal end of instrumentation to pelvic bony structures) other than sacrum (List separately in addition to code for primary procedure)

➔ *CPT Assistant* Feb 96:6, Sep 97:8, Feb 02:6; *CPT Changes: An Insider's View* 2008

▶(Use 22848 in conjunction with 22100-22102, 22110-22114, 22206-22208, 22210-22214, 22220-22224, 22305-22327, 22532-22533, 22548-22558, 22590-22612, 22630, 22800-22812, 63001-63030, 63040-63042, 63045-63047, 63050-63056, 63064, 63075, 63077, 63081, 63085, 63087, 63090, 63101-63102, 63170-63290, 63300-63307)◀

22849 Reinsertion of spinal fixation device

➔ *CPT Assistant* Feb 96:6, Sep 97:8, Feb 02:6, Nov 02:3

22850 Removal of posterior nonsegmental instrumentation (eg, Harrington rod)

➔ *CPT Assistant* Feb 96:6, Sep 97:8, Feb 02:6

+▲ 22851 Application of intervertebral biomechanical device(s) (eg, synthetic cage(s), threaded bone dowel(s), methylmethacrylate) to vertebral defect or interspace (List separately in addition to code for primary procedure)

➔ *CPT Assistant* Feb 96:6, Sep 97:8, Nov 99:12, Dec 99:2, May 00:11, Mar 01:2, Feb 02:6, Feb 05:14-15; *CPT Changes: An Insider's View* 2002, 2008

▶(Use 22851 in conjunction with 22100-22102, 22110-22114, 22206-22208, 22210-22214, 22220-22224, 22305-22327, 22532-22533, 22548-22558, 22590-22612, 22630, 22800-22812, 63001-63030, 63040-63042, 63045-63047, 63050-63056, 63064, 63075, 63077, 63081, 63085, 63087, 63090, 63101-63102, 63170-63290, 63300-63307)◀

▶(For insertion of posterior spinous process distraction devices, see 0171T, 0172T)◀

Spinal Prosthetic Devices
22851

Application of prosthetic device

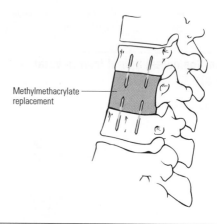

Methylmethacrylate replacement

22852 Removal of posterior segmental instrumentation

➔ *CPT Assistant* Feb 96:6, Sep 97:8, Feb 02:6, May 06:16

22855 Removal of anterior instrumentation

➔ *CPT Assistant* Feb 96:6, Sep 97:8, Feb 02:6, Nov 02:2

22857 Total disc arthroplasty (artificial disc), anterior approach, including discectomy to prepare interspace (other than for decompression), lumbar, single interspace

➔ *CPT Changes: An Insider's View* 2007

(Do not report 22857 in conjunction with 22558, 22845, 22851, 49010 when performed at the same level)

(For additional interspace, use Category III code 0163T)

22862 Revision including replacement of total disc arthroplasty (artificial disc) anterior approach, lumbar, single interspace

➔ *CPT Changes: An Insider's View* 2007

(Do not report 22862 in conjunction with 22558, 22845, 22851, 22865, 49010 when performed at the same level)

(For additional interspace, use Category III code 0165T)

22865 Removal of total disc arthroplasty (artificial disc), anterior approach, lumbar, single interspace

➔ *CPT Changes: An Insider's View* 2007

(Do not report 22865 in conjunction with 49010)

(For additional interspace, see Category III code 0164T)

(22857-22865 include fluoroscopy when performed)

(For decompression, see 63001-63048)

Other Procedures

22899   Unlisted procedure, spine
➜ *CPT Assistant* May 00:11, Sep 00:10, Jul 06:19

Abdomen

Excision

22900   Excision, abdominal wall tumor, subfascial (eg, desmoid)

Other Procedures

22999   Unlisted procedure, abdomen, musculoskeletal system

Shoulder

The area known as the shoulder is made up of the clavicle, scapula, humerus head and neck, sterno-clavicular joint, acromioclavicular joint, and shoulder joint.

Incision

23000   Removal of subdeltoid calcareous deposits, open
➜ *CPT Changes: An Insider's View* 2002, 2003

(For arthroscopic removal of bursal deposits, use 29999)

23020   Capsular contracture release (eg, Sever type procedure)

(For incision and drainage procedures, superficial, see 10040-10160)

23030   Incision and drainage, shoulder area; deep abscess or hematoma

23031   infected bursa

23035   Incision, bone cortex (eg, osteomyelitis or bone abscess), shoulder area

23040   Arthrotomy, glenohumeral joint, including exploration, drainage, or removal of foreign body
➜ *CPT Assistant* Nov 98:8

23044   Arthrotomy, acromioclavicular, sternoclavicular joint, including exploration, drainage, or removal of foreign body
➜ *CPT Assistant* Nov 98:8

Excision

23065   Biopsy, soft tissue of shoulder area; superficial

23066   deep

(For needle biopsy of soft tissue, use 20206)

23075   Excision, soft tissue tumor, shoulder area; subcutaneous
➜ *CPT Assistant* Summer 92:22, Nov 98:8

23076   deep, subfascial, or intramuscular
➜ *CPT Assistant* Summer 92:22

23077   Radical resection of tumor (eg, malignant neoplasm), soft tissue of shoulder area

23100   Arthrotomy, glenohumeral joint, including biopsy
➜ *CPT Assistant* Nov 98:8

23101   Arthrotomy, acromioclavicular joint or sternoclavicular joint, including biopsy and/or excision of torn cartilage
➜ *CPT Assistant* Nov 98:8

23105   Arthrotomy; glenohumeral joint, with synovectomy, with or without biopsy
➜ *CPT Assistant* Nov 98:8

23106   sternoclavicular joint, with synovectomy, with or without biopsy

23107   Arthrotomy, glenohumeral joint, with joint exploration, with or without removal of loose or foreign body

23120   Claviculectomy; partial

(For arthroscopic procedure, use 29824)

23125   total

23130   Acromioplasty or acromionectomy, partial, with or without coracoacromial ligament release
➜ *CPT Assistant* Aug 01:11

23140   Excision or curettage of bone cyst or benign tumor of clavicle or scapula;

23145   with autograft (includes obtaining graft)

23146   with allograft

23150   Excision or curettage of bone cyst or benign tumor of proximal humerus;

23155   with autograft (includes obtaining graft)

23156   with allograft

23170   Sequestrectomy (eg, for osteomyelitis or bone abscess), clavicle

23172   Sequestrectomy (eg, for osteomyelitis or bone abscess), scapula

23174   Sequestrectomy (eg, for osteomyelitis or bone abscess), humeral head to surgical neck

23180   Partial excision (craterization, saucerization, or diaphysectomy) bone (eg, osteomyelitis), clavicle
➜ *CPT Assistant* Nov 98:9

23182   Partial excision (craterization, saucerization, or diaphysectomy) bone (eg, osteomyelitis), scapula
➜ *CPT Assistant* Nov 98:9

23184   Partial excision (craterization, saucerization, or diaphysectomy) bone (eg, osteomyelitis), proximal humerus
➜ *CPT Assistant* Nov 98:9

23190   Ostectomy of scapula, partial (eg, superior medial angle)

23195   Resection, humeral head

(For replacement with implant, use 23470)

23200   Radical resection for tumor; clavicle

23210   scapula

23220 Radical resection of bone tumor, proximal humerus;
➜ *CPT Assistant* Nov 98:8

23221 with autograft (includes obtaining graft)

23222 with prosthetic replacement

Introduction or Removal

(For arthrocentesis or needling of bursa, use 20610)

(For K-wire or pin insertion or removal, see 20650, 20670, 20680)

23330 Removal of foreign body, shoulder; subcutaneous
➜ *CPT Assistant* Aug 99:3

23331 deep (eg, Neer hemiarthroplasty removal)
➜ *CPT Assistant* Aug 99:3

23332 complicated (eg, total shoulder)
➜ *CPT Assistant* Jun 96:10, Nov 98:8, Aug 99:3

23350 Injection procedure for shoulder arthrography or enhanced CT/MRI shoulder arthrography
➜ *CPT Assistant* Jul 01:3; *CPT Changes: An Insider's View* 2002
➜ *Clinical Examples in Radiology* Spring 05:5

(For radiographic arthrography, radiological supervision and interpretation, use 73040. Fluoroscopy [77002] is inclusive of radiographic arthrography)

(When fluoroscopic guided injection is performed for enhanced CT arthrography, use 23350, 77002, and 73201 or 73202)

(When fluoroscopic guided injection is performed for enhanced MR arthrography, use 23350, 77002, and 73222 or 73223)

(For enhanced CT or enhanced MRI arthrography, use 77002 and either 73201, 73202, 73222, or 73223)

(To report biopsy of the shoulder and joint, see 29805-29826)

Repair, Revision, and/or Reconstruction

23395 Muscle transfer, any type, shoulder or upper arm; single

23397 multiple

23400 Scapulopexy (eg, Sprengels deformity or for paralysis)

23405 Tenotomy, shoulder area; single tendon
➜ *CPT Assistant* Nov 98:8

23406 multiple tendons through same incision
➜ *CPT Assistant* Nov 98:8

23410 Repair of ruptured musculotendinous cuff (eg, rotator cuff) open; acute
➜ *CPT Assistant* Aug 01:11, Feb 02:11; *CPT Changes: An Insider's View* 2003

23412 chronic
➜ *CPT Assistant* Feb 02:11

(For arthroscopic procedure, use 29827)

23415 Coracoacromial ligament release, with or without acromioplasty

(For arthroscopic procedure, use 29826)

23420 Reconstruction of complete shoulder (rotator) cuff avulsion, chronic (includes acromioplasty)
➜ *CPT Assistant* Feb 02:11, Oct 05:23

23430 Tenodesis of long tendon of biceps

►(For arthroscopic biceps tenodesis, use 29828)◄

23440 Resection or transplantation of long tendon of biceps

23450 Capsulorrhaphy, anterior; Putti-Platt procedure or Magnuson type operation

(To report arthroscopic thermal capsulorrhaphy, use 29999)

23455 with labral repair (eg, Bankart procedure)
➜ *CPT Assistant* Nov 98:8

(For arthroscopic procedure, use 29806)

23460 Capsulorrhaphy, anterior, any type; with bone block

23462 with coracoid process transfer

(To report open thermal capsulorrhaphy, use 23929)

23465 Capsulorrhaphy, glenohumeral joint, posterior, with or without bone block
➜ *CPT Assistant* Nov 98:8

(For sternoclavicular and acromioclavicular reconstruction, see 23530, 23550)

23466 Capsulorrhaphy, glenohumeral joint, any type multi-directional instability
➜ *CPT Assistant* Nov 98:8

23470 Arthroplasty, glenohumeral joint; hemiarthroplasty
➜ *CPT Assistant* Nov 98:8

23472 total shoulder (glenoid and proximal humeral replacement (eg, total shoulder))
➜ *CPT Assistant* Jun 96:10, Nov 98:8

(For removal of total shoulder implants, see 23331, 23332)

(For osteotomy, proximal humerus, use 24400)

23480 Osteotomy, clavicle, with or without internal fixation;

23485 with bone graft for nonunion or malunion (includes obtaining graft and/or necessary fixation)

23490 Prophylactic treatment (nailing, pinning, plating or wiring) with or without methylmethacrylate; clavicle

23491 proximal humerus
➜ *CPT Assistant* Nov 98:8

Fracture and/or Dislocation

23500 Closed treatment of clavicular fracture; without manipulation

23505 with manipulation

▲ **23515**   Open treatment of clavicular fracture, includes internal fixation, when performed
➔ *CPT Changes: An Insider's View* 2008

23520   Closed treatment of sternoclavicular dislocation; without manipulation

23525   with manipulation

23530   Open treatment of sternoclavicular dislocation, acute or chronic;

23532   with fascial graft (includes obtaining graft)

23540   Closed treatment of acromioclavicular dislocation; without manipulation

23545   with manipulation

23550   Open treatment of acromioclavicular dislocation, acute or chronic;

23552   with fascial graft (includes obtaining graft)

23570   Closed treatment of scapular fracture; without manipulation

23575   with manipulation, with or without skeletal traction (with or without shoulder joint involvement)

23585   Open treatment of scapular fracture (body, glenoid or acromion) with or without internal fixation
➔ *CPT Assistant* Oct 04:10

23600   Closed treatment of proximal humeral (surgical or anatomical neck) fracture; without manipulation

23605   with manipulation, with or without skeletal traction

▲ **23615**   Open treatment of proximal humeral (surgical or anatomical neck) fracture, includes internal fixation, when performed, includes repair of tuberosity(s), when performed;
➔ *CPT Changes: An Insider's View* 2008

▲ **23616**   with proximal humeral prosthetic replacement
➔ *CPT Changes: An Insider's View* 2008

23620   Closed treatment of greater humeral tuberosity fracture; without manipulation
➔ *CPT Assistant* Nov 98:8

23625   with manipulation

▲ **23630**   Open treatment of greater humeral tuberosity fracture, includes internal fixation, when performed
➔ *CPT Assistant* Nov 98:8; *CPT Changes: An Insider's View* 2008

23650   Closed treatment of shoulder dislocation, with manipulation; without anesthesia

23655   requiring anesthesia

23660   Open treatment of acute shoulder dislocation
➔ *CPT Assistant* Feb 96:5

(Repairs for recurrent dislocations, see 23450-23466)

23665   Closed treatment of shoulder dislocation, with fracture of greater humeral tuberosity, with manipulation
➔ *CPT Assistant* Nov 98:8

▲ **23670**   Open treatment of shoulder dislocation, with fracture of greater humeral tuberosity, includes internal fixation, when performed
➔ *CPT Assistant* Nov 98:8; *CPT Changes: An Insider's View* 2008

23675   Closed treatment of shoulder dislocation, with surgical or anatomical neck fracture, with manipulation

▲ **23680**   Open treatment of shoulder dislocation, with surgical or anatomical neck fracture, includes internal fixation, when performed
➔ *CPT Changes: An Insider's View* 2008

Manipulation

23700   Manipulation under anesthesia, shoulder joint, including application of fixation apparatus (dislocation excluded)
➔ *CPT Assistant* Jan 99:10, Apr 05:14

Arthrodesis

23800   Arthrodesis, glenohumeral joint;
➔ *CPT Assistant* Nov 98:8

23802   with autogenous graft (includes obtaining graft)

Amputation

23900   Interthoracoscapular amputation (forequarter)

23920   Disarticulation of shoulder;

23921   secondary closure or scar revision

Other Procedures

23929   Unlisted procedure, shoulder

Humerus (Upper Arm) and Elbow

The elbow area includes the head and neck of the radius and olecranon process.

Incision

(For incision and drainage procedures, superficial, see 10040-10160)

23930   Incision and drainage, upper arm or elbow area; deep abscess or hematoma

23931   bursa
➔ *CPT Assistant* Nov 98:8

23935   Incision, deep, with opening of bone cortex (eg, for osteomyelitis or bone abscess), humerus or elbow

24000   Arthrotomy, elbow, including exploration, drainage, or removal of foreign body
➔ *CPT Assistant* Nov 98:8-9

24006   Arthrotomy of the elbow, with capsular excision for capsular release (separate procedure)

Excision

24065 Biopsy, soft tissue of upper arm or elbow area; superficial

24066   deep (subfascial or intramuscular)

(For needle biopsy of soft tissue, use 20206)

24075 Excision, tumor, soft tissue of upper arm or elbow area; subcutaneous
➲ *CPT Changes: An Insider's View* 2002

24076   deep (subfascial or intramuscular)

24077 Radical resection of tumor (eg, malignant neoplasm), soft tissue of upper arm or elbow area

24100 Arthrotomy, elbow; with synovial biopsy only

24101   with joint exploration, with or without biopsy, with or without removal of loose or foreign body

24102   with synovectomy

24105 Excision, olecranon bursa

24110 Excision or curettage of bone cyst or benign tumor, humerus;

24115   with autograft (includes obtaining graft)

24116   with allograft

24120 Excision or curettage of bone cyst or benign tumor of head or neck of radius or olecranon process;

24125   with autograft (includes obtaining graft)

24126   with allograft

24130 Excision, radial head

(For replacement with implant, use 24366)

24134 Sequestrectomy (eg, for osteomyelitis or bone abscess), shaft or distal humerus

24136 Sequestrectomy (eg, for osteomyelitis or bone abscess), radial head or neck

24138 Sequestrectomy (eg, for osteomyelitis or bone abscess), olecranon process

24140 Partial excision (craterization, saucerization, or diaphysectomy) bone (eg, osteomyelitis), humerus
➲ *CPT Assistant* Nov 98:9

24145 Partial excision (craterization, saucerization, or diaphysectomy) bone (eg, osteomyelitis), radial head or neck
➲ *CPT Assistant* Nov 98:9

24147 Partial excision (craterization, saucerization, or diaphysectomy) bone (eg, osteomyelitis), olecranon process
➲ *CPT Assistant* Nov 98:9

24149 Radical resection of capsule, soft tissue, and heterotopic bone, elbow, with contracture release (separate procedure)
➲ *CPT Assistant* Nov 96:4

(For capsular and soft tissue release only, use 24006)

24150 Radical resection for tumor, shaft or distal humerus;

24151   with autograft (includes obtaining graft)

24152 Radical resection for tumor, radial head or neck;

24153   with autograft (includes obtaining graft)

24155 Resection of elbow joint (arthrectomy)

Introduction or Removal

(For K-wire or pin insertion or removal, see 20650, 20670, 20680)

(For arthrocentesis or needling of bursa or joint, use 20605)

24160 Implant removal; elbow joint

24164   radial head

24200 Removal of foreign body, upper arm or elbow area; subcutaneous

24201   deep (subfascial or intramuscular)
➲ *CPT Assistant* Nov 98:8

24220 Injection procedure for elbow arthrography

(For radiological supervision and interpretation, use 73085. Do not report 77002 in conjunction with 73085)

(For injection for tennis elbow, use 20550)

Repair, Revision, and/or Reconstruction

24300 Manipulation, elbow, under anesthesia
➲ *CPT Changes: An Insider's View* 2002

(For application of external fixation, see 20690 or 20692)

24301 Muscle or tendon transfer, any type, upper arm or elbow, single (excluding 24320-24331)

24305 Tendon lengthening, upper arm or elbow, each tendon
➲ *CPT Assistant* Nov 98:8

24310 Tenotomy, open, elbow to shoulder, each tendon
➲ *CPT Assistant* Nov 98:8

24320 Tenoplasty, with muscle transfer, with or without free graft, elbow to shoulder, single (Seddon-Brookes type procedure)

24330 Flexor-plasty, elbow (eg, Steindler type advancement);

24331   with extensor advancement

24332 Tenolysis, triceps
➲ *CPT Changes: An Insider's View* 2002

24340 Tenodesis of biceps tendon at elbow (separate procedure)

24341 Repair, tendon or muscle, upper arm or elbow, each tendon or muscle, primary or secondary (excludes rotator cuff)
➲ *CPT Assistant* Nov 96:4

24342 Reinsertion of ruptured biceps or triceps tendon, distal, with or without tendon graft
➲ *CPT Assistant* Nov 96:4

24343 Repair lateral collateral ligament, elbow, with local tissue
→ *CPT Changes: An Insider's View* 2002

24344 Reconstruction lateral collateral ligament, elbow, with tendon graft (includes harvesting of graft)
→ *CPT Changes: An Insider's View* 2002

24345 Repair medial collateral ligament, elbow, with local tissue
→ *CPT Changes: An Insider's View* 2002

24346 Reconstruction medial collateral ligament, elbow, with tendon graft (includes harvesting of graft)
→ *CPT Changes: An Insider's View* 2002

▶(24350-24356 have been deleted. To report, see 24357-24359)◀

● **24357** Tenotomy, elbow, lateral or medial (eg, epicondylitis, tennis elbow, golfer's elbow); percutaneous
→ *CPT Changes: An Insider's View* 2008

● **24358** debridement, soft tissue and/or bone, open
→ *CPT Changes: An Insider's View* 2008

● **24359** debridement, soft tissue and/or bone, open with tendon repair or reattachment
→ *CPT Changes: An Insider's View* 2008

▶(Do not report 24357-24359 in conjunction with 29837, 29838)◀

24360 Arthroplasty, elbow; with membrane (eg, fascial)
→ *CPT Assistant* Nov 98:8

24361 with distal humeral prosthetic replacement

24362 with implant and fascia lata ligament reconstruction

24363 with distal humerus and proximal ulnar prosthetic replacement (eg, total elbow)

24365 Arthroplasty, radial head;

24366 with implant

24400 Osteotomy, humerus, with or without internal fixation

24410 Multiple osteotomies with realignment on intramedullary rod, humeral shaft (Sofield type procedure)

24420 Osteoplasty, humerus (eg, shortening or lengthening) (excluding 64876)

24430 Repair of nonunion or malunion, humerus; without graft (eg, compression technique)

24435 with iliac or other autograft (includes obtaining graft)

(For proximal radius and/or ulna, see 25400-25420)

24470 Hemiepiphyseal arrest (eg, cubitus varus or valgus, distal humerus)

24495 Decompression fasciotomy, forearm, with brachial artery exploration

24498 Prophylactic treatment (nailing, pinning, plating or wiring), with or without methylmethacrylate, humeral shaft
→ *CPT Assistant* Nov 98:8

Fracture and/or Dislocation

24500 Closed treatment of humeral shaft fracture; without manipulation

24505 with manipulation, with or without skeletal traction

24515 Open treatment of humeral shaft fracture with plate/screws, with or without cerclage

24516 Treatment of humeral shaft fracture, with insertion of intramedullary implant, with or without cerclage and/or locking screws
→ *CPT Assistant* Feb 96:4; *CPT Changes: An Insider's View* 2003

24530 Closed treatment of supracondylar or transcondylar humeral fracture, with or without intercondylar extension; without manipulation

24535 with manipulation, with or without skin or skeletal traction

24538 Percutaneous skeletal fixation of supracondylar or transcondylar humeral fracture, with or without intercondylar extension
→ *CPT Assistant* Winter 92:10

▲ **24545** Open treatment of humeral supracondylar or transcondylar fracture, includes internal fixation, when performed; without intercondylar extension
→ *CPT Changes: An Insider's View* 2008

▲ **24546** with intercondylar extension
→ *CPT Changes: An Insider's View* 2008

24560 Closed treatment of humeral epicondylar fracture, medial or lateral; without manipulation

24565 with manipulation

24566 Percutaneous skeletal fixation of humeral epicondylar fracture, medial or lateral, with manipulation

▲ **24575** Open treatment of humeral epicondylar fracture, medial or lateral, includes internal fixation, when performed
→ *CPT Changes: An Insider's View* 2008

24576 Closed treatment of humeral condylar fracture, medial or lateral; without manipulation

24577 with manipulation

▲ **24579** Open treatment of humeral condylar fracture, medial or lateral, includes internal fixation, when performed
→ *CPT Changes: An Insider's View* 2008

(To report closed treatment of fractures without manipulation, see 24530, 24560, 24576, 24650, 24670)

(To report closed treatment of fractures with manipulation, see 24535, 24565, 24577, 24675)

24582 Percutaneous skeletal fixation of humeral condylar fracture, medial or lateral, with manipulation

24586 Open treatment of periarticular fracture and/or dislocation of the elbow (fracture distal humerus and proximal ulna and/or proximal radius);

24587 with implant arthroplasty

(See also 24361)

24600 Treatment of closed elbow dislocation; without anesthesia

24605 requiring anesthesia

24615 Open treatment of acute or chronic elbow dislocation

24620 Closed treatment of Monteggia type of fracture dislocation at elbow (fracture proximal end of ulna with dislocation of radial head), with manipulation

▲ **24635** Open treatment of Monteggia type of fracture dislocation at elbow (fracture proximal end of ulna with dislocation of radial head), includes internal fixation, when performed

➔ *CPT Changes: An Insider's View* 2008

24640 Closed treatment of radial head subluxation in child, nursemaid elbow, with manipulation

24650 Closed treatment of radial head or neck fracture; without manipulation

24655 with manipulation

▲ **24665** Open treatment of radial head or neck fracture, includes internal fixation or radial head excision, when performed;

➔ *CPT Changes: An Insider's View* 2008

▲ **24666** with radial head prosthetic replacement

➔ *CPT Changes: An Insider's View* 2008

▲ **24670** Closed treatment of ulnar fracture, proximal end (eg, olecranon or coronoid process[es]); without manipulation

➔ *CPT Changes: An Insider's View* 2008

▲ **24675** with manipulation

➔ *CPT Changes: An Insider's View* 2008

▲ **24685** Open treatment of ulnar fracture, proximal end (eg, olecranon or coronoid process[es]), includes internal fixation, when performed

➔ *CPT Changes: An Insider's View* 2008

▶(Do not report 24685 in conjunction with 24100-24102)◀

Arthrodesis

24800 Arthrodesis, elbow joint; local

24802 with autogenous graft (includes obtaining graft)

Amputation

24900 Amputation, arm through humerus; with primary closure

24920 open, circular (guillotine)

24925 secondary closure or scar revision

24930 re-amputation

24931 with implant

24935 Stump elongation, upper extremity

24940 Cineplasty, upper extremity, complete procedure

Other Procedures

24999 Unlisted procedure, humerus or elbow

Forearm and Wrist

Radius, ulna, carpal bones, and joints.

Incision

25000 Incision, extensor tendon sheath, wrist (eg, deQuervains disease)

➔ *CPT Assistant* Nov 98:8

(For decompression median nerve or for carpal tunnel syndrome, use 64721)

25001 Incision, flexor tendon sheath, wrist (eg, flexor carpi radialis)

➔ *CPT Changes: An Insider's View* 2002

25020 Decompression fasciotomy, forearm and/or wrist, flexor OR extensor compartment; without debridement of nonviable muscle and/or nerve

➔ *CPT Changes: An Insider's View* 2002

25023 with debridement of nonviable muscle and/or nerve

(For decompression fasciotomy with brachial artery exploration, use 24495)

(For incision and drainage procedures, superficial, see 10060-10160)

(For debridement, see also 11000-11044)

25024 Decompression fasciotomy, forearm and/or wrist, flexor AND extensor compartment; without debridement of nonviable muscle and/or nerve

➔ *CPT Changes: An Insider's View* 2002

25025 with debridement of nonviable muscle and/or nerve

➔ *CPT Changes: An Insider's View* 2002

25028 Incision and drainage, forearm and/or wrist; deep abscess or hematoma

25031 bursa

➔ *CPT Assistant* Nov 98:9

25035 Incision, deep, bone cortex, forearm and/or wrist (eg, osteomyelitis or bone abscess)

25040 Arthrotomy, radiocarpal or midcarpal joint, with exploration, drainage, or removal of foreign body

Excision

25065 Biopsy, soft tissue of forearm and/or wrist; superficial

25066 deep (subfascial or intramuscular)

➔ *CPT Assistant* Nov 98:8

(For needle biopsy of soft tissue, use 20206)

25075 Excision, tumor, soft tissue of forearm and/or wrist area; subcutaneous

➔ *CPT Changes: An Insider's View* 2002

25076 deep (subfascial or intramuscular)

25077 Radical resection of tumor (eg, malignant neoplasm), soft tissue of forearm and/or wrist area

25085 Capsulotomy, wrist (eg, contracture)

25100 Arthrotomy, wrist joint; with biopsy

25101 with joint exploration, with or without biopsy, with or without removal of loose or foreign body

25105 with synovectomy

25107 Arthrotomy, distal radioulnar joint including repair of triangular cartilage, complex

25109 Excision of tendon, forearm and/or wrist, flexor or extensor, each
➔ *CPT Changes: An Insider's View* 2007

25110 Excision, lesion of tendon sheath, forearm and/or wrist

25111 Excision of ganglion, wrist (dorsal or volar); primary

25112 recurrent

(For hand or finger, use 26160)

25115 Radical excision of bursa, synovia of wrist, or forearm tendon sheaths (eg, tenosynovitis, fungus, Tbc, or other granulomas, rheumatoid arthritis); flexors

25116 extensors, with or without transposition of dorsal retinaculum

(For finger synovectomies, use 26145)

25118 Synovectomy, extensor tendon sheath, wrist, single compartment;

25119 with resection of distal ulna

25120 Excision or curettage of bone cyst or benign tumor of radius or ulna (excluding head or neck of radius and olecranon process);

(For head or neck of radius or olecranon process, see 24120-24126)

25125 with autograft (includes obtaining graft)

25126 with allograft

25130 Excision or curettage of bone cyst or benign tumor of carpal bones;

25135 with autograft (includes obtaining graft)

25136 with allograft

25145 Sequestrectomy (eg, for osteomyelitis or bone abscess), forearm and/or wrist

25150 Partial excision (craterization, saucerization, or diaphysectomy) of bone (eg, for osteomyelitis); ulna

25151 radius

(For head or neck of radius or olecranon process, see 24145, 24147)

25170 Radical resection for tumor, radius or ulna

25210 Carpectomy; one bone

(For carpectomy with implant, see 25441-25445)

25215 all bones of proximal row

25230 Radial styloidectomy (separate procedure)

25240 Excision distal ulna partial or complete (eg, Darrach type or matched resection)

(For implant replacement, distal ulna, use 25442)

(For obtaining fascia for interposition, see 20920, 20922)

Introduction or Removal

(For K-wire, pin or rod insertion or removal, see 20650, 20670, 20680)

25246 Injection procedure for wrist arthrography

(For radiological supervision and interpretation, use 73115. Do not report 77002 in conjunction with 73115)

(For foreign body removal, superficial use 20520)

25248 Exploration with removal of deep foreign body, forearm or wrist

25250 Removal of wrist prosthesis; (separate procedure)

25251 complicated, including total wrist

25259 Manipulation, wrist, under anesthesia
➔ *CPT Assistant* Jan 04:27, Jun 05:12; *CPT Changes: An Insider's View* 2002

(For application of external fixation, see 20690 or 20692)

Repair, Revision, and/or Reconstruction

25260 Repair, tendon or muscle, flexor, forearm and/or wrist; primary, single, each tendon or muscle

25263 secondary, single, each tendon or muscle

25265 secondary, with free graft (includes obtaining graft), each tendon or muscle

25270 Repair, tendon or muscle, extensor, forearm and/or wrist; primary, single, each tendon or muscle

25272 secondary, single, each tendon or muscle

25274 secondary, with free graft (includes obtaining graft), each tendon or muscle
➔ *CPT Changes: An Insider's View* 2002

25275 Repair, tendon sheath, extensor, forearm and/or wrist, with free graft (includes obtaining graft) (eg, for extensor carpi ulnaris subluxation)
➔ *CPT Changes: An Insider's View* 2002

25280 Lengthening or shortening of flexor or extensor tendon, forearm and/or wrist, single, each tendon

25290 Tenotomy, open, flexor or extensor tendon, forearm and/or wrist, single, each tendon

25295 Tenolysis, flexor or extensor tendon, forearm and/or wrist, single, each tendon
➔ *CPT Assistant* Apr 97:11, Aug 98:10

25300 Tenodesis at wrist; flexors of fingers

25301 extensors of fingers

25310 Tendon transplantation or transfer, flexor or extensor, forearm and/or wrist, single; each tendon
> *CPT Assistant Jun 02:11*

25312   with tendon graft(s) (includes obtaining graft), each tendon

25315 Flexor origin slide (eg, for cerebral palsy, Volkmann contracture), forearm and/or wrist;

25316   with tendon(s) transfer

25320 Capsulorrhaphy or reconstruction, wrist, open (eg, capsulodesis, ligament repair, tendon transfer or graft) (includes synovectomy, capsulotomy and open reduction) for carpal instability
> *CPT Changes: An Insider's View 2003*

25332 Arthroplasty, wrist, with or without interposition, with or without external or internal fixation
> *CPT Assistant Nov 96:5, Jan 05:8*

(For obtaining fascia for interposition, see 20920, 20922)

(For prosthetic replacement arthroplasty, see 25441-25446)

25335 Centralization of wrist on ulna (eg, radial club hand)

25337 Reconstruction for stabilization of unstable distal ulna or distal radioulnar joint, secondary by soft tissue stabilization (eg, tendon transfer, tendon graft or weave, or tenodesis) with or without open reduction of distal radioulnar joint

(For harvesting of fascia lata graft, see 20920, 20922)

25350 Osteotomy, radius; distal third

25355   middle or proximal third

25360 Osteotomy; ulna

25365   radius AND ulna

25370 Multiple osteotomies, with realignment on intramedullary rod (Sofield type procedure); radius OR ulna

25375   radius AND ulna

25390 Osteoplasty, radius OR ulna; shortening

25391   lengthening with autograft

25392 Osteoplasty, radius AND ulna; shortening (excluding 64876)

25393   lengthening with autograft

25394 Osteoplasty, carpal bone, shortening
> *CPT Changes: An Insider's View 2002*

25400 Repair of nonunion or malunion, radius OR ulna; without graft (eg, compression technique)

25405   with autograft (includes obtaining graft)
> *CPT Changes: An Insider's View 2002*

25415 Repair of nonunion or malunion, radius AND ulna; without graft (eg, compression technique)

25420   with autograft (includes obtaining graft)
> *CPT Changes: An Insider's View 2002*

25425 Repair of defect with autograft; radius OR ulna

25426   radius AND ulna

25430 Insertion of vascular pedicle into carpal bone (eg, Hori procedure)
> *CPT Changes: An Insider's View 2002*

25431 Repair of nonunion of carpal bone (excluding carpal scaphoid (navicular)) (includes obtaining graft and necessary fixation), each bone
> *CPT Changes: An Insider's View 2002*

25440 Repair of nonunion, scaphoid carpal (navicular) bone, with or without radial styloidectomy (includes obtaining graft and necessary fixation)
> *CPT Changes: An Insider's View 2002*

25441 Arthroplasty with prosthetic replacement; distal radius
> *CPT Assistant Jan 05:8-9*

25442   distal ulna
> *CPT Assistant Jan 05:8-9*

25443   scaphoid carpal (navicular)
> *CPT Assistant Jan 05:8-9; CPT Changes: An Insider's View 2002*

25444   lunate
> *CPT Assistant Jan 05:8, 10*

25445   trapezium
> *CPT Assistant Jan 05:8, 10*

25446   distal radius and partial or entire carpus (total wrist)
> *CPT Assistant Jan 05:8, 11*

25447 Arthroplasty, interposition, intercarpal or carpometacarpal joints
> *CPT Assistant Nov 98:8, Jan 05:8, 11-12*

(For wrist arthroplasty, use 25332)

25449 Revision of arthroplasty, including removal of implant, wrist joint

25450 Epiphyseal arrest by epiphysiodesis or stapling; distal radius OR ulna

25455   distal radius AND ulna

25490 Prophylactic treatment (nailing, pinning, plating or wiring) with or without methylmethacrylate; radius

25491   ulna

25492   radius AND ulna

Fracture and/or Dislocation

(For application of external fixation in addition to internal fixation, use 20690 and the appropriate internal fixation code)

25500 Closed treatment of radial shaft fracture; without manipulation

25505   with manipulation

▲ **25515** Open treatment of radial shaft fracture, includes internal fixation, when performed
> *CPT Changes: An Insider's View 2008*

25520 Closed treatment of radial shaft fracture and closed treatment of dislocation of distal radioulnar joint (Galeazzi fracture/dislocation)
➔ *CPT Changes: An Insider's View* 2002

▲ **25525** Open treatment of radial shaft fracture, includes internal fixation, when performed, and closed treatment of distal radioulnar joint dislocation (Galeazzi fracture/ dislocation), includes percutaneous skeletal fixation, when performed
➔ *CPT Changes: An Insider's View* 2008

▲ **25526** Open treatment of radial shaft fracture, includes internal fixation, when performed, and open treatment of distal radioulnar joint dislocation (Galeazzi fracture/ dislocation), includes internal fixation, when performed, includes repair of triangular fibrocartilage complex
➔ *CPT Changes: An Insider's View* 2002, 2008

25530 Closed treatment of ulnar shaft fracture; without manipulation
➔ *CPT Assistant* Apr 02:14

25535   with manipulation

▲ **25545** Open treatment of ulnar shaft fracture, includes internal fixation, when performed
➔ *CPT Assistant* Fall 93:23, Oct 99:5; *CPT Changes: An Insider's View* 2008

25560 Closed treatment of radial and ulnar shaft fractures; without manipulation

25565   with manipulation

▲ **25574** Open treatment of radial AND ulnar shaft fractures, with internal fixation, when performed; of radius OR ulna
➔ *CPT Assistant* Fall 93:23, Oct 99:5; *CPT Changes: An Insider's View* 2008

▲ **25575**   of radius AND ulna
➔ *CPT Changes: An Insider's View* 2008

25600 Closed treatment of distal radial fracture (eg, Colles or Smith type) or epiphyseal separation, includes closed treatment of fracture of ulnar styloid, when performed; without manipulation
➔ *CPT Changes: An Insider's View* 2007

25605   with manipulation

(Do not report 25600, 25605 in conjunction with 25650)

25606 Percutaneous skeletal fixation of distal radial fracture or epiphyseal separation
➔ *CPT Changes: An Insider's View* 2007

(Do not report 25606 in conjunction with 25650)

(For percutaneous treatment of ulnar styloid fracture, use 25651)

(For open treatment of ulnar styloid fracture, use 25652)

25607 Open treatment of distal radial extra-articular fracture or epiphyseal separation, with internal fixation
➔ *CPT Changes: An Insider's View* 2007

(Do not report 25607 in conjunction with 25650)

(For percutaneous treatment of ulnar styloid fracture, use 25651)

(For open treatment of ulnar styloid fracture, use 25652)

25608 Open treatment of distal radial intra-articular fracture or epiphyseal separation; with internal fixation of 2 fragments
➔ *CPT Changes: An Insider's View* 2007

(Do not report 25608 in conjunction with 25609)

25609   with internal fixation of 3 or more fragments
➔ *CPT Changes: An Insider's View* 2007

(Do not report 25608, 25609 in conjunction with 25650)

(For percutaneous treatment of ulnar styloid fracture, use 25651)

(For open treatment of ulnar styloid fracture, use 25652)

(25611 has been deleted. To report, use 25606)

(25620 has been deleted. To report, see 25607-25609)

25622 Closed treatment of carpal scaphoid (navicular) fracture; without manipulation

25624   with manipulation

▲ **25628** Open treatment of carpal scaphoid (navicular) fracture, includes internal fixation, when performed
➔ *CPT Changes: An Insider's View* 2008

25630 Closed treatment of carpal bone fracture (excluding carpal scaphoid (navicular)); without manipulation, each bone

25635   with manipulation, each bone

25645 Open treatment of carpal bone fracture (other than carpal scaphoid (navicular)), each bone
➔ *CPT Changes: An Insider's View* 2002

25650 Closed treatment of ulnar styloid fracture

(Do not report 25650 in conjunction with 25600, 25605, 25607-25609)

25651 Percutaneous skeletal fixation of ulnar styloid fracture
➔ *CPT Changes: An Insider's View* 2002

25652 Open treatment of ulnar styloid fracture
➔ *CPT Changes: An Insider's View* 2002

25660 Closed treatment of radiocarpal or intercarpal dislocation, one or more bones, with manipulation

25670 Open treatment of radiocarpal or intercarpal dislocation, one or more bones

25671 Percutaneous skeletal fixation of distal radioulnar dislocation
➔ *CPT Changes: An Insider's View* 2002

25675 Closed treatment of distal radioulnar dislocation with manipulation

25676 Open treatment of distal radioulnar dislocation, acute or chronic

25680 Closed treatment of trans-scaphoperilunar type of fracture dislocation, with manipulation

25685 Open treatment of trans-scaphoperilunar type of fracture dislocation

25690 Closed treatment of lunate dislocation, with manipulation

25695 Open treatment of lunate dislocation

Arthrodesis

25800 Arthrodesis, wrist; complete, without bone graft (includes radiocarpal and/or intercarpal and/or carpometacarpal joints)
→ *CPT Assistant* Nov 98:8

25805 with sliding graft

25810 with iliac or other autograft (includes obtaining graft)

25820 Arthrodesis, wrist; limited, without bone graft (eg, intercarpal or radiocarpal)
→ *CPT Assistant* Nov 98:8

25825 with autograft (includes obtaining graft)

25830 Arthrodesis, distal radioulnar joint with segmental resection of ulna, with or without bone graft (eg, Sauve-Kapandji procedure)
→ *CPT Assistant* Nov 98:8

Amputation

25900 Amputation, forearm, through radius and ulna;

25905 open, circular (guillotine)

25907 secondary closure or scar revision

25909 re-amputation

25915 Krukenberg procedure

25920 Disarticulation through wrist;

25922 secondary closure or scar revision

25924 re-amputation

25927 Transmetacarpal amputation;

25929 secondary closure or scar revision

25931 re-amputation

Other Procedures

25999 Unlisted procedure, forearm or wrist

Hand and Fingers

Incision

26010 Drainage of finger abscess; simple

26011 complicated (eg, felon)

26020 Drainage of tendon sheath, digit and/or palm, each

26025 Drainage of palmar bursa; single, bursa
→ *CPT Assistant* Nov 98:8

26030 multiple bursa
→ *CPT Assistant* Nov 98:8

26034 Incision, bone cortex, hand or finger (eg, osteomyelitis or bone abscess)
→ *CPT Assistant* Nov 98:8

26035 Decompression fingers and/or hand, injection injury (eg, grease gun)

26037 Decompressive fasciotomy, hand (excludes 26035)

(For injection injury, use 26035)

26040 Fasciotomy, palmar (eg, Dupuytren's contracture); percutaneous
→ *CPT Assistant* Nov 98:8

26045 open, partial

(For fasciectomy, see 26121-26125)

26055 Tendon sheath incision (eg, for trigger finger)

26060 Tenotomy, percutaneous, single, each digit

26070 Arthrotomy, with exploration, drainage, or removal of loose or foreign body; carpometacarpal joint
→ *CPT Assistant* Nov 98:10

26075 metacarpophalangeal joint, each

26080 interphalangeal joint, each

Excision

26100 Arthrotomy with biopsy; carpometacarpal joint, each

26105 metacarpophalangeal joint, each

26110 interphalangeal joint, each

26115 Excision, tumor or vascular malformation, soft tissue of hand or finger; subcutaneous
→ *CPT Changes: An Insider's View* 2002

26116 deep (subfascial or intramuscular)
→ *CPT Changes: An Insider's View* 2002

26117 Radical resection of tumor (eg, malignant neoplasm), soft tissue of hand or finger

26121 Fasciectomy, palm only, with or without Z-plasty, other local tissue rearrangement, or skin grafting (includes obtaining graft)

26123 Fasciectomy, partial palmar with release of single digit including proximal interphalangeal joint, with or without Z-plasty, other local tissue rearrangement, or skin grafting (includes obtaining graft);
→ *CPT Assistant* Jan 05:8

+ 26125 each additional digit (List separately in addition to code for primary procedure)
→ *CPT Assistant* Jan 05:8

(Use 26125 in conjunction with 26123)

(For fasciotomy, see 26040, 26045)

26130 Synovectomy, carpometacarpal joint

26135 Synovectomy, metacarpophalangeal joint including intrinsic release and extensor hood reconstruction, each digit

26140 Synovectomy, proximal interphalangeal joint, including extensor reconstruction, each interphalangeal joint

26145 Synovectomy, tendon sheath, radical (tenosynovectomy), flexor tendon, palm and/or finger, each tendon
> *CPT Assistant* Nov 98:8

(For tendon sheath synovectomies at wrist, see 25115, 25116)

26160 Excision of lesion of tendon sheath or joint capsule (eg, cyst, mucous cyst, or ganglion), hand or finger
> *CPT Changes: An Insider's View* 2002

(For wrist ganglion, see 25111, 25112)

(For trigger digit, use 26055)

26170 Excision of tendon, palm, flexor or extensor, single, each tendon
> *CPT Changes: An Insider's View* 2007

(Do not report 26170 in conjunction with 26390, 26415)

26180 Excision of tendon, finger, flexor or extensor, each tendon
> *CPT Assistant* Nov 98:8; *CPT Changes: An Insider's View* 2007

(Do not report 26180 in conjunction with 26390, 26415)

26185 Sesamoidectomy, thumb or finger (separate procedure)

26200 Excision or curettage of bone cyst or benign tumor of metacarpal;

26205 with autograft (includes obtaining graft)

26210 Excision or curettage of bone cyst or benign tumor of proximal, middle, or distal phalanx of finger;

26215 with autograft (includes obtaining graft)

26230 Partial excision (craterization, saucerization, or diaphysectomy) bone (eg, osteomyelitis); metacarpal

26235 proximal or middle phalanx of finger

26236 distal phalanx of finger

26250 Radical resection, metacarpal (eg, tumor);
> *CPT Assistant* Nov 98:8

26255 with autograft (includes obtaining graft)

26260 Radical resection, proximal or middle phalanx of finger (eg, tumor);
> *CPT Assistant* Nov 98:8

26261 with autograft (includes obtaining graft)

26262 Radical resection, distal phalanx of finger (eg, tumor)
> *CPT Assistant* Nov 98:8

Introduction or Removal

26320 Removal of implant from finger or hand

(For removal of foreign body in hand or finger, see 20520, 20525)

Repair, Revision, and/or Reconstruction

26340 Manipulation, finger joint, under anesthesia, each joint
> *CPT Assistant* Nov 02:10; *CPT Changes: An Insider's View* 2002

(For application of external fixation, see 20690 or 20692)

26350 Repair or advancement, flexor tendon, not in zone 2 digital flexor tendon sheath (eg, no man's land); primary or secondary without free graft, each tendon
> *CPT Assistant* Nov 98:8; *CPT Changes: An Insider's View* 2002

26352 secondary with free graft (includes obtaining graft), each tendon

26356 Repair or advancement, flexor tendon, in zone 2 digital flexor tendon sheath (eg, no man's land); primary, without free graft, each tendon
> *CPT Assistant* Nov 98:8, Dec 98:9; *CPT Changes: An Insider's View* 2002, 2004

26357 secondary, without free graft, each tendon
> *CPT Changes: An Insider's View* 2004

26358 secondary, with free graft (includes obtaining graft), each tendon

26370 Repair or advancement of profundus tendon, with intact superficialis tendon; primary, each tendon
> *CPT Assistant* Nov 98:8

26372 secondary with free graft (includes obtaining graft), each tendon
> *CPT Assistant* Nov 98:8

26373 secondary without free graft, each tendon
> *CPT Assistant* Nov 98:8

26390 Excision flexor tendon, with implantation of synthetic rod for delayed tendon graft, hand or finger, each rod
> *CPT Assistant* Nov 98:8; *CPT Changes: An Insider's View* 2002

26392 Removal of synthetic rod and insertion of flexor tendon graft, hand or finger (includes obtaining graft), each rod
> *CPT Assistant* Nov 98:8; *CPT Changes: An Insider's View* 2002

26410 Repair, extensor tendon, hand, primary or secondary; without free graft, each tendon
> *CPT Assistant* Nov 98:8

26412 with free graft (includes obtaining graft), each tendon
> *CPT Assistant* Nov 98:8

26415 Excision of extensor tendon, with implantation of synthetic rod for delayed tendon graft, hand or finger, each rod
> *CPT Assistant* Nov 98:8; *CPT Changes: An Insider's View* 2002

26416 Removal of synthetic rod and insertion of extensor tendon graft (includes obtaining graft), hand or finger, each rod
> *CPT Assistant* Nov 99:12; *CPT Changes: An Insider's View* 2000, 2002

26418 Repair, extensor tendon, finger, primary or secondary; without free graft, each tendon
> *CPT Assistant* Nov 98:8, Dec 99:10, Dec 00:14

26420 with free graft (includes obtaining graft) each tendon

26426 Repair of extensor tendon, central slip, secondary (eg, boutonniere deformity); using local tissue(s), including lateral band(s), each finger
> *CPT Assistant* Nov 98:8; *CPT Changes: An Insider's View* 2002

26428 with free graft (includes obtaining graft), each finger
> *CPT Changes: An Insider's View* 2002

26432 Closed treatment of distal extensor tendon insertion, with or without percutaneous pinning (eg, mallet finger)
> *CPT Assistant* Nov 98:8

26433 Repair of extensor tendon, distal insertion, primary or secondary; without graft (eg, mallet finger)
> *CPT Assistant* Nov 98:8

26434 with free graft (includes obtaining graft)

(For tenovaginotomy for trigger finger, use 26055)

26437 Realignment of extensor tendon, hand, each tendon
> *CPT Assistant* Nov 98:8

26440 Tenolysis, flexor tendon; palm OR finger, each tendon
> *CPT Assistant* Apr 02:18; *CPT Changes: An Insider's View* 2003

26442 palm AND finger, each tendon

26445 Tenolysis, extensor tendon, hand OR finger, each tendon
> *CPT Assistant* Nov 98:8, Dec 02:11, Mar 03:20; *CPT Changes: An Insider's View* 2002

26449 Tenolysis, complex, extensor tendon, finger, including forearm, each tendon
> *CPT Assistant* Nov 98:8

26450 Tenotomy, flexor, palm, open, each tendon
> *CPT Assistant* Nov 98:8

26455 Tenotomy, flexor, finger, open, each tendon
> *CPT Assistant* Nov 98:8

26460 Tenotomy, extensor, hand or finger, open, each tendon
> *CPT Assistant* Nov 98:8

26471 Tenodesis; of proximal interphalangeal joint, each joint
> *CPT Assistant* Nov 98:8

26474 of distal joint, each joint
> *CPT Assistant* Nov 98:8

26476 Lengthening of tendon, extensor, hand or finger, each tendon
> *CPT Assistant* Nov 98:8

26477 Shortening of tendon, extensor, hand or finger, each tendon
> *CPT Assistant* Nov 98:8

26478 Lengthening of tendon, flexor, hand or finger, each tendon
> *CPT Assistant* Nov 98:8

26479 Shortening of tendon, flexor, hand or finger, each tendon
> *CPT Assistant* Nov 98:8

26480 Transfer or transplant of tendon, carpometacarpal area or dorsum of hand; without free graft, each tendon
> *CPT Assistant* Nov 98:8

26483 with free tendon graft (includes obtaining graft), each tendon

26485 Transfer or transplant of tendon, palmar; without free tendon graft, each tendon
> *CPT Assistant* Nov 98:8

26489 with free tendon graft (includes obtaining graft), each tendon

26490 Opponensplasty; superficialis tendon transfer type, each tendon

26492 tendon transfer with graft (includes obtaining graft), each tendon

26494 hypothenar muscle transfer

26496 other methods

(For thumb fusion in opposition, use 26820)

26497 Transfer of tendon to restore intrinsic function; ring and small finger
> *CPT Assistant* Nov 98:8

26498 all four fingers

26499 Correction claw finger, other methods

26500 Reconstruction of tendon pulley, each tendon; with local tissues (separate procedure)
> *CPT Assistant* Nov 98:8

26502 with tendon or fascial graft (includes obtaining graft) (separate procedure)

(26504 has been deleted. To report, use 26390)

26508 Release of thenar muscle(s) (eg, thumb contracture)
> *CPT Assistant* Nov 98:8

26510 Cross intrinsic transfer, each tendon
> *CPT Changes: An Insider's View* 2002

26516 Capsulodesis, metacarpophalangeal joint; single digit
> *CPT Assistant* Nov 98:8

26517 two digits

26518 three or four digits

26520 Capsulectomy or capsulotomy; metacarpophalangeal joint, each joint
> *CPT Assistant* Nov 98:8

26525 interphalangeal joint, each joint
> *CPT Assistant* Nov 98:8, Apr 02:18, Mar 03:20

(To report carpometacarpal joint arthroplasty, use 25447)

26530 Arthroplasty, metacarpophalangeal joint; each joint
> *CPT Assistant* Nov 98:8

26531 with prosthetic implant, each joint
> *CPT Assistant* Nov 98:8

26535 Arthroplasty, interphalangeal joint; each joint
> *CPT Assistant* Nov 98:8

26536 with prosthetic implant, each joint
> *CPT Assistant* Nov 98:8

26540 Repair of collateral ligament, metacarpophalangeal or interphalangeal joint
> *CPT Assistant* Nov 96:6

26541 Reconstruction, collateral ligament, metacarpophalangeal joint, single; with tendon or fascial graft (includes obtaining graft)
➔ *CPT Assistant* Jan 97:3

26542 with local tissue (eg, adductor advancement)
➔ *CPT Assistant* Jan 97:3

26545 Reconstruction, collateral ligament, interphalangeal joint, single, including graft, each joint

26546 Repair non-union, metacarpal or phalanx (includes obtaining bone graft with or without external or internal fixation)
➔ *CPT Assistant* Nov 96:6

26548 Repair and reconstruction, finger, volar plate, interphalangeal joint

26550 Pollicization of a digit

26551 Transfer, toe-to-hand with microvascular anastomosis; great toe wrap-around with bone graft
➔ *CPT Assistant* Nov 96:6, Apr 97:7, Jun 97:9, Nov 98:8, 10-11

(For great toe with web space, use 20973)

26553 other than great toe, single
➔ *CPT Assistant* Nov 96:6, Apr 97:7, Jun 97:9, Nov 98:8, 10-11

26554 other than great toe, double
➔ *CPT Assistant* Nov 96:6, Apr 97:7, Jun 97:9, Nov 98:8, 10-11

(Do not report code 69990 in addition to codes 26551-26554)

26555 Transfer, finger to another position without microvascular anastomosis
➔ *CPT Assistant* Nov 98:8, 10-11

26556 Transfer, free toe joint, with microvascular anastomosis
➔ *CPT Assistant* Nov 96:6, Apr 97:7, Jun 97:9, Nov 98:8

(Do not report code 69990 in addition to code 26556)

(To report great toe-to-hand transfer, use 20973)

26560 Repair of syndactyly (web finger) each web space; with skin flaps

26561 with skin flaps and grafts

26562 complex (eg, involving bone, nails)

26565 Osteotomy; metacarpal, each
➔ *CPT Assistant* Nov 98:9

26567 phalanx of finger, each

26568 Osteoplasty, lengthening, metacarpal or phalanx

26580 Repair cleft hand

26587 Reconstruction of polydactylous digit, soft tissue and bone
➔ *CPT Assistant* Oct 01:10, Aug 03:14, May 04:16; *CPT Changes: An Insider's View* 2002

(For excision of polydactylous digit, soft tissue only, use 11200)

26590 Repair macrodactylia, each digit
➔ *CPT Assistant* Oct 01:10, Aug 03:14, May 04:16; *CPT Changes: An Insider's View* 2002

26591 Repair, intrinsic muscles of hand, each muscle
➔ *CPT Assistant* May 98:11, Jul 98:11, Nov 98:8, 11

26593 Release, intrinsic muscles of hand, each muscle
➔ *CPT Assistant* Nov 98:8, 11

26596 Excision of constricting ring of finger, with multiple Z-plasties

(To report release of scar contracture or graft repairs see 11041-11042, 14040-14041, or 15120, 15240)

Fracture and/or Dislocation

26600 Closed treatment of metacarpal fracture, single; without manipulation, each bone

26605 with manipulation, each bone

26607 Closed treatment of metacarpal fracture, with manipulation, with external fixation, each bone
➔ *CPT Changes: An Insider's View* 2002

26608 Percutaneous skeletal fixation of metacarpal fracture, each bone

▲ **26615** Open treatment of metacarpal fracture, single, includes internal fixation, when performed, each bone
➔ *CPT Changes: An Insider's View* 2008

26641 Closed treatment of carpometacarpal dislocation, thumb, with manipulation

26645 Closed treatment of carpometacarpal fracture dislocation, thumb (Bennett fracture), with manipulation

▲ **26650** Percutaneous skeletal fixation of carpometacarpal fracture dislocation, thumb (Bennett fracture), with manipulation
➔ *CPT Changes: An Insider's View* 2008

▲ **26665** Open treatment of carpometacarpal fracture dislocation, thumb (Bennett fracture), includes internal fixation, when performed
➔ *CPT Changes: An Insider's View* 2008

26670 Closed treatment of carpometacarpal dislocation, other than thumb, with manipulation, each joint; without anesthesia
➔ *CPT Changes: An Insider's View* 2002

26675 requiring anesthesia

26676 Percutaneous skeletal fixation of carpometacarpal dislocation, other than thumb, with manipulation, each joint
➔ *CPT Changes: An Insider's View* 2002

▲ **26685** Open treatment of carpometacarpal dislocation, other than thumb; includes internal fixation, when performed, each joint
➔ *CPT Changes: An Insider's View* 2002, 2008

26686 complex, multiple, or delayed reduction

26700   Closed treatment of metacarpophalangeal dislocation, single, with manipulation; without anesthesia

26705   requiring anesthesia

26706   Percutaneous skeletal fixation of metacarpophalangeal dislocation, single, with manipulation

▲ **26715**   Open treatment of metacarpophalangeal dislocation, single, includes internal fixation, when performed
➔ *CPT Changes: An Insider's View* 2008

26720   Closed treatment of phalangeal shaft fracture, proximal or middle phalanx, finger or thumb; without manipulation, each

26725   with manipulation, with or without skin or skeletal traction, each

26727   Percutaneous skeletal fixation of unstable phalangeal shaft fracture, proximal or middle phalanx, finger or thumb, with manipulation, each

▲ **26735**   Open treatment of phalangeal shaft fracture, proximal or middle phalanx, finger or thumb, includes internal fixation, when performed, each
➔ *CPT Changes: An Insider's View* 2008

26740   Closed treatment of articular fracture, involving metacarpophalangeal or interphalangeal joint; without manipulation, each

26742   with manipulation, each

▲ **26746**   Open treatment of articular fracture, involving metacarpophalangeal or interphalangeal joint, includes internal fixation, when performed, each
➔ *CPT Changes: An Insider's View* 2008

26750   Closed treatment of distal phalangeal fracture, finger or thumb; without manipulation, each

26755   with manipulation, each

26756   Percutaneous skeletal fixation of distal phalangeal fracture, finger or thumb, each

▲ **26765**   Open treatment of distal phalangeal fracture, finger or thumb, includes internal fixation, when performed, each
➔ *CPT Changes: An Insider's View* 2008

26770   Closed treatment of interphalangeal joint dislocation, single, with manipulation; without anesthesia

26775   requiring anesthesia

26776   Percutaneous skeletal fixation of interphalangeal joint dislocation, single, with manipulation

▲ **26785**   Open treatment of interphalangeal joint dislocation, includes internal fixation, when performed, single
➔ *CPT Changes: An Insider's View* 2008

Arthrodesis

26820   Fusion in opposition, thumb, with autogenous graft (includes obtaining graft)

26841   Arthrodesis, carpometacarpal joint, thumb, with or without internal fixation;

26842   with autograft (includes obtaining graft)

26843   Arthrodesis, carpometacarpal joint, digit, other than thumb, each;
➔ *CPT Changes: An Insider's View* 2002

26844   with autograft (includes obtaining graft)

26850   Arthrodesis, metacarpophalangeal joint, with or without internal fixation;

26852   with autograft (includes obtaining graft)

26860   Arthrodesis, interphalangeal joint, with or without internal fixation;

✛ **26861**   each additional interphalangeal joint (List separately in addition to code for primary procedure)

(Use 26861 in conjunction with 26860)

26862   with autograft (includes obtaining graft)

✛ **26863**   with autograft (includes obtaining graft), each additional joint (List separately in addition to code for primary procedure)

(Use 26863 in conjunction with 26862)

Amputation

(For hand through metacarpal bones, use 25927)

26910   Amputation, metacarpal, with finger or thumb (ray amputation), single, with or without interosseous transfer

(For repositioning, see 26550, 26555)

26951   Amputation, finger or thumb, primary or secondary, any joint or phalanx, single, including neurectomies; with direct closure

26952   with local advancement flaps (V-Y, hood)

(For repair of soft tissue defect requiring split or full thickness graft or other pedicle flaps, see 15050-15758)

Other Procedures

26989   Unlisted procedure, hands or fingers

Pelvis and Hip Joint

Including head and neck of femur.

Incision

(For incision and drainage procedures, superficial, see 10040-10160)

26990   Incision and drainage, pelvis or hip joint area; deep abscess or hematoma

26991   infected bursa

26992   Incision, bone cortex, pelvis and/or hip joint (eg, osteomyelitis or bone abscess)
➔ *CPT Assistant* Jan 02:10

27000   Tenotomy, adductor of hip, percutaneous (separate procedure)

27001   Tenotomy, adductor of hip, open

(To report bilateral procedures, report 27001 with modifier 50)

27003   Tenotomy, adductor, subcutaneous, open, with obturator neurectomy

(To report bilateral procedures, report 27003 with modifier 50)

27005   Tenotomy, hip flexor(s), open (separate procedure)

27006   Tenotomy, abductors and/or extensor(s) of hip, open (separate procedure)

27025   Fasciotomy, hip or thigh, any type

(To report bilateral procedures, report 27025 with modifier 50)

27030   Arthrotomy, hip, with drainage (eg, infection)
➔ *CPT Assistant* Nov 98:8

27033   Arthrotomy, hip, including exploration or removal of loose or foreign body
➔ *CPT Assistant* Spring 92:11

27035   Denervation, hip joint, intrapelvic or extrapelvic intra-articular branches of sciatic, femoral, or obturator nerves
➔ *CPT Assistant* Nov 98:8

(For obturator neurectomy, see 64763, 64766)

27036   Capsulectomy or capsulotomy, hip, with or without excision of heterotopic bone, with release of hip flexor muscles (ie, gluteus medius, gluteus minimus, tensor fascia latae, rectus femoris, sartorius, iliopsoas)
➔ *CPT Assistant* Jan 05:8

Excision

27040   Biopsy, soft tissue of pelvis and hip area; superficial

27041   deep, subfascial or intramuscular
➔ *CPT Assistant* Nov 98:8

(For needle biopsy of soft tissue, use 20206)

27047   Excision, tumor, pelvis and hip area; subcutaneous tissue
➔ *CPT Assistant* Nov 98:8

27048   deep, subfascial, intramuscular

27049   Radical resection of tumor, soft tissue of pelvis and hip area (eg, malignant neoplasm)
➔ *CPT Assistant* Nov 98:8

27050   Arthrotomy, with biopsy; sacroiliac joint

27052   hip joint

27054   Arthrotomy with synovectomy, hip joint

27060   Excision; ischial bursa

27062   trochanteric bursa or calcification

(For arthrocentesis or needling of bursa, use 20610)

27065   Excision of bone cyst or benign tumor; superficial (wing of ilium, symphysis pubis, or greater trochanter of femur) with or without autograft

27066   deep, with or without autograft

27067   with autograft requiring separate incision

27070   Partial excision (craterization, saucerization) (eg, osteomyelitis or bone abscess); superficial (eg, wing of ilium, symphysis pubis, or greater trochanter of femur)

27071   deep (subfascial or intramuscular)

27075   Radical resection of tumor or infection; wing of ilium, one pubic or ischial ramus or symphysis pubis

27076   ilium, including acetabulum, both pubic rami, or ischium and acetabulum

27077   innominate bone, total

27078   ischial tuberosity and greater trochanter of femur

27079   ischial tuberosity and greater trochanter of femur, with skin flaps

27080   Coccygectomy, primary

(For pressure (decubitus) ulcer, see 15920, 15922 and 15931-15958)

Introduction or Removal

27086   Removal of foreign body, pelvis or hip; subcutaneous tissue
➔ *CPT Assistant* Jul 98:8

27087   deep (subfascial or intramuscular)
➔ *CPT Assistant* Nov 98:8

27090   Removal of hip prosthesis; (separate procedure)

27091   complicated, including total hip prosthesis, methylmethacrylate with or without insertion of spacer

27093   Injection procedure for hip arthrography; without anesthesia

(For radiological supervision and interpretation, use 73525. Do not report 77002 in conjunction with 73525)

27095   with anesthesia

(For radiological supervision and interpretation, use 73525. Do not report 77002 in conjunction with 73525)

27096   Injection procedure for sacroiliac joint, arthrography and/or anesthetic/steroid
➔ *CPT Assistant* Nov 99:12, Apr 03:8, Apr 04:15; *CPT Changes: An Insider's View* 2000

(27096 is to be used only with imaging confirmation of intra-articular needle positioning)

(For radiological supervision and interpretation of sacroiliac joint arthrography, use 73542)

(For fluoroscopic guidance without formal arthrography, use 77003)

(Code 27096 is a unilateral procedure. For bilateral procedure, use modifier 50)

Repair, Revision, and/or Reconstruction

27097 Release or recession, hamstring, proximal

⮕ *CPT Assistant* Nov 98:8

27098 Transfer, adductor to ischium

⮕ *CPT Assistant* Nov 98:8

27100 Transfer external oblique muscle to greater trochanter including fascial or tendon extension (graft)

27105 Transfer paraspinal muscle to hip (includes fascial or tendon extension graft)

27110 Transfer iliopsoas; to greater trochanter of femur

⮕ *CPT Changes: An Insider's View* 2002

27111 to femoral neck

27120 Acetabuloplasty; (eg, Whitman, Colonna, Haygroves, or cup type)

27122 resection, femoral head (eg, Girdlestone procedure)

27125 Hemiarthroplasty, hip, partial (eg, femoral stem prosthesis, bipolar arthroplasty)

⮕ *CPT Assistant* Spring 92:8, Feb 98:11, Nov 98:8

(For prosthetic replacement following fracture of the hip, use 27236)

Partial Hip Replacement With or Without Bipolar Prosthesis
27125

The femoral neck is excised so the physician can measure and then replace the femoral stem.

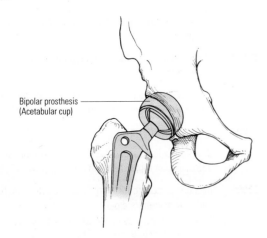

Bipolar prosthesis
(Acetabular cup)

27130 Arthroplasty, acetabular and proximal femoral prosthetic replacement (total hip arthroplasty), with or without autograft or allograft

⮕ *CPT Assistant* Spring 92:8, Jan 07:1; *CPT Changes: An Insider's View* 2002

Total Hip Replacement
27130

The femoral head is excised, osteophytes are removed, and acetabulum is reamed out before replacement is inserted in the femoral shaft.

Acetabular component

Femoral component

Femoral shaft

27132 Conversion of previous hip surgery to total hip arthroplasty, with or without autograft or allograft

⮕ *CPT Assistant* Spring 92:11; *CPT Changes: An Insider's View* 2002

27134 Revision of total hip arthroplasty; both components, with or without autograft or allograft

⮕ *CPT Assistant* Spring 92:7

27137 acetabular component only, with or without autograft or allograft

⮕ *CPT Assistant* Spring 92:7

27138 femoral component only, with or without allograft

⮕ *CPT Assistant* Spring 92:7

27140 Osteotomy and transfer of greater trochanter of femur (separate procedure)

⮕ *CPT Changes: An Insider's View* 2002

27146   Osteotomy, iliac, acetabular or innominate bone;
> *CPT Assistant* Feb 99:10

27147   with open reduction of hip

27151   with femoral osteotomy

27156   with femoral osteotomy and with open reduction of hip

27158   Osteotomy, pelvis, bilateral (eg, congenital malformation)

27161   Osteotomy, femoral neck (separate procedure)

27165   Osteotomy, intertrochanteric or subtrochanteric including internal or external fixation and/or cast
> *CPT Assistant* Spring 92:11

27170   Bone graft, femoral head, neck, intertrochanteric or subtrochanteric area (includes obtaining bone graft)
> *CPT Assistant* Spring 92:11

27175   Treatment of slipped femoral epiphysis; by traction, without reduction

27176   by single or multiple pinning, in situ

27177   Open treatment of slipped femoral epiphysis; single or multiple pinning or bone graft (includes obtaining graft)

27178   closed manipulation with single or multiple pinning

27179   osteoplasty of femoral neck (Heyman type procedure)

27181   osteotomy and internal fixation

27185   Epiphyseal arrest by epiphysiodesis or stapling, greater trochanter of femur
> *CPT Changes: An Insider's View* 2002

27187   Prophylactic treatment (nailing, pinning, plating or wiring) with or without methylmethacrylate, femoral neck and proximal femur

Fracture and/or Dislocation

27193   Closed treatment of pelvic ring fracture, dislocation, diastasis or subluxation; without manipulation

27194   with manipulation, requiring more than local anesthesia

27200   Closed treatment of coccygeal fracture

27202   Open treatment of coccygeal fracture

27215   Open treatment of iliac spine(s), tuberosity avulsion, or iliac wing fracture(s) (eg, pelvic fracture(s) which do not disrupt the pelvic ring), with internal fixation

27216   Percutaneous skeletal fixation of posterior pelvic ring fracture and/or dislocation (includes ilium, sacroiliac joint and/or sacrum)

27217   Open treatment of anterior ring fracture and/or dislocation with internal fixation (includes pubic symphysis and/or rami)

27218   Open treatment of posterior ring fracture and/or dislocation with internal fixation (includes ilium, sacroiliac joint and/or sacrum)

27220   Closed treatment of acetabulum (hip socket) fracture(s); without manipulation

27222   with manipulation, with or without skeletal traction

27226   Open treatment of posterior or anterior acetabular wall fracture, with internal fixation

27227   Open treatment of acetabular fracture(s) involving anterior or posterior (one) column, or a fracture running transversely across the acetabulum, with internal fixation

27228   Open treatment of acetabular fracture(s) involving anterior and posterior (two) columns, includes T-fracture and both column fracture with complete articular detachment, or single column or transverse fracture with associated acetabular wall fracture, with internal fixation

27230   Closed treatment of femoral fracture, proximal end, neck; without manipulation

27232   with manipulation, with or without skeletal traction

27235   Percutaneous skeletal fixation of femoral fracture, proximal end, neck
> *CPT Changes: An Insider's View* 2003

Percutaneous Treatment of Femoral Fracture
27235

Femoral fracture treatment without fracture exposure

Head of femur

Fracture site

Femoral shaft

27236 Open treatment of femoral fracture, proximal end, neck, internal fixation or prosthetic replacement

➔ *CPT Assistant* Spring 92:10, Feb 98:11, Jan 07:1; *CPT Changes: An Insider's View* 2000

Open Treatment of Femoral Fracture
27236

A. Femoral fracture treatment by internal fixation device (with fracture exposure)

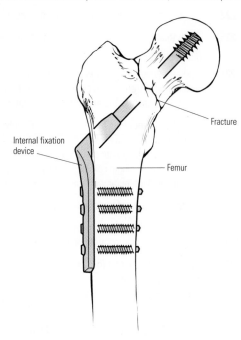

B. Femoral fracture treatment by prosthetic replacement

27238 Closed treatment of intertrochanteric, peritrochanteric, or subtrochanteric femoral fracture; without manipulation

➔ *CPT Assistant* Summer 93:12

27240 with manipulation, with or without skin or skeletal traction

➔ *CPT Assistant* Summer 93:12

27244 Treatment of intertrochanteric, peritrochanteric, or subtrochanteric femoral fracture; with plate/screw type implant, with or without cerclage

➔ *CPT Assistant* Summer 93:12; *CPT Changes: An Insider's View* 2003

27245 with intramedullary implant, with or without interlocking screws and/or cerclage

➔ *CPT Assistant* Summer 93:12

27246 Closed treatment of greater trochanteric fracture, without manipulation

▲ **27248** Open treatment of greater trochanteric fracture, includes internal fixation, when performed

➔ *CPT Changes: An Insider's View* 2008

27250 Closed treatment of hip dislocation, traumatic; without anesthesia

27252 requiring anesthesia

27253 Open treatment of hip dislocation, traumatic, without internal fixation

27254 Open treatment of hip dislocation, traumatic, with acetabular wall and femoral head fracture, with or without internal or external fixation

(For treatment of acetabular fracture with fixation, see 27226, 27227)

27256 Treatment of spontaneous hip dislocation (developmental, including congenital or pathological), by abduction, splint or traction; without anesthesia, without manipulation

27257 with manipulation, requiring anesthesia

27258 Open treatment of spontaneous hip dislocation (developmental, including congenital or pathological), replacement of femoral head in acetabulum (including tenotomy, etc);

27259 with femoral shaft shortening

27265 Closed treatment of post hip arthroplasty dislocation; without anesthesia

27266 requiring regional or general anesthesia

● **27267** Closed treatment of femoral fracture, proximal end, head; without manipulation

➔ *CPT Changes: An Insider's View* 2008

● **27268** with manipulation

➔ *CPT Changes: An Insider's View* 2008

● **27269** Open treatment of femoral fracture, proximal end, head, includes internal fixation, when performed

➔ *CPT Changes: An Insider's View* 2008

▶(Do not report 27269 in conjunction with 27033, 27253)◀

Manipulation

27275   Manipulation, hip joint, requiring general anesthesia

Arthrodesis

27280   Arthrodesis, sacroiliac joint (including obtaining graft)

(To report bilateral procedures, report 27280 with modifier 50)

27282   Arthrodesis, symphysis pubis (including obtaining graft)

27284   Arthrodesis, hip joint (including obtaining graft);

27286   with subtrochanteric osteotomy

Amputation

27290   Interpelviabdominal amputation (hindquarter amputation)

27295   Disarticulation of hip

Other Procedures

27299   Unlisted procedure, pelvis or hip joint
➔ *CPT Assistant* Jan 02:10, Dec 05:9

Femur (Thigh Region) and Knee Joint

Including tibial plateaus.

Incision

(For incision and drainage of abscess or hematoma, superficial, see 10040-10160)

27301   Incision and drainage, deep abscess, bursa, or hematoma, thigh or knee region
➔ *CPT Assistant* Nov 98:9

27303   Incision, deep, with opening of bone cortex, femur or knee (eg, osteomyelitis or bone abscess)
➔ *CPT Assistant* Nov 98:8

27305   Fasciotomy, iliotibial (tenotomy), open

(For combined Ober-Yount fasciotomy, use 27025)

27306   Tenotomy, percutaneous, adductor or hamstring; single tendon (separate procedure)
➔ *CPT Assistant* Nov 98:8

27307   multiple tendons
➔ *CPT Assistant* Nov 98:8

27310   Arthrotomy, knee, with exploration, drainage, or removal of foreign body (eg, infection)
➔ *CPT Assistant* Nov 98:8

(27315 has been deleted. To report, use 27325)

(27320 has been deleted. To report, use 27326)

Excision

27323   Biopsy, soft tissue of thigh or knee area; superficial
➔ *CPT Assistant* Jun 97:12

27324   deep (subfascial or intramuscular)
➔ *CPT Assistant* Mar 97:4, Nov 98:8

(For needle biopsy of soft tissue, use 20206)

27325   Neurectomy, hamstring muscle
➔ *CPT Changes: An Insider's View* 2007

27326   Neurectomy, popliteal (gastrocnemius)
➔ *CPT Changes: An Insider's View* 2007

27327   Excision, tumor, thigh or knee area; subcutaneous

27328   deep, subfascial, or intramuscular

27329   Radical resection of tumor (eg, malignant neoplasm), soft tissue of thigh or knee area

27330   Arthrotomy, knee; with synovial biopsy only

27331   including joint exploration, biopsy, or removal of loose or foreign bodies
➔ *CPT Assistant* May 96:6, Nov 98:8

27332   Arthrotomy, with excision of semilunar cartilage (meniscectomy) knee; medial OR lateral
➔ *CPT Assistant* Nov 98:8

27333   medial AND lateral

27334   Arthrotomy, with synovectomy, knee; anterior OR posterior
➔ *CPT Assistant* Nov 98:8

27335   anterior AND posterior including popliteal area

27340   Excision, prepatellar bursa

27345   Excision of synovial cyst of popliteal space (eg, Baker's cyst)

27347   Excision of lesion of meniscus or capsule (eg, cyst, ganglion), knee
➔ *CPT Assistant* Nov 98:11

27350   Patellectomy or hemipatellectomy

27355   Excision or curettage of bone cyst or benign tumor of femur;

27356   with allograft

27357   with autograft (includes obtaining graft)
➔ *CPT Assistant* Dec 02:11

+ 27358   with internal fixation (List in addition to code for primary procedure)

(Use 27358 in conjunction with 27355, 27356, or 27357)

27360   Partial excision (craterization, saucerization, or diaphysectomy) bone, femur, proximal tibia and/or fibula (eg, osteomyelitis or bone abscess)
➔ *CPT Assistant* Nov 98:8

27365   Radical resection of tumor, bone, femur or knee

(For radical resection of tumor, soft tissue, use 27329)

▲=Revised code   ●=New code   ▶◀=Contains new or revised text   ⊘=Modifier 51 exempt

Introduction or Removal

27370 Injection procedure for knee arthrography

(For radiological supervision and interpretation, use 73580. Do not report 77002 in conjunction with 73580)

27372 Removal of foreign body, deep, thigh region or knee area

(For removal of knee prosthesis including "total knee," use 27488)

(For surgical arthroscopic knee procedures, see 29870-29887)

Repair, Revision, and/or Reconstruction

27380 Suture of infrapatellar tendon; primary

27381 secondary reconstruction, including fascial or tendon graft

27385 Suture of quadriceps or hamstring muscle rupture; primary

27386 secondary reconstruction, including fascial or tendon graft

27390 Tenotomy, open, hamstring, knee to hip; single tendon
➔ *CPT Assistant* Nov 98:8

27391 multiple tendons, one leg
➔ *CPT Assistant* Nov 98:8

27392 multiple tendons, bilateral
➔ *CPT Assistant* Nov 98:8

27393 Lengthening of hamstring tendon; single tendon
➔ *CPT Assistant* Nov 98:8

27394 multiple tendons, one leg
➔ *CPT Assistant* Nov 98:8

27395 multiple tendons, bilateral
➔ *CPT Assistant* Nov 98:8

27396 Transplant, hamstring tendon to patella; single tendon
➔ *CPT Assistant* Nov 98:8

27397 multiple tendons
➔ *CPT Assistant* Nov 98:8

27400 Transfer, tendon or muscle, hamstrings to femur (eg, Egger's type procedure)
➔ *CPT Assistant* Nov 98:8

27403 Arthrotomy with meniscus repair, knee
➔ *CPT Assistant* Nov 98:8

(For arthroscopic repair, use 29882)

27405 Repair, primary, torn ligament and/or capsule, knee; collateral

27407 cruciate

(For cruciate ligament reconstruction, use 27427)

27409 collateral and cruciate ligaments

(For ligament reconstruction, see 27427-27429)

27412 Autologous chondrocyte implantation, knee
➔ *CPT Changes: An Insider's View* 2005

(Do not report 27412 in conjunction with 20926, 27331, 27570)

(For harvesting of chondrocytes, use 29870)

27415 Osteochondral allograft, knee, open
➔ *CPT Changes: An Insider's View* 2005

(For arthroscopic implant of osteochondral allograft, use 29867)

▶(Do not report 27415 in conjunction with 27416)◄

● **27416** Osteochondral autograft(s), knee, open (eg, mosaicplasty) (includes harvesting of autograft[s])
➔ *CPT Changes: An Insider's View* 2008

▶(Do not report 27416 in conjunction with 27415, 29870, 29871, 29875, 29884 when performed at the same session and/or 29874, 29877, 29879, 29885-29887 when performed in the same compartment)◄

▶(For arthroscopic osteochondral autograft of knee, use 29866)◄

27418 Anterior tibial tubercleplasty (eg, Maquet type procedure)

27420 Reconstruction of dislocating patella; (eg, Hauser type procedure)

27422 with extensor realignment and/or muscle advancement or release (eg, Campbell, Goldwaite type procedure)

27424 with patellectomy

27425 Lateral retinacular release, open
➔ *CPT Assistant* Nov 00:11; *CPT Changes: An Insider's View* 2002, 2003

(For arthroscopic lateral release, use 29873)

27427 Ligamentous reconstruction (augmentation), knee; extra-articular
➔ *CPT Assistant* Nov 99:13; *CPT Changes: An Insider's View* 2000

27428 intra-articular (open)
➔ *CPT Assistant* Nov 99:13; *CPT Changes: An Insider's View* 2000

27429 intra-articular (open) and extra-articular
➔ *CPT Assistant* Nov 99:13; *CPT Changes: An Insider's View* 2000

(For primary repair of ligament(s) performed in conjunction with reconstruction, report 27405, 27407 or 27409 in conjunction with 27427, 27428 or 27429)

27430 Quadricepsplasty (eg, Bennett or Thompson type)

27435 Capsulotomy, posterior capsular release, knee
➔ *CPT Assistant* Nov 98:8

27437 Arthroplasty, patella; without prosthesis

27438 with prosthesis

27440 Arthroplasty, knee, tibial plateau;

27441 with debridement and partial synovectomy

27442 Arthroplasty, femoral condyles or tibial plateau(s), knee;
➔ *CPT Assistant* Nov 99:13

27443 with debridement and partial synovectomy

27445 Arthroplasty, knee, hinge prosthesis (eg, Walldius type)
➔ *CPT Assistant* Nov 98:8

27446 Arthroplasty, knee, condyle and plateau; medial OR lateral compartment

27447 medial AND lateral compartments with or without patella resurfacing (total knee arthroplasty)
➔ *CPT Changes: An Insider's View* 2002

(For revision of total knee arthroplasty, use 27487)

(For removal of total knee prosthesis, use 27488)

27448 Osteotomy, femur, shaft or supracondylar; without fixation

(To report bilateral procedures, report 27448 with modifier 50)

27450 with fixation

(To report bilateral procedures, report 27450 with modifier 50)

27454 Osteotomy, multiple, with realignment on intramedullary rod, femoral shaft (eg, Sofield type procedure)
➔ *CPT Assistant* Nov 98:8

27455 Osteotomy, proximal tibia, including fibular excision or osteotomy (includes correction of genu varus (bowleg) or genu valgus (knock-knee)); before epiphyseal closure

(To report bilateral procedures, report 27455 with modifier 50)

27457 after epiphyseal closure

(To report bilateral procedures, report 27457 with modifier 50)

27465 Osteoplasty, femur; shortening (excluding 64876)

27466 lengthening

27468 combined, lengthening and shortening with femoral segment transfer

27470 Repair, nonunion or malunion, femur, distal to head and neck; without graft (eg, compression technique)

27472 with iliac or other autogenous bone graft (includes obtaining graft)

27475 Arrest, epiphyseal, any method (eg, epiphysiodesis); distal femur
➔ *CPT Assistant* Nov 98:8

27477 tibia and fibula, proximal

27479 combined distal femur, proximal tibia and fibula

27485 Arrest, hemiepiphyseal, distal femur or proximal tibia or fibula (eg, genu varus or valgus)
➔ *CPT Assistant* Nov 98:8

27486 Revision of total knee arthroplasty, with or without allograft; one component

27487 femoral and entire tibial component
➔ *CPT Assistant* Nov 98:8

27488 Removal of prosthesis, including total knee prosthesis, methylmethacrylate with or without insertion of spacer, knee
➔ *CPT Assistant* Nov 98:8

27495 Prophylactic treatment (nailing, pinning, plating, or wiring) with or without methylmethacrylate, femur

27496 Decompression fasciotomy, thigh and/or knee, one compartment (flexor or extensor or adductor);

27497 with debridement of nonviable muscle and/or nerve

27498 Decompression fasciotomy, thigh and/or knee, multiple compartments;

27499 with debridement of nonviable muscle and/or nerve

Fracture and/or Dislocation

(For arthroscopic treatment of intercondylar spine[s] and tuberosity fracture[s] of the knee, see 29850, 29851)

(For arthroscopic treatment of tibial fracture, see 29855, 29856)

27500 Closed treatment of femoral shaft fracture, without manipulation

27501 Closed treatment of supracondylar or transcondylar femoral fracture with or without intercondylar extension, without manipulation

27502 Closed treatment of femoral shaft fracture, with manipulation, with or without skin or skeletal traction
➔ *CPT Assistant* Fall 93:22, Oct 99:5

27503 Closed treatment of supracondylar or transcondylar femoral fracture with or without intercondylar extension, with manipulation, with or without skin or skeletal traction

27506 Open treatment of femoral shaft fracture, with or without external fixation, with insertion of intramedullary implant, with or without cerclage and/or locking screws
➔ *CPT Assistant* Winter 92:10

27507 Open treatment of femoral shaft fracture with plate/screws, with or without cerclage

27508 Closed treatment of femoral fracture, distal end, medial or lateral condyle, without manipulation

27509 Percutaneous skeletal fixation of femoral fracture, distal end, medial or lateral condyle, or supracondylar or transcondylar, with or without intercondylar extension, or distal femoral epiphyseal separation

27510 Closed treatment of femoral fracture, distal end, medial or lateral condyle, with manipulation

▲ **27511**   Open treatment of femoral supracondylar or transcondylar fracture without intercondylar extension, includes internal fixation, when performed
→ *CPT Assistant* May 96:6; *CPT Changes: An Insider's View* 2008

▲ **27513**   Open treatment of femoral supracondylar or transcondylar fracture with intercondylar extension, includes internal fixation, when performed
→ *CPT Changes: An Insider's View* 2008

▲ **27514**   Open treatment of femoral fracture, distal end, medial or lateral condyle, includes internal fixation, when performed
→ *CPT Changes: An Insider's View* 2008

27516   Closed treatment of distal femoral epiphyseal separation; without manipulation

27517   with manipulation, with or without skin or skeletal traction

▲ **27519**   Open treatment of distal femoral epiphyseal separation, includes internal fixation, when performed
→ *CPT Changes: An Insider's View* 2008

27520   Closed treatment of patellar fracture, without manipulation

27524   Open treatment of patellar fracture, with internal fixation and/or partial or complete patellectomy and soft tissue repair

27530   Closed treatment of tibial fracture, proximal (plateau); without manipulation

27532   with or without manipulation, with skeletal traction

(For arthroscopic treatment, see 29855, 29856)

▲ **27535**   Open treatment of tibial fracture, proximal (plateau); unicondylar, includes internal fixation, when performed
→ *CPT Changes: An Insider's View* 2008

27536   bicondylar, with or without internal fixation

(For arthroscopic treatment, see 29855, 29856)

27538   Closed treatment of intercondylar spine(s) and/or tuberosity fracture(s) of knee, with or without manipulation

(For arthroscopic treatment, see 29850, 29851)

▲ **27540**   Open treatment of intercondylar spine(s) and/or tuberosity fracture(s) of the knee, includes internal fixation, when performed
→ *CPT Changes: An Insider's View* 2008

27550   Closed treatment of knee dislocation; without anesthesia

27552   requiring anesthesia

▲ **27556**   Open treatment of knee dislocation, includes internal fixation, when performed; without primary ligamentous repair or augmentation/reconstruction
→ *CPT Changes: An Insider's View* 2008

▲ **27557**   with primary ligamentous repair
→ *CPT Changes: An Insider's View* 2008

▲ **27558**   with primary ligamentous repair, with augmentation/reconstruction
→ *CPT Changes: An Insider's View* 2008

27560   Closed treatment of patellar dislocation; without anesthesia
→ *CPT Assistant* Apr 02:15

(For recurrent dislocation, see 27420-27424)

27562   requiring anesthesia

27566   Open treatment of patellar dislocation, with or without partial or total patellectomy

Manipulation

27570   Manipulation of knee joint under general anesthesia (includes application of traction or other fixation devices)

Arthrodesis

27580   Arthrodesis, knee, any technique

Amputation

27590   Amputation, thigh, through femur, any level;

27591   immediate fitting technique including first cast

27592   open, circular (guillotine)

27594   secondary closure or scar revision

27596   re-amputation

27598   Disarticulation at knee

Other Procedures

27599   Unlisted procedure, femur or knee

Leg (Tibia and Fibula) and Ankle Joint

Incision

27600   Decompression fasciotomy, leg; anterior and/or lateral compartments only

27601   posterior compartment(s) only

27602   anterior and/or lateral, and posterior compartment(s)

(For incision and drainage procedures, superficial, see 10040-10160)

(For decompression fasciotomy with debridement, see 27892-27894)

27603   Incision and drainage, leg or ankle; deep abscess or hematoma

27604   infected bursa

27605   Tenotomy, percutaneous, Achilles tendon (separate procedure); local anesthesia

27606   general anesthesia

27607   Incision (eg, osteomyelitis or bone abscess), leg or ankle

27610   Arthrotomy, ankle, including exploration, drainage, or removal of foreign body
➔ *CPT Assistant* Nov 98:9

27612   Arthrotomy, posterior capsular release, ankle, with or without Achilles tendon lengthening
➔ *CPT Assistant* Nov 98:8

(See also 27685)

Excision

27613   Biopsy, soft tissue of leg or ankle area; superficial

27614   deep (subfascial or intramuscular)
➔ *CPT Assistant* Nov 98:8

(For needle biopsy of soft tissue, use 20206)

27615   Radical resection of tumor (eg, malignant neoplasm), soft tissue of leg or ankle area

27618   Excision, tumor, leg or ankle area; subcutaneous tissue

27619   deep (subfascial or intramuscular)

27620   Arthrotomy, ankle, with joint exploration, with or without biopsy, with or without removal of loose or foreign body

27625   Arthrotomy, with synovectomy, ankle;
➔ *CPT Assistant* Nov 98:8

27626   including tenosynovectomy

27630   Excision of lesion of tendon sheath or capsule (eg, cyst or ganglion), leg and/or ankle

27635   Excision or curettage of bone cyst or benign tumor, tibia or fibula;

27637   with autograft (includes obtaining graft)

27638   with allograft

27640   Partial excision (craterization, saucerization, or diaphysectomy) bone (eg, osteomyelitis or exostosis); tibia

27641   fibula

27645   Radical resection of tumor, bone; tibia

27646   fibula

27647   talus or calcaneus

Introduction or Removal

27648   Injection procedure for ankle arthrography

(For radiological supervision and interpretation, use 73615. Do not report 77002 in conjunction with 73615)

(For ankle arthroscopy, see 29894-29898)

Repair, Revision, and/or Reconstruction

27650   Repair, primary, open or percutaneous, ruptured Achilles tendon;

27652   with graft (includes obtaining graft)

27654   Repair, secondary, Achilles tendon, with or without graft

27656   Repair, fascial defect of leg

27658   Repair, flexor tendon, leg; primary, without graft, each tendon
➔ *CPT Assistant* Nov 98:8

27659   secondary, with or without graft, each tendon

27664   Repair, extensor tendon, leg; primary, without graft, each tendon
➔ *CPT Assistant* Nov 98:8

27665   secondary, with or without graft, each tendon
➔ *CPT Assistant* Nov 98:8

27675   Repair, dislocating peroneal tendons; without fibular osteotomy

27676   with fibular osteotomy

27680   Tenolysis, flexor or extensor tendon, leg and/or ankle; single, each tendon
➔ *CPT Assistant* Nov 98:8

27681   multiple tendons (through separate incision(s))
➔ *CPT Assistant* Nov 98:8

27685   Lengthening or shortening of tendon, leg or ankle; single tendon (separate procedure)
➔ *CPT Assistant* Nov 98:8

27686   multiple tendons (through same incision), each
➔ *CPT Assistant* Nov 98:8

27687   Gastrocnemius recession (eg, Strayer procedure)

(Toe extensors are considered as a group to be a single tendon when transplanted into midfoot)

27690   Transfer or transplant of single tendon (with muscle redirection or rerouting); superficial (eg, anterior tibial extensors into midfoot)

27691   deep (eg, anterior tibial or posterior tibial through interosseous space, flexor digitorum longus, flexor hallucis longus, or peroneal tendon to midfoot or hindfoot)

+ 27692   each additional tendon (List separately in addition to code for primary procedure)

(Use 27692 in conjunction with 27690, 27691)

27695   Repair, primary, disrupted ligament, ankle; collateral

27696   both collateral ligaments

27698   Repair, secondary, disrupted ligament, ankle, collateral (eg, Watson-Jones procedure)

27700   Arthroplasty, ankle;

27702   with implant (total ankle)

27703   revision, total ankle

27704   Removal of ankle implant

27705   Osteotomy; tibia

27707   fibula

27709   tibia and fibula

27712   multiple, with realignment on intramedullary rod (eg, Sofield type procedure)

(For osteotomy to correct genu varus (bowleg) or genu valgus (knock-knee), see 27455-27457)

27715   Osteoplasty, tibia and fibula, lengthening or shortening

27720   Repair of nonunion or malunion, tibia; without graft, (eg, compression technique)

27722   with sliding graft

27724   with iliac or other autograft (includes obtaining graft)

27725   by synostosis, with fibula, any method

● **27726**   Repair of fibula nonunion and/or malunion with internal fixation
       → *CPT Changes: An Insider's View* 2008

       ▶(Do not report 27726 in conjunction with 27707)◀

27727   Repair of congenital pseudarthrosis, tibia

27730   Arrest, epiphyseal (epiphysiodesis), open; distal tibia
       → *CPT Assistant* Nov 98:8; *CPT Changes: An Insider's View* 2003

27732   distal fibula

27734   distal tibia and fibula

27740   Arrest, epiphyseal (epiphysiodesis), any method, combined, proximal and distal tibia and fibula;
       → *CPT Assistant* Nov 98:8

27742   and distal femur

(For epiphyseal arrest of proximal tibia and fibula, use 27477)

27745   Prophylactic treatment (nailing, pinning, plating or wiring) with or without methylmethacrylate, tibia

Fracture and/or Dislocation

27750   Closed treatment of tibial shaft fracture (with or without fibular fracture); without manipulation
       → *CPT Assistant* Winter 92:10, Fall 93:21, Mar 96:10

27752   with manipulation, with or without skeletal traction
           → *CPT Assistant* Winter 92:10, Fall 93:21, Feb 96:3, Mar 96:10

27756   Percutaneous skeletal fixation of tibial shaft fracture (with or without fibular fracture) (eg, pins or screws)
       → *CPT Assistant* Winter 92:10

27758   Open treatment of tibial shaft fracture (with or without fibular fracture), with plate/screws, with or without cerclage
       → *CPT Assistant* Winter 92:10, Mar 00:11

27759   Treatment of tibial shaft fracture (with or without fibular fracture) by intramedullary implant, with or without interlocking screws and/or cerclage
       → *CPT Assistant* Winter 92:10; *CPT Changes: An Insider's View* 2003

27760   Closed treatment of medial malleolus fracture; without manipulation

27762   with manipulation, with or without skin or skeletal traction

▲ **27766**   Open treatment of medial malleolus fracture, includes internal fixation, when performed
       → *CPT Changes: An Insider's View* 2008

● **27767**   Closed treatment of posterior malleolus fracture; without manipulation
       → *CPT Changes: An Insider's View* 2008

● **27768**   with manipulation
           → *CPT Changes: An Insider's View* 2008

● **27769**   Open treatment of posterior malleolus fracture, includes internal fixation, when performed
       → *CPT Changes: An Insider's View* 2008

       ▶(Do not report 27767-27769 in conjunction with 27808-27823)◀

27780   Closed treatment of proximal fibula or shaft fracture; without manipulation
       → *CPT Assistant* Winter 92:11

27781   with manipulation

▲ **27784**   Open treatment of proximal fibula or shaft fracture, includes internal fixation, when performed
       → *CPT Assistant* Mar 00:11; *CPT Changes: An Insider's View* 2008

27786   Closed treatment of distal fibular fracture (lateral malleolus); without manipulation

27788   with manipulation

▲ **27792**   Open treatment of distal fibular fracture (lateral malleolus), includes internal fixation, when performed
       → *CPT Changes: An Insider's View* 2008

(For treatment of tibia and fibula shaft fractures, see 27750-27759)

▲ **27808**   Closed treatment of bimalleolar ankle fracture (eg, lateral and medial malleoli, or lateral and posterior malleoli or medial and posterior malleoli); without manipulation
       → *CPT Changes: An Insider's View* 2008

▲ **27810**   with manipulation
           → *CPT Changes: An Insider's View* 2008

▲ **27814**   Open treatment of bimalleolar ankle fracture (eg, lateral and medial malleoli, or lateral and posterior malleoli, or medial and posterior malleoli), includes internal fixation, when performed
       → *CPT Changes: An Insider's View* 2008

27816   Closed treatment of trimalleolar ankle fracture; without manipulation

27818   with manipulation

▲ **27822** Open treatment of trimalleolar ankle fracture, includes internal fixation, when performed, medial and/or lateral malleolus; without fixation of posterior lip
➜ *CPT Changes: An Insider's View* 2008

▲ **27823** with fixation of posterior lip
➜ *CPT Changes: An Insider's View* 2008

27824 Closed treatment of fracture of weight bearing articular portion of distal tibia (eg, pilon or tibial plafond), with or without anesthesia; without manipulation

27825 with skeletal traction and/or requiring manipulation

▲ **27826** Open treatment of fracture of weight bearing articular surface/portion of distal tibia (eg, pilon or tibial plafond), with internal fixation, when performed; of fibula only
➜ *CPT Changes: An Insider's View* 2008

▲ **27827** of tibia only
➜ *CPT Changes: An Insider's View* 2008

▲ **27828** of both tibia and fibula
➜ *CPT Changes: An Insider's View* 2008

▲ **27829** Open treatment of distal tibiofibular joint (syndesmosis) disruption, includes internal fixation, when performed
➜ *CPT Assistant* Winter 92:11; *CPT Changes: An Insider's View* 2008

27830 Closed treatment of proximal tibiofibular joint dislocation; without anesthesia

27831 requiring anesthesia

▲ **27832** Open treatment of proximal tibiofibular joint dislocation, includes internal fixation, when performed, or with excision of proximal fibula
➜ *CPT Changes: An Insider's View* 2008

27840 Closed treatment of ankle dislocation; without anesthesia

27842 requiring anesthesia, with or without percutaneous skeletal fixation

27846 Open treatment of ankle dislocation, with or without percutaneous skeletal fixation; without repair or internal fixation

27848 with repair or internal or external fixation

(For surgical or diagnostic arthroscopic procedures, see 29894-29898)

Manipulation

27860 Manipulation of ankle under general anesthesia (includes application of traction or other fixation apparatus)

Arthrodesis

27870 Arthrodesis, ankle, open
➜ *CPT Changes: An Insider's View* 2003

(For arthroscopic ankle arthrodesis, use 29899)

27871 Arthrodesis, tibiofibular joint, proximal or distal

Amputation

27880 Amputation, leg, through tibia and fibula;

27881 with immediate fitting technique including application of first cast

27882 open, circular (guillotine)

27884 secondary closure or scar revision

27886 re-amputation

27888 Amputation, ankle, through malleoli of tibia and fibula (eg, Syme, Pirogoff type procedures), with plastic closure and resection of nerves

27889 Ankle disarticulation

Other Procedures

27892 Decompression fasciotomy, leg; anterior and/or lateral compartments only, with debridement of nonviable muscle and/or nerve

(For decompression fasciotomy of the leg without debridement, use 27600)

27893 posterior compartment(s) only, with debridement of nonviable muscle and/or nerve

(For decompression fasciotomy of the leg without debridement, use 27601)

27894 anterior and/or lateral, and posterior compartment(s), with debridement of nonviable muscle and/or nerve

(For decompression fasciotomy of the leg without debridement, use 27602)

27899 Unlisted procedure, leg or ankle
➜ *CPT Assistant* Aug 00:11

Foot and Toes

Incision

(For incision and drainage procedures, superficial, see 10040-10160)

28001 Incision and drainage, bursa, foot
➜ *CPT Assistant* Nov 98:9

28002 Incision and drainage below fascia, with or without tendon sheath involvement, foot; single bursal space
➜ *CPT Assistant* Nov 98:8

28003 multiple areas
➜ *CPT Assistant* Nov 98:9

28005 Incision, bone cortex (eg, osteomyelitis or bone abscess), foot
➜ *CPT Assistant* Nov 98:9

28008 Fasciotomy, foot and/or toe

(See also 28060, 28062, 28250)

28010 Tenotomy, percutaneous, toe; single tendon
➔ *CPT Assistant* Nov 98:8

28011 multiple tendons
➔ *CPT Assistant* Nov 98:8

(For open tenotomy, see 28230-28234)

28020 Arthrotomy, including exploration, drainage, or removal of loose or foreign body; intertarsal or tarsometatarsal joint

28022 metatarsophalangeal joint

28024 interphalangeal joint

(28030 has been deleted. To report, use 28055)

28035 Release, tarsal tunnel (posterior tibial nerve decompression)
➔ *CPT Assistant* Nov 98:8

(For other nerve entrapments, see 64704, 64722)

Excision

28043 Excision, tumor, foot; subcutaneous tissue

28045 deep, subfascial, intramuscular

28046 Radical resection of tumor (eg, malignant neoplasm), soft tissue of foot

28050 Arthrotomy with biopsy; intertarsal or tarsometatarsal joint

28052 metatarsophalangeal joint

28054 interphalangeal joint

28055 Neurectomy, intrinsic musculature of foot
➔ *CPT Changes: An Insider's View* 2007

28060 Fasciectomy, plantar fascia; partial (separate procedure)

28062 radical (separate procedure)

(For plantar fasciotomy, see 28008, 28250)

28070 Synovectomy; intertarsal or tarsometatarsal joint, each

28072 metatarsophalangeal joint, each

28080 Excision, interdigital (Morton) neuroma, single, each

28086 Synovectomy, tendon sheath, foot; flexor

28088 extensor

28090 Excision of lesion, tendon, tendon sheath, or capsule (including synovectomy) (eg, cyst or ganglion); foot
➔ *CPT Assistant* Nov 98:8

28092 toe(s), each

28100 Excision or curettage of bone cyst or benign tumor, talus or calcaneus;

28102 with iliac or other autograft (includes obtaining graft)

28103 with allograft

28104 Excision or curettage of bone cyst or benign tumor, tarsal or metatarsal, except talus or calcaneus;
➔ *CPT Changes: An Insider's View* 2002

28106 with iliac or other autograft (includes obtaining graft)

28107 with allograft

28108 Excision or curettage of bone cyst or benign tumor, phalanges of foot

(For ostectomy, partial (eg, hallux valgus, Silver type procedure), use 28290)

28110 Ostectomy, partial excision, fifth metatarsal head (bunionette) (separate procedure)
➔ *CPT Assistant* Oct 98:10, Sep 00:9

28111 Ostectomy, complete excision; first metatarsal head

28112 other metatarsal head (second, third or fourth)

28113 fifth metatarsal head

28114 all metatarsal heads, with partial proximal phalangectomy, excluding first metatarsal (eg, Clayton type procedure)

28116 Ostectomy, excision of tarsal coalition

28118 Ostectomy, calcaneus;

28119 for spur, with or without plantar fascial release

28120 Partial excision (craterization, saucerization, sequestrectomy, or diaphysectomy) bone (eg, osteomyelitis or bossing); talus or calcaneus

28122 tarsal or metatarsal bone, except talus or calcaneus
➔ *CPT Assistant* Nov 98:11

(For partial excision of talus or calcaneus, use 28120)

(For cheilectomy for hallux rigidus, use 28289)

28124 phalanx of toe

28126 Resection, partial or complete, phalangeal base, each toe
➔ *CPT Assistant* Nov 98:8

28130 Talectomy (astragalectomy)

(For calcanectomy, use 28118)

28140 Metatarsectomy

28150 Phalangectomy, toe, each toe
➔ *CPT Assistant* Nov 98:8

28153 Resection, condyle(s), distal end of phalanx, each toe
➔ *CPT Assistant* Nov 98:8

28160 Hemiphalangectomy or interphalangeal joint excision, toe, proximal end of phalanx, each
➔ *CPT Assistant* Nov 98:8

28171 Radical resection of tumor, bone; tarsal (except talus or calcaneus)

28173 metatarsal

28175 phalanx of toe

(For talus or calcaneus, use 27647)

Introduction or Removal

28190   Removal of foreign body, foot; subcutaneous

28192   deep

28193   complicated

Repair, Revision, and/or Reconstruction

28200   Repair, tendon, flexor, foot; primary or secondary, without free graft, each tendon
> *CPT Assistant* Nov 98:8

28202   secondary with free graft, each tendon (includes obtaining graft)

28208   Repair, tendon, extensor, foot; primary or secondary, each tendon
> *CPT Assistant* Nov 98:8

28210   secondary with free graft, each tendon (includes obtaining graft)

28220   Tenolysis, flexor, foot; single tendon
> *CPT Assistant* Nov 98:8

28222   multiple tendons
> *CPT Assistant* Nov 98:8

28225   Tenolysis, extensor, foot; single tendon
> *CPT Assistant* Nov 98:8

28226   multiple tendons
> *CPT Assistant* Nov 98:8

28230   Tenotomy, open, tendon flexor; foot, single or multiple tendon(s) (separate procedure)
> *CPT Assistant* Nov 98:8

28232   toe, single tendon (separate procedure)
> *CPT Assistant* Nov 98:8

28234   Tenotomy, open, extensor, foot or toe, each tendon
> *CPT Assistant* Nov 98:8

(For tendon transfer to midfoot or hindfoot, see 27690, 27691)

28238   Reconstruction (advancement), posterior tibial tendon with excision of accessory tarsal navicular bone (eg, Kidner type procedure)
> *CPT Changes: An Insider's View* 2002

(For subcutaneous tenotomy, see 28010, 28011)

(For transfer or transplant of tendon with muscle redirection or rerouting, see 27690-27692)

(For extensor hallucis longus transfer with great toe IP fusion (Jones procedure), use 28760)

28240   Tenotomy, lengthening, or release, abductor hallucis muscle

28250   Division of plantar fascia and muscle (eg, Steindler stripping) (separate procedure)

28260   Capsulotomy, midfoot; medial release only (separate procedure)

28261   with tendon lengthening

28262   extensive, including posterior talotibial capsulotomy and tendon(s) lengthening (eg, resistant clubfoot deformity)

28264   Capsulotomy, midtarsal (eg, Heyman type procedure)

28270   Capsulotomy; metatarsophalangeal joint, with or without tenorrhaphy, each joint (separate procedure)

28272   interphalangeal joint, each joint (separate procedure)
> *CPT Assistant* Dec 02:11

28280   Syndactylization, toes (eg, webbing or Kelikian type procedure)
> *CPT Assistant* Nov 98:8

28285   Correction, hammertoe (eg, interphalangeal fusion, partial or total phalangectomy)
> *CPT Assistant* Nov 98:8, May 06:18

28286   Correction, cock-up fifth toe, with plastic skin closure (eg, Ruiz-Mora type procedure)
> *CPT Assistant* Nov 98:8

28288   Ostectomy, partial, exostectomy or condylectomy, metatarsal head, each metatarsal head

28289   Hallux rigidus correction with cheilectomy, debridement and capsular release of the first metatarsophalangeal joint
> *CPT Assistant* Nov 98:11

28290   Correction, hallux valgus (bunion), with or without sesamoidectomy; simple exostectomy (eg, Silver type procedure)
> *CPT Assistant* Dec 96:5, Nov 98:8, Jan 07:31

Hallux Valgus Correction
28290

Simple resection of the medial eminence (Silver-type procedure)

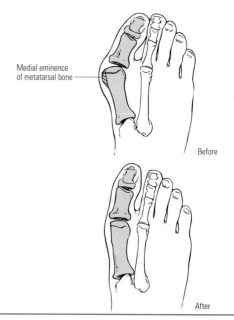

Medial eminence of metatarsal bone

Before

After

28292   Keller, McBride, or Mayo type procedure
> *CPT Assistant* Dec 96:5, Sep 00:9, Jan 07:31

Keller-Type Procedure
28292

Simple resection of the base of the proximal phalanx is accompanied by removal of the medial eminence. A hemi implant is optional.

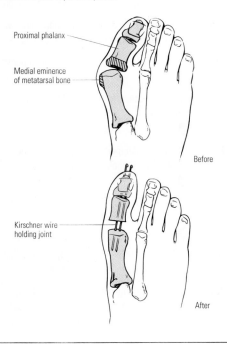

Proximal phalanx

Medial eminence of metatarsal bone

Before

Kirschner wire holding joint

After

28293   resection of joint with implant
> *CPT Assistant* Dec 96:6, Jan 07:31

Keller-Mayo Procedure With Implant
28293

A total double stem implant is usually used.

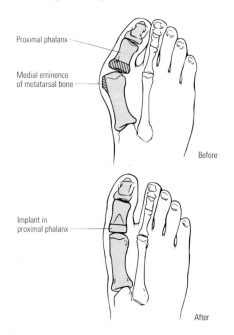

Proximal phalanx

Medial eminence of metatarsal bone

Before

Implant in proximal phalanx

After

28294   with tendon transplants (eg, Joplin type procedure)
> *CPT Assistant* Dec 96:6, Jan 07:31

Joplin Procedure
28294

A tendon transplant is an important part of the procedure.

Extensor tendon of great toe

Medial eminence of metatarsal bone

Before

Fusion of proximal phalanx and metatarsal bone

Extensor tendon transplanted to head of metatarsal bone

After

28296   with metatarsal osteotomy (eg, Mitchell, Chevron, or concentric type procedures)
> *CPT Assistant* Dec 96:6, Jan 97:10, Jan 07:31

Mitchell Procedure
28296

A complex, biplanar, double step-cut osteotomy through the neck of the first metatarsal is also known as the Mitchell Chevron (Austin) procedure.

Medial eminence of metatarsal bone

Osteotomy

Before

Wirelink

After

28297	Lapidus-type procedure

→ *CPT Assistant* Dec 96:6, Jan 07:31

Lapidus-Type Procedure
28297

A metatarsocuneiform fusion of bones and a distal bunion repair to correct valgus deformity

Medial eminence of metatarsal bone

Before

Tenotomy

Arthrodesis of the first metatarsal and first cuneiform joint and the first and second metatarsal bases

After

28298	by phalanx osteotomy

→ *CPT Assistant* Dec 96:7, Jan 07:31

Phalanx Osteotomy
28298

The Akin procedure involves removal of a bony wedge from the base of the proximal phalanx to reorient the axis.

Proximal phalanx

Medial eminence of metatarsal bone

Before

Kirschner wire

After

28299	by double osteotomy

→ *CPT Assistant* Dec 96:7, Jan 07:31; *CPT Changes: An Insider's View* 2002

Double Osteotomy
28299

A. This technique depicts a medial resection of the first metatarsal, osteotomy of the distal first metatarsal with correction of the hallux valgus, followed by an osteotomy of the proximal phalanx to correct additional angular deformity, with placement of appropriate internal fixation (eg, wire[s], pin[s], screw[s]).

PREOP

Angular deformity of proximal phalanx

Medial eminence of metatarsal bone

POSTOP

Osteotomy proximal phalanx

Osteotomy distal first metatarsal

Note: Internal fixation is not depicted but would include screw(s), pin(s), wire(s), as needed.

B. This technique depicts hallux valgus correction (without the medial resection of the base of the proximal phalanx) with double osteotomy of the first metatarsal and placement of appropriate internal fixation (eg, wire[s], pin[s], screw[s]).

PREOP

Medial eminence of metatarsal bone

POSTOP

Double osteotomy of the metatarsal with internal fixation (eg, wire[s], pin[s], screw[s])

Note: Internal fixation depicted is for illustrative purpose only and does not suggest to limit choice of fixation options required.

28300	Osteotomy; calcaneus (eg, Dwyer or Chambers type procedure), with or without internal fixation
28302	talus
28304	Osteotomy, tarsal bones, other than calcaneus or talus;

→ *CPT Assistant* Nov 98:8

28305	with autograft (includes obtaining graft) (eg, Fowler type)
28306	Osteotomy, with or without lengthening, shortening or angular correction, metatarsal; first metatarsal

→ *CPT Assistant* Nov 98:8, Dec 99:7

28307	first metatarsal with autograft (other than first toe)

→ *CPT Assistant* Nov 98:9

28308	other than first metatarsal, each
28309	multiple (eg, Swanson type cavus foot procedure)

→ *CPT Assistant* Nov 98:8, Dec 99:7

28310 Osteotomy, shortening, angular or rotational correction; proximal phalanx, first toe (separate procedure)

28312   other phalanges, any toe

28313 Reconstruction, angular deformity of toe, soft tissue procedures only (eg, overlapping second toe, fifth toe, curly toes)
➔*CPT Assistant* Nov 98:8

28315 Sesamoidectomy, first toe (separate procedure)

28320 Repair, nonunion or malunion; tarsal bones
➔*CPT Assistant* Nov 98:9

28322   metatarsal, with or without bone graft (includes obtaining graft)

28340 Reconstruction, toe, macrodactyly; soft tissue resection

28341   requiring bone resection

28344 Reconstruction, toe(s); polydactyly

28345   syndactyly, with or without skin graft(s), each web

28360 Reconstruction, cleft foot

Fracture and/or Dislocation

28400 Closed treatment of calcaneal fracture; without manipulation

28405   with manipulation

28406 Percutaneous skeletal fixation of calcaneal fracture, with manipulation

▲ **28415** Open treatment of calcaneal fracture, includes internal fixation, when performed;
➔*CPT Changes: An Insider's View* 2008

▲ **28420**   with primary iliac or other autogenous bone graft (includes obtaining graft)
➔*CPT Changes: An Insider's View* 2008

28430 Closed treatment of talus fracture; without manipulation

28435   with manipulation

28436 Percutaneous skeletal fixation of talus fracture, with manipulation

▲ **28445** Open treatment of talus fracture, includes internal fixation, when performed
➔*CPT Changes: An Insider's View* 2008

● **28446** Open osteochondral autograft, talus (includes obtaining graft[s])
➔*CPT Changes: An Insider's View* 2008

    ▶(Do not report 28446 in conjunction with 27705, 27707)◀

    ▶(For arthroscopic osteochondral talus graft, use 29892)◀

    ▶(For open osteochondral allograft or repairs with industrial grafts, use 27599)◀

28450 Treatment of tarsal bone fracture (except talus and calcaneus); without manipulation, each
➔*CPT Assistant* Dec 01:7

28455   with manipulation, each

28456 Percutaneous skeletal fixation of tarsal bone fracture (except talus and calcaneus), with manipulation, each

▲ **28465** Open treatment of tarsal bone fracture (except talus and calcaneus), includes internal fixation, when performed, each
➔*CPT Changes: An Insider's View* 2008

28470 Closed treatment of metatarsal fracture; without manipulation, each

28475   with manipulation, each

28476 Percutaneous skeletal fixation of metatarsal fracture, with manipulation, each

▲ **28485** Open treatment of metatarsal fracture, includes internal fixation, when performed, each
➔*CPT Changes: An Insider's View* 2008

28490 Closed treatment of fracture great toe, phalanx or phalanges; without manipulation

28495   with manipulation

28496 Percutaneous skeletal fixation of fracture great toe, phalanx or phalanges, with manipulation

▲ **28505** Open treatment of fracture, great toe, phalanx or phalanges, includes internal fixation, when performed
➔*CPT Changes: An Insider's View* 2008

28510 Closed treatment of fracture, phalanx or phalanges, other than great toe; without manipulation, each

28515   with manipulation, each

▲ **28525** Open treatment of fracture, phalanx or phalanges, other than great toe, includes internal fixation, when performed, each
➔*CPT Changes: An Insider's View* 2008

28530 Closed treatment of sesamoid fracture

28531 Open treatment of sesamoid fracture, with or without internal fixation

28540 Closed treatment of tarsal bone dislocation, other than talotarsal; without anesthesia

28545   requiring anesthesia

28546 Percutaneous skeletal fixation of tarsal bone dislocation, other than talotarsal, with manipulation

▲ **28555** Open treatment of tarsal bone dislocation, includes internal fixation, when performed
➔*CPT Changes: An Insider's View* 2008

28570 Closed treatment of talotarsal joint dislocation; without anesthesia

28575   requiring anesthesia

28576   Percutaneous skeletal fixation of talotarsal joint
        dislocation, with manipulation

▲ 28585   Open treatment of talotarsal joint dislocation, includes
         internal fixation, when performed
         ➔ *CPT Changes: An Insider's View* 2008

28600   Closed treatment of tarsometatarsal joint dislocation;
        without anesthesia

28605   requiring anesthesia

28606   Percutaneous skeletal fixation of tarsometatarsal joint
        dislocation, with manipulation

▲ 28615   Open treatment of tarsometatarsal joint dislocation,
         includes internal fixation, when performed
         ➔ *CPT Changes: An Insider's View* 2008

28630   Closed treatment of metatarsophalangeal joint
        dislocation; without anesthesia

28635   requiring anesthesia

28636   Percutaneous skeletal fixation of metatarsophalangeal
        joint dislocation, with manipulation

▲ 28645   Open treatment of metatarsophalangeal joint dislocation,
         includes internal fixation, when performed
         ➔ *CPT Changes: An Insider's View* 2008

28660   Closed treatment of interphalangeal joint dislocation;
        without anesthesia

28665   requiring anesthesia

28666   Percutaneous skeletal fixation of interphalangeal joint
        dislocation, with manipulation

▲ 28675   Open treatment of interphalangeal joint dislocation,
         includes internal fixation, when performed
         ➔ *CPT Changes: An Insider's View* 2008

Arthrodesis

28705   Arthrodesis; pantalar

28715   triple

28725   subtalar

28730   Arthrodesis, midtarsal or tarsometatarsal, multiple or
        transverse;

28735   with osteotomy (eg, flatfoot correction)

28737   Arthrodesis, with tendon lengthening and advancement,
        midtarsal, tarsal navicular-cuneiform (eg, Miller type
        procedure)
        ➔ *CPT Changes: An Insider's View* 2002

28740   Arthrodesis, midtarsal or tarsometatarsal, single joint

28750   Arthrodesis, great toe; metatarsophalangeal joint
        ➔ *CPT Assistant* Dec 96:7

28755   interphalangeal joint

28760   Arthrodesis, with extensor hallucis longus transfer to first
        metatarsal neck, great toe, interphalangeal joint (eg,
        Jones type procedure)
        ➔ *CPT Assistant* Nov 98:8

        (For hammertoe operation or interphalangeal fusion, use
        28285)

Amputation

28800   Amputation, foot; midtarsal (eg, Chopart type procedure)

28805   transmetatarsal
            ➔ *CPT Assistant* May 97:8

28810   Amputation, metatarsal, with toe, single

28820   Amputation, toe; metatarsophalangeal joint
        ➔ *CPT Assistant* May 97:8

28825   interphalangeal joint

        (For amputation of tuft of distal phalanx, use 11752)

Other Procedures

28890   Extracorporeal shock wave, high energy, performed by a
        physician, requiring anesthesia other than local, including
        ultrasound guidance, involving the plantar fascia
        ➔ *CPT Assistant* Dec 05:10, Mar 06:1; *CPT Changes: An Insider's
          View* 2006

        (For extracorporeal shock wave therapy involving
        musculoskeletal system not otherwise specified, see
        Category III codes 0019T, 0101T, 0102T)

28899   Unlisted procedure, foot or toes

Application of Casts and Strapping

The listed procedures apply when the cast application or
strapping is a replacement procedure used during or after
the period of follow-up care, or when the cast application
or strapping is an initial service performed without a
restorative treatment or procedure(s) to stabilize or
protect a fracture, injury, or dislocation and/or to afford
comfort to a patient. Restorative treatment or
procedure(s) rendered by another physician following the
application of the initial cast/splint/strap may be reported
with a treatment of fracture and/or dislocation code.

A physician who applies the initial cast, strap or splint
and also assumes all of the subsequent fracture,
dislocation, or injury care cannot use the application of
casts and strapping codes as an initial service, since the
first cast/splint or strap application is included in the
treatment of fracture and/or dislocation codes. (See notes
under Musculoskeletal System, page 75.) A temporary
cast/splint/strap is not considered to be part of the
preoperative care, and the use of the modifier 56 is not
applicable. Additional evaluation and management
services are reportable only if significant identifiable
further services are provided at the time of the cast
application or strapping.

If cast application or strapping is provided as an initial service (eg, casting of a sprained ankle or knee) in which no other procedure or treatment (eg, surgical repair, reduction of a fracture or joint dislocation) is performed or is expected to be performed by a physician rendering the initial care only, use the casting, strapping and/or supply code (99070) in addition to an evaluation and management code as appropriate.

Listed procedures include removal of cast or strapping.

> (For orthotics management and training, see 97760-97762)

Body and Upper Extremity

Casts

29000 Application of halo type body cast (see 20661-20663 for insertion)
➔ *CPT Assistant* Feb 96:3, 5, Apr 02:13

29010 Application of Risser jacket, localizer, body; only
➔ *CPT Assistant* Feb 96:3, Apr 02:13

29015 including head
➔ *CPT Assistant* Feb 96:3, Apr 02:13

29020 Application of turnbuckle jacket, body; only
➔ *CPT Assistant* Feb 96:3, Apr 02:13

29025 including head
➔ *CPT Assistant* Feb 96:3, Apr 02:13

29035 Application of body cast, shoulder to hips;
➔ *CPT Assistant* Feb 96:3, Apr 02:13

29040 including head, Minerva type
➔ *CPT Assistant* Feb 96:3, Apr 02:13

29044 including one thigh
➔ *CPT Assistant* Feb 96:3, Apr 02:13

29046 including both thighs
➔ *CPT Assistant* Feb 96:3, Apr 02:13

29049 Application, cast; figure-of-eight
➔ *CPT Assistant* Feb 96:3, Apr 02:13; *CPT Changes: An Insider's View* 2002

29055 shoulder spica
➔ *CPT Assistant* Feb 96:3, Apr 02:13

29058 plaster Velpeau
➔ *CPT Assistant* Feb 96:3, Apr 02:13

29065 shoulder to hand (long arm)
➔ *CPT Assistant* Feb 96:3, Apr 02:13

29075 elbow to finger (short arm)
➔ *CPT Assistant* Feb 96:3-4, Apr 02:13

29085 hand and lower forearm (gauntlet)
➔ *CPT Assistant* Feb 96:3, Apr 02:13, Dec 02:11

29086 finger (eg, contracture)
➔ *CPT Assistant* Apr 02:13; *CPT Changes: An Insider's View* 2002

Splints

29105 Application of long arm splint (shoulder to hand)
➔ *CPT Assistant* Feb 96:3, Apr 02:13

29125 Application of short arm splint (forearm to hand); static
➔ *CPT Assistant* Feb 96:3-4, Apr 02:13

29126 dynamic
➔ *CPT Assistant* Feb 96:3, Apr 02:13

29130 Application of finger splint; static
➔ *CPT Assistant* Feb 96:3, Apr 02:13

29131 dynamic
➔ *CPT Assistant* Feb 96:3, Apr 02:13

Strapping—Any Age

29200 Strapping; thorax
➔ *CPT Assistant* Feb 96:3, Apr 02:13

29220 low back
➔ *CPT Assistant* Feb 96:3, Apr 02:13

29240 shoulder (eg, Velpeau)
➔ *CPT Assistant* Feb 96:3, Apr 02:13

29260 elbow or wrist
➔ *CPT Assistant* Feb 96:3, Apr 02:13

29280 hand or finger
➔ *CPT Assistant* Feb 96:3, Apr 02:13

Lower Extremity

Casts

29305 Application of hip spica cast; one leg
➔ *CPT Assistant* Feb 96:3, Apr 02:13

29325 one and one-half spica or both legs
➔ *CPT Assistant* Feb 96:3, Apr 02:13

> (For hip spica (body) cast, including thighs only, use 29046)

29345 Application of long leg cast (thigh to toes);
➔ *CPT Assistant* Feb 96:3, Apr 02:13

29355 walker or ambulatory type
➔ *CPT Assistant* Feb 96:3, Apr 02:13

29358 Application of long leg cast brace
➔ *CPT Assistant* Feb 96:3, Apr 02:13

29365 Application of cylinder cast (thigh to ankle)
➔ *CPT Assistant* Feb 96:3, Apr 02:13

29405 Application of short leg cast (below knee to toes);
➔ *CPT Assistant* Feb 96:3, Apr 02:13, Mar 03:17

29425 walking or ambulatory type
➔ *CPT Assistant* Feb 96:3, Apr 02:13

29435 Application of patellar tendon bearing (PTB) cast
➔ *CPT Assistant* Feb 96:3, Apr 02:13

29440 Adding walker to previously applied cast
➔ *CPT Assistant* Feb 96:3, Apr 02:13

29445 Application of rigid total contact leg cast
➔ *CPT Assistant* Feb 96:3, Apr 02:13

29450 Application of clubfoot cast with molding or manipulation, long or short leg
➔ *CPT Assistant* Feb 96:3, Apr 02:13

(To report bilateral procedure, use 29450 with modifier 50)

Splints

29505 Application of long leg splint (thigh to ankle or toes)
➔ *CPT Assistant* Feb 96:3, Apr 02:13

29515 Application of short leg splint (calf to foot)
➔ *CPT Assistant* Feb 96:3, Apr 02:13, Mar 03:18

Strapping—Any Age

29520 Strapping; hip
➔ *CPT Assistant* Feb 96:3, Apr 02:13

29530 knee
➔ *CPT Assistant* Feb 96:3, Apr 02:13

29540 ankle and/or foot
➔ *CPT Assistant* Feb 96:3, Apr 02:13, Mar 03:17; *CPT Changes: An Insider's View* 2003

29550 toes
➔ *CPT Assistant* Feb 96:3, Apr 02:13

29580 Unna boot
➔ *CPT Assistant* Feb 96:3, Jul 99:10, Apr 02:13

29590 Denis-Browne splint strapping
➔ *CPT Assistant* Feb 96:3, Apr 02:13

Removal or Repair

Codes for cast removals should be employed only for casts applied by another physician.

29700 Removal or bivalving; gauntlet, boot or body cast
➔ *CPT Assistant* Apr 02:13

29705 full arm or full leg cast
➔ *CPT Assistant* Apr 02:13

29710 shoulder or hip spica, Minerva, or Risser jacket, etc.
➔ *CPT Assistant* Apr 02:13

29715 turnbuckle jacket
➔ *CPT Assistant* Apr 02:13

29720 Repair of spica, body cast or jacket
➔ *CPT Assistant* Apr 02:13

29730 Windowing of cast
➔ *CPT Assistant* Apr 02:13

29740 Wedging of cast (except clubfoot casts)
➔ *CPT Assistant* Apr 02:13

29750 Wedging of clubfoot cast
➔ *CPT Assistant* Apr 02:13

(To report bilateral procedure, use 29750 with modifier 50)

Other Procedures

29799 Unlisted procedure, casting or strapping

Endoscopy/Arthroscopy

Surgical endoscopy/arthroscopy always includes a diagnostic endoscopy/arthroscopy.

When arthroscopy is performed in conjunction with arthrotomy, add modifier 51.

29800 Arthroscopy, temporomandibular joint, diagnostic, with or without synovial biopsy (separate procedure)

29804 Arthroscopy, temporomandibular joint, surgical

(For open procedure, use 21010)

29805 Arthroscopy, shoulder, diagnostic, with or without synovial biopsy (separate procedure)
➔ *CPT Changes: An Insider's View* 2002

(For open procedure, see 23065-23066, 23100-23101)

29806 Arthroscopy, shoulder, surgical; capsulorrhaphy
➔ *CPT Changes: An Insider's View* 2002

(For open procedure, see 23450-23466)

(To report thermal capsulorrhaphy, use 29999)

29807 repair of SLAP lesion
➔ *CPT Changes: An Insider's View* 2002

29819 with removal of loose body or foreign body
➔ *CPT Changes: An Insider's View* 2002

(For open procedure, see 23040-23044, 23107)

29820 synovectomy, partial

(For open procedure, see 23105)

29821 synovectomy, complete

(For open procedure, see 23105)

29822 debridement, limited
➔ *CPT Assistant* May 01:9

(For open procedure, see specific open shoulder procedure performed)

29823 debridement, extensive

(For open procedure, see specific open shoulder procedure performed)

29824   distal claviculectomy including distal articular surface (Mumford procedure)

→ *CPT Changes: An Insider's View* 2002

Arthroscopy, Shoulder, Distal Claviculectomy (Mumford Procedure)
29824

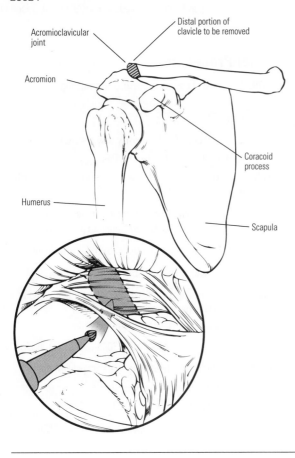

Acromioclavicular joint

Distal portion of clavicle to be removed

Acromion

Humerus

Coracoid process

Scapula

(For open procedure, use 23120)

29825   with lysis and resection of adhesions, with or without manipulation

(For open procedure, see specific open shoulder procedure performed)

29826   decompression of subacromial space with partial acromioplasty, with or without coracoacromial release

→ *CPT Assistant* May 01:9, Aug 02:10

(For open procedure, use 23130 or 23415)

29827   with rotator cuff repair

→ *CPT Changes: An Insider's View* 2003

(For open or mini-open rotator cuff repair, use 23412)

(When arthroscopic subacromial decompression is performed at the same setting, use 29826 and append modifier 51)

(When arthroscopic distal clavicle resection is performed at the same setting, use 29824 and append modifier 51)

● **29828**   biceps tenodesis

→ *CPT Changes: An Insider's View* 2008

►(Do not report 29828 in conjunction with 29805, 29820, 29822)◄

►(For open biceps tenodesis, use 23430)◄

29830   Arthroscopy, elbow, diagnostic, with or without synovial biopsy (separate procedure)

29834   Arthroscopy, elbow, surgical; with removal of loose body or foreign body

29835   synovectomy, partial

29836   synovectomy, complete

29837   debridement, limited

29838   debridement, extensive

29840   Arthroscopy, wrist, diagnostic, with or without synovial biopsy (separate procedure)

29843   Arthroscopy, wrist, surgical; for infection, lavage and drainage

29844   synovectomy, partial

29845   synovectomy, complete

→ *CPT Assistant* Dec 03:11

29846   excision and/or repair of triangular fibrocartilage and/or joint debridement

→ *CPT Assistant* Dec 03:11

29847   internal fixation for fracture or instability

29848   Endoscopy, wrist, surgical, with release of transverse carpal ligament

→ *CPT Assistant* Dec 99:7

(For open procedure, use 64721)

29850   Arthroscopically aided treatment of intercondylar spine(s) and/or tuberosity fracture(s) of the knee, with or without manipulation; without internal or external fixation (includes arthroscopy)

29851   with internal or external fixation (includes arthroscopy)

(For bone graft, use 20900, 20902)

▲ **29855**   Arthroscopically aided treatment of tibial fracture, proximal (plateau); unicondylar, includes internal fixation, when performed (includes arthroscopy)

→ *CPT Changes: An Insider's View* 2008

▲ **29856**   bicondylar, includes internal fixation, when performed (includes arthroscopy)

→ *CPT Changes: An Insider's View* 2008

(For bone graft, use 20900, 20902)

29860   Arthroscopy, hip, diagnostic with or without synovial biopsy (separate procedure)

→ *CPT Assistant* Nov 97:15, Jul 98:8

29861   Arthroscopy, hip, surgical; with removal of loose body or foreign body

→ *CPT Assistant* Nov 97:15, Jul 98:8

29862   with debridement/shaving of articular cartilage (chondroplasty), abrasion arthroplasty, and/or resection of labrum

→ *CPT Assistant* Nov 97:15, Jul 98:8

29863   with synovectomy

→ *CPT Assistant* Nov 97:15, Jul 98:8

Arthroscopy of the Knee
29866-29887

Portal incisions are made on either side of the patellar tendon and compartments of the knee are examined using the arthroscope and a probe. Additional treatment is performed as needed.

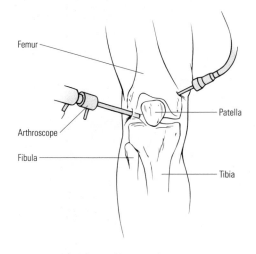

▲ **29866**   Arthroscopy, knee, surgical; osteochondral autograft(s) (eg, mosaicplasty) (includes harvesting of the autograft[s])

→ *CPT Changes: An Insider's View* 2005, 2008

(Do not report 29866 in conjunction with 29870, 29871, 29875, 29884 when performed at the same session and/or 29874, 29877, 29879, 29885-29887 when performed in the same compartment)

▶(For open osteochondral autograft of knee, use 27416)◀

29867   osteochondral allograft (eg, mosaicplasty)

→ *CPT Changes: An Insider's View* 2005

(Do not report 29867 in conjunction with 27570, 29870, 29871, 29875, 29884 when performed at the same session and/or 29874, 29877, 29879, 29885-29887 when performed in the same compartment)

(Do not report 29867 in conjunction with 27415)

29868   meniscal transplantation (includes arthrotomy for meniscal insertion), medial or lateral

→ *CPT Changes: An Insider's View* 2005

(Do not report 29868 in conjunction with 29870, 29871, 29875, 29880, 29883, 29884 when performed at the same session or 29874, 29877, 29881, 29882 when performed in the same compartment)

29870   Arthroscopy, knee, diagnostic, with or without synovial biopsy (separate procedure)

(For open autologous chondrocyte implantation of the knee, use 27412)

29871   Arthroscopy, knee, surgical; for infection, lavage and drainage

→ *CPT Assistant* Aug 01:6

(For implantation of osteochondral graft for treatment of articular surface defect, see 27412, 27415, 29866, 29867)

29873   with lateral release

→ *CPT Changes: An Insider's View* 2003

(For open lateral release, use 27425)

29874   for removal of loose body or foreign body (eg, osteochondritis dissecans fragmentation, chondral fragmentation)

→ *CPT Assistant* Aug 01:6, Apr 03:12

29875   synovectomy, limited (eg, plica or shelf resection) (separate procedure)

→ *CPT Assistant* Aug 01:6

29876   synovectomy, major, two or more compartments (eg, medial or lateral)

→ *CPT Assistant* Aug 01:6

29877   debridement/shaving of articular cartilage (chondroplasty)

→ *CPT Assistant* Feb 96:9, Jun 99:11, Aug 01:7, Apr 03:7, Apr 05:14

29879   abrasion arthroplasty (includes chondroplasty where necessary) or multiple drilling or microfracture

→ *CPT Assistant* Nov 99:13, Aug 01:7; *CPT Changes: An Insider's View* 2000

29880   with meniscectomy (medial AND lateral, including any meniscal shaving)

→ *CPT Assistant* Jun 99:11, Aug 01:7

29881   with meniscectomy (medial OR lateral, including any meniscal shaving)

→ *CPT Assistant* Feb 96:9, Jun 99:11, Aug 01:7, Oct 03:11, Apr 05:14

29882   with meniscus repair (medial OR lateral)

→ *CPT Assistant* Aug 01:7, Sep 04:12

29883   with meniscus repair (medial AND lateral)

→ *CPT Assistant* Aug 01:7, Sep 04:12

(For meniscal transplantation, medial or lateral, knee, use 29868)

29884   with lysis of adhesions, with or without manipulation (separate procedure)

→ *CPT Assistant* Aug 01:7

29885   drilling for osteochondritis dissecans with bone grafting, with or without internal fixation (including debridement of base of lesion)
➔ *CPT Assistant* Aug 01:7

29886   drilling for intact osteochondritis dissecans lesion
➔ *CPT Assistant* Aug 01:12

29887   drilling for intact osteochondritis dissecans lesion with internal fixation
➔ *CPT Assistant* Aug 01:12

29888   Arthroscopically aided anterior cruciate ligament repair/augmentation or reconstruction
➔ *CPT Assistant* Oct 03:11

29889   Arthroscopically aided posterior cruciate ligament repair/augmentation or reconstruction
➔ *CPT Assistant* Sep 96:9, Oct 98:11, Aug 01:8

(Procedures 29888 and 29889 should not be used with reconstruction procedures 27427-27429)

29891   Arthroscopy, ankle, surgical, excision of osteochondral defect of talus and/or tibia, including drilling of the defect
➔ *CPT Assistant* Nov 97:15

29892   Arthroscopically aided repair of large osteochondritis dissecans lesion, talar dome fracture, or tibial plafond fracture, with or without internal fixation (includes arthroscopy)
➔ *CPT Assistant* Nov 97:15

29893   Endoscopic plantar fasciotomy
➔ *CPT Assistant* Nov 97:15

29894   Arthroscopy, ankle (tibiotalar and fibulotalar joints), surgical; with removal of loose body or foreign body

Arthroscopy of the Ankle
29894-29899

Incisions are made allowing the ankle to be examined using the arthroscope and a probe. Additional treatment is performed as needed.

Tibia

Arthroscope

Fibula

Talus

29895   synovectomy, partial

29897   debridement, limited

29898   debridement, extensive

29899   with ankle arthrodesis
➔ *CPT Changes: An Insider's View* 2003

(For open ankle arthrodesis, use 27870)

29900   Arthroscopy, metacarpophalangeal joint, diagnostic, includes synovial biopsy
➔ *CPT Changes: An Insider's View* 2002

(Do not report 29900 with 29901, 29902)

29901   Arthroscopy, metacarpophalangeal joint, surgical; with debridement
➔ *CPT Changes: An Insider's View* 2002

29902   with reduction of displaced ulnar collateral ligament (eg, Stener lesion)
➔ *CPT Changes: An Insider's View* 2002

● **29904**   Arthroscopy, subtalar joint, surgical; with removal of loose body or foreign body
➔ *CPT Changes: An Insider's View* 2008

● **29905**   with synovectomy
➔ *CPT Changes: An Insider's View* 2008

● **29906**   with debridement
➔ *CPT Changes: An Insider's View* 2008

● **29907**   with subtalar arthrodesis
➔ *CPT Changes: An Insider's View* 2008

29999   Unlisted procedure, arthroscopy
➔ *CPT Assistant* Aug 02:10, Sep 04:12; *CPT Changes: An Insider's View* 2002

Respiratory System

Nose

Incision

30000   Drainage abscess or hematoma, nasal, internal approach

(For external approach, see 10060, 10140)

30020   Drainage abscess or hematoma, nasal septum

(For lateral rhinotomy, see specific application (eg, 30118, 30320))

Excision

30100   Biopsy, intranasal

(For biopsy skin of nose, see 11100, 11101)

30110   Excision, nasal polyp(s), simple

(30110 would normally be completed in an office setting)

(To report bilateral procedure, use 30110 with modifier 50)

30115   Excision, nasal polyp(s), extensive

(30115 would normally require the facilities available in a hospital setting)

(To report bilateral procedure, use 30115 with modifier 50)

30117   Excision or destruction (eg, laser), intranasal lesion; internal approach
➔ *CPT Changes: An Insider's View* 2002

30118   external approach (lateral rhinotomy)
➔ *CPT Changes: An Insider's View* 2002

30120   Excision or surgical planing of skin of nose for rhinophyma

30124   Excision dermoid cyst, nose; simple, skin, subcutaneous

30125   complex, under bone or cartilage

30130   Excision inferior turbinate, partial or complete, any method
➔ *CPT Assistant* Feb 98:11, Nov 98:11, Sep 01:10, May 03:5; *CPT Changes: An Insider's View* 2006

(For excision of superior or middle turbinate, use 30999)

30140   Submucous resection inferior turbinate, partial or complete, any method
➔ *CPT Assistant* Nov 98:11, Dec 02:10, Apr 03:26, May 03:5, Dec 04:18; *CPT Changes: An Insider's View* 2006

(Do not report 30130 or 30140 in conjunction with 30801, 30802, 30930)

(For submucous resection of superior or middle turbinate, use 30999)

(For endoscopic resection of concha bullosa of middle turbinate, use 31240)

(For submucous resection of nasal septum, use 30520)

(For reduction of turbinates, use 30140 with modifier 52)

30150   Rhinectomy; partial

30160   total

(For closure and/or reconstruction, primary or delayed, see **Integumentary System,** 13150-13160, 14060-14300, 15120, 15121, 15260, 15261, 15760, 20900-20912)

Introduction

30200   Injection into turbinate(s), therapeutic
➔ *CPT Assistant* Dec 04:19

30210   Displacement therapy (Proetz type)

30220   Insertion, nasal septal prosthesis (button)

Removal of Foreign Body

30300   Removal foreign body, intranasal; office type procedure

30310   requiring general anesthesia

30320   by lateral rhinotomy

Repair

(For obtaining tissues for graft, see 20900-20926, 21210)

30400   Rhinoplasty, primary; lateral and alar cartilages and/or elevation of nasal tip

(For columellar reconstruction, see 13150 et seq)

30410   complete, external parts including bony pyramid, lateral and alar cartilages, and/or elevation of nasal tip

30420   including major septal repair

30430   Rhinoplasty, secondary; minor revision (small amount of nasal tip work)

30435   intermediate revision (bony work with osteotomies)

30450   major revision (nasal tip work and osteotomies)

30460   Rhinoplasty for nasal deformity secondary to congenital cleft lip and/or palate, including columellar lengthening; tip only

30462   tip, septum, osteotomies

30465 Repair of nasal vestibular stenosis (eg, spreader grafting, lateral nasal wall reconstruction)

➔ *CPT Changes: An Insider's View* 2001

(30465 excludes obtaining graft. For graft procedure, see 20900-20926, 21210)

(30465 is used to report a bilateral procedure. For unilateral procedure, use modifier 52)

Surgical Repair of Vestibular Stenosis
30465

An incision is made in the upper lateral cartilage and continued as an osteotomy of the medial aspect of the nasal bones. The spreader graft is placed to widen the nasal vestibule.

Nasal bone
Osteotomy site
Lateral nasal cartilage
Incision line
Greater alar cartilage
Spreader graft providing separation of upper lateral cartilage from septum

30520 Septoplasty or submucous resection, with or without cartilage scoring, contouring or replacement with graft

➔ *CPT Assistant* Oct 97:11, Dec 02:10

(For submucous resection of turbinates, use 30140)

30540 Repair choanal atresia; intranasal

30545 transpalatine

(Do not report modifier 63 in conjunction with 30540, 30545)

30560 Lysis intranasal synechia

30580 Repair fistula; oromaxillary (combine with 31030 if antrotomy is included)

30600 oronasal

30620 Septal or other intranasal dermatoplasty (does not include obtaining graft)

30630 Repair nasal septal perforations

Destruction

30801 Cautery and/or ablation, mucosa of inferior turbinates, unilateral or bilateral, any method; superficial

➔ *CPT Changes: An Insider's View* 2002, 2006

(For cautery and ablation of superior or middle turbinates, use 30999)

30802 intramural

(Do not report 30801, 30802, 30930 in conjunction with 30130 or 30140)

(For cautery performed for control of nasal hemorrhage, see 30901-30906)

Other Procedures

30901 Control nasal hemorrhage, anterior, simple (limited cautery and/or packing) any method

(To report bilateral procedure, use 30901 with modifier 50)

30903 Control nasal hemorrhage, anterior, complex (extensive cautery and/or packing) any method

(To report bilateral procedure, use 30903 with modifier 50)

30905 Control nasal hemorrhage, posterior, with posterior nasal packs and/or cautery, any method; initial

➔ *CPT Changes: An Insider's View* 2002

30906 subsequent

30915 Ligation arteries; ethmoidal

30920 internal maxillary artery, transantral

(For ligation external carotid artery, use 37600)

30930 Fracture nasal inferior turbinate(s), therapeutic

➔ *CPT Assistant* Jul 01:11, Dec 02:10, Jul 03:15, Aug 03:14, Dec 04:18; *CPT Changes: An Insider's View* 2006

(Do not report 30801, 30802, 30930 in conjunction with 30130 or 30140)

(For fracture of superior or middle turbinate(s), use 30999)

30999 Unlisted procedure, nose

Accessory Sinuses

Incision

31000 Lavage by cannulation; maxillary sinus (antrum puncture or natural ostium)

(To report bilateral procedure, use 31000 with modifier 50)

31002 sphenoid sinus

31020 Sinusotomy, maxillary (antrotomy); intranasal

(To report bilateral procedure, use 31020 with modifier 50)

31030   radical (Caldwell-Luc) without removal of antrochoanal polyps

(To report bilateral procedure, use 31030 with modifier 50)

31032   radical (Caldwell-Luc) with removal of antrochoanal polyps

(To report bilateral procedure, use 31032 with modifier 50)

31040   Pterygomaxillary fossa surgery, any approach

(For transantral ligation of internal maxillary artery, use 30920)

31050   Sinusotomy, sphenoid, with or without biopsy;

31051   with mucosal stripping or removal of polyp(s)

31070   Sinusotomy frontal; external, simple (trephine operation)

(For frontal intranasal sinusotomy, use 31276)

Sinusotomy, Frontal
31070

A trephine is used to access the frontal sinus.

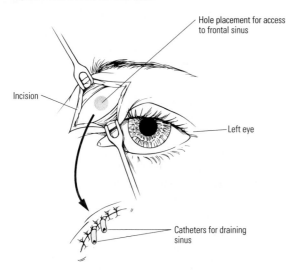

31075   transorbital, unilateral (for mucocele or osteoma, Lynch type)

31080   obliterative without osteoplastic flap, brow incision (includes ablation)

31081   obliterative, without osteoplastic flap, coronal incision (includes ablation)

31084   obliterative, with osteoplastic flap, brow incision

31085   obliterative, with osteoplastic flap, coronal incision

31086   nonobliterative, with osteoplastic flap, brow incision

31087   nonobliterative, with osteoplastic flap, coronal incision

31090   Sinusotomy, unilateral, three or more paranasal sinuses (frontal, maxillary, ethmoid, sphenoid)
         CPT Assistant Nov 97:15, Nov 98:11

Excision

31200   Ethmoidectomy; intranasal, anterior

31201   intranasal, total

31205   extranasal, total

31225   Maxillectomy; without orbital exenteration

31230   with orbital exenteration (en bloc)

(For orbital exenteration only, see 65110 et seq)

(For skin grafts, see 15120 et seq)

Endoscopy

A surgical sinus endoscopy includes a sinusotomy (when appropriate) and diagnostic endoscopy.

Codes 31231-31294 are used to report unilateral procedures unless otherwise specified.

The codes 31231-31235 for diagnostic evaluation refer to employing a nasal/sinus endoscope to inspect the interior of the nasal cavity and the middle and superior meatus, the turbinates, and the spheno-ethmoid recess. Any time a diagnostic evaluation is performed all these areas would be inspected and a separate code is not reported for each area.

Sinus Endoscopy
31231-31294

The physician uses an endoscope for visualizing and magnifying the internal structure of the sinuses.

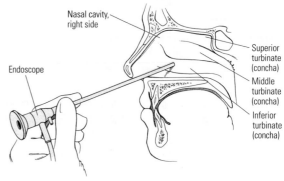

31231 Nasal endoscopy, diagnostic, unilateral or bilateral (separate procedure)
> *CPT Assistant* Winter 93:22, Jan 97:4

31233 Nasal/sinus endoscopy, diagnostic with maxillary sinusoscopy (via inferior meatus or canine fossa puncture)
> *CPT Assistant* Winter 93:22, Jan 97:4

31235 Nasal/sinus endoscopy, diagnostic with sphenoid sinusoscopy (via puncture of sphenoidal face or cannulation of ostium)
> *CPT Assistant* Winter 93:22, Jan 97:4

31237 Nasal/sinus endoscopy, surgical; with biopsy, polypectomy or debridement (separate procedure)
> *CPT Assistant* Winter 93:23, Jan 97:4, Dec 01:6, May 03:5

31238 with control of nasal hemorrhage
> *CPT Assistant* Winter 93:23, Jan 97:4; *CPT Changes: An Insider's View* 2002

31239 with dacryocystorhinostomy
> *CPT Assistant* Winter 93:23, Jan 97:4

31240 with concha bullosa resection
> *CPT Assistant* Winter 93:23, Jan 97:4, May 03:5

(For endoscopic osteomeatal complex (OMC) resection with antrostomy and/or anterior ethmoidectomy, with or without removal of polyp(s), use 31254 and 31256)

(For endoscopic osteomeatal complex (OMC) resection with antrostomy, removal of antral mucosal disease, and/or anterior ethmoidectomy, with or without removal of polyp(s), use 31254 and 31267)

(For endoscopic frontal sinus exploration, osteomeatal complex (OMC) resection and/or anterior ethmoidectomy, with or without removal of polyp(s), use 31254 and 31276)

(For endoscopic frontal sinus exploration, osteomeatal complex (OMC) resection, antrostomy, and/or anterior ethmoidectomy, with or without removal of polyp(s), use 31254, 31256, and 31276)

(For endoscopic nasal diagnostic endoscopy, see 31231-31235)

(For endoscopic osteomeatal complex (OMC) resection, frontal sinus exploration, antrostomy, removal of antral mucosal disease, and/or anterior ethmoidectomy, with or without removal of polyp(s), use 31254, 31267, and 31276)

31254 Nasal/sinus endoscopy, surgical; with ethmoidectomy, partial (anterior)
> *CPT Assistant* Winter 93:23, Jan 97:4, Sep 97:10, Oct 97:5, Dec 01:6, May 03:5

31255 with ethmoidectomy, total (anterior and posterior)
> *CPT Assistant* Winter 93:23, Jan 97:4, Dec 02:10, May 03:5

31256 Nasal/sinus endoscopy, surgical, with maxillary antrostomy;
> *CPT Assistant* Winter 93:23, Jan 97:4

(For endoscopic anterior and posterior ethmoidectomy (APE) and antrostomy, with or without removal of polyp(s), use 31255 and 31256)

(For endoscopic anterior and posterior ethmoidectomy (APE), antrostomy and removal of antral mucosal disease, with or without removal of polyp(s), use 31255 and 31267)

(For endoscopic anterior and posterior ethmoidectomy (APE), and frontal sinus exploration, with or without removal of polyp(s), use 31255 and 31276)

31267 with removal of tissue from maxillary sinus
> *CPT Assistant* Jan 97:4, Dec 01:6

(For endoscopic anterior and posterior ethmoidectomy (APE), and frontal sinus exploration and antrostomy, with or without removal of polyp(s), use 31255, 31256, and 31276)

(For endoscopic anterior and posterior ethmoidectomy (APE), frontal sinus exploration, antrostomy, and removal of antral mucosal disease, with or without removal of polyp(s), use 31255, 31267, and 31276)

31276 Nasal/sinus endoscopy, surgical with frontal sinus exploration, with or without removal of tissue from frontal sinus
> *CPT Assistant* Winter 93:24, Jan 97:4

(For endoscopic anterior and posterior ethmoidectomy and sphenoidotomy (APS), with or without removal of polyp(s), use 31255, 31287 or 31288)

(For endoscopic anterior and posterior ethmoidectomy and sphenoidotomy (APS), and antrostomy, with or without removal of polyp(s), use 31255, 31256, and 31287 or 31288)

(For endoscopic anterior and posterior ethmoidectomy and sphenoidotomy (APS), antrostomy and removal of antral mucosal disease, with or without removal of polyp(s), use 31255, 31267, and 31287 or 31288)

(For endoscopic anterior and posterior ethmoidectomy and sphenoidotomy (APS), and frontal sinus exploration with or without removal of polyp(s), use 31255, 31287 or 31288, and 31276)

(For endoscopic anterior and posterior ethmoidectomy and sphenoidotomy (APS), with or without removal of polyp(s), with frontal sinus exploration and antrostomy, use 31255, 31256, 31287 or 31288, and 31276)

(For unilateral endoscopy of two or more sinuses, see 31231-31235)

(For endoscopic anterior and posterior ethmoidectomy and sphenoidotomy (APS), frontal sinus exploration, antrostomy and removal of antral mucosal disease, with or without removal of polyp(s), see 31255, 31267, 31287 or 31288 and 31276)

31287   Nasal/sinus endoscopy, surgical, with sphenoidotomy;
      ➲ *CPT Assistant* Winter 93:24, Jan 97:4

31288   with removal of tissue from the sphenoid sinus
      ➲ *CPT Assistant* Winter 93:24, Jan 97:4

31290   Nasal/sinus endoscopy, surgical, with repair of cerebrospinal fluid leak; ethmoid region
      ➲ *CPT Assistant* Winter 93:24, Jan 97:4

31291   sphenoid region
      ➲ *CPT Assistant* Winter 93:24, Jan 97:4

31292   Nasal/sinus endoscopy, surgical; with medial or inferior orbital wall decompression
      ➲ *CPT Assistant* Winter 93:24, Jan 97:4

31293   with medial orbital wall and inferior orbital wall decompression
      ➲ *CPT Assistant* Winter 93:24, Jan 97:4

31294   with optic nerve decompression
      ➲ *CPT Assistant* Winter 93:24, Jan 97:4

Other Procedures

(For hypophysectomy, transantral or transeptal approach, use 61548)

(For transcranial hypophysectomy, use 61546)

31299   Unlisted procedure, accessory sinuses

Larynx

Excision

31300   Laryngotomy (thyrotomy, laryngofissure); with removal of tumor or laryngocele, cordectomy

31320   diagnostic

31360   Laryngectomy; total, without radical neck dissection

31365   total, with radical neck dissection
      ➲ *CPT Assistant* Oct 01:10

31367   subtotal supraglottic, without radical neck dissection

31368   subtotal supraglottic, with radical neck dissection

31370   Partial laryngectomy (hemilaryngectomy); horizontal

31375   laterovertical

31380   anterovertical

31382   antero-latero-vertical

31390   Pharyngolaryngectomy, with radical neck dissection; without reconstruction

31395   with reconstruction

31400   Arytenoidectomy or arytenoidopexy, external approach

(For endoscopic arytenoidectomy, use 31560)

31420   Epiglottidectomy

Introduction

⊘ **31500**   Intubation, endotracheal, emergency procedure
      ➲ *CPT Assistant* Nov 99:32-33, Oct 03:2, Aug 04:8, Jul 06:4

(For injection procedure for segmental bronchography, use 31656)

31502   Tracheotomy tube change prior to establishment of fistula tract
      ➲ *CPT Assistant* Winter 90:6

Endoscopy

For endoscopic procedures, code appropriate endoscopy of each anatomic site examined. If using operating microscope, telescope, or both, use the applicable code only once per operative session.

31505   Laryngoscopy, indirect; diagnostic (separate procedure)
      ➲ *CPT Assistant* Nov 99:13; *CPT Changes: An Insider's View* 2000

31510   with biopsy
      ➲ *CPT Assistant* Nov 99:13

31511   with removal of foreign body
      ➲ *CPT Assistant* Nov 99:13

31512   with removal of lesion
      ➲ *CPT Assistant* Nov 99:13

31513   with vocal cord injection
      ➲ *CPT Assistant* Nov 99:13

31515   Laryngoscopy direct, with or without tracheoscopy; for aspiration

31520   diagnostic, newborn

(Do not report modifier 63 in conjunction with 31520)

31525   diagnostic, except newborn

31526   diagnostic, with operating microscope or telescope
      ➲ *CPT Assistant* Nov 98:11-12; *CPT Changes: An Insider's View* 2006

(Do not report code 69990 in addition to code 31526)

31527   with insertion of obturator

31528   with dilation, initial
      ➲ *CPT Changes: An Insider's View* 2002

31529   with dilation, subsequent
      ➲ *CPT Changes: An Insider's View* 2002

31530   Laryngoscopy, direct, operative, with foreign body removal;

31531   with operating microscope or telescope
      ➲ *CPT Assistant* Nov 98:11-12; *CPT Changes: An Insider's View* 2006

(Do not report code 69990 in addition to code 31531)

31535   Laryngoscopy, direct, operative, with biopsy;

▲=Revised code   ●=New code   ▶ ◀=Contains new or revised text   ⊘=Modifier 51 exempt   American Medical Association   **135**

31536   with operating microscope or telescope
> *CPT Assistant* Nov 98:11-12; *CPT Changes: An Insider's View* 2006

(Do not report code 69990 in addition to code 31536)

31540   Laryngoscopy, direct, operative, with excision of tumor and/or stripping of vocal cords or epiglottis;

31541   with operating microscope or telescope
> *CPT Assistant* Nov 98:11-12; *CPT Changes: An Insider's View* 2006

(Do not report code 69990 in addition to code 31541)

31545   Laryngoscopy, direct, operative, with operating microscope or telescope, with submucosal removal of non-neoplastic lesion(s) of vocal cord; reconstruction with local tissue flap(s)
> *CPT Changes: An Insider's View* 2005

31546   reconstruction with graft(s) (includes obtaining autograft)
> *CPT Changes: An Insider's View* 2005

(Do not report 31546 in addition to 20926 for graft harvest)

(For reconstruction of vocal cord with allograft, use 31599)

(Do not report 31545 or 31546 in conjunction with 31540, 31541, 69990)

31560   Laryngoscopy, direct, operative, with arytenoidectomy;

31561   with operating microscope or telescope
> *CPT Assistant* Nov 98:11-12; *CPT Changes: An Insider's View* 2006

(Do not report code 69990 in addition to code 31561)

31570   Laryngoscopy, direct, with injection into vocal cord(s), therapeutic;

31571   with operating microscope or telescope
> *CPT Assistant* Nov 98:11-12; *CPT Changes: An Insider's View* 2006

(Do not report code 69990 in addition to code 31571)

31575   Laryngoscopy, flexible fiberoptic; diagnostic

31576   with biopsy

31577   with removal of foreign body

31578   with removal of lesion

(To report flexible fiberoptic endoscopic evaluation of swallowing, see 92612-92613)

(To report flexible fiberoptic endoscopic evaluation with sensory testing, see 92614-92615)

(To report flexible fiberoptic endoscopic evaluation of swallowing with sensory testing, see 92616-92617)

(For flexible fiberoptic laryngoscopy as part of flexible fiberoptic endoscopic evaluation of swallowing and/or laryngeal sensory testing by cine or video recording, see 92612-92617)

31579   Laryngoscopy, flexible or rigid fiberoptic, with stroboscopy

Repair

31580   Laryngoplasty; for laryngeal web, two stage, with keel insertion and removal

31582   for laryngeal stenosis, with graft or core mold, including tracheotomy

31584   with open reduction of fracture

(31585 and 31586 have been deleted. To report, use the appropriate Evaluation and Management codes)

31587   Laryngoplasty, cricoid split

31588   Laryngoplasty, not otherwise specified (eg, for burns, reconstruction after partial laryngectomy)
> *CPT Assistant* Aug 04:11

31590   Laryngeal reinnervation by neuromuscular pedicle

Destruction

31595   Section recurrent laryngeal nerve, therapeutic (separate procedure), unilateral

Other Procedures

31599   Unlisted procedure, larynx

Trachea and Bronchi

Incision

31600   Tracheostomy, planned (separate procedure);

31601   younger than two years

31603   Tracheostomy, emergency procedure; transtracheal

31605   cricothyroid membrane

31610   Tracheostomy, fenestration procedure with skin flaps

(For endotracheal intubation, use 31500)

(For tracheal aspiration under direct vision, use 31515)

31611   Construction of tracheoesophageal fistula and subsequent insertion of an alaryngeal speech prosthesis (eg, voice button, Blom-Singer prosthesis)

31612   Tracheal puncture, percutaneous with transtracheal aspiration and/or injection

31613   Tracheostoma revision; simple, without flap rotation

31614   complex, with flap rotation

Endoscopy

For endoscopy procedures, code appropriate endoscopy of each anatomic site examined. Surgical bronchoscopy always includes diagnostic bronchoscopy when performed by the same physician. Codes 31622-31646 include fluoroscopic guidance, when performed.

(For tracheoscopy, see laryngoscopy codes 31515-31578)

⊙ **31615** Tracheobronchoscopy through established tracheostomy incision

⊙+ **31620** Endobronchial ultrasound (EBUS) during bronchoscopic diagnostic or therapeutic intervention(s) (List separately in addition to code for primary procedure(s))

➔ *CPT Assistant* Aug 05:4; *CPT Changes: An Insider's View* 2005

(Use 31620 in conjunction with 31622-31646)

⊙ **31622** Bronchoscopy, rigid or flexible, with or without fluoroscopic guidance; diagnostic, with or without cell washing (separate procedure)

➔ *CPT Assistant* Jul 96:11, Nov 98:12, Dec 98:8, Mar 99:3, Apr 00:10, Jun 01:10, Jan 02:10, Sep 04:8, 12, Aug 05:4; *CPT Changes: An Insider's View* 2004

⊙ **31623** with brushing or protected brushings

➔ *CPT Assistant* Nov 98:12, Mar 99:3, Nov 99:13, Jan 02:10, Sep 04:8, Aug 05:4

⊙ **31624** with bronchial alveolar lavage

➔ *CPT Assistant* Nov 98:12, Feb 99:9, Mar 99:3, 11, Jan 02:10, Sep 04:8, Aug 05:4

⊙ **31625** with bronchial or endobronchial biopsy(s), single or multiple sites

➔ *CPT Assistant* Spring 91:2, Jan 02:10, Jun 02:10, Sep 03:15, Sep 04:9, Aug 05:4; *CPT Changes: An Insider's View* 2004

Bronchoscopy
31622-31656

A rigid or flexible bronchoscope is inserted through the oropharynx and vocal cords and beyond the trachea into the right or left bronchi.

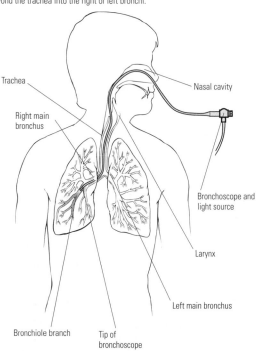

Trachea

Nasal cavity

Right main bronchus

Bronchoscope and light source

Larynx

Left main bronchus

Bronchiole branch

Tip of bronchoscope

⊙ **31628** with transbronchial lung biopsy(s), single lobe

➔ *CPT Assistant* Jun 01:10, Jan 02:10, Sep 04:9, Aug 05:4; *CPT Changes: An Insider's View* 2004

(31628 should be reported only once regardless of how many transbronchial lung biopsies are performed in a lobe)

(To report transbronchial lung biopsies performed on additional lobe, use 31632)

⊙ **31629** with transbronchial needle aspiration biopsy(s), trachea, main stem and/or lobar bronchus(i)

➔ *CPT Assistant* Apr 00:10, Jan 02:10, Sep 03:15, May 04:15, Jul 04:13, Aug 05:4; *CPT Changes: An Insider's View* 2004

(31629 should be reported only once for upper airway biopsies regardless of how many transbronchial needle aspiration biopsies are performed in the upper airway or in a lobe)

(To report transbronchial needle aspiration biopsies performed on additional lobe(s), use 31633)

31630 with tracheal/bronchial dilation or closed reduction of fracture

➔ *CPT Assistant* Jan 02:10, Aug 05:4; *CPT Changes: An Insider's View* 2005

31631 with placement of tracheal stent(s) (includes tracheal/bronchial dilation as required)

➔ *CPT Assistant* Jan 02:10, Aug 05:4; *CPT Changes: An Insider's View* 2005

(For placement of bronchial stent, see 31636, 31637)

(For revision of tracheal/bronchial stent, use 31638)

+ **31632** with transbronchial lung biopsy(s), each additional lobe (List separately in addition to code for primary procedure)

➔ *CPT Assistant* Jan 02:10, Sep 04:9, Aug 05:4; *CPT Changes: An Insider's View* 2004

(Use 31632 in conjunction with 31628)

(31632 should be reported only once regardless of how many transbronchial lung biopsies are performed in a lobe)

+ **31633** with transbronchial needle aspiration biopsy(s), each additional lobe (List separately in addition to code for primary procedure)

➔ *CPT Assistant* Jan 02:10, May 04:15, Jul 04:13, Sep 04:10, Aug 05:4; *CPT Changes: An Insider's View* 2004

(Use 31633 in conjunction with 31629)

(31633 should be reported only once regardless of how many transbronchial needle aspiration biopsies are performed in the trachea or the additional lobe)

⊙ **31635** with removal of foreign body

➔ *CPT Assistant* Jan 02:10, Jun 02:10

31636 with placement of bronchial stent(s) (includes tracheal/bronchial dilation as required), initial bronchus

➔ *CPT Assistant* Aug 05:4; *CPT Changes: An Insider's View* 2005

+ 31637   each additional major bronchus stented (List separately in addition to code for primary procedure)
> *CPT Assistant* Aug 05:4; *CPT Changes: An Insider's View* 2005

(Use 31637 in conjunction with 31636)

31638   with revision of tracheal or bronchial stent inserted at previous session (includes tracheal/bronchial dilation as required)
> *CPT Assistant* Aug 05:4; *CPT Changes: An Insider's View* 2005

31640   with excision of tumor
> *CPT Assistant* Jan 02:10, Aug 05:4

31641   Bronchoscopy (rigid or flexible); with destruction of tumor or relief of stenosis by any method other than excision (eg, laser therapy, cryotherapy)
> *CPT Assistant* Nov 99:13, Sep 00:5, Jan 02:10, Aug 05:4; *CPT Changes: An Insider's View* 2002

(For bronchoscopic photodynamic therapy, report 31641 in addition to 96570, 96571 as appropriate)

31643   with placement of catheter(s) for intracavitary radioelement application
> *CPT Assistant* Nov 98:12, Mar 99:3, Jan 02:10, Aug 05:4

(For intracavitary radioelement application, see 77761-77763, 77781-77784)

⊙ 31645   with therapeutic aspiration of tracheobronchial tree, initial (eg, drainage of lung abscess)
> *CPT Assistant* Jan 02:10, Aug 05:4

⊙ 31646   with therapeutic aspiration of tracheobronchial tree, subsequent
> *CPT Assistant* Jan 02:10, Aug 05:4

(For catheter aspiration of tracheobronchial tree at bedside, use 31725)

⊙ 31656   with injection of contrast material for segmental bronchography (fiberscope only)
> *CPT Assistant* Jan 02:10

(For radiological supervision and interpretation, see 71040, 71060)

Introduction

(For endotracheal intubation, use 31500)

(For tracheal aspiration under direct vision, see 31515)

(31700, 31708, 31710 have been deleted)

31715   Transtracheal injection for bronchography

(For radiological supervision and interpretation, see 71040, 71060)

(For prolonged services, see 99354-99360)

31717   Catheterization with bronchial brush biopsy
> *CPT Assistant* Feb 01:11

31720   Catheter aspiration (separate procedure); nasotracheal

⊙ 31725   tracheobronchial with fiberscope, bedside

31730   Transtracheal (percutaneous) introduction of needle wire dilator/stent or indwelling tube for oxygen therapy

Excision, Repair

31750   Tracheoplasty; cervical

31755   tracheopharyngeal fistulization, each stage

31760   intrathoracic

31766   Carinal reconstruction

31770   Bronchoplasty; graft repair

31775   excision stenosis and anastomosis

(For lobectomy and bronchoplasty, use 32501)

31780   Excision tracheal stenosis and anastomosis; cervical

31781   cervicothoracic

31785   Excision of tracheal tumor or carcinoma; cervical

31786   thoracic

31800   Suture of tracheal wound or injury; cervical

31805   intrathoracic

31820   Surgical closure tracheostomy or fistula; without plastic repair

31825   with plastic repair

(For repair tracheoesophageal fistula, see 43305, 43312)

31830   Revision of tracheostomy scar

Other Procedures

31899   Unlisted procedure, trachea, bronchi

Lungs and Pleura

Incision

►(32000 has been deleted. To report, use 32421)◄

►(32002 has been deleted. To report, use 32422)◄

►(32005 has been deleted. To report, use 32560)◄

►(32019 has been deleted. To report, use 32550)◄

►(32020 has been deleted. To report, use 32551)◄

32035   Thoracostomy; with rib resection for empyema

32036   with open flap drainage for empyema

32095   Thoracotomy, limited, for biopsy of lung or pleura

(To report wound exploration due to penetrating trauma without thoractomy, use 20102)

32100   Thoracotomy, major; with exploration and biopsy

(Do not report 32100 in conjunction with 19260, 19271, 19272, 32503, 32504)

32110	with control of traumatic hemorrhage and/or repair of lung tear
32120	for postoperative complications
32124	with open intrapleural pneumonolysis
32140	with cyst(s) removal, with or without a pleural procedure
32141	with excision-plication of bullae, with or without any pleural procedure

(For lung volume reduction, use 32491)

32150	with removal of intrapleural foreign body or fibrin deposit
32151	with removal of intrapulmonary foreign body
32160	with cardiac massage

(For segmental or other resections of lung, see 32480-32504)

32200 Pneumonostomy; with open drainage of abscess or cyst
➔ *CPT Assistant* Nov 97:15

⊙ **32201** with percutaneous drainage of abscess or cyst
➔ *CPT Assistant* Nov 97:15-16, Mar 98:8

(For radiological supervision and interpretation, use 75989)

32215 Pleural scarification for repeat pneumothorax

32220 Decortication, pulmonary (separate procedure); total

32225 partial

Excision

32310 Pleurectomy, parietal (separate procedure)

32320 Decortication and parietal pleurectomy

32400 Biopsy, pleura; percutaneous needle
➔ *CPT Assistant* Fall 94:1-2

(If imaging guidance is performed, see 76942, 77002, 77012, 77021)

(For fine needle aspiration, use 10021 or 10022)

(For evaluation of fine needle aspirate, see 88172, 88173)

32402 open
➔ *CPT Assistant* Fall 94:1-2

32405 Biopsy, lung or mediastinum, percutaneous needle
➔ *CPT Assistant* Fall 94:1-2, Mar 97:4, Aug 02:10

(For radiological supervision and interpretation, see 76942, 77002, 77012, 77021)

(For fine needle aspiration, use 10022)

(For evaluation of fine needle aspirate, see 88172, 88173)

Removal

32420 Pneumocentesis, puncture of lung for aspiration
➔ *CPT Assistant* Fall 94:1-2; *CPT Changes: An Insider's View* 2002

● **32421** Thoracentesis, puncture of pleural cavity for aspiration, initial or subsequent
➔ *CPT Changes: An Insider's View* 2008

▶(If imaging guidance is performed, see 76942, 77002, 77012)◀

▶(For total lung lavage, use 32997)◀

● **32422** Thoracentesis with insertion of tube, includes water seal (eg, for pneumothorax), when performed (separate procedure)
➔ *CPT Changes: An Insider's View* 2008

▶(Do not report 32422 in conjunction with 19260, 19271, 19272, 32503, 32504)◀

▶(If imaging guidance is performed, see 76942, 77002, 77012)◀

Thoracentesis
32421-32422

Accumulated fluid or air is removed from the pleural space by puncturing space between the ribs. In 32421, a tube is inserted and a syringe attached to the catheter for the removal of fluid and/or air.

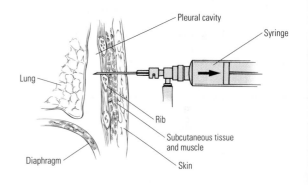

32440 Removal of lung, total pneumonectomy;
➔ *CPT Assistant* Fall 94:1

32442 with resection of segment of trachea followed by broncho-tracheal anastomosis (sleeve pneumonectomy)
➔ *CPT Assistant* Fall 94:1, 3

32445 extrapleural
➔ *CPT Assistant* Fall 94:1, 3

(For extrapleural pneumonectomy, with empyemectomy, use 32445 and 32540)

(If lung resection is performed with chest wall tumor resection, report the appropriate chest wall tumor resection code, 19260-19272, in addition to lung resection code 32440-32445)

32480 Removal of lung, other than total pneumonectomy; single lobe (lobectomy)

> *CPT Assistant* Spring 91:5, Fall 94:1, 4

32482 two lobes (bilobectomy)

> *CPT Assistant* Fall 94:1, 4, Jan 07:31

32484 single segment (segmentectomy)

> *CPT Assistant* Fall 94:1, 4

(For removal of lung with bronchoplasty, use 32501)

32486 with circumferential resection of segment of bronchus followed by broncho-bronchial anastomosis (sleeve lobectomy)

> *CPT Assistant* Fall 94:1, 4

32488 all remaining lung following previous removal of a portion of lung (completion pneumonectomy)

> *CPT Assistant* Fall 94:1, 4

(For total or segmental lobectomy, with concomitant decortication, use 32320 and the appropriate removal of lung code)

32491 excision-plication of emphysematous lung(s) (bullous or non-bullous) for lung volume reduction, sternal split or transthoracic approach, with or without any pleural procedure

> *CPT Assistant* Nov 96:7

32500 wedge resection, single or multiple

> *CPT Assistant* Fall 94:1, 5, Mar 97:4

(If lung resection is performed with chest wall tumor resection, report the appropriate chest wall tumor resection code, 19260-19272, in addition to lung resection code 32480-32500)

+ 32501 Resection and repair of portion of bronchus (bronchoplasty) when performed at time of lobectomy or segmentectomy (List separately in addition to code for primary procedure)

(Use 32501 in conjunction with 32480, 32482, 32484)

(32501 is to be used when a portion of the bronchus to preserved lung is removed and requires plastic closure to preserve function of that preserved lung. It is not to be used for closure for the proximal end of a resected bronchus)

32503 Resection of apical lung tumor (eg, Pancoast tumor), including chest wall resection, rib(s) resection(s), neurovascular dissection, when performed; without chest wall reconstruction(s)

> *CPT Changes: An Insider's View* 2006

32504 with chest wall reconstruction

> *CPT Changes: An Insider's View* 2006

▶(Do not report 32503, 32504 in conjunction with 19260, 19271, 19272, 32100, 32422, 32551)◀

(32520, 32522, and 32525 have been deleted)

(For performance of lung resection in conjunction with chest wall resection, see 19260, 19271, 19272 and 32480-32500, 32503, 32504)

32540 Extrapleural enucleation of empyema (empyemectomy)

(For extrapleural enucleation of empyema (empyemectomy) with lobectomy, use 32540 and the appropriate removal of lung code)

▶Introduction◀

32550 Insertion of indwelling tunneled pleural catheter with cuff

> *CPT Changes: An Insider's View* 2008

▶(Do not report 32550 in conjunction with 32421, 32422, 32551, 32560, 36000, 36410, 62318, 62319, 64450, 64470, 64475)◀

▶(If imaging guidance is performed, use 75989)◀

32551 Tube thoracostomy, includes water seal (eg, for abscess, hemothorax, empyema), when performed (separate procedure)

> *CPT Changes: An Insider's View* 2008

▶(Do not report 32551 in conjunction with 19260, 19271, 19272, 32503, 32504)◀

▶(If imaging guidance is performed, use 75989)◀

Insertion of Chest Tube
32551

A trocar is used to puncture through the space between the ribs into the pleural cavity for the insertion of a chest tube via a thoracic drainage system to drain air and/or fluid from the pleural space, promoting lung re-expansion.

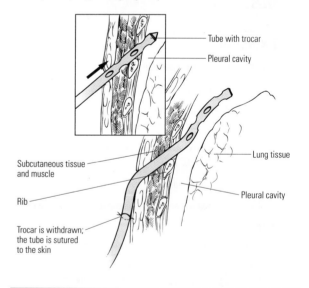

Tube with trocar
Pleural cavity
Lung tissue
Pleural cavity
Subcutaneous tissue and muscle
Rib
Trocar is withdrawn; the tube is sutured to the skin

▶Destruction◀

32560 Chemical pleurodesis (eg, for recurrent or persistent pneumothorax)

> *CPT Changes: An Insider's View* 2008

Endoscopy

Surgical thoracoscopy always includes diagnostic thoracoscopy.

For endoscopic procedures, code appropriate endoscopy of each anatomic site examined.

Thoracoscopy
32601-32665

The inside of the chest cavity is examined through a fiberoptic endoscope.

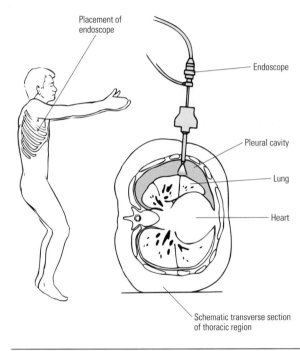

Placement of endoscope

Endoscope

Pleural cavity

Lung

Heart

Schematic transverse section of thoracic region

32601   Thoracoscopy, diagnostic (separate procedure); lungs and pleural space, without biopsy
⊃ *CPT Assistant* Fall 94:1, 4

32602   lungs and pleural space, with biopsy
⊃ *CPT Assistant* Fall 94:1, 4, Jun 97:5

32603   pericardial sac, without biopsy
⊃ *CPT Assistant* Fall 94:1, 4

32604   pericardial sac, with biopsy
⊃ *CPT Assistant* Fall 94:1, 4

32605   mediastinal space, without biopsy
⊃ *CPT Assistant* Fall 94:1, 4

32606   mediastinal space, with biopsy
⊃ *CPT Assistant* Fall 94:1, 5

(Surgical thoracoscopy always includes diagnostic thoracoscopy)

32650   Thoracoscopy, surgical; with pleurodesis (eg, mechanical or chemical)
⊃ *CPT Assistant* Fall 94:1, 6; *CPT Changes: An Insider's View* 2002

32651   with partial pulmonary decortication
⊃ *CPT Assistant* Fall 94:1, 6

32652   with total pulmonary decortication, including intrapleural pneumonolysis
⊃ *CPT Assistant* Fall 94:1, 6

32653   with removal of intrapleural foreign body or fibrin deposit
⊃ *CPT Assistant* Fall 94:1, 6

32654   with control of traumatic hemorrhage
⊃ *CPT Assistant* Fall 94:1, 6

32655   with excision-plication of bullae, including any pleural procedure
⊃ *CPT Assistant* Fall 94:1, 6, Aug 05:15

32656   with parietal pleurectomy
⊃ *CPT Assistant* Fall 94:1, 6

32657   with wedge resection of lung, single or multiple
⊃ *CPT Assistant* Fall 94:1, 6

32658   with removal of clot or foreign body from pericardial sac
⊃ *CPT Assistant* Fall 94:1, 6

32659   with creation of pericardial window or partial resection of pericardial sac for drainage
⊃ *CPT Assistant* Fall 94:1, 6

32660   with total pericardiectomy
⊃ *CPT Assistant* Fall 94:1, 6

32661   with excision of pericardial cyst, tumor, or mass
⊃ *CPT Assistant* Fall 94:1, 6

32662   with excision of mediastinal cyst, tumor, or mass
⊃ *CPT Assistant* Fall 94:1, 6

32663   with lobectomy, total or segmental
⊃ *CPT Assistant* Fall 94:1, 6

32664   with thoracic sympathectomy
⊃ *CPT Assistant* Fall 94:1, Oct 99:10

32665   with esophagomyotomy (Heller type)
⊃ *CPT Assistant* Fall 94:1, 6

(For exploratory thoracoscopy, and exploratory thoracoscopy with biopsy, see 32601-32606)

Repair

32800   Repair lung hernia through chest wall

32810   Closure of chest wall following open flap drainage for empyema (Clagett type procedure)

32815   Open closure of major bronchial fistula

32820   Major reconstruction, chest wall (posttraumatic)

Lung Transplantation

Lung allotransplantation involves three distinct components of physician work:

1) *Cadaver donor pneumonectomy(s)*, which include(s) harvesting the allograft and cold preservation of the allograft (perfusing with cold preservation solution and cold maintenance) (use 32850).

2) *Backbench work*:

Preparation of a cadaver donor single lung allograft prior to transplantation, including dissection of the allograft from surrounding soft tissues to prepare the pulmonary venous/atrial cuff, pulmonary artery, and bronchus unilaterally (use 32855).

Preparation of a cadaver donor double lung allograft prior to transplantation, including dissection of the allograft from surrounding soft tissues to prepare the pulmonary venous/atrial cuff, pulmonary artery, and bronchus bilaterally (use 32856).

3) *Recipient lung allotransplantation*, which includes transplantation of a single or double lung allograft and care of the recipient (see 32851-32854).

32850   Donor pneumonectomy(s) (including cold preservation), from cadaver donor
> *CPT Changes: An Insider's View* 2005

32851   Lung transplant, single; without cardiopulmonary bypass

32852   with cardiopulmonary bypass

32853   Lung transplant, double (bilateral sequential or en bloc); without cardiopulmonary bypass

32854   with cardiopulmonary bypass

32855   Backbench standard preparation of cadaver donor lung allograft prior to transplantation, including dissection of allograft from surrounding soft tissues to prepare pulmonary venous/atrial cuff, pulmonary artery, and bronchus; unilateral
> *CPT Changes: An Insider's View* 2005

32856   bilateral
> *CPT Changes: An Insider's View* 2005

(For repair or resection procedures on the donor lung, see 32491, 32500, 35216, or 35276)

Surgical Collapse Therapy; Thoracoplasty

(See also 32503, 32504)

32900   Resection of ribs, extrapleural, all stages

32905   Thoracoplasty, Schede type or extrapleural (all stages);

32906   with closure of bronchopleural fistula

(For open closure of major bronchial fistula, use 32815)

(For resection of first rib for thoracic outlet compression, see 21615, 21616)

32940   Pneumonolysis, extraperiosteal, including filling or packing procedures

32960   Pneumothorax, therapeutic, intrapleural injection of air

Other Procedures

32997   Total lung lavage (unilateral)
> *CPT Assistant* Nov 98:13, Nov 99:14; *CPT Changes: An Insider's View* 2000, 2002

(For bronchoscopic bronchial alveolar lavage, use 31624)

32998   Ablation therapy for reduction or eradication of one or more pulmonary tumor(s) including pleura or chest wall when involved by tumor extension, percutaneous, radiofrequency, unilateral
> *CPT Changes: An Insider's View* 2007

(For imaging guidance and monitoring, see 76940, 77013, 77022)

32999   Unlisted procedure, lungs and pleura
> *CPT Assistant* Jan 02:11, Feb 02:11
> *Clinical Examples in Radiology* Spring 06:8-9

Cardiovascular System

Selective vascular catheterizations should be coded to include introduction and all lesser order selective catheterizations used in the approach (eg, the description for a selective right middle cerebral artery catheterization includes the introduction and placement catheterization of the right common and internal carotid arteries).

Additional second and/or third order arterial catheterizations within the same family of arteries supplied by a single first order artery should be expressed by 36218 or 36248. Additional first order or higher catheterizations in vascular families supplied by a first order vessel different from a previously selected and coded family should be separately coded using the conventions described above.

> (For monitoring, operation of pump and other nonsurgical services, see 99190-99192, 99291, 99292, 99354-99360)

> (For other medical or laboratory related services, see appropriate section)

> (For radiological supervision and interpretation, see 75600-75978)

Heart and Pericardium

Pericardium

⊙ **33010**   Pericardiocentesis; initial

> (For radiological supervision and interpretation, use 76930)

⊙ **33011**   subsequent

> (For radiological supervision and interpretation, use 76930)

33015   Tube pericardiostomy

33020   Pericardiotomy for removal of clot or foreign body (primary procedure)

33025   Creation of pericardial window or partial resection for drainage

33030   Pericardiectomy, subtotal or complete; without cardiopulmonary bypass

33031   with cardiopulmonary bypass

33050   Excision of pericardial cyst or tumor

Cardiac Tumor

33120   Excision of intracardiac tumor, resection with cardiopulmonary bypass

33130   Resection of external cardiac tumor

Transmyocardial Revascularization

33140   Transmyocardial laser revascularization, by thoracotomy; (separate procedure)

> ⟳ *CPT Assistant* Nov 99:14, Nov 00:5, Apr 01:7; *CPT Changes: An Insider's View* 2000, 2001, 2002

+ **33141**   performed at the time of other open cardiac procedure(s) (List separately in addition to code for primary procedure)

> ⟳ *CPT Assistant* Apr 01:7; *CPT Changes: An Insider's View* 2001

> (Use 33141 in conjunction with 33400-33496, 33510-33536, 33542)

Pacemaker or Pacing Cardioverter-Defibrillator

A pacemaker system includes a pulse generator containing electronics, a battery, and one or more electrodes (leads). Pulse generators are placed in a subcutaneous "pocket" created in either a subclavicular site or underneath the abdominal muscles just below the ribcage. Electrodes may be inserted through a vein (transvenous) or they may be placed on the surface of the heart (epicardial). The epicardial location of electrodes requires a thoracotomy for electrode insertion.

A single chamber pacemaker system includes a pulse generator and one electrode inserted in either the atrium or ventricle. A dual chamber pacemaker system includes a pulse generator and one electrode inserted in the right atrium and one electrode inserted in the right ventricle. In certain circumstances, an additional electrode may be required to achieve pacing of the left ventricle (bi-ventricular pacing). In this event, transvenous (cardiac vein) placement of the electrode should be separately reported using code 33224 or 33225. Epicardial placement of the electrode should be separately reported using 33202-33203.

Like a pacemaker system, a pacing cardioverter-defibrillator system includes a pulse generator and electrodes, although pacing cardioverter-defibrillators may require multiple leads, even when only a single chamber is being paced. A pacing cardioverter-defibrillator system may be inserted in a single chamber (pacing in the ventricle) or in dual chambers (pacing in atrium and ventricle). These devices use a combination of antitachycardia pacing, low-energy cardioversion or defibrillating shocks to treat ventricular tachycardia or ventricular fibrillation.

Pacing cardioverter-defibrillator pulse generators may be implanted in a subcutaneous infraclavicular pocket or in an abdominal pocket. Removal of a pacing cardioverter-defibrillator pulse generator requires opening of the existing subcutaneous pocket and disconnection of the pulse generator from its electrode(s). A thoracotomy (or laparotomy in the case of abdominally placed pulse generators) is not required to remove the pulse generator.

The electrodes (leads) of a pacing cardioverter-defibrillator system are positioned in the heart via the venous system (transvenously), in most circumstances. In certain circumstances, an additional electrode may be required to achieve pacing of the left ventricle (bi-ventricular pacing). In this event, transvenous (cardiac vein) placement of the electrode should be separately reported using code 33224 or 33225. Epicardial placement of the electrode should be separately reported using 33202-33203.

Electrode positioning on the epicardial surface of the heart requires thoracotomy, or thoracoscopic placement of the leads. Removal of electrode(s) may first be attempted by transvenous extraction (code 33244). However, if transvenous extraction is unsuccessful, a thoracotomy may be required to remove the electrodes (code 33243). Use codes 33212, 33213, 33240 as appropriate in addition to the thoracotomy or endoscopic epicardial lead placement codes to report the insertion of the generator if done by the same physician during the same session.

When the "battery" of a pacemaker or pacing cardioverter-defibrillator is changed, it is actually the pulse generator that is changed. Replacement of a pulse generator should be reported with a code for removal of the pulse generator and another code for insertion of a pulse generator.

Repositioning of a pacemaker electrode, pacing cardioverter-defibrillator electrode(s), or a left ventricular pacing electrode is reported using 33215 or 33226, as appropriate. Replacement of a pacemaker electrode, pacing cardioverter-defibrillator electrode(s), or a left ventricular pacing electrode is reported using 33206-33208, 33210-33213, or 33224, as appropriate.

> (For electronic, telephonic analysis of internal pacemaker system, see 93731-93736)

> (For radiological supervision and interpretation with insertion of pacemaker, use 71090)

> (33200, 33201 have been deleted)

33202 Insertion of epicardial electrode(s); open incision (eg, thoracotomy, median sternotomy, subxiphoid approach)
> ➔ *CPT Changes: An Insider's View* 2007

33203 endoscopic approach (eg, thoracoscopy, pericardioscopy)
> ➔ *CPT Changes: An Insider's View* 2007

> (When epicardial lead placement is performed by the same physician at the same session as insertion of the generator, report 33202, 33203 in conjunction with 33212, 33213, as appropriate)

⊙ 33206 Insertion or replacement of permanent pacemaker with transvenous electrode(s); atrial
> ➔ *CPT Assistant* Summer 94:10, 17, Oct 96:9, Nov 99:15

⊙ 33207 ventricular
> ➔ *CPT Assistant* Summer 94:10, 17, Oct 96:9, Nov 99:15

⊙ 33208 atrial and ventricular
> ➔ *CPT Assistant* Summer 94:10, 17, Jul 96:10, Nov 99:15

> (Codes 33206-33208 include subcutaneous insertion of the pulse generator and transvenous placement of electrode(s))

⊙ 33210 Insertion or replacement of temporary transvenous single chamber cardiac electrode or pacemaker catheter (separate procedure)
> ➔ *CPT Assistant* Summer 94:10, 17, Mar 07:1

Temporary Pacemaker
33210

The pacemaker pulse generator with the electrodes transvenously placed

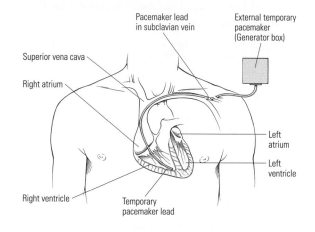

Pacemaker lead in subclavian vein

External temporary pacemaker (Generator box)

Superior vena cava

Right atrium

Left atrium

Left ventricle

Right ventricle

Temporary pacemaker lead

⊙ 33211 Insertion or replacement of temporary transvenous dual chamber pacing electrodes (separate procedure)
> ➔ *CPT Assistant* Summer 94:10, 17, Mar 07:1

⊙ 33212 Insertion or replacement of pacemaker pulse generator only; single chamber, atrial or ventricular
> ➔ *CPT Assistant* Summer 94:10, 18, Fall 94:24, May 04:15

⊙ 33213 dual chamber
> ➔ *CPT Assistant* Summer 94:10, 18, Oct 96:10, Feb 98:11

> (Use 33212, 33213, as appropriate, in conjunction with the epicardial lead placement codes 33202, 33203 to report the insertion of the generator when done by the same physician during the same session)

Implanted Pacemaker
33212-33214

A. In 33212, a pacemaker pulse generator is inserted or replaced in a single chamber.

A

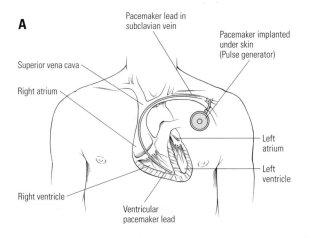

B. In 33213, a pacemaker pulse generator is inserted or replaced in two chambers. In 33214, an upgrade to an existing pacemaker system is done.

B

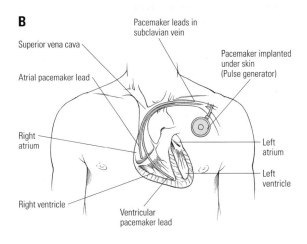

⊙ **33214**   Upgrade of implanted pacemaker system, conversion of single chamber system to dual chamber system (includes removal of previously placed pulse generator, testing of existing lead, insertion of new lead, insertion of new pulse generator)

➔ *CPT Assistant* Summer 94:10, 18, Fall 94:24

(When epicardial electrode placement is performed, report 33214 in conjunction with 33202, 33203)

33215   Repositioning of previously implanted transvenous pacemaker or pacing cardioverter-defibrillator (right atrial or right ventricular) electrode

➔ *CPT Changes: An Insider's View* 2003

⊙ **33216**   Insertion of a transvenous electrode; single chamber (one electrode) permanent pacemaker or single chamber pacing cardioverter-defibrillator

➔ *CPT Assistant* Summer 94:10, 18, Jul 96:10, Nov 99:15-16; *CPT Changes: An Insider's View* 2000, 2003

⊙ **33217**   dual chamber (two electrodes) permanent pacemaker or dual chamber pacing cardioverter-defibrillator

➔ *CPT Assistant* Summer 94:10, 18, Jul 96:10, Nov 99:15-16, Jul 00:5; *CPT Changes: An Insider's View* 2000

(Do not report 33216-33217 in conjunction with 33214)

⊙ **33218**   Repair of single transvenous electrode for a single chamber, permanent pacemaker or single chamber pacing cardioverter-defibrillator

➔ *CPT Assistant* Summer 94:10, 19, Oct 96:9, Nov 99:15-16; *CPT Changes: An Insider's View* 2000

(For atrial or ventricular single chamber repair of pacemaker electrode(s) with replacement of pulse generator, see 33212 or 33213 and 33218 or 33220)

⊙ **33220**   Repair of two transvenous electrodes for a dual chamber permanent pacemaker or dual chamber pacing cardioverter-defibrillator

➔ *CPT Assistant* Summer 94:10, 19, Oct 96:9, Nov 99:15-16; *CPT Changes: An Insider's View* 2000

⊙ **33222**   Revision or relocation of skin pocket for pacemaker

➔ *CPT Assistant* Spring 94:30, Summer 94:10, Nov 99:15-16; *CPT Changes: An Insider's View* 2000

⊙ **33223**   Revision of skin pocket for single or dual chamber pacing cardioverter-defibrillator

➔ *CPT Assistant* Summer 94:10, 19, Nov 99:15-16; *CPT Changes: An Insider's View* 2000

33224   Insertion of pacing electrode, cardiac venous system, for left ventricular pacing, with attachment to previously placed pacemaker or pacing cardioverter-defibrillator pulse generator (including revision of pocket, removal, insertion, and/or replacement of generator)

➔ *CPT Changes: An Insider's View* 2003

(When epicardial electrode placement is performed, report 33224 in conjunction with 33202, 33203)

Biventricular Pacing
33224-33226

Insertion or repositioning of venous pacing electrode

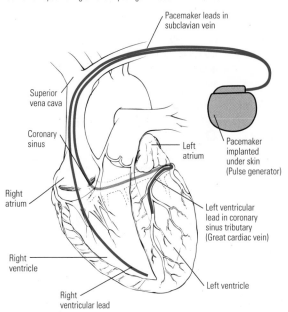

+ 33225 Insertion of pacing electrode, cardiac venous system, for left ventricular pacing, at time of insertion of pacing cardioverter-defibrillator or pacemaker pulse generator (including upgrade to dual chamber system) (List separately in addition to code for primary procedure)

➔ *CPT Changes: An Insider's View* 2003

(Use 33225 in conjunction with 33206, 33207, 33208, 33212, 33213, 33214, 33216, 33217, 33222, 33233, 33234, 33235, 33240, 33249)

33226 Repositioning of previously implanted cardiac venous system (left ventricular) electrode (including removal, insertion and/or replacement of generator)

➔ *CPT Changes: An Insider's View* 2003

⊙ **33233** Removal of permanent pacemaker pulse generator

➔ *CPT Assistant* Summer 94:10, 19, Fall 94:24, Oct 96:10; *CPT Changes: An Insider's View* 2000

⊙ **33234** Removal of transvenous pacemaker electrode(s); single lead system, atrial or ventricular

➔ *CPT Assistant* Summer 94:10, 19, Nov 99:16; *CPT Changes: An Insider's View* 2000

⊙ **33235** dual lead system

➔ *CPT Assistant* Summer 94:10, 19, Nov 99:16; *CPT Changes: An Insider's View* 2000

33236 Removal of permanent epicardial pacemaker and electrodes by thoracotomy; single lead system, atrial or ventricular

➔ *CPT Assistant* Summer 94:10, 19, Nov 99:16; *CPT Changes: An Insider's View* 2000

33237 dual lead system

➔ *CPT Assistant* Summer 94:10, 19, Nov 99:16; *CPT Changes: An Insider's View* 2000

33238 Removal of permanent transvenous electrode(s) by thoracotomy

➔ *CPT Assistant* Summer 94:10, 19, Nov 99:16; *CPT Changes: An Insider's View* 2000

⊙ **33240** Insertion of single or dual chamber pacing cardioverter-defibrillator pulse generator

➔ *CPT Assistant* Summer 94:40, Jun 96:10, Nov 99:16-17, Jul 00:5, Apr 04:6; *CPT Changes: An Insider's View* 2000

(Use 33240, as appropriate, in addition to the epicardial lead placement codes to report the insertion of the generator when done by the same physician during the same session)

⊙ **33241** Subcutaneous removal of single or dual chamber pacing cardioverter-defibrillator pulse generator

➔ *CPT Assistant* Summer 94:40, Nov 99:16-17; *CPT Changes: An Insider's View* 2000

(For removal of electrode(s) by thoracotomy, use 33243 in conjunction with 33241)

(For removal of electrode(s) by transvenous extraction, use 33244 in conjunction with 33241)

(For removal and reinsertion of a pacing cardioverter-defibrillator system (pulse generator and electrodes), report 33241 and 33243 or 33244 and 33249)

(For repair of implantable cardioverter-defibrillator pulse generator and/or leads, see 33218, 33220)

33243 Removal of single or dual chamber pacing cardioverter-defibrillator electrode(s); by thoracotomy

➔ *CPT Assistant* Summer 94:40, Nov 99:16-17; *CPT Changes: An Insider's View* 2000

⊙ **33244** by transvenous extraction

➔ *CPT Assistant* Summer 94:40, Nov 99:16-17, Jul 00:5; *CPT Changes: An Insider's View* 2000

(For subcutaneous removal of the pulse generator, use 33241 in conjunction with 33243 or 33244)

(33245, 33246 have been deleted)

⊙ **33249** Insertion or repositioning of electrode lead(s) for single or dual chamber pacing cardioverter-defibrillator and insertion of pulse generator

➔ *CPT Assistant* Summer 94:21, Nov 99:16-17, Apr 04:6; *CPT Changes: An Insider's View* 2000

(For removal and reinsertion of a pacing cardioverter-defibrillator system (pulse generator and electrodes), report 33241 and 33243 or 33244 and 33249)

(For insertion of implantable cardioverter-defibrillator lead(s), without thoracotomy, use 33216)

Electrophysiologic Operative Procedures

▶This family of codes describes the surgical treatment of supraventricular dysrhythmias. Tissue ablation, disruption, and reconstruction can be accomplished by many methods including surgical incision or through the use of a variety of energy sources (eg, radiofrequency, cryotherapy, microwave, ultrasound, laser). If excision or isolation of the left atrial appendage by any method, including stapling, oversewing, ligation, or plication, is performed in conjunction with any of the atrial tissue ablation and reconstruction (maze) procedures (33254-33259, 33265-33266), it is considered part of the procedure. Codes 33254-33256 are only to be reported when there is no concurrently performed procedure that requires median sternotomy or cardiopulmonary bypass. The appropriate atrial tissue ablation add-on code, 33257, 33258, 33259 should be reported in addition to an open cardiac procedure requiring sternotomy or cardiopulmonary bypass if performed concurrently.◀

Definitions

Limited operative ablation and reconstruction includes:

Surgical isolation of triggers of supraventricular dysrhythmias by operative ablation that isolates the pulmonary veins or other anatomically defined triggers in the left or right atrium.

Extensive operative ablation and reconstruction includes:

1. The services included in "*limited*"

2. Additional ablation of atrial tissue to eliminate sustained supraventricular dysrhythmias. This must include operative ablation that involves either the right atrium, the atrial septum, or left atrium in continuity with the atrioventricular annulus.

Incision

33250 Operative ablation of supraventricular arrhythmogenic focus or pathway (eg, Wolff-Parkinson-White, atrioventricular node re-entry), tract(s) and/or focus (foci); without cardiopulmonary bypass

> *CPT Assistant* Summer 94:16, Nov 99:17-18; *CPT Changes: An Insider's View* 2000, 2002

33251 with cardiopulmonary bypass

> *CPT Assistant* Summer 94:16, Nov 99:17-18; *CPT Changes: An Insider's View* 2000

(33253 has been deleted. To report, use 33254–33256)

33254 Operative tissue ablation and reconstruction of atria, limited (eg, modified maze procedure)

> *CPT Changes: An Insider's View* 2007

33255 Operative tissue ablation and reconstruction of atria, extensive (eg, maze procedure); without cardiopulmonary bypass

> *CPT Changes: An Insider's View* 2007

33256 with cardiopulmonary bypass

> *CPT Changes: An Insider's View* 2007

▶(Do not report 33254-33256 in conjunction with 32100, 32551, 33120, 33130, 33210, 33211, 33400-33507, 33510-33523, 33533-33548, 33600-33853, 33860-33863, 33910-33920)◀

+● 33257 Operative tissue ablation and reconstruction of atria, performed at the time of other cardiac procedure(s), limited (eg, modified maze procedure) (List separately in addition to code for primary procedure)

> *CPT Changes: An Insider's View* 2008

▶(Use 33257 in conjunction with 33120-33130, 33250-33251, 33261, 33300-33335, 33400-33496, 33500-33507, 33510-33516, 33533-33548, 33600-33619, 33641-33697, 33702-33732, 33735-33767, 33770-33814, 33840-33877, 33910-33922, 33925-33926, 33935, 33945, 33975-33980)◀

+● 33258 Operative tissue ablation and reconstruction of atria, performed at the time of other cardiac procedure(s), extensive (eg, maze procedure), without cardiopulmonary bypass (List separately in addition to code for primary procedure)

> *CPT Changes: An Insider's View* 2008

▶(Use 33258 in conjunction with 33130, 33250, 33300, 33310, 33320, 33321, 33330, 33332, 33401, 33414-33417, 33420, 33470-33472, 33501-33503, 33510-33516, 33533-33536, 33690, 33735, 33737, 33800-33813, 33840-33852, 33915, 33925 when the procedure is performed without cardiopulmonary bypass)◀

+● 33259 Operative tissue ablation and reconstruction of atria, performed at the time of other cardiac procedure(s), extensive (eg, maze procedure), with cardiopulmonary bypass (List separately in addition to code for primary procedure)

> *CPT Changes: An Insider's View* 2008

▶(Use 33259 in conjunction with 33120, 33251, 33261, 33305, 33315, 33322, 33335, 33400, 33403-33413, 33422-33468, 33474-33478, 33496, 33500, 33504-33507, 33510-33516, 33533-33548, 33600-33688, 33692-33722, 33730, 33732, 33736, 33750-33767, 33770-33781, 33786-33788, 33814, 33853, 33860-33877, 33910, 33916-33922, 33926, 33935, 33945, 33975-33980 when the procedure is performed with cardiopulmonary bypass)◀

▶(Do not report 33257, 33258 and 33259 in conjunction with 32551, 33210, 33211, 33254-33256, 33265, 33266)◀

33261 Operative ablation of ventricular arrhythmogenic focus with cardiopulmonary bypass

> *CPT Assistant* Summer 94:16

Endoscopy

33265 Endoscopy, surgical; operative tissue ablation and reconstruction of atria, limited (eg, modified maze procedure), without cardiopulmonary bypass

> *CPT Changes: An Insider's View* 2007

33266 operative tissue ablation and reconstruction of atria, extensive (eg, maze procedure), without cardiopulmonary bypass

> *CPT Changes: An Insider's View* 2007

▶(Do not report 33265-33266 in conjunction with 32551, 33210, 33211)◀

Patient-Activated Event Recorder

33282 Implantation of patient-activated cardiac event recorder

> *CPT Assistant* Nov 99:17-18, Jul 00:5; *CPT Changes: An Insider's View* 2000

(Initial implantation includes programming. For subsequent electronic analysis and/or reprogramming, use 93727)

33284 Removal of an implantable, patient-activated cardiac event recorder

> *CPT Assistant* Nov 99:17-18, Jul 00:5; *CPT Changes: An Insider's View* 2000

Wounds of the Heart and Great Vessels

33300   Repair of cardiac wound; without bypass

33305   with cardiopulmonary bypass

33310   Cardiotomy, exploratory (includes removal of foreign body, atrial or ventricular thrombus); without bypass
> *CPT Changes: An Insider's View* 2004

33315   with cardiopulmonary bypass

(Do not report removal of thrombus (33310-33315) in conjunction with other cardiac procedures unless a separate incision in the heart is required to remove the atrial or ventricular thrombus)

(If removal of thrombus with cardiopulmonary bypass (33315) is reported in conjunction with 33120, 33130, 33420-33430, 33460-33468, 33496, 33542, 33545, 33641-33647, 33670, 33681, 33975-33980 which requires a separate heart incision, report 33315 with modifier 59)

33320   Suture repair of aorta or great vessels; without shunt or cardiopulmonary bypass
> *CPT Assistant* Fall 91:7

33321   with shunt bypass
> *CPT Assistant* Fall 91:7

33322   with cardiopulmonary bypass
> *CPT Assistant* Fall 91:7

33330   Insertion of graft, aorta or great vessels; without shunt, or cardiopulmonary bypass

33332   with shunt bypass

33335   with cardiopulmonary bypass

Cardiac Valves

(For multiple valve procedures, see 33400-33478 and add modifier 51 to the secondary valve procedure code)

Aortic Valve

33400   Valvuloplasty, aortic valve; open, with cardiopulmonary bypass
> *CPT Assistant* Feb 05:14, Mar 07:1

33401   open, with inflow occlusion
> *CPT Assistant* Feb 05:14

33403   using transventricular dilation, with cardiopulmonary bypass
> *CPT Assistant* Feb 05:14

(Do not report modifier 63 in conjunction with 33401, 33403)

33404   Construction of apical-aortic conduit
> *CPT Assistant* Jan 04:28, Feb 05:14

33405   Replacement, aortic valve, with cardiopulmonary bypass; with prosthetic valve other than homograft or stentless valve
> *CPT Assistant* Nov 99:18, Feb 05:14; *CPT Changes: An Insider's View* 2000

33406   with allograft valve (freehand)
> *CPT Assistant* Nov 99:18, Feb 05:14; *CPT Changes: An Insider's View* 2002

(For aortic valve valvotomy, (commissurotomy) with inflow occlusion, use 33401)

(For aortic valve valvotomy, (commissurotomy) with cardiopulmonary bypass, use 33403)

33410   with stentless tissue valve
> *CPT Assistant* Nov 99:18, Feb 05:14; *CPT Changes: An Insider's View* 2000

33411   Replacement, aortic valve; with aortic annulus enlargement, noncoronary cusp
> *CPT Assistant* Feb 05:14

33412   with transventricular aortic annulus enlargement (Konno procedure)
> *CPT Assistant* Feb 05:14

33413   by translocation of autologous pulmonary valve with allograft replacement of pulmonary valve (Ross procedure)
> *CPT Assistant* Feb 05:14; *CPT Changes: An Insider's View* 2002

33414   Repair of left ventricular outflow tract obstruction by patch enlargement of the outflow tract
> *CPT Assistant* Feb 05:14

33415   Resection or incision of subvalvular tissue for discrete subvalvular aortic stenosis
> *CPT Assistant* Feb 05:14

33416   Ventriculomyotomy (-myectomy) for idiopathic hypertrophic subaortic stenosis (eg, asymmetric septal hypertrophy)
> *CPT Assistant* Feb 05:14

33417   Aortoplasty (gusset) for supravalvular stenosis
> *CPT Assistant* Feb 05:14

Mitral Valve

33420   Valvotomy, mitral valve; closed heart
> *CPT Assistant* Feb 05:14

33422   open heart, with cardiopulmonary bypass
> *CPT Assistant* Feb 05:14

33425   Valvuloplasty, mitral valve, with cardiopulmonary bypass;
> *CPT Assistant* May 03:19, Feb 05:14

33426   with prosthetic ring
> *CPT Assistant* Feb 05:14

33427   radical reconstruction, with or without ring
> *CPT Assistant* Feb 05:14

33430   Replacement, mitral valve, with cardiopulmonary bypass
> *CPT Assistant* Feb 05:14

Tricuspid Valve

33460 Valvectomy, tricuspid valve, with cardiopulmonary bypass
➔ *CPT Assistant* Feb 05:14

33463 Valvuloplasty, tricuspid valve; without ring insertion
➔ *CPT Assistant* Feb 05:14

33464 with ring insertion
➔ *CPT Assistant* Feb 05:14

33465 Replacement, tricuspid valve, with cardiopulmonary bypass
➔ *CPT Assistant* Feb 05:14

33468 Tricuspid valve repositioning and plication for Ebstein anomaly
➔ *CPT Assistant* Feb 05:14

Pulmonary Valve

33470 Valvotomy, pulmonary valve, closed heart; transventricular
➔ *CPT Assistant* Feb 05:14

(Do not report modifier 63 in conjunction with 33470)

33471 via pulmonary artery
➔ *CPT Assistant* Feb 05:14

(To report percutaneous valvuloplasty of pulmonary valve, use 92990)

33472 Valvotomy, pulmonary valve, open heart; with inflow occlusion
➔ *CPT Assistant* Feb 05:14

(Do not report modifier 63 in conjunction with 33472)

33474 with cardiopulmonary bypass
➔ *CPT Assistant* Feb 05:14

33475 Replacement, pulmonary valve
➔ *CPT Assistant* Feb 05:14

33476 Right ventricular resection for infundibular stenosis, with or without commissurotomy
➔ *CPT Assistant* Feb 05:14

33478 Outflow tract augmentation (gusset), with or without commissurotomy or infundibular resection
➔ *CPT Assistant* Feb 05:14

(Use 33478 in conjunction with 33768 when a cavopulmonary anastomosis to a second superior vena cava is performed)

Other Valvular Procedures

33496 Repair of non-structural prosthetic valve dysfunction with cardiopulmonary bypass (separate procedure)
➔ *CPT Assistant* Nov 97:16, Feb 05:14

(For reoperation, use 33530 in addition to 33496)

Coronary Artery Anomalies

Basic procedures include endarterectomy or angioplasty.

33500 Repair of coronary arteriovenous or arteriocardiac chamber fistula; with cardiopulmonary bypass

33501 without cardiopulmonary bypass

33502 Repair of anomalous coronary artery from pulmonary artery origin; by ligation
➔ *CPT Changes: An Insider's View* 2006

33503 by graft, without cardiopulmonary bypass

(Do not report modifier 63 in conjunction with 33502, 33503)

33504 by graft, with cardiopulmonary bypass

33505 with construction of intrapulmonary artery tunnel (Takeuchi procedure)

33506 by translocation from pulmonary artery to aorta

(Do not report modifier 63 in conjunction with 33505, 33506)

33507 Repair of anomalous (eg, intramural) aortic origin of coronary artery by unroofing or translocation
➔ *CPT Changes: An Insider's View* 2006

Endoscopy

Surgical vascular endoscopy always includes diagnostic endoscopy.

+ 33508 Endoscopy, surgical, including video-assisted harvest of vein(s) for coronary artery bypass procedure (List separately in addition to code for primary procedure)
➔ *CPT Changes: An Insider's View* 2003

(Use 33508 in conjunction with 33510-33523)

(For open harvest of upper extremity vein procedure, use 35500)

Venous Grafting Only for Coronary Artery Bypass

The following codes are used to report coronary artery bypass procedures using venous grafts only. These codes should NOT be used to report the performance of coronary artery bypass procedures using arterial grafts and venous grafts during the same procedure. See 33517-33523 and 33533-33536 for reporting combined arterial-venous grafts.

Procurement of the saphenous vein graft is included in the description of the work for 33510-33516 and should not be reported as a separate service or co-surgery. To report harvesting of an upper extremity vein, use 35500 in addition to the bypass procedure. To report harvesting of a femoropopliteal vein segment, report 35572 in addition to the bypass procedure. When surgical assistant performs graft procurement, add modifier 80 to 33510-33516.

Coronary Artery Bypass—Venous Grafting Only
33510-33516

A. Use 33510 to report a single coronary venous graft.

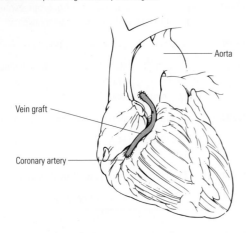

B. Report 33512 when three coronary venous grafts are performed.

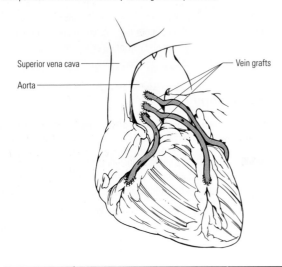

Combined Arterial-Venous Grafting for Coronary Bypass

The following codes are used to report coronary artery bypass procedures using venous grafts and arterial grafts during the same procedure. These codes may NOT be used alone.

To report combined arterial-venous grafts it is necessary to report two codes: 1) the appropriate combined arterial-venous graft code (33517-33523); and 2) the appropriate arterial graft code (33533-33536).

Procurement of the saphenous vein graft is included in the description of the work for 33517-33523 and should not be reported as a separate service or co-surgery. Procurement of the artery for grafting is included in the description of the work for 33533-33536 and should not be reported as a separate service or co-surgery, except when an upper extremity artery (eg, radial artery) is procured. To report harvesting of an upper extremity artery, use 35600 in addition to the bypass procedure. To report harvesting of an upper extremity vein, use 35500 in addition to the bypass procedure. To report harvesting of a femoropopliteal vein segment, report 35572 in addition to the bypass procedure. When surgical assistant performs arterial and/or venous graft procurement, add modifier 80 to 33517-33523, 33533-33536, as appropriate.

Coronary Artery Bypass—Combined Arterial-Venous Grafting
33517-33530

Both venous and arterial grafts are used in these bypass procedures. The appropriate arterial graft codes (33533-33536) must also be reported in conjunction with codes 33517-33530.

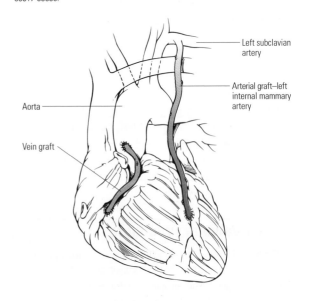

33510 Coronary artery bypass, vein only; single coronary venous graft

➔ *CPT Assistant* Fall 91:5, Winter 92:12, Jul 99:11, Apr 01:7, Feb 05:14, Jan 07:7, Mar 07:1

33511 two coronary venous grafts

➔ *CPT Assistant* Fall 91:5, Winter 92:12, Jul 99:11, Apr 01:7, Feb 05:14, Jan 07:7, Mar 07:1

33512 three coronary venous grafts

➔ *CPT Assistant* Fall 91:5, Winter 92:12, Apr 01:7, Feb 05:14, Jan 07:7, Mar 07:1

33513 four coronary venous grafts

➔ *CPT Assistant* Fall 91:5, Winter 92:12, Apr 01:7, Feb 05:14, Jan 07:7, Mar 07:1

33514 five coronary venous grafts

➔ *CPT Assistant* Fall 91:5, Winter 92:12, Apr 01:7, Feb 05:14, Jan 07:7, Mar 07:1

33516 six or more coronary venous grafts

➔ *CPT Assistant* Fall 91:5, Winter 92:12, Jul 99:11, Apr 01:7, Feb 05:14, Jan 07:7, Mar 07:1

Coronary Artery Bypass—Sequential Combined Arterial-Venous Grafting
33517-33530

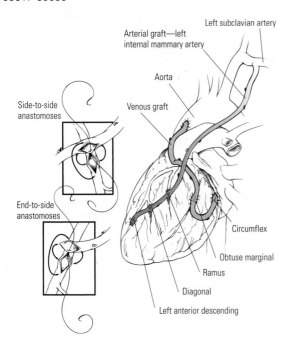

Left subclavian artery

Arterial graft—left internal mammary artery

Aorta

Venous graft

Side-to-side anastomoses

End-to-side anastomoses

Circumflex

Obtuse marginal

Ramus

Diagonal

Left anterior descending

Note: To determine the number of bypass grafts in a coronary artery bypass (CABG), count the number of distal anastomoses (contact point[s]) where the bypass graft artery or vein is sutured to the diseased coronary artery(s).

+▲ 33517 Coronary artery bypass, using venous graft(s) and arterial graft(s); single vein graft (List separately in addition to code for primary procedure)

> *CPT Assistant* Fall 91:5, Winter 92:13, Nov 99:18, Apr 01:7, Feb 05:14; *CPT Changes: An Insider's View* 2000, 2008

▶(Use 33517 in conjunction with 33533-33536)◀

+▲ 33518 two venous grafts (List separately in addition to code for primary procedure)

> *CPT Assistant* Fall 91:5, Winter 92:13, Apr 01:7, Feb 05:14, Jan 07:7, Mar 07:1; *CPT Changes: An Insider's View* 2008

▶(Use 33518 in conjunction with 33533-33536)◀

+▲ 33519 three venous grafts (List separately in addition to code for primary procedure)

> *CPT Assistant* Fall 91:5, Winter 92:13, Apr 01:7, Feb 05:14, Jan 07:7, Mar 07:1; *CPT Changes: An Insider's View* 2008

▶(Use 33519 in conjunction with 33533-33536)◀

+▲ 33521 four venous grafts (List separately in addition to code for primary procedure)

> *CPT Assistant* Fall 91:5, Winter 92:13, Apr 01:7, Feb 05:14, Jan 07:7, Mar 07:1; *CPT Changes: An Insider's View* 2008

▶(Use 33521 in conjunction with 33533-33536)◀

+▲ 33522 five venous grafts (List separately in addition to code for primary procedure)

> *CPT Assistant* Fall 91:5, Winter 92:13, Apr 01:7, Feb 05:14, Jan 07:7, Mar 07:1; *CPT Changes: An Insider's View* 2008

▶(Use 33522 in conjunction with 33533-33536)◀

+▲ 33523 six or more venous grafts (List separately in addition to code for primary procedure)

> *CPT Assistant* Fall 91:5, Winter 92:13, Apr 01:7, Feb 05:14, Jan 07:7, Mar 07:1; *CPT Changes: An Insider's View* 2008

▶(Use 33523 in conjunction with 33533-33536)◀

+ 33530 Reoperation, coronary artery bypass procedure or valve procedure, more than one month after original operation (List separately in addition to code for primary procedure)

> *CPT Assistant* Winter 90:6, Fall 91:5, Winter 92:13, Apr 01:7, Jul 01:11, Feb 05:13-14, Jan 07:7

(Use 33530 in conjunction with 33400-33496; 33510-33536, 33863)

Arterial Grafting for Coronary Artery Bypass

The following codes are used to report coronary artery bypass procedures using either arterial grafts only or a combination of arterial-venous grafts. The codes include the use of the internal mammary artery, gastroepiploic artery, epigastric artery, radial artery, and arterial conduits procured from other sites.

To report combined arterial-venous grafts it is necessary to report two codes: 1) the appropriate arterial graft code (33533-33536); and 2) the appropriate combined arterial-venous graft code (33517-33523).

Procurement of the artery for grafting is included in the description of the work for 33533-33536 and should not be reported as a separate service or co-surgery, except when an upper extremity artery (eg, radial artery) is procured. To report harvesting of an upper extremity artery, use 35600 in addition to the bypass procedure. To report harvesting of an upper extremity vein, use 35500 in addition to the bypass procedure. To report harvesting of a femoropopliteal vein segment, report 35572 in addition to the bypass procedure. When surgical assistant performs arterial and/or venous graft procurement, add modifier 80 to 33517-33523, 33533-33536, as appropriate.

33533 Coronary artery bypass, using arterial graft(s); single arterial graft

> *CPT Assistant* Winter 92:12, Nov 99:18, Apr 01:7, Feb 05:14, Jan 07:7, Mar 07:1; *CPT Changes: An Insider's View* 2000

33534 two coronary arterial grafts

> *CPT Assistant* Winter 92:12, Apr 01:7, Feb 05:14, Jan 07:7, Mar 07:1

33535 three coronary arterial grafts

> *CPT Assistant* Winter 92:12, Apr 01:7, Feb 05:14, Jan 07:7, Mar 07:1

33536 four or more coronary arterial grafts

> *CPT Assistant* Winter 92:12, Apr 01:7, Feb 05:14, Jan 07:7, Mar 07:1

33542 Myocardial resection (eg, ventricular aneurysmectomy)

33545 Repair of postinfarction ventricular septal defect, with or without myocardial resection

33548 Surgical ventricular restoration procedure, includes prosthetic patch, when performed (eg, ventricular remodeling, SVR, SAVER, Dor procedures)

➔ *CPT Changes: An Insider's View* 2006

▶(Do not report 33548 in conjunction with 32551, 33210, 33211, 33310, 33315)◀

(For Batista procedure or pachopexy, use 33999)

Coronary Endarterectomy

+ 33572 Coronary endarterectomy, open, any method, of left anterior descending, circumflex, or right coronary artery performed in conjunction with coronary artery bypass graft procedure, each vessel (List separately in addition to primary procedure)

(Use 33572 in conjunction with 33510-33516, 33533-33536)

Single Ventricle and Other Complex Cardiac Anomalies

33600 Closure of atrioventricular valve (mitral or tricuspid) by suture or patch

33602 Closure of semilunar valve (aortic or pulmonary) by suture or patch

33606 Anastomosis of pulmonary artery to aorta (Damus-Kaye-Stansel procedure)

33608 Repair of complex cardiac anomaly other than pulmonary atresia with ventricular septal defect by construction or replacement of conduit from right or left ventricle to pulmonary artery

(For repair of pulmonary artery arborization anomalies by unifocalization, see 33925-33926)

33610 Repair of complex cardiac anomalies (eg, single ventricle with subaortic obstruction) by surgical enlargement of ventricular septal defect

➔ *CPT Changes: An Insider's View* 2002

(Do not report modifier 63 in conjunction with 33610)

33611 Repair of double outlet right ventricle with intraventricular tunnel repair;

(Do not report modifier 63 in conjunction with 33611)

33612 with repair of right ventricular outflow tract obstruction

33615 Repair of complex cardiac anomalies (eg, tricuspid atresia) by closure of atrial septal defect and anastomosis of atria or vena cava to pulmonary artery (simple Fontan procedure)

33617 Repair of complex cardiac anomalies (eg, single ventricle) by modified Fontan procedure

(Use 33617 in conjunction with 33768 when a cavopulmonary anastomosis to a second superior vena cava is performed)

33619 Repair of single ventricle with aortic outflow obstruction and aortic arch hypoplasia (hypoplastic left heart syndrome) (eg, Norwood procedure)

(Do not report modifier 63 in conjunction with 33619)

Septal Defect

33641 Repair atrial septal defect, secundum, with cardiopulmonary bypass, with or without patch

33645 Direct or patch closure, sinus venosus, with or without anomalous pulmonary venous drainage

(Do not report 33645 in conjunction with 33724, 33726)

33647 Repair of atrial septal defect and ventricular septal defect, with direct or patch closure

(Do not report modifier 63 in conjunction with 33647)

(For repair of tricuspid atresia (eg, Fontan, Gago procedures), use 33615)

33660 Repair of incomplete or partial atrioventricular canal (ostium primum atrial septal defect), with or without atrioventricular valve repair

33665 Repair of intermediate or transitional atrioventricular canal, with or without atrioventricular valve repair

33670 Repair of complete atrioventricular canal, with or without prosthetic valve

(Do not report modifier 63 in conjunction with 33670)

33675 Closure of multiple ventricular septal defects;
➔ *CPT Changes: An Insider's View* 2007

33676 with pulmonary valvotomy or infundibular resection (acyanotic)
➔ *CPT Changes: An Insider's View* 2007

33677 with removal of pulmonary artery band, with or without gusset
➔ *CPT Changes: An Insider's View* 2007

▶(Do not report 33675-33677 in conjunction with 32100, 32422, 33210, 32551, 33681, 33684, 33688)◀

(For transmyocardial closure, see Category III codes 0166T and 0167T)

(For percutaneous closure, use 93581)

33681 Closure of single ventricular septal defect, with or without patch;
➔ *CPT Changes: An Insider's View* 2007

33684 with pulmonary valvotomy or infundibular resection (acyanotic)

33688   with removal of pulmonary artery band, with or without gusset

(For pulmonary vein repair requiring creation of atrial septal defect, use 33724)

33690   Banding of pulmonary artery

(Do not report modifier 63 in conjunction with 33690)

33692   Complete repair tetralogy of Fallot without pulmonary atresia;

33694   with transannular patch

(Do not report modifier 63 in conjunction with 33694)

(For ligation and takedown of a systemic-to-pulmonary artery shunt, performed in conjunction with a congenital heart procedure; see 33924)

33697   Complete repair tetralogy of Fallot with pulmonary atresia including construction of conduit from right ventricle to pulmonary artery and closure of ventricular septal defect

(For ligation and takedown of a systemic-to-pulmonary artery shunt, performed in conjunction with a congenital heart procedure; see 33924)

Sinus of Valsalva

33702   Repair sinus of Valsalva fistula, with cardiopulmonary bypass;

33710   with repair of ventricular septal defect

33720   Repair sinus of Valsalva aneurysm, with cardiopulmonary bypass

33722   Closure of aortico-left ventricular tunnel

Venous Anomalies

33724   Repair of isolated partial anomalous pulmonary venous return (eg, Scimitar Syndrome)
➔ *CPT Changes: An Insider's View* 2007

▶(Do not report 33724 in conjunction with 32551, 33210, 33211)◀

33726   Repair of pulmonary venous stenosis
➔ *CPT Changes: An Insider's View* 2007

▶(Do not report 33726 in conjunction with 32551, 33210, 33211)◀

33730   Complete repair of anomalous pulmonary venous return (supracardiac, intracardiac, or infracardiac types)

(Do not report modifier 63 in conjunction with 33730)

(For partial anomalous pulmonary venous return, use 33724; for repair of pulmonary venous stenosis, use 33726)

33732   Repair of cor triatriatum or supravalvular mitral ring by resection of left atrial membrane

(Do not report modifier 63 in conjunction with 33732)

Shunting Procedures

33735   Atrial septectomy or septostomy; closed heart (Blalock-Hanlon type operation)

33736   open heart with cardiopulmonary bypass

(Do not report modifier 63 in conjunction with 33735, 33736)

33737   open heart, with inflow occlusion

(For transvenous method cardiac catheterization balloon atrial septectomy or septostomy (Rashkind type), use 92992)

(For blade method cardiac catheterization atrial septectomy or septostomy (Sang-Park septostomy), use 92993)

33750   Shunt; subclavian to pulmonary artery (Blalock-Taussig type operation)

33755   ascending aorta to pulmonary artery (Waterston type operation)

33762   descending aorta to pulmonary artery (Potts-Smith type operation)

(Do not report modifier 63 in conjunction with 33750, 33755, 33762)

33764   central, with prosthetic graft

33766   superior vena cava to pulmonary artery for flow to one lung (classical Glenn procedure)

33767   superior vena cava to pulmonary artery for flow to both lungs (bidirectional Glenn procedure)

+ 33768   Anastomosis, cavopulmonary, second superior vena cava (List separately in addition to primary procedure)
➔ *CPT Changes: An Insider's View* 2006

(Use 33768 in conjunction with 33478, 33617, 33767)

▶(Do not report 33768 in conjunction with 32551, 33210, 33211)◀

Transposition of the Great Vessels

33770   Repair of transposition of the great arteries with ventricular septal defect and subpulmonary stenosis; without surgical enlargement of ventricular septal defect

33771   with surgical enlargement of ventricular septal defect

33774   Repair of transposition of the great arteries, atrial baffle procedure (eg, Mustard or Senning type) with cardiopulmonary bypass;

33775   with removal of pulmonary band

33776   with closure of ventricular septal defect

33777   with repair of subpulmonic obstruction

33778   Repair of transposition of the great arteries, aortic pulmonary artery reconstruction (eg, Jatene type);

(Do not report modifier 63 in conjunction with 33778)

33779   with removal of pulmonary band

33780   with closure of ventricular septal defect

33781   with repair of subpulmonic obstruction

Truncus Arteriosus

33786   Total repair, truncus arteriosus (Rastelli type operation)

(Do not report modifier 63 in conjunction with 33786)

33788   Reimplantation of an anomalous pulmonary artery

(For pulmonary artery band, use 33690)

Aortic Anomalies

33800   Aortic suspension (aortopexy) for tracheal decompression (eg, for tracheomalacia) (separate procedure)

33802   Division of aberrant vessel (vascular ring);

33803   with reanastomosis

33813   Obliteration of aortopulmonary septal defect; without cardiopulmonary bypass

33814   with cardiopulmonary bypass

33820   Repair of patent ductus arteriosus; by ligation

Patent Ductus Arteriosus
33820

The tissues surrounding the ductus are dissected away and then several heavy ligatures are passed around the ductus and tied off on both ends.

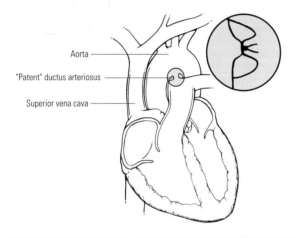

Aorta

"Patent" ductus arteriosus

Superior vena cava

33822   by division, younger than 18 years

33824   by division, 18 years and older

33840   Excision of coarctation of aorta, with or without associated patent ductus arteriosus; with direct anastomosis

33845   with graft

33851   repair using either left subclavian artery or prosthetic material as gusset for enlargement

33852   Repair of hypoplastic or interrupted aortic arch using autogenous or prosthetic material; without cardiopulmonary bypass

33853   with cardiopulmonary bypass

(For repair of hypoplastic left heart syndrome (eg, Norwood type), via excision of coarctation of aorta, use 33619)

Thoracic Aortic Aneurysm

33860   Ascending aorta graft, with cardiopulmonary bypass, with or without valve suspension;

33861   with coronary reconstruction

33863   with aortic root replacement using composite prosthesis and coronary reconstruction
➔ *CPT Assistant* Feb 05:14, Mar 07:1

(For graft of ascending aorta, with cardiopulmonary bypass and valve replacement, with or without coronary implant or valve suspension; use 33860 or 33861 and 33405 or 33406)

● **33864**   Ascending aorta graft, with cardiopulmonary bypass with valve suspension, with coronary reconstruction and valve sparing aortic annulus remodeling (eg, David Procedure, Yacoub Procedure)
➔ *CPT Changes: An Insider's View* 2008

▶(Do not report 33864 in conjunction with 32551, 33210, 33211, 33400, 33860, 33863)◀

33870   Transverse arch graft, with cardiopulmonary bypass

33875   Descending thoracic aorta graft, with or without bypass

33877   Repair of thoracoabdominal aortic aneurysm with graft, with or without cardiopulmonary bypass

Endovascular Repair of Descending Thoracic Aorta

Codes 33880-33891 represent a family of procedures to report placement of an endovascular graft for repair of the descending thoracic aorta. These codes include all device introduction, manipulation, positioning, and deployment. All balloon angioplasty and/or stent deployment within the target treatment zone for the endoprosthesis, either before or after endograft deployment, are not separately reportable. Open arterial exposure and associated closure of the arteriotomy sites (eg, 34812, 34820, 34833, 34834), introduction of guidewires and catheters (eg, 36140, 36200-36218), and extensive repair or replacement of an artery (eg, 35226, 35286) should be additionally reported. Transposition of subclavian artery to carotid, and carotid-carotid bypass performed in conjunction with endovascular repair of the descending thoracic aorta (eg, 33889, 33891) should be separately reported. The primary codes, 33880 and 33881, include placement of all distal extensions, if required, in the distal thoracic aorta, while proximal extensions, if needed, are reported separately.

For fluoroscopic guidance in conjunction with endovascular repair of the thoracic aorta, see codes 75956-75959 as appropriate. Codes 75956 and 75957 include all angiography of the thoracic aorta and its branches for diagnostic imaging prior to deployment of the primary endovascular devices (including all routine components of modular devices), fluoroscopic guidance in the delivery of the endovascular components, and intraprocedural arterial angiography (eg, confirm position, detect endoleak, evaluate runoff). Code 75958 includes the analogous services for placement of each proximal thoracic endovascular extension. Code 75959 includes the analogous services for placement of a distal thoracic endovascular extension(s) placed during a procedure after the primary repair.

Other interventional procedures performed at the time of endovascular repair of the descending thoracic aorta should be additionally reported (eg, innominate, carotid, subclavian, visceral, or iliac artery transluminal angioplasty or stenting, arterial embolization, intravascular ultrasound) when performed before or after deployment of the aortic prostheses.

▶(For transcatheter placement of wireless physiologic sensor in aneurysmal sac, use 34806)◀

▶(For analysis, interpretation, and report of implanted wireless pressure sensor in aneurysmal sac, use 93982)◀

33880 Endovascular repair of descending thoracic aorta (eg, aneurysm, pseudoaneurysm, dissection, penetrating ulcer, intramural hematoma, or traumatic disruption); involving coverage of left subclavian artery origin, initial endoprosthesis plus descending thoracic aortic extension(s), if required, to level of celiac artery origin
→ *CPT Changes: An Insider's View* 2006
→ *Clinical Examples in Radiology* Winter 06:14

(For radiological supervision and interpretation, use 75956 in conjunction with 33880)

33881 not involving coverage of left subclavian artery origin, initial endoprosthesis plus descending thoracic aortic extension(s), if required, to level of celiac artery origin
→ *CPT Changes: An Insider's View* 2006
→ *Clinical Examples in Radiology* Winter 06:14

(For radiological supervision and interpretation, use 75957 in conjunction with 33881)

33883 Placement of proximal extension prosthesis for endovascular repair of descending thoracic aorta (eg, aneurysm, pseudoaneurysm, dissection, penetrating ulcer, intramural hematoma, or traumatic disruption); initial extension
→ *CPT Changes: An Insider's View* 2006
→ *Clinical Examples in Radiology* Winter 06:14

(For radiological supervision and interpretation, use 75958 in conjunction with 33883)

(Do not report 33881, 33883 when extension placement converts repair to cover left subclavian origin. Use only 33880)

+ 33884 each additional proximal extension (List separately in addition to code for primary procedure)
→ *CPT Changes: An Insider's View* 2006
→ *Clinical Examples in Radiology* Winter 06:14

(Use 33884 in conjunction with 33883)

(For radiological supervision and interpretation, use 75958 in conjunction with 33884)

33886 Placement of distal extension prosthesis(s) delayed after endovascular repair of descending thoracic aorta
→ *CPT Changes: An Insider's View* 2006
→ *Clinical Examples in Radiology* Winter 06:14

(Do not report 33886 in conjunction with 33880, 33881)

(Report 33886 once, regardless of number of modules deployed)

(For radiological supervision and interpretation, use 75959 in conjunction with 33886)

33889 Open subclavian to carotid artery transposition performed in conjunction with endovascular repair of descending thoracic aorta, by neck incision, unilateral
→ *CPT Changes: An Insider's View* 2006
→ *Clinical Examples in Radiology* Winter 06:15

(Do not report 33889 in conjunction with 35694)

33891 Bypass graft, with other than vein, transcervical retropharyngeal carotid-carotid, performed in conjunction with endovascular repair of descending thoracic aorta, by neck incision
→ *CPT Changes: An Insider's View* 2006
→ *Clinical Examples in Radiology* Winter 06:15

(Do not report 33891 in conjunction with 35509, 35601)

Pulmonary Artery

33910 Pulmonary artery embolectomy; with cardiopulmonary bypass

33915 without cardiopulmonary bypass

33916 Pulmonary endarterectomy, with or without embolectomy, with cardiopulmonary bypass

33917 Repair of pulmonary artery stenosis by reconstruction with patch or graft

(33918, 33919 have been deleted. To report, see 33925, 33926)

33920 Repair of pulmonary atresia with ventricular septal defect, by construction or replacement of conduit from right or left ventricle to pulmonary artery

(For repair of other complex cardiac anomalies by construction or replacement of right or left ventricle to pulmonary artery conduit, use 33608)

33922 Transection of pulmonary artery with cardiopulmonary bypass

(Do not report modifier 63 in conjunction with 33922)

+ 33924   Ligation and takedown of a systemic-to-pulmonary artery shunt, performed in conjunction with a congenital heart procedure (List separately in addition to code for primary procedure)

(Use 33924 in conjunction with 33470-33475, 33600-33619, 33684-33688, 33692-33697, 33735-33767, 33770-33781, 33786, 33920-33922)

33925   Repair of pulmonary artery arborization anomalies by unifocalization; without cardiopulmonary bypass

➔ *CPT Changes: An Insider's View* 2006

33926   with cardiopulmonary bypass

➔ *CPT Changes: An Insider's View* 2006

Heart/Lung Transplantation

Heart with or without lung allotransplantation involves three distinct components of physician work:

1) ***Cadaver donor cardiectomy with or without pneumonectomy***, which includes harvesting the allograft and cold preservation of the allograft (perfusing with cold preservation solution and cold maintenance) (see 33930, 33940).

2) ***Backbench work***:

Preparation of a cadaver donor heart and lung allograft prior to transplantation, including dissection of the allograft from surrounding soft tissues to prepare the aorta, superior vena cava, inferior vena cava, and trachea for implantation (use 33933).

Preparation of a cadaver donor heart allograft prior to transplantation, including dissection of the allograft from surrounding soft tissues to prepare aorta, superior vena cava, inferior vena cava, pulmonary artery, and left atrium for implantation (use 33944).

3) ***Recipient heart with or without lung allotransplantation***, which includes transplantation of allograft and care of the recipient (see 33935, 33945).

(For implantation of a total replacement heart system (artificial heart) with recipient cardiectomy or heart replacement system components, see Category III codes 0051T-0053T)

33930   Donor cardiectomy-pneumonectomy (including cold preservation)

➔ *CPT Changes: An Insider's View* 2005

33933   Backbench standard preparation of cadaver donor heart/lung allograft prior to transplantation, including dissection of allograft from surrounding soft tissues to prepare aorta, superior vena cava, inferior vena cava, and trachea for implantation

➔ *CPT Changes: An Insider's View* 2005

33935   Heart-lung transplant with recipient cardiectomy-pneumonectomy

33940   Donor cardiectomy (including cold preservation)

➔ *CPT Assistant* Apr 05:10-11; *CPT Changes: An Insider's View* 2005

33944   Backbench standard preparation of cadaver donor heart allograft prior to transplantation, including dissection of allograft from surrounding soft tissues to prepare aorta, superior vena cava, inferior vena cava, pulmonary artery, and left atrium for implantation

➔ *CPT Changes: An Insider's View* 2005

(For repair or resection procedures on the donor heart, see 33300, 33310, 33320, 33400, 33463, 33464, 33510, 33641, 35216, 35276 or 35685)

33945   Heart transplant, with or without recipient cardiectomy

➔ *CPT Assistant* Fall 92:20

Cardiac Assist

(For percutaneous implantation of extracorporeal ventricular assist device or for removal of percutaneously implanted extracorporeal ventricular assist device, see Category III codes 0048T-0050T)

33960   Prolonged extracorporeal circulation for cardiopulmonary insufficiency; initial 24 hours

+ 33961   each additional 24 hours (List separately in addition to code for primary procedure)

(Do not report modifier 63 in conjunction with 33960, 33961)

(Use 33961 in conjunction with 33960)

(For insertion of cannula for prolonged extracorporeal circulation, use 36822)

33967   Insertion of intra-aortic balloon assist device, percutaneous

➔ *CPT Assistant* Feb 02:2; *CPT Changes: An Insider's View* 2002

33968   Removal of intra-aortic balloon assist device, percutaneous

➔ *CPT Assistant* Nov 99:19, Jan 00:10; *CPT Changes: An Insider's View* 2000

33970   Insertion of intra-aortic balloon assist device through the femoral artery, open approach

➔ *CPT Assistant* Nov 99:19; *CPT Changes: An Insider's View* 2000

33971   Removal of intra-aortic balloon assist device including repair of femoral artery, with or without graft

33973   Insertion of intra-aortic balloon assist device through the ascending aorta

33974   Removal of intra-aortic balloon assist device from the ascending aorta, including repair of the ascending aorta, with or without graft

33975   Insertion of ventricular assist device; extracorporeal, single ventricle

➔ *CPT Assistant* Feb 92:2, Jan 04:28; *CPT Changes: An Insider's View* 2002

33976   extracorporeal, biventricular

➔ *CPT Assistant* Feb 02:2; *CPT Changes: An Insider's View* 2002

33977   Removal of ventricular assist device; extracorporeal, single ventricle

➔ *CPT Assistant* Feb 02:2; *CPT Changes: An Insider's View* 2002

33978   extracorporeal, biventricular

➔ *CPT Assistant* Feb 02:2; *CPT Changes: An Insider's View* 2002

33979   Insertion of ventricular assist device, implantable intracorporeal, single ventricle

➔ *CPT Assistant* Feb 02:3, Jan 04:28; *CPT Changes: An Insider's View* 2002

Insertion of Implantable Single Ventricle Assist Device
33979

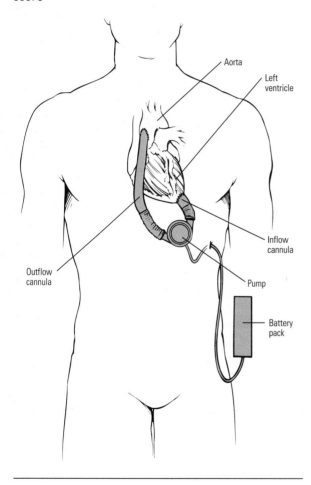

33980   Removal of ventricular assist device, implantable intracorporeal, single ventricle

➔ *CPT Assistant* Feb 02:3; *CPT Changes: An Insider's View* 2002

Other Procedures

33999   Unlisted procedure, cardiac surgery

➔ *CPT Assistant* Oct 99:11, Jan 04:7, Mar 07:1

Arteries and Veins

Primary vascular procedure listings include establishing both inflow and outflow by whatever procedures necessary. Also included is that portion of the operative arteriogram performed by the surgeon, as indicated. Sympathectomy, when done, is included in the listed aortic procedures. For unlisted vascular procedure, use 37799.

Embolectomy/Thrombectomy

Arterial, With or Without Catheter

34001   Embolectomy or thrombectomy, with or without catheter; carotid, subclavian or innominate artery, by neck incision

34051   innominate, subclavian artery, by thoracic incision

34101   axillary, brachial, innominate, subclavian artery, by arm incision

34111   radial or ulnar artery, by arm incision

34151   renal, celiac, mesentery, aortoiliac artery, by abdominal incision

34201   femoropopliteal, aortoiliac artery, by leg incision

34203   popliteal-tibio-peroneal artery, by leg incision

Venous, Direct or With Catheter

34401   Thrombectomy, direct or with catheter; vena cava, iliac vein, by abdominal incision

34421   vena cava, iliac, femoropopliteal vein, by leg incision

➔ *CPT Assistant* Spring 94:30

34451   vena cava, iliac, femoropopliteal vein, by abdominal and leg incision

34471   subclavian vein, by neck incision

34490   axillary and subclavian vein, by arm incision

Venous Reconstruction

34501   Valvuloplasty, femoral vein

34502   Reconstruction of vena cava, any method

34510   Venous valve transposition, any vein donor

34520   Cross-over vein graft to venous system

34530   Saphenopopliteal vein anastomosis

Endovascular Repair of Abdominal Aortic Aneurysm

Codes 34800-34826 represent a family of component procedures to report placement of an endovascular graft for abdominal aortic aneurysm repair. These codes describe open femoral or iliac artery exposure, device manipulation and deployment, and closure of the arteriotomy sites. Balloon angioplasty and/or stent deployment within the target treatment zone for the endoprosthesis, either before or after endograft deployment, are not separately reportable. Introduction of guidewires and catheters should be reported separately (eg, 36200, 36245-36248, 36140). Extensive repair or replacement of an artery should be additionally reported (eg, 35226 or 35286).

For fluoroscopic guidance in conjunction with endovascular aneurysm repair, see code 75952 or 75953, as appropriate. Code 75952 includes angiography of the aorta and its branches for diagnostic imaging prior to deployment of the endovascular device (including all routine components of modular devices), fluoroscopic guidance in the delivery of the endovascular components, and intraprocedural arterial angiography (eg, confirm position, detect endoleak, evaluate runoff). Code 75953 includes the analogous services for placement of additional extension prostheses (not for routine components of modular devices).

Other interventional procedures performed at the time of endovascular abdominal aortic aneurysm repair should be additionally reported (eg, renal transluminal angioplasty, arterial embolization, intravascular ultrasound, balloon angioplasty or stenting of native artery(s) outside the endoprosthesis target zone, when done before or after deployment of graft).

▶(For transcatheter placement of wireless physiologic sensor in aneurysmal sac, use 34806)◀

▶(For analysis, interpretation and report of implanted wireless pressure sensor in aneurysmal sac, use 93982)◀

34800   Endovascular repair of infrarenal abdominal aortic aneurysm or dissection; using aorto-aortic tube prosthesis

➔ *CPT Assistant* Dec 00:1, 4, Sep 02:3, Feb 03:2, Nov 03:5, Dec 04:18; *CPT Changes: An Insider's View* 2001

34802   using modular bifurcated prosthesis (one docking limb)

➔ *CPT Assistant* Dec 00:1, 4, Sep 02:3, Feb 03:2, Dec 04:18; *CPT Changes: An Insider's View* 2001

Endovascular Repair of Abdominal Aortic Aneurysm
34802

Using fluoroscopic guidance, a "compressed" prosthesis is introduced through arteries in the groin and advanced into position with the aneurysm. Once in the aorta, the prosthesis is expanded.

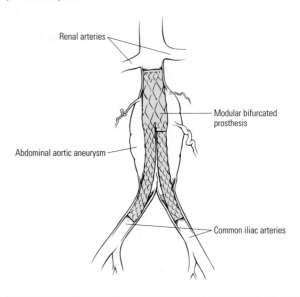

Renal arteries

Modular bifurcated prosthesis

Abdominal aortic aneurysm

Common iliac arteries

34803   using modular bifurcated prosthesis (two docking limbs)

➔ *CPT Changes: An Insider's View* 2005

(For endovascular repair of abdominal aortic aneurysm or dissection involving visceral vessels using a fenestrated modular bifurcated prosthesis (two docking limbs), use Category III codes 0078T, 0079T)

34804   using unibody bifurcated prosthesis

➔ *CPT Assistant* Dec 00:5, Sep 02:3, Feb 03:2; *CPT Changes: An Insider's View* 2001

34805   using aorto-uniiliac or aorto-unifemoral prosthesis

➔ *CPT Assistant* Jun 04:9, Dec 04:18; *CPT Changes: An Insider's View* 2004

✛● **34806**   Transcatheter placement of wireless physiologic sensor in aneurysmal sac during endovascular repair, including radiological supervision and interpretation, instrument calibration, and collection of pressure data

➔ *CPT Changes: An Insider's View* 2008

▶(Use 34806 in conjunction with 33880, 33881, 33886, 34800-34805, 34825, 34900)◀

▶(Do not report 34806 in conjunction with 93982)◀

+ 34808   Endovascular placement of iliac artery occlusion device
(List separately in addition to code for primary procedure)

➲ *CPT Assistant* Dec 00:6, Sep 02:3; *CPT Changes: An Insider's View* 2001

(Use 34808 in conjunction with 34800, 34805, 34813, 34825, 34826)

(For radiological supervision and interpretation, use 75952 in conjunction with 34800-34808)

(For open arterial exposure, report 34812, 34820, 34833, 34834 as appropriate, in addition to 34800-34808)

34812   Open femoral artery exposure for delivery of endovascular prosthesis, by groin incision, unilateral

➲ *CPT Assistant* Dec 00:6, Sep 02:3, Feb 03:2, Mar 04:10, Jul 06:7; *CPT Changes: An Insider's View* 2001, 2003

(For bilateral procedure, use modifier 50)

+ 34813   Placement of femoral-femoral prosthetic graft during endovascular aortic aneurysm repair (List separately in addition to code for primary procedure)

➲ *CPT Assistant* Dec 00:6, Sep 02:3; *CPT Changes: An Insider's View* 2001

(Use 34813 in conjunction with 34812)

(For femoral artery grafting, see 35521, 35533, 35539, 35540, 35551-35558, 35566, 35621, 35646, 35651-35661, 35666, 35700)

34820   Open iliac artery exposure for delivery of endovascular prosthesis or iliac occlusion during endovascular therapy, by abdominal or retroperitoneal incision, unilateral

➲ *CPT Assistant* Dec 00:7-8, Sep 02:3, Feb 03:4, Aug 04:10, Jul 06:7; *CPT Changes: An Insider's View* 2001

(For bilateral procedure, use modifier 50)

34825   Placement of proximal or distal extension prosthesis for endovascular repair of infrarenal abdominal aortic or iliac aneurysm, false aneurysm, or dissection; initial vessel

➲ *CPT Assistant* Dec 00:5, Sep 02:3, Feb 03:3; *CPT Changes: An Insider's View* 2001, 2003

+ 34826   each additional vessel (List separately in addition to code for primary procedure)

➲ *CPT Assistant* Dec 00:6, Sep 02:3, Feb 03:3; *CPT Changes: An Insider's View* 2001

(Use 34826 in conjunction with 34825)

(Use 34825, 34826 in addition to 34800-34808, 34900 as appropriate)

(For staged procedure, use modifier 58)

(For radiological supervision and interpretation, use 75953)

34830   Open repair of infrarenal aortic aneurysm or dissection, plus repair of associated arterial trauma, following unsuccessful endovascular repair; tube prosthesis

➲ *CPT Assistant* Dec 00:6, Sep 02:3; *CPT Changes: An Insider's View* 2001

34831   aorto-bi-iliac prosthesis

➲ *CPT Assistant* Dec 00:6, Sep 02:3; *CPT Changes: An Insider's View* 2001

34832   aorto-bifemoral prosthesis

➲ *CPT Assistant* Dec 00:6, Sep 02:3; *CPT Changes: An Insider's View* 2001

34833   Open iliac artery exposure with creation of conduit for delivery of aortic or iliac endovascular prosthesis, by abdominal or retroperitoneal incision, unilateral

➲ *CPT Assistant* Aug 04:10, Feb 03:4, Jul 06:7; *CPT Changes: An Insider's View* 2003, 2006

➲ *Clinical Examples in Radiology* Winter 06:19

(For bilateral procedure, use modifier 50)

(Do not report 34833 in addition to 34820)

34834   Open brachial artery exposure to assist in the deployment of aortic or iliac endovascular prosthesis by arm incision, unilateral

➲ *CPT Assistant* Feb 03:4, Jul 06:7; *CPT Changes: An Insider's View* 2003, 2006

➲ *Clinical Examples in Radiology* Winter 06:19

(For bilateral procedure, use modifier 50)

Endovascular Repair of Iliac Aneurysm

Code 34900 represents a procedure to report introduction, positioning, and deployment of an endovascular graft for treatment of aneurysm, pseudoaneurysm, or arteriovenous malformation or trauma of the iliac artery (common, hypogastric, external). All balloon angioplasty and/or stent deployments within the target treatment zone for the endoprosthesis, either before or after endograft deployment, are included in the work of 34900 and are not separately reportable. Open femoral or iliac artery exposure (eg, 34812, 34820), introduction of guidewires and catheters (eg, 36200, 36215-36218), and extensive repair or replacement of an artery (eg, 35206-35286) should be additionally reported.

For fluoroscopic guidance in conjunction with endovascular iliac aneurysm repair, see code 75954. Code 75954 includes angiography of the aorta and iliac arteries for diagnostic imaging prior to deployment of the endovascular device (including all routine components), fluoroscopic guidance in the delivery of the endovascular components, and intraprocedural arterial angiography to confirm appropriate position of the graft, detect endoleaks, and evaluate the status of the runoff vessels (eg, evaluation for dissection, stenosis, thrombosis, distal embolization, or iatrogenic injury).

Other interventional procedures performed at the time of endovascular iliac aneurysm repair should be additionally reported (eg, transluminal angioplasty outside the aneurysm target zone, arterial embolization, intravascular ultrasound).

34900 Endovascular graft placement for repair of iliac artery (eg, aneurysm, pseudoaneurysm, arteriovenous malformation, trauma)

⮕ CPT Assistant Feb 93:2; CPT Changes: An Insider's View 2003

(For radiological supervision and interpretation, use 75954)

(For placement of extension prosthesis during endovascular iliac artery repair, use 34825)

(For bilateral procedure, use modifier 50)

Direct Repair of Aneurysm or Excision (Partial or Total) and Graft Insertion for Aneurysm, Pseudoaneurysm, Ruptured Aneurysm, and Associated Occlusive Disease

Procedures 35001-35152 include preparation of artery for anastomosis including endarterectomy.

(For direct repairs associated with occlusive disease only, see 35201-35286)

(For intracranial aneurysm, see 61700 et seq)

(For endovascular repair of abdominal aortic aneurysm, see 34800-34826)

(For endovascular repair of iliac artery aneurysm, see 34900)

(For thoracic aortic aneurysm, see 33860-33875)

(For endovascular repair of descending thoracic aorta, involving coverage of left subclavian artery origin, use 33880)

35001 Direct repair of aneurysm, pseudoaneurysm, or excision (partial or total) and graft insertion, with or without patch graft; for aneurysm and associated occlusive disease, carotid, subclavian artery, by neck incision

⮕ CPT Changes: An Insider's View 2002

35002 for ruptured aneurysm, carotid, subclavian artery, by neck incision

35005 for aneurysm, pseudoaneurysm, and associated occlusive disease, vertebral artery

⮕ CPT Changes: An Insider's View 2002

35011 for aneurysm and associated occlusive disease, axillary-brachial artery, by arm incision

35013 for ruptured aneurysm, axillary-brachial artery, by arm incision

35021 for aneurysm, pseudoaneurysm, and associated occlusive disease, innominate, subclavian artery, by thoracic incision

⮕ CPT Changes: An Insider's View 2002

35022 for ruptured aneurysm, innominate, subclavian artery, by thoracic incision

35045 for aneurysm, pseudoaneurysm, and associated occlusive disease, radial or ulnar artery

⮕ CPT Changes: An Insider's View 2002

35081 for aneurysm, pseudoaneurysm, and associated occlusive disease, abdominal aorta

⮕ CPT Assistant Dec 00:2, Dec 01:7; CPT Changes: An Insider's View 2002

35082 for ruptured aneurysm, abdominal aorta

35091 for aneurysm, pseudoaneurysm, and associated occlusive disease, abdominal aorta involving visceral vessels (mesenteric, celiac, renal)

⮕ CPT Assistant Dec 00:2; CPT Changes: An Insider's View 2002

35092 for ruptured aneurysm, abdominal aorta involving visceral vessels (mesenteric, celiac, renal)

35102 for aneurysm, pseudoaneurysm, and associated occlusive disease, abdominal aorta involving iliac vessels (common, hypogastric, external)

⮕ CPT Changes: An Insider's View 2002

35103 for ruptured aneurysm, abdominal aorta involving iliac vessels (common, hypogastric, external)

35111 for aneurysm, pseudoaneurysm, and associated occlusive disease, splenic artery

⮕ CPT Changes: An Insider's View 2002

35112 for ruptured aneurysm, splenic artery

35121 for aneurysm, pseudoaneurysm, and associated occlusive disease, hepatic, celiac, renal, or mesenteric artery

⮕ CPT Changes: An Insider's View 2002

35122 for ruptured aneurysm, hepatic, celiac, renal, or mesenteric artery

35131 for aneurysm, pseudoaneurysm, and associated occlusive disease, iliac artery (common, hypogastric, external)

⮕ CPT Assistant Feb 03:2; CPT Changes: An Insider's View 2002

35132 for ruptured aneurysm, iliac artery (common, hypogastric, external)

35141 for aneurysm, pseudoaneurysm, and associated occlusive disease, common femoral artery (profunda femoris, superficial femoral)

⮕ CPT Changes: An Insider's View 2002

35142 for ruptured aneurysm, common femoral artery (profunda femoris, superficial femoral)

35151 for aneurysm, pseudoaneurysm, and associated occlusive disease, popliteal artery

⮕ CPT Changes: An Insider's View 2002

35152 for ruptured aneurysm, popliteal artery

Repair Arteriovenous Fistula

35180 Repair, congenital arteriovenous fistula; head and neck

35182   thorax and abdomen

35184   extremities

35188   Repair, acquired or traumatic arteriovenous fistula; head and neck

35189   thorax and abdomen

35190   extremities

Repair Blood Vessel Other Than for Fistula, With or Without Patch Angioplasty

(For AV fistula repair, see 35180-35190)

35201   Repair blood vessel, direct; neck

35206   upper extremity
   → CPT Assistant Oct 00:3, Nov 03:5

35207   hand, finger

35211   intrathoracic, with bypass

35216   intrathoracic, without bypass
   → CPT Assistant Apr 05:10-11

35221   intra-abdominal

35226   lower extremity

35231   Repair blood vessel with vein graft; neck

35236   upper extremity
   → CPT Assistant Oct 04:8

35241   intrathoracic, with bypass

35246   intrathoracic, without bypass

35251   intra-abdominal

35256   lower extremity

35261   Repair blood vessel with graft other than vein; neck

35266   upper extremity

35271   intrathoracic, with bypass

35276   intrathoracic, without bypass

35281   intra-abdominal

35286   lower extremity

Thromboendarterectomy

(For coronary artery, see 33510-33536 and 33572)

(35301-35372 include harvest of saphenous or upper extremity vein when performed)

35301   Thromboendarterectomy, including patch graft, if performed; carotid, vertebral, subclavian, by neck incision
   → CPT Changes: An Insider's View 2007

35302   superficial femoral artery
   → CPT Changes: An Insider's View 2007

35303   popliteal artery
   → CPT Changes: An Insider's View 2007

(Do not report 35302, 35303 in conjunction with 35483, 35500)

35304   tibioperoneal trunk artery
   → CPT Changes: An Insider's View 2007

35305   tibial or peroneal artery, initial vessel
   → CPT Changes: An Insider's View 2007

+ 35306   each additional tibial or peroneal artery (List separately in addition to code for primary procedure)
   → CPT Changes: An Insider's View 2007

(Use 35306 in conjunction with 35305)

(Do not report 35304, 35305, 35306 in conjunction with 35485, 35500)

35311   subclavian, innominate, by thoracic incision

35321   axillary-brachial

35331   abdominal aorta

35341   mesenteric, celiac, or renal

35351   iliac

35355   iliofemoral

35361   combined aortoiliac

35363   combined aortoiliofemoral

35371   common femoral

35372   deep (profunda) femoral

(35381 has been deleted. For thromboendarterectomy of the superficial femoral artery, use 35302; of the popliteal artery, use 35303; of the tibioperoneal trunk, use 35304; of the tibial or peroneal artery, see 35305, 35306)

Thromboendarterectomy
35371-35372

The common femoral artery (35371) or the deep (profunda) femoral artery (35372) is incised and the plaque and lining are removed, enlarging the diameter of the artery.

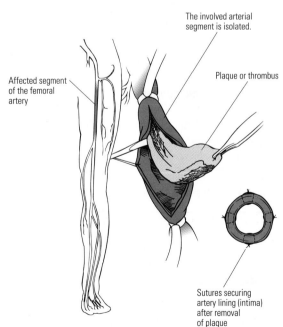

The involved arterial segment is isolated.

Plaque or thrombus

Affected segment of the femoral artery

Sutures securing artery lining (intima) after removal of plaque

+ **35390** Reoperation, carotid, thromboendarterectomy, more than one month after original operation (List separately in addition to code for primary procedure)

 → *CPT Assistant* Nov 97:16

 (Use 35390 in conjunction with 35301)

Angioscopy

+ **35400** Angioscopy (non-coronary vessels or grafts) during therapeutic intervention (List separately in addition to code for primary procedure)

 → *CPT Assistant* Nov 97:16

Transluminal Angioplasty

If done as part of another operation, use modifier 51 or use modifier 52.

 (For radiological supervision and interpretation, see 75962-75968 and 75978)

Open

35450 Transluminal balloon angioplasty, open; renal or other visceral artery

 → *CPT Assistant* Feb 97:2-3

35452 aortic

 → *CPT Assistant* Feb 97:2-3

35454 iliac

 → *CPT Assistant* Feb 97:2-3, Dec 00:1, 4, Feb 03:3

35456 femoral-popliteal

 → *CPT Assistant* Feb 97:2-3

35458 brachiocephalic trunk or branches, each vessel

 → *CPT Assistant* Feb 97:2-3, May 01:11

35459 tibioperoneal trunk and branches

 → *CPT Assistant* Feb 97:2-3

35460 venous

 → *CPT Assistant* Feb 97:2-3

Percutaneous

Codes for catheter placement and the radiologic supervision and interpretation should also be reported, in addition to the code(s) for the therapeutic aspect of the procedure.

⊙ **35470** Transluminal balloon angioplasty, percutaneous; tibioperoneal trunk or branches, each vessel

 → *CPT Assistant* Aug 96:3, Feb 97:2-3

⊙ **35471** renal or visceral artery

 → *CPT Assistant* Aug 96:3, Feb 97:2-3

⊙ **35472** aortic

 → *CPT Assistant* Aug 96:3, Feb 97:2-3

⊙ **35473** iliac

 → *CPT Assistant* Fall 93:11, Aug 96:3, Feb 97:2-3, May 01:4, Feb 03:3

Transluminal Balloon Angioplasty
35473

A balloon catheter is passed into the iliac artery and inflated to stretch the blood vessel to a larger diameter.

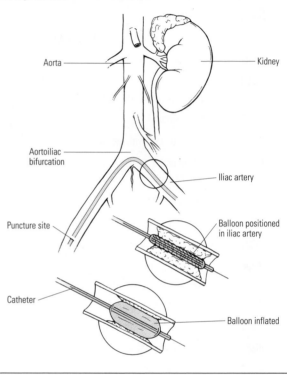

⊙ **35474** femoral-popliteal

 → *CPT Assistant* Aug 96:3, Feb 97:2-3, May 01:4, Aug 06:10

⊙ **35475** brachiocephalic trunk or branches, each vessel

 → *CPT Assistant* Aug 96:3, Feb 97:2-3, May 01:4

⊙ **35476** venous

 → *CPT Assistant* Aug 96:3, Feb 97:2-3, May 01:4, Dec 03:2

 → *Clinical Examples in Radiology* Spring 05:8-10, Spring 07:1-3

 (For radiological supervision and interpretation, use 75978)

Transluminal Atherectomy

If done as part of another operation, use modifier 51 or use modifier 52.

 (For radiological supervision and interpretation, see 75992-75996)

Open

35480 Transluminal peripheral atherectomy, open; renal or other visceral artery

 → *CPT Assistant* Feb 97:2-3

35481 aortic

 → *CPT Assistant* Feb 97:2

35482 iliac
→ *CPT Assistant* Feb 97:2

35483 femoral-popliteal
→ *CPT Assistant* Feb 97:2

35484 brachiocephalic trunk or branches, each vessel
→ *CPT Assistant* Feb 97:2

35485 tibioperoneal trunk and branches
→ *CPT Assistant* Feb 97:2

Percutaneous

Codes for catheter placement and the radiologic supervision and interpretation should also be reported, in addition to the code(s) for the therapeutic aspect of the procedure.

35490 Transluminal peripheral atherectomy, percutaneous; renal or other visceral artery
→ *CPT Assistant* Feb 97:2

35491 aortic
→ *CPT Assistant* Feb 97:2

35492 iliac
→ *CPT Assistant* Feb 97:2

35493 femoral-popliteal
→ *CPT Assistant* Feb 97:2

35494 brachiocephalic trunk or branches, each vessel
→ *CPT Assistant* Feb 97:2

35495 tibioperoneal trunk and branches
→ *CPT Assistant* Feb 97:2

Bypass Graft

Vein

Procurement of the saphenous vein graft is included in the description of the work for 35501-35587 and should not be reported as a separate service or co-surgery. To report harvesting of an upper extremity vein, use 35500 in addition to the bypass procedure. To report harvesting of a femoropopliteal vein segment, use 35572 in addition to the bypass procedure. To report harvesting and construction of an autogenous composite graft of two segments from two distant locations, report 35682 in addition to the bypass procedure, for autogenous composite of three or more segments from distant sites, report 35683.

+ 35500 Harvest of upper extremity vein, one segment, for lower extremity or coronary artery bypass procedure (List separately in addition to code for primary procedure)
→ *CPT Assistant* Nov 98:13, Mar 99:6, Nov 99:19, Jan 07:7; *CPT Changes: An Insider's View* 2000

(Use 35500 in conjunction with 33510-33536, 35556, 35566, 35571, 35583-35587)

(For harvest of more than one vein segment, see 35682, 35683)

(For endoscopic procedure, use 33508)

35501 Bypass graft, with vein; common carotid-ipsilateral internal carotid
→ *CPT Assistant* Apr 99:11; *CPT Changes: An Insider's View* 2007

35506 carotid-subclavian or subclavian-carotid
→ *CPT Assistant* Oct 04:6, Jan 07:7; *CPT Changes: An Insider's View* 2007

(35507 has been deleted. For subclavian-carotid bypass with vein, use 35506)

35508 carotid-vertebral

35509 carotid-contralateral carotid
→ *CPT Changes: An Insider's View* 2007

35510 carotid-brachial
→ *CPT Assistant* Oct 04:6; *CPT Changes: An Insider's View* 2004

35511 subclavian-subclavian

35512 subclavian-brachial
→ *CPT Assistant* Oct 04:7; *CPT Changes: An Insider's View* 2004

35515 subclavian-vertebral

35516 subclavian-axillary

35518 axillary-axillary
→ *CPT Assistant* Oct 04:9

35521 axillary-femoral

(For bypass graft performed with synthetic graft, use 35621)

35522 axillary-brachial
→ *CPT Assistant* Oct 04:9; *CPT Changes: An Insider's View* 2004

● **35523** brachial-ulnar or -radial
→ *CPT Changes: An Insider's View* 2008

►(Do not report 35523 in conjunction with 35206, 35500, 35525, 36838)◄

►(For bypass graft performed with synthetic conduit, use 37799)◄

35525 brachial-brachial
→ *CPT Assistant* Oct 04:10; *CPT Changes: An Insider's View* 2004

35526 aortosubclavian or carotid

(For bypass graft performed with synthetic graft, use 35626)

35531 aortoceliac or aortomesenteric

35533 axillary-femoral-femoral

(For bypass graft performed with synthetic graft, use 35654)

35536 splenorenal
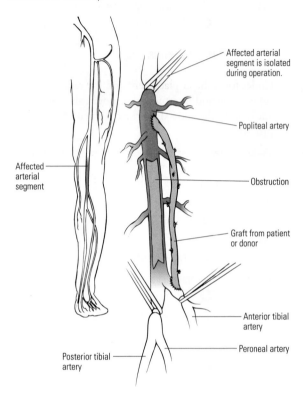 *CPT Assistant* Jun 99:10

35537 aortoiliac
CPT Changes: An Insider's View 2007

(For bypass graft performed with synthetic graft, use 35637)

(Do not report 35537 in conjunction with 35538)

35538 aortobi-iliac
CPT Changes: An Insider's View 2007

(For bypass graft performed with synthetic graft, use 35638)

(Do not report 35538 in conjunction with 35537)

35539 aortofemoral
CPT Changes: An Insider's View 2007

(For bypass graft performed with synthetic graft, use 35647)

(Do not report 35539 in conjunction with 35540)

35540 aortobifemoral
CPT Changes: An Insider's View 2007

(For bypass graft performed with synthetic graft, use 35646)

(Do not report 35540 in conjunction with 35539)

(35541 has been deleted. For aortoiliac graft with vein, use 35537. For aortobi-iliac graft with vein, use 35538)

(35546 has been deleted. For aortofemoral graft with vein use 35539. For aortobifemoral graft with vein, use 35540)

35548 aortoiliofemoral, unilateral

(For bypass graft performed with synthetic graft, use 37799)

35549 aortoiliofemoral, bilateral

(For bypass graft performed with synthetic graft, use 37799)

35551 aortofemoral-popliteal

35556 femoral-popliteal
CPT Assistant Fall 92:20, May 97:10, Jan 07:7

35558 femoral-femoral

35560 aortorenal
CPT Assistant Jun 99:10

35563 ilioiliac

35565 iliofemoral
CPT Assistant Oct 04:8

35566 femoral-anterior tibial, posterior tibial, peroneal artery or other distal vessels

35571 popliteal-tibial, -peroneal artery or other distal vessels

Bypass Graft, Vein
35571

The physician creates a bypass around the popliteal artery, using a harvested vein that is sutured to the tibial artery.

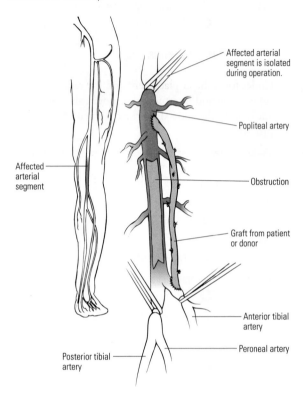

Affected arterial segment is isolated during operation.

Popliteal artery

Affected arterial segment

Obstruction

Graft from patient or donor

Anterior tibial artery

Peroneal artery

Posterior tibial artery

+ 35572 Harvest of femoropopliteal vein, one segment, for vascular reconstruction procedure (eg, aortic, vena caval, coronary, peripheral artery) (List separately in addition to code for primary procedure)
CPT Changes: An Insider's View 2003

(Use 35572 in conjunction with 33510-33516, 33517-33523, 33533-33536, 34502, 34520, 35001, 35002, 35011-35022, 35102, 35103, 35121-35152, 35231-35256, 35501-35587, 35879-35907)

(For bilateral procedure, use modifier 50)

In-Situ Vein

(To report aortobifemoral bypass using synthetic conduit, and femoral-popliteal bypass with vein conduit in-situ, use 35646 and 35583. To report aorto(uni)femoral bypass with synthetic conduit, and femoral-popliteal bypass with vein conduit in-situ, use 35647 and 35583. To report aortofemoral bypass using vein conduit, and femoral-popliteal bypass with vein conduit in-situ, use 35539 and 35583)

35583   In-situ vein bypass; femoral-popliteal

35585   femoral-anterior tibial, posterior tibial, or peroneal artery

35587   popliteal-tibial, peroneal
    → *CPT Assistant* Apr 99:11, Jan 07:7

Other Than Vein

(For arterial transposition and/or reimplantation, see 35691-35695)

+▲ 35600   Harvest of upper extremity artery, one segment, for coronary artery bypass procedure (List separately in addition to code for primary procedure)
    → *CPT Changes: An Insider's View* 2001, 2008

   ▶(Use 35600 in conjunction with 33533–33536)◀

Harvest of Upper Extremity Artery
35600

Open procurement of a radial artery to secure conduit for construction of a coronary artery bypass graft

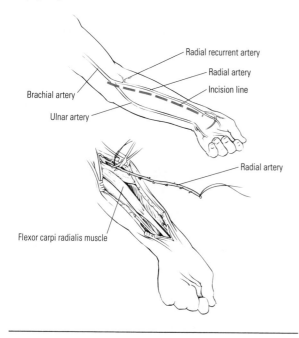

Radial recurrent artery
Radial artery
Incision line
Brachial artery
Ulnar artery
Radial artery
Flexor carpi radialis muscle

35601   Bypass graft, with other than vein; common carotid-ipsilateral internal carotid
    → *CPT Changes: An Insider's View* 2007

35606   carotid-subclavian

(For open transcervical common carotid-common carotid bypass performed in conjunction with endovascular repair of descending thoracic aorta, use 33891)

(For open subclavian to carotid artery transposition performed in conjunction with endovascular thoracic aneurysm repair by neck incision, use 33889)

35612   subclavian-subclavian

35616   subclavian-axillary

35621   axillary-femoral

35623   axillary-popliteal or -tibial

35626   aortosubclavian or carotid

35631   aortoceliac, aortomesenteric, aortorenal

35636   splenorenal (splenic to renal arterial anastomosis)

35637   aortoiliac
    → *CPT Changes: An Insider's View* 2007

(Do not report 35637 in conjunction with 35638, 35646)

35638   aortobi-iliac
    → *CPT Changes: An Insider's View* 2007

(Do not report 35638 in conjunction with 35637, 35646)

(35641 has been deleted. For aortoiliac graft constructed with conduit other than vein, use 35637. For aortobi-iliac graft with other than vein, use 35638)

(For open placement of aortobi-iliac prosthesis following unsuccessful endovascular repair, use 34831)

35642   carotid-vertebral

35645   subclavian-vertebral

35646   aortobifemoral
    → *CPT Changes: An Insider's View* 2002

(For bypass graft performed with vein graft, use 35540)

(For open placement of aortobifemoral prosthesis following unsuccessful endovascular repair, use 34832)

35647   aortofemoral
    → *CPT Changes: An Insider's View* 2002

(For bypass graft performed with vein graft, use 35539)

35650   axillary-axillary

35651   aortofemoral-popliteal

35654   axillary-femoral-femoral

35656   femoral-popliteal

35661   femoral-femoral

35663   ilioiliac

35665   iliofemoral

35666   femoral-anterior tibial, posterior tibial, or peroneal artery

35671   popliteal-tibial or -peroneal artery

Composite Grafts

Codes 35682-35683 are used to report harvest and anastomosis of multiple vein segments from distant sites for use as arterial bypass graft conduits. These codes are intended for use when the two or more vein segments are harvested from a limb other than that undergoing bypass. Add-on codes 35682 and 35683 may be reported in addition to codes 35556, 35566, 35571, 35583-35587, as appropriate.

+ **35681** Bypass graft; composite, prosthetic and vein (List separately in addition to code for primary procedure)

➔ *CPT Assistant* Nov 98:13-14, Mar 99:6, Apr 99:11

(Do not report 35681 in addition to 35682, 35683)

+ **35682** autogenous composite, two segments of veins from two locations (List separately in addition to code for primary procedure)

➔ *CPT Assistant* Nov 98:13-14, Mar 99:6, Apr 99:11, Sep 02:4

(Do not report 35682 in addition to 35681, 35683)

+ **35683** autogenous composite, three or more segments of vein from two or more locations (List separately in addition to code for primary procedure)

➔ *CPT Assistant* Nov 98:13-14, Mar 99:6, Apr 99:11, Sep 02:4

(Do not report 35683 in addition to 35681, 35682)

Adjuvant Techniques

Adjuvant (additional) technique(s) may be required at the time a bypass graft is created to improve patency of the lower extremity autogenous or synthetic bypass graft (eg, femoral-popliteal, femoral-tibial, or popliteal-tibial arteries). Code 35685 should be reported in addition to the primary synthetic bypass graft procedure, when an interposition of venous tissue (vein patch or cuff) is placed at the anastomosis between the synthetic bypass conduit and the involved artery (includes harvest).

Code 35686 should be reported in addition to the primary bypass graft procedure, when autogenous vein is used to create a fistula between the tibial or peroneal artery and vein at or beyond the distal bypass anastomosis site of the involved artery.

(For composite graft(s), see 35681-35683)

+ **35685** Placement of vein patch or cuff at distal anastomosis of bypass graft, synthetic conduit (List separately in addition to code for primary procedure)

➔ *CPT Assistant* Sep 02:3; *CPT Changes: An Insider's View* 2002

(Use 35685 in conjunction with 35656, 35666, or 35671)

+ **35686** Creation of distal arteriovenous fistula during lower extremity bypass surgery (non-hemodialysis) (List separately in addition to code for primary procedure)

➔ *CPT Assistant* Sep 02:3; *CPT Changes: An Insider's View* 2002

(Use 35686 in conjunction with 35556, 35566, 35571, 35583-35587, 35623, 35656, 35666, 35671)

Arterial Transposition

35691 Transposition and/or reimplantation; vertebral to carotid artery

35693 vertebral to subclavian artery

35694 subclavian to carotid artery

(For open subclavian to carotid artery transposition performed in conjunction with endovascular repair of descending thoracic aorta, use 33889)

35695 carotid to subclavian artery

+ **35697** Reimplantation, visceral artery to infrarenal aortic prosthesis, each artery (List separately in addition to code for primary procedure)

➔ *CPT Changes: An Insider's View* 2004

(Do not report 35697 in conjunction with 33877)

Excision, Exploration, Repair, Revision

+ **35700** Reoperation, femoral-popliteal or femoral (popliteal)-anterior tibial, posterior tibial, peroneal artery, or other distal vessels, more than one month after original operation (List separately in addition to code for primary procedure)

(Use 35700 in conjunction with 35556, 35566, 35571, 35583, 35585, 35587, 35656, 35666, 35671)

35701 Exploration (not followed by surgical repair), with or without lysis of artery; carotid artery

35721 femoral artery

➔ *CPT Assistant* Jun 96:8

35741 popliteal artery

35761 other vessels

35800 Exploration for postoperative hemorrhage, thrombosis or infection; neck

35820 chest

35840 abdomen

➔ *CPT Assistant* May 97:8

35860 extremity

➔ *CPT Assistant* Fall 92:21

35870   Repair of graft-enteric fistula

35875   Thrombectomy of arterial or venous graft (other than hemodialysis graft or fistula);
➡ *CPT Assistant* Nov 98:14, Feb 99:6, Mar 99:6, Apr 00:10

35876   with revision of arterial or venous graft
➡ *CPT Assistant* Nov 98:14

(For thrombectomy of hemodialysis graft or fistula, see 36831, 36833)

Codes 35879 and 35881 describe open revision of graft-threatening stenoses of lower extremity arterial bypass graft(s) (previously constructed with autogenous vein conduit) using vein patch angioplasty or segmental vein interposition techniques. For thrombectomy with revision of any non-coronary arterial or venous graft, including those of the lower extremity, (other than hemodialysis graft or fistula), use 35876. For direct repair (other than for fistula) of a lower extremity blood vessel (with or without patch angioplasty), use 35226. For repair (other than for fistula) of a lower extremity blood vessel using a vein graft, use 35256.

35879   Revision, lower extremity arterial bypass, without thrombectomy, open; with vein patch angioplasty
➡ *CPT Assistant* Nov 99:19; *CPT Changes: An Insider's View* 2000

35881   with segmental vein interposition
➡ *CPT Assistant* Nov 99:19; *CPT Changes: An Insider's View* 2000

(For revision of femoral anastomosis of synthetic arterial bypass graft, see 35883, 35884)

(For excision of infected graft, see 35901-35907 and appropriate revascularization code)

35883   Revision, femoral anastomosis of synthetic arterial bypass graft in groin, open; with nonautogenous patch graft (eg, Dacron, ePTFE, bovine pericardium)
➡ *CPT Changes: An Insider's View* 2007

(For bilateral procedure, use modifier 50)

(Do not report 35883 in conjunction with 35700, 35875, 35876, 35884)

35884   with autogenous vein patch graft
➡ *CPT Changes: An Insider's View* 2007

(For bilateral procedure, use modifier 50)

(Do not report 35884 in conjunction with 35700, 35875, 35876, 35883)

35901   Excision of infected graft; neck

35903   extremity

35905   thorax

35907   abdomen

Vascular Injection Procedures

Listed services for injection procedures include necessary local anesthesia, introduction of needles or catheter, injection of contrast media with or without automatic power injection, and/or necessary pre- and postinjection care specifically related to the injection procedure.

Catheters, drugs, and contrast media are not included in the listed service for the injection procedures.

Selective vascular catheterization should be coded to include introduction and all lesser order selective catheterization used in the approach (eg, the description for a selective right middle cerebral artery catheterization includes the introduction and placement catheterization of the right common and internal carotid arteries).

Additional second and/or third order arterial catheterization within the same family of arteries or veins supplied by a single first order vessel should be expressed by 36012, 36218, or 36248.

Additional first order or higher catheterization in vascular families supplied by a first order vessel different from a previously selected and coded family should be separately coded using the conventions described above.

(For radiological supervision and interpretation, see **Radiology**)

(For injection procedures in conjunction with cardiac catheterization, see 93541-93545)

(For chemotherapy of malignant disease, see 96401-96549)

Intravenous

An intracatheter is a sheathed combination of needle and short catheter.

36000   Introduction of needle or intracatheter, vein
➡ *CPT Assistant* Summer 95:2, Apr 98:1, 3, 7, Jul 98:1, Apr 03:26, Oct 03:2, Jul 06:4, Feb 07:10

36002 Injection procedures (eg, thrombin) for percutaneous treatment of extremity pseudoaneurysm

➲ *CPT Changes: An Insider's View* 2002

(For imaging guidance, see 76942, 77002, 77012, 77021)

(For ultrasound guided compression repair of pseudoaneurysms, use 76936)

(Do not report 36002 for vascular sealant of an arteriotomy site)

Injection Procedure (eg, Thrombin) for Percutaneous Treatment of Extremity Pseudoaneurysm
36002

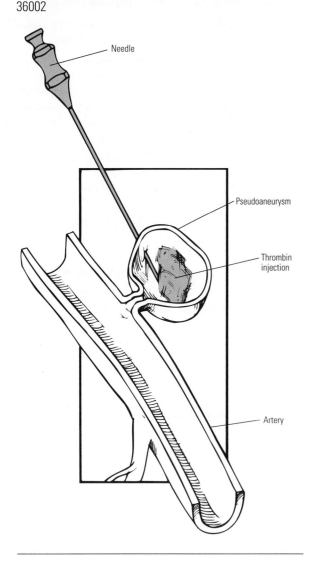

Needle

Pseudoaneurysm

Thrombin injection

Artery

36005 Injection procedure for extremity venography (including introduction of needle or intracatheter)

➲ *CPT Changes: An Insider's View* 2002

(For radiological supervision and interpretation, see 75820, 75822)

36010 Introduction of catheter, superior or inferior vena cava

➲ *CPT Assistant* Aug 96:2, Apr 98:7, Sep 00:11, May 01:10, Jul 03:12

➲ *Clinical Examples in Radiology* Winter 05:5-6

36011 Selective catheter placement, venous system; first order branch (eg, renal vein, jugular vein)

➲ *CPT Assistant* Aug 96:11, Apr 98:7, Jul 03:12, Dec 03:2

36012 second order, or more selective, branch (eg, left adrenal vein, petrosal sinus)

➲ *CPT Assistant* Aug 96:11, Sep 98:7, Jul 03:12

36013 Introduction of catheter, right heart or main pulmonary artery

➲ *CPT Assistant* Aug 96:11

36014 Selective catheter placement, left or right pulmonary artery

➲ *CPT Assistant* Aug 96:11, Apr 98:7

36015 Selective catheter placement, segmental or subsegmental pulmonary artery

➲ *CPT Assistant* Aug 96:11, Sep 00:11

(For insertion of flow directed catheter (eg, Swan-Ganz), use 93503)

(For venous catheterization for selective organ blood sampling, use 36500)

Intra-Arterial—Intra-Aortic

(For radiological supervision and interpretation, see **Radiology**)

36100 Introduction of needle or intracatheter, carotid or vertebral artery

➲ *CPT Assistant* Aug 96:11

(For bilateral procedure, report 36100 with modifier 50)

36120 Introduction of needle or intracatheter; retrograde brachial artery

➲ *CPT Assistant* Fall 93:16, Aug 96:3

36140 extremity artery

➲ *CPT Assistant* Fall 93:16, Aug 96:3, Nov 99:32-33, Oct 03:2, Jul 06:4,7

36145 arteriovenous shunt created for dialysis (cannula, fistula, or graft)

➲ *CPT Assistant* Aug 96:3, Feb 97:2, May 01:4

➲ *Clinical Examples in Radiology* Spring 05:8-10, Spring 07:1-3

(For insertion of arteriovenous cannula, see 36810-36821)

36160 Introduction of needle or intracatheter, aortic, translumbar

➲ *CPT Assistant* Aug 96:3

36200 Introduction of catheter, aorta

➲ *CPT Assistant* Fall 93:16, Aug 96:3, Jul 06:7

36215 Selective catheter placement, arterial system; each first order thoracic or brachiocephalic branch, within a vascular family

➲ *CPT Assistant* Fall 93:15, Aug 96:3, Nov 97:16, Apr 98:9, Sep 00:11, Oct 00:4, Feb 03:3

(For catheter placement for coronary angiography, use 93508)

36216   initial second order thoracic or brachiocephalic branch, within a vascular family
➔ *CPT Assistant* Fall 93:15, Aug 96:3, Oct 00:4

36217   initial third order or more selective thoracic or brachiocephalic branch, within a vascular family
➔ *CPT Assistant* Fall 93:15, Aug 96:3, Oct 00:4

+ 36218   additional second order, third order, and beyond, thoracic or brachiocephalic branch, within a vascular family (List in addition to code for initial second or third order vessel as appropriate)
➔ *CPT Assistant* Fall 93:15, Aug 96:3, Oct 00:4, Jul 06:7

(Use 36218 in conjunction with 36216, 36217)

(For angiography, see 75600-75790)

(For angioplasty, see 35470-35475)

(For transcatheter therapies, see 37200-37208, 61624, 61626)

(When coronary artery, arterial conduit (eg, internal mammary, inferior epigastric or free radical artery) or venous bypass graft angiography is performed in conjunction with cardiac catheterization, see the appropriate cardiac catheterization, injection procedure, and imaging supervision code(s) (93501-93556) in the **Medicine** section of the CPT codebook. When coronary artery, arterial coronary conduit or venous bypass graft angiography is performed without concomitant left heart cardiac catheterization, use 93508. When internal mammary artery angiography only is performed without a concomitant left heart cardiac catheterization, use 36216 or 36217 as appropriate.)

36245   Selective catheter placement, arterial system; each first order abdominal, pelvic, or lower extremity artery branch, within a vascular family
➔ *CPT Assistant* Fall 93:15, Aug 96:3, Jan 01:14, Jan 07:7

36246   initial second order abdominal, pelvic, or lower extremity artery branch, within a vascular family
➔ *CPT Assistant* Fall 93:15, Aug 96:3, Jan 01:14, Jan 07:7

36247   initial third order or more selective abdominal, pelvic, or lower extremity artery branch, within a vascular family
➔ *CPT Assistant* Fall 93:15, Aug 96:3, Jan 01:14, Jan 07:7

+ 36248   additional second order, third order, and beyond, abdominal, pelvic, or lower extremity artery branch, within a vascular family (List in addition to code for initial second or third order vessel as appropriate)
➔ *CPT Assistant* Fall 93:15, Aug 96:3, Apr 98:1, 7, Oct 00:4, Jan 01:14, Jan 07:7

(Use 36248 in conjunction with 36246, 36247)

36260   Insertion of implantable intra-arterial infusion pump (eg, for chemotherapy of liver)
➔ *CPT Assistant* Fall 95:5

36261   Revision of implanted intra-arterial infusion pump

36262   Removal of implanted intra-arterial infusion pump

36299   Unlisted procedure, vascular injection

Venous

▶Venipuncture, needle or catheter for diagnostic study or intravenous therapy, percutaneous. These codes are also used to report the therapy as specified. For collection of a specimen from an established catheter, use 36592. For collection of a specimen from a completely implantable venous access device, use 36591.◀

36400   Venipuncture, younger than age 3 years, necessitating physician's skill, not to be used for routine venipuncture; femoral or jugular vein
➔ *CPT Changes: An Insider's View* 2002, 2004

36405   scalp vein

36406   other vein

36410   Venipuncture, age 3 years or older, necessitating physician's skill (separate procedure), for diagnostic or therapeutic purposes (not to be used for routine venipuncture)
➔ *CPT Assistant* Jun 96:10, May 01:11, Aug 02:2, Oct 03:10, Feb 07:10; *CPT Changes: An Insider's View* 2004

36415   Collection of venous blood by venipuncture
➔ *CPT Assistant* Jun 96:10, Mar 98:10, Oct 99:11, Aug 00:2, Feb 07:10; *CPT Changes: An Insider's View* 2003

(Do not report modifier 63 in conjunction with 36415)

36416   Collection of capillary blood specimen (eg, finger, heel, ear stick)
➔ *CPT Changes: An Insider's View* 2003

36420   Venipuncture, cutdown; younger than age 1 year
➔ *CPT Assistant* Nov 99:32-33, Aug 00:2, Oct 03:2, Jul 06:4

(Do not report modifier 63 in conjunction with 36420)

36425   age 1 or over

36430   Transfusion, blood or blood components
➔ *CPT Assistant* Aug 97:18, Nov 99:32-33, Aug 00:2, Mar 01:10, Oct 03:2, Jul 06:4

36440   Push transfusion, blood, 2 years or younger
➔ *CPT Assistant* Aug 00:2, Oct 03:2, Jul 06:4

36450   Exchange transfusion, blood; newborn

(Do not report modifier 63 in conjunction with 36450)

36455   other than newborn

36460   Transfusion, intrauterine, fetal

(Do not report modifier 63 in conjunction with 36460)

(For radiological supervision and interpretation, use 76941)

36468   Single or multiple injections of sclerosing solutions, spider veins (telangiectasia); limb or trunk

36469   face

36470   Injection of sclerosing solution; single vein

36471   multiple veins, same leg

36475 Endovenous ablation therapy of incompetent vein, extremity, inclusive of all imaging guidance and monitoring, percutaneous, radiofrequency; first vein treated

➲ *CPT Changes: An Insider's View* 2005

+ 36476 second and subsequent veins treated in a single extremity, each through separate access sites (List separately in addition to code for primary procedure)

➲ *CPT Changes: An Insider's View* 2005

(Use 36476 in conjunction with 36475)

(Do not report 36475, 36476 in conjunction with 36000-36005, 36410, 36425, 36478, 36479, 37204, 75894, 76000, 76001, 76937, 76942, 77022, 93970, 93971)

36478 Endovenous ablation therapy of incompetent vein, extremity, inclusive of all imaging guidance and monitoring, percutaneous, laser; first vein treated

➲ *CPT Changes: An Insider's View* 2005

+ 36479 second and subsequent veins treated in a single extremity, each through separate access sites (List separately in addition to code for primary procedure)

➲ *CPT Changes: An Insider's View* 2005

(Use 36479 in conjunction with 36478)

(Do not report 36478, 36479 in conjunction with 36000-36005, 36410, 36425, 36475, 36476, 37204, 75894, 76000, 76001, 76937, 76942, 77022, 93970, 93971)

36481 Percutaneous portal vein catheterization by any method

➲ *CPT Assistant* Oct 96:1, Mar 02:10, Dec 03:2

(For radiological supervision and interpretation, see 75885, 75887)

36500 Venous catheterization for selective organ blood sampling

(For catheterization in superior or inferior vena cava, use 36010)

(For radiological supervision and interpretation, use 75893)

36510 Catheterization of umbilical vein for diagnosis or therapy, newborn

➲ *CPT Assistant* Nov 99:5-6, Aug 00:2, Oct 03:2, Jul 06:4

(Do not report modifier 63 in conjunction with 36510)

36511 Therapeutic apheresis; for white blood cells

➲ *CPT Changes: An Insider's View* 2003

36512 for red blood cells

➲ *CPT Changes: An Insider's View* 2003

36513 for platelets

➲ *CPT Changes: An Insider's View* 2003

36514 for plasma pheresis

➲ *CPT Changes: An Insider's View* 2003

36515 with extracorporeal immunoadsorption and plasma reinfusion

➲ *CPT Changes: An Insider's View* 2003

36516 with extracorporeal selective adsorption or selective filtration and plasma reinfusion

➲ *CPT Changes: An Insider's View* 2003

(For physician evaluation, use modifier 26)

36522 Photopheresis, extracorporeal

➲ *CPT Assistant* Fall 93:25

▶(36540 has been deleted. To report, use 36591)◀

▶(36550 has been deleted. To report, use 36593)◀

Central Venous Access Procedures

To qualify as a central venous access catheter or device, the tip of the catheter/device must terminate in the subclavian, brachiocephalic (innominate) or iliac veins, the superior or inferior vena cava, or the right atrium. The venous access device may be either centrally inserted (jugular, subclavian, femoral vein or inferior vena cava catheter entry site) or peripherally inserted (eg, basilic or cephalic vein). The device may be accessed for use either via exposed catheter (external to the skin), via a subcutaneous port or via a subcutaneous pump.

The procedures involving these types of devices fall into five categories:

1) ***Insertion*** (placement of catheter through a newly established venous access)

2) ***Repair*** (fixing device without replacement of either catheter or port/pump, other than pharmacologic or mechanical correction of intracatheter or pericatheter occlusion (see 36595 or 36596))

3) ***Partial replacement*** of only the catheter component associated with a port/pump device, but not entire device

4) ***Complete replacement*** of entire device via same venous access site (complete exchange)

5) ***Removal*** of entire device.

There is no coding distinction between venous access achieved percutaneously versus by cutdown or based on catheter size.

For the repair, partial (catheter only) replacement, complete replacement, or removal of both catheters (placed from separate venous access sites) of a multi-catheter device, with or without subcutaneous ports/pumps, use the appropriate code describing the service with a frequency of two.

If an existing central venous access device is removed and a new one placed via a separate venous access site, appropriate codes for both procedures (removal of old, if code exists, and insertion of new device) should be reported.

When imaging is used for these procedures, either for gaining access to the venous entry site or for manipulating the catheter into final central position, use 76937, 77001.

(For refilling and maintenance of an implantable pump or reservoir for intravenous or intra-arterial drug delivery, use 96522)

Insertion of Central Venous Access Device

⊙ **36555**   Insertion of non-tunneled centrally inserted central venous catheter; younger than 5 years of age

➡ *CPT Assistant* Dec 04:7, Jul 06:4; *CPT Changes: An Insider's View* 2004

➡ *Clinical Examples in Radiology* Summer 06:8-9

(For peripherally inserted non-tunneled central venous catheter, younger than 5 years of age, use 36568)

Insertion of Non-Tunneled Centrally Inserted Central Venous Catheter
36555

During placement of a central venous catheter, a short tract is developed as the catheter is advanced from the skin entry site to the point of venous cannulation. The catheter tip must reside in the subclavian, innominate or iliac veins, the inferior or superior vena cava, or right atrium to be considered a "central venous" catheter.

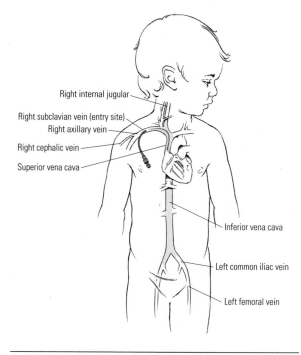

36556   age 5 years or older

➡ *CPT Assistant* Dec 04:7; *CPT Changes: An Insider's View* 2004

➡ *Clinical Examples in Radiology* Summer 06:8-9

(For peripherally inserted non-tunneled central venous catheter, age 5 years or older, use 36569)

Insertion of Non-Tunneled Centrally Inserted Central Venous Catheter
36556

During placement of a central venous catheter, a short tract is developed as the catheter is advanced from the skin entry site to the point of venous cannulation. The catheter tip must reside in the subclavian, innominate or iliac veins, the inferior or superior vena cava, or right atrium, to be considered a "central venous" catheter.

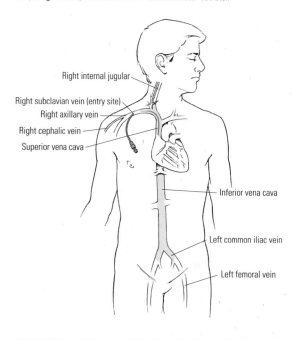

⊙ **36557**   Insertion of tunneled centrally inserted central venous catheter, without subcutaneous port or pump; younger than 5 years of age

➡ *CPT Assistant* Dec 04:7; *CPT Changes: An Insider's View* 2004

⊙ **36558**   age 5 years or older

➡ *CPT Assistant* Dec 04:7; *CPT Changes: An Insider's View* 2004

(For peripherally inserted central venous catheter with port, 5 years or older, use 36571)

Insertion of Tunneled Central Venous Catheter
36557-36558

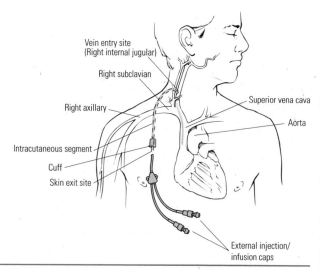

⊙ **36560** Insertion of tunneled centrally inserted central venous access device, with subcutaneous port; younger than 5 years of age

➲ *CPT Assistant* Dec 04:7; *CPT Changes: An Insider's View* 2004

(For peripherally inserted central venous access device with subcutaneous port, younger than 5 years of age, use 36570)

⊙ **36561** age 5 years or older

➲ *CPT Assistant* Dec 04:7; *CPT Changes: An Insider's View* 2004

(For peripherally inserted central venous catheter with subcutaneous port, 5 years or older, use 36571)

⊙ **36563** Insertion of tunneled centrally inserted central venous access device with subcutaneous pump

➲ *CPT Assistant* Dec 04:8; *CPT Changes: An Insider's View* 2004

⊙ **36565** Insertion of tunneled centrally inserted central venous access device, requiring two catheters via two separate venous access sites; without subcutaneous port or pump (eg, Tesio type catheter)

➲ *CPT Assistant* Dec 04:8; *CPT Changes: An Insider's View* 2004

⊙ **36566** with subcutaneous port(s)

➲ *CPT Assistant* Dec 04:8; *CPT Changes: An Insider's View* 2004

⊙ **36568** Insertion of peripherally inserted central venous catheter (PICC), without subcutaneous port or pump; younger than 5 years of age

➲ *CPT Assistant* Oct 04:14, Dec 04:8, May 05:13; *CPT Changes: An Insider's View* 2004

(For placement of centrally inserted non-tunneled central venous catheter, without subcutaneous port or pump, younger than 5 years of age, use 36555)

36569 age 5 years or older

➲ *CPT Assistant* Oct 04:14, Dec 04:8, May 05:13; *CPT Changes: An Insider's View* 2004

➲ *Clinical Examples in Radiology* Inaugural 04:1-2

(For placement of centrally inserted non-tunneled central venous catheter, without subcutaneous port or pump, age 5 years or older, use 36556)

⊙ **36570** Insertion of peripherally inserted central venous access device, with subcutaneous port; younger than 5 years of age

➲ *CPT Assistant* Dec 04:8; *CPT Changes: An Insider's View* 2004

(For insertion of tunneled centrally inserted central venous access device with subcutaneous port, younger than 5 years of age, use 36560)

⊙ **36571** age 5 years or older

➲ *CPT Assistant* Dec 04:9; *CPT Changes: An Insider's View* 2004

(For insertion of tunneled centrally inserted central venous access device with subcutaneous port, age 5 years or older, use 36561)

Implantable Venous Access Port
36570-36571, 36576, 36578

Noncoring needle

Venous access port

Central vein

Repair of Central Venous Access Device

(For mechanical removal of pericatheter obstructive material, use 36595)

(For mechanical removal of intracatheter obstructive material, use 36596)

36575 Repair of tunneled or non-tunneled central venous access catheter, without subcutaneous port or pump, central or peripheral insertion site

➲ *CPT Changes: An Insider's View* 2004

⊙ **36576** Repair of central venous access device, with subcutaneous port or pump, central or peripheral insertion site

➲ *CPT Assistant* Dec 04:9; *CPT Changes: An Insider's View* 2004

Partial Replacement of Central Venous Access Device (Catheter Only)

⊙ **36578** Replacement, catheter only, of central venous access device, with subcutaneous port or pump, central or peripheral insertion site

➲ *CPT Assistant* Dec 04:10; *CPT Changes: An Insider's View* 2004

(For complete replacement of entire device through same venous access, use 36582 or 36583)

Complete Replacement of Central Venous Access Device Through Same Venous Access Site

36580 Replacement, complete, of a non-tunneled centrally inserted central venous catheter, without subcutaneous port or pump, through same venous access
➔ *CPT Assistant* Dec 04:10; *CPT Changes: An Insider's View* 2004

⊙ **36581** Replacement, complete, of a tunneled centrally inserted central venous catheter, without subcutaneous port or pump, through same venous access
➔ *CPT Assistant* Dec 04:10; *CPT Changes: An Insider's View* 2004

⊙ **36582** Replacement, complete, of a tunneled centrally inserted central venous access device, with subcutaneous port, through same venous access
➔ *CPT Assistant* Dec 04:10; *CPT Changes: An Insider's View* 2004

⊙ **36583** Replacement, complete, of a tunneled centrally inserted central venous access device, with subcutaneous pump, through same venous access
➔ *CPT Assistant* Dec 04:10-11; *CPT Changes: An Insider's View* 2004

36584 Replacement, complete, of a peripherally inserted central venous catheter (PICC), without subcutaneous port or pump, through same venous access
➔ *CPT Assistant* Dec 04:11; *CPT Changes: An Insider's View* 2004

⊙ **36585** Replacement, complete, of a peripherally inserted central venous access device, with subcutaneous port, through same venous access
➔ *CPT Assistant* Dec 04:11; *CPT Changes: An Insider's View* 2004

Removal of Central Venous Access Device

36589 Removal of tunneled central venous catheter, without subcutaneous port or pump
➔ *CPT Assistant* Dec 04:11; *CPT Changes: An Insider's View* 2004

⊙ **36590** Removal of tunneled central venous access device, with subcutaneous port or pump, central or peripheral insertion
➔ *CPT Assistant* Dec 04:11; *CPT Changes: An Insider's View* 2004

(Do not report 36589 or 36590 for removal of non-tunneled central venous catheters)

▶ Other Central Venous Access Procedures◄

● **36591** Collection of blood specimen from a completely implantable venous access device
➔ *CPT Changes: An Insider's View* 2008

▶(Do not report 36591 in conjunction with any other service)◄

▶(For collection of venous blood specimen by venipuncture, use 36415)◄

▶(For collection of capillary blood specimen, use 36416)◄

● **36592** Collection of blood specimen using established central or peripheral catheter, venous, not otherwise specified
➔ *CPT Changes: An Insider's View* 2008

▶(For blood collection from an established arterial catheter, use 37799)◄

▶(Do not report 36592 in conjunction with any other service)◄

● **36593** Declotting by thrombolytic agent of implanted vascular access device or catheter
➔ *CPT Changes: An Insider's View* 2008

36595 Mechanical removal of pericatheter obstructive material (eg, fibrin sheath) from central venous device via separate venous access
➔ *CPT Assistant* Dec 04:9, 12; *CPT Changes: An Insider's View* 2004

▶(Do not report 36595 in conjunction with 36593)◄

(For venous catheterization, see 36010-36012)

(For radiological supervision and interpretation, use 75901)

36596 Mechanical removal of intraluminal (intracatheter) obstructive material from central venous device through device lumen
➔ *CPT Assistant* Dec 04:9, 12; *CPT Changes: An Insider's View* 2004

▶(Do not report 36596 in conjunction with 36593)◄

(For venous catheterization, see 36010-36012)

(For radiological supervision and interpretation, use 75902)

36597 Repositioning of previously placed central venous catheter under fluoroscopic guidance
➔ *CPT Assistant* Dec 04:12; *CPT Changes: An Insider's View* 2004

(For fluoroscopic guidance, use 76000)

36598 Contrast injection(s) for radiologic evaluation of existing central venous access device, including fluoroscopy, image documentation and report
➔ *CPT Changes: An Insider's View* 2006
➔ *Clinical Examples in Radiology* Winter 06:15

(Do not report 36598 in conjunction with 76000)

(Do not report 36598 in conjunction with 36595, 36596)

(For complete diagnostic studies, see 75820, 75825, 75827)

Arterial

36600 Arterial puncture, withdrawal of blood for diagnosis
➔ *CPT Assistant* Fall 95:7, Aug 00:2, Oct 03:2, Jul 05:11, Jul 06:4, Feb 07:10

⊘ **36620** Arterial catheterization or cannulation for sampling, monitoring or transfusion (separate procedure); percutaneous
➔ *CPT Assistant* Fall 95:7, Apr 98:3, Nov 99:32-33, Aug 00:2, Oct 03:2, Jul 06:4

36625   cutdown
➔ *CPT Assistant* Fall 95:7

36640 Arterial catheterization for prolonged infusion therapy (chemotherapy), cutdown
➔ *CPT Assistant* Fall 95:7

(See also 96420-96425)

(For arterial catheterization for occlusion therapy, see 75894)

▲ **36660** Catheterization, umbilical artery, newborn, for diagnosis or therapy
➔ *CPT Assistant* Fall 95:8, Oct 03:2, Jul 06:4; *CPT Changes: An Insider's View* 2008

(Do not report modifier 63 in conjunction with 36660)

Intraosseous

36680 Placement of needle for intraosseous infusion

Hemodialysis Access, Intervascular Cannulation for Extracorporeal Circulation, or Shunt Insertion

36800 Insertion of cannula for hemodialysis, other purpose (separate procedure); vein to vein
➔ *CPT Assistant* Fall 93:3

36810   arteriovenous, external (Scribner type)
➔ *CPT Assistant* Fall 93:3, May 97:10

36815   arteriovenous, external revision, or closure
➔ *CPT Assistant* Fall 93:3

36818 Arteriovenous anastomosis, open; by upper arm cephalic vein transposition
➔ *CPT Assistant* Jul 05:9; *CPT Changes: An Insider's View* 2005

(Do not report 36818 in conjunction with 36819, 36820, 36821, 36830 during a unilateral upper extremity procedure. For bilateral upper extremity open arteriovenous anastomoses performed at the same operative session, use modifier 50 or 59 as appropriate)

36819   by upper arm basilic vein transposition
➔ *CPT Assistant* Nov 99:20, Jul 05:9; *CPT Changes: An Insider's View* 2000, 2002

(Do not report 36819 in conjunction with 36818, 36820, 36821, 36830 during a unilateral upper extremity procedure. For bilateral upper extremity open arteriovenous anastomoses performed at the same operative session, use modifier 50 or 59 as appropriate)

36820   by forearm vein transposition
➔ *CPT Assistant* Fall 93:4, Jul 05:9; *CPT Changes: An Insider's View* 2002

36821   direct, any site (eg, Cimino type) (separate procedure)
➔ *CPT Assistant* Fall 93:3, Feb 97:2, Nov 99:20, Jul 05:9; *CPT Changes: An Insider's View* 2000

Arteriovenous Anastomosis, Direct
36821

A section of artery and a neighboring vein are joined, allowing blood to flow down the artery and into the vein for the purpose of increasing blood flow, usually in hemodialysis.

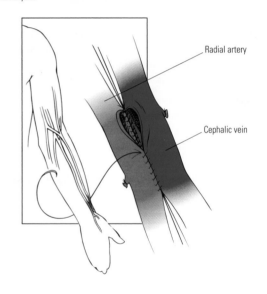

Radial artery

Cephalic vein

36822   Insertion of cannula(s) for prolonged extracorporeal circulation for cardiopulmonary insufficiency (ECMO) (separate procedure)
➔ *CPT Assistant* Feb 97:11

Insertion of Cannulas for Prolonged Extracorporeal Circulation Membrane Oxygenation (ECMO)
36822

The patient's venous blood is shunted and oxygenated outside of the body, bypassing the lungs. The treated blood is returned to body tissues through the femoral artery.

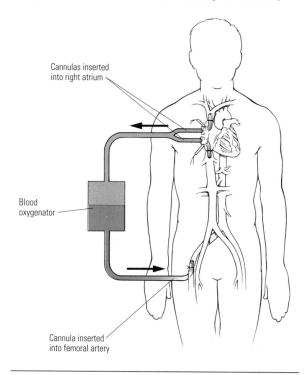

Cannulas inserted into right atrium

Blood oxygenator

Cannula inserted into femoral artery

(For maintenance of prolonged extracorporeal circulation, see 33960, 33961)

36823   Insertion of arterial and venous cannula(s) for isolated extracorporeal circulation including regional chemotherapy perfusion to an extremity, with or without hyperthermia, with removal of cannula(s) and repair of arteriotomy and venotomy sites
➔ *CPT Assistant* Nov 98:14-15; *CPT Changes: An Insider's View* 2002

(36823 includes chemotherapy perfusion supported by a membrane oxygenator/perfusion pump. Do not report 96409-96425 in conjunction with 36823)

36825   Creation of arteriovenous fistula by other than direct arteriovenous anastomosis (separate procedure); autogenous graft
➔ *CPT Assistant* Fall 93:3, Feb 97:2, Jul 05:9

(For direct arteriovenous anastomosis, use 36821)

36830   nonautogenous graft (eg, biological collagen, thermoplastic graft)
➔ *CPT Assistant* Fall 93:3, Feb 97:2, Jul 05:9; *CPT Changes: An Insider's View* 2003

(For direct arteriovenous anastomosis, use 36821)

Arteriovenous Fistula
36825-36830

A donor's vein (36825) or a synthetic vein (36830) is used to connect an artery and vein.

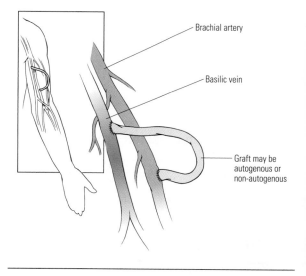

Brachial artery

Basilic vein

Graft may be autogenous or non-autogenous

36831   Thrombectomy, open, arteriovenous fistula without revision, autogenous or nonautogenous dialysis graft (separate procedure)
➔ *CPT Assistant* Nov 98:14-15, Feb 99:6, Mar 99:6, Apr 99:11; *CPT Changes: An Insider's View* 2001

36832   Revision, open, arteriovenous fistula; without thrombectomy, autogenous or nonautogenous dialysis graft (separate procedure)
➔ *CPT Assistant* Fall 93:3, Feb 97:2, Nov 98:15, Feb 99:6, Mar 99:6, Apr 99:11, Nov 99:20-21; *CPT Changes: An Insider's View* 2000, 2001

36833   with thrombectomy, autogenous or nonautogenous dialysis graft (separate procedure)
➔ *CPT Assistant* Nov 98:15, Feb 99:6, Apr 99:11

36834   Plastic repair of arteriovenous aneurysm (separate procedure)
➔ *CPT Assistant* Fall 93:3

36835   Insertion of Thomas shunt (separate procedure)

36838 Distal revascularization and interval ligation (DRIL), upper extremity hemodialysis access (steal syndrome)
> *CPT Changes: An Insider's View* 2004

▶(Do not report 36838 in conjunction with 35512, 35522, 35523, 36832, 37607, 37618)◀

36860 External cannula declotting (separate procedure); without balloon catheter
> *CPT Assistant* Fall 93:3, Feb 97:2, Nov 98:15, Feb 99:6, May 01:3

36861 with balloon catheter
> *CPT Assistant* Fall 93:3, Feb 97:2, May 01:3

(If imaging guidance is performed, use 76000)

⊙ **36870** Thrombectomy, percutaneous, arteriovenous fistula, autogenous or nonautogenous graft (includes mechanical thrombus extraction and intra-graft thrombolysis)
> *CPT Assistant* May 01:3; *CPT Changes: An Insider's View* 2001
> *Clinical Examples in Radiology* Spring 05:8-10, Summer 06:7, 12

▶(Do not report 36870 in conjunction with 36593)◀

(For catheterization, use 36145)

(For radiological supervision and interpretation, use 75790)

Portal Decompression Procedures

37140 Venous anastomosis, open; portocaval
> *CPT Changes: An Insider's View* 2003

(For peritoneal-venous shunt, use 49425)

37145 renoportal

37160 caval-mesenteric

37180 splenorenal, proximal

37181 splenorenal, distal (selective decompression of esophagogastric varices, any technique)

(For percutaneous procedure, use 37182)

37182 Insertion of transvenous intrahepatic portosystemic shunt(s) (TIPS) (includes venous access, hepatic and portal vein catheterization, portography with hemodynamic evaluation, intrahepatic tract formation/dilatation, stent placement and all associated imaging guidance and documentation)
> *CPT Assistant* Dec 03:2; *CPT Changes: An Insider's View* 2003

(Do not report 75885 or 75887 in conjunction with 37182)

(For open procedure, use 37140)

37183 Revision of transvenous intrahepatic portosystemic shunt(s) (TIPS) (includes venous access, hepatic and portal vein catheterization, portography with hemodynamic evaluation, intrahepatic tract recanulization/dilatation, stent placement and all associated imaging guidance and documentation)
> *CPT Assistant* Dec 03:2; *CPT Changes: An Insider's View* 2003

(Do not report 75885 or 75887 in conjunction with 37183)

(For repair of arteriovenous aneurysm, use 36834)

Transcatheter Procedures

Codes for catheter placement and the radiologic supervision and interpretation should also be reported, in addition to the code(s) for the therapeutic aspect of the procedure.

Mechanical Thrombectomy

Code(s) for catheter placement(s), diagnostic studies, and other percutaneous interventions (eg, transluminal balloon angioplasty, stent placement) provided are separately reportable.

Codes 37184-37188 specifically include intraprocedural fluoroscopic radiological supervision and interpretation services for guidance of the procedure.

Intraprocedural injection(s) of a thrombolytic agent is an included service and not separately reportable in conjunction with mechanical thrombectomy. However, subsequent or prior continuous infusion of a thrombolytic is not an included service and is separately reportable (see 37201, 75896, 75898).

For coronary mechanical thrombectomy, use 92973.

For mechanical thrombectomy for dialysis fistula, use 36870.

Arterial Mechanical Thrombectomy

▶Arterial mechanical thrombectomy may be performed as a "primary" transcatheter procedure with pretreatment planning, performance of the procedure, and postprocedure evaluation focused on providing this service. Typically, the diagnosis of thrombus has been made prior to the procedure, and a mechanical thrombectomy is planned preoperatively. Primary mechanical thrombectomy is reported per vascular family using 37184 for the initial vessel treated and 37185 for second or all subsequent vessel(s) within the same vascular family. To report mechanical thrombectomy of an additional vascular family treated through a separate access site, use modifier 51 in conjunction with 37184-37185.

Primary mechanical thrombectomy may precede or follow another percutaneous intervention. Most commonly primary mechanical thrombectomy will precede another percutaneous intervention with the decision regarding the need for other services not made until after mechanical thrombectomy has been performed. Occasionally, the performance of primary mechanical thrombectomy may follow another percutaneous intervention.

Do **NOT** report 37184-37185 for mechanical thrombectomy performed for the retrieval of short segments of thrombus or embolus evident during other percutaneous interventional procedures. See 37186 for these procedures.◀

Arterial mechanical thrombectomy is considered a "secondary" transcatheter procedure for removal or retrieval of short segments of thrombus or embolus when performed either before or after another percutaneous intervention (eg, percutaneous transluminal balloon angioplasty, stent placement). Secondary mechanical thrombectomy is reported using 37186. Do **NOT** report 37186 in conjunction with 37184-37185.

Venous Mechanical Thrombectomy

Use 37187 to report the initial application of venous mechanical thrombectomy. To report bilateral venous mechanical thrombectomy performed through a separate access site(s), use modifier 50 in conjunction with 37187. For repeat treatment on a subsequent day during a course of thrombolytic therapy, use 37188.

Arterial Mechanical Thrombectomy

⊙ **37184** Primary percutaneous transluminal mechanical thrombectomy, noncoronary, arterial or arterial bypass graft, including fluoroscopic guidance and intraprocedural pharmacological thrombolytic injection(s); initial vessel

➔ CPT Changes: An Insider's View 2006
➔ Clinical Examples in Radiology Winter 06:15

(Do not report 37184 in conjunction with 76000, 76001, 90774, 99143-99150)

⊙**+ 37185** second and all subsequent vessel(s) within the same vascular family (List separately in addition to code for primary mechanical thrombectomy procedure)

➔ CPT Changes: An Insider's View 2006
➔ Clinical Examples in Radiology Winter 06:15

(Do not report 37185 in conjunction with 76000, 76001, 90775)

⊙**+ 37186** Secondary percutaneous transluminal thrombectomy (eg, nonprimary mechanical, snare basket, suction technique), noncoronary, arterial or arterial bypass graft, including fluoroscopic guidance and intraprocedural pharmacological thrombolytic injections, provided in conjunction with another percutaneous intervention other than primary mechanical thrombectomy (List separately in addition to code for primary procedure)

➔ CPT Changes: An Insider's View 2006
➔ Clinical Examples in Radiology Winter 06:15

(Do not report 37186 in conjunction with 76000, 76001, 90775)

Venous Mechanical Thrombectomy

⊙ **37187** Percutaneous transluminal mechanical thrombectomy, vein(s), including intraprocedural pharmacological thrombolytic injections and fluoroscopic guidance

➔ CPT Changes: An Insider's View 2006
➔ Clinical Examples in Radiology Winter 06:15

(Do not report 37187 in conjunction with 76000, 76001, 90775)

⊙ **37188** Percutaneous transluminal mechanical thrombectomy, vein(s), including intraprocedural pharmacological thrombolytic injections and fluoroscopic guidance, repeat treatment on subsequent day during course of thrombolytic therapy

➔ CPT Changes: An Insider's View 2006
➔ Clinical Examples in Radiology Winter 06:15

(Do not report 37188 in conjunction with 76000, 76001, 90775)

Other Procedures

37195 Thrombolysis, cerebral, by intravenous infusion
➔ CPT Assistant Nov 97:16

37200 Transcatheter biopsy

(For radiological supervision and interpretation, use 75970)

37201 Transcatheter therapy, infusion for thrombolysis other than coronary
➔ CPT Assistant Feb 97:2, Feb 01:10, May 01:4

(For radiological supervision and interpretation, use 75896)

37202 Transcatheter therapy, infusion other than for thrombolysis, any type (eg, spasmolytic, vasoconstrictive)
➔ CPT Assistant Oct 96:11, Jan 98:11, Apr 98:3, 9

(For thrombolysis of coronary vessels, see 92975, 92977)

(For radiological supervision and interpretation, use 75896)

⊙ **37203** Transcatheter retrieval, percutaneous, of intravascular foreign body (eg, fractured venous or arterial catheter)

(For radiological supervision and interpretation, use 75961)

37204 Transcatheter occlusion or embolization (eg, for tumor destruction, to achieve hemostasis, to occlude a vascular malformation), percutaneous, any method, non-central nervous system, non-head or neck
➔ CPT Assistant Sep 98:2, Oct 98:10
➔ Clinical Examples in Radiology Winter 07:1-3

(See also 61624, 61626)

(For radiological supervision and interpretation, use 75894)

(For uterine fibroid embolization [uterine artery embolization performed to treat uterine fibroids], use 37210)

(For obstetrical and gynecologic embolization procedures other than uterine fibroid embolization [eg, embolization to treat obstetrical or postpartum hemorrhage], use 37204)

37205   Transcatheter placement of an intravascular stent(s) (except coronary, carotid, and vertebral vessel), percutaneous; initial vessel

> *CPT Assistant* Fall 93:18, Feb 97:2, May 01:4, Feb 03:3, Dec 03:2; *CPT Changes: An Insider's View* 2005

> *Clinical Examples in Radiology* Winter 06:19

(For radiological supervision and interpretation, use 75960)

(For coronary stent placement, see 92980, 92981; intracranial, use 61635)

+ 37206   each additional vessel (List separately in addition to code for primary procedure)

> *CPT Assistant* Fall 93:18, Feb 97:2, Feb 03:3

(Use 37206 in conjunction with 37205)

(For transcatheter placement of intravascular cervical carotid artery stent(s), see 37215, 37216)

(For transcatheter placement of extracranial vertebral or intrathoracic carotid artery stent(s), see Category III codes 0075T, 0076T)

(For radiological supervision and interpretation, use 75960)

37207   Transcatheter placement of an intravascular stent(s) (non-coronary vessel), open; initial vessel

> *CPT Assistant* Feb 97:2, Feb 03:3

+ 37208   each additional vessel (List separately in addition to code for primary procedure)

> *CPT Assistant* Feb 97:2, Feb 03:3

(Use 37208 in conjunction with 37207)

(For radiological supervision and interpretation, use 75960)

(For catheterizations, see 36215-36248)

(For transcatheter placement of intracoronary stent(s), see 92980, 92981)

37209   Exchange of a previously placed intravascular catheter during thrombolytic therapy

> *CPT Changes: An Insider's View* 2006

> *Clinical Examples in Radiology* Winter 06:19

(For radiological supervision and interpretation, use 75900)

⊙ **37210**   Uterine fibroid embolization (UFE, embolization of the uterine arteries to treat uterine fibroids, leiomyomata), percutaneous approach inclusive of vascular access, vessel selection, embolization, and all radiological supervision and interpretation, intraprocedural roadmapping, and imaging guidance necessary to complete the procedure

> *CPT Changes: An Insider's View* 2007

(37210 includes all catheterizations and intraprocedural imaging required for a UFE procedure to confirm the presence of previously known fibroids and to roadmap vascular anatomy to enable appropriate therapy)

(Do not report 37210 in conjunction with 36200, 36245-36248, 37204, 75894, 75898)

(For all other non-central nervous system (CNS) embolization procedures, use 37204)

⊙ **37215**   Transcatheter placement of intravascular stent(s), cervical carotid artery, percutaneous; with distal embolic protection

> *CPT Assistant* May 05:7; *CPT Changes: An Insider's View* 2005

⊙ **37216**   without distal embolic protection

> *CPT Assistant* May 05:7; *CPT Changes: An Insider's View* 2005

(37215 and 37216 include all ipsilateral selective carotid catheterization, all diagnostic imaging for ipsilateral, cervical and cerebral carotid arteriography, and all related radiological supervision and interpretation. When ipsilateral carotid arteriogram (including imaging and selective catheterization) confirms the need for carotid stenting, 37215 and 37216 are inclusive of these services. If carotid stenting is not indicated, then the appropriate codes for carotid catheterization and imaging should be reported in lieu of 37215 and 37216)

(Do not report 37215, 37216 in conjunction with 75671, 75680)

(For transcatheter placement of extracranial vertebral or intrathoracic carotid artery stent(s), see Category III codes 0075T, 0076T)

(For percutaneous transcatheter placement of intravascular stents other than coronary, carotid, or vertebral, see 37205, 37206)

Intravascular Ultrasound Services

Intravascular ultrasound services include all transducer manipulations and repositioning within the specific vessel being examined, both before and after therapeutic intervention (eg, stent placement).

Vascular access for intravascular ultrasound performed during a therapeutic intervention is not reported separately.

+ 37250 Intravascular ultrasound (non-coronary vessel) during diagnostic evaluation and/or therapeutic intervention; initial vessel (List separately in addition to code for primary procedure)

➔ *CPT Assistant* Nov 96:7, Nov 97:17, Nov 99:20; *CPT Changes: An Insider's View* 2000

+ 37251 each additional vessel (List separately in addition to code for primary procedure)

➔ *CPT Assistant* Nov 96:7, Nov 97:17, Nov 99:20; *CPT Changes: An Insider's View* 2000

(Use 37251 in conjunction with 37250)

(For catheterizations, see 36215-36248)

(For transcatheter therapies, see 37200-37208, 61624, 61626)

(For radiological supervision and interpretation see 75945, 75946)

Endoscopy

Surgical vascular endoscopy always includes diagnostic endoscopy.

37500 Vascular endoscopy, surgical, with ligation of perforator veins, subfascial (SEPS)

➔ *CPT Changes: An Insider's View* 2003

(For open procedure, use 37760)

37501 Unlisted vascular endoscopy procedure

➔ *CPT Changes: An Insider's View* 2003

Ligation

(For phleborraphy and arteriorraphy, see 35201-35286)

37565 Ligation, internal jugular vein

37600 Ligation; external carotid artery

37605 internal or common carotid artery

37606 internal or common carotid artery, with gradual occlusion, as with Selverstone or Crutchfield clamp

(For transcatheter permanent arterial occlusion or embolization, see 61624-61626)

(For endovascular temporary arterial balloon occlusion, use 61623)

(For ligation treatment of intracranial aneurysm, use 61703)

37607 Ligation or banding of angioaccess arteriovenous fistula

37609 Ligation or biopsy, temporal artery

37615 Ligation, major artery (eg, post-traumatic, rupture); neck

37616 chest

37617 abdomen

37618 extremity

37620 Interruption, partial or complete, of inferior vena cava by suture, ligation, plication, clip, extravascular, intravascular (umbrella device)

➔ *CPT Assistant* Nov 00:10, May 01:10

➔ *Clinical Examples in Radiology* Winter 05:5-6

(For radiological supervision and interpretation, use 75940)

37650 Ligation of femoral vein

(For bilateral procedure, report 37650 with modifier 50)

37660 Ligation of common iliac vein

37700 Ligation and division of long saphenous vein at saphenofemoral junction, or distal interruptions

➔ *CPT Assistant* Aug 96:10

(Do not report 37700 in conjunction with 37718, 37722)

(For bilateral procedure, report 37700 with modifier 50)

Ligation and Division of Long Saphenous Vein
37700

The physician ligates sections of the saphenous vein along the leg.

Femoral vein

Great saphenous vein

37718 Ligation, division, and stripping, short saphenous vein

➔ *CPT Changes: An Insider's View* 2006

(For bilateral procedure, use modifier 50)

(Do not report 37718 in conjunction with 37735, 37780)

(37720 has been deleted)

37722   Ligation, division, and stripping, long (greater) saphenous veins from saphenofemoral junction to knee or below

➲ *CPT Changes: An Insider's View* 2006

(For ligation and stripping of the short saphenous vein, use 37718)

(For bilateral procedure, report 37722 with modifier 50)

(Do not report 37722 in conjunction with 37700, 37735)

(37730 has been deleted. For ligation, division, and stripping of the greater saphenous vein, use 37722. For ligation, division, and stripping of the short saphenous vein, use 37718)

37735   Ligation and division and complete stripping of long or short saphenous veins with radical excision of ulcer and skin graft and/or interruption of communicating veins of lower leg, with excision of deep fascia

(Do not report 37735 in conjunction with 37700, 37718, 37722, 37780)

(For bilateral procedure, report 37735 with modifier 50)

37760   Ligation of perforator veins, subfascial, radical (Linton type), with or without skin graft, open

➲ *CPT Changes: An Insider's View* 2003

(For endoscopic procedure, use 37500)

37765   Stab phlebectomy of varicose veins, one extremity; 10-20 stab incisions

➲ *CPT Assistant* Aug 04:6; *CPT Changes: An Insider's View* 2004

(For less than 10 incisions, use 37799)

(For more than 20 incisions, use 37766)

37766   more than 20 incisions

➲ *CPT Assistant* Aug 04:6; *CPT Changes: An Insider's View* 2004

37780   Ligation and division of short saphenous vein at saphenopopliteal junction (separate procedure)

➲ *CPT Assistant* Aug 96:10

(For bilateral procedure, report 37780 with modifier 50)

37785   Ligation, division, and/or excision of varicose vein cluster(s), one leg

➲ *CPT Assistant* Aug 04:5; *CPT Changes: An Insider's View* 2004

(For bilateral procedure, report 37785 with modifier 50)

Other Procedures

37788   Penile revascularization, artery, with or without vein graft

37790   Penile venous occlusive procedure

37799   Unlisted procedure, vascular surgery

➲ *CPT Assistant* Spring 93:12, Fall 93:3, Feb 97:10, Sep 97:10, May 01:11, Oct 04:16

Hemic and Lymphatic Systems

Spleen

Excision

38100   Splenectomy; total (separate procedure)

➲ *CPT Assistant* Jul 93:9, Summer 93:10

38101   partial (separate procedure)

➲ *CPT Assistant* Summer 93:10

+ 38102   total, en bloc for extensive disease, in conjunction with other procedure (List in addition to code for primary procedure)

➲ *CPT Assistant* Summer 93:10

Repair

38115   Repair of ruptured spleen (splenorrhaphy) with or without partial splenectomy

➲ *CPT Assistant* Summer 93:10

Laparoscopy

Surgical laparoscopy always includes diagnostic laparoscopy. To report a diagnostic laparoscopy (peritoneoscopy) (separate procedure), use 49320.

38120   Laparoscopy, surgical, splenectomy

➲ *CPT Assistant* Nov 99:20-21, Mar 00:8; *CPT Changes: An Insider's View* 2000

38129   Unlisted laparoscopy procedure, spleen

➲ *CPT Assistant* Nov 99:20-21, Mar 00:8; *CPT Changes: An Insider's View* 2000

Introduction

38200   Injection procedure for splenoportography

(For radiological supervision and interpretation, use 75810)

General

Bone Marrow or Stem Cell Services/Procedures

Codes 38207-38215 describe various steps used to preserve, prepare and purify bone marrow/stem cells prior to transplantation or reinfusion. Each code may be reported only once per day regardless of the quantity of bone marrow/stem cells manipulated.

38204   Management of recipient hematopoietic progenitor cell donor search and cell acquisition

➲ *CPT Changes: An Insider's View* 2003

38205 Blood-derived hematopoietic progenitor cell harvesting for transplantation, per collection; allogenic
➔ *CPT Changes: An Insider's View* 2003

38206 autologous
➔ *CPT Changes: An Insider's View* 2003

38207 Transplant preparation of hematopoietic progenitor cells; cryopreservation and storage
➔ *CPT Assistant* Jul 03:9; *CPT Changes: An Insider's View* 2003

(For diagnostic cryopreservation and storage, see 88240)

38208 thawing of previously frozen harvest, without washing
➔ *CPT Assistant* Jul 03:9; *CPT Changes: An Insider's View* 2003, 2004

(For diagnostic thawing and expansion of frozen cells, see 88241)

38209 thawing of previously frozen harvest, with washing
➔ *CPT Changes: An Insider's View* 2003, 2004

38210 specific cell depletion within harvest, T-cell depletion
➔ *CPT Changes: An Insider's View* 2003

38211 tumor cell depletion
➔ *CPT Changes: An Insider's View* 2003

38212 red blood cell removal
➔ *CPT Changes: An Insider's View* 2003

38213 platelet depletion
➔ *CPT Changes: An Insider's View* 2003

38214 plasma (volume) depletion
➔ *CPT Changes: An Insider's View* 2003

38215 cell concentration in plasma, mononuclear, or buffy coat layer
➔ *CPT Changes: An Insider's View* 2003

(Do not report 38207-38215 in conjunction with 88182, 88184-88189)

38220 Bone marrow; aspiration only
➔ *CPT Assistant* Jan 04:26; *CPT Changes: An Insider's View* 2002, 2003

38221 biopsy, needle or trocar
➔ *CPT Changes: An Insider's View* 2002, 2003

(For bone marrow biopsy interpretation, use 88305)

38230 Bone marrow harvesting for transplantation
➔ *CPT Assistant* Apr 96:1

(For autologous and allogenic blood-derived peripheral stem cell harvesting for transplantation, see 38205-38206)

Bone Marrow Harvesting for Transplantation
38230

A biopsy needle is inserted into the marrow cavity of the iliac crest and bone marrow is removed from the donor.

Placement of biopsy needle · Posterior iliac spine

Biopsy needle · Bone marrow

38240 Bone marrow or blood-derived peripheral stem cell transplantation; allogenic
➔ *CPT Assistant* Apr 96:2, Nov 98:15, Nov 99:21; *CPT Changes: An Insider's View* 2000

38241 autologous
➔ *CPT Assistant* Apr 96:2, Nov 98:15, Nov 99:21; *CPT Changes: An Insider's View* 2000

38242 allogeneic donor lymphocyte infusions
➔ *CPT Changes: An Insider's View* 2003

(For bone marrow aspiration, use 38220)

(For modification, treatment, and processing of bone marrow or blood-derived stem cell specimens for transplantation, use 38210-38213)

(For cryopreservation, freezing and storage of blood-derived stem cells for transplantation, use 88240)

(For thawing and expansion of blood-derived stem cells for transplantation, use 88241)

(For compatibility studies, see 86812-86822)

Lymph Nodes and Lymphatic Channels

Incision

38300 Drainage of lymph node abscess or lymphadenitis; simple

38305 extensive

38308 Lymphangiotomy or other operations on lymphatic channels

38380 Suture and/or ligation of thoracic duct; cervical approach

38381 thoracic approach

38382 abdominal approach

Excision

(For injection for sentinel node identification, use 38792)

38500 Biopsy or excision of lymph node(s); open, superficial
➔ *CPT Assistant* Jun 97:5, Jul 99:7, Oct 05:23; *CPT Changes: An Insider's View* 2001

(Do not report 38500 with 38700-38780)

38505 by needle, superficial (eg, cervical, inguinal, axillary)
➔ *CPT Assistant* Jul 99:6

(If imaging guidance is performed, see 76942, 77012, 77021)

(For fine needle aspiration, use 10021 or 10022)

(For evaluation of fine needle aspirate, see 88172, 88173)

38510 open, deep cervical node(s)
➔ *CPT Assistant* May 98:10, Jul 99:6; *CPT Changes: An Insider's View* 2001

38520 open, deep cervical node(s) with excision scalene fat pad
➔ *CPT Assistant* May 98:10, Jul 99:6; *CPT Changes: An Insider's View* 2001

38525 open, deep axillary node(s)
➔ *CPT Assistant* May 98:10, Jul 99:7, Oct 05:23; *CPT Changes: An Insider's View* 2001

38530 open, internal mammary node(s)
➔ *CPT Assistant* May 98:10, Jul 99:6; *CPT Changes: An Insider's View* 2001

(Do not report 38530 with 38720-38746)

(For percutaneous needle biopsy, retroperitoneal lymph node or mass, use 49180. For fine needle aspiration, use 10022)

38542 Dissection, deep jugular node(s)
➔ *CPT Assistant* Jul 99:7

(For radical cervical neck dissection, use 38720)

38550 Excision of cystic hygroma, axillary or cervical; without deep neurovascular dissection

38555 with deep neurovascular dissection

Limited Lymphadenectomy for Staging

38562 Limited lymphadenectomy for staging (separate procedure); pelvic and para-aortic
➔ *CPT Assistant* Mar 01:10

(When combined with prostatectomy, use 55812 or 55842)

(When combined with insertion of radioactive substance into prostate, use 55862)

38564 retroperitoneal (aortic and/or splenic)

Laparoscopy

Surgical laparoscopy always includes diagnostic laparoscopy. To report a diagnostic laparoscopy (peritoneoscopy) (separate procedure), use 49320.

38570 Laparoscopy, surgical; with retroperitoneal lymph node sampling (biopsy), single or multiple
➔ *CPT Assistant* Nov 99:21, Mar 00:8; *CPT Changes: An Insider's View* 2000

38571 with bilateral total pelvic lymphadenectomy
➔ *CPT Assistant* Nov 99:21, Mar 00:8; *CPT Changes: An Insider's View* 2000

38572 with bilateral total pelvic lymphadenectomy and peri-aortic lymph node sampling (biopsy), single or multiple
➔ *CPT Assistant* Nov 99:21; *CPT Changes: An Insider's View* 2000

(For drainage of lymphocele to peritoneal cavity, use 49323)

38589 Unlisted laparoscopy procedure, lymphatic system
➔ *CPT Assistant* Nov 99:21, Mar 00:8; *CPT Changes: An Insider's View* 2000

Radical Lymphadenectomy (Radical Resection of Lymph Nodes)

(For limited pelvic and retroperitoneal lymphadenectomies, see 38562, 38564)

38700 Suprahyoid lymphadenectomy
➔ *CPT Assistant* Aug 02:8

(For bilateral procedure, report 38700 with modifier 50)

38720 Cervical lymphadenectomy (complete)
➔ *CPT Assistant* Oct 01:10, Aug 02:8

(For bilateral procedure, report 38720 with modifier 50)

38724 Cervical lymphadenectomy (modified radical neck dissection)
> *CPT Assistant* Jan 01:13, Aug 02:8

38740 Axillary lymphadenectomy; superficial

38745   complete

+ 38746 Thoracic lymphadenectomy, regional, including mediastinal and peritracheal nodes (List separately in addition to code for primary procedure)

+ 38747 Abdominal lymphadenectomy, regional, including celiac, gastric, portal, peripancreatic, with or without para-aortic and vena caval nodes (List separately in addition to code for primary procedure)
> *CPT Assistant* Nov 98:15

38760 Inguinofemoral lymphadenectomy, superficial, including Cloquets node (separate procedure)

(For bilateral procedure, report 38760 with modifier 50)

38765 Inguinofemoral lymphadenectomy, superficial, in continuity with pelvic lymphadenectomy, including external iliac, hypogastric, and obturator nodes (separate procedure)

(For bilateral procedure, report 38765 with modifier 50)

38770 Pelvic lymphadenectomy, including external iliac, hypogastric, and obturator nodes (separate procedure)

(For bilateral procedure, report 38770 with modifier 50)

38780 Retroperitoneal transabdominal lymphadenectomy, extensive, including pelvic, aortic, and renal nodes (separate procedure)

(For excision and repair of lymphedematous skin and subcutaneous tissue, see 15004-15005, 15570-15650)

Introduction

38790 Injection procedure; lymphangiography
> *CPT Assistant* Jul 99:6

(For bilateral procedure, report 38790 with modifier 50)

(For radiological supervision and interpretation, see 75801-75807)

▲ 38792   for identification of sentinel node
> *CPT Assistant* Nov 98:15, Jul 99:6, Dec 99:8; *CPT Changes: An Insider's View* 2008

(For excision of sentinel node, see 38500-38542)

(For nuclear medicine lymphatics and lymph gland imaging, use 78195)

38794 Cannulation, thoracic duct

Other Procedures

38999 Unlisted procedure, hemic or lymphatic system
> *CPT Assistant* May 98:10

Mediastinum and Diaphragm

Mediastinum

Incision

39000 Mediastinotomy with exploration, drainage, removal of foreign body, or biopsy; cervical approach

39010   transthoracic approach, including either transthoracic or median sternotomy

Excision

39200 Excision of mediastinal cyst

39220 Excision of mediastinal tumor

(For substernal thyroidectomy, use 60270)

(For thymectomy, use 60520)

Endoscopy

39400 Mediastinoscopy, with or without biopsy

Other Procedures

39499 Unlisted procedure, mediastinum

Diaphragm

Repair

(For transabdominal repair of diaphragmatic (esophageal hiatal) hernia, see 43324, 43325)

39501 Repair, laceration of diaphragm, any approach
> *CPT Assistant* Nov 00:3

39502 Repair, paraesophageal hiatus hernia, transabdominal, with or without fundoplasty, vagotomy, and/or pyloroplasty, except neonatal

39503 Repair, neonatal diaphragmatic hernia, with or without chest tube insertion and with or without creation of ventral hernia

(Do not report modifier 63 in conjunction with 39503)

39520 Repair, diaphragmatic hernia (esophageal hiatal); transthoracic

39530   combined, thoracoabdominal

39531   combined, thoracoabdominal, with dilation of stricture (with or without gastroplasty)

39540   Repair, diaphragmatic hernia (other than neonatal), traumatic; acute

→ *CPT Assistant* Nov 00:9, Nov 03

39541   chronic

39545   Imbrication of diaphragm for eventration, transthoracic or transabdominal, paralytic or nonparalytic

→ *CPT Assistant* Nov 00:3

39560   Resection, diaphragm; with simple repair (eg, primary suture)

→ *CPT Assistant* Nov 99:21, Nov 00:3; *CPT Changes: An Insider's View* 2000

39561   with complex repair (eg, prosthetic material, local muscle flap)

→ *CPT Assistant* Nov 99:21, Nov 00:3; *CPT Changes: An Insider's View* 2000

Other Procedures

39599   Unlisted procedure, diaphragm

Digestive System

Lips

(For procedures on skin of lips, see 10040 et seq)

Excision

40490   Biopsy of lip

40500   Vermilionectomy (lip shave), with mucosal advancement

40510   Excision of lip; transverse wedge excision with primary closure

40520   V-excision with primary direct linear closure

(For excision of mucous lesions, see 40810-40816)

40525   full thickness, reconstruction with local flap (eg, Estlander or fan)

40527   full thickness, reconstruction with cross lip flap (Abbe-Estlander)

40530   Resection of lip, more than one-fourth, without reconstruction

(For reconstruction, see 13131 et seq)

Repair (Cheiloplasty)

40650   Repair lip, full thickness; vermilion only
→ *CPT Assistant* Jul 00:10

40652   up to half vertical height
→ *CPT Assistant* Jul 00:10

40654   over one-half vertical height, or complex

40700   Plastic repair of cleft lip/nasal deformity; primary, partial or complete, unilateral

40701   primary bilateral, one stage procedure

40702   primary bilateral, one of two stages

40720   secondary, by recreation of defect and reclosure

(For bilateral procedure, report 40720 with modifier 50)

(To report rhinoplasty only for nasal deformity secondary to congenital cleft lip, see 30460, 30462)

(For repair of cleft lip, with cross lip pedicle flap (Abbe-Estlander type), use 40527)

40761   with cross lip pedicle flap (Abbe-Estlander type), including sectioning and inserting of pedicle

(For repair cleft palate, see 42200 et seq)

(For other reconstructive procedures, see 14060, 14061, 15120-15261, 15574, 15576, 15630)

Other Procedures

40799   Unlisted procedure, lips

Vestibule of Mouth

The vestibule is the part of the oral cavity outside the dentoalveolar structures; it includes the mucosal and submucosal tissue of lips and cheeks.

Incision

40800   Drainage of abscess, cyst, hematoma, vestibule of mouth; simple

40801   complicated

40804   Removal of embedded foreign body, vestibule of mouth; simple

40805   complicated

40806   Incision of labial frenum (frenotomy)

Excision, Destruction

40808   Biopsy, vestibule of mouth

40810   Excision of lesion of mucosa and submucosa, vestibule of mouth; without repair

40812   with simple repair

40814   with complex repair

40816   complex, with excision of underlying muscle

40818   Excision of mucosa of vestibule of mouth as donor graft

40819   Excision of frenum, labial or buccal (frenumectomy, frenulectomy, frenectomy)

40820   Destruction of lesion or scar of vestibule of mouth by physical methods (eg, laser, thermal, cryo, chemical)

Repair

40830   Closure of laceration, vestibule of mouth; 2.5 cm or less

40831   over 2.5 cm or complex

40840   Vestibuloplasty; anterior

40842   posterior, unilateral

40843   posterior, bilateral

40844   entire arch

40845   complex (including ridge extension, muscle repositioning)

(For skin grafts, see 15002 et seq)

Other Procedures

40899   Unlisted procedure, vestibule of mouth

Tongue and Floor of Mouth

Incision

41000 Intraoral incision and drainage of abscess, cyst, or hematoma of tongue or floor of mouth; lingual

41005 sublingual, superficial

41006 sublingual, deep, supramylohyoid

41007 submental space

41008 submandibular space

41009 masticator space

41010 Incision of lingual frenum (frenotomy)

41015 Extraoral incision and drainage of abscess, cyst, or hematoma of floor of mouth; sublingual

41016 submental

41017 submandibular

41018 masticator space

(For frenoplasty, use 41520)

● **41019** Placement of needles, catheters, or other device(s) into the head and/or neck region (percutaneous, transoral, or transnasal) for subsequent interstitial radioelement application

➔ *CPT Changes: An Insider's View* 2008

▶(For imaging guidance, see 76942, 77002, 77012, 77021)◀

▶(For stereotactic insertion of intracranial brachytherapy radiation sources, use 61770)◀

▶(For interstitial radioelement application, see 77776-77784)◀

Excision

41100 Biopsy of tongue; anterior two-thirds

41105 posterior one-third

41108 Biopsy of floor of mouth

41110 Excision of lesion of tongue without closure

41112 Excision of lesion of tongue with closure; anterior two-thirds

41113 posterior one-third

41114 with local tongue flap

(List 41114 in addition to code 41112 or 41113)

41115 Excision of lingual frenum (frenectomy)

41116 Excision, lesion of floor of mouth

41120 Glossectomy; less than one-half tongue

41130 hemiglossectomy

41135 partial, with unilateral radical neck dissection

41140 complete or total, with or without tracheostomy, without radical neck dissection

41145 complete or total, with or without tracheostomy, with unilateral radical neck dissection

41150 composite procedure with resection floor of mouth and mandibular resection, without radical neck dissection

41153 composite procedure with resection floor of mouth, with suprahyoid neck dissection

41155 composite procedure with resection floor of mouth, mandibular resection, and radical neck dissection (Commando type)

➔ *CPT Assistant* Jan 01:13

Repair

41250 Repair of laceration 2.5 cm or less; floor of mouth and/or anterior two-thirds of tongue

41251 posterior one-third of tongue

41252 Repair of laceration of tongue, floor of mouth, over 2.6 cm or complex

Other Procedures

41500 Fixation of tongue, mechanical, other than suture (eg, K-wire)

41510 Suture of tongue to lip for micrognathia (Douglas type procedure)

41520 Frenoplasty (surgical revision of frenum, eg, with Z-plasty)

(For frenotomy, see 40806, 41010)

41599 Unlisted procedure, tongue, floor of mouth

➔ *CPT Assistant* Dec 00:14

Dentoalveolar Structures

Incision

41800 Drainage of abscess, cyst, hematoma from dentoalveolar structures

41805 Removal of embedded foreign body from dentoalveolar structures; soft tissues

41806 bone

Excision, Destruction

41820 Gingivectomy, excision gingiva, each quadrant

41821 Operculectomy, excision pericoronal tissues

41822 Excision of fibrous tuberosities, dentoalveolar structures

41823 Excision of osseous tuberosities, dentoalveolar structures

41825   Excision of lesion or tumor (except listed above), dentoalveolar structures; without repair

41826   with simple repair

41827   with complex repair

         (For nonexcisional destruction, use 41850)

41828   Excision of hyperplastic alveolar mucosa, each quadrant (specify)

41830   Alveolectomy, including curettage of osteitis or sequestrectomy

41850   Destruction of lesion (except excision), dentoalveolar structures

Other Procedures

41870   Periodontal mucosal grafting

41872   Gingivoplasty, each quadrant (specify)

41874   Alveoloplasty, each quadrant (specify)

         (For closure of lacerations, see 40830, 40831)

         (For segmental osteotomy, use 21206)

         (For reduction of fractures, see 21421-21490)

41899   Unlisted procedure, dentoalveolar structures

Palate and Uvula

Incision

42000   Drainage of abscess of palate, uvula

Excision, Destruction

42100   Biopsy of palate, uvula

42104   Excision, lesion of palate, uvula; without closure

42106   with simple primary closure

42107   with local flap closure

         (For skin graft, see 14040-14300)

         (For mucosal graft, use 40818)

42120   Resection of palate or extensive resection of lesion

         (For reconstruction of palate with extraoral tissue, see 14040-14300, 15050, 15120, 15240, 15576)

42140   Uvulectomy, excision of uvula

42145   Palatopharyngoplasty (eg, uvulopalatopharyngoplasty, uvulopharyngoplasty)
         ➔ *CPT Assistant* Dec 04:19

         (For removal of exostosis of the bony palate, see 21031, 21032)

42160   Destruction of lesion, palate or uvula (thermal, cryo or chemical)

Repair

42180   Repair, laceration of palate; up to 2 cm

42182   over 2 cm or complex

42200   Palatoplasty for cleft palate, soft and/or hard palate only

42205   Palatoplasty for cleft palate, with closure of alveolar ridge; soft tissue only

42210   with bone graft to alveolar ridge (includes obtaining graft)

42215   Palatoplasty for cleft palate; major revision

42220   secondary lengthening procedure

42225   attachment pharyngeal flap

42226   Lengthening of palate, and pharyngeal flap

42227   Lengthening of palate, with island flap

42235   Repair of anterior palate, including vomer flap

         (For repair of oronasal fistula, use 30600)

42260   Repair of nasolabial fistula

         (For repair of cleft lip, see 40700 et seq)

42280   Maxillary impression for palatal prosthesis

42281   Insertion of pin-retained palatal prosthesis

Other Procedures

42299   Unlisted procedure, palate, uvula
         ➔ *CPT Assistant* Dec 04:19

Salivary Gland and Ducts

Incision

42300   Drainage of abscess; parotid, simple

42305   parotid, complicated

42310   Drainage of abscess; submaxillary or sublingual, intraoral
         ➔ *CPT Changes: An Insider's View* 2003

42320   submaxillary, external

         (42325, 42326 have been deleted)

42330   Sialolithotomy; submandibular (submaxillary), sublingual or parotid, uncomplicated, intraoral

42335   submandibular (submaxillary), complicated, intraoral

42340   parotid, extraoral or complicated intraoral

Excision

42400	Biopsy of salivary gland; needle

(For fine needle aspiration, see 10021, 10022)

(For evaluation of fine needle aspirate, see 88172, 88173)

(If imaging guidance is performed, see 76942, 77002, 77012, 77021)

42405	incisional

(If imaging guidance is performed, see 76942, 77002, 77012, 77021)

42408	Excision of sublingual salivary cyst (ranula)
42409	Marsupialization of sublingual salivary cyst (ranula)
42410	Excision of parotid tumor or parotid gland; lateral lobe, without nerve dissection
42415	lateral lobe, with dissection and preservation of facial nerve
42420	total, with dissection and preservation of facial nerve
42425	total, en bloc removal with sacrifice of facial nerve
42426	total, with unilateral radical neck dissection

(For suture or grafting of facial nerve, see 64864, 64865, 69740, 69745)

42440	Excision of submandibular (submaxillary) gland
42450	Excision of sublingual gland

Repair

42500	Plastic repair of salivary duct, sialodochoplasty; primary or simple
42505	secondary or complicated
42507	Parotid duct diversion, bilateral (Wilke type procedure);
42508	with excision of one submandibular gland
42509	with excision of both submandibular glands
42510	with ligation of both submandibular (Wharton's) ducts

Other Procedures

42550	Injection procedure for sialography

(For radiological supervision and interpretation, use 70390)

42600	Closure salivary fistula
42650	Dilation salivary duct
42660	Dilation and catheterization of salivary duct, with or without injection
42665	Ligation salivary duct, intraoral
42699	Unlisted procedure, salivary glands or ducts

Pharynx, Adenoids, and Tonsils

Incision

42700	Incision and drainage abscess; peritonsillar
42720	retropharyngeal or parapharyngeal, intraoral approach
42725	retropharyngeal or parapharyngeal, external approach

Excision, Destruction

42800	Biopsy; oropharynx
42802	hypopharynx
42804	nasopharynx, visible lesion, simple
42806	nasopharynx, survey for unknown primary lesion

(For laryngoscopic biopsy, see 31510, 31535, 31536)

42808	Excision or destruction of lesion of pharynx, any method
42809	Removal of foreign body from pharynx
42810	Excision branchial cleft cyst or vestige, confined to skin and subcutaneous tissues
42815	Excision branchial cleft cyst, vestige, or fistula, extending beneath subcutaneous tissues and/or into pharynx
42820	Tonsillectomy and adenoidectomy; younger than age 12
	➔ *CPT Assistant* Feb 98:11
42821	age 12 or over
42825	Tonsillectomy, primary or secondary; younger than age 12
42826	age 12 or over
42830	Adenoidectomy, primary; younger than age 12
42831	age 12 or over
42835	Adenoidectomy, secondary; younger than age 12
42836	age 12 or over
	➔ *CPT Assistant* Feb 98:11
42842	Radical resection of tonsil, tonsillar pillars, and/or retromolar trigone; without closure
42844	closure with local flap (eg, tongue, buccal)
42845	closure with other flap

(For closure with other flap(s), use appropriate number for flap(s))

(When combined with radical neck dissection, use also 38720)

42860	Excision of tonsil tags
42870	Excision or destruction lingual tonsil, any method (separate procedure)

(For resection of the nasopharynx (eg, juvenile angiofibroma) by bicoronal and/or transzygomatic approach, see 61586 and 61600)

42890   Limited pharyngectomy

42892   Resection of lateral pharyngeal wall or pyriform sinus, direct closure by advancement of lateral and posterior pharyngeal walls

(When combined with radical neck dissection, use also 38720)

42894   Resection of pharyngeal wall requiring closure with myocutaneous flap

(When combined with radical neck dissection, use also 38720)

(For limited pharyngectomy with radical neck dissection, use 38720 with 42890)

Repair

42900   Suture pharynx for wound or injury

42950   Pharyngoplasty (plastic or reconstructive operation on pharynx)

(For pharyngeal flap, use 42225)

42953   Pharyngoesophageal repair

(For closure with myocutaneous or other flap, use appropriate number in addition)

Other Procedures

42955   Pharyngostomy (fistulization of pharynx, external for feeding)

42960   Control oropharyngeal hemorrhage, primary or secondary (eg, post-tonsillectomy); simple

42961   complicated, requiring hospitalization

42962   with secondary surgical intervention

42970   Control of nasopharyngeal hemorrhage, primary or secondary (eg, postadenoidectomy); simple, with posterior nasal packs, with or without anterior packs and/or cautery
➔ *CPT Changes: An Insider's View* 2002

42971   complicated, requiring hospitalization

42972   with secondary surgical intervention

42999   Unlisted procedure, pharynx, adenoids, or tonsils

Esophagus

Incision

(For esophageal intubation with laparotomy, use 43510)

43020   Esophagotomy, cervical approach, with removal of foreign body

43030   Cricopharyngeal myotomy

43045   Esophagotomy, thoracic approach, with removal of foreign body

Excision

(For gastrointestinal reconstruction for previous esophagectomy, see 43360, 43361)

43100   Excision of lesion, esophagus, with primary repair; cervical approach

43101   thoracic or abdominal approach

(For wide excision of malignant lesion of cervical esophagus, with total laryngectomy without radical neck dissection, see 43107, 43116, 43124, and 31360)

(For wide excision of malignant lesion of cervical esophagus, with total laryngectomy with radical neck dissection, see 43107, 43116, 43124, and 31365)

43107   Total or near total esophagectomy, without thoracotomy; with pharyngogastrostomy or cervical esophagogastrostomy, with or without pyloroplasty (transhiatal)

43108   with colon interposition or small intestine reconstruction, including intestine mobilization, preparation and anastomosis(es)
➔ *CPT Changes: An Insider's View* 2002

43112   Total or near total esophagectomy, with thoracotomy; with pharyngogastrostomy or cervical esophagogastrostomy, with or without pyloroplasty

43113   with colon interposition or small intestine reconstruction, including intestine mobilization, preparation, and anastomosis(es)
➔ *CPT Changes: An Insider's View* 2002

43116   Partial esophagectomy, cervical, with free intestinal graft, including microvascular anastomosis, obtaining the graft and intestinal reconstruction
➔ *CPT Assistant* Nov 97:17, Nov 98:16

(Do not report 43116 in conjunction with 69990)

(Report 43116 with the modifier 52 appended if intestinal or free jejunal graft with microvascular anastomosis is performed by another physician)

(For free jejunal graft with microvascular anastomosis performed by another physician, use 43496)

43117   Partial esophagectomy, distal two-thirds, with thoracotomy and separate abdominal incision, with or without proximal gastrectomy; with thoracic esophagogastrostomy, with or without pyloroplasty (Ivor Lewis)

43118   with colon interposition or small intestine reconstruction, including intestine mobilization, preparation, and anastomosis(es)
➔ *CPT Changes: An Insider's View* 2002

(For total esophagectomy with gastropharyngostomy, see 43107, 43124)

(For esophagogastrectomy (lower third) and vagotomy, use 43122)

43121 Partial esophagectomy, distal two-thirds, with thoracotomy only, with or without proximal gastrectomy, with thoracic esophagogastrostomy, with or without pyloroplasty

43122 Partial esophagectomy, thoracoabdominal or abdominal approach, with or without proximal gastrectomy; with esophagogastrostomy, with or without pyloroplasty

43123 with colon interposition or small intestine reconstruction, including intestine mobilization, preparation, and anastomosis(es)
➡ *CPT Changes: An Insider's View* 2002

43124 Total or partial esophagectomy, without reconstruction (any approach), with cervical esophagostomy

43130 Diverticulectomy of hypopharynx or esophagus, with or without myotomy; cervical approach

43135 thoracic approach

Endoscopy

For endoscopic procedures, code appropriate endoscopy of each anatomic site examined.

Surgical endoscopy always includes diagnostic endoscopy.

⊙ **43200** Esophagoscopy, rigid or flexible; diagnostic, with or without collection of specimen(s) by brushing or washing (separate procedure)
➡ *CPT Assistant* Spring 91:7, Spring 94:1, Jun 98:10, Nov 99:21, Sep 03:3; *CPT Changes: An Insider's View* 2000

⊙ **43201** with directed submucosal injection(s), any substance
➡ *CPT Changes: An Insider's View* 2003

(For injection sclerosis of esophageal varices, use 43204)

⊙ **43202** with biopsy, single or multiple
➡ *CPT Assistant* Spring 94:1

⊙ **43204** with injection sclerosis of esophageal varices
➡ *CPT Assistant* Spring 94:1

⊙ **43205** with band ligation of esophageal varices
➡ *CPT Assistant* Spring 94:1

⊙ **43215** with removal of foreign body
➡ *CPT Assistant* Spring 94:1

(For radiological supervision and interpretation, use 74235)

⊙ **43216** with removal of tumor(s), polyp(s), or other lesion(s) by hot biopsy forceps or bipolar cautery
➡ *CPT Assistant* Spring 94:1

⊙ **43217** with removal of tumor(s), polyp(s), or other lesion(s) by snare technique
➡ *CPT Assistant* Spring 94:1

⊙ **43219** with insertion of plastic tube or stent
➡ *CPT Assistant* Spring 94:2

⊙ **43220** with balloon dilation (less than 30 mm diameter)
➡ *CPT Assistant* Spring 94:2, Jan 97:10, May 05:3

(If imaging guidance is performed, use 74360)

(For endoscopic dilation with balloon 30 mm diameter or larger, use 43458)

(For dilation without visualization, use 43450-43453)

(For diagnostic fiberoptic esophagogastroscopy, use 43200, 43235)

(For fiberoptic esophagogastroscopy with biopsy or collection of specimen, use 43200, 43202, 43235, 43239)

(For fiberoptic esophagogastroscopy with removal of foreign body, use 43215, 43247)

(For fiberoptic esophagogastroscopy with removal of polyp(s), use 43217, 43251)

⊙ **43226** with insertion of guide wire followed by dilation over guide wire
➡ *CPT Assistant* Spring 94:2

(For radiological supervision and interpretation, use 74360)

⊙ **43227** with control of bleeding (eg, injection, bipolar cautery, unipolar cautery, laser, heater probe, stapler, plasma coagulator)
➡ *CPT Assistant* Spring 94:2; *CPT Changes: An Insider's View* 2002

⊙ **43228** with ablation of tumor(s), polyp(s), or other lesion(s), not amenable to removal by hot biopsy forceps, bipolar cautery or snare technique
➡ *CPT Assistant* Spring 94:2, Nov 98:21

(For esophagoscopic photodynamic therapy, report 43228 in addition to 96570, 96571 as appropriate)

⊙ **43231** with endoscopic ultrasound examination
➡ *CPT Assistant* Oct 01:4, May 04:6; *CPT Changes: An Insider's View* 2001

(Do not report 43231 in conjunction with 76975)

⊙ **43232** with transendoscopic ultrasound-guided intramural or transmural fine needle aspiration/biopsy(s)
➡ *CPT Assistant* Oct 01:4, Mar 04:11, May 04:6; *CPT Changes: An Insider's View* 2001

(Do not report 43232 in conjunction with 76942, 76975)

(For interpretation of specimen, see 88172-88173)

⊙ **43234** Upper gastrointestinal endoscopy, simple primary examination (eg, with small diameter flexible endoscope) (separate procedure)

⊙ **43235**   Upper gastrointestinal endoscopy including esophagus, stomach, and either the duodenum and/or jejunum as appropriate; diagnostic, with or without collection of specimen(s) by brushing or washing (separate procedure)
➔ *CPT Assistant* Spring 94:4, Dec 97:11, Jun 03:11, Sep 03:3

Upper Gastrointestinal Endoscopy
43235

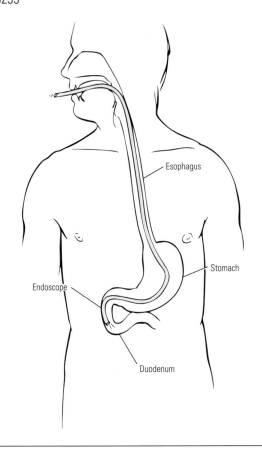

Esophagus

Stomach

Endoscope

Duodenum

⊙ **43236**   with directed submucosal injection(s), any substance
➔ *CPT Changes: An Insider's View* 2003

(For injection sclerosis of esophageal and/or gastric varices, use 43243)

⊙ **43237**   with endoscopic ultrasound examination limited to the esophagus
➔ *CPT Changes: An Insider's View* 2004

(Do not report 43237 in conjunction with 76942, 76975)

⊙ **43238**   with transendoscopic ultrasound-guided intramural or transmural fine needle aspiration/biopsy(s), esophagus (includes endoscopic ultrasound examination limited to the esophagus)
➔ *CPT Changes: An Insider's View* 2004

(Do not report 43238 in conjunction with 76942 or 76975)

⊙ **43239**   with biopsy, single or multiple
➔ *CPT Assistant* Spring 94:4, Apr 98:14, Feb 99:11, Oct 01:4

⊙ **43240**   with transmural drainage of pseudocyst
➔ *CPT Assistant* Oct 01:4; *CPT Changes: An Insider's View* 2001

⊙ **43241**   with transendoscopic intraluminal tube or catheter placement
➔ *CPT Assistant* Spring 94:4, Nov 01:7; *CPT Changes: An Insider's View* 2001

⊙ **43242**   with transendoscopic ultrasound-guided intramural or transmural fine needle aspiration/biopsy(s) (includes endoscopic ultrasound examination of the esophagus, stomach, and either the duodenum and/or jejunum as appropriate)
➔ *CPT Assistant* Oct 01:4; *CPT Changes: An Insider's View* 2001, 2004

(Do not report 43242 in conjunction with 76942, 76975)

(For transendoscopic fine needle aspiration/biopsy limited to esophagus, use 43238)

(For interpretation of specimen, see 88172-88173)

⊙ **43243**   with injection sclerosis of esophageal and/or gastric varices
➔ *CPT Assistant* Spring 94:4

⊙ **43244**   with band ligation of esophageal and/or gastric varices
➔ *CPT Assistant* Spring 94:4

⊙ **43245**   with dilation of gastric outlet for obstruction (eg, balloon, guide wire, bougie)
➔ *CPT Assistant* Spring 94:4, Oct 01:4, Jan 04:26; *CPT Changes: An Insider's View* 2002, 2003

(Do not report 43245 in conjunction with 43256)

⊙ **43246**   with directed placement of percutaneous gastrostomy tube
➔ *CPT Assistant* Spring 94:4, Feb 97:10

▶(For nonendoscopic percutaneous placement of gastrostomy tube, see 49440)◀

⊙ **43247**   with removal of foreign body
➔ *CPT Assistant* Spring 94:4

(For radiological supervision and interpretation, use 74235)

⊙ **43248**   with insertion of guide wire followed by dilation of esophagus over guide wire
➔ *CPT Assistant* Spring 94:4, Dec 97:11

⊙ **43249**   with balloon dilation of esophagus (less than 30 mm diameter)
➔ *CPT Assistant* May 05:3

⊙ **43250**   with removal of tumor(s), polyp(s), or other lesion(s) by hot biopsy forceps or bipolar cautery
➔ *CPT Assistant* Spring 94:4, Feb 99:11

⊙ **43251**   with removal of tumor(s), polyp(s), or other lesion(s) by snare technique
➔ *CPT Assistant* Spring 94:4, Oct 04:12

⊙ **43255**   with control of bleeding, any method
➔ *CPT Assistant* Spring 94:4

⊙ **43256** with transendoscopic stent placement (includes predilation)

➔ *CPT Changes: An Insider's View* 2001

⊙ **43257** with delivery of thermal energy to the muscle of lower esophageal sphincter and/or gastric cardia, for treatment of gastroesophageal reflux disease

➔ *CPT Assistant* May 05:3; *CPT Changes: An Insider's View* 2005

⊙ **43258** with ablation of tumor(s), polyp(s), or other lesion(s) not amenable to removal by hot biopsy forceps, bipolar cautery or snare technique

➔ *CPT Assistant* Spring 94:4

(For injection sclerosis of esophageal varices, use 43204, 43243)

⊙ **43259** with endoscopic ultrasound examination, including the esophagus, stomach, and either the duodenum and/or jejunum as appropriate

➔ *CPT Assistant* Spring 94:4, May 04:7; *CPT Changes: An Insider's View* 2004

(Do not report 43259 in conjunction with 76975)

⊙ **43260** Endoscopic retrograde cholangiopancreatography (ERCP); diagnostic, with or without collection of specimen(s) by brushing or washing (separate procedure)

➔ *CPT Assistant* Spring 94:5, Oct 04:13

(For radiological supervision and interpretation, see 74328, 74329, 74330)

Endoscopic Retrograde Cholangiopancreatography (ERCP)
43260

Examination of the hepatobiliary system (pancreatic ducts, hepatic ducts, common bile ducts, duodenal papilla [ampulla of Vater] and gallbladder [if present]) is performed through a side-viewing flexible fiberoptic endoscope.

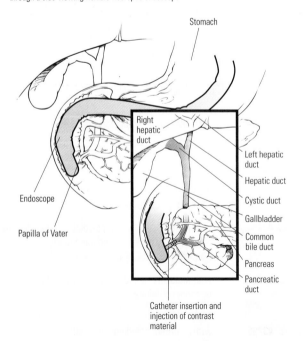

Stomach

Endoscope

Papilla of Vater

Right hepatic duct

Left hepatic duct

Hepatic duct

Cystic duct

Gallbladder

Common bile duct

Pancreas

Pancreatic duct

Catheter insertion and injection of contrast material

⊙ **43261** with biopsy, single or multiple

➔ *CPT Assistant* Spring 94:5

(For radiological supervision and interpretation, see 74328, 74329, 74330)

⊙ **43262** with sphincterotomy/papillotomy

➔ *CPT Assistant* Spring 94:5, Oct 04:13

(For radiological supervision and interpretation, see 74328, 74329, 74330)

⊙ **43263** with pressure measurement of sphincter of Oddi (pancreatic duct or common bile duct)

➔ *CPT Assistant* Spring 94:5, Oct 04:13

(For radiological supervision and interpretation, see 74328, 74329, 74330)

⊙ **43264** with endoscopic retrograde removal of calculus/calculi from biliary and/or pancreatic ducts

➔ *CPT Assistant* Spring 94:5; *CPT Changes: An Insider's View* 2002

(When done with sphincterotomy, also use 43262)

(For radiological supervision and interpretation, see 74328, 74329, 74330)

⊙ **43265** with endoscopic retrograde destruction, lithotripsy of calculus/calculi, any method

➔ *CPT Assistant* Spring 94:5; *CPT Changes: An Insider's View* 2002

(When done with sphincterotomy, also use 43262)

(For radiological supervision and interpretation, see 74328, 74329, 74330)

⊙ **43267** with endoscopic retrograde insertion of nasobiliary or nasopancreatic drainage tube

➔ *CPT Assistant* Spring 94:6

(When done with sphincterotomy, also use 43262)

(For radiological supervision and interpretation, see 74328, 74329, 74330)

⊙ **43268** with endoscopic retrograde insertion of tube or stent into bile or pancreatic duct

➔ *CPT Assistant* Spring 94:6, Sep 04:13, Oct 04:12

(When done with sphincterotomy, also use 43262)

(For radiological supervision and interpretation, see 74328, 74329, 74330)

⊙ **43269** with endoscopic retrograde removal of foreign body and/or change of tube or stent

➔ *CPT Assistant* Spring 94:6

(When done with sphincterotomy, also use 43262)

(For radiological supervision and interpretation, see 74328, 74329, 74330)

⊙ **43271**   with endoscopic retrograde balloon dilation of ampulla, biliary and/or pancreatic duct(s)

➔ *CPT Assistant* Spring 94:6

(When done with sphincterotomy, also use 43262)

(For radiological supervision and interpretation, see 74328, 74329, 74330)

⊙ **43272**   with ablation of tumor(s), polyp(s), or other lesion(s) not amenable to removal by hot biopsy forceps, bipolar cautery or snare technique

(For radiological supervision and interpretation, see 74328, 74329, 74330)

Laparoscopy

Surgical laparoscopy always includes diagnostic laparoscopy. To report a diagnostic laparoscopy (peritoneoscopy) (separate procedure), use 49320.

43280   Laparoscopy, surgical, esophagogastric fundoplasty (eg, Nissen, Toupet procedures)

➔ *CPT Assistant* Nov 99:22, Mar 00:8, Dec 02:2; *CPT Changes: An Insider's View* 2000

(For open approach, use 43324)

Laparoscopic Fundoplasty
43280

With the esophagus and fundus held aside, sutures are placed in both crus diaphragmatis muscles below the esophagus to bring them together to close the hiatal hernia, and the anterior and posterior walls of the fundus are wrapped and stitched around the esophagus to complete the laparoscopic fundoplasty.

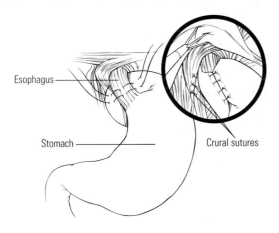

Esophagus

Stomach

Crural sutures

43289   Unlisted laparoscopy procedure, esophagus

➔ *CPT Assistant* Nov 99:22, Mar 00:8; *CPT Changes: An Insider's View* 2000

Repair

43300   Esophagoplasty (plastic repair or reconstruction), cervical approach; without repair of tracheoesophageal fistula

43305   with repair of tracheoesophageal fistula

43310   Esophagoplasty (plastic repair or reconstruction), thoracic approach; without repair of tracheoesophageal fistula

43312   with repair of tracheoesophageal fistula

43313   Esophagoplasty for congenital defect (plastic repair or reconstruction), thoracic approach; without repair of congenital tracheoesophageal fistula

➔ *CPT Changes: An Insider's View* 2002

43314   with repair of congenital tracheoesophageal fistula

➔ *CPT Changes: An Insider's View* 2002

(Do not report modifier 63 in conjunction with 43313, 43314)

43320   Esophagogastrostomy (cardioplasty), with or without vagotomy and pyloroplasty, transabdominal or transthoracic approach

43324   Esophagogastric fundoplasty (eg, Nissen, Belsey IV, Hill procedures)

➔ *CPT Assistant* Sep 96:10, Nov 99:22, May 05:3; *CPT Changes: An Insider's View* 2000

(For laparoscopic procedure, use 43280)

Nissen Fundoplasty
43324

The lower esophagus is accessed through an upper abdominal or lower thoracic incision. The fundus of the stomach is mobilized and wrapped around the lower esophageal sphincter, and the wrap is sutured into place.

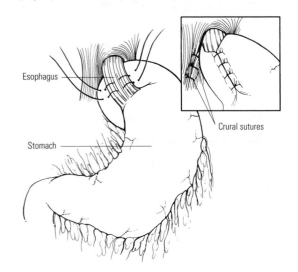

Esophagus

Stomach

Crural sutures

43325 Esophagogastric fundoplasty; with fundic patch (Thal-Nissen procedure)
➔ *CPT Assistant* Winter 90:6

(For cricopharyngeal myotomy, use 43030)

43326 with gastroplasty (eg, Collis)
➔ *CPT Assistant* Winter 90:6

43330 Esophagomyotomy (Heller type); abdominal approach
➔ *CPT Assistant* Nov 99:22; *CPT Changes: An Insider's View* 2000

43331 thoracic approach
➔ *CPT Assistant* Nov 99:22; *CPT Changes: An Insider's View* 2000

(For thoracoscopic esophagomyotomy, use 32665)

43340 Esophagojejunostomy (without total gastrectomy); abdominal approach

43341 thoracic approach

43350 Esophagostomy, fistulization of esophagus, external; abdominal approach

43351 thoracic approach

43352 cervical approach

43360 Gastrointestinal reconstruction for previous esophagectomy, for obstructing esophageal lesion or fistula, or for previous esophageal exclusion; with stomach, with or without pyloroplasty

43361 with colon interposition or small intestine reconstruction, including intestine mobilization, preparation, and anastomosis(es)
➔ *CPT Changes: An Insider's View* 2002

43400 Ligation, direct, esophageal varices

43401 Transection of esophagus with repair, for esophageal varices

43405 Ligation or stapling at gastroesophageal junction for pre-existing esophageal perforation

43410 Suture of esophageal wound or injury; cervical approach
➔ *CPT Assistant* Jun 96:7

43415 transthoracic or transabdominal approach

43420 Closure of esophagostomy or fistula; cervical approach

43425 transthoracic or transabdominal approach

(For repair of esophageal hiatal hernia, see 39520 et seq)

Manipulation

(For associated esophagogram, use 74220)

43450 Dilation of esophagus, by unguided sound or bougie, single or multiple passes
➔ *CPT Assistant* Spring 94:1, Jan 97:10, Apr 98:14, Jun 98:10

(For radiological supervision and interpretation, use 74360)

⊙ **43453** Dilation of esophagus, over guide wire
➔ *CPT Assistant* Spring 94:1, Jan 97:10, Dec 97:11

(For dilation with direct visualization, use 43220)

(For dilation of esophagus, by balloon or dilator, see 43220, 43458, and 74360)

(For radiological supervision and interpretation, use 74360)

⊙ **43456** Dilation of esophagus, by balloon or dilator, retrograde
➔ *CPT Assistant* Spring 94:3, Jan 97:10, May 05:3

(For radiological supervision and interpretation, use 74360)

⊙ **43458** Dilation of esophagus with balloon (30 mm diameter or larger) for achalasia
➔ *CPT Assistant* Spring 94:3, Jan 97:10, May 05:3

(For dilation with balloon less than 30 mm diameter, use 43220)

(For radiological supervision and interpretation, use 74360)

43460 Esophagogastric tamponade, with balloon (Sengstaaken type)

(For removal of esophageal foreign body by balloon catheter, see 43215, 43247, 74235)

Other Procedures

43496 Free jejunum transfer with microvascular anastomosis
➔ *CPT Assistant* Nov 96:8, Apr 97:4, Jun 97:10, Nov 97:17, Nov 98:16

(Do not report code 69990 in addition to code 43496)

43499 Unlisted procedure, esophagus

Stomach

Incision

43500 Gastrotomy; with exploration or foreign body removal

43501 with suture repair of bleeding ulcer

43502 with suture repair of pre-existing esophagogastric laceration (eg, Mallory-Weiss)

43510 with esophageal dilation and insertion of permanent intraluminal tube (eg, Celestin or Mousseaux-Barbin)

43520   Pyloromyotomy, cutting of pyloric muscle (Fredet-Ramstedt type operation)

(Do not report modifier 63 in conjunction with 43520)

Excision

43600   Biopsy of stomach; by capsule, tube, peroral (one or more specimens)

43605   by laparotomy

43610   Excision, local; ulcer or benign tumor of stomach

43611   malignant tumor of stomach

43620   Gastrectomy, total; with esophagoenterostomy

43621   with Roux-en-Y reconstruction

43622   with formation of intestinal pouch, any type

43631   Gastrectomy, partial, distal; with gastroduodenostomy

43632   with gastrojejunostomy

43633   with Roux-en-Y reconstruction

43634   with formation of intestinal pouch

+ 43635   Vagotomy when performed with partial distal gastrectomy (List separately in addition to code(s) for primary procedure)
   → *CPT Assistant* Nov 97:17

(Use 43635 in conjunction with 43631, 43632, 43633, 43634)

(43638, 43639 have been deleted)

43640   Vagotomy including pyloroplasty, with or without gastrostomy; truncal or selective

(For pyloroplasty, use 43800)

(For vagotomy, see 64752-64760)

43641   parietal cell (highly selective)

(For upper gastrointestinal endoscopy, see 43234-43259)

Laparoscopy

Surgical laparoscopy always includes diagnostic laparoscopy. To report a diagnostic laparoscopy (peritoneoscopy) (separate procedure), use 49320.

(For upper gastrointestinal endoscopy including esophagus, stomach, and either the duodenum and/or jejunum, see 43235-43259)

43644   Laparoscopy, surgical, gastric restrictive procedure; with gastric bypass and Roux-en-Y gastroenterostomy (roux limb 150 cm or less)
   → *CPT Assistant* May 05:3; *CPT Changes: An Insider's View* 2005

(Do not report 43644 in conjunction with 43846, 49320)

(Esophagogastroduodenoscopy (EGD) performed for a separate condition should be reported with modifier 59)

(For greater than 150 cm, use 43645)

(For open procedure, use 43846)

43645   with gastric bypass and small intestine reconstruction to limit absorption
   → *CPT Assistant* May 05:3; *CPT Changes: An Insider's View* 2005

(Do not report 43645 in conjunction with 49320, 43847)

43647   Laparoscopy, surgical; implantation or replacement of gastric neurostimulator electrodes, antrum
   → *CPT Changes: An Insider's View* 2007

43648   revision or removal of gastric neurostimulator electrodes, antrum
   → *CPT Changes: An Insider's View* 2007

(For open approach, see 43881, 43882)

(For insertion of gastric neurostimulator pulse generator, use 64590)

(For revision or removal of gastric neurostimulator pulse generator, use 64595)

►(For electronic analysis and programming of gastric neurostimulator pulse generator, see 95980-95982)◄

(For laparoscopic implantation, revision, or removal of gastric neurostimulator electrodes, lesser curvature [morbid obesity], see Category III codes 0155T, 0156T)

►(For electronic analysis and programming of gastric neurostimulator, lesser curvature, use Category III code 0162T)◄

43651   Laparoscopy, surgical; transection of vagus nerves, truncal
   → *CPT Assistant* Nov 99:22, Mar 00:8; *CPT Changes: An Insider's View* 2000

43652   transection of vagus nerves, selective or highly selective
   → *CPT Assistant* Nov 99:22, Mar 00:8; *CPT Changes: An Insider's View* 2000

43653   gastrostomy, without construction of gastric tube (eg, Stamm procedure) (separate procedure)
   → *CPT Assistant* Nov 99:22, Mar 00:8; *CPT Changes: An Insider's View* 2000

43659   Unlisted laparoscopy procedure, stomach
   → *CPT Assistant* Nov 99:22, Mar 00:8, Apr 06:19, Jun 06:16; *CPT Changes: An Insider's View* 2000

Introduction

▶(43750 has been deleted. To report percutaneous gastrostomy tube insertion, use 43246)◀

43752 Naso- or oro-gastric tube placement, requiring physician's skill and fluoroscopic guidance (includes fluoroscopy, image documentation and report)

➔ *CPT Assistant* Jan 02:11, Apr 03:7, Oct 03:2, Jul 06:4, Feb 07:10; *CPT Changes: An Insider's View* 2001, 2004

▶(For percutaneous placement of gastrostomy tube, use 49440)◀

(For enteric tube placement, see 44500, 74340)

(Do not report 43752 in conjunction with critical care codes 99291-99292, neonatal critical care codes 99295-99296, pediatric critical care codes 99293-99294 or low birth weight intensive care service codes 99298-99299)

▲ **43760** Change of gastrostomy tube, percutaneous, without imaging or endoscopic guidance

➔ *CPT Changes: An Insider's View* 2008

▶(To report fluoroscopically guided gastrostomy, use 49450)◀

(For endoscopic placement of gastrostomy tube, use 43246)

▲ **43761** Repositioning of the gastric feeding tube, through the duodenum for enteric nutrition

➔ *CPT Assistant* Oct 96:9, Nov 99:22; *CPT Changes: An Insider's View* 2000, 2008

▶(If imaging guidance is performed, use 76000)◀

▶(For endoscopic conversion of a gastrostomy tube to jejunostomy tube, use 44373)◀

▶(For placement of a long gastrointestinal tube into the duodenum, use 44500)◀

▶(Do not report 43761 in conjunction with 44500, 49446)◀

Bariatric Surgery

Bariatric surgical procedures may involve the stomach, duodenum, jejunum, and/or the ileum.

Laparoscopy

Surgical laparoscopy always includes diagnostic laparoscopy. To report a diagnostic laparoscopy (separate procedure), use 49320.

▶Typical postoperative follow-up care (see Surgery Guidelines, CPT Surgical Package Definition) after gastric restriction using the adjustable gastric restrictive device includes subsequent restrictive device adjustment(s) through the postoperative period for the typical patient. Adjustment consists of changing the gastric restrictive device component diameter by injection or aspiration of fluid through the subcutaneous port component.◀

▲ **43770** Laparoscopy, surgical, gastric restrictive procedure; placement of adjustable gastric restrictive device (eg, gastric band and subcutaneous port components)

➔ *CPT Changes: An Insider's View* 2006, 2008

(For individual component placement, report 43770 with modifier 52)

▲ **43771** revision of adjustable gastric restrictive device component only

➔ *CPT Changes: An Insider's View* 2006, 2008

▲ **43772** removal of adjustable gastric restrictive device component only

➔ *CPT Changes: An Insider's View* 2006, 2008

▲ **43773** removal and replacement of adjustable gastric restrictive device component only

➔ *CPT Changes: An Insider's View* 2006, 2008

(Do not report 43773 in conjunction with 43772)

▲ **43774** removal of adjustable gastric restrictive device and subcutaneous port components

➔ *CPT Changes: An Insider's View* 2006, 2008

(For removal and replacement of both gastric band and subcutaneous port components, use 43659)

Other Procedures

43800 Pyloroplasty

(For pyloroplasty and vagotomy, use 43640)

43810 Gastroduodenostomy

43820 Gastrojejunostomy; without vagotomy

43825 with vagotomy, any type

43830 Gastrostomy, open; without construction of gastric tube (eg, Stamm procedure) (separate procedure)

➔ *CPT Assistant* Nov 99:22; *CPT Changes: An Insider's View* 2000

43831 neonatal, for feeding

➔ *CPT Assistant* Nov 99:22; *CPT Changes: An Insider's View* 2000

(For change of gastrostomy tube, use 43760)

(Do not report modifier 63 in conjunction with 43831)

43832 with construction of gastric tube (eg, Janeway procedure)

➔ *CPT Assistant* Nov 99:22; *CPT Changes: An Insider's View* 2000

(For percutaneous endoscopic gastrostomy, use 43246)

43840   Gastrorrhaphy, suture of perforated duodenal or gastric ulcer, wound, or injury

43842   Gastric restrictive procedure, without gastric bypass, for morbid obesity; vertical-banded gastroplasty

➔ *CPT Assistant* May 98:5

43843   other than vertical-banded gastroplasty

➔ *CPT Assistant* May 98:5

43845   Gastric restrictive procedure with partial gastrectomy, pylorus-preserving duodenoileostomy and ileoileostomy (50 to 100 cm common channel) to limit absorption (biliopancreatic diversion with duodenal switch)

➔ *CPT Assistant* May 05:3; *CPT Changes: An Insider's View* 2005

(Do not report 43845 in conjunction with 43633, 43847, 44130, 49000)

43846   Gastric restrictive procedure, with gastric bypass for morbid obesity; with short limb (150 cm or less) Roux-en-Y gastroenterostomy

➔ *CPT Assistant* May 98:5, May 05:3; *CPT Changes: An Insider's View* 2005

(For greater than 150 cm, use 43847)

(For laparoscopic procedure, use 43644)

Gastric Bypass for Morbid Obesity
43846

The stomach is partitioned with a staple line on the lesser curvature (no band, no gastric transection). A short limb of small bowel (less than 100 cm) is divided and anastomosed to the small upper stomach pouch.

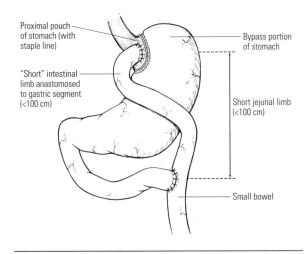

43847   with small intestine reconstruction to limit absorption

➔ *CPT Assistant* May 98:5, May 02:7; *CPT Changes: An Insider's View* 2002

▲ **43848**   Revision, open, of gastric restrictive procedure for morbid obesity, other than adjustable gastric restrictive device (separate procedure)

➔ *CPT Assistant* May 98:5, Apr 06:1; *CPT Changes: An Insider's View* 2006, 2008

▶(For laparoscopic adjustable gastric restrictive procedures, see 43770-43774)◀

▶(For gastric restrictive port procedures, see 43886-43888)◀

43850   Revision of gastroduodenal anastomosis (gastroduodenostomy) with reconstruction; without vagotomy

43855   with vagotomy

43860   Revision of gastrojejunal anastomosis (gastrojejunostomy) with reconstruction, with or without partial gastrectomy or intestine resection; without vagotomy

➔ *CPT Changes: An Insider's View* 2002

43865   with vagotomy

43870   Closure of gastrostomy, surgical

43880   Closure of gastrocolic fistula

43881   Implantation or replacement of gastric neurostimulator electrodes, antrum, open

➔ *CPT Changes: An Insider's View* 2007

43882   Revision or removal of gastric neurostimulator electrodes, antrum, open

➔ *CPT Changes: An Insider's View* 2007

(For laparoscopic approach, see 43647, 43648)

(For insertion of gastric neurostimulator pulse generator, use 64590)

(For revision or removal of gastric neurostimulator pulse generator, use 64595)

(For electronic analysis and programming of gastric neurostimulator pulse generator, use 95999)

(For open implantation, revision, or removal of gastric neurostimulator electrodes, lesser curvature [morbid obesity], see Category III codes 0157T, 0158T)

(For electronic analysis and programming of gastric neurostimulator, lesser curvature, use Category III code 0162T)

43886   Gastric restrictive procedure, open; revision of subcutaneous port component only
> *CPT Changes: An Insider's View* 2006

43887   removal of subcutaneous port component only
> *CPT Changes: An Insider's View* 2006

43888   removal and replacement of subcutaneous port component only
> *CPT Changes: An Insider's View* 2006

(Do not report 43888 in conjunction with 43774, 43887)

►(For laparoscopic removal of both gastric restrictive device and subcutaneous port components, use 43774)◄

►(For removal and replacement of both gastric restrictive device and subcutaneous port components, use 43659)◄

43999   Unlisted procedure, stomach

Intestines (Except Rectum)

Incision

44005   Enterolysis (freeing of intestinal adhesion) (separate procedure)
> *CPT Assistant* Winter 90:6, Nov 97:17, Nov 99:23, Jan 00:11, Apr 00:10; *CPT Changes: An Insider's View* 2000

(Do not report 44005 in addition to 45136)

(For laparoscopic approach, use 44180)

44010   Duodenotomy, for exploration, biopsy(s), or foreign body removal

+ 44015   Tube or needle catheter jejunostomy for enteral alimentation, intraoperative, any method (List separately in addition to primary procedure)
> *CPT Assistant* Mar 02:10

44020   Enterotomy, small intestine, other than duodenum; for exploration, biopsy(s), or foreign body removal
> *CPT Changes: An Insider's View* 2002

44021   for decompression (eg, Baker tube)

44025   Colotomy, for exploration, biopsy(s), or foreign body removal

(For exteriorization of intestine (Mikulicz resection with crushing of spur), see 44602-44605)

44050   Reduction of volvulus, intussusception, internal hernia, by laparotomy

44055   Correction of malrotation by lysis of duodenal bands and/or reduction of midgut volvulus (eg, Ladd procedure)

(Do not report modifier 63 in conjunction with 44055)

Excision

Intestinal allotransplantation involves three distinct components of physician work:

1) ***Cadaver donor enterectomy***, which includes harvesting the intestine graft and cold preservation of the graft (perfusing with cold preservation solution and cold maintenance) (use 44132). ***Living donor enterectomy***, which includes harvesting the intestine graft, cold preservation of the graft (perfusing with cold preservation solution and cold maintenance), and care of the donor (use 44133).

2) ***Backbench work***:

   Standard preparation of an intestine allograft prior to transplantation includes mobilization and fashioning of the superior mesenteric artery and vein (see 44715).

   Additional reconstruction of an intestine allograft prior to transplantation may include venous and/or arterial anastomosis(es) (see 44720-44721).

3) ***Recipient intestinal allotransplantation with or without recipient enterectomy***, which includes transplantation of allograft and care of the recipient (see 44135, 44136).

44100   Biopsy of intestine by capsule, tube, peroral (one or more specimens)

44110   Excision of one or more lesions of small or large intestine not requiring anastomosis, exteriorization, or fistulization; single enterotomy
> *CPT Changes: An Insider's View* 2002

44111   multiple enterotomies

44120   Enterectomy, resection of small intestine; single resection and anastomosis
> *CPT Assistant* Mar 04:3

(Do not report 44120 in addition to 45136)

+ 44121   each additional resection and anastomosis (List separately in addition to code for primary procedure)

(Use 44121 in conjunction with 44120)

44125   with enterostomy

44126   Enterectomy, resection of small intestine for congenital atresia, single resection and anastomosis of proximal segment of intestine; without tapering
> *CPT Changes: An Insider's View* 2002

44127   with tapering

➔ *CPT Changes: An Insider's View* 2002

Enterectomy, Resection for Congenital Atresia
44127

Proximal intestine

90 degrees

End to oblique anastomosis

45 degrees

+ 44128   each additional resection and anastomosis (List separately in addition to code for primary procedure)

➔ *CPT Changes: An Insider's View* 2002

(Use 44128 in conjunction with 44126, 44127)

(Do not report modifier 63 in conjunction with 44126, 44127, 44128)

44130   Enteroenterostomy, anastomosis of intestine, with or without cutaneous enterostomy (separate procedure)

44132   Donor enterectomy (including cold preservation), open; from cadaver donor

➔ *CPT Changes: An Insider's View* 2001, 2005

44133   partial, from living donor

➔ *CPT Changes: An Insider's View* 2001

(For backbench intestinal graft preparation or reconstruction, see 44715, 44720, 44721)

44135   Intestinal allotransplantation; from cadaver donor

➔ *CPT Changes: An Insider's View* 2001

44136   from living donor

➔ *CPT Changes: An Insider's View* 2001

44137   Removal of transplanted intestinal allograft, complete

➔ *CPT Changes: An Insider's View* 2005

(For partial removal of transplant allograft, see 44120, 44121, 44140)

+ 44139   Mobilization (take-down) of splenic flexure performed in conjunction with partial colectomy (List separately in addition to primary procedure)

(Use 44139 in conjunction with 44140-44147)

44140   Colectomy, partial; with anastomosis

➔ *CPT Assistant* Fall 92:23

(For laparoscopic procedure, use 44204)

Colectomy, Partial
44140

A segment of the colon is resected and an anastomosis is performed between the remaining ends of the colon.

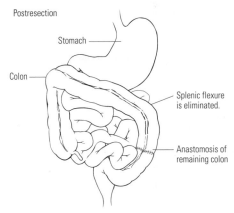

Postresection

Stomach

Colon

Splenic flexure is eliminated.

Anastomosis of remaining colon

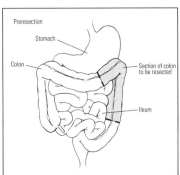

Preresection

Stomach

Colon

Section of colon to be resected

Ileum

44141	with skin level cecostomy or colostomy
	➔ *CPT Assistant* Fall 92:24
44143	with end colostomy and closure of distal segment (Hartmann type procedure)
	➔ *CPT Assistant* Fall 92:24
	(For laparoscopic procedure, use 44206)
44144	with resection, with colostomy or ileostomy and creation of mucofistula
	➔ *CPT Assistant* Fall 92:24
44145	with coloproctostomy (low pelvic anastomosis)
	➔ *CPT Assistant* Fall 92:24
	(For laparoscopic procedure, use 44207)
44146	with coloproctostomy (low pelvic anastomosis), with colostomy
	➔ *CPT Assistant* Fall 92:24
	(For laparoscopic procedure, use 44208)
44147	abdominal and transanal approach
	➔ *CPT Assistant* Fall 92:24
44150	Colectomy, total, abdominal, without proctectomy; with ileostomy or ileoproctostomy
	(For laparoscopic procedure, use 44210)
44151	with continent ileostomy
	(44152 and 44153 have been deleted. To report, use 44799)
44155	Colectomy, total, abdominal, with proctectomy; with ileostomy
	(For laparoscopic procedure, use 44212)
44156	with continent ileostomy
44157	with ileoanal anastomosis, includes loop ileostomy, and rectal mucosectomy, when performed
	➔ *CPT Changes: An Insider's View* 2007
44158	with ileoanal anastomosis, creation of ileal reservoir (S or J), includes loop ileostomy, and rectal mucosectomy, when performed
	➔ *CPT Changes: An Insider's View* 2007
	(For laparoscopic procedure, use 44211)
44160	Colectomy, partial, with removal of terminal ileum with ileocolostomy
	➔ *CPT Changes: An Insider's View* 2002
	(For laparoscopic procedure, use 44205)

Colectomy With Removal of Terminal Ileum and Ileocolostomy
44160

A segment of the colon and terminal ileum is removed and an anastomosis is performed between the remaining ileum and colon.

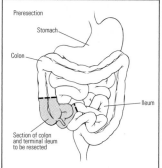

Laparoscopy

Surgical laparoscopy always includes diagnostic laparoscopy. To report a diagnostic laparoscopy (peritoneoscopy) (separate procedure), use 49320.

Incision

44180	Laparoscopy, surgical, enterolysis (freeing of intestinal adhesion) (separate procedure)
	➔ *CPT Changes: An Insider's View* 2006
	(For laparoscopy with salpingolysis, ovariolysis, use 58660)

Enterostomy—External Fistulization of Intestines

44186	Laparoscopy, surgical; jejunostomy (eg, for decompression or feeding)
	➔ *CPT Changes: An Insider's View* 2006
44187	ileostomy or jejunostomy, non-tube
	➔ *CPT Changes: An Insider's View* 2006
	(For open procedure, use 44310)

44188   Laparoscopy, surgical, colostomy or skin level cecostomy

➔ *CPT Changes: An Insider's View* 2006

(For open procedure, use 44320)

(Do not report 44188 in conjunction with 44970)

(44200 has been deleted. To report, use 44180)

(44201 has been deleted. To report, use 44186)

Excision

44202   Laparoscopy, surgical; enterectomy, resection of small intestine, single resection and anastomosis

➔ *CPT Assistant* Nov 99:23, Mar 00:9, May 03:2, Apr 06:1; *CPT Changes: An Insider's View* 2000, 2002, 2006

+ 44203   each additional small intestine resection and anastomosis (List separately in addition to code for primary procedure)

➔ *CPT Assistant* May 03:2; *CPT Changes: An Insider's View* 2002

(Use 44203 in conjunction with 44202)

(For open procedure, see 44120, 44121)

44204   colectomy, partial, with anastomosis

➔ *CPT Assistant* May 03:3, Apr 06:1, 19; *CPT Changes: An Insider's View* 2002

(For open procedure, use 44140)

44205   colectomy, partial, with removal of terminal ileum with ileocolostomy

➔ *CPT Assistant* May 03:3, Apr 06:1; *CPT Changes: An Insider's View* 2002

(For open procedure, use 44160)

44206   colectomy, partial, with end colostomy and closure of distal segment (Hartmann type procedure)

➔ *CPT Assistant* May 03:3, Apr 06:1; *CPT Changes: An Insider's View* 2003

(For open procedure, use 44143)

44207   colectomy, partial, with anastomosis, with coloproctostomy (low pelvic anastomosis)

➔ *CPT Assistant* May 03:3, Apr 06:1; *CPT Changes: An Insider's View* 2003

(For open procedure, use 44145)

44208   colectomy, partial, with anastomosis, with coloproctostomy (low pelvic anastomosis) with colostomy

➔ *CPT Assistant* May 03:3, Apr 06:1; *CPT Changes: An Insider's View* 2003

(For open procedure, use 44146)

44210   colectomy, total, abdominal, without proctectomy, with ileostomy or ileoproctostomy

➔ *CPT Assistant* May 03:3; *CPT Changes: An Insider's View* 2003

(For open procedure, use 44150)

44211   colectomy, total, abdominal, with proctectomy, with ileoanal anastomosis, creation of ileal reservoir (S or J), with loop ileostomy, includes rectal mucosectomy, when performed

➔ *CPT Assistant* May 03:3; *CPT Changes: An Insider's View* 2003, 2007

(For open procedure, see 44157, 44158)

44212   colectomy, total, abdominal, with proctectomy, with ileostomy

➔ *CPT Assistant* May 03:3; *CPT Changes: An Insider's View* 2003

(For open procedure, use 44155)

+ 44213   Laparoscopy, surgical, mobilization (take-down) of splenic flexure performed in conjunction with partial colectomy (List separately in addition to primary procedure)

➔ *CPT Changes: An Insider's View* 2006

(Use 44213 in conjunction with 44204-44208)

(For open procedure, use 44139)

Repair

44227   Laparoscopy, surgical, closure of enterostomy, large or small intestine, with resection and anastomosis

➔ *CPT Changes: An Insider's View* 2006

(For open procedure, see 44625, 44626)

Other Procedures

44238   Unlisted laparoscopy procedure, intestine (except rectum)

➔ *CPT Assistant* May 03:4; *CPT Changes: An Insider's View* 2003

(44239 has been deleted. To report, use 45499)

Enterostomy—External Fistulization of Intestines

▲ **44300**   Placement, enterostomy or cecostomy, tube open (eg, for feeding or decompression) (separate procedure)

➔ *CPT Assistant* Mar 02:10; *CPT Changes: An Insider's View* 2008

▶(For percutaneous placement of duodenostomy, jejunostomy, gastro-jejunostomy or cecostomy [or other colonic] tube including fluoroscopic imaging guidance, see 49441-49442)◀

44310   Ileostomy or jejunostomy, non-tube

➔ *CPT Assistant* Mar 02:10, Apr 06:1; *CPT Changes: An Insider's View* 2006

(For laparoscopic procedure, use 44187)

(Do not report 44310 in conjunction with 44144, 44150-44151, 44155, 44156, 45113, 45119, 45136)

44312   Revision of ileostomy; simple (release of superficial scar) (separate procedure)

➔ *CPT Assistant* Spring 93:35

44314   complicated (reconstruction in-depth) (separate procedure)

44316   Continent ileostomy (Kock procedure) (separate procedure)

(For fiberoptic evaluation, use 44385)

44320   Colostomy or skin level cecostomy;
⮕ *CPT Changes: An Insider's View* 2006

(For laparoscopic procedure, use 44188)

(Do not report 44320 in conjunction with 44141, 44144, 44146, 44605, 45110, 45119, 45126, 45563, 45805, 45825, 50810, 51597, 57307, or 58240)

44322   with multiple biopsies (eg, for congenital megacolon) (separate procedure)
⮕ *CPT Changes: An Insider's View* 2002

44340   Revision of colostomy; simple (release of superficial scar) (separate procedure)

44345   complicated (reconstruction in-depth) (separate procedure)

44346   with repair of paracolostomy hernia (separate procedure)

Endoscopy, Small Intestine and Stomal

Surgical endoscopy always includes diagnostic endoscopy.

(For upper gastrointestinal endoscopy, see 43234-43258)

⊙ **44360**   Small intestinal endoscopy, enteroscopy beyond second portion of duodenum, not including ileum; diagnostic, with or without collection of specimen(s) by brushing or washing (separate procedure)
⮕ *CPT Assistant* Spring 94:7

⊙ **44361**   with biopsy, single or multiple

⊙ **44363**   with removal of foreign body

⊙ **44364**   with removal of tumor(s), polyp(s), or other lesion(s) by snare technique

⊙ **44365**   with removal of tumor(s), polyp(s), or other lesion(s) by hot biopsy forceps or bipolar cautery

⊙ **44366**   with control of bleeding (eg, injection, bipolar cautery, unipolar cautery, laser, heater probe, stapler, plasma coagulator)
⮕ *CPT Changes: An Insider's View* 2002

⊙ **44369**   with ablation of tumor(s), polyp(s), or other lesion(s) not amenable to removal by hot biopsy forceps, bipolar cautery or snare technique

⊙ **44370**   with transendoscopic stent placement (includes predilation)
⮕ *CPT Assistant* Nov 01:7; *CPT Changes: An Insider's View* 2001

⊙ **44372**   with placement of percutaneous jejunostomy tube
⮕ *CPT Assistant* Spring 94:7

⊙ **44373**   with conversion of percutaneous gastrostomy tube to percutaneous jejunostomy tube
⮕ *CPT Assistant* Spring 94:7

(For fiberoptic jejunostomy through stoma, use 43235)

⊙ **44376**   Small intestinal endoscopy, enteroscopy beyond second portion of duodenum, including ileum; diagnostic, with or without collection of specimen(s) by brushing or washing (separate procedure)
⮕ *CPT Assistant* Spring 94:7

⊙ **44377**   with biopsy, single or multiple
⮕ *CPT Assistant* Spring 94:7

⊙ **44378**   with control of bleeding (eg, injection, bipolar cautery, unipolar cautery, laser, heater probe, stapler, plasma coagulator)
⮕ *CPT Assistant* Spring 94:7; *CPT Changes: An Insider's View* 2002

⊙ **44379**   with transendoscopic stent placement (includes predilation)
⮕ *CPT Assistant* Nov 01:7; *CPT Changes: An Insider's View* 2001

⊙ **44380**   Ileoscopy, through stoma; diagnostic, with or without collection of specimen(s) by brushing or washing (separate procedure)

⊙ **44382**   with biopsy, single or multiple

⊙ **44383**   with transendoscopic stent placement (includes predilation)
⮕ *CPT Assistant* Nov 01:7; *CPT Changes: An Insider's View* 2001

⊙ **44385**   Endoscopic evaluation of small intestinal (abdominal or pelvic) pouch; diagnostic, with or without collection of specimen(s) by brushing or washing (separate procedure)

⊙ **44386**   with biopsy, single or multiple

⊙ **44388**   Colonoscopy through stoma; diagnostic, with or without collection of specimen(s) by brushing or washing (separate procedure)

⊙ **44389**   with biopsy, single or multiple

⊙ **44390**   with removal of foreign body

⊙ **44391**   with control of bleeding (eg, injection, bipolar cautery, unipolar cautery, laser, heater probe, stapler, plasma coagulator)
⮕ *CPT Changes: An Insider's View* 2002

⊙ **44392**   with removal of tumor(s), polyp(s), or other lesion(s) by hot biopsy forceps or bipolar cautery

⊙ **44393**   with ablation of tumor(s), polyp(s), or other lesion(s) not amenable to removal by hot biopsy forceps, bipolar cautery or snare technique

⊙ **44394**   with removal of tumor(s), polyp(s), or other lesion(s) by snare technique

(For colonoscopy per rectum, see 45330-45385)

⊙ **44397**   with transendoscopic stent placement (includes predilation)
⮕ *CPT Assistant* Nov 01:7; *CPT Changes: An Insider's View* 2001

Introduction

⊙⊘ **44500**   Introduction of long gastrointestinal tube (eg, Miller-Abbott) (separate procedure)

(For radiological supervision and interpretation, use 74340)

(For naso- or oro-gastric tube placement, use 43752)

Repair

44602   Suture of small intestine (enterorrhaphy) for perforated ulcer, diverticulum, wound, injury or rupture; single perforation

44603   multiple perforations

44604   Suture of large intestine (colorrhaphy) for perforated ulcer, diverticulum, wound, injury or rupture (single or multiple perforations); without colostomy

44605   with colostomy

44615   Intestinal stricturoplasty (enterotomy and enterorrhaphy) with or without dilation, for intestinal obstruction

44620   Closure of enterostomy, large or small intestine;
⊃ *CPT Assistant* Nov 97:17, May 02:7

44625   with resection and anastomosis other than colorectal
⊃ *CPT Assistant* Nov 97:17

44626   with resection and colorectal anastomosis (eg, closure of Hartmann type procedure)
⊃ *CPT Assistant* Nov 97:17

(For laparoscopic procedure, use 44227)

44640   Closure of intestinal cutaneous fistula

44650   Closure of enteroenteric or enterocolic fistula

44660   Closure of enterovesical fistula; without intestinal or bladder resection

44661   with intestine and/or bladder resection
⊃ *CPT Changes: An Insider's View* 2002

(For closure of renocolic fistula, see 50525, 50526)

(For closure of gastrocolic fistula, use 43880)

(For closure of rectovesical fistula, see 45800, 45805)

44680   Intestinal plication (separate procedure)

Other Procedures

44700   Exclusion of small intestine from pelvis by mesh or other prosthesis, or native tissue (eg, bladder or omentum)
⊃ *CPT Assistant* Nov 97:18; *CPT Changes: An Insider's View* 2002

(For therapeutic radiation clinical treatment, see **Radiation Oncology** section)

+ **44701**   Intraoperative colonic lavage (List separately in addition to code for primary procedure)
⊃ *CPT Changes: An Insider's View* 2003

(Use 44701 in conjunction with 44140, 44145, 44150, or 44604 as appropriate)

(Do not report 44701 in conjunction with 44300, 44950-44960)

44715   Backbench standard preparation of cadaver or living donor intestine allograft prior to transplantation, including mobilization and fashioning of the superior mesenteric artery and vein
⊃ *CPT Changes: An Insider's View* 2005

44720   Backbench reconstruction of cadaver or living donor intestine allograft prior to transplantation; venous anastomosis, each
⊃ *CPT Changes: An Insider's View* 2005

44721   arterial anastomosis, each
⊃ *CPT Assistant* Apr 05:10-11; *CPT Changes: An Insider's View* 2005

44799   Unlisted procedure, intestine
⊃ *CPT Assistant* Dec 00:14

(For unlisted laparoscopic procedure, intestine except rectum, use 44238)

Meckel's Diverticulum and the Mesentery

Excision

44800   Excision of Meckel's diverticulum (diverticulectomy) or omphalomesenteric duct

44820   Excision of lesion of mesentery (separate procedure)

(With intestine resection, see 44120 or 44140 et seq)

Suture

44850   Suture of mesentery (separate procedure)

(For reduction and repair of internal hernia, use 44050)

Other Procedures

44899   Unlisted procedure, Meckel's diverticulum and the mesentery

Appendix

Incision

44900   Incision and drainage of appendiceal abscess; open
⊃ *CPT Assistant* Nov 97:18

⊙ **44901**   percutaneous
⊃ *CPT Assistant* Nov 97:18, Mar 98:8

(For radiological supervision and interpretation, use 75989)

Excision

44950 Appendectomy;

→ *CPT Assistant* Feb 92:22, Sep 96:4, Aug 02:2

(Incidental appendectomy during intra-abdominal surgery does not usually warrant a separate identification. If necessary to report, add modifier 52)

+ 44955 when done for indicated purpose at time of other major procedure (not as separate procedure) (List separately in addition to code for primary procedure)

→ *CPT Assistant* Fall 92:22, Sep 96:4, Apr 97:3

44960 for ruptured appendix with abscess or generalized peritonitis

→ *CPT Assistant* Fall 92:22

Laparoscopy

Surgical laparoscopy always includes diagnostic laparoscopy. To report a diagnostic laparoscopy (peritoneoscopy) (separate procedure), use 49320.

44970 Laparoscopy, surgical, appendectomy

→ *CPT Assistant* Nov 99:23, Mar 00:9, Apr 06:1, 20; *CPT Changes: An Insider's View* 2000

44979 Unlisted laparoscopy procedure, appendix

→ *CPT Assistant* Nov 99:23, Mar 00:9; *CPT Changes: An Insider's View* 2000

Rectum

Incision

45000 Transrectal drainage of pelvic abscess

45005 Incision and drainage of submucosal abscess, rectum

45020 Incision and drainage of deep supralevator, pelvirectal, or retrorectal abscess

(See also 46050, 46060)

Excision

45100 Biopsy of anorectal wall, anal approach (eg, congenital megacolon)

(For endoscopic biopsy, use 45305)

45108 Anorectal myomectomy

45110 Proctectomy; complete, combined abdominoperineal, with colostomy

(For laparoscopic procedure, use 45395)

45111 partial resection of rectum, transabdominal approach

45112 Proctectomy, combined abdominoperineal, pull-through procedure (eg, colo-anal anastomosis)

→ *CPT Assistant* Nov 97:18

(For colo-anal anastomosis with colonic reservoir or pouch, use 45119)

45113 Proctectomy, partial, with rectal mucosectomy, ileoanal anastomosis, creation of ileal reservoir (S or J), with or without loop ileostomy

45114 Proctectomy, partial, with anastomosis; abdominal and transsacral approach

45116 transsacral approach only (Kraske type)

45119 Proctectomy, combined abdominoperineal pull-through procedure (eg, colo-anal anastomosis), with creation of colonic reservoir (eg, J-pouch), with diverting enterostomy when performed

→ *CPT Assistant* Nov 97:18, Apr 06:1; *CPT Changes: An Insider's View* 2006

(For laparoscopic procedure, use 45397)

45120 Proctectomy, complete (for congenital megacolon), abdominal and perineal approach; with pull-through procedure and anastomosis (eg, Swenson, Duhamel, or Soave type operation)

45121 with subtotal or total colectomy, with multiple biopsies

45123 Proctectomy, partial, without anastomosis, perineal approach

45126 Pelvic exenteration for colorectal malignancy, with proctectomy (with or without colostomy), with removal of bladder and ureteral transplantations, and/or hysterectomy, or cervicectomy, with or without removal of tube(s), with or without removal of ovary(s), or any combination thereof

→ *CPT Assistant* Nov 98:16

45130 Excision of rectal procidentia, with anastomosis; perineal approach

45135 abdominal and perineal approach

45136 Excision of ileoanal reservoir with ileostomy

→ *CPT Changes: An Insider's View* 2002

(Do not report 45136 in addition to 44005, 44120, 44310)

45150 Division of stricture of rectum

45160 Excision of rectal tumor by proctotomy, transsacral or transcoccygeal approach

45170 Excision of rectal tumor, transanal approach

Destruction

45190 Destruction of rectal tumor (eg, electrodesiccation, electrosurgery, laser ablation, laser resection, cryosurgery) transanal approach

→ *CPT Changes: An Insider's View* 2002

Endoscopy

Definitions

Proctosigmoidoscopy is the examination of the rectum and sigmoid colon.

Sigmoidoscopy is the examination of the entire rectum, sigmoid colon and may include examination of a portion of the descending colon.

Colonoscopy is the examination of the entire colon, from the rectum to the cecum, and may include the examination of the terminal ileum.

For an incomplete colonoscopy, with full preparation for a colonoscopy, use a colonoscopy code with the modifier 52 and provide documentation.

Surgical endoscopy always includes diagnostic endoscopy.

45300 Proctosigmoidoscopy, rigid; diagnostic, with or without collection of specimen(s) by brushing or washing (separate procedure)
➔ *CPT Assistant* Spring 94:8, Oct 97:6, Apr 06:1

⊙ **45303** with dilation (eg, balloon, guide wire, bougie)
➔ *CPT Assistant* Spring 94:8, Oct 97:6, Apr 06:1; *CPT Changes: An Insider's View* 2002

(For radiological supervision and interpretation, use 74360)

⊙ **45305** with biopsy, single or multiple
➔ *CPT Assistant* Spring 94:8, Oct 97:6, Apr 06:1

⊙ **45307** with removal of foreign body
➔ *CPT Assistant* Spring 94:8, Oct 97:6, Apr 06:1

⊙ **45308** with removal of single tumor, polyp, or other lesion by hot biopsy forceps or bipolar cautery
➔ *CPT Assistant* Spring 94:8, Oct 97:6, Apr 06:1

⊙ **45309** with removal of single tumor, polyp, or other lesion by snare technique
➔ *CPT Assistant* Spring 94:8, Oct 97:6, Apr 06:1

⊙ **45315** with removal of multiple tumors, polyps, or other lesions by hot biopsy forceps, bipolar cautery or snare technique
➔ *CPT Assistant* Spring 94:8, Oct 97:6, Apr 06:1

⊙ **45317** with control of bleeding (eg, injection, bipolar cautery, unipolar cautery, laser, heater probe, stapler, plasma coagulator)
➔ *CPT Assistant* Spring 94:8, Oct 97:6, Apr 06:1; *CPT Changes: An Insider's View* 2002

⊙ **45320** with ablation of tumor(s), polyp(s), or other lesion(s) not amenable to removal by hot biopsy forceps, bipolar cautery or snare technique (eg, laser)
➔ *CPT Assistant* Spring 94:8, Oct 97:6, Apr 06:1

⊙ **45321** with decompression of volvulus
➔ *CPT Assistant* Spring 94:8, Oct 97:6, Apr 06:1

⊙ **45327** with transendoscopic stent placement (includes predilation)
➔ *CPT Assistant* Nov 01:7, Apr 06:1; *CPT Changes: An Insider's View* 2001

45330 Sigmoidoscopy, flexible; diagnostic, with or without collection of specimen(s) by brushing or washing (separate procedure)
➔ *CPT Assistant* Spring 94:9, May 05:3

45331 with biopsy, single or multiple
➔ *CPT Assistant* Spring 94:9, Sep 96:6, Jan 07:28

⊙ **45332** with removal of foreign body
➔ *CPT Assistant* Winter 90:3, Spring 94:9

⊙ **45333** with removal of tumor(s), polyp(s), or other lesion(s) by hot biopsy forceps or bipolar cautery
➔ *CPT Assistant* Winter 90:3, Spring 94:9

⊙ **45334** with control of bleeding (eg, injection, bipolar cautery, unipolar cautery, laser, heater probe, stapler, plasma coagulator)
➔ *CPT Assistant* Spring 94:9, Sep 96:6, Jan 07:28; *CPT Changes: An Insider's View* 2002

⊙ **45335** with directed submucosal injection(s), any substance
➔ *CPT Assistant* Mar 03:22; *CPT Changes: An Insider's View* 2003

⊙ **45337** with decompression of volvulus, any method
➔ *CPT Assistant* Spring 94:9

⊙ **45338** with removal of tumor(s), polyp(s), or other lesion(s) by snare technique
➔ *CPT Assistant* Spring 94:9

⊙ **45339** with ablation of tumor(s), polyp(s), or other lesion(s) not amenable to removal by hot biopsy forceps, bipolar cautery or snare technique
➔ *CPT Assistant* Spring 94:9

⊙ **45340** with dilation by balloon, 1 or more strictures
➔ *CPT Changes: An Insider's View* 2003

(Do not report 45340 in conjunction with 45345)

⊙ **45341** with endoscopic ultrasound examination
➔ *CPT Assistant* Oct 01:4, May 05:3; *CPT Changes: An Insider's View* 2001

⊙ **45342** with transendoscopic ultrasound guided intramural or transmural fine needle aspiration/biopsy(s)
➔ *CPT Assistant* Oct 01:4, May 05:3; *CPT Changes: An Insider's View* 2001

(Do not report 45341, 45342 in conjunction with 76942, 76975)

(For interpretation of specimen, see 88172-88173)

(For transrectal ultrasound utilizing rigid probe device, use 76872)

⊙ **45345** with transendoscopic stent placement (includes predilation)
➔ *CPT Assistant* Nov 01:7; *CPT Changes: An Insider's View* 2001

⊙ **45355** Colonoscopy, rigid or flexible, transabdominal via colotomy, single or multiple

(For fiberoptic colonoscopy beyond 25cm to splenic flexure, see 45330-45345)

⊙ **45378**   Colonoscopy, flexible, proximal to splenic flexure; diagnostic, with or without collection of specimen(s) by brushing or washing, with or without colon decompression (separate procedure)

➜ *CPT Assistant* Spring 94:9, Aug 99:3, Jan 02:12, Jan 04:4, May 05:3

Colonoscopy
45378

A colonoscope is inserted in the anus and moved through the colon past the splenic flexure in order to visualize the lumen of the rectum and colon.

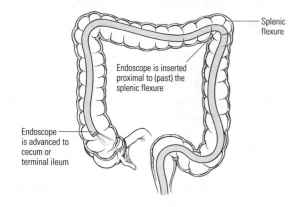

Splenic flexure

Endoscope is inserted proximal to (past) the splenic flexure

Endoscope is advanced to cecum or terminal ileum

⊙ **45379**   with removal of foreign body

➜ *CPT Assistant* Spring 94:9, Aug 99:3

⊙ **45380**   with biopsy, single or multiple

➜ *CPT Assistant* Spring 94:9, Jan 96:7, Feb 99:11, Aug 99:3, Jan 04:7, Jul 04:15

⊙ **45381**   with directed submucosal injection(s), any substance

➜ *CPT Assistant* Mar 03:22, Jan 04:7; *CPT Changes: An Insider's View* 2003

⊙ **45382**   with control of bleeding (eg, injection, bipolar cautery, unipolar cautery, laser, heater probe, stapler, plasma coagulator)

➜ *CPT Assistant* Spring 94:9, Aug 99:3; *CPT Changes: An Insider's View* 2002

⊙ **45383**   with ablation of tumor(s), polyp(s), or other lesion(s) not amenable to removal by hot biopsy forceps, bipolar cautery or snare technique

➜ *CPT Assistant* Spring 94:9, Aug 99:3, Jan 04:4

Colonoscopy With Lesion Ablation or Removal
45383, 45385

Insertion and advancement of a colonoscope through the colon and past the splenic flexure for ablation (45383) or removal (45385) of tumors, polyps, or other lesions

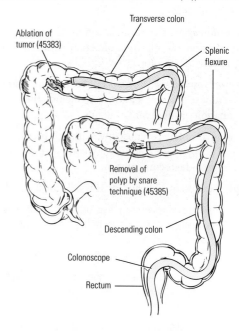

Transverse colon

Ablation of tumor (45383)

Splenic flexure

Removal of polyp by snare technique (45385)

Descending colon

Colonoscope

Rectum

⊙ **45384**   with removal of tumor(s), polyp(s), or other lesion(s) by hot biopsy forceps or bipolar cautery

➜ *CPT Assistant* Spring 94:9, Jul 98:10, Feb 99:11, Aug 99:3, Jan 04:6, Jul 04:15

⊙ **45385**   with removal of tumor(s), polyp(s), or other lesion(s) by snare technique

➜ *CPT Assistant* Spring 94:9, Jan 96:7, Jul 98:10, Aug 99:3, Jan 04:5, Jul 04:15

(For small intestine and stomal endoscopy, see 44360-44393)

⊙ **45386**   with dilation by balloon, 1 or more strictures

➜ *CPT Changes: An Insider's View* 2003

(Do not report 45386 in conjunction with 45387)

⊙ **45387**   with transendoscopic stent placement (includes predilation)

➜ *CPT Assistant* Nov 01:7; *CPT Changes: An Insider's View* 2001

⊙ **45391**   with endoscopic ultrasound examination

➜ *CPT Assistant* May 05:3; *CPT Changes: An Insider's View* 2005

(Do not report 45391 in conjunction with 45330, 45341, 45342, 45378, 76872)

⊙ **45392**   with transendoscopic ultrasound guided intramural or transmural fine needle aspiration/biopsy(s)

➔ *CPT Assistant* May 05:3; *CPT Changes: An Insider's View* 2005

(Do not report 45392 in conjunction with 45330, 45341, 45342, 45378, 76872)

Laparoscopy

Surgical laparoscopy always includes diagnostic laparoscopy. To report a diagnostic laparoscopy (peritoneoscopy) (separate procedure), use 49320.

Excision

45395   Laparoscopy, surgical; proctectomy, complete, combined abdominoperineal, with colostomy

➔ *CPT Changes: An Insider's View* 2006

(For open procedure, use 45110)

45397   proctectomy, combined abdominoperineal pull-through procedure (eg, colo-anal anastomosis), with creation of colonic reservoir (eg, J-pouch), with diverting enterostomy, when performed

➔ *CPT Changes: An Insider's View* 2006

(For open procedure, use 45119)

Repair

45400   Laparoscopy, surgical; proctopexy (for prolapse)

➔ *CPT Changes: An Insider's View* 2006

(For open procedure, use 45540, 45541)

45402   proctopexy (for prolapse), with sigmoid resection

➔ *CPT Changes: An Insider's View* 2006

(For open procedure, use 45550)

45499   Unlisted laparoscopy procedure, rectum

➔ *CPT Changes: An Insider's View* 2006

Repair

45500   Proctoplasty; for stenosis

45505   for prolapse of mucous membrane

45520   Perirectal injection of sclerosing solution for prolapse

➔ *CPT Assistant* Jul 01:11, Aug 01:10

45540   Proctopexy (eg, for prolapse); abdominal approach

➔ *CPT Changes: An Insider's View* 2006

(For laparoscopic procedure, use 45400)

45541   perineal approach

45550   with sigmoid resection, abdominal approach

➔ *CPT Changes: An Insider's View* 2006

(For laparoscopic procedure, use 45402)

45560   Repair of rectocele (separate procedure)

(For repair of rectocele with posterior colporrhaphy, use 57250)

45562   Exploration, repair, and presacral drainage for rectal injury;

45563   with colostomy

45800   Closure of rectovesical fistula;

45805   with colostomy

45820   Closure of rectourethral fistula;

45825   with colostomy

(For rectovaginal fistula closure, see 57300-57308)

Manipulation

45900   Reduction of procidentia (separate procedure) under anesthesia

45905   Dilation of anal sphincter (separate procedure) under anesthesia other than local

45910   Dilation of rectal stricture (separate procedure) under anesthesia other than local

45915   Removal of fecal impaction or foreign body (separate procedure) under anesthesia

➔ *CPT Changes: An Insider's View* 2003

Other Procedures

Surgical diagnostic anorectal exam (45990) includes the following elements: external perineal exam, digital rectal exam, pelvic exam (when performed), diagnostic anoscopy, and diagnostic rigid proctoscopy.

45990   Anorectal exam, surgical, requiring anesthesia (general, spinal, or epidural), diagnostic

➔ *CPT Changes: An Insider's View* 2006

(Do not report 45990 in conjunction with 45300-45327, 46600, 57410, 99170)

45999   Unlisted procedure, rectum

(For unlisted laparoscopic procedure, rectum, use 45499)

Anus

Incision

(For subcutaneous fistulotomy, use 46270)

46020 Placement of seton

➤ *CPT Changes: An Insider's View* 2002

(Do not report 46020 in addition to 46060, 46280, 46600)

Placement of Seton
46020

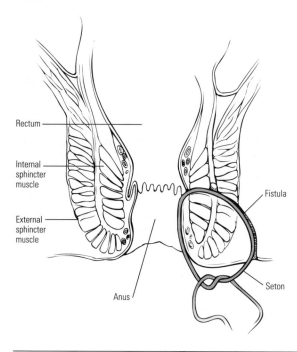

Rectum

Internal sphincter muscle

External sphincter muscle

Anus

Fistula

Seton

46030 Removal of anal seton, other marker

46040 Incision and drainage of ischiorectal and/or perirectal abscess (separate procedure)

46045 Incision and drainage of intramural, intramuscular, or submucosal abscess, transanal, under anesthesia

46050 Incision and drainage, perianal abscess, superficial

(See also 45020, 46060)

46060 Incision and drainage of ischiorectal or intramural abscess, with fistulectomy or fistulotomy, submuscular, with or without placement of seton

(Do not report 46060 in addition to 46020)

(See also 45020)

46070 Incision, anal septum (infant)

(For anoplasty, see 46700-46705)

(Do not report modifier 63 in conjunction with 46070)

46080 Sphincterotomy, anal, division of sphincter (separate procedure)

46083 Incision of thrombosed hemorrhoid, external

➤ *CPT Assistant* Jun 97:10

Excision

46200 Fissurectomy, with or without sphincterotomy

46210 Cryptectomy; single

46211 multiple (separate procedure)

46220 Papillectomy or excision of single tag, anus (separate procedure)

46221 Hemorrhoidectomy, by simple ligature (eg, rubber band)

➤ *CPT Assistant* Oct 97:8

46230 Excision of external hemorrhoid tags and/or multiple papillae

46250 Hemorrhoidectomy, external, complete

46255 Hemorrhoidectomy, internal and external, simple;

46257 with fissurectomy

46258 with fistulectomy, with or without fissurectomy

46260 Hemorrhoidectomy, internal and external, complex or extensive;

46261 with fissurectomy

46262 with fistulectomy, with or without fissurectomy

➤ *CPT Assistant* May 05:3

(For injection of hemorrhoids, use 46500; for destruction, see 46934-46936; for ligation, see 46945, 46946; for hemorrhoidopexy, use 46947)

46270 Surgical treatment of anal fistula (fistulectomy/fistulotomy); subcutaneous

46275 submuscular

46280 complex or multiple, with or without placement of seton

(Do not report 46280 in addition to 46020)

46285 second stage

46288 Closure of anal fistula with rectal advancement flap

46320 Enucleation or excision of external thrombotic hemorrhoid

Introduction

46500 Injection of sclerosing solution, hemorrhoids

➤ *CPT Assistant* May 05:3

(For excision of hemorrhoids, see 46250-46262; for destruction, see 46934-46936; for ligation, see 46945, 46946; for hemorrhoidopexy, use 46947)

46505   Chemodenervation of internal anal sphincter
> *CPT Changes: An Insider's View* 2006

(For chemodenervation of other muscles, see 64612-64614, 64640)

(Report the specific service in conjunction with the specific substance(s) or drug(s) provided)

Endoscopy

Surgical endoscopy always includes diagnostic endoscopy.

46600   Anoscopy; diagnostic, with or without collection of specimen(s) by brushing or washing (separate procedure)
> *CPT Assistant* Spring 94:9, Oct 97:6, Apr 06:1

(Do not report 46600 in addition to 46020)

46604   with dilation (eg, balloon, guide wire, bougie)
> *CPT Assistant* Spring 94:9, Oct 97:6; *CPT Changes: An Insider's View* 2002

46606   with biopsy, single or multiple
> *CPT Assistant* Spring 94:9, Oct 97:6

46608   with removal of foreign body
> *CPT Assistant* Spring 94:9, Oct 97:6

46610   with removal of single tumor, polyp, or other lesion by hot biopsy forceps or bipolar cautery
> *CPT Assistant* Spring 94:10, Oct 97:6

46611   with removal of single tumor, polyp, or other lesion by snare technique
> *CPT Assistant* Spring 94:10, Oct 97:6

46612   with removal of multiple tumors, polyps, or other lesions by hot biopsy forceps, bipolar cautery or snare technique
> *CPT Assistant* Spring 94:10, Oct 97:6

46614   with control of bleeding (eg, injection, bipolar cautery, unipolar cautery, laser, heater probe, stapler, plasma coagulator)
> *CPT Assistant* Spring 94:10, Oct 97:6; *CPT Changes: An Insider's View* 2002

46615   with ablation of tumor(s), polyp(s), or other lesion(s) not amenable to removal by hot biopsy forceps, bipolar cautery or snare technique
> *CPT Assistant* Spring 94:10, Oct 97:6

Repair

46700   Anoplasty, plastic operation for stricture; adult

46705   infant

(For simple incision of anal septum, use 46070)

(Do not report modifier 63 in conjunction with 46705)

46706   Repair of anal fistula with fibrin glue
> *CPT Changes: An Insider's View* 2003

46710   Repair of ileoanal pouch fistula/sinus (eg, perineal or vaginal), pouch advancement; transperineal approach
> *CPT Changes: An Insider's View* 2006

46712   combined transperineal and transabdominal approach
> *CPT Changes: An Insider's View* 2006

46715   Repair of low imperforate anus; with anoperineal fistula (cut-back procedure)

46716   with transposition of anoperineal or anovestibular fistula

(Do not report modifier 63 in conjunction with 46715, 46716)

46730   Repair of high imperforate anus without fistula; perineal or sacroperineal approach

46735   combined transabdominal and sacroperineal approaches

(Do not report modifier 63 in conjunction with 46730, 46735)

46740   Repair of high imperforate anus with rectourethral or rectovaginal fistula; perineal or sacroperineal approach

46742   combined transabdominal and sacroperineal approaches

(Do not report modifier 63 in conjunction with 46740, 46742)

46744   Repair of cloacal anomaly by anorectovaginoplasty and urethroplasty, sacroperineal approach

(Do not report modifier 63 in conjunction with 46744)

46746   Repair of cloacal anomaly by anorectovaginoplasty and urethroplasty, combined abdominal and sacroperineal approach;

46748   with vaginal lengthening by intestinal graft or pedicle flaps

46750   Sphincteroplasty, anal, for incontinence or prolapse; adult

46751   child

46753   Graft (Thiersch operation) for rectal incontinence and/or prolapse

46754   Removal of Thiersch wire or suture, anal canal

46760   Sphincteroplasty, anal, for incontinence, adult; muscle transplant

46761   levator muscle imbrication (Park posterior anal repair)

46762   implantation artificial sphincter

Destruction

46900 Destruction of lesion(s), anus (eg, condyloma, papilloma, molluscum contagiosum, herpetic vesicle), simple; chemical

46910 electrodesiccation

46916 cryosurgery

46917 laser surgery

46922 surgical excision

46924 Destruction of lesion(s), anus (eg, condyloma, papilloma, molluscum contagiosum, herpetic vesicle), extensive (eg, laser surgery, electrosurgery, cryosurgery, chemosurgery)
➲ *CPT Changes: An Insider's View* 2002

46934 Destruction of hemorrhoids, any method; internal

46935 external

46936 internal and external
➲ *CPT Assistant* May 05:3

(For excision of hemorrhoids, see 46250-46262; for injection, use 46500; for ligation, see 46945, 46946; for hemorrhoidopexy, use 46947)

46937 Cryosurgery of rectal tumor; benign

46938 malignant

46940 Curettage or cautery of anal fissure, including dilation of anal sphincter (separate procedure); initial
➲ *CPT Changes: An Insider's View* 2002

46942 subsequent

Suture

46945 Ligation of internal hemorrhoids; single procedure

46946 multiple procedures

46947 Hemorrhoidopexy (eg, for prolapsing internal hemorrhoids) by stapling
➲ *CPT Assistant* May 05:3, 14; *CPT Changes: An Insider's View* 2005

(For excision of hemorrhoids, see 46250-46262; for injection, use 46500; for destruction, see 46934-46936)

Other Procedures

46999 Unlisted procedure, anus
➲ *CPT Assistant* Oct 97:8

Liver

Incision

47000 Biopsy of liver, needle; percutaneous
➲ *CPT Assistant* Fall 93:12

(If imaging guidance is performed, see 76942, 77002, 77012, 77021)

+ 47001 when done for indicated purpose at time of other major procedure (List separately in addition to code for primary procedure)

(If imaging guidance is performed, see 76942, 77002)

(For fine needle aspiration in conjunction with 47000, 47001, see 10021, 10022)

(For evaluation of fine needle aspirate in conjunction with 47000, 47001, see 88172, 88173)

47010 Hepatotomy; for open drainage of abscess or cyst, one or two stages
➲ *CPT Assistant* Nov 97:18

⊙ **47011** for percutaneous drainage of abscess or cyst, one or two stages
➲ *CPT Assistant* Nov 97:18, Mar 98:8

(For radiological supervision and interpretation, use 75989)

47015 Laparotomy, with aspiration and/or injection of hepatic parasitic (eg, amoebic or echinococcal) cyst(s) or abscess(es)

Excision

47100 Biopsy of liver, wedge

47120 Hepatectomy, resection of liver; partial lobectomy
➲ *CPT Assistant* May 98:10

47122 trisegmentectomy

47125 total left lobectomy

47130 total right lobectomy

Liver Transplantation

Liver allotransplantation involves three distinct components of physician work:

1) ***Cadaver donor hepatectomy***, which includes harvesting the graft and cold preservation of the graft (perfusing with cold preservation solution and cold maintenance) (use 47133). ***Living donor hepatectomy***, which includes harvesting the graft, cold preservation of the graft (perfusing with cold preservation solution and cold maintenance), and care of the donor (see 47140-47142).

2) ***Backbench work***:

Standard preparation of the whole liver graft will include one of the following:

Preparation of whole liver graft (including cholecystectomy, if necessary, and dissection and removal of surrounding soft tissues to prepare vena cava, portal vein, hepatic artery, and common bile duct for implantation) (use 47143).

Preparation as described for whole liver graft, plus trisegment split into two partial grafts (use 47144).

Preparation as described for whole liver graft, plus lobe split into two partial grafts (use 47145).

Additional reconstruction of the liver graft may include venous and/or arterial anastomosis(es) (see 47146, 47147).

3) ***Recipient liver allotransplantation***, which includes recipient hepatectomy (partial or whole), transplantation of the allograft (partial or whole), and care of the recipient (see 47135, 47136).

47133   Donor hepatectomy (including cold preservation), from cadaver donor
   ➔ *CPT Changes: An Insider's View* 2005

47135   Liver allotransplantation; orthotopic, partial or whole, from cadaver or living donor, any age

47136   heterotopic, partial or whole, from cadaver or living donor, any age

47140   Donor hepatectomy (including cold preservation), from living donor; left lateral segment only (segments II and III)
   ➔ *CPT Changes: An Insider's View* 2004, 2005

47141   total left lobectomy (segments II, III and IV)
   ➔ *CPT Changes: An Insider's View* 2004

47142   total right lobectomy (segments V, VI, VII and VIII)
   ➔ *CPT Changes: An Insider's View* 2004

47143   Backbench standard preparation of cadaver donor whole liver graft prior to allotransplantation, including cholecystectomy, if necessary, and dissection and removal of surrounding soft tissues to prepare the vena cava, portal vein, hepatic artery, and common bile duct for implantation; without trisegment or lobe split
   ➔ *CPT Assistant* Apr 05:10, 12; *CPT Changes: An Insider's View* 2005

47144   with trisegment split of whole liver graft into two partial liver grafts (ie, left lateral segment (segments II and III) and right trisegment (segments I and IV through VIII))
   ➔ *CPT Changes: An Insider's View* 2005

47145   with lobe split of whole liver graft into two partial liver grafts (ie, left lobe (segments II, III, and IV) and right lobe (segments I and V through VIII))
   ➔ *CPT Changes: An Insider's View* 2005

47146   Backbench reconstruction of cadaver or living donor liver graft prior to allotransplantation; venous anastomosis, each
   ➔ *CPT Changes: An Insider's View* 2005

47147   arterial anastomosis, each
   ➔ *CPT Changes: An Insider's View* 2005

   (Do not report 47143-47147 in conjunction with 47120-47125, 47600, 47610)

Repair

47300   Marsupialization of cyst or abscess of liver

47350   Management of liver hemorrhage; simple suture of liver wound or injury

47360   complex suture of liver wound or injury, with or without hepatic artery ligation

47361   exploration of hepatic wound, extensive debridement, coagulation and/or suture, with or without packing of liver

47362   re-exploration of hepatic wound for removal of packing

Laparoscopy

Surgical laparoscopy always includes diagnostic laparoscopy. To report a diagnostic laparoscopy (peritoneoscopy) (separate procedure), use 49320.

47370   Laparoscopy, surgical, ablation of one or more liver tumor(s); radiofrequency
   ➔ *CPT Assistant* Oct 02:2; *CPT Changes: An Insider's View* 2002

   (For imaging guidance, use 76940)

47371   cryosurgical
   ➔ *CPT Changes: An Insider's View* 2002

   (For imaging guidance, use 76940)

47379   Unlisted laparoscopic procedure, liver
   ➔ *CPT Changes: An Insider's View* 2001

Other Procedures

47380   Ablation, open, of one or more liver tumor(s); radiofrequency
   ➔ *CPT Assistant* Oct 02:1; *CPT Changes: An Insider's View* 2002

   (For imaging guidance, use 76940)

47381   cryosurgical
   ➔ *CPT Changes: An Insider's View* 2002

   (For imaging guidance, use 76940)

47382   Ablation, one or more liver tumor(s), percutaneous, radiofrequency

➔ *CPT Assistant* Oct 02:1; *CPT Changes: An Insider's View* 2002

(For imaging guidance and monitoring, see 76940, 77013, 77022)

47399   Unlisted procedure, liver

Biliary Tract

Incision

47400   Hepaticotomy or hepaticostomy with exploration, drainage, or removal of calculus

47420   Choledochotomy or choledochostomy with exploration, drainage, or removal of calculus, with or without cholecystotomy; without transduodenal sphincterotomy or sphincteroplasty

47425   with transduodenal sphincterotomy or sphincteroplasty

47460   Transduodenal sphincterotomy or sphincteroplasty, with or without transduodenal extraction of calculus (separate procedure)

47480   Cholecystotomy or cholecystostomy with exploration, drainage, or removal of calculus (separate procedure)

47490   Percutaneous cholecystostomy

(For radiological supervision and interpretation, use 75989)

Introduction

47500   Injection procedure for percutaneous transhepatic cholangiography

(For radiological supervision and interpretation, use 74320)

47505   Injection procedure for cholangiography through an existing catheter (eg, percutaneous transhepatic or T-tube)

(For radiological supervision and interpretation, use 74305)

47510   Introduction of percutaneous transhepatic catheter for biliary drainage

(For radiological supervision and interpretation, use 75980)

47511   Introduction of percutaneous transhepatic stent for internal and external biliary drainage

(For radiological supervision and interpretation, use 75982)

47525   Change of percutaneous biliary drainage catheter

(For radiological supervision and interpretation, use 75984)

47530   Revision and/or reinsertion of transhepatic tube

(For radiological supervision and interpretation, use 75984)

Endoscopy

Surgical endoscopy always includes diagnostic endoscopy.

+ 47550   Biliary endoscopy, intraoperative (choledochoscopy) (List separately in addition to code for primary procedure)

47552   Biliary endoscopy, percutaneous via T-tube or other tract; diagnostic, with or without collection of specimen(s) by brushing and/or washing (separate procedure)

47553   with biopsy, single or multiple

47554   with removal of calculus/calculi

➔ *CPT Changes: An Insider's View* 2002

47555   with dilation of biliary duct stricture(s) without stent

47556   with dilation of biliary duct stricture(s) with stent

(For ERCP, see 43260-43272, 74363)

(If imaging guidance is performed, see 74363, 75982)

Laparoscopy

Surgical laparoscopy always includes diagnostic laparoscopy. To report a diagnostic laparoscopy (peritoneoscopy) (separate procedure), use 49320.

47560   Laparoscopy, surgical; with guided transhepatic cholangiography, without biopsy

➔ *CPT Assistant* Nov 99:23, Mar 00:9; *CPT Changes: An Insider's View* 2000

47561   with guided transhepatic cholangiography with biopsy

➔ *CPT Assistant* Nov 99:23, Mar 00:9; *CPT Changes: An Insider's View* 2000

47562   cholecystectomy
> *CPT Assistant* Nov 99:23, Mar 00:9, Sep 03:3; *CPT Changes: An Insider's View* 2000

Laparoscopic Cholecystectomy
47562

The gallbladder is dissected and removed from the liver bed under laparoscopic guidance.

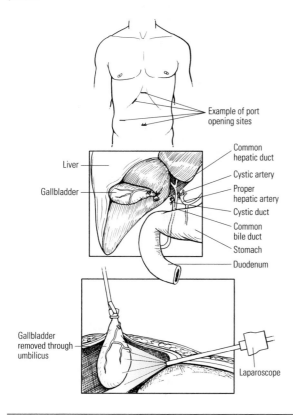

Liver
Gallbladder

Example of port opening sites

Common hepatic duct
Cystic artery
Proper hepatic artery
Cystic duct
Common bile duct
Stomach
Duodenum

Gallbladder removed through umbilicus

Laparoscope

47563   cholecystectomy with cholangiography
> *CPT Assistant* Nov 99:23, Mar 00:9, Dec 00:14; *CPT Changes: An Insider's View* 2000

47564   cholecystectomy with exploration of common duct
> *CPT Assistant* Nov 99:23, Mar 00:9; *CPT Changes: An Insider's View* 2000

47570   cholecystoenterostomy
> *CPT Assistant* Nov 99:23, Mar 00:9; *CPT Changes: An Insider's View* 2000

47579   Unlisted laparoscopy procedure, biliary tract
> *CPT Assistant* Nov 99:23, Mar 00:9; *CPT Changes: An Insider's View* 2000

Excision

47600   Cholecystectomy;
> *CPT Assistant* Fall 92:19, Nov 99:24; *CPT Changes: An Insider's View* 2000

47605   with cholangiography
> *CPT Assistant* Nov 99:24, Apr 02:19; *CPT Changes: An Insider's View* 2000

(For laparoscopic approach, see 47562-47564)

47610   Cholecystectomy with exploration of common duct;
> *CPT Assistant* Apr 02:19

(For cholecystectomy with exploration of common duct with biliary endoscopy, use 47610 with 47550)

47612   with choledochoenterostomy

47620   with transduodenal sphincterotomy or sphincteroplasty, with or without cholangiography

47630   Biliary duct stone extraction, percutaneous via T-tube tract, basket, or snare (eg, Burhenne technique)
> *CPT Assistant* Jun 98:10

(For radiological supervision and interpretation, use 74327)

47700   Exploration for congenital atresia of bile ducts, without repair, with or without liver biopsy, with or without cholangiography

(Do not report modifier 63 in conjunction with 47700)

47701   Portoenterostomy (eg, Kasai procedure)

(Do not report modifier 63 in conjunction with 47701)

47711   Excision of bile duct tumor, with or without primary repair of bile duct; extrahepatic

47712   intrahepatic

(For anastomosis, see 47760-47800)

47715   Excision of choledochal cyst

Repair

▶(47719 has been deleted)◀

47720   Cholecystoenterostomy; direct
> *CPT Assistant* Nov 99:24; *CPT Changes: An Insider's View* 2000

(For laparoscopic approach, use 47570)

47721   with gastroenterostomy

47740   Roux-en-Y

47741   Roux-en-Y with gastroenterostomy

47760   Anastomosis, of extrahepatic biliary ducts and gastrointestinal tract

47765   Anastomosis, of intrahepatic ducts and gastrointestinal tract

47780   Anastomosis, Roux-en-Y, of extrahepatic biliary ducts and gastrointestinal tract

47785   Anastomosis, Roux-en-Y, of intrahepatic biliary ducts and gastrointestinal tract

47800   Reconstruction, plastic, of extrahepatic biliary ducts with end-to-end anastomosis

47801   Placement of choledochal stent

47802	U-tube hepaticoenterostomy
47900	Suture of extrahepatic biliary duct for pre-existing injury (separate procedure)

Other Procedures

47999	Unlisted procedure, biliary tract

Pancreas

(For peroral pancreatic endoscopic procedures, see 43260-43272)

Incision

48000	Placement of drains, peripancreatic, for acute pancreatitis;
48001	with cholecystostomy, gastrostomy, and jejunostomy

(48005 has been deleted. To report, see 48105)

48020	Removal of pancreatic calculus

➔ *CPT Assistant* Spring 91:7

Excision

48100	Biopsy of pancreas, open (eg, fine needle aspiration, needle core biopsy, wedge biopsy)

➔ *CPT Changes: An Insider's View* 2002

48102	Biopsy of pancreas, percutaneous needle

(For radiological supervision and interpretation, see 76942, 77002, 77012, 77021)

(For fine needle aspiration, use 10022)

(For evaluation of fine needle aspirate, see 88172, 88173)

48105	Resection or debridement of pancreas and peripancreatic tissue for acute necrotizing pancreatitis

➔ *CPT Changes: An Insider's View* 2007

48120	Excision of lesion of pancreas (eg, cyst, adenoma)
48140	Pancreatectomy, distal subtotal, with or without splenectomy; without pancreaticojejunostomy
48145	with pancreaticojejunostomy
48146	Pancreatectomy, distal, near-total with preservation of duodenum (Child-type procedure)
48148	Excision of ampulla of Vater
48150	Pancreatectomy, proximal subtotal with total duodenectomy, partial gastrectomy, choledochoenterostomy and gastrojejunostomy (Whipple-type procedure); with pancreatojejunostomy
48152	without pancreatojejunostomy

48153	Pancreatectomy, proximal subtotal with near-total duodenectomy, choledochoenterostomy and duodenojejunostomy (pylorus-sparing, Whipple-type procedure); with pancreatojejunostomy
48154	without pancreatojejunostomy
48155	Pancreatectomy, total
48160	Pancreatectomy, total or subtotal, with autologous transplantation of pancreas or pancreatic islet cells

➔ *CPT Changes: An Insider's View* 2002

(48180 has been deleted. To report, see 48548)

Introduction

✚ 48400	Injection procedure for intraoperative pancreatography (List separately in addition to code for primary procedure)

(For radiological supervision and interpretation, see 74300-74305)

Repair

48500	Marsupialization of pancreatic cyst

➔ *CPT Changes: An Insider's View* 2002

48510	External drainage, pseudocyst of pancreas; open

➔ *CPT Assistant* Nov 97:18

⊙ 48511	percutaneous

➔ *CPT Assistant* Nov 97:18, Mar 98:8

(For radiological supervision and interpretation, use 75989)

48520	Internal anastomosis of pancreatic cyst to gastrointestinal tract; direct
48540	Roux-en-Y
48545	Pancreatorrhaphy for injury

➔ *CPT Changes: An Insider's View* 2002

48547	Duodenal exclusion with gastrojejunostomy for pancreatic injury

➔ *CPT Changes: An Insider's View* 2002

48548	Pancreaticojejunostomy, side-to-side anastomosis (Puestow-type operation)

➔ *CPT Changes: An Insider's View* 2007

Pancreas Transplantation

Pancreas allotransplantation involves three distinct components of physician work:

1) **Cadaver donor pancreatectomy**, which includes harvesting the pancreas graft, with or without duodenal segment, and cold preservation of the graft (perfusing with cold preservation solution and cold maintenance) (use 48550).

2) ***Backbench work***:

Standard preparation of a cadaver donor pancreas allograft prior to transplantation includes dissection of the allograft from surrounding soft tissues, splenectomy, duodenotomy, ligation of bile duct, ligation of mesenteric vessels, and Y-graft arterial anastomoses from the iliac artery to the superior mesenteric artery and to the splenic artery (use 48551).

Additional reconstruction of a cadaver donor pancreas allograft prior to transplantation may include venous anastomosis(es) (use 48552).

3) ***Recipient pancreas allotransplantation***, which includes transplantation of allograft, and care of the recipient (use 48554).

48550 Donor pancreatectomy (including cold preservation), with or without duodenal segment for transplantation
> *CPT Assistant* Apr 05:10, 12; *CPT Changes: An Insider's View* 2005

48551 Backbench standard preparation of cadaver donor pancreas allograft prior to transplantation, including dissection of allograft from surrounding soft tissues, splenectomy, duodenotomy, ligation of bile duct, ligation of mesenteric vessels, and Y-graft arterial anastomoses from iliac artery to superior mesenteric artery and to splenic artery
> *CPT Changes: An Insider's View* 2005

48552 Backbench reconstruction of cadaver donor pancreas allograft prior to transplantation, venous anastomosis, each
> *CPT Changes: An Insider's View* 2005

(Do not report 48551 and 48552 in conjunction with 35531, 35563, 35685, 38100-38102, 44010, 44820, 44850, 47460, 47505-47525, 47550-47556, 48100-48120, 48545)

48554 Transplantation of pancreatic allograft

48556 Removal of transplanted pancreatic allograft

Other Procedures

48999 Unlisted procedure, pancreas

Abdomen, Peritoneum, and Omentum

Incision

49000 Exploratory laparotomy, exploratory celiotomy with or without biopsy(s) (separate procedure)
> *CPT Assistant* Fall 92:23, Mar 01:10

(To report wound exploration due to penetrating trauma without laparotomy, use 20102)

49002 Reopening of recent laparotomy
> *CPT Assistant* Fall 92:23

(To report re-exploration of hepatic wound for removal of packing, use 47362)

49010 Exploration, retroperitoneal area with or without biopsy(s) (separate procedure)

(To report wound exploration due to penetrating trauma without laparotomy, use 20102)

49020 Drainage of peritoneal abscess or localized peritonitis, exclusive of appendiceal abscess; open

(For appendiceal abscess, use 44900)

⊙ **49021** percutaneous

(For radiological supervision and interpretation, use 75989)

49040 Drainage of subdiaphragmatic or subphrenic abscess; open
> *CPT Assistant* Nov 97:18

⊙ **49041** percutaneous
> *CPT Assistant* Nov 97:18, Mar 98:8

(For radiological supervision and interpretation, use 75989)

49060 Drainage of retroperitoneal abscess; open
> *CPT Assistant* Nov 97:18, Nov 99:24, Jul 01:11, Aug 01:10; *CPT Changes: An Insider's View* 2000

⊙ **49061** percutaneous
> *CPT Assistant* Nov 97:18, Mar 98:8, Nov 99:24, Jul 01:11, Aug 01:10; *CPT Changes: An Insider's View* 2000

(For laparoscopic drainage, use 49323)

(For radiological supervision and interpretation, use 75989)

49062 Drainage of extraperitoneal lymphocele to peritoneal cavity, open
> *CPT Assistant* Nov 97:19, Jul 01:11, Aug 01:10

49080 Peritoneocentesis, abdominal paracentesis, or peritoneal lavage (diagnostic or therapeutic); initial

49081 subsequent

(If imaging guidance is performed, see 76942, 77012)

(49085 has been deleted. To report, see 49402)

Excision, Destruction

(For lysis of intestinal adhesions, use 44005)

49180 Biopsy, abdominal or retroperitoneal mass, percutaneous needle
> *CPT Assistant* Fall 93:11

(If imaging guidance is performed, see 76942, 77002, 77012, 77021)

(For fine needle aspiration, use 10021 or 10022)

(For evaluation of fine needle aspirate, see 88172, 88173)

▶(49200, 49201 have been deleted. To report, see 49203-49205, 58957, 58958)◀

● **49203** Excision or destruction, open, intra-abdominal tumors, cysts or endometriomas, 1 or more peritoneal, mesenteric, or retroperitoneal primary or secondary tumors; largest tumor 5 cm diameter or less
→ CPT Changes: An Insider's View 2008

● **49204** largest tumor 5.1-10.0 cm diameter
→ CPT Changes: An Insider's View 2008

● **49205** largest tumor greater than 10.0 cm diameter
→ CPT Changes: An Insider's View 2008

▶(Do not report 49203-49205 in conjunction with 38770, 38780, 49000, 49010, 49215, 50010, 50205, 50225, 50236, 50250, 50290, 58900-58960)◀

▶(For partial or total nephrectomy, use 50220 or 50240 in conjunction with 49203-49205)◀

▶(For colectomy, use 44140 in conjunction with 49203-49205)◀

▶(For small bowel resection, use 44120 in conjunction with 49203-49205)◀

▶(For vena caval resection with reconstruction, use 49203-49205 in conjunction with 37799)◀

(For resection of recurrent ovarian, tubal, primary peritoneal, or uterine malignancy, see 58957, 58958)

▶(For cryoablation of renal tumors, see 50250, 50593)◀

49215 Excision of presacral or sacrococcygeal tumor

(Do not report modifier 63 in conjunction with 49215)

49220 Staging laparotomy for Hodgkins disease or lymphoma (includes splenectomy, needle or open biopsies of both liver lobes, possibly also removal of abdominal nodes, abdominal node and/or bone marrow biopsies, ovarian repositioning)
→ CPT Changes: An Insider's View 2002

49250 Umbilectomy, omphalectomy, excision of umbilicus (separate procedure)

49255 Omentectomy, epiploectomy, resection of omentum (separate procedure)
→ CPT Assistant Nov 99:24; CPT Changes: An Insider's View 2000

Laparoscopy

Surgical laparoscopy always includes diagnostic laparoscopy. To report a diagnostic laparoscopy (peritoneoscopy), (separate procedure), use 49320.

For laparoscopic fulguration or excision of lesions of the ovary, pelvic viscera, or peritoneal surface use 58662.

49320 Laparoscopy, abdomen, peritoneum, and omentum, diagnostic, with or without collection of specimen(s) by brushing or washing (separate procedure)
→ CPT Assistant Nov 99:24, Mar 00:9, Apr 06:19, Mar 07:4; CPT Changes: An Insider's View 2000, 2001

Laparoscopy
49320

The physician inserts a fiberoptic laparoscope to observe the necessary organs in these procedures.

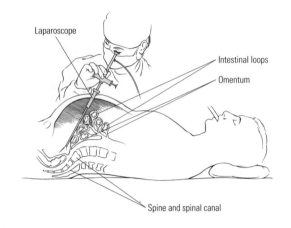

Laparoscope

Intestinal loops

Omentum

Spine and spinal canal

49321 Laparoscopy, surgical; with biopsy (single or multiple)
→ CPT Assistant Nov 99:24, Mar 00:9; CPT Changes: An Insider's View 2000, 2001

49322 with aspiration of cavity or cyst (eg, ovarian cyst) (single or multiple)
→ CPT Assistant Nov 99:24, Mar 00:9; CPT Changes: An Insider's View 2000

49323 with drainage of lymphocele to peritoneal cavity
→ CPT Assistant Nov 99:24, Mar 00:9, May 00:4, Jul 01:11, Aug 01:10; CPT Changes: An Insider's View 2000

(For percutaneous or open drainage, see 49060, 49061)

49324 with insertion of intraperitoneal cannula or catheter, permanent
→ CPT Changes: An Insider's View 2007

(For subcutaneous extension of intraperitoneal catheter with remote chest exit site, use 49435 in conjunction with 49324)

(For open insertion of permanent intraperitoneal cannula or catheter, use 49421)

49325 with revision of previously placed intraperitoneal cannula or catheter, with removal of intraluminal obstructive material if performed
→ CPT Changes: An Insider's View 2007

✚ **49326** with omentopexy (omental tacking procedure) (List separately in addition to code for primary procedure)
→ CPT Changes: An Insider's View 2007

(Use 49326 in conjunction with 49324, 49325)

49329   Unlisted laparoscopy procedure, abdomen, peritoneum and omentum

> *CPT Assistant* Nov 99:24, Mar 00:9, Feb 06:16; *CPT Changes: An Insider's View* 2000

Introduction, Revision, Removal

49400   Injection of air or contrast into peritoneal cavity (separate procedure)

(For radiological supervision and interpretation, use 74190)

49402   Removal of peritoneal foreign body from peritoneal cavity

> *CPT Changes: An Insider's View* 2007

(For lysis of intestinal adhesions, use 44005)

49419   Insertion of intraperitoneal cannula or catheter, with subcutaneous reservoir, permanent (ie, totally implantable)

> *CPT Changes: An Insider's View* 2003

(For removal, use 49422)

49420   Insertion of intraperitoneal cannula or catheter for drainage or dialysis; temporary

> *CPT Assistant* Fall 93:2

49421   permanent

> *CPT Assistant* Fall 93:2, Jul 06:19

(For laparoscopic insertion of permanent intraperitoneal cannula or catheter, use 49324)

(For subcutaneous extension of intraperitoneal catheter with remote chest exit site, use 49435 in conjunction with 49421)

49422   Removal of permanent intraperitoneal cannula or catheter

(For removal of a temporary catheter/cannula, use appropriate E/M code)

49423   Exchange of previously placed abscess or cyst drainage catheter under radiological guidance (separate procedure)

> *CPT Assistant* Nov 97:19, Mar 98:8

(For radiological supervision and interpretation, use 75984)

49424   Contrast injection for assessment of abscess or cyst via previously placed drainage catheter or tube (separate procedure)

> *CPT Assistant* Nov 97:19, Mar 98:8, Nov 03:14; *CPT Changes: An Insider's View* 2002

(For radiological supervision and interpretation, use 76080)

49425   Insertion of peritoneal-venous shunt

49426   Revision of peritoneal-venous shunt

(For shunt patency test, use 78291)

49427   Injection procedure (eg, contrast media) for evaluation of previously placed peritoneal-venous shunt

(For radiological supervision and interpretation, see 75809, 78291)

49428   Ligation of peritoneal-venous shunt

49429   Removal of peritoneal-venous shunt

+ 49435   Insertion of subcutaneous extension to intraperitoneal cannula or catheter with remote chest exit site (List separately in addition to code for primary procedure)

> *CPT Changes: An Insider's View* 2007

(Use 49435 in conjunction with 49324, 49421)

49436   Delayed creation of exit site from embedded subcutaneous segment of intraperitoneal cannula or catheter

> *CPT Changes: An Insider's View* 2007

▶Initial Placement◀

▶Do not additionally report 43752 for placement of a nasogastric (NG) or orogastric (OG) tube to insufflate the stomach prior to percutaneous gastrointestinal tube placement. NG or OG tube placement is considered part of the procedure in this family of codes.◀

⊙● **49440**   Insertion of gastrostomy tube, percutaneous, under fluoroscopic guidance including contrast injection(s), image documentation and report

> *CPT Changes: An Insider's View* 2008

▶(For conversion to a gastro-jejunostomy tube at the time of initial gastrostomy tube placement, use 49440 in conjunction with 49446)◀

⊙● **49441**   Insertion of duodenostomy or jejunostomy tube, percutaneous, under fluoroscopic guidance including contrast injection(s), image documentation and report

> *CPT Changes: An Insider's View* 2008

▶(For conversion of gastrostomy tube to gastro-jejunostomy tube, use 49446)◀

⊙● **49442**   Insertion of cecostomy or other colonic tube, percutaneous, under fluoroscopic guidance including contrast injection(s), image documentation and report

> *CPT Changes: An Insider's View* 2008

▶Conversion◀

⊙● **49446**   Conversion of gastrostomy tube to gastro-jejunostomy tube, percutaneous, under fluoroscopic guidance including contrast injection(s), image documentation and report

> *CPT Changes: An Insider's View* 2008

▶(For conversion to a gastro-jejunostomy tube at the time of initial gastrostomy tube placement, use 49446 in conjunction with 49440)◀

►Replacement◄

►If an existing gastrostomy, duodenostomy, jejunostomy, gastro-jejunostomy, or cecostomy (or other colonic) tube is removed and a new tube is placed via a separate percutaneous access site, the placement of the new tube is not considered a replacement and would be reported using the appropriate initial placement codes 49440-49442.◄

● **49450** Replacement of gastrostomy or cecostomy (or other colonic) tube, percutaneous, under fluoroscopic guidance including contrast injection(s), image documentation and report

   ⮕ *CPT Changes: An Insider's View* 2008

● **49451** Replacement of duodenostomy or jejunostomy tube, percutaneous, under fluoroscopic guidance including contrast injection(s), image documentation and report

   ⮕ *CPT Changes: An Insider's View* 2008

● **49452** Replacement of gastro-jejunostomy tube, percutaneous, under fluoroscopic guidance including contrast injection(s), image documentation and report

   ⮕ *CPT Changes: An Insider's View* 2008

►Mechanical Removal of Obstructive Material◄

● **49460** Mechanical removal of obstructive material from gastrostomy, duodenostomy, jejunostomy, gastro-jejunostomy, or cecostomy (or other colonic) tube, any method, under fluoroscopic guidance including contrast injection(s), if performed, image documentation and report

   ⮕ *CPT Changes: An Insider's View* 2008

   ►(Do not report 49460 in conjunction with 49450-49452, 49465)◄

►Other◄

● **49465** Contrast injection(s) for radiological evaluation of existing gastrostomy, duodenostomy, jejunostomy, gastro-jejunostomy, or cecostomy (or other colonic) tube, from a percutaneous approach including image documentation and report

   ⮕ *CPT Changes: An Insider's View* 2008

   ►(Do not report 49465 in conjunction with 49450-49460)◄

Repair

Hernioplasty, Herniorrhaphy, Herniotomy

The hernia repair codes in this section are categorized primarily by the type of hernia (inguinal, femoral, incisional, etc).

Some types of hernias are further categorized as "initial" or "recurrent" based on whether or not the hernia has required previous repair(s).

Additional variables accounted for by some of the codes include patient age and clinical presentation (reducible vs. incarcerated or strangulated).

With the exception of the incisional hernia repairs (see 49560-49566) the use of mesh or other prostheses is not separately reported.

The excision/repair of strangulated organs or structures such as testicle(s), intestine, ovaries are reported by using the appropriate code for the excision/repair (eg, 44120, 54520, and 58940) in addition to the appropriate code for the repair of the strangulated hernia.

   (For reduction and repair of intra-abdominal hernia, use 44050)

   (For debridement of abdominal wall, see 11042, 11043)

   (Codes 49491-49651 are unilateral procedures. To report bilateral procedures, report modifier 50 with the appropriate procedure code)

49491 Repair, initial inguinal hernia, preterm infant (younger than 37 weeks gestation at birth), performed from birth up to 50 weeks postconception age, with or without hydrocelectomy; reducible

   ⮕ *CPT Assistant* Mar 04:2; *CPT Changes: An Insider's View* 2002

49492   incarcerated or strangulated

   ⮕ *CPT Assistant* Mar 04:2; *CPT Changes: An Insider's View* 2002

   (Do not report modifier 63 in conjunction with 49491, 49492)

   (Postconception age equals gestational age at birth plus age of infant in weeks at the time of the hernia repair. Initial inguinal hernia repairs that are performed on preterm infants who are older than 50 weeks postconception age and younger than age 6 months at the time of surgery, should be reported using codes 49495, 49496)

49495 Repair, initial inguinal hernia, full term infant younger than age 6 months, or preterm infant older than 50 weeks postconception age and younger than age 6 months at the time of surgery, with or without hydrocelectomy; reducible

   ⮕ *CPT Assistant* Winter 93:6, Winter 94:13, Jan 04:27, Mar 04:10, May 04:14; *CPT Changes: An Insider's View* 2002

49496   incarcerated or strangulated
➔ *CPT Assistant* Winter 93:6, Winter 94:13, Jan 04:27,
Mar 04:10, May 04:14

(Do not report modifier 63 in conjunction with 49495,
49496)

(Postconception age equals gestational age at birth plus
age in weeks at the time of the hernia repair. Initial
inguinal hernia repairs that are performed on preterm
infants who are younger than or up to 50 weeks
postconception age but younger than 6 months of age
since birth, should be reported using codes 49491, 49492.
Inguinal hernia repairs on infants age 6 months to
younger than 5 years should be reported using codes
49500-49501)

49500   Repair initial inguinal hernia, age 6 months to younger
than 5 years, with or without hydrocelectomy; reducible
➔ *CPT Assistant* Winter 94:13, Jan 04:27, Mar 04:10;
CPT Changes: An Insider's View 2002

49501   incarcerated or strangulated
➔ *CPT Assistant* Winter 94:13, Jan 04:27, Mar 04:12;
CPT Changes: An Insider's View 2002

49505   Repair initial inguinal hernia, age 5 years or older;
reducible
➔ *CPT Assistant* Winter 94:13, Sep 00:10, Jan 04:27, Mar 04:12

49507   incarcerated or strangulated
➔ *CPT Assistant* Winter 94:13, Jan 04:27, Mar 04:10

(For inguinal hernia repair, with simple orchiectomy, see
49505 or 49507 and 54520)

(For inguinal hernia repair, with excision of hydrocele or
spermatocele, see 49505 or 49507 and 54840 or 55040)

49520   Repair recurrent inguinal hernia, any age; reducible
➔ *CPT Assistant* Winter 94:13, Sep 03:3, Jan 04:27, Mar 04:3

49521   incarcerated or strangulated
➔ *CPT Assistant* Winter 94:13, Jan 04:27, Mar 04:10

49525   Repair inguinal hernia, sliding, any age
➔ *CPT Assistant* Winter 94:14, Jan 04:27, Mar 04:10

(For incarcerated or strangulated inguinal hernia repair,
see 49496, 49501, 49507, 49521)

49540   Repair lumbar hernia
➔ *CPT Assistant* Winter 94:14

49550   Repair initial femoral hernia, any age; reducible
➔ *CPT Assistant* Winter 94:14

49553   incarcerated or strangulated
➔ *CPT Assistant* Winter 94:14

49555   Repair recurrent femoral hernia; reducible
➔ *CPT Assistant* Winter 94:14

49557   incarcerated or strangulated
➔ *CPT Assistant* Winter 94:14

49560   Repair initial incisional or ventral hernia; reducible
➔ *CPT Assistant* Winter 93:6, Winter 94:14, Nov 97:19

49561   incarcerated or strangulated
➔ *CPT Assistant* Winter 94:14

49565   Repair recurrent incisional or ventral hernia; reducible
➔ *CPT Assistant* Winter 94:14, Nov 97:19

49566   incarcerated or strangulated
➔ *CPT Assistant* Winter 94:14

+▲ **49568**   Implantation of mesh or other prosthesis for incisional or
ventral hernia repair or mesh for closure of debridement
for necrotizing soft tissue infection (List separately in
addition to code for the incisional or ventral hernia repair)
➔ *CPT Assistant* Winter 94:14, Nov 97:19, Sep 01:11, Nov 05:15;
CPT Changes: An Insider's View 2008

▶(Use 49568 in conjunction with 11004-11006, 49560-
49566)◀

49570   Repair epigastric hernia (eg, preperitoneal fat); reducible
(separate procedure)
➔ *CPT Assistant* Winter 94:15

49572   incarcerated or strangulated
➔ *CPT Assistant* Winter 94:15

49580   Repair umbilical hernia, younger than age 5 years;
reducible
➔ *CPT Assistant* Winter 94:15

49582   incarcerated or strangulated
➔ *CPT Assistant* Winter 94:15

49585   Repair umbilical hernia, age 5 years or older; reducible
➔ *CPT Assistant* Winter 94:15

49587   incarcerated or strangulated
➔ *CPT Assistant* Winter 94:15

49590   Repair spigelian hernia
➔ *CPT Assistant* Winter 94:15

49600   Repair of small omphalocele, with primary closure
➔ *CPT Assistant* Winter 94:15

(Do not report modifier 63 in conjunction with 49600)

49605   Repair of large omphalocele or gastroschisis; with or
without prosthesis
➔ *CPT Assistant* Winter 94:15

49606   with removal of prosthesis, final reduction and
closure, in operating room
➔ *CPT Assistant* Winter 94:15

(Do not report modifier 63 in conjunction with 49605,
49606)

49610   Repair of omphalocele (Gross type operation); first stage
➔ *CPT Assistant* Winter 94:15

49611   second stage
➔ *CPT Assistant* Winter 94:15

(Do not report modifier 63 in conjunction with 49610,
49611)

(For diaphragmatic or hiatal hernia repair, see 39502-
39541)

(For surgical repair of omentum, use 49999)

▲=Revised code   ●=New code   ▶◀=Contains new or revised text   ⊘=Modifier 51 exempt

Laparoscopy

Surgical laparoscopy always includes diagnostic laparoscopy. To report a diagnostic laparoscopy (peritoneoscopy) (separate procedure), use 49320.

49650 Laparoscopy, surgical; repair initial inguinal hernia

➡*CPT Assistant* Nov 99:24, Mar 00:9; *CPT Changes: An Insider's View* 2000

49651 repair recurrent inguinal hernia

➡*CPT Assistant* Nov 99:24, Mar 00:9; *CPT Changes: An Insider's View* 2000

49659 Unlisted laparoscopy procedure, hernioplasty, herniorrhaphy, herniotomy

➡*CPT Assistant* Nov 99:25, Mar 00:9, Sep 01:11, Nov 05:15, Feb 06:16; *CPT Changes: An Insider's View* 2000

Suture

49900 Suture, secondary, of abdominal wall for evisceration or dehiscence

(For suture of ruptured diaphragm, see 39540, 39541)

(For debridement of abdominal wall, see 11042, 11043)

Other Procedures

49904 Omental flap, extra-abdominal (eg, for reconstruction of sternal and chest wall defects)

➡*CPT Changes: An Insider's View* 2003

(Code 49904 includes harvest and transfer. If a second surgeon harvests the omental flap, then the two surgeons should code 49904 as co-surgeons, using modifier 62)

+ 49905 Omental flap, intra-abdominal (List separately in addition to code for primary procedure)

➡*CPT Assistant* Nov 00:11; *CPT Changes: An Insider's View* 2003

(Do not report 49905 in conjunction with 44700)

49906 Free omental flap with microvascular anastomosis

➡*CPT Assistant* Nov 96:8, Apr 97:8, Nov 98:16

(Do not report code 69990 in addition to 49906)

49999 Unlisted procedure, abdomen, peritoneum and omentum

Urinary System

(For provision of chemotherapeutic agents, report both the specific service in addition to code(s) for the specific substance(s) or drug(s) provided)

Kidney

Incision

▶(For retroperitoneal exploration, abscess, tumor, or cyst, see 49010, 49060, 49203-49205)◀

50010   Renal exploration, not necessitating other specific procedures

(For laparoscopic ablation of renal mass lesion(s), use 50542)

50020   Drainage of perirenal or renal abscess; open
➲ *CPT Assistant* Nov 97:19, Oct 01:8

Drainage of Renal Abscess
50020

An incision is made to the abscess cavity and the site is irrigated and drained.

⊙ 50021   percutaneous
➲ *CPT Assistant* Nov 97:19, Mar 98:8, Oct 01:8

(For radiological supervision and interpretation, use 75989)

50040   Nephrostomy, nephrotomy with drainage
➲ *CPT Assistant* Spring 93:35, Oct 01:8

50045   Nephrotomy, with exploration
➲ *CPT Assistant* Oct 01:8

(For renal endoscopy performed in conjunction with this procedure, see 50570-50580)

50060   Nephrolithotomy; removal of calculus
➲ *CPT Assistant* Oct 01:8

Nephrolithotomy With Calculus Removal
50060-50075

A kidney stone (calculus) is removed by an incision in the kidney. Use 50070 if complicated by a congenital kidney abnormality.

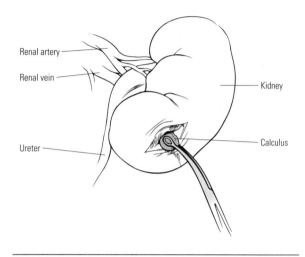

50065   secondary surgical operation for calculus
➲ *CPT Assistant* Oct 01:8

50070   complicated by congenital kidney abnormality
➲ *CPT Assistant* Oct 01:8

50075   removal of large staghorn calculus filling renal pelvis and calyces (including anatrophic pyelolithotomy)
➲   *CPT Assistant* Oct 01:8

50080   Percutaneous nephrostolithotomy or pyelostolithotomy, with or without dilation, endoscopy, lithotripsy, stenting, or basket extraction; up to 2 cm
➲ *CPT Assistant* Oct 01:8

50081   over 2 cm
➲   *CPT Assistant* Oct 01:8

(For establishment of nephrostomy without nephrostolithotomy, see 50040, 50395, 52334)

(For fluoroscopic guidance, see 76000, 76001)

50100   Transection or repositioning of aberrant renal vessels (separate procedure)
➲ *CPT Assistant* Oct 01:8

50120   Pyelotomy; with exploration
➲ *CPT Assistant* Oct 01:8

(For renal endoscopy performed in conjunction with this procedure, see 50570-50580)

50125   with drainage, pyelostomy
➲ *CPT Assistant* Oct 01:8

50130   with removal of calculus (pyelolithotomy, pelviolithotomy, including coagulum pyelolithotomy)
➲ *CPT Assistant* Oct 01:8

50135   complicated (eg, secondary operation, congenital kidney abnormality)

→ *CPT Assistant* Oct 01:8

(For supply of anticarcinogenic agents, use 99070 in addition to code for primary procedure)

Excision

►(For excision of retroperitoneal tumor or cyst, see 49203-49205)◄

(For laparoscopic ablation of renal mass lesion(s), use 50542)

50200   Renal biopsy; percutaneous, by trocar or needle

→ *CPT Assistant* Fall 93:13, Oct 01:8

(For radiological supervision and interpretation, see 76942, 77002, 77012, 77021)

(For fine needle aspiration, use 10022)

(For evaluation of fine needle aspirate, see 88172, 88173)

50205   by surgical exposure of kidney

→ *CPT Assistant* Oct 01:8

50220   Nephrectomy, including partial ureterectomy, any open approach including rib resection;

→ *CPT Assistant* Oct 01:8, Nov 02:3; *CPT Changes: An Insider's View* 2002

50225   complicated because of previous surgery on same kidney

→ *CPT Assistant* Oct 01:8, Nov 02:3

50230   radical, with regional lymphadenectomy and/or vena caval thrombectomy

→ *CPT Assistant* Oct 01:8, Nov 02:3

(When vena caval resection with reconstruction is necessary, use 37799)

50234   Nephrectomy with total ureterectomy and bladder cuff; through same incision

→ *CPT Assistant* Oct 01:8, Nov 02:3

50236   through separate incision

→ *CPT Assistant* Oct 01:8, Nov 02:3

50240   Nephrectomy, partial

→ *CPT Assistant* Oct 01:8, Nov 02:3, Jan 03:20, Apr 05:10, 12

(For laparoscopic partial nephrectomy, use 50543)

50250   Ablation, open, one or more renal mass lesion(s), cryosurgical, including intraoperative ultrasound, if performed

→ *CPT Changes: An Insider's View* 2006

(For laparoscopic ablation of renal mass lesions, use 50542)

►(For cryoablation of renal tumors, use 50593)◄

50280   Excision or unroofing of cyst(s) of kidney

→ *CPT Assistant* Nov 99:25, Oct 01:8; *CPT Changes: An Insider's View* 2000

(For laparoscopic ablation of renal cysts, use 50541)

50290   Excision of perinephric cyst

→ *CPT Assistant* Oct 01:8

Renal Transplantation

Renal *auto*transplantation includes reimplantation of the autograft as the primary procedure, along with secondary extra-corporeal procedure(s) (eg, partial nephrectomy, nephrolithotomy) reported with modifier 51 (see 50380 and applicable secondary procedure(s)).

Renal *allo*transplantation involves three distinct components of physician work:

1) ***Cadaver donor nephrectomy, unilateral or bilateral***, which includes harvesting the graft(s) and cold preservation of the graft(s) (perfusing with cold preservation solution and cold maintenance) (use 50300). ***Living donor nephrectomy***, which includes harvesting the graft, cold preservation of the graft (perfusing with cold preservation solution and cold maintenance), and care of the donor (see 50320, 50547).

2) ***Backbench work***:

Standard preparation of a cadaver donor renal allograft prior to transplantation including dissection and removal of perinephric fat, diaphragmatic and retroperitoneal attachments; excision of adrenal gland; and preparation of ureter(s), renal vein(s), and renal artery(s), ligating branches, as necessary (use 50323).

Standard preparation of a living donor renal allograft (open or laparoscopic) prior to transplantation including dissection and removal of perinephric fat and preparation of ureter(s), renal vein(s), and renal artery(s), ligating branches, as necessary (use 50325).

Additional reconstruction of a cadaver or living donor renal allograft prior to transplantation may include venous, arterial, and/or ureteral anastomosis(es) necessary for implantation (see 50327-50329).

3) ***Recipient renal allotransplantation***, which includes transplantation of the allograft (with or without recipient nephrectomy) and care of the recipient (see 50360, 50365).

(For dialysis, see 90935-90999)

(For laparoscopic donor nephrectomy, use 50547)

(For laparoscopic drainage of lymphocele to peritoneal cavity, use 49323)

50300   Donor nephrectomy (including cold preservation); from cadaver donor, unilateral or bilateral

➔ *CPT Assistant* Nov 99:25, Apr 05:10-12; *CPT Changes: An Insider's View* 2000, 2005

50320   open, from living donor

➔ *CPT Assistant* Nov 99:25, May 00:4; *CPT Changes: An Insider's View* 2000, 2005

50323   Backbench standard preparation of cadaver donor renal allograft prior to transplantation, including dissection and removal of perinephric fat, diaphragmatic and retroperitoneal attachments, excision of adrenal gland, and preparation of ureter(s), renal vein(s), and renal artery(s), ligating branches, as necessary

➔ *CPT Assistant* Apr 05:10-11; *CPT Changes: An Insider's View* 2005

(Do not report 50323 in conjunction with 60540, 60545)

50325   Backbench standard preparation of living donor renal allograft (open or laparoscopic) prior to transplantation, including dissection and removal of perinephric fat and preparation of ureter(s), renal vein(s), and renal artery(s), ligating branches, as necessary

➔ *CPT Changes: An Insider's View* 2005

50327   Backbench reconstruction of cadaver or living donor renal allograft prior to transplantation; venous anastomosis, each

➔ *CPT Changes: An Insider's View* 2005

50328   arterial anastomosis, each

➔ *CPT Changes: An Insider's View* 2005

50329   ureteral anastomosis, each

➔ *CPT Changes: An Insider's View* 2005

50340   Recipient nephrectomy (separate procedure)

(For bilateral procedure, report 50340 with modifier 50)

50360   Renal allotransplantation, implantation of graft; without recipient nephrectomy

➔ *CPT Changes: An Insider's View* 2005

50365   with recipient nephrectomy

➔ *CPT Assistant* Apr 05:10-11

(For bilateral procedure, report 50365 with modifier 50)

50370   Removal of transplanted renal allograft

50380   Renal autotransplantation, reimplantation of kidney

➔ *CPT Assistant* Apr 05:10, 12

(For renal autotransplantation extra-corporeal (bench) surgery, use autotransplantation as the primary procedure and report secondary procedure(s) (eg, partial nephrectomy, nephrolithotomy) with modifier 51)

Introduction

Renal Pelvis Catheter Procedures

Internally Dwelling

⊙ **50382**   Removal (via snare/capture) and replacement of internally dwelling ureteral stent via percutaneous approach, including radiological supervision and interpretation

➔ *CPT Changes: An Insider's View* 2006

➔ *Clinical Examples in Radiology* Winter 06:15

(For bilateral procedure, use modifier 50)

▶(For removal and replacement of an internally dwelling ureteral stent via a transurethral approach, use 50385)◀

⊙ **50384**   Removal (via snare/capture) of internally dwelling ureteral stent via percutaneous approach, including radiological supervision and interpretation

➔ *CPT Changes: An Insider's View* 2006

➔ *Clinical Examples in Radiology* Winter 06:16

(For bilateral procedure, use modifier 50)

(Do not report 50382, 50384 in conjunction with 50395)

▶(For removal of an internally dwelling ureteral stent via a transurethral approach, use 50386)◀

⊙● **50385**   Removal (via snare/capture) and replacement of internally dwelling ureteral stent via transurethral approach, without use of cystoscopy, including radiological supervision and interpretation

➔ *CPT Changes: An Insider's View* 2008

⊙● **50386**   Removal (via snare/capture) of internally dwelling ureteral stent via transurethral approach, without use of cystoscopy, including radiological supervision and interpretation

➔ *CPT Changes: An Insider's View* 2008

Externally Accessible

⊙ **50387**   Removal and replacement of externally accessible transnephric ureteral stent (eg, external/internal stent) requiring fluoroscopic guidance, including radiological supervision and interpretation

➔ *CPT Changes: An Insider's View* 2006

➔ *Clinical Examples in Radiology* Winter 06:16

(For bilateral procedure, use modifier 50)

(For removal and replacement of externally accessible ureteral stent via ureterostomy or ilieal conduit, use 50688)

(For removal without replacement of an externally accessible ureteral stent not requiring fluoroscopic guidance, see **Evaluation and Management** services codes)

50389   Removal of nephrostomy tube, requiring fluoroscopic guidance (eg, with concurrent indwelling ureteral stent)

➔ *CPT Changes: An Insider's View* 2006

➔ *Clinical Examples in Radiology* Winter 06:16

(Removal of nephrostomy tube not requiring fluoroscopic guidance is considered inherent to E/M services. Report the appropriate level of E/M service provided)

Other Introduction Procedures

50390   Aspiration and/or injection of renal cyst or pelvis by needle, percutaneous

➔ *CPT Assistant* Fall 93:14, Dec 97:7, Oct 01:8, Oct 05:18

(For radiological supervision and interpretation, see 74425, 74470, 76942, 77002, 77012, 77021)

(For evaluation of fine needle aspirate, see 88172, 88173)

50391   Instillation(s) of therapeutic agent into renal pelvis and/or ureter through established nephrostomy, pyelostomy or ureterostomy tube (eg, anticarcinogenic or antifungal agent)

➔ *CPT Assistant* Oct 05:18; *CPT Changes: An Insider's View* 2005

50392   Introduction of intracatheter or catheter into renal pelvis for drainage and/or injection, percutaneous

➔ *CPT Assistant* Dec 97:7, Oct 01:8, Oct 05:18

(For radiological supervision and interpretation, see 74475, 76942, 77012)

Introduction of Catheter Into Renal Pelvis
50392

The physician inserts a catheter into the renal pelvis in order to drain urine and/or give an injection.

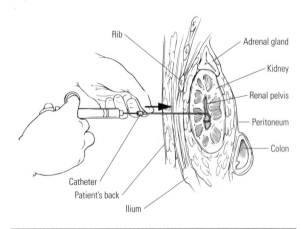

Rib
Adrenal gland
Kidney
Renal pelvis
Peritoneum
Colon
Catheter
Patient's back
Ilium

50393   Introduction of ureteral catheter or stent into ureter through renal pelvis for drainage and/or injection, percutaneous

➔ *CPT Assistant* Fall 93:14, Oct 01:8, Oct 05:18

➔ *Clinical Examples in Radiology* Summer 06:1-3

(For radiological supervision and interpretation, see 74480, 76942, 77002, 77012)

50394   Injection procedure for pyelography (as nephrostogram, pyelostogram, antegrade pyeloureterograms) through nephrostomy or pyelostomy tube, or indwelling ureteral catheter

➔ *CPT Assistant* Fall 93:15, Dec 97:7, Oct 01:8, Oct 05:18

➔ *Clinical Examples in Radiology* Summer 06:1-3

(For radiological supervision and interpretation, use 74425)

50395   Introduction of guide into renal pelvis and/or ureter with dilation to establish nephrostomy tract, percutaneous

➔ *CPT Assistant* Oct 01:8, Oct 05:18, Sep 06:1

(For radiological supervision and interpretation, see 74475, 74480, 74485)

(For nephrostolithotomy, see 50080, 50081)

(For retrograde percutaneous nephrostomy, use 52334)

(For endoscopic surgery, see 50551-50561)

50396   Manometric studies through nephrostomy or pyelostomy tube, or indwelling ureteral catheter

➔ *CPT Assistant* Fall 93:16, Dec 97:7, Oct 01:8

(For radiological supervision and interpretation, see 74425, 74475, 74480)

50398   Change of nephrostomy or pyelostomy tube

➔ *CPT Assistant* Oct 01:8

(For radiological supervision and interpretation, use 75984)

Repair

50400   Pyeloplasty (Foley Y-pyeloplasty), plastic operation on renal pelvis, with or without plastic operation on ureter, nephropexy, nephrostomy, pyelostomy, or ureteral splinting; simple

➔ *CPT Assistant* Nov 99:25, May 00:4, Oct 01:8; *CPT Changes: An Insider's View* 2000

50405   complicated (congenital kidney abnormality, secondary pyeloplasty, solitary kidney, calycoplasty)

➔ *CPT Assistant* Nov 99:25, May 00:4, Oct 01:8; *CPT Changes: An Insider's View* 2000

(For laparoscopic approach, use 50544)

50500   Nephrorrhaphy, suture of kidney wound or injury

50520   Closure of nephrocutaneous or pyelocutaneous fistula

50525   Closure of nephrovisceral fistula (eg, renocolic), including visceral repair; abdominal approach

50526   thoracic approach

50540   Symphysiotomy for horseshoe kidney with or without pyeloplasty and/or other plastic procedure, unilateral or bilateral (one operation)

Laparoscopy

Surgical laparoscopy always includes diagnostic laparoscopy. To report a diagnostic laparoscopy (peritoneoscopy) (separate procedure), use 49320.

50541   Laparoscopy, surgical; ablation of renal cysts
➔ *CPT Assistant* Nov 99:25, May 00:4, Oct 01:8, Nov 02:3, Jan 03:20; *CPT Changes: An Insider's View* 2000

50542   ablation of renal mass lesion(s)
➔ *CPT Assistant* Nov 02:3, Jan 03:21, Aug 04:12; *CPT Changes: An Insider's View* 2003

(For open procedure, see 50220-50240)

▶(For cryosurgical ablation, see 50250, 50593)◀

50543   partial nephrectomy
➔ *CPT Assistant* Nov 02:3, Jan 03:21; *CPT Changes: An Insider's View* 2003

(For open procedure, use 50240)

50544   pyeloplasty
➔ *CPT Assistant* Nov 99:25, May 00:4, Oct 01:8; *CPT Changes: An Insider's View* 2000

50545   radical nephrectomy (includes removal of Gerota's fascia and surrounding fatty tissue, removal of regional lymph nodes, and adrenalectomy)
➔ *CPT Assistant* Oct 01:8; *CPT Changes: An Insider's View* 2001

(For open procedure, use 50230)

Laparoscopic Radical Nephrectomy
50545

Radical nephrectomy (includes removal of Gerota's fascia and surrounding fatty tissue, removal of regional lymph nodes, and adrenalectomy)

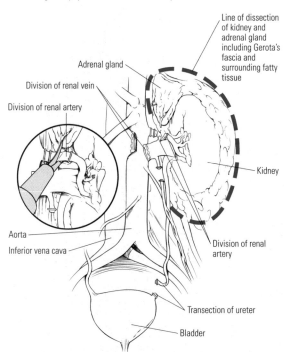

50546   nephrectomy, including partial ureterectomy
➔ *CPT Assistant* Nov 99:25, May 00:4, Oct 01:8; *CPT Changes: An Insider's View* 2000, 2001

Laparoscopic Nephrectomy
50546

A kidney is dissected and removed under laparoscopic guidance.

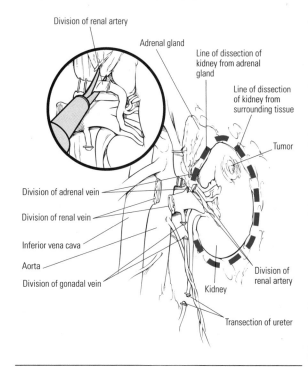

50547   donor nephrectomy (including cold preservation), from living donor
➔ *CPT Assistant* Nov 99:25, May 00:4, Oct 01:8; *CPT Changes: An Insider's View* 2000, 2005

(For open procedure, use 50320)

(For backbench renal allograft standard preparation prior to transplantation, use 50325)

(For backbench renal allograft reconstruction prior to transplantation, see 50327-50329)

50548   nephrectomy with total ureterectomy
➔ *CPT Assistant* Nov 99:25, May 00:4, Oct 01:8; *CPT Changes: An Insider's View* 2000, 2001

(For open procedure, see 50234, 50236)

50549   Unlisted laparoscopy procedure, renal
➔ *CPT Assistant* Nov 99:25, Mar 00:9, May 00:4, Feb 06:16; *CPT Changes: An Insider's View* 2000

(For laparoscopic drainage of lymphocele to peritoneal cavity, use 49323)

Endoscopy

(For supplies and materials, use 99070)

50551 Renal endoscopy through established nephrostomy or pyelostomy, with or without irrigation, instillation, or ureteropyelography, exclusive of radiologic service;

➔ *CPT Assistant* Oct 01:8, Jan 03:21

50553 with ureteral catheterization, with or without dilation of ureter

➔ *CPT Assistant* Oct 01:8

50555 with biopsy

➔ *CPT Assistant* Oct 01:8

50557 with fulguration and/or incision, with or without biopsy

➔ *CPT Assistant* Oct 01:8

50561 with removal of foreign body or calculus

➔ *CPT Assistant* Oct 01:8, Jan 03:21

50562 with resection of tumor

➔ *CPT Assistant* Jan 03:21; *CPT Changes: An Insider's View* 2003

(When procedures 50570-50580 provide a significant identifiable service, they may be added to 50045 and 50120)

50570 Renal endoscopy through nephrotomy or pyelotomy, with or without irrigation, instillation, or ureteropyelography, exclusive of radiologic service;

➔ *CPT Assistant* Oct 01:8

(For nephrotomy, use 50045)

(For pyelotomy, use 50120)

50572 with ureteral catheterization, with or without dilation of ureter

➔ *CPT Assistant* Oct 01:8

50574 with biopsy

➔ *CPT Assistant* Oct 01:8

50575 with endopyelotomy (includes cystoscopy, ureteroscopy, dilation of ureter and ureteral pelvic junction, incision of ureteral pelvic junction and insertion of endopyelotomy stent)

➔ *CPT Assistant* Oct 01:8, Aug 02:11

50576 with fulguration and/or incision, with or without biopsy

➔ *CPT Assistant* Oct 01:8

50580 with removal of foreign body or calculus

➔ *CPT Assistant* Oct 01:8

Other Procedures

50590 Lithotripsy, extracorporeal shock wave

➔ *CPT Assistant* Jul 01:11, Aug 01:10, Oct 01:8, Jul 03:16, Aug 03:14

Lithotripsy
50590

The physician breaks up a kidney stone (calculus) by directing shock waves through a liquid surrounding the patient.

Kidney stone (calculus) · Radiologic monitors for guidance · Medium · Shock waves are concentrated on stone · Electrode · Patient, transverse section

⊙ **50592** Ablation, one or more renal tumor(s), percutaneous, unilateral, radiofrequency

➔ *CPT Changes: An Insider's View* 2006

➔ *Clinical Examples in Radiology* Winter 06:16

(50592 is a unilateral procedure. For bilateral procedure, report 50592 with modifier 50)

(For imaging guidance and monitoring, see 76940, 77013, 77022)

⊙● **50593** Ablation, renal tumor(s), unilateral, percutaneous, cryotherapy

➔ *CPT Changes: An Insider's View* 2008

▶(50593 is a unilateral procedure. For bilateral procedure, report 50593 with modifier 50)◀

▶(For imaging guidance and monitoring, see codes 76940, 77013, 77022)◀

Ureter

Incision

50600 Ureterotomy with exploration or drainage (separate procedure)

(For ureteral endoscopy performed in conjunction with this procedure, see 50970-50980)

50605 Ureterotomy for insertion of indwelling stent, all types

➔ *CPT Assistant* Oct 01:8

Indwelling Ureteral Stent
50605

The physician makes an incision in the ureter (ureterotomy) and inserts a stent. For placement using cystourethroscopic technique, use 52332.

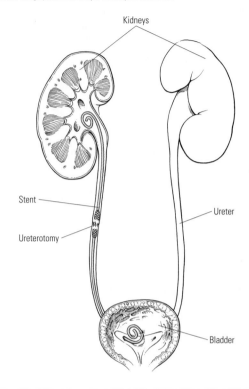

Kidneys

Stent

Ureterotomy

Ureter

Bladder

50610 Ureterolithotomy; upper one-third of ureter

➔ *CPT Assistant* Nov 99:26, Oct 01:8; *CPT Changes: An Insider's View* 2000

50620 middle one-third of ureter

➔ *CPT Assistant* Nov 99:26, Oct 01:8; *CPT Changes: An Insider's View* 2000

50630 lower one-third of ureter

➔ *CPT Assistant* Nov 99:26, Oct 01:8; *CPT Changes: An Insider's View* 2000

(For laparoscopic approach, use 50945)

(For transvesical ureterolithotomy, use 51060)

(For cystotomy with stone basket extraction of ureteral calculus, use 51065)

(For endoscopic extraction or manipulation of ureteral calculus, see 50080, 50081, 50561, 50961, 50980, 52320-52330, 52352, 52353)

Excision

(For ureterocele, see 51535, 52300)

50650 Ureterectomy, with bladder cuff (separate procedure)

50660 Ureterectomy, total, ectopic ureter, combination abdominal, vaginal and/or perineal approach

Introduction

50684 Injection procedure for ureterography or ureteropyelography through ureterostomy or indwelling ureteral catheter

(For radiological supervision and interpretation, use 74425)

50686 Manometric studies through ureterostomy or indwelling ureteral catheter

50688 Change of ureterostomy tube or externally accessible ureteral stent via ileal conduit

➔ *CPT Changes: An Insider's View* 2006

➔ *Clinical Examples in Radiology* Winter 06:20

(If imaging guidance is performed, use 75984)

50690 Injection procedure for visualization of ileal conduit and/or ureteropyelography, exclusive of radiologic service

(For radiological supervision and interpretation, use 74425)

Repair

50700 Ureteroplasty, plastic operation on ureter (eg, stricture)

50715 Ureterolysis, with or without repositioning of ureter for retroperitoneal fibrosis

(For bilateral procedure, report 50715 with modifier 50)

50722 Ureterolysis for ovarian vein syndrome

50725 Ureterolysis for retrocaval ureter, with reanastomosis of upper urinary tract or vena cava

50727 Revision of urinary-cutaneous anastomosis (any type urostomy);

50728 with repair of fascial defect and hernia

50740 Ureteropyelostomy, anastomosis of ureter and renal pelvis

➔ *CPT Assistant* Oct 01:8

50750 Ureterocalycostomy, anastomosis of ureter to renal calyx

➔ *CPT Assistant* Oct 01:8

50760 Ureteroureterostomy

➔ *CPT Assistant* Oct 01:8

50770 Transureteroureterostomy, anastomosis of ureter to contralateral ureter

(Codes 50780-50785 include minor procedures to prevent vesicoureteral reflux)

50780 Ureteroneocystostomy; anastomosis of single ureter to bladder

➔ *CPT Assistant* Oct 01:8

(For bilateral procedure, report 50780 with modifier 50)

(When combined with cystourethroplasty or vesical neck revision, use 51820)

50782 anastomosis of duplicated ureter to bladder

➔ *CPT Assistant* Oct 01:8

50783 with extensive ureteral tailoring
> *CPT Assistant* Oct 01:8

50785 with vesico-psoas hitch or bladder flap
> *CPT Assistant* Oct 01:8

(For bilateral procedure, report 50785 with modifier 50)

50800 Ureteroenterostomy, direct anastomosis of ureter to intestine
> *CPT Assistant* Oct 01:8

(For bilateral procedure, report 50800 with modifier 50)

50810 Ureterosigmoidostomy, with creation of sigmoid bladder and establishment of abdominal or perineal colostomy, including intestine anastomosis
> *CPT Assistant* Oct 01:8; *CPT Changes: An Insider's View* 2002

50815 Ureterocolon conduit, including intestine anastomosis
> *CPT Assistant* Oct 01:8

(For bilateral procedure, report 50815 with modifier 50)

50820 Ureteroileal conduit (ileal bladder), including intestine anastomosis (Bricker operation)
> *CPT Assistant* Oct 01:8; *CPT Changes: An Insider's View* 2002

(For bilateral procedure, report 50820 with modifier 50)

(For combination of 50800-50820 with cystectomy, see 51580-51595)

Ureteroileal Conduit
50820

The ureters are connected to a segment of intestine to divert urine flow through an opening in the skin.

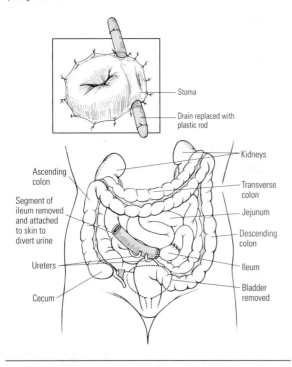

50825 Continent diversion, including intestine anastomosis using any segment of small and/or large intestine (Kock pouch or Camey enterocystoplasty)
> *CPT Assistant* Oct 01:8; *CPT Changes: An Insider's View* 2002

50830 Urinary undiversion (eg, taking down of ureteroileal conduit, ureterosigmoidostomy or ureteroenterostomy with ureteroureterostomy or ureteroneocystostomy)
> *CPT Assistant* Oct 01:8

50840 Replacement of all or part of ureter by intestine segment, including intestine anastomosis
> *CPT Assistant* Oct 01:8; *CPT Changes: An Insider's View* 2002

(For bilateral procedure, report 50840 with modifier 50)

50845 Cutaneous appendico-vesicostomy

50860 Ureterostomy, transplantation of ureter to skin

(For bilateral procedure, report 50860 with modifier 50)

50900 Ureterorrhaphy, suture of ureter (separate procedure)

50920 Closure of ureterocutaneous fistula

50930 Closure of ureterovisceral fistula (including visceral repair)

50940 Deligation of ureter

(For ureteroplasty, ureterolysis, see 50700-50860)

Laparoscopy

Surgical laparoscopy always includes diagnostic laparoscopy. To report a diagnostic laparoscopy (peritoneoscopy) (separate procedure), use 49320.

50945 Laparoscopy, surgical; ureterolithotomy
> *CPT Assistant* Nov 99:26, May 00:4, Oct 01:8, Sep 06:13; *CPT Changes: An Insider's View* 2000

50947 ureteroneocystostomy with cystoscopy and ureteral stent placement
> *CPT Assistant* Oct 01:8; *CPT Changes: An Insider's View* 2001

Laparoscopic Ureteroneocystostomy
50947

Ureteroneocystostomy with cystoscopy and ureteral stent placement

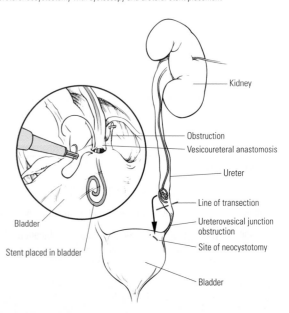

50948   ureteroneocystostomy without cystoscopy and
              ureteral stent placement
              → *CPT Assistant* Oct 01:8; *CPT Changes: An Insider's View*
                2001

              (For open ureteroneocystostomy, see 50780-50785)

50949   Unlisted laparoscopy procedure, ureter
              → *CPT Assistant* Oct 01:8; *CPT Changes: An Insider's View* 2001

Endoscopy

50951   Ureteral endoscopy through established ureterostomy,
              with or without irrigation, instillation, or
              ureteropyelography, exclusive of radiologic service;
              → *CPT Assistant* Oct 01:8

50953   with ureteral catheterization, with or without dilation
                  of ureter
                  → *CPT Assistant* Oct 01:8

50955   with biopsy
                  → *CPT Assistant* Oct 01:8

50957   with fulguration and/or incision, with or without
                  biopsy
                  → *CPT Assistant* Oct 01:8

50961   with removal of foreign body or calculus
                  → *CPT Assistant* Oct 01:8, Mar 07:10, Apr 07:12

              (When procedures 50970-50980 provide a significant
              identifiable service, they may be added to 50600)

50970   Ureteral endoscopy through ureterotomy, with or without
              irrigation, instillation, or ureteropyelography, exclusive of
              radiologic service;
              → *CPT Assistant* Oct 01:8

              (For ureterotomy, use 50600)

50972   with ureteral catheterization, with or without dilation
                  of ureter
                  → *CPT Assistant* Oct 01:8

50974   with biopsy
                  → *CPT Assistant* Oct 01:8

50976   with fulguration and/or incision, with or without
                  biopsy
                  → *CPT Assistant* Oct 01:8

50980   with removal of foreign body or calculus
                  → *CPT Assistant* Oct 01:8

Bladder

Incision

              ►(51000 has been deleted. To report, use 51100)◄

              ►(51005 has been deleted. To report, use 51101)◄

              ►(51010 has been deleted. To report, use 51102)◄

51020   Cystotomy or cystostomy; with fulguration and/or
              insertion of radioactive material

51030   with cryosurgical destruction of intravesical lesion

51040   Cystostomy, cystotomy with drainage

51045   Cystotomy, with insertion of ureteral catheter or stent
              (separate procedure)

51050   Cystolithotomy, cystotomy with removal of calculus,
              without vesical neck resection

51060   Transvesical ureterolithotomy

51065   Cystotomy, with calculus basket extraction and/or
              ultrasonic or electrohydraulic fragmentation of ureteral
              calculus
              → *CPT Changes: An Insider's View* 2002

51080   Drainage of perivesical or prevesical space abscess

►Removal◄

● **51100**   Aspiration of bladder; by needle
              → *CPT Changes: An Insider's View* 2008

● **51101**   by trocar or intracatheter
                  → *CPT Changes: An Insider's View* 2008

● **51102**   with insertion of suprapubic catheter
                  → *CPT Changes: An Insider's View* 2008

              ►(For imaging guidance, see 76942, 77002, 77012)◄

Excision

51500   Excision of urachal cyst or sinus, with or without
              umbilical hernia repair

51520   Cystotomy; for simple excision of vesical neck (separate
              procedure)

51525   for excision of bladder diverticulum, single or multiple
                  (separate procedure)

51530   for excision of bladder tumor

              (For transurethral resection, see 52234-52240, 52305)

51535   Cystotomy for excision, incision, or repair of ureterocele

              (For bilateral procedure, report 51535 with modifier 50)

              (For transurethral excision, use 52300)

51550   Cystectomy, partial; simple

51555   complicated (eg, postradiation, previous surgery,
                  difficult location)

51565   Cystectomy, partial, with reimplantation of ureter(s) into
              bladder (ureteroneocystostomy)

51570   Cystectomy, complete; (separate procedure)
              → *CPT Assistant* Spring 93:35

51575   with bilateral pelvic lymphadenectomy, including
                  external iliac, hypogastric, and obturator nodes
                  → *CPT Assistant* Spring 93:35

51580   Cystectomy, complete, with ureterosigmoidostomy or
              ureterocutaneous transplantations;

51585   with bilateral pelvic lymphadenectomy, including
                  external iliac, hypogastric, and obturator nodes

---

51590 Cystectomy, complete, with ureteroileal conduit or sigmoid bladder, including intestine anastomosis;

➔ *CPT Changes: An Insider's View* 2002

51595 with bilateral pelvic lymphadenectomy, including external iliac, hypogastric, and obturator nodes

51596 Cystectomy, complete, with continent diversion, any open technique, using any segment of small and/or large intestine to construct neobladder

➔ *CPT Changes: An Insider's View* 2002

51597 Pelvic exenteration, complete, for vesical, prostatic or urethral malignancy, with removal of bladder and ureteral transplantations, with or without hysterectomy and/or abdominoperineal resection of rectum and colon and colostomy, or any combination thereof

(For pelvic exenteration for gynecologic malignancy, use 58240)

Introduction

51600 Injection procedure for cystography or voiding urethrocystography

(For radiological supervision and interpretation, see 74430, 74455)

51605 Injection procedure and placement of chain for contrast and/or chain urethrocystography

(For radiological supervision and interpretation, use 74430)

51610 Injection procedure for retrograde urethrocystography

(For radiological supervision and interpretation, use 74450)

51700 Bladder irrigation, simple, lavage and/or instillation

(Codes 51701-51702 are reported only when performed independently. Do not report 51701-51702 when catheter insertion is an inclusive component of another procedure.)

51701 Insertion of non-indwelling bladder catheter (eg, straight catheterization for residual urine)

➔ *CPT Changes: An Insider's View* 2003

51702 Insertion of temporary indwelling bladder catheter; simple (eg, Foley)

➔ *CPT Assistant* Oct 03:10, Jul 06:4, Jan 07:31; *CPT Changes: An Insider's View* 2003

51703 complicated (eg, altered anatomy, fractured catheter/balloon)

➔ *CPT Changes: An Insider's View* 2003

51705 Change of cystostomy tube; simple

51710 complicated

(If imaging guidance is performed, use 75984)

51715 Endoscopic injection of implant material into the submucosal tissues of the urethra and/or bladder neck

51720 Bladder instillation of anticarcinogenic agent (including retention time)

➔ *CPT Assistant* Nov 02:11; *CPT Changes: An Insider's View* 2007

Urodynamics

The following section (51725-51797) lists procedures that may be used separately or in many and varied combinations.

When multiple procedures are performed in the same investigative session, modifier 51 should be employed.

All procedures in this section imply that these services are performed by, or are under the direct supervision of, a physician and that all instruments, equipment, fluids, gases, probes, catheters, technician's fees, medications, gloves, trays, tubing and other sterile supplies be provided by the physician. When the physician only interprets the results and/or operates the equipment, a professional component, modifier 26, should be used to identify physicians' services.

51725 Simple cystometrogram (CMG) (eg, spinal manometer)

➔ *CPT Assistant* Sep 02:6

51726 Complex cystometrogram (eg, calibrated electronic equipment)

➔ *CPT Assistant* Sep 02:6

51736 Simple uroflowmetry (UFR) (eg, stop-watch flow rate, mechanical uroflowmeter)

➔ *CPT Assistant* Sep 02:6

51741 Complex uroflowmetry (eg, calibrated electronic equipment)

➔ *CPT Assistant* Sep 02:6

51772 Urethral pressure profile studies (UPP) (urethral closure pressure profile), any technique

➔ *CPT Assistant* Sep 02:6, Nov 05:15

51784 Electromyography studies (EMG) of anal or urethral sphincter, other than needle, any technique

➔ *CPT Assistant* Sep 02:6

51785 Needle electromyography studies (EMG) of anal or urethral sphincter, any technique

➔ *CPT Assistant* Apr 02:6, Sep 02:6, Jul 04:13

51792 Stimulus evoked response (eg, measurement of bulbocavernosus reflex latency time)

➔ *CPT Assistant* Apr 02:6, Sep 02:6

51795 Voiding pressure studies (VP); bladder voiding pressure, any technique

➔ *CPT Assistant* Dec 01:7, Sep 02:6

+▲ **51797** intra-abdominal voiding pressure (AP) (rectal, gastric, intraperitoneal) (List separately in addition to code for primary procedure)

➔ *CPT Assistant* Dec 01:7, Sep 02:6; *CPT Changes: An Insider's View* 2008

▶(Use 51797 in conjuncton with 51795)◀

51798   Measurement of post-voiding residual urine and/or bladder capacity by ultrasound, non-imaging

> *CPT Assistant* Dec 05:3; *CPT Changes: An Insider's View* 2003

Measurement of Postvoiding
51798

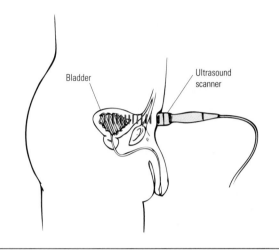

Bladder

Ultrasound scanner

Repair

51800   Cystoplasty or cystourethroplasty, plastic operation on bladder and/or vesical neck (anterior Y-plasty, vesical fundus resection), any procedure, with or without wedge resection of posterior vesical neck

51820   Cystourethroplasty with unilateral or bilateral ureteroneocystostomy

51840   Anterior vesicourethropexy, or urethropexy (eg, Marshall-Marchetti-Krantz, Burch); simple

> *CPT Assistant* Jan 97:1, Nov 97:19, Apr 98:15, Jun 02:7, May 06:17

51841   complicated (eg, secondary repair)

> *CPT Assistant* Jan 97:1, Jun 02:7

(For urethropexy (Pereyra type), use 57289)

51845   Abdomino-vaginal vesical neck suspension, with or without endoscopic control (eg, Stamey, Raz, modified Pereyra)

> *CPT Assistant* Jan 97:3

51860   Cystorrhaphy, suture of bladder wound, injury or rupture; simple

51865   complicated

51880   Closure of cystostomy (separate procedure)

51900   Closure of vesicovaginal fistula, abdominal approach

(For vaginal approach, see 57320-57330)

51920   Closure of vesicouterine fistula;

51925   with hysterectomy

(For closure of vesicoenteric fistula, see 44660, 44661)

(For closure of rectovesical fistula, see 45800-45805)

51940   Closure, exstrophy of bladder

> *CPT Changes: An Insider's View* 2002

(See also 54390)

51960   Enterocystoplasty, including intestinal anastomosis

> *CPT Changes: An Insider's View* 2002

51980   Cutaneous vesicostomy

Laparoscopy

Surgical laparoscopy always includes diagnostic laparoscopy. To report a diagnostic laparoscopy (peritoneoscopy) (separate procedure), use 49320.

51990   Laparoscopy, surgical; urethral suspension for stress incontinence

> *CPT Assistant* Nov 99:26, May 00:4; *CPT Changes: An Insider's View* 2000

51992   sling operation for stress incontinence (eg, fascia or synthetic)

> *CPT Assistant* Nov 99:26, May 00:4; *CPT Changes: An Insider's View* 2000

(For open sling operation for stress incontinence, use 57288)

(For reversal or removal of sling operation for stress incontinence, use 57287)

Laparoscopic Sling Suspension Urinary Incontinence
51990

Nonabsorbable sutures are placed laparoscopically into the endopelvic fascia at the bladder neck region on each side and secured to the ipsilateral pectineal ligament. The sutures are tied using extra vaginal-urethral knots so as to create a hammock type suspension of the bladder neck, without urethral occlusion.

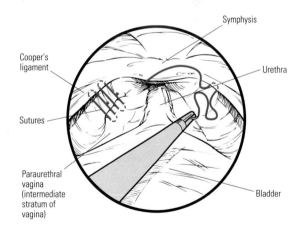

Symphysis

Cooper's ligament

Urethra

Sutures

Paraurethral vagina (intermediate stratum of vagina)

Bladder

51999   Unlisted laparoscopy procedure, bladder

> *CPT Changes: An Insider's View* 2006

Endoscopy—Cystoscopy, Urethroscopy, Cystourethroscopy

Endoscopic descriptions are listed so that the main procedure can be identified without having to list all the minor related functions performed at the same time. For example: meatotomy, urethral calibration and/or dilation, urethro-scopy, and cystoscopy prior to a transurethral resection of prostate; ureteral catheterization following extraction of ureteral calculus; internal urethrotomy and bladder neck fulguration when performing a cystourethroscopy for the female urethral syndrome. When the secondary procedure requires significant additional time and effort, it may be identified by the addition of modifier 22.

For example: urethrotomy performed for a documented pre-existing stricture or bladder neck contracture.

52000 Cystourethroscopy (separate procedure)
> *CPT Assistant* Oct 00:7, May 01:5, Sep 04:11, Oct 05:23

52001 Cystourethroscopy with irrigation and evacuation of multiple obstructing clots
> *CPT Changes: An Insider's View* 2002, 2003

(Do not report 52001 in conjunction with 52000)

52005 Cystourethroscopy, with ureteral catheterization, with or without irrigation, instillation, or ureteropyelography, exclusive of radiologic service;
> *CPT Assistant* Sep 00:11, Jan 01:13, May 01:5, Oct 01:8

Cystourethroscopy With Ureteral Catheterization 52005

A cystourethroscope is passed through the urethra and bladder in order to view the urinary collecting system.

52007 with brush biopsy of ureter and/or renal pelvis
> *CPT Assistant* May 01:5, Oct 01:8

52010 Cystourethroscopy, with ejaculatory duct catheterization, with or without irrigation, instillation, or duct radiography, exclusive of radiologic service
> *CPT Assistant* May 01:5

(For radiological supervision and interpretation, use 74440)

Transurethral Surgery

Urethra and Bladder

52204 Cystourethroscopy, with biopsy(s)
> *CPT Assistant* May 01:5, Sep 01:1, Sep 03:16; *CPT Changes: An Insider's View* 2007

52214 Cystourethroscopy, with fulguration (including cryosurgery or laser surgery) of trigone, bladder neck, prostatic fossa, urethra, or periurethral glands
> *CPT Assistant* May 01:5, Sep 01:1

52224 Cystourethroscopy, with fulguration (including cryosurgery or laser surgery) or treatment of MINOR (less than 0.5 cm) lesion(s) with or without biopsy
> *CPT Assistant* May 01:5, Sep 01:1

52234 Cystourethroscopy, with fulguration (including cryosurgery or laser surgery) and/or resection of; SMALL bladder tumor(s) (0.5 up to 2.0 cm)
> *CPT Assistant* May 01:5, Sep 01:1, Oct 02:12, Jan 03:21; *CPT Changes: An Insider's View* 2005

52235 MEDIUM bladder tumor(s) (2.0 to 5.0 cm)
> *CPT Assistant* May 01:5, Sep 01:1, Oct 02:12, Jan 03:21

52240 LARGE bladder tumor(s)
> *CPT Assistant* May 01:5, Sep 01:1

52250 Cystourethroscopy with insertion of radioactive substance, with or without biopsy or fulguration
> *CPT Assistant* May 01:5, Sep 01:1

52260 Cystourethroscopy, with dilation of bladder for interstitial cystitis; general or conduction (spinal) anesthesia
> *CPT Assistant* May 01:5, Sep 01:1, Oct 05:23

52265 local anesthesia
> *CPT Assistant* May 01:5, Sep 01:1

52270 Cystourethroscopy, with internal urethrotomy; female
> *CPT Assistant* May 01:5, Sep 01:1

52275 male
> *CPT Assistant* May 01:5, Sep 01:1

52276 Cystourethroscopy with direct vision internal urethrotomy
> *CPT Assistant* May 01:5, Sep 01:1

52277 Cystourethroscopy, with resection of external sphincter (sphincterotomy)
> *CPT Assistant* May 01:5, Sep 01:1

52281 Cystourethroscopy, with calibration and/or dilation of urethral stricture or stenosis, with or without meatotomy, with or without injection procedure for cystography, male or female
> *CPT Assistant* Nov 97:20, May 01:5, Sep 01:1

52282 Cystourethroscopy, with insertion of urethral stent
➡ *CPT Assistant* Nov 97:20, May 01:5, Sep 01:1

52283 Cystourethroscopy, with steroid injection into stricture
➡ *CPT Assistant* May 01:5, Sep 01:1

52285 Cystourethroscopy for treatment of the female urethral syndrome with any or all of the following: urethral meatotomy, urethral dilation, internal urethrotomy, lysis of urethrovaginal septal fibrosis, lateral incisions of the bladder neck, and fulguration of polyp(s) of urethra, bladder neck, and/or trigone
➡ *CPT Assistant* May 01:5, Sep 01:1

52290 Cystourethroscopy; with ureteral meatotomy, unilateral or bilateral
➡ *CPT Assistant* May 01:5, Sep 01:1

52300 with resection or fulguration of orthotopic ureterocele(s), unilateral or bilateral
➡ *CPT Assistant* May 01:5, Sep 01:1

52301 with resection or fulguration of ectopic ureterocele(s), unilateral or bilateral
➡ *CPT Assistant* May 01:5, Sep 01:1

52305 with incision or resection of orifice of bladder diverticulum, single or multiple
➡ *CPT Assistant* May 01:5, Sep 01:1

52310 Cystourethroscopy, with removal of foreign body, calculus, or ureteral stent from urethra or bladder (separate procedure); simple
➡ *CPT Assistant* May 01:5, Sep 01:1

52315 complicated
➡ *CPT Assistant* May 01:5, Sep 01:1

52317 Litholapaxy: crushing or fragmentation of calculus by any means in bladder and removal of fragments; simple or small (less than 2.5 cm)
➡ *CPT Assistant* May 01:5, Sep 01:1

52318 complicated or large (over 2.5 cm)
➡ *CPT Assistant* May 01:5, Sep 01:1

Ureter and Pelvis

Therapeutic cystourethroscopy always includes diagnostic cystourethroscopy. To report a diagnostic cystourethroscopy, use 52000. Therapeutic cystourethroscopy with ureteroscopy and/or pyeloscopy always includes diagnostic cystourethroscopy with ureteroscopy and/or pyeloscopy. To report a diagnostic cystourethroscopy with ureteroscopy and/or pyeloscopy, use 52351.

Do not report 52000 in conjunction with 52320-52343.

Do not report 52351 in conjunction with 52344-52346, 52352-52355.

The insertion and removal of a temporary ureteral catheter (52005) during diagnostic or therapeutic cystourethroscopic with ureteroscopy and/or pyeloscopy is included in 52320-52355 and should not be reported separately.

To report insertion of a self-retaining, indwelling stent performed during diagnostic or therapeutic cystourethroscopy with ureteroscopy and/or pyeloscopy, report 52332, in addition to primary procedure(s) performed (52320-52355), and append modifier 51. 52332 is used to report a unilateral procedure unless otherwise specified.

For bilateral insertion of self-retaining, indwelling ureteral stents, use code 52332, and append modifier 50.

To report cystourethroscopic removal of a self-retaining, indwelling ureteral stent, see 52310, 52315, and append modifier 58, if appropriate.

52320 Cystourethroscopy (including ureteral catheterization); with removal of ureteral calculus
➡ *CPT Assistant* Mar 96:1, May 96:11, Jan 01:13, May 01:5, Sep 01:1, Oct 01:8

52325 with fragmentation of ureteral calculus (eg, ultrasonic or electro-hydraulic technique)
➡ *CPT Assistant* Mar 96:1, May 96:11, May 01:5, Sep 01:1, Oct 01:8

52327 with subureteric injection of implant material
➡ *CPT Assistant* Mar 96:1, May 96:11, May 01:5, Sep 01:1, Oct 01:8

52330 with manipulation, without removal of ureteral calculus
➡ *CPT Assistant* Mar 96:1, May 96:11, Sep 00:11, May 01:5, Sep 01:1, Oct 01:8

52332 Cystourethroscopy, with insertion of indwelling ureteral stent (eg, Gibbons or double-J type)
➡ *CPT Assistant* Mar 96:1, May 96:11, Nov 96:8, Jan 01:13, May 01:5, Sep 01:1, Oct 01:8, Oct 05:18

52334 Cystourethroscopy with insertion of ureteral guide wire through kidney to establish a percutaneous nephrostomy, retrograde
➡ *CPT Assistant* Mar 96:11, May 96:11, May 01:5, Sep 01:1, Oct 01:8

(For percutaneous nephrostolithotomy, see 50080, 50081; for establishment of nephrostomy tract only, use 50395)

(For cystourethroscopy, with ureteroscopy and/or pyeloscopy, see 52351-52355)

(For cystourethroscopy with incision, fulguration, or resection of congenital posterior urethral valves or obstructive hypertrophic mucosal folds, use 52400)

52341 Cystourethroscopy; with treatment of ureteral stricture (eg, balloon dilation, laser, electrocautery, and incision)
➡ *CPT Assistant* Nov 96:9, Apr 01:4, May 01:5, Sep 01:1, Oct 01:8; *CPT Changes: An Insider's View* 2001

52342 with treatment of ureteropelvic junction stricture (eg, balloon dilation, laser, electrocautery, and incision)
➡ *CPT Assistant* Apr 01:4, May 01:5, Sep 01:1, Oct 01:8, Aug 02:11; *CPT Changes: An Insider's View* 2001

52343 with treatment of intra-renal stricture (eg, balloon dilation, laser, electrocautery, and incision)
➡ *CPT Assistant* Apr 01:4, May 01:5, Sep 01:1, Oct 01:8; *CPT Changes: An Insider's View* 2001

52344 Cystourethroscopy with ureteroscopy; with treatment of ureteral stricture (eg, balloon dilation, laser, electrocautery, and incision)

> *CPT Assistant* Apr 01:4, May 01:5, Sep 01:1, Oct 01:8; *CPT Changes: An Insider's View* 2001

52345 with treatment of ureteropelvic junction stricture (eg, balloon dilation, laser, electrocautery, and incision)

> *CPT Assistant* Apr 01:4, May 01:5, Sep 01:1, Oct 01:8; *CPT Changes: An Insider's View* 2001

52346 with treatment of intra-renal stricture (eg, balloon dilation, laser, electrocautery, and incision)

> *CPT Assistant* Apr 01:4, May 01:5, Sep 01:1, Oct 01:8; *CPT Changes: An Insider's View* 2001

(For transurethral resection or incision of ejaculatory ducts, use 52402)

52351 Cystourethroscopy, with ureteroscopy and/or pyeloscopy; diagnostic

> *CPT Assistant* Apr 01:4, May 01:5, Sep 01:1, Oct 01:8; *CPT Changes: An Insider's View* 2001

(For radiological supervision and interpretation, use 74485)

(Do not report 52351 in conjunction with 52341-52346, 52352-52355)

52352 with removal or manipulation of calculus (ureteral catheterization is included)

> *CPT Assistant* Apr 01:4, May 01:5, Sep 01:1, Oct 01:8; *CPT Changes: An Insider's View* 2001

52353 with lithotripsy (ureteral catheterization is included)

> *CPT Assistant* Apr 01:4, May 01:5, Sep 01:1, Oct 01:8; *CPT Changes: An Insider's View* 2001

52354 with biopsy and/or fulguration of ureteral or renal pelvic lesion

> *CPT Assistant* Apr 01:4, May 01:5, Sep 01:1, Oct 01:8; *CPT Changes: An Insider's View* 2001, 2003

52355 with resection of ureteral or renal pelvic tumor

> *CPT Assistant* Apr 01:4, May 01:5, Sep 01:1, Oct 01:8, Jan 03:21; *CPT Changes: An Insider's View* 2001, 2003

Vesical Neck and Prostate

52400 Cystourethroscopy with incision, fulguration, or resection of congenital posterior urethral valves, or congenital obstructive hypertrophic mucosal folds

> *CPT Assistant* Apr 01:4; *CPT Changes: An Insider's View* 2001

52402 Cystourethroscopy with transurethral resection or incision of ejaculatory ducts

> *CPT Changes: An Insider's View* 2005

52450 Transurethral incision of prostate

> *CPT Assistant* Apr 01:4, Jul 05:15

52500 Transurethral resection of bladder neck (separate procedure)

> *CPT Assistant* Apr 01:4, Jan 04:27, Jul 05:15

▶(52510 has been deleted)◀

52601 Transurethral electrosurgical resection of prostate, including control of postoperative bleeding, complete (vasectomy, meatotomy, cystourethroscopy, urethral calibration and/or dilation, and internal urethrotomy are included)

> *CPT Assistant* Nov 97:20, Apr 01:4, Jun 03:6

(For other approaches, see 55801-55845)

Transurethral Resection of Prostate, Complete
52601

The physician removes the prostate gland using an electrocautery knife.

52606 Transurethral fulguration for postoperative bleeding occurring after the usual follow-up time

> *CPT Assistant* Apr 01:4

52612 Transurethral resection of prostate; first stage of two-stage resection (partial resection)

> *CPT Assistant* Apr 01:4

52614 second stage of two-stage resection (resection completed)

> *CPT Assistant* Apr 01:4

52620 Transurethral resection; of residual obstructive tissue after 90 days postoperative

> *CPT Assistant* Apr 01:4

52630 of regrowth of obstructive tissue longer than one year postoperative

> *CPT Assistant* Apr 01:4

52640 of postoperative bladder neck contracture

> *CPT Assistant* Apr 01:4

52647 Laser coagulation of prostate, including control of postoperative bleeding, complete (vasectomy, meatotomy, cystourethroscopy, urethral calibration and/or dilation, and internal urethrotomy are included if performed)

> *CPT Assistant* Nov 97:20, Mar 98:11, Apr 01:4, Nov 06:21; *CPT Changes: An Insider's View* 2006

52648 Laser vaporization of prostate, including control of postoperative bleeding, complete (vasectomy, meatotomy, cystourethroscopy, urethral calibration and/or dilation, internal urethrotomy and transurethral resection of prostate are included if performed)

➔ *CPT Assistant* Mar 98:11, Apr 01:5, Jul 05:15, Nov 06:21; *CPT Changes: An Insider's View* 2006

Contact Laser Vaporization of Prostate
52648

A laser is used to vaporize the prostate.

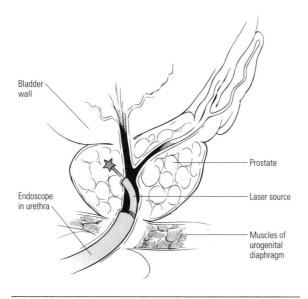

Bladder wall

Prostate

Laser source

Endoscope in urethra

Muscles of urogenital diaphragm

● **52649** Laser enucleation of the prostate with morcellation, including control of postoperative bleeding, complete (vasectomy, meatotomy, cystourethroscopy, urethral calibration and/or dilation, internal urethrotomy and transurethral resection of prostate are included if performed)

➔ *CPT Changes: An Insider's View* 2008

►(Do not report 52649 in conjunction with 52000, 52276, 52281, 52601, 52647, 52648, 53020, 55250)◄

52700 Transurethral drainage of prostatic abscess

➔ *CPT Assistant* Apr 01:4

(For litholapaxy, use 52317, 52318)

Urethra

(For endoscopy, see cystoscopy, urethroscopy, cystourethroscopy, 52000-52700)

(For injection procedure for urethrocystography, see 51600-51610)

Incision

53000 Urethrotomy or urethrostomy, external (separate procedure); pendulous urethra

53010 perineal urethra, external

53020 Meatotomy, cutting of meatus (separate procedure); except infant

53025 infant

(Do not report modifier 63 in conjunction with 53025)

53040 Drainage of deep periurethral abscess

(For subcutaneous abscess, see 10060, 10061)

53060 Drainage of Skene's gland abscess or cyst

53080 Drainage of perineal urinary extravasation; uncomplicated (separate procedure)

53085 complicated

Excision

53200 Biopsy of urethra

53210 Urethrectomy, total, including cystostomy; female

53215 male

53220 Excision or fulguration of carcinoma of urethra

53230 Excision of urethral diverticulum (separate procedure); female

53235 male

53240 Marsupialization of urethral diverticulum, male or female

53250 Excision of bulbourethral gland (Cowper's gland)

53260 Excision or fulguration; urethral polyp(s), distal urethra

(For endoscopic approach, see 52214, 52224)

53265 urethral caruncle

53270 Skene's glands

53275 urethral prolapse

Repair

(For hypospadias, see 54300-54352)

53400 Urethroplasty; first stage, for fistula, diverticulum, or stricture (eg, Johannsen type)

53405 second stage (formation of urethra), including urinary diversion

53410 Urethroplasty, one-stage reconstruction of male anterior urethra

53415 Urethroplasty, transpubic or perineal, one stage, for reconstruction or repair of prostatic or membranous urethra

53420 Urethroplasty, two-stage reconstruction or repair of prostatic or membranous urethra; first stage

53425 second stage

53430 Urethroplasty, reconstruction of female urethra

53431 Urethroplasty with tubularization of posterior urethra and/or lower bladder for incontinence (eg, Tenago, Leadbetter procedure)

➔ *CPT Changes: An Insider's View* 2002

53440 Sling operation for correction of male urinary incontinence (eg, fascia or synthetic)
↪ *CPT Changes: An Insider's View* 2003

53442 Removal or revision of sling for male urinary incontinence (eg, fascia or synthetic)
↪ *CPT Changes: An Insider's View* 2003

53444 Insertion of tandem cuff (dual cuff)
↪ *CPT Changes: An Insider's View* 2002

53445 Insertion of inflatable urethral/bladder neck sphincter, including placement of pump, reservoir, and cuff
↪ *CPT Changes: An Insider's View* 2002

53446 Removal of inflatable urethral/bladder neck sphincter, including pump, reservoir, and cuff
↪ *CPT Changes: An Insider's View* 2002

53447 Removal and replacement of inflatable urethral/bladder neck sphincter including pump, reservoir, and cuff at the same operative session
↪ *CPT Changes: An Insider's View* 2002

53448 Removal and replacement of inflatable urethral/bladder neck sphincter including pump, reservoir, and cuff through an infected field at the same operative session including irrigation and debridement of infected tissue
↪ *CPT Changes: An Insider's View* 2002

(Do not report 11040-11043 in addition to 53448)

53449 Repair of inflatable urethral/bladder neck sphincter, including pump, reservoir, and cuff
↪ *CPT Changes: An Insider's View* 2002

53450 Urethromeatoplasty, with mucosal advancement

(For meatotomy, see 53020, 53025)

53460 Urethromeatoplasty, with partial excision of distal urethral segment (Richardson type procedure)

53500 Urethrolysis, transvaginal, secondary, open, including cystourethroscopy (eg, postsurgical obstruction, scarring)
↪ *CPT Assistant* Sep 04:11; *CPT Changes: An Insider's View* 2004

(For urethrolysis by retropubic approach, use 53899)

(Do not report 53500 in conjunction with 52000)

53502 Urethrorrhaphy, suture of urethral wound or injury, female

53505 Urethrorrhaphy, suture of urethral wound or injury; penile

53510 perineal

53515 prostatomembranous

53520 Closure of urethrostomy or urethrocutaneous fistula, male (separate procedure)

(For closure of urethrovaginal fistula, use 57310)

(For closure of urethrorectal fistula, see 45820, 45825)

Manipulation

(For radiological supervision and interpretation, use 74485)

53600 Dilation of urethral stricture by passage of sound or urethral dilator, male; initial

53601 subsequent

53605 Dilation of urethral stricture or vesical neck by passage of sound or urethral dilator, male, general or conduction (spinal) anesthesia

53620 Dilation of urethral stricture by passage of filiform and follower, male; initial

53621 subsequent

53660 Dilation of female urethra including suppository and/or instillation; initial

53661 subsequent

53665 Dilation of female urethra, general or conduction (spinal) anesthesia

(For urethral catheterization, see 51701-51703)

Other Procedures

(For two or three glass urinalysis, use 81020)

53850 Transurethral destruction of prostate tissue; by microwave thermotherapy
↪ *CPT Assistant* Nov 97:20, Apr 01:6

53852 by radiofrequency thermotherapy
↪ *CPT Assistant* Nov 97:20, Apr 01:6

53853 by water-induced thermotherapy
↪ *CPT Assistant* Aug 04:12, Sep 04:11; *CPT Changes: An Insider's View* 2002

53899 Unlisted procedure, urinary system
↪ *CPT Assistant* Aug 04:12, Sep 04:11, Oct 05:18, 23-24, Feb 06:14
↪ *Clinical Examples in Radiology* Summer 06:1-3

Male Genital System

Penis

Incision

(For abdominal perineal gangrene debridement, see 11004-11006)

54000 Slitting of prepuce, dorsal or lateral (separate procedure); newborn

(Do not report modifier 63 in conjunction with 54000)

54001 except newborn

54015 Incision and drainage of penis, deep

(For skin and subcutaneous abscess, see 10060-10160)

Destruction

54050 Destruction of lesion(s), penis (eg, condyloma, papilloma, molluscum contagiosum, herpetic vesicle), simple; chemical

54055 electrodesiccation

54056 cryosurgery

54057 laser surgery

54060 surgical excision

54065 Destruction of lesion(s), penis (eg, condyloma, papilloma, molluscum contagiosum, herpetic vesicle), extensive (eg, laser surgery, electrosurgery, cryosurgery, chemosurgery)
➔ *CPT Changes: An Insider's View 2002*

(For destruction or excision of other lesions, see **Integumentary System**)

Excision

54100 Biopsy of penis; (separate procedure)
➔ *CPT Assistant Nov 99:26; CPT Changes: An Insider's View 2000*

54105 deep structures

54110 Excision of penile plaque (Peyronie disease);

54111 with graft to 5 cm in length
➔ *CPT Assistant Aug 99:5*

54112 with graft greater than 5 cm in length

54115 Removal foreign body from deep penile tissue (eg, plastic implant)

54120 Amputation of penis; partial

54125 complete

54130 Amputation of penis, radical; with bilateral inguinofemoral lymphadenectomy

54135 in continuity with bilateral pelvic lymphadenectomy, including external iliac, hypogastric and obturator nodes

(For lymphadenectomy (separate procedure), see 38760-38770)

54150 Circumcision, using clamp or other device with regional dorsal penile or ring block
➔ *CPT Assistant Sep 96:11, May 98:11, Apr 03:27, Aug 03:6; CPT Changes: An Insider's View 2007*

(Do not report modifier 63 in conjunction with 54150)

(Report 54150 with modifier 52 when performed without dorsal penile or ring block)

(54152 has been deleted. To report, use 54150)

54160 Circumcision, surgical excision other than clamp, device, or dorsal slit; neonate (28 days of age or less)
➔ *CPT Assistant Sep 96:11, May 98:11; CPT Changes: An Insider's View 2007*

(Do not report modifier 63 in conjunction with 54160)

54161 older than 28 days of age
➔ *CPT Assistant Sep 96:11, Dec 96:10, May 98:11; CPT Changes: An Insider's View 2007*

54162 Lysis or excision of penile post-circumcision adhesions
➔ *CPT Changes: An Insider's View 2002*

54163 Repair incomplete circumcision
➔ *CPT Changes: An Insider's View 2002*

54164 Frenulotomy of penis
➔ *CPT Changes: An Insider's View 2002*

(Do not report 54164 with circumcision codes 54150-54161, 54162, 54163)

Introduction

54200 Injection procedure for Peyronie disease;

54205 with surgical exposure of plaque

54220 Irrigation of corpora cavernosa for priapism

54230 Injection procedure for corpora cavernosography

(For radiological supervision and interpretation, use 74445)

54231 Dynamic cavernosometry, including intracavernosal injection of vasoactive drugs (eg, papaverine, phentolamine)

54235 Injection of corpora cavernosa with pharmacologic agent(s) (eg, papaverine, phentolamine)
➔ *CPT Assistant Sep 96:10*

54240 Penile plethysmography

54250 Nocturnal penile tumescence and/or rigidity test

Repair

(For other urethroplasties, see 53400-53430)

(For penile revascularization, use 37788)

54300 Plastic operation of penis for straightening of chordee (eg, hypospadias), with or without mobilization of urethra

54304 Plastic operation on penis for correction of chordee or for first stage hypospadias repair with or without transplantation of prepuce and/or skin flaps

54308 Urethroplasty for second stage hypospadias repair (including urinary diversion); less than 3 cm

54312   greater than 3 cm

54316 Urethroplasty for second stage hypospadias repair (including urinary diversion) with free skin graft obtained from site other than genitalia

54318 Urethroplasty for third stage hypospadias repair to release penis from scrotum (eg, third stage Cecil repair)

54322 One stage distal hypospadias repair (with or without chordee or circumcision); with simple meatal advancement (eg, Magpi, V-flap)

54324   with urethroplasty by local skin flaps (eg, flip-flap, prepucial flap)

54326   with urethroplasty by local skin flaps and mobilization of urethra

54328   with extensive dissection to correct chordee and urethroplasty with local skin flaps, skin graft patch, and/or island flap

> *CPT Assistant* Oct 04:15

(For urethroplasty and straightening of chordee, use 54308)

54332 One stage proximal penile or penoscrotal hypospadias repair requiring extensive dissection to correct chordee and urethroplasty by use of skin graft tube and/or island flap

> *CPT Assistant* Mar 04:11, Sep 04:12

54336 One stage perineal hypospadias repair requiring extensive dissection to correct chordee and urethroplasty by use of skin graft tube and/or island flap

> *CPT Assistant* Oct 04:15

54340 Repair of hypospadias complications (ie, fistula, stricture, diverticula); by closure, incision, or excision, simple

54344   requiring mobilization of skin flaps and urethroplasty with flap or patch graft

54348   requiring extensive dissection and urethroplasty with flap, patch or tubed graft (includes urinary diversion)

54352 Repair of hypospadias cripple requiring extensive dissection and excision of previously constructed structures including re-release of chordee and reconstruction of urethra and penis by use of local skin as grafts and island flaps and skin brought in as flaps or grafts

54360 Plastic operation on penis to correct angulation

54380 Plastic operation on penis for epispadias distal to external sphincter;

54385   with incontinence

54390   with exstrophy of bladder

54400 Insertion of penile prosthesis; non-inflatable (semi-rigid)

54401   inflatable (self-contained)

(For removal or replacement of penile prosthesis, see 54415, 54416)

54405 Insertion of multi-component, inflatable penile prosthesis, including placement of pump, cylinders, and reservoir

> *CPT Changes: An Insider's View* 2002

(For reduced services, report 54405 with modifier 52)

54406 Removal of all components of a multi-component, inflatable penile prosthesis without replacement of prosthesis

> *CPT Changes: An Insider's View* 2002

(For reduced services, report 54406 with modifier 52)

54408 Repair of component(s) of a multi-component, inflatable penile prosthesis

> *CPT Changes: An Insider's View* 2002

54410 Removal and replacement of all component(s) of a multi-component, inflatable penile prosthesis at the same operative session

> *CPT Changes: An Insider's View* 2002

54411 Removal and replacement of all components of a multi-component inflatable penile prosthesis through an infected field at the same operative session, including irrigation and debridement of infected tissue

> *CPT Changes: An Insider's View* 2002

(For reduced services, report 54411 with modifier 52)

(Do not report 11040-11043 in addition to 54411)

54415 Removal of non-inflatable (semi-rigid) or inflatable (self-contained) penile prosthesis, without replacement of prosthesis

> *CPT Changes: An Insider's View* 2002

54416 Removal and replacement of non-inflatable (semi-rigid) or inflatable (self-contained) penile prosthesis at the same operative session

> *CPT Changes: An Insider's View* 2002

54417 Removal and replacement of non-inflatable (semi-rigid) or inflatable (self-contained) penile prosthesis through an infected field at the same operative session, including irrigation and debridement of infected tissue

> *CPT Changes: An Insider's View* 2002

(Do not report 11040-11043 in addition to 54417)

54420 Corpora cavernosa-saphenous vein shunt (priapism operation), unilateral or bilateral

54430 Corpora cavernosa-corpus spongiosum shunt (priapism operation), unilateral or bilateral

54435 Corpora cavernosa-glans penis fistulization (eg, biopsy needle, Winter procedure, rongeur, or punch) for priapism

54440 Plastic operation of penis for injury

Manipulation

54450   Foreskin manipulation including lysis of preputial adhesions and stretching

Testis

Excision

(For abdominal perineal gangrene debridement, see 11004-11006)

54500   Biopsy of testis, needle (separate procedure)

(For fine needle aspiration, see 10021, 10022)

(For evaluation of fine needle aspirate, see 88172, 88173)

54505   Biopsy of testis, incisional (separate procedure)
➔ *CPT Assistant* Oct 01:8

(For bilateral procedure, report 54505 with modifier 50)

(When combined with vasogram, seminal vesiculogram, or epididymogram, use 55300)

54512   Excision of extraparenchymal lesion of testis
➔ *CPT Assistant* Oct 01:8, Aug 05:13; *CPT Changes: An Insider's View* 2001

54520   Orchiectomy, simple (including subcapsular), with or without testicular prosthesis, scrotal or inguinal approach
➔ *CPT Assistant* Winter 94:13, Oct 01:8, Mar 04:3

(For bilateral procedure, report 54520 with modifier 50)

54522   Orchiectomy, partial
➔ *CPT Assistant* Oct 01:8; *CPT Changes: An Insider's View* 2001

54530   Orchiectomy, radical, for tumor; inguinal approach
➔ *CPT Assistant* Oct 01:8

54535   with abdominal exploration
➔   *CPT Assistant* Oct 01:8

(For orchiectomy with repair of hernia, see 49505 or 49507 and 54520)

(For radical retroperitoneal lymphadenectomy, use 38780)

Exploration

54550   Exploration for undescended testis (inguinal or scrotal area)
➔ *CPT Assistant* Oct 01:8

(For bilateral procedure, report 54550 with modifier 50)

54560   Exploration for undescended testis with abdominal exploration
➔ *CPT Assistant* Oct 01:8

(For bilateral procedure, report 54560 with modifier 50)

Repair

54600   Reduction of torsion of testis, surgical, with or without fixation of contralateral testis
➔ *CPT Assistant* Aug 05:13

54620   Fixation of contralateral testis (separate procedure)

54640   Orchiopexy, inguinal approach, with or without hernia repair
➔ *CPT Assistant* Oct 01:8, Jan 04:27, Mar 04:10

(For bilateral procedure, report 54640 with modifier 50)

(For inguinal hernia repair performed in conjunction with inguinal orchiopexy, see 49495-49525)

54650   Orchiopexy, abdominal approach, for intra-abdominal testis (eg, Fowler-Stephens)
➔ *CPT Assistant* Nov 99:26, May 00:4, Oct 01:8; *CPT Changes: An Insider's View* 2000

(For laparoscopic approach, use 54692)

54660   Insertion of testicular prosthesis (separate procedure)
➔ *CPT Assistant* Oct 01:8

(For bilateral procedure, report 54660 with modifier 50)

54670   Suture or repair of testicular injury
➔ *CPT Assistant* Oct 01:8

54680   Transplantation of testis(es) to thigh (because of scrotal destruction)
➔ *CPT Assistant* Oct 01:8

Laparoscopy

Surgical laparoscopy always includes diagnostic laparoscopy. To report a diagnostic laparoscopy (peritoneoscopy) (separate procedure), use 49320.

54690   Laparoscopy, surgical; orchiectomy
➔ *CPT Assistant* Nov 99:26, Mar 00:5, Oct 01:8; *CPT Changes: An Insider's View* 2000

54692   orchiopexy for intra-abdominal testis
➔ *CPT Assistant* Nov 99:27, May 00:4, Oct 01:8; *CPT Changes: An Insider's View* 2000

Laparoscopic Orchiopexy
54692

Surgical fixation of an undescended testis in the scrotum under laparoscopic guidance

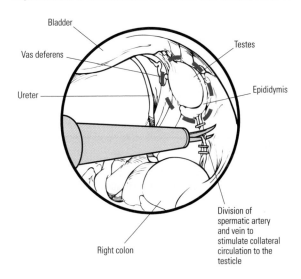

54699 Unlisted laparoscopy procedure, testis
➔ *CPT Assistant* Nov 99:27, Mar 00:9; *CPT Changes: An Insider's View* 2000

Epididymis

Incision

54700 Incision and drainage of epididymis, testis and/or scrotal space (eg, abscess or hematoma)
➔ *CPT Assistant* Oct 01:8

▶(For debridement of necrotizing soft tissue infection of external genitalia, see 11004-11006)◀

Excision

54800 Biopsy of epididymis, needle
➔ *CPT Assistant* Oct 01:8

(For fine needle aspiration, see 10021, 10022)

(For evaluation of fine needle aspirate, see 88172, 88173)

(54820 has been deleted. To report, use 54865)

54830 Excision of local lesion of epididymis
➔ *CPT Assistant* Oct 01:8

54840 Excision of spermatocele, with or without epididymectomy
➔ *CPT Assistant* Oct 01:8

54860 Epididymectomy; unilateral

54861 bilateral

Exploration

54865 Exploration of epididymis, with or without biopsy
➔ *CPT Changes: An Insider's View* 2007

Repair

54900 Epididymovasostomy, anastomosis of epididymis to vas deferens; unilateral
➔ *CPT Assistant* Nov 98:16

54901 bilateral
➔ *CPT Assistant* Nov 98:16

(For operating microscope, use 69990)

Tunica Vaginalis

Incision

55000 Puncture aspiration of hydrocele, tunica vaginalis, with or without injection of medication

Excision

55040 Excision of hydrocele; unilateral

55041 bilateral

(With hernia repair, see 49495-49501)

Repair

55060 Repair of tunica vaginalis hydrocele (Bottle type)

Scrotum

Incision

55100 Drainage of scrotal wall abscess

(See also 54700)

▶(For debridement of necrotizing soft tissue infection of external genitalia, see 11004-11006)◀

55110 Scrotal exploration

55120 Removal of foreign body in scrotum

Excision

(For excision of local lesion of skin of scrotum, see **Integumentary System**)

55150 Resection of scrotum

Repair

55175 Scrotoplasty; simple

55180 complicated

Vas Deferens

Incision

55200 Vasotomy, cannulization with or without incision of vas, unilateral or bilateral (separate procedure)

Excision

55250 Vasectomy, unilateral or bilateral (separate procedure), including postoperative semen examination(s)
➔ *CPT Assistant* Jun 98:10, Jul 98:10

Introduction

55300 Vasotomy for vasograms, seminal vesiculograms, or epididymograms, unilateral or bilateral

(For radiological supervision and interpretation, use 74440)

(When combined with biopsy of testis, see 54505 and use modifier 51)

Repair

55400   Vasovasostomy, vasovasorrhaphy
> *CPT Assistant* Nov 98:16, Oct 01:8

(For bilateral procedure, report 55400 with modifier 50)

(For operating microscope, use 69990)

Suture

55450   Ligation (percutaneous) of vas deferens, unilateral or bilateral (separate procedure)

Spermatic Cord

Excision

55500   Excision of hydrocele of spermatic cord, unilateral (separate procedure)
> *CPT Assistant* Oct 01:8

55520   Excision of lesion of spermatic cord (separate procedure)
> *CPT Assistant* Sep 00:10, Oct 01:8

55530   Excision of varicocele or ligation of spermatic veins for varicocele; (separate procedure)
> *CPT Assistant* Oct 01:8

55535   abdominal approach
> *CPT Assistant* Oct 01:8

55540   with hernia repair
> *CPT Assistant* Oct 01:8

Laparoscopy

Surgical laparoscopy always includes diagnostic laparoscopy. To report a diagnostic laparoscopy (peritoneoscopy) (separate procedure), use 49320.

55550   Laparoscopy, surgical, with ligation of spermatic veins for varicocele
> *CPT Assistant* Nov 99:27, Mar 00:9, Oct 01:8; *CPT Changes: An Insider's View* 2000

55559   Unlisted laparoscopy procedure, spermatic cord
> *CPT Assistant* Nov 99:27, Mar 00:9; *CPT Changes: An Insider's View* 2000

Seminal Vesicles

Incision

55600   Vesiculotomy;

(For bilateral procedure, report 55600 with modifier 50)

55605   complicated

Excision

55650   Vesiculectomy, any approach

(For bilateral procedure, report 55650 with modifier 50)

55680   Excision of Mullerian duct cyst

(For injection procedure, see 52010, 55300)

Prostate

Incision

55700   Biopsy, prostate; needle or punch, single or multiple, any approach
> *CPT Assistant* May 96:3

(For prostate needle biopsy saturation sampling for prostate mapping, use Category III code 0137T)

(If imaging guidance is performed, use 76942)

(For fine needle aspiration, see 10021, 10022)

(For evaluation of fine needle aspirate, see 88172, 88173)

55705   incisional, any approach

55720   Prostatotomy, external drainage of prostatic abscess, any approach; simple

55725   complicated

(For transurethral drainage, use 52700)

Excision

(For transurethral removal of prostate, see 52601-52640)

(For transurethral destruction of prostate, see 53850-53852)

(For limited pelvic lymphadenectomy for staging (separate procedure), use 38562)

(For independent node dissection, see 38770-38780)

55801   Prostatectomy, perineal, subtotal (including control of postoperative bleeding, vasectomy, meatotomy, urethral calibration and/or dilation, and internal urethrotomy)
> *CPT Assistant* Jun 03:6-7

55810   Prostatectomy, perineal radical;

55812   with lymph node biopsy(s) (limited pelvic lymphadenectomy)

55815   with bilateral pelvic lymphadenectomy, including external iliac, hypogastric and obturator nodes

(If 55815 is carried out on separate days, use 38770 with modifier 50 and 55810)

55821   Prostatectomy (including control of postoperative bleeding, vasectomy, meatotomy, urethral calibration and/or dilation, and internal urethrotomy); suprapubic, subtotal, one or two stages
➔ *CPT Assistant* Jun 03:6

55831   retropubic, subtotal
➔ *CPT Assistant* Jun 03:7

55840   Prostatectomy, retropubic radical, with or without nerve sparing;
➔ *CPT Assistant* Jun 03:8

55842   with lymph node biopsy(s) (limited pelvic lymphadenectomy)
➔ *CPT Assistant* Jun 03:8

55845   with bilateral pelvic lymphadenectomy, including external iliac, hypogastric, and obturator nodes
➔ *CPT Assistant* Jun 03:8

(If 55845 is carried out on separate days, use 38770 with modifier 50 and 55840)

(For laparoscopic retropubic radical prostatectomy, use 55866)

(55859 has been deleted. To report, use 55875)

55860   Exposure of prostate, any approach, for insertion of radioactive substance;

(For application of interstitial radioelement, see 77776-77778)

55862   with lymph node biopsy(s) (limited pelvic lymphadenectomy)

55865   with bilateral pelvic lymphadenectomy, including external iliac, hypogastric and obturator nodes

Laparoscopy

Surgical laparoscopy always includes diagnostic laparoscopy. To report a diagnostic laparoscopy (peritoneoscopy) (separate procedure), use 49320.

55866   Laparoscopy, surgical prostatectomy, retropubic radical, including nerve sparing
➔ *CPT Assistant* Jun 03:8; *CPT Changes: An Insider's View* 2003

(For open procedure, use 55840)

Other Procedures

(For artificial insemination, see 58321, 58322)

55870   Electroejaculation

55873   Cryosurgical ablation of the prostate (includes ultrasonic guidance for interstitial cryosurgical probe placement)
➔ *CPT Assistant* Apr 01:4, Sep 02:9, Jun 03:8; *CPT Changes: An Insider's View* 2001

55875   Transperineal placement of needles or catheters into prostate for interstitial radioelement application, with or without cystoscopy
➔ *CPT Changes: An Insider's View* 2007

▶(For placement of needles or catheters into pelvic organs and/or genitalia [except prostate] for interstitial radioelement application, use 55920)◀

(For interstitial radioelement application, see 77776-77784)

(For ultrasonic guidance for interstitial radioelement application, use 76965)

55876   Placement of interstitial device(s) for radiation therapy guidance (eg, fiducial markers, dosimeter), prostate (via needle, any approach), single or multiple
➔ *CPT Changes: An Insider's View* 2007

(Report supply of device separately)

(For imaging guidance, see 76942, 77002, 77012, 77021)

55899   Unlisted procedure, male genital system
➔ *CPT Assistant* Jun 03:8
➔ *Clinical Examples in Radiology* Spring 06:8-9

▶Reproductive System Procedures◀

● **55920**   Placement of needles or catheters into pelvic organs and/or genitalia (except prostate) for subsequent interstitial radioelement application
➔ *CPT Changes: An Insider's View* 2008

▶(For placement of needles or catheters into prostate, use 55875)◀

▶(For insertion of uterine tandems and/or vaginal ovoids for clinical brachytherapy, use 57155)◀

▶(For insertion of Heyman capsules for clinical brachytherapy, use 58346)◀

Intersex Surgery

55970   Intersex surgery; male to female

55980   female to male

Female Genital System

(For pelvic laparotomy, use 49000)

►(For excision or destruction of endometriomas, open method, see 49203-49205, 58957, 58958)◄

(For paracentesis, see 49080, 49081)

(For secondary closure of abdominal wall evisceration or disruption, use 49900)

(For fulguration or excision of lesions, laparoscopic approach, use 58662)

(For chemotherapy, see 96401-96549)

Vulva, Perineum, and Introitus

Definitions

The following definitions apply to the vulvectomy codes (56620-56640).

A *simple* procedure is the removal of skin and superficial subcutaneous tissues.

A *radical* procedure is the removal of skin and deep subcutaneous tissue.

A *partial* procedure is the removal of less than 80% of the vulvar area.

A *complete* procedure is the removal of greater than 80% of the vulvar area.

Incision

(For incision and drainage of sebaceous cyst, furuncle, or abscess, see 10040, 10060, 10061)

56405   Incision and drainage of vulva or perineal abscess

56420   Incision and drainage of Bartholin's gland abscess

(For incision and drainage of Skene's gland abscess or cyst, use 53060)

56440   Marsupialization of Bartholin's gland cyst

56441   Lysis of labial adhesions
➔ *CPT Assistant* Winter 90:7

56442   Hymenotomy, simple incision
➔ *CPT Changes: An Insider's View* 2007

Destruction

56501   Destruction of lesion(s), vulva; simple (eg, laser surgery, electrosurgery, cryosurgery, chemosurgery)
➔ *CPT Changes: An Insider's View* 2002

56515   extensive (eg, laser surgery, electrosurgery, cryosurgery, chemosurgery)
➔ *CPT Changes: An Insider's View* 2002

(For destruction of Skene's gland cyst or abscess, use 53270)

(For cautery destruction of urethral caruncle, use 53265)

Excision

56605   Biopsy of vulva or perineum (separate procedure); one lesion
➔ *CPT Assistant* Sep 00:9

+ 56606   each separate additional lesion (List separately in addition to code for primary procedure)

(Use 56606 in conjunction with 56605)

(For excision of local lesion, see 11420-11426, 11620-11626)

56620   Vulvectomy simple; partial

56625   complete

(For skin graft, see 15002 et seq)

56630   Vulvectomy, radical, partial;

(For skin graft, if used, see 15004-15005, 15120, 15121, 15240, 15241)

56631   with unilateral inguinofemoral lymphadenectomy

56632   with bilateral inguinofemoral lymphadenectomy

56633   Vulvectomy, radical, complete;

56634   with unilateral inguinofemoral lymphadenectomy

56637   with bilateral inguinofemoral lymphadenectomy

56640   Vulvectomy, radical, complete, with inguinofemoral, iliac, and pelvic lymphadenectomy

(For bilateral procedure, report 56640 with modifier 50)

(For lymphadenectomy, see 38760-38780)

56700   Partial hymenectomy or revision of hymenal ring

(56720 has been deleted. To report, use 56442)

56740   Excision of Bartholin's gland or cyst

(For excision of Skene's gland, use 53270)

(For excision of urethral caruncle, use 53265)

(For excision or fulguration of urethral carcinoma, use 53220)

(For excision or marsupialization of urethral diverticulum, see 53230, 53240)

Repair

(For repair of urethra for mucosal prolapse, use 53275)

56800   Plastic repair of introitus

56805   Clitoroplasty for intersex state

56810 Perineoplasty, repair of perineum, nonobstetrical (separate procedure)

(See also 56800)

(For repair of wounds to genitalia, see 12001-12007, 12041-12047, 13131-13133)

(For repair of recent injury of vagina and perineum, nonobstetrical, use 57210)

(For anal sphincteroplasty, see 46750, 46751)

(For episiorrhaphy, episioperineorrhaphy for recent injury of vulva and/or perineum, nonobstetrical, use 57210)

Endoscopy

56820 Colposcopy of the vulva;
→ *CPT Assistant* Feb 03:5; *CPT Changes: An Insider's View* 2003

56821 with biopsy(s)
→ *CPT Assistant* Feb 03:5, Jun 03:11; *CPT Changes: An Insider's View* 2003

(For colposcopic examinations/procedures involving the vagina, see 57420, 57421; cervix, see 57452-57461)

Vagina

Incision

57000 Colpotomy; with exploration

57010 with drainage of pelvic abscess

57020 Colpocentesis (separate procedure)

57022 Incision and drainage of vaginal hematoma; obstetrical/postpartum
→ *CPT Changes: An Insider's View* 2001, 2002

57023 non-obstetrical (eg, post-trauma, spontaneous bleeding)
→ *CPT Changes: An Insider's View* 2001

Destruction

57061 Destruction of vaginal lesion(s); simple (eg, laser surgery, electrosurgery, cryosurgery, chemosurgery)
→ *CPT Assistant* Apr 96:11; *CPT Changes: An Insider's View* 2002

57065 extensive (eg, laser surgery, electrosurgery, cryosurgery, chemosurgery)
→ *CPT Assistant* Apr 96:11; *CPT Changes: An Insider's View* 2002

Excision

57100 Biopsy of vaginal mucosa; simple (separate procedure)

57105 extensive, requiring suture (including cysts)

57106 Vaginectomy, partial removal of vaginal wall;
→ *CPT Assistant* Nov 98:17, Oct 99:5

Vaginectomy, Partial Removal of Vaginal Wall
57106

A specific portion of the upper or lower vaginal wall is excised.

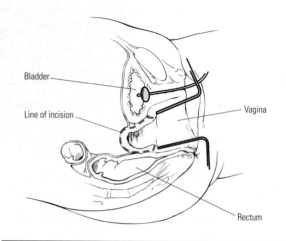

57107 with removal of paravaginal tissue (radical vaginectomy)
→ *CPT Assistant* Nov 98:17, Oct 99:5

57109 with removal of paravaginal tissue (radical vaginectomy) with bilateral total pelvic lymphadenectomy and para-aortic lymph node sampling (biopsy)
→ *CPT Assistant* Nov 98:17, Oct 99:5

57110 Vaginectomy, complete removal of vaginal wall;
→ *CPT Assistant* Nov 98:17, Oct 99:5

57111 with removal of paravaginal tissue (radical vaginectomy)
→ *CPT Assistant* Nov 98:17, Oct 99:5

Vaginectomy, Complete Removal of Vaginal Wall (Radical Vaginectomy)
57111

Removal of all of the vaginal wall and removal of paravaginal tissue (the highly vascular supporting connective tissue next to the vagina)

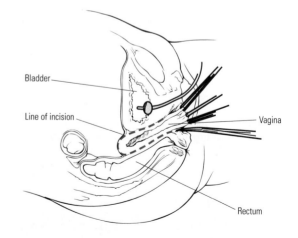

57112   with removal of paravaginal tissue (radical vaginectomy) with bilateral total pelvic lymphadenectomy and para-aortic lymph node sampling (biopsy)
> *CPT Assistant* Nov 98:17, Oct 99:5

57120   Colpocleisis (Le Fort type)

57130   Excision of vaginal septum

57135   Excision of vaginal cyst or tumor

Introduction

57150   Irrigation of vagina and/or application of medicament for treatment of bacterial, parasitic, or fungoid disease

57155   Insertion of uterine tandems and/or vaginal ovoids for clinical brachytherapy
> *CPT Assistant* Feb 02:8; *CPT Changes: An Insider's View* 2002

▶(For placement of needles or catheters into pelvic organs and/or genitalia [except prostate] for interstitial radioelement application, use 55920)◀

(For insertion of radioelement sources or ribbons, see 77761-77763, 77781-77784)

57160   Fitting and insertion of pessary or other intravaginal support device
> *CPT Assistant* Nov 96:9, Oct 98:11, Jun 00:11

57170   Diaphragm or cervical cap fitting with instructions

57180   Introduction of any hemostatic agent or pack for spontaneous or traumatic nonobstetrical vaginal hemorrhage (separate procedure)

Repair

(For urethral suspension, Marshall-Marchetti-Krantz type, abdominal approach, see 51840, 51841)

(For laparoscopic suspension, use 51990)

57200   Colporrhaphy, suture of injury of vagina (nonobstetrical)

57210   Colpoperineorrhaphy, suture of injury of vagina and/or perineum (nonobstetrical)

57220   Plastic operation on urethral sphincter, vaginal approach (eg, Kelly urethral plication)
> *CPT Assistant* Winter 90:7

57230   Plastic repair of urethrocele
> *CPT Assistant* Winter 90:7

57240   Anterior colporrhaphy, repair of cystocele with or without repair of urethrocele
> *CPT Assistant* Winter 90:7, Jan 97:3, Jun 02:5

57250   Posterior colporrhaphy, repair of rectocele with or without perineorrhaphy
> *CPT Assistant* Winter 90:7, Jun 02:4

(For repair of rectocele (separate procedure) without posterior colporrhaphy, use 45560)

57260   Combined anteroposterior colporrhaphy;
> *CPT Assistant* Jun 02:5

57265   with enterocele repair
> *CPT Assistant* Jun 02:6

+ 57267   Insertion of mesh or other prosthesis for repair of pelvic floor defect, each site (anterior, posterior compartment), vaginal approach (List separately in addition to code for primary procedure)
> *CPT Assistant* Jul 05:16; *CPT Changes: An Insider's View* 2005

(Use 57267 in addition to 45560, 57240-57265)

57268   Repair of enterocele, vaginal approach (separate procedure)
> *CPT Assistant* Jun 02:6

57270   Repair of enterocele, abdominal approach (separate procedure)
> *CPT Assistant* Jun 02:6

57280   Colpopexy, abdominal approach
> *CPT Assistant* Jan 97:3, Jun 02:6

57282   Colpopexy, vaginal; extra-peritoneal approach (sacrospinous, iliococcygeus)
> *CPT Assistant* Jan 97:3, Jun 02:6; *CPT Changes: An Insider's View* 2005

57283   intra-peritoneal approach (uterosacral, levator myorrhaphy)
> *CPT Changes: An Insider's View* 2005

▲ **57284**   Paravaginal defect repair (including repair of cystocele, if performed); open abdominal approach
> *CPT Assistant* Jan 97:1, Jun 02:7, Jul 05:16; *CPT Changes: An Insider's View* 2008

▶(Do not report 57284 in conjunction with 51840, 51841, 51990, 57240, 57260, 57265, 58152, 58267)◀

● **57285**   vaginal approach
> *CPT Changes: An Insider's View* 2008

▶(Do not report 57285 in conjunction with 51990, 57240, 57260, 57265, 58267)◀

57287   Removal or revision of sling for stress incontinence (eg, fascia or synthetic)
> *CPT Assistant* Jun 02:7; *CPT Changes: An Insider's View* 2001

57288   Sling operation for stress incontinence (eg, fascia or synthetic)
> *CPT Assistant* Nov 99:28, May 00:4, Oct 00:7, Apr 02:18, Jun 02:7; *CPT Changes: An Insider's View* 2000

(For laparoscopic approach, use 51992)

57289   Pereyra procedure, including anterior colporrhaphy
> *CPT Assistant* Jan 97:3, Jun 02:7

57291   Construction of artificial vagina; without graft

57292   with graft

57295   Revision (including removal) of prosthetic vaginal graft; vaginal approach
> *CPT Changes: An Insider's View* 2006

57296   open abdominal approach
> *CPT Changes: An Insider's View* 2007

57300 Closure of rectovaginal fistula; vaginal or transanal approach
> *CPT Assistant* Nov 97:21

57305 abdominal approach
> *CPT Assistant* Nov 97:21

57307 abdominal approach, with concomitant colostomy
> *CPT Assistant* Nov 97:21

57308 transperineal approach, with perineal body reconstruction, with or without levator plication
> *CPT Assistant* Nov 97:21

57310 Closure of urethrovaginal fistula;

57311 with bulbocavernosus transplant

57320 Closure of vesicovaginal fistula; vaginal approach

▶(For concomitant cystostomy, see 51020-51040, 51101, 51102)◀

57330 transvesical and vaginal approach

(For abdominal approach, use 51900)

57335 Vaginoplasty for intersex state

Manipulation

57400 Dilation of vagina under anesthesia

57410 Pelvic examination under anesthesia
> *CPT Assistant* Spring 93:34, Apr 06:1

57415 Removal of impacted vaginal foreign body (separate procedure) under anesthesia

(For removal without anesthesia of an impacted vaginal foreign body, use the appropriate E/M code)

Endoscopy

(For speculoscopy, see Category III codes 0031T, 0032T)

57420 Colposcopy of the entire vagina, with cervix if present;
> *CPT Assistant* Feb 03:5; *CPT Changes: An Insider's View* 2003

57421 with biopsy(s) of vagina/cervix
> *CPT Assistant* Feb 03:5, Jun 03:11, Jun 06:16; *CPT Changes: An Insider's View* 2003, 2006

(For colposcopic visualization of cervix and adjacent upper vagina, use 57452)

(When reporting colposcopies of multiple sites, use modifier 51 as appropriate. For colposcopic examinations/procedures involving the vulva, see 56820, 56821; cervix, see 57452-57461)

(For endometrial sampling (biopsy) performed in conjunction with colposcopy, use 58110)

● **57423** Paravaginal defect repair (including repair of cystocele, if performed), laparoscopic approach
> *CPT Changes: An Insider's View* 2008

▶(Do not report 57423 in conjunction with 49320, 51840, 51841, 51990, 57240, 57260, 58152, 58267)◀

57425 Laparoscopy, surgical, colpopexy (suspension of vaginal apex)
> *CPT Changes: An Insider's View* 2004

Cervix Uteri

(For cervicography, see Category III code 0003T)

Endoscopy

(For colposcopic examinations/procedures involving the vulva, see 56820, 56821; vagina, see 57420, 57421)

57452 Colposcopy of the cervix including upper/adjacent vagina;
> *CPT Assistant* Apr 00:5, Feb 03:5, Jun 03:10; *CPT Changes: An Insider's View* 2003

(Do not report 57452 in addition to 57454-57461)

57454 with biopsy(s) of the cervix and endocervical curettage
> *CPT Assistant* Apr 00:5, Feb 03:5, Jun 03:10; *CPT Changes: An Insider's View* 2003

57455 with biopsy(s) of the cervix
> *CPT Assistant* Apr 00:5, Feb 03:5, Jun 03:10; *CPT Changes: An Insider's View* 2003

57456 with endocervical curettage
> *CPT Assistant* Apr 00:5, Jan 03:23, Feb 03:5, Jun 03:10; *CPT Changes: An Insider's View* 2003

57460 with loop electrode biopsy(s) of the cervix
> *CPT Assistant* Apr 00:5, Jan 03:23, Feb 03:5, Jun 03:10, Jul 05:15; *CPT Changes: An Insider's View* 2003

57461 with loop electrode conization of the cervix
> *CPT Assistant* Jan 03:23, Feb 03:5, Jun 03:10, Dec 06:15; *CPT Changes: An Insider's View* 2003

(Do not report 57456 in addition to 57461)

(For endometrial sampling (biopsy) performed in conjunction with colposcopy, use 58110)

Excision

(For radical surgical procedures, see 58200-58240)

▲ **57500** Biopsy of cervix, single or multiple, or local excision of lesion, with or without fulguration (separate procedure)
> *CPT Changes: An Insider's View* 2008

57505 Endocervical curettage (not done as part of a dilation and curettage)
> *CPT Assistant* Jul 05:15

57510 Cautery of cervix; electro or thermal
> *CPT Changes: An Insider's View* 2002

57511 cryocautery, initial or repeat

57513 laser ablation

57520 Conization of cervix, with or without fulguration, with or without dilation and curettage, with or without repair; cold knife or laser
> *CPT Assistant* Apr 00:5

(See also 58120)

57522   loop electrode excision
> *CPT Assistant* Apr 00:5, Mar 03:22, Jul 03:15

57530   Trachelectomy (cervicectomy), amputation of cervix (separate procedure)

57531   Radical trachelectomy, with bilateral total pelvic lymphadenectomy and para-aortic lymph node sampling biopsy, with or without removal of tube(s), with or without removal of ovary(s)
> *CPT Assistant* Nov 97:21

(For radical abdominal hysterectomy, use 58210)

57540   Excision of cervical stump, abdominal approach;

57545   with pelvic floor repair

57550   Excision of cervical stump, vaginal approach;

57555   with anterior and/or posterior repair

57556   with repair of enterocele

(For insertion of intrauterine device, use 58300)

(For insertion of any hemostatic agent or pack for control of spontaneous non-obstetrical hemorrhage, see 57180)

57558   Dilation and curettage of cervical stump
> *CPT Changes: An Insider's View* 2007

Repair

57700   Cerclage of uterine cervix, nonobstetrical

57720   Trachelorrhaphy, plastic repair of uterine cervix, vaginal approach

Manipulation

57800   Dilation of cervical canal, instrumental (separate procedure)

(57820 has been deleted. To report, use 57558)

Corpus Uteri

Excision

58100   Endometrial sampling (biopsy) with or without endocervical sampling (biopsy), without cervical dilation, any method (separate procedure)

(For endocervical curettage only, use 57505)

(For endometrial sampling (biopsy) performed in conjunction with colposcopy (57420, 57421, 57452-57461), use 58110)

+ 58110   Endometrial sampling (biopsy) performed in conjunction with colposcopy (List separately in addition to code for primary procedure)
> *CPT Changes: An Insider's View* 2006

(Use 58110 in conjunction with 57420, 57421, 57452-57461)

58120   Dilation and curettage, diagnostic and/or therapeutic (nonobstetrical)
> *CPT Assistant* Fall 95:16, Nov 97:21, May 03:19

(For postpartum hemorrhage, use 59160)

58140   Myomectomy, excision of fibroid tumor(s) of uterus, 1 to 4 intramural myoma(s) with total weight of 250 g or less and/or removal of surface myomas; abdominal approach
> *CPT Assistant* Feb 03:15, Jun 03:5; *CPT Changes: An Insider's View* 2002, 2003

58145   vaginal approach

58146   Myomectomy, excision of fibroid tumor(s) of uterus, 5 or more intramural myomas and/or intramural myomas with total weight greater than 250 g, abdominal approach
> *CPT Assistant* Feb 03:15, Jun 03:5; *CPT Changes: An Insider's View* 2003

(Do not report 58146 in addition to 58140-58145, 58150-58240)

Hysterectomy Procedures

58150   Total abdominal hysterectomy (corpus and cervix), with or without removal of tube(s), with or without removal of ovary(s);
> *CPT Assistant* Dec 96:10, Apr 97:3, Nov 97:21, Sep 00:9, Aug 01:11

58152   with colpo-urethrocystopexy (eg, Marshall-Marchetti-Krantz, Burch)
> *CPT Assistant* Jan 97:1, Nov 97:22

(For urethrocystopexy without hysterectomy, see 51840, 51841)

58180   Supracervical abdominal hysterectomy (subtotal hysterectomy), with or without removal of tube(s), with or without removal of ovary(s)

58200   Total abdominal hysterectomy, including partial vaginectomy, with para-aortic and pelvic lymph node sampling, with or without removal of tube(s), with or without removal of ovary(s)

58210   Radical abdominal hysterectomy, with bilateral total pelvic lymphadenectomy and para-aortic lymph node sampling (biopsy), with or without removal of tube(s), with or without removal of ovary(s)
> *CPT Assistant* Fall 92:21

(For radical hysterectomy with ovarian transposition, use also 58825)

58240   Pelvic exenteration for gynecologic malignancy, with total abdominal hysterectomy or cervicectomy, with or without removal of tube(s), with or without removal of ovary(s), with removal of bladder and ureteral transplantations, and/or abdominoperineal resection of rectum and colon and colostomy, or any combination thereof

(For pelvic exenteration for lower urinary tract or male genital malignancy, use 51597)

58260   Vaginal hysterectomy, for uterus 250 g or less;
             ➡ *CPT Changes: An Insider's View* 2003

58262   with removal of tube(s), and/or ovary(s)

58263   with removal of tube(s), and/or ovary(s), with repair of
               enterocele

             (Do not report 58263 in addition to 57283)

58267   with colpo-urethrocystopexy (Marshall-Marchetti-
               Krantz type, Pereyra type) with or without endoscopic
               control

58270   with repair of enterocele

             (For repair of enterocele with removal of tubes and/or
             ovaries, use 58263)

58275   Vaginal hysterectomy, with total or partial vaginectomy;
             ➡ *CPT Changes: An Insider's View* 2002

58280   with repair of enterocele

58285   Vaginal hysterectomy, radical (Schauta type operation)

58290   Vaginal hysterectomy, for uterus greater than 250 g;
             ➡ *CPT Changes: An Insider's View* 2003

58291   with removal of tube(s) and/or ovary(s)
             ➡ *CPT Changes: An Insider's View* 2003

58292   with removal of tube(s) and/or ovary(s), with repair of
               enterocele
             ➡ *CPT Changes: An Insider's View* 2003

58293   with colpo-urethrocystopexy (Marshall-Marchetti-
               Krantz type, Pereyra type) with or without endoscopic
               control
             ➡ *CPT Changes: An Insider's View* 2003

58294   with repair of enterocele
             ➡ *CPT Changes: An Insider's View* 2003

Introduction

             (For insertion/removal of implantable contraceptive
             capsules, see 11975, 11976, 11977)

58300   Insertion of intrauterine device (IUD)
             ➡ *CPT Assistant* Apr 98:14

58301   Removal of intrauterine device (IUD)
             ➡ *CPT Assistant* Apr 98:14

58321   Artificial insemination; intra-cervical

58322   intra-uterine

58323   Sperm washing for artificial insemination
             ➡ *CPT Assistant* Jan 98:6

58340   Catheterization and introduction of saline or contrast
             material for saline infusion sonohysterography (SIS) or
             hysterosalpingography
             ➡ *CPT Assistant* Nov 97:22, Jul 99:8; *CPT Changes: An Insider's
               View* 2004

             (For radiological supervision and interpretation of saline
             infusion sonohysterography, use 76831)

             (For radiological supervision and interpretation of
             hysterosalpingography, use 74740)

58345   Transcervical introduction of fallopian tube catheter for
             diagnosis and/or re-establishing patency (any method),
             with or without hysterosalpingography
             ➡ *CPT Assistant* Nov 97:22

             (For radiological supervision and interpretation, use
             74742)

58346   Insertion of Heyman capsules for clinical brachytherapy
             ➡ *CPT Assistant* Feb 02:8; *CPT Changes: An Insider's View* 2002

             ►(For placement of needles or catheters into pelvic
             organs and/or genitalia [except prostate] for interstitial
             radioelement application, use 55920)◄

             (For insertion of radioelement sources or ribbons, see
             77761-77763, 77781-77784)

58350   Chromotubation of oviduct, including materials
             ➡ *CPT Assistant* May 02:19

             (For materials supplied by physician, use 99070)

58353   Endometrial ablation, thermal, without hysteroscopic
             guidance
             ➡ *CPT Assistant* Mar 02:11, Apr 02:19; *CPT Changes: An Insider's
               View* 2001

             (For hysteroscopic procedure, use 58563)

58356   Endometrial cryoablation with ultrasonic guidance,
             including endometrial curettage, when performed
             ➡ *CPT Changes: An Insider's View* 2005

             (Do not report 58356 in conjunction with 58100, 58120,
             58340, 76700, 76856)

Repair

58400   Uterine suspension, with or without shortening of round
             ligaments, with or without shortening of sacrouterine
             ligaments; (separate procedure)

58410   with presacral sympathectomy

             (For anastomosis of tubes to uterus, use 58752)

58520   Hysterorrhaphy, repair of ruptured uterus (nonobstetrical)

58540   Hysteroplasty, repair of uterine anomaly (Strassman type)

             (For closure of vesicouterine fistula, use 51920)

Laparoscopy/Hysteroscopy

Surgical laparoscopy always includes diagnostic
laparoscopy. To report a diagnostic laparoscopy
(peritoneoscopy) (separate procedure), use 49320. To
report a diagnostic hysteroscopy (separate procedure), use
58555.

58541   Laparoscopy, surgical, supracervical hysterectomy, for
             uterus 250 g or less;
             ➡ *CPT Changes: An Insider's View* 2007

58542   with removal of tube(s) and/or ovary(s)

➔ *CPT Changes: An Insider's View* 2007

▶(Do not report 58541-58542 in conjunction with 49320, 57000, 57180, 57410, 58140-58146, 58545, 58546, 58561, 58661, 58670, 58671)◀

58543   Laparoscopy, surgical, supracervical hysterectomy, for uterus greater than 250 g;

➔ *CPT Changes: An Insider's View* 2007

58544   with removal of tube(s) and/or ovary(s)

➔ *CPT Changes: An Insider's View* 2007

▶(Do not report 58543-58544 in conjunction with 49320, 57000, 57180, 57410, 58140-58146, 58545, 58546, 58561, 58661, 58670, 58671)◀

58545   Laparoscopy, surgical, myomectomy, excision; 1 to 4 intramural myomas with total weight of 250 g or less and/or removal of surface myomas

➔ *CPT Assistant* Jun 03:5, 12; *CPT Changes: An Insider's View* 2003

58546   5 or more intramural myomas and/or intramural myomas with total weight greater than 250 g

➔ *CPT Assistant* Jun 03:12, Jan 04:26; *CPT Changes: An Insider's View* 2003

58548   Laparoscopy, surgical, with radical hysterectomy, with bilateral total pelvic lymphadenectomy and para-aortic lymph node sampling (biopsy), with removal of tube(s) and ovary(s), if performed

➔ *CPT Changes: An Insider's View* 2007

(Do not report 58548 in conjunction with 38570-38572, 58210, 58285, 58550-58554)

58550   Laparoscopy, surgical, with vaginal hysterectomy, for uterus 250 g or less;

➔ *CPT Assistant* Nov 99:28, Mar 00:9; *CPT Changes: An Insider's View* 2000, 2003

58552   with removal of tube(s) and/or ovary(s)

➔ *CPT Changes: An Insider's View* 2003

▶(Do not report 58550-58552 in conjunction with 49320, 57000, 57180, 57410, 58140-58146, 58545, 58546, 58561, 58661, 58670, 58671)◀

58553   Laparoscopy, surgical, with vaginal hysterectomy, for uterus greater than 250 g;

➔ *CPT Changes: An Insider's View* 2003

58554   with removal of tube(s) and/or ovary(s)

➔ *CPT Changes: An Insider's View* 2003

▶(Do not report 58553-58554 in conjunction with 49320, 57000, 57180, 57410, 58140-58146, 58545, 58546, 58561, 58661, 58670, 58671)◀

58555   Hysteroscopy, diagnostic (separate procedure)

➔ *CPT Assistant* Nov 99:28, Mar 00:10; *CPT Changes: An Insider's View* 2000

58558   Hysteroscopy, surgical; with sampling (biopsy) of endometrium and/or polypectomy, with or without D & C

➔ *CPT Assistant* Nov 99:28, Mar 00:10, Sep 02:10, Jan 03:7, May 03:19; *CPT Changes: An Insider's View* 2000

58559   with lysis of intrauterine adhesions (any method)

➔ *CPT Assistant* Nov 99:28, Mar 00:10; *CPT Changes: An Insider's View* 2000

58560   with division or resection of intrauterine septum (any method)

➔ *CPT Assistant* Nov 99:28, Mar 00:10; *CPT Changes: An Insider's View* 2000

58561   with removal of leiomyomata

➔ *CPT Assistant* Nov 99:28, Mar 00:10, Jan 03:7; *CPT Changes: An Insider's View* 2000

58562   with removal of impacted foreign body

➔ *CPT Assistant* Nov 99:28, Mar 00:10; *CPT Changes: An Insider's View* 2000

58563   with endometrial ablation (eg, endometrial resection, electrosurgical ablation, thermoablation)

➔ *CPT Assistant* Nov 99:28, Mar 00:10, Mar 02:11, Apr 02:19, Jan 03:7; *CPT Changes: An Insider's View* 2000, 2002

Hysteroscopy
58563

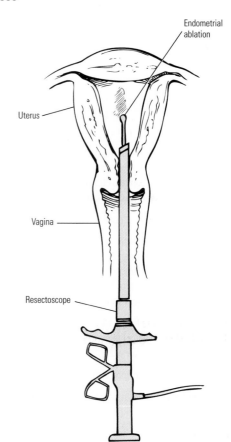

Endometrial ablation

Uterus

Vagina

Resectoscope

58565   with bilateral fallopian tube cannulation to induce occlusion by placement of permanent implants

➔ *CPT Changes: An Insider's View* 2005

(Do not report 58565 in conjunction with 58555 or 57800)

(For unilateral procedure, use modifier 52)

▲=Revised code   ●=New code   ▶ ◀=Contains new or revised text   ⊘=Modifier 51 exempt

● **58570** Laparoscopy, surgical, with total hysterectomy, for uterus 250 g or less;
> *CPT Changes: An Insider's View* 2008

● **58571** with removal of tube(s) and/or ovary(s)
> *CPT Changes: An Insider's View* 2008

● **58572** Laparoscopy, surgical, with total hysterectomy, for uterus greater than 250 g;
> *CPT Changes: An Insider's View* 2008

● **58573** with removal of tube(s) and/or ovary(s)
> *CPT Changes: An Insider's View* 2008

▶(Do not report 58570-58573 in conjunction with 49320, 57000, 57180, 57410, 58140-58146, 58150, 58545, 58546, 58561, 58661, 58670, 58671)◀

58578 Unlisted laparoscopy procedure, uterus
> *CPT Assistant* Nov 99:28, Mar 00:10, Mar 07:9; *CPT Changes: An Insider's View* 2000

58579 Unlisted hysteroscopy procedure, uterus
> *CPT Assistant* Nov 99:28, Mar 00:10; *CPT Changes: An Insider's View* 2000

Oviduct/Ovary

Incision

58600 Ligation or transection of fallopian tube(s), abdominal or vaginal approach, unilateral or bilateral
> *CPT Assistant* Nov 99:28; *CPT Changes: An Insider's View* 2000

58605 Ligation or transection of fallopian tube(s), abdominal or vaginal approach, postpartum, unilateral or bilateral, during same hospitalization (separate procedure)
> *CPT Assistant* Nov 99:28; *CPT Changes: An Insider's View* 2000

(For laparoscopic procedures, use 58670, 58671)

+ **58611** Ligation or transection of fallopian tube(s) when done at the time of cesarean delivery or intra-abdominal surgery (not a separate procedure) (List separately in addition to code for primary procedure)
> *CPT Changes: An Insider's View* 2002

58615 Occlusion of fallopian tube(s) by device (eg, band, clip, Falope ring) vaginal or suprapubic approach
> *CPT Assistant* Nov 99:28; *CPT Changes: An Insider's View* 2000

(For laparoscopic approach, use 58671)

(For lysis of adnexal adhesions, use 58740)

Laparoscopy

Surgical laparoscopy always includes diagnostic laparoscopy. To report a diagnostic laparoscopy (peritoneoscopy) (separate procedure), use 49320.

58660 Laparoscopy, surgical; with lysis of adhesions (salpingolysis, ovariolysis) (separate procedure)
> *CPT Assistant* Nov 99:28, Mar 00:10, Mar 03:22; *CPT Changes: An Insider's View* 2000

58661 with removal of adnexal structures (partial or total oophorectomy and/or salpingectomy)
> *CPT Assistant* Nov 99:28, Mar 00:10, Jan 02:11; *CPT Changes: An Insider's View* 2000

58662 with fulguration or excision of lesions of the ovary, pelvic viscera, or peritoneal surface by any method
> *CPT Assistant* Nov 99:28, Mar 00:10; *CPT Changes: An Insider's View* 2000

58670 with fulguration of oviducts (with or without transection)
> *CPT Assistant* Nov 99:29, Mar 00:10; *CPT Changes: An Insider's View* 2000

58671 with occlusion of oviducts by device (eg, band, clip, or Falope ring)
> *CPT Assistant* Nov 99:29, Mar 00:10; *CPT Changes: An Insider's View* 2000

58672 with fimbrioplasty
> *CPT Assistant* Nov 99:29, Mar 00:10; *CPT Changes: An Insider's View* 2000

58673 with salpingostomy (salpingoneostomy)
> *CPT Assistant* Nov 99:29, Mar 00:10, May 02:19; *CPT Changes: An Insider's View* 2000

(Codes 58672 and 58673 are used to report unilateral procedures. For bilateral procedure, use modifier 50)

58679 Unlisted laparoscopy procedure, oviduct, ovary
> *CPT Assistant* Nov 99:29, Mar 00:10; *CPT Changes: An Insider's View* 2000

(For laparoscopic aspiration of ovarian cyst, use 49322)

(For laparoscopic biopsy of the ovary or fallopian tube, use 49321)

Excision

58700 Salpingectomy, complete or partial, unilateral or bilateral (separate procedure)

58720 Salpingo-oophorectomy, complete or partial, unilateral or bilateral (separate procedure)
> *CPT Assistant* Sep 00:9, Jul 06:19

Repair

58740 Lysis of adhesions (salpingolysis, ovariolysis)
> *CPT Assistant* Sep 96:9, Nov 99:29; *CPT Changes: An Insider's View* 2000

(For laparoscopic approach, use 58660)

▶(For excision or destruction of endometriomas, open method, see 49203-49205, 58957, 58958)◀

(For fulguration or excision of lesions, laparoscopic approach, use 58662)

58750 Tubotubal anastomosis

58752 Tubouterine implantation

58760 Fimbrioplasty
> *CPT Assistant* Nov 99:29; *CPT Changes: An Insider's View* 2000

(For laparoscopic approach, use 58672)

58770   Salpingostomy (salpingoneostomy)

➲ *CPT Assistant* Nov 99:29; *CPT Changes: An Insider's View* 2000

(For laparoscopic approach, use 58673)

Ovary

Incision

58800   Drainage of ovarian cyst(s), unilateral or bilateral (separate procedure); vaginal approach

58805   abdominal approach

58820   Drainage of ovarian abscess; vaginal approach, open

➲ *CPT Assistant* Nov 97:22

58822   abdominal approach

➲ *CPT Assistant* Nov 97:22

⊙ **58823**   Drainage of pelvic abscess, transvaginal or transrectal approach, percutaneous (eg, ovarian, pericolic)

➲ *CPT Assistant* Nov 97:22, Mar 98:8

(For radiological supervision and interpretation, use 75989)

58825   Transposition, ovary(s)

Excision

58900   Biopsy of ovary, unilateral or bilateral (separate procedure)

➲ *CPT Assistant* Nov 99:29; *CPT Changes: An Insider's View* 2000

(For laparoscopic biopsy of the ovary or fallopian tube, use 49321)

58920   Wedge resection or bisection of ovary, unilateral or bilateral

58925   Ovarian cystectomy, unilateral or bilateral

58940   Oophorectomy, partial or total, unilateral or bilateral;

➲ *CPT Assistant* Mar 04:3

(For oophorectomy with concomitant debulking for ovarian malignancy, use 58952)

58943   for ovarian, tubal or primary peritoneal malignancy, with para-aortic and pelvic lymph node biopsies, peritoneal washings, peritoneal biopsies, diaphragmatic assessments, with or without salpingectomy(s), with or without omentectomy

➲ *CPT Changes: An Insider's View* 2001

58950   Resection (initial) of ovarian, tubal or primary peritoneal malignancy with bilateral salpingo-oophorectomy and omentectomy;

➲ *CPT Changes: An Insider's View* 2001, 2007

58951   with total abdominal hysterectomy, pelvic and limited para-aortic lymphadenectomy

➲ *CPT Assistant* Aug 01:11

58952   with radical dissection for debulking (ie, radical excision or destruction, intra-abdominal or retroperitoneal tumors)

➲ *CPT Assistant* Dec 96:10, Aug 01:11; *CPT Changes: An Insider's View* 2001

(For resection of recurrent ovarian, tubal, primary peritoneal, or uterine malignancy, see 58957, 58958)

58953   Bilateral salpingo-oophorectomy with omentectomy, total abdominal hysterectomy and radical dissection for debulking;

➲ *CPT Assistant* Feb 02:8; *CPT Changes: An Insider's View* 2002

58954   with pelvic lymphadenectomy and limited para-aortic lymphadenectomy

➲ *CPT Assistant* Feb 02:9; *CPT Changes: An Insider's View* 2002

58956   Bilateral salpingo-oophorectomy with total omentectomy, total abdominal hysterectomy for malignancy

➲ *CPT Changes: An Insider's View* 2005

(Do not report 58956 in conjunction with 49255, 58150, 58180, 58262, 58263, 58550, 58661, 58700, 58720, 58900, 58925, 58940, 58957, 58958)

58957   Resection (tumor debulking) of recurrent ovarian, tubal, primary peritoneal, uterine malignancy (intra-abdominal, retroperitoneal tumors), with omentectomy, if performed;

➲ *CPT Changes: An Insider's View* 2007

58958   with pelvic lymphadenectomy and limited para-aortic lymphadenectomy

➲ *CPT Changes: An Insider's View* 2007

▶(Do not report 58957, 58958 in conjunction with 38770, 38780, 44005, 49000, 49203-49215, 49255, 58900-58960)◀

58960   Laparotomy, for staging or restaging of ovarian, tubal, or primary peritoneal malignancy (second look), with or without omentectomy, peritoneal washing, biopsy of abdominal and pelvic peritoneum, diaphragmatic assessment with pelvic and limited para-aortic lymphadenectomy

➲ *CPT Changes: An Insider's View* 2001

(Do not report 58960 in conjunction with 58957, 58958)

In Vitro Fertilization

58970   Follicle puncture for oocyte retrieval, any method

(For radiological supervision and interpretation, use 76948)

58974   Embryo transfer, intrauterine

58976   Gamete, zygote, or embryo intrafallopian transfer, any method

➲ *CPT Assistant* Nov 99:29; *CPT Changes: An Insider's View* 2000

(For laparoscopic adnexal procedures, see 58660-58673)

Other Procedures

58999   Unlisted procedure, female genital system (nonobstetrical)

Maternity Care and Delivery

The services normally provided in uncomplicated maternity cases include antepartum care, delivery, and postpartum care.

Antepartum care includes the initial and subsequent history, physical examinations, recording of weight, blood pressures, fetal heart tones, routine chemical urinalysis, and monthly visits up to 28 weeks gestation, biweekly visits to 36 weeks gestation, and weekly visits until delivery. Any other visits or services within this time period should be coded separately.

Delivery services include admission to the hospital, the admission history and physical examination, management of uncomplicated labor, vaginal delivery (with or without episiotomy, with or without forceps), or cesarean delivery. Medical problems complicating labor and delivery management may require additional resources and should be identified by utilizing the codes in the **Medicine** and **Evaluation and Management Services** section in addition to codes for maternity care.

Postpartum care includes hospital and office visits following vaginal or cesarean section delivery.

For medical complications of pregnancy (eg, cardiac problems, neurological problems, diabetes, hypertension, toxemia, hyperemesis, pre-term labor, premature rupture of membranes), see services in the **Medicine** and **Evaluation and Management Services** section.

For surgical complications of pregnancy (eg, appendectomy, hernia, ovarian cyst, Bartholin cyst), see services in the **Surgery** section.

If a physician provides all or part of the antepartum and/or postpartum patient care but does not perform delivery due to termination of pregnancy by abortion or referral to another physician for delivery, see the antepartum and postpartum care codes 59425-59426 and 59430.

(For circumcision of newborn, see 54150, 54160)

Antepartum Services

59000 Amniocentesis; diagnostic
➔ *CPT Assistant* Apr 97:2, Feb 02:7, Aug 02:2, May 04:2; *CPT Changes: An Insider's View* 2002

(For radiological supervision and interpretation, use 76946)

59001 therapeutic amniotic fluid reduction (includes ultrasound guidance)
➔ *CPT Assistant* Feb 02:7, Aug 02:2; *CPT Changes: An Insider's View* 2002

Amniocentesis, Therapeutic Amniotic Fluid Reduction
59001

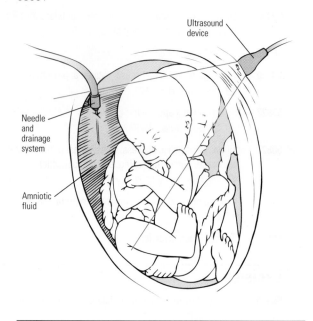

Ultrasound device

Needle and drainage system

Amniotic fluid

59012 Cordocentesis (intrauterine), any method
➔ *CPT Assistant* Aug 02:2

(For radiological supervision and interpretation, use 76941)

59015 Chorionic villus sampling, any method
➔ *CPT Assistant* Apr 97:2, Aug 02:2

(For radiological supervision and interpretation, use 76945)

59020 Fetal contraction stress test
➔ *CPT Assistant* Apr 97:2, Aug 02:2

59025 Fetal non-stress test
➔ *CPT Assistant* Apr 97:2, May 98:10, Oct 04:10

59030 Fetal scalp blood sampling
➔ *CPT Assistant* Aug 02:3

(For repeat fetal scalp blood sampling, use 59030 and see modifiers 76 and 77)

59050 Fetal monitoring during labor by consulting physician (ie, non-attending physician) with written report; supervision and interpretation
➔ *CPT Assistant* Nov 97:22

59051 interpretation only
➔ *CPT Assistant* Nov 97:22

59070 Transabdominal amnioinfusion, including ultrasound guidance
➔ *CPT Assistant* May 04:2; *CPT Changes: An Insider's View* 2004

59072   Fetal umbilical cord occlusion, including ultrasound guidance

➔ *CPT Assistant* May 04:2; *CPT Changes: An Insider's View* 2004

59074   Fetal fluid drainage (eg, vesicocentesis, thoracocentesis, paracentesis), including ultrasound guidance

➔ *CPT Assistant* May 04:2, 4, Dec 04:19; *CPT Changes: An Insider's View* 2004

59076   Fetal shunt placement, including ultrasound guidance

➔ *CPT Assistant* May 04:2, 4, Dec 04:19; *CPT Changes: An Insider's View* 2004

(For unlisted fetal invasive procedure, use 59897)

Excision

59100   Hysterotomy, abdominal (eg, for hydatidiform mole, abortion)

(When tubal ligation is performed at the same time as hysterotomy, use 58611 in addition to 59100)

59120   Surgical treatment of ectopic pregnancy; tubal or ovarian, requiring salpingectomy and/or oophorectomy, abdominal or vaginal approach

59121   tubal or ovarian, without salpingectomy and/or oophorectomy

59130   abdominal pregnancy

59135   interstitial, uterine pregnancy requiring total hysterectomy

59136   interstitial, uterine pregnancy with partial resection of uterus

59140   cervical, with evacuation

59150   Laparoscopic treatment of ectopic pregnancy; without salpingectomy and/or oophorectomy

➔ *CPT Assistant* Sep 96:9

Laparoscopic Treatment of Ectopic Pregnancy
59150

The site of gestation is located with a laparoscope and a small incision is made above the site. The ectopic pregnancy is then removed.

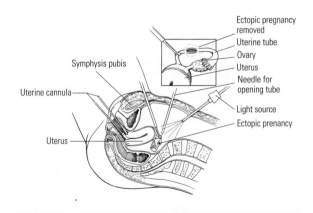

59151   with salpingectomy and/or oophorectomy

59160   Curettage, postpartum

➔ *CPT Assistant* Nov 97:22, Sep 02:11

Introduction

(For intrauterine fetal transfusion, use 36460)

(For introduction of hypertonic solution and/or prostaglandins to initiate labor, see 59850-59857)

59200   Insertion of cervical dilator (eg, laminaria, prostaglandin) (separate procedure)

➔ *CPT Assistant* Fall 93:9, Apr 97:3

Repair

(For tracheloplasty, use 57700)

59300   Episiotomy or vaginal repair, by other than attending physician

59320   Cerclage of cervix, during pregnancy; vaginal

➔ *CPT Assistant* Aug 02:2, Nov 06:21, Feb 07:10

59325   abdominal

➔ *CPT Assistant* Aug 02:2, Nov 06:21, Feb 07:10

59350   Hysterorrhaphy of ruptured uterus

➔ *CPT Assistant* Aug 02:2

Vaginal Delivery, Antepartum and Postpartum Care

59400   Routine obstetric care including antepartum care, vaginal delivery (with or without episiotomy, and/or forceps) and postpartum care

➔ *CPT Assistant* Feb 96:1, Mar 96:11, Feb 97:11, Apr 97:3, Apr 98:15, Jun 98:10, Aug 02:3, Feb 03:15

Vaginal Delivery
59400-59410

59409 Vaginal delivery only (with or without episiotomy and/or forceps);

> *CPT Assistant* Feb 96:1, Mar 96:11, Jul 96:11, Sep 96:4, Feb 97:11, Apr 97:1, Aug 02:3

59410 including postpartum care

59412 External cephalic version, with or without tocolysis

> *CPT Assistant* Fall 94:21, Feb 96:1, Aug 02:2-3

(Use 59412 in addition to code(s) for delivery)

59414 Delivery of placenta (separate procedure)

> *CPT Assistant* Jun 96:10, Jun 98:10, Aug 02:3

(For antepartum care only, see 59425, 59426 or appropriate E/M code(s))

(For 1-3 antepartum care visits, see appropriate E/M code(s))

59425 Antepartum care only; 4-6 visits

> *CPT Assistant* Fall 94:21, Apr 97:11, Aug 02:3

59426 7 or more visits

> *CPT Assistant* Fall 94:21, Apr 97:11, Aug 02:3

59430 Postpartum care only (separate procedure)

> *CPT Assistant* Jun 96:10, Aug 02:3

Cesarean Delivery

(For standby attendance for infant, use 99360)

(For low cervical cesarean section, see 59510, 59515, 59525)

Cesarean Delivery
59510-59515

Vertical incision

Transverse incision

59510 Routine obstetric care including antepartum care, cesarean delivery, and postpartum care

> *CPT Assistant* Jul 96:11, Sep 96:4, Oct 96:10, Feb 97:11, Apr 97:2, Aug 02:3

59514 Cesarean delivery only;

> *CPT Assistant* Oct 96:10, Feb 97:11

59515 including postpartum care

(For classic cesarean section, see 59510, 59515, 59525)

+ 59525 Subtotal or total hysterectomy after cesarean delivery (List separately in addition to code for primary procedure)

(Use 59525 in conjunction with 59510, 59514, 59515, 59618, 59620, 59622)

(For extraperitoneal cesarean section, or cesarean section with subtotal or total hysterectomy, see 59510, 59515, 59525)

Delivery After Previous Cesarean Delivery

Patients who have had a previous cesarean delivery and now present with the expectation of a vaginal delivery are coded using codes 59610-59622. If the patient has a successful vaginal delivery after a previous cesarean delivery (VBAC), use codes 59610-59614. If the attempt is unsuccessful and another cesarean delivery is carried out, use codes 59618-59622. To report elective cesarean deliveries use code 59510, 59514 or 59515.

59610 Routine obstetric care including antepartum care, vaginal delivery (with or without episiotomy, and/or forceps) and postpartum care, after previous cesarean delivery

> *CPT Assistant* Feb 96:2, Apr 97:3, Aug 02:3

59612 Vaginal delivery only, after previous cesarean delivery (with or without episiotomy and/or forceps);

> *CPT Assistant* Feb 96:2, Aug 02:3

59614 including postpartum care

> *CPT Assistant* Feb 96:2

59618 Routine obstetric care including antepartum care, cesarean delivery, and postpartum care, following attempted vaginal delivery after previous cesarean delivery

> *CPT Assistant* Feb 96:2, Aug 02:4

59620 Cesarean delivery only, following attempted vaginal delivery after previous cesarean delivery;

> *CPT Assistant* Feb 96:2

59622 including postpartum care

> *CPT Assistant* Feb 96:2

Abortion

(For medical treatment of spontaneous complete abortion, any trimester, use E/M codes 99201-99233)

(For surgical treatment of spontaneous abortion, use 59812)

59812   Treatment of incomplete abortion, any trimester, completed surgically

> *CPT Assistant* Fall 93:9, Fall 95:16

59820   Treatment of missed abortion, completed surgically; first trimester

> *CPT Assistant* Fall 93:9, Fall 95:16, Feb 99:10

59821   second trimester

> *CPT Assistant* Fall 93:9, Fall 95:16

59830   Treatment of septic abortion, completed surgically

> *CPT Assistant* Fall 93:9

59840   Induced abortion, by dilation and curettage

> *CPT Assistant* Fall 93:9, Sep 03:16

59841   Induced abortion, by dilation and evacuation

> *CPT Assistant* Fall 93:9

59850   Induced abortion, by one or more intra-amniotic injections (amniocentesis-injections), including hospital admission and visits, delivery of fetus and secundines;

> *CPT Assistant* Fall 93:10

59851   with dilation and curettage and/or evacuation

> *CPT Assistant* Fall 93:10

59852   with hysterotomy (failed intra-amniotic injection)

> *CPT Assistant* Fall 93:10

(For insertion of cervical dilator, use 59200)

59855   Induced abortion, by one or more vaginal suppositories (eg, prostaglandin) with or without cervical dilation (eg, laminaria), including hospital admission and visits, delivery of fetus and secundines;

59856   with dilation and curettage and/or evacuation

59857   with hysterotomy (failed medical evacuation)

Other Procedures

59866   Multifetal pregnancy reduction(s) (MPR)

59870   Uterine evacuation and curettage for hydatidiform mole

> *CPT Assistant* Feb 99:10

59871   Removal of cerclage suture under anesthesia (other than local)

> *CPT Assistant* Nov 97:22, Nov 06:21, Feb 07:10

59897   Unlisted fetal invasive procedure, including ultrasound guidance

> *CPT Assistant* May 04:5; *CPT Changes: An Insider's View* 2004

59898   Unlisted laparoscopy procedure, maternity care and delivery

> *CPT Assistant* Nov 99:29, Mar 00:10; *CPT Changes: An Insider's View* 2000

59899   Unlisted procedure, maternity care and delivery

> *CPT Assistant* Jun 97:10

Endocrine System

(For pituitary and pineal surgery, see **Nervous System**)

Thyroid Gland

Incision

60000   Incision and drainage of thyroglossal duct cyst, infected

> *CPT Changes: An Insider's View* 2002

Excision

▶(60001 has been deleted. To report, use 60300)◄

60100   Biopsy thyroid, percutaneous core needle

> *CPT Assistant* Jun 97:5

(If imaging guidance is performed, see 76942, 77002, 77012, 77021)

(For fine needle aspiration, use 10021 or 10022)

(For evaluation of fine needle aspirate, see 88172, 88173)

60200   Excision of cyst or adenoma of thyroid, or transection of isthmus

60210   Partial thyroid lobectomy, unilateral; with or without isthmusectomy

60212   with contralateral subtotal lobectomy, including isthmusectomy

60220   Total thyroid lobectomy, unilateral; with or without isthmusectomy

Thyroid Lobectomy
60220

The thyroid is exposed via a transverse cervical incision. The superior and inferior thyroid vessels serving the lobe are ligated, the isthmus is severed, and the entire thyroid lobe is resected.

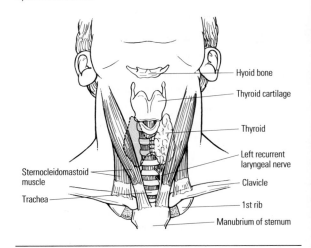

60225   with contralateral subtotal lobectomy, including isthmusectomy

60240 Thyroidectomy, total or complete

(For thyroidectomy, subtotal or partial, use 60271)

60252 Thyroidectomy, total or subtotal for malignancy; with limited neck dissection
➔ *CPT Assistant* Nov 00:10

60254 with radical neck dissection
➔ *CPT Assistant* Nov 00:10

60260 Thyroidectomy, removal of all remaining thyroid tissue following previous removal of a portion of thyroid

(For bilateral procedure, report 60260 with modifier 50)

60270 Thyroidectomy, including substernal thyroid; sternal split or transthoracic approach
➔ *CPT Changes: An Insider's View* 2002

60271 cervical approach

60280 Excision of thyroglossal duct cyst or sinus;

60281 recurrent

(For thyroid ultrasonography, use 76536)

►Removal◄

● **60300** Aspiration and/or injection, thyroid cyst
➔ *CPT Changes: An Insider's View* 2008

►(For fine needle aspiration, see 10021, 10022)◄

►(If imaging guidance is performed, see 76942, 77012)◄

Parathyroid, Thymus, Adrenal Glands, Pancreas, and Carotid Body

Excision

(For pituitary and pineal surgery, see **Nervous System**)

60500 Parathyroidectomy or exploration of parathyroid(s);

60502 re-exploration

60505 with mediastinal exploration, sternal split or transthoracic approach

✛ **60512** Parathyroid autotransplantation (List separately in addition to code for primary procedure)

(Use 60512 in conjunction with 60500, 60502, 60505, 60212, 60225, 60240, 60252, 60254, 60260, 60270, 60271)

Posterior View of the Pharynx
60512

60520 Thymectomy, partial or total; transcervical approach (separate procedure)

60521 sternal split or transthoracic approach, without radical mediastinal dissection (separate procedure)

60522 sternal split or transthoracic approach, with radical mediastinal dissection (separate procedure)

60540 Adrenalectomy, partial or complete, or exploration of adrenal gland with or without biopsy, transabdominal, lumbar or dorsal (separate procedure);
➔ *CPT Assistant* Nov 98:17

60545 with excision of adjacent retroperitoneal tumor
➔ *CPT Assistant* Nov 98:17

(Do not report 60540, 60545 in conjunction with 50323)

(For bilateral procedure, report 60540 with modifier 50)

►(For excision of remote or disseminated pheochromocytoma, see 49203-49205)◄

(For laparoscopic approach, use 60650)

60600 Excision of carotid body tumor; without excision of carotid artery

60605 with excision of carotid artery

Laparoscopy

Surgical laparoscopy always includes diagnostic laparoscopy. To report a diagnostic laparoscopy (peritoneoscopy) (separate procedure), use 49320.

60650 Laparoscopy, surgical, with adrenalectomy, partial or complete, or exploration of adrenal gland with or without biopsy, transabdominal, lumbar or dorsal

➔ *CPT Assistant* Nov 99:30, Mar 00:10, Nov 01:8; *CPT Changes: An Insider's View* 2000

Laparoscopic Adrenalectomy
60650

An adrenal gland is dissected and removed under laparoscopic guidance. Multiple small blood vessels from the vena cava and the aorta do not follow standard anatomic pattern, requiring intricate dissection.

Left

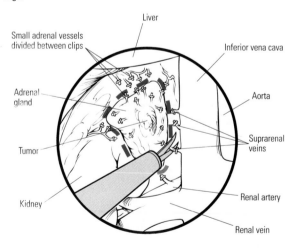

Right

60659 Unlisted laparoscopy procedure, endocrine system

➔ *CPT Assistant* Nov 99:30, Mar 00:10; *CPT Changes: An Insider's View* 2000

Other Procedures

60699 Unlisted procedure, endocrine system

➔ *CPT Assistant* Feb 06:16

Notes

⊙=Moderate sedation   ✚=Add-on code   ✗=FDA approval pending   ➔➔=See p xvii for details

Nervous System

Skull, Meninges, and Brain

(For injection procedure for cerebral angiography, see 36100-36218)

(For injection procedure for ventriculography, see 61026, 61120)

(For injection procedure for pneumoencephalography, use 61055)

Injection, Drainage, or Aspiration

61000   Subdural tap through fontanelle, or suture, infant, unilateral or bilateral; initial

61001   subsequent taps

61020   Ventricular puncture through previous burr hole, fontanelle, suture, or implanted ventricular catheter/reservoir; without injection

61026   with injection of medication or other substance for diagnosis or treatment
➔ *CPT Changes: An Insider's View* 2002

61050   Cisternal or lateral cervical (C1-C2) puncture; without injection (separate procedure)

61055   with injection of medication or other substance for diagnosis or treatment (eg, C1-C2)
➔ *CPT Changes: An Insider's View* 2002

(For radiological supervision and interpretation, see **Radiology**)

61070   Puncture of shunt tubing or reservoir for aspiration or injection procedure

(For radiological supervision and interpretation, use 75809)

Twist Drill, Burr Hole(s), or Trephine

61105   Twist drill hole for subdural or ventricular puncture

⊘ **61107**   Twist drill hole(s) for subdural, intracerebral, or ventricular puncture; for implanting ventricular catheter, pressure recording device, or other intracerebral monitoring device
➔ *CPT Changes: An Insider's View* 2007

(For intracranial neuroendoscopic ventricular catheter placement, use 62160)

(For twist drill or burr hole performed to place thermal perfusion probe, use Category III code 0077T)

61108   for evacuation and/or drainage of subdural hematoma

61120   Burr hole(s) for ventricular puncture (including injection of gas, contrast media, dye, or radioactive material)

61140   Burr hole(s) or trephine; with biopsy of brain or intracranial lesion

61150   with drainage of brain abscess or cyst

61151   with subsequent tapping (aspiration) of intracranial abscess or cyst

61154   Burr hole(s) with evacuation and/or drainage of hematoma, extradural or subdural

(For bilateral procedure, report 61154 with modifier 50)

61156   Burr hole(s); with aspiration of hematoma or cyst, intracerebral

▲ **61210**   for implanting ventricular catheter, reservoir, EEG electrode(s), pressure recording device, or other cerebral monitoring device (separate procedure)
➔ *CPT Changes: An Insider's View* 2007, 2008

(For intracranial neuroendoscopic ventricular catheter placement, use 62160)

61215   Insertion of subcutaneous reservoir, pump or continuous infusion system for connection to ventricular catheter
➔ *CPT Assistant* Spring 93:13

(For refilling and maintenance of an implantable infusion pump for spinal or brain drug therapy, use 95990)

(For chemotherapy, use 96450)

61250   Burr hole(s) or trephine, supratentorial, exploratory, not followed by other surgery

(For bilateral procedure, report 61250 with modifier 50)

61253   Burr hole(s) or trephine, infratentorial, unilateral or bilateral
➔ *CPT Assistant* Sep 02:10

(If burr hole(s) or trephine are followed by craniotomy at same operative session, use 61304-61321; do not use 61250 or 61253)

Craniectomy or Craniotomy

61304   Craniectomy or craniotomy, exploratory; supratentorial

61305   infratentorial (posterior fossa)

61312   Craniectomy or craniotomy for evacuation of hematoma, supratentorial; extradural or subdural

61313   intracerebral

61314   Craniectomy or craniotomy for evacuation of hematoma, infratentorial; extradural or subdural

61315   intracerebellar

+ **61316**   Incision and subcutaneous placement of cranial bone graft (List separately in addition to code for primary procedure)
➔ *CPT Changes: An Insider's View* 2003

(Use 61316 in conjunction with 61304, 61312, 61313, 61322, 61323, 61340, 61570, 61571, 61680-61705)

61320 Craniectomy or craniotomy, drainage of intracranial abscess; supratentorial

61321 infratentorial

61322 Craniectomy or craniotomy, decompressive, with or without duraplasty, for treatment of intracranial hypertension, without evacuation of associated intraparenchymal hematoma; without lobectomy
➔ *CPT Changes: An Insider's View* 2003

(Do not report 61313 in addition to 61322)

(For subtemporal decompression, use 61340)

61323 with lobectomy
➔ *CPT Changes: An Insider's View* 2003

(Do not report 61313 in addition to 61323)

(For subtemporal decompression, use 61340)

61330 Decompression of orbit only, transcranial approach

(For bilateral procedure, report 61330 with modifier 50)

61332 Exploration of orbit (transcranial approach); with biopsy

61333 with removal of lesion

61334 with removal of foreign body

61340 Subtemporal cranial decompression (pseudotumor cerebri, slit ventricle syndrome)
➔ *CPT Changes: An Insider's View* 2003

(For bilateral procedure, report 61340 with modifier 50)

(For decompressive craniotomy or craniectomy for intracranial hypertension, without hematoma evacuation, see 61322, 61323)

61343 Craniectomy, suboccipital with cervical laminectomy for decompression of medulla and spinal cord, with or without dural graft (eg, Arnold-Chiari malformation)

61345 Other cranial decompression, posterior fossa

(For orbital decompression by lateral wall approach, Kroenlein type, use 67445)

61440 Craniotomy for section of tentorium cerebelli (separate procedure)

61450 Craniectomy, subtemporal, for section, compression, or decompression of sensory root of gasserian ganglion

61458 Craniectomy, suboccipital; for exploration or decompression of cranial nerves

61460 for section of one or more cranial nerves

61470 for medullary tractotomy

61480 for mesencephalic tractotomy or pedunculotomy

61490 Craniotomy for lobotomy, including cingulotomy

(For bilateral procedure, report 61490 with modifier 50)

61500 Craniectomy; with excision of tumor or other bone lesion of skull

61501 for osteomyelitis

61510 Craniectomy, trephination, bone flap craniotomy; for excision of brain tumor, supratentorial, except meningioma

61512 for excision of meningioma, supratentorial

61514 for excision of brain abscess, supratentorial

61516 for excision or fenestration of cyst, supratentorial

(For excision of pituitary tumor or craniopharyngioma, see 61545, 61546, 61548)

+ 61517 Implantation of brain intracavitary chemotherapy agent (List separately in addition to code for primary procedure)
➔ *CPT Changes: An Insider's View* 2003

(Use 61517 only in conjunction with 61510 or 61518)

(Do not report 61517 for brachytherapy insertion. For intracavitary insertion of radioelement sources or ribbons, see 77781-77784)

61518 Craniectomy for excision of brain tumor, infratentorial or posterior fossa; except meningioma, cerebellopontine angle tumor, or midline tumor at base of skull

61519 meningioma

61520 cerebellopontine angle tumor

61521 midline tumor at base of skull

61522 Craniectomy, infratentorial or posterior fossa; for excision of brain abscess

61524 for excision or fenestration of cyst

61526 Craniectomy, bone flap craniotomy, transtemporal (mastoid) for excision of cerebellopontine angle tumor;
➔ *CPT Assistant* Summer 91:8

61530 combined with middle/posterior fossa craniotomy/craniectomy

61531 Subdural implantation of strip electrodes through one or more burr or trephine hole(s) for long-term seizure monitoring

(For stereotactic implantation of electrodes, use 61760)

(For craniotomy for excision of intracranial arteriovenous malformation, see 61680-61692)

61533 Craniotomy with elevation of bone flap; for subdural implantation of an electrode array, for long-term seizure monitoring

(For continuous EEG monitoring, see 95950-95954)

61534 for excision of epileptogenic focus without electrocorticography during surgery

61535 for removal of epidural or subdural electrode array, without excision of cerebral tissue (separate procedure)

61536 for excision of cerebral epileptogenic focus, with electrocorticography during surgery (includes removal of electrode array)

61537   for lobectomy, temporal lobe, without electrocorticography during surgery
➔ *CPT Changes: An Insider's View* 2004

61538   for lobectomy, temporal lobe, with electrocorticography during surgery
➔ *CPT Changes: An Insider's View* 2004

61539   for lobectomy, other than temporal lobe, partial or total, with electrocorticography during surgery
➔ *CPT Changes: An Insider's View* 2004

61540   for lobectomy, other than temporal lobe, partial or total, without electrocorticography during surgery
➔ *CPT Changes: An Insider's View* 2004

61541   for transection of corpus callosum

61542   for total hemispherectomy

61543   for partial or subtotal (functional) hemispherectomy
➔ *CPT Changes: An Insider's View* 2004

61544   for excision or coagulation of choroid plexus

61545   for excision of craniopharyngioma

(For craniotomy for selective amygdalohippocampectomy, use 61566)

(For craniotomy for multiple subpial transections during surgery, use 61567)

61546   Craniotomy for hypophysectomy or excision of pituitary tumor, intracranial approach

61548   Hypophysectomy or excision of pituitary tumor, transnasal or transseptal approach, nonstereotactic
➔ *CPT Assistant* Nov 98:17

(Do not report code 69990 in addition to code 61548)

61550   Craniectomy for craniosynostosis; single cranial suture

61552   multiple cranial sutures

(For cranial reconstruction for orbital hypertelorism, see 21260-21263)

(For reconstruction, see 21172-21180)

61556   Craniotomy for craniosynostosis; frontal or parietal bone flap

61557   bifrontal bone flap

61558   Extensive craniectomy for multiple cranial suture craniosynostosis (eg, cloverleaf skull); not requiring bone grafts

61559   recontouring with multiple osteotomies and bone autografts (eg, barrel-stave procedure) (includes obtaining grafts)

(For reconstruction, see 21172-21180)

61563   Excision, intra and extracranial, benign tumor of cranial bone (eg, fibrous dysplasia); without optic nerve decompression

61564   with optic nerve decompression

(For reconstruction, see 21181-21183)

61566   Craniotomy with elevation of bone flap; for selective amygdalohippocampectomy
➔ *CPT Changes: An Insider's View* 2004

61567   for multiple subpial transections, with electrocorticography during surgery
➔ *CPT Changes: An Insider's View* 2004

61570   Craniectomy or craniotomy; with excision of foreign body from brain

61571   with treatment of penetrating wound of brain

(For sequestrectomy for osteomyelitis, use 61501)

61575   Transoral approach to skull base, brain stem or upper spinal cord for biopsy, decompression or excision of lesion;

61576   requiring splitting of tongue and/or mandible (including tracheostomy)

(For arthrodesis, use 22548)

Surgery of Skull Base

The surgical management of lesions involving the skull base (base of anterior, middle, and posterior cranial fossae) often requires the skills of several surgeons of different surgical specialties working together or in tandem during the operative session. These operations are usually not staged because of the need for definitive closure of dura, subcutaneous tissues, and skin to avoid serious infections such as osteomyelitis and/or meningitis.

The procedures are categorized according to (1) *approach procedure* necessary to obtain adequate exposure to the lesion (pathologic entity), (2) *definitive procedure(s)* necessary to biopsy, excise or otherwise treat the lesion, and (3) *repair/reconstruction* of the defect present following the definitive procedure(s).

The *approach procedure* is described according to anatomical area involved, ie, anterior cranial fossa, middle cranial fossa, posterior cranial fossa, and brain stem or upper spinal cord.

The *definitive procedure(s)* describes the repair, biopsy, resection, or excision of various lesions of the skull base and, when appropriate, primary closure of the dura, mucous membranes, and skin.

The *repair/reconstruction procedure(s)* is reported separately if extensive dural grafting, cranioplasty, local or regional myocutaneous pedicle flaps, or extensive skin grafts are required.

For primary closure, see the appropriate codes, ie, 15732, 15756-15758.

When one surgeon performs the approach procedure, another surgeon performs the definitive procedure, and another surgeon performs the repair/reconstruction procedure, each surgeon reports only the code for the specific procedure performed.

If one surgeon performs more than one procedure (ie, approach procedure and definitive procedure), then both codes are reported, adding modifier 51 to the secondary, additional procedure(s).

Approach Procedures

Anterior Cranial Fossa

61580 Craniofacial approach to anterior cranial fossa; extradural, including lateral rhinotomy, ethmoidectomy, sphenoidectomy, without maxillectomy or orbital exenteration
➔ *CPT Assistant* Winter 93:17, Spring 94:11

61581 extradural, including lateral rhinotomy, orbital exenteration, ethmoidectomy, sphenoidectomy and/or maxillectomy
➔ *CPT Assistant* Winter 93:17, Spring 94:11

61582 extradural, including unilateral or bifrontal craniotomy, elevation of frontal lobe(s), osteotomy of base of anterior cranial fossa
➔ *CPT Assistant* Winter 93:17, Spring 94:11

61583 intradural, including unilateral or bifrontal craniotomy, elevation or resection of frontal lobe, osteotomy of base of anterior cranial fossa
➔ *CPT Assistant* Winter 93:17, Spring 94:11

61584 Orbitocranial approach to anterior cranial fossa, extradural, including supraorbital ridge osteotomy and elevation of frontal and/or temporal lobe(s); without orbital exenteration
➔ *CPT Assistant* Winter 93:18

61585 with orbital exenteration
➔ *CPT Assistant* Winter 93:18

61586 Bicoronal, transzygomatic and/or LeFort I osteotomy approach to anterior cranial fossa with or without internal fixation, without bone graft
➔ *CPT Assistant* Winter 93:18, Nov 96:12

Middle Cranial Fossa

61590 Infratemporal pre-auricular approach to middle cranial fossa (parapharyngeal space, infratemporal and midline skull base, nasopharynx), with or without disarticulation of the mandible, including parotidectomy, craniotomy, decompression and/or mobilization of the facial nerve and/or petrous carotid artery
➔ *CPT Assistant* Winter 93:18

61591 Infratemporal post-auricular approach to middle cranial fossa (internal auditory meatus, petrous apex, tentorium, cavernous sinus, parasellar area, infratemporal fossa) including mastoidectomy, resection of sigmoid sinus, with or without decompression and/or mobilization of contents of auditory canal or petrous carotid artery
➔ *CPT Assistant* Winter 93:18

61592 Orbitocranial zygomatic approach to middle cranial fossa (cavernous sinus and carotid artery, clivus, basilar artery or petrous apex) including osteotomy of zygoma, craniotomy, extra- or intradural elevation of temporal lobe
➔ *CPT Assistant* Winter 93:18

Posterior Cranial Fossa

61595 Transtemporal approach to posterior cranial fossa, jugular foramen or midline skull base, including mastoidectomy, decompression of sigmoid sinus and/or facial nerve, with or without mobilization
➔ *CPT Assistant* Winter 93:18

61596 Transcochlear approach to posterior cranial fossa, jugular foramen or midline skull base, including labyrinthectomy, decompression, with or without mobilization of facial nerve and/or petrous carotid artery
➔ *CPT Assistant* Winter 93:18

61597 Transcondylar (far lateral) approach to posterior cranial fossa, jugular foramen or midline skull base, including occipital condylectomy, mastoidectomy, resection of C1-C3 vertebral body(s), decompression of vertebral artery, with or without mobilization
➔ *CPT Assistant* Winter 93:18

61598 Transpetrosal approach to posterior cranial fossa, clivus or foramen magnum, including ligation of superior petrosal sinus and/or sigmoid sinus
➔ *CPT Assistant* Winter 93:18

Definitive Procedures

Base of Anterior Cranial Fossa

61600 Resection or excision of neoplastic, vascular or infectious lesion of base of anterior cranial fossa; extradural
➔ *CPT Assistant* Winter 93:19, Spring 94:12, Nov 96:12

61601 intradural, including dural repair, with or without graft
➔ *CPT Assistant* Winter 93:19, Spring 94:12

Base of Middle Cranial Fossa

61605 Resection or excision of neoplastic, vascular or infectious lesion of infratemporal fossa, parapharyngeal space, petrous apex; extradural
➔ *CPT Assistant* Winter 93:19

61606 intradural, including dural repair, with or without graft
➔ *CPT Assistant* Winter 93:20

61607   Resection or excision of neoplastic, vascular or infectious lesion of parasellar area, cavernous sinus, clivus or midline skull base; extradural
➔ *CPT Assistant* Winter 93:20

61608   intradural, including dural repair, with or without graft
➔ *CPT Assistant* Winter 93:20

Codes 61609-61612 are reported in addition to code(s) for primary procedure(s) 61605-61608. Report only one transection or ligation of carotid artery code per operative session.

+ 61609   Transection or ligation, carotid artery in cavernous sinus; without repair (List separately in addition to code for primary procedure)
➔ *CPT Assistant* Winter 93:20

+ 61610   with repair by anastomosis or graft (List separately in addition to code for primary procedure)
➔ *CPT Assistant* Winter 93:20

+ 61611   Transection or ligation, carotid artery in petrous canal; without repair (List separately in addition to code for primary procedure)
➔ *CPT Assistant* Winter 93:20

+ 61612   with repair by anastomosis or graft (List separately in addition to code for primary procedure)
➔ *CPT Assistant* Winter 93:20

61613   Obliteration of carotid aneurysm, arteriovenous malformation, or carotid-cavernous fistula by dissection within cavernous sinus
➔ *CPT Assistant* Winter 93:20

Base of Posterior Cranial Fossa

61615   Resection or excision of neoplastic, vascular or infectious lesion of base of posterior cranial fossa, jugular foramen, foramen magnum, or C1-C3 vertebral bodies; extradural
➔ *CPT Assistant* Winter 93:20

61616   intradural, including dural repair, with or without graft

Repair and/or Reconstruction of Surgical Defects of Skull Base

61618   Secondary repair of dura for cerebrospinal fluid leak, anterior, middle or posterior cranial fossa following surgery of the skull base; by free tissue graft (eg, pericranium, fascia, tensor fascia lata, adipose tissue, homologous or synthetic grafts)
➔ *CPT Assistant* Winter 93:20, Spring 94:19, Mar 00:11

61619   by local or regionalized vascularized pedicle flap or myocutaneous flap (including galea, temporalis, frontalis or occipitalis muscle)
➔ *CPT Assistant* Winter 93:20, Spring 94:19, Mar 00:11

Endovascular Therapy

61623   Endovascular temporary balloon arterial occlusion, head or neck (extracranial/intracranial) including selective catheterization of vessel to be occluded, positioning and inflation of occlusion balloon, concomitant neurological monitoring, and radiologic supervision and interpretation of all angiography required for balloon occlusion and to exclude vascular injury post occlusion
➔ *CPT Changes: An Insider's View* 2003

(If selective catheterization and angiography of arteries other than artery to be occluded is performed, use appropriate catheterization and radiologic supervision and interpretation codes)

(If complete diagnostic angiography of the artery to be occluded is performed immediately prior to temporary occlusion, use appropriate radiologic supervision and interpretation codes only)

61624   Transcatheter permanent occlusion or embolization (eg, for tumor destruction, to achieve hemostasis, to occlude a vascular malformation), percutaneous, any method; central nervous system (intracranial, spinal cord)
➔ *CPT Assistant* Jun 99:10, Nov 06:8; *CPT Changes: An Insider's View* 2003

(See also 37204)

(For radiological supervision and interpretation, use 75894)

61626   non-central nervous system, head or neck (extracranial, brachiocephalic branch)

(See also 37204)

(For radiological supervision and interpretation, use 75894)

61630   Balloon angioplasty, intracranial (eg, atherosclerotic stenosis), percutaneous
➔ *CPT Changes: An Insider's View* 2006
➔ *Clinical Examples in Radiology* Winter 06:16

61635   Transcatheter placement of intravascular stent(s), intracranial (eg, atherosclerotic stenosis), including balloon angioplasty, if performed
➔ *CPT Changes: An Insider's View* 2006
➔ *Clinical Examples in Radiology* Winter 06:16

(61630 and 61635 include all selective vascular catheterization of the target vascular family, all diagnostic imaging for arteriography of the target vascular family, and all related radiological supervision and interpretation. When diagnostic arteriogram (including imaging and selective catheterization) confirms the need for angioplasty or stent placement, 61630 and 61635 are inclusive of these services. If angioplasty or stenting are not indicated, then the appropriate codes for selective catheterization and imaging should be reported in lieu of 61630 and 61635)

61640 Balloon dilatation of intracranial vasospasm, percutaneous; initial vessel

→ *CPT Changes: An Insider's View* 2006
→ *Clinical Examples in Radiology* Winter 06:16

+ 61641 each additional vessel in same vascular family (List separately in addition to code for primary procedure)

→ *CPT Changes: An Insider's View* 2006
→ *Clinical Examples in Radiology* Winter 06:16

+ 61642 each additional vessel in different vascular family (List separately in addition to code for primary procedure)

→ *CPT Changes: An Insider's View* 2006
→ *Clinical Examples in Radiology* Winter 06:16

(Use 61641 and 61642 in conjunction with 61640)

(61640, 61641, 61642 include all selective vascular catheterization of the target vessel, contrast injection(s), vessel measurement, roadmapping, postdilatation angiography, and fluoroscopic guidance for the balloon dilatation)

Surgery for Aneurysm, Arteriovenous Malformation or Vascular Disease

Includes craniotomy when appropriate for procedure.

61680 Surgery of intracranial arteriovenous malformation; supratentorial, simple

61682 supratentorial, complex

61684 infratentorial, simple

61686 infratentorial, complex

61690 dural, simple

61692 dural, complex

61697 Surgery of complex intracranial aneurysm, intracranial approach; carotid circulation

→ *CPT Changes: An Insider's View* 2001

61698 vertebrobasilar circulation

→ *CPT Changes: An Insider's View* 2001

(61697, 61698 involve aneurysms that are larger than 15 mm or with calcification of the aneurysm neck, or with incorporation of normal vessels into the aneurysm neck, or a procedure requiring temporary vessel occlusion, trapping or cardiopulmonary bypass to successfully treat the aneurysm)

61700 Surgery of simple intracranial aneurysm, intracranial approach; carotid circulation

→ *CPT Assistant* Jun 99:11, Jul 99:10; *CPT Changes: An Insider's View* 2001

Intracranial Aneurysm, Intracranial Approach
61700

Placement of ligating clip across the neck of an intracranial aneurysm

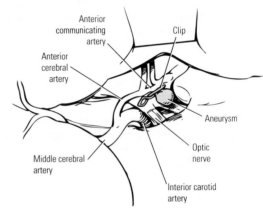

61702 vertebrobasilar circulation

→ *CPT Changes: An Insider's View* 2001

61703 Surgery of intracranial aneurysm, cervical approach by application of occluding clamp to cervical carotid artery (Selverstone-Crutchfield type)

(For cervical approach for direct ligation of carotid artery, see 37600-37606)

61705 Surgery of aneurysm, vascular malformation or carotid-cavernous fistula; by intracranial and cervical occlusion of carotid artery

61708 by intracranial electrothrombosis

(For ligation or gradual occlusion of internal/common carotid artery, see 37605, 37606)

61710 by intra-arterial embolization, injection procedure, or balloon catheter

61711   Anastomosis, arterial, extracranial-intracranial (eg, middle cerebral/cortical) arteries

(For carotid or vertebral thromboendarterectomy, use 35301)

(Use 69990 when the surgical microscope is employed for the microsurgical procedure. Do not use 69990 for visualization with magnifying loupes or corrected vision)

Stereotaxis

61720   Creation of lesion by stereotactic method, including burr hole(s) and localizing and recording techniques, single or multiple stages; globus pallidus or thalamus

61735   subcortical structure(s) other than globus pallidus or thalamus

61750   Stereotactic biopsy, aspiration, or excision, including burr hole(s), for intracranial lesion;
➔ *CPT Assistant* Nov 99:30; *CPT Changes: An Insider's View* 2000

61751   with computed tomography and/or magnetic resonance guidance
➔ *CPT Assistant* Jun 96:10, Nov 99:30, Dec 04:20; *CPT Changes: An Insider's View* 2000, 2003

(For radiological supervision and interpretation of computerized tomography, see 70450, 70460, or 70470 as appropriate)

(For radiological supervision and interpretation of magnetic resonance imaging, see 70551, 70552, or 70553 as appropriate)

61760   Stereotactic implantation of depth electrodes into the cerebrum for long-term seizure monitoring

61770   Stereotactic localization, including burr hole(s), with insertion of catheter(s) or probe(s) for placement of radiation source
➔ *CPT Changes: An Insider's View* 2001

61790   Creation of lesion by stereotactic method, percutaneous, by neurolytic agent (eg, alcohol, thermal, electrical, radiofrequency); gasserian ganglion

61791   trigeminal medullary tract

61793   Stereotactic radiosurgery (particle beam, gamma ray or linear accelerator), one or more sessions
➔ *CPT Assistant* Nov 97:23, May 03:19, Apr 04:15, Jan 06:46

(For intensity modulated beam delivery plan and treatment, see 77301, 77418)

+ 61795   Stereotactic computer-assisted volumetric (navigational) procedure, intracranial, extracranial, or spinal (List separately in addition to code for primary procedure)
➔ *CPT Assistant* Nov 99:30, Oct 01:10, Jan 06:46; *CPT Changes: An Insider's View* 2000

Neurostimulators (Intracranial)

Codes 61850-61888 apply to both simple and complex neurostimulators. For initial or subsequent electronic analysis and programming of neurostimulator pulse generators, see codes 95970-95975.

Microelectrode recording, when performed by the operating surgeon in association with implantation of neurostimulator electrode arrays, is an inclusive service and should not be reported separately. If another physician participates in neurophysiological mapping during a deep brain stimulator implantation procedure, this service may be reported by the other physician with codes 95961-95962.

61850   Twist drill or burr hole(s) for implantation of neurostimulator electrodes, cortical
➔ *CPT Assistant* Sep 99:5, Nov 99:30; *CPT Changes: An Insider's View* 2000

61860   Craniectomy or craniotomy for implantation of neurostimulator electrodes, cerebral, cortical
➔ *CPT Assistant* Sep 99:5, Nov 99:30; *CPT Changes: An Insider's View* 2000

61863   Twist drill, burr hole, craniotomy, or craniectomy with stereotactic implantation of neurostimulator electrode array in subcortical site (eg, thalamus, globus pallidus, subthalamic nucleus, periventricular, periaqueductal gray), without use of intraoperative microelectrode recording; first array
➔ *CPT Assistant* Sep 99:5; *CPT Changes: An Insider's View* 2004

+ 61864   each additional array (List separately in addition to primary procedure)
➔ *CPT Assistant* Sep 99:5; *CPT Changes: An Insider's View* 2004

(Use 61864 in conjunction with 61863)

61867   Twist drill, burr hole, craniotomy, or craniectomy with stereotactic implantation of neurostimulator electrode array in subcortical site (eg, thalamus, globus pallidus, subthalamic nucleus, periventricular, periaqueductal gray), with use of intraoperative microelectrode recording; first array
➔ *CPT Changes: An Insider's View* 2004

+ 61868   each additional array (List separately in addition to primary procedure)

     → *CPT Changes: An Insider's View* 2004

     (Use 61868 in conjunction with 61867)

Placement of Cranial Neurostimulator
61867-61868, 61885

Placement of subcortical (eg, thalamic) neurostimulator electrode via burr hole (61867-61868) with connection of the electrode to an implanted programmable pulse generator (61885) in the infraclavicular area

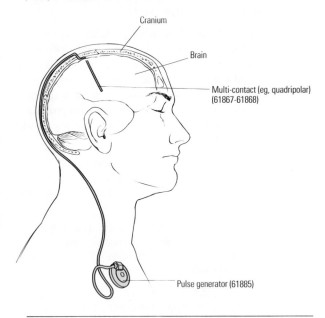

Cranium

Brain

Multi-contact (eg, quadripolar) (61867-61868)

Pulse generator (61885)

61870   Craniectomy for implantation of neurostimulator electrodes, cerebellar; cortical

61875   subcortical

61880   Revision or removal of intracranial neurostimulator electrodes

61885   Insertion or replacement of cranial neurostimulator pulse generator or receiver, direct or inductive coupling; with connection to a single electrode array

     → *CPT Assistant* Sep 99:5, Nov 99:30, Jun 00:3, Apr 01:8, Sep 03:3; *CPT Changes: An Insider's View* 2000, 2005

61886   with connection to two or more electrode arrays

     → *CPT Assistant* Nov 99:30, Jun 00:3, Apr 01:8; *CPT Changes: An Insider's View* 2000

(For open placement of cranial nerve (eg, vagal, trigeminal) neurostimulator electrode(s), use 64573)

(For percutaneous placement of cranial nerve (eg, vagal, trigeminal) neurostimulator electrode(s), use 64553)

(For revision or removal of cranial nerve (eg, vagal, trigeminal) neurostimulator electrode(s), use 64585)

61888   Revision or removal of cranial neurostimulator pulse generator or receiver

(Do not report 61888 in conjunction with 61885 or 61886 for the same pulse generator)

Repair

62000   Elevation of depressed skull fracture; simple, extradural

62005   compound or comminuted, extradural

62010   with repair of dura and/or debridement of brain

62100   Craniotomy for repair of dural/cerebrospinal fluid leak, including surgery for rhinorrhea/otorrhea

     → *CPT Changes: An Insider's View* 2002

(For repair of spinal dural/CSF leak, see 63707, 63709)

62115   Reduction of craniomegalic skull (eg, treated hydrocephalus); not requiring bone grafts or cranioplasty

62116   with simple cranioplasty

62117   requiring craniotomy and reconstruction with or without bone graft (includes obtaining grafts)

62120   Repair of encephalocele, skull vault, including cranioplasty

62121   Craniotomy for repair of encephalocele, skull base

62140   Cranioplasty for skull defect; up to 5 cm diameter

62141   larger than 5 cm diameter

62142   Removal of bone flap or prosthetic plate of skull

62143   Replacement of bone flap or prosthetic plate of skull

62145   Cranioplasty for skull defect with reparative brain surgery

62146   Cranioplasty with autograft (includes obtaining bone grafts); up to 5 cm diameter

62147   larger than 5 cm diameter

+ 62148   Incision and retrieval of subcutaneous cranial bone graft for cranioplasty (List separately in addition to code for primary procedure)

     → *CPT Changes: An Insider's View* 2003

(Use 62148 in conjunction with 62140-62147)

Neuroendoscopy

Surgical endoscopy always includes diagnostic endoscopy.

+ 62160   Neuroendoscopy, intracranial, for placement or replacement of ventricular catheter and attachment to shunt system or external drainage (List separately in addition to code for primary procedure)

     → *CPT Changes: An Insider's View* 2003

(Use 62160 only in conjunction with 61107, 61210, 62220-62230, 62258)

62161 Neuroendoscopy, intracranial; with dissection of adhesions, fenestration of septum pellucidum or intraventricular cysts (including placement, replacement, or removal of ventricular catheter)

➔ *CPT Changes: An Insider's View* 2003

62162 with fenestration or excision of colloid cyst, including placement of external ventricular catheter for drainage

➔ *CPT Changes: An Insider's View* 2003

62163 with retrieval of foreign body

➔ *CPT Changes: An Insider's View* 2003

62164 with excision of brain tumor, including placement of external ventricular catheter for drainage

➔ *CPT Changes: An Insider's View* 2003

62165 with excision of pituitary tumor, transnasal or trans-sphenoidal approach

➔ *CPT Changes: An Insider's View* 2003

Cerebrospinal Fluid (CSF) Shunt

62180 Ventriculocisternostomy (Torkildsen type operation)

62190 Creation of shunt; subarachnoid/subdural-atrial, -jugular, -auricular

62192 subarachnoid/subdural-peritoneal, -pleural, other terminus

62194 Replacement or irrigation, subarachnoid/subdural catheter

62200 Ventriculocisternostomy, third ventricle;

62201 stereotactic, neuroendoscopic method

➔ *CPT Changes: An Insider's View* 2003

(For intracranial neuroendoscopic procedures, see 62161-62165)

62220 Creation of shunt; ventriculo-atrial, -jugular, -auricular

(For intracranial neuroendoscopic ventricular catheter placement, use 62160)

62223 ventriculo-peritoneal, -pleural, other terminus

(For intracranial neuroendoscopic ventricular catheter placement, use 62160)

Cerebrospinal Fluid (CSF) Shunt (Ventricular Peritoneal)
62223

A ventriculostomy is performed to drain CSF into the peritoneal cavity.

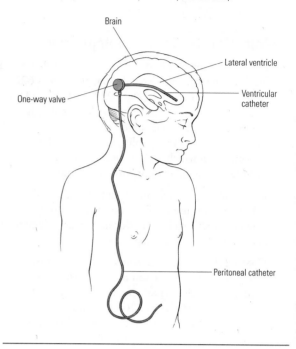

Brain

Lateral ventricle

Ventricular catheter

One-way valve

Peritoneal catheter

62225 Replacement or irrigation, ventricular catheter

(For intracranial neuroendoscopic ventricular catheter placement, use 62160)

62230 Replacement or revision of cerebrospinal fluid shunt, obstructed valve, or distal catheter in shunt system

➔ *CPT Changes: An Insider's View* 2002

(For intracranial neuroendoscopic ventricular catheter placement, use 62160)

62252 Reprogramming of programmable cerebrospinal shunt

➔ *CPT Changes: An Insider's View* 2001, 2002

62256 Removal of complete cerebrospinal fluid shunt system; without replacement

➔ *CPT Changes: An Insider's View* 2002

62258 with replacement by similar or other shunt at same operation

(For percutaneous irrigation or aspiration of shunt reservoir, use 61070)

(For reprogramming of programmable CSF shunt, use 62252)

(For intracranial neuroendoscopic ventricular catheter placement, use 62160)

Spine and Spinal Cord

(For application of caliper or tongs, use 20660)

(For treatment of fracture or dislocation of spine, see 22305-22327)

Injection, Drainage, or Aspiration

Injection of contrast during fluoroscopic guidance and localization is an inclusive component of codes 62263-62264, 62270-62273, 62280-62282, 62310-62319, 0027T. Fluoroscopic guidance and localization is reported by code 77003, unless a formal contrast study (myelography, epidurography, or arthrography) is performed, in which case the use of fluoroscopy is included in the supervision and interpretation codes.

For radiologic supervision and interpretation of epidurography, use 72275. Code 72275 is only to be used when an epidurogram is performed, images documented, and a formal radiologic report is issued.

Code 62263 describes a catheter-based treatment involving targeted injection of various substances (eg, hypertonic saline, steroid, anesthetic) via an indwelling epidural catheter. Code 62263 includes percutaneous insertion and removal of an epidural catheter (remaining in place over a several-day period), for the administration of multiple injections of a neurolytic agent(s) performed during serial treatment sessions (ie, spanning two or more treatment days). If required, adhesions or scarring may also be lysed by mechanical means. Code 62263 is NOT reported for each adhesiolysis treatment, but should be reported ONCE to describe the entire series of injections/infusions spanning two or more treatment days. For endoscopic lysis of adhesions, use 0027T.

Code 62264 describes multiple adhesiolysis treatment sessions performed on the same day. Adhesions or scarring may be lysed by injections of neurolytic agent(s). If required, adhesions or scarring may also be lysed mechanically using a percutaneously-deployed catheter.

Codes 62263 and 62264 include the procedure of injections of contrast for epidurography (72275) and fluoroscopic guidance and localization (77003) during initial or subsequent sessions.

(Report 01996 for daily hospital management of continuous epidural or subarachnoid drug administration performed in conjunction with 62318-62319)

(For endoscopic lysis of epidural adhesions, use Category III code 0027T)

62263 Percutaneous lysis of epidural adhesions using solution injection (eg, hypertonic saline, enzyme) or mechanical means (eg, catheter) including radiologic localization (includes contrast when administered), multiple adhesiolysis sessions; 2 or more days

➔ *CPT Assistant* Nov 99:33, Dec 99:11, Mar 02:11, Dec 02:10, Nov 05:14; *CPT Changes: An Insider's View* 2000, 2003

(62263 includes codes 72275 and 77003)

62264 1 day

➔ *CPT Assistant* Nov 05:14; *CPT Changes: An Insider's View* 2003

(Do not report 62264 with 62263)

(62264 includes codes 72275 and 77003)

62268 Percutaneous aspiration, spinal cord cyst or syrinx

(For radiological supervision and interpretation, see 76942, 77002, 77012)

62269 Biopsy of spinal cord, percutaneous needle

(For radiological supervision and interpretation, see 76942, 77002, 77012)

(For fine needle aspiration, see 10021, 10022)

(For evaluation of fine needle aspirate, see 88172, 88173)

62270 Spinal puncture, lumbar, diagnostic

➔ *CPT Assistant* Nov 99:32-33, Oct 03:2, Jul 06:4; *CPT Changes: An Insider's View* 2000, 2002

62272 Spinal puncture, therapeutic, for drainage of cerebrospinal fluid (by needle or catheter)

➔ *CPT Assistant* Nov 99:32-33; *CPT Changes: An Insider's View* 2000

62273 Injection, epidural, of blood or clot patch

➔ *CPT Assistant* Nov 99:32-34; *CPT Changes: An Insider's View* 2000

(For injection of diagnostic or therapeutic substance(s), see 62310, 62311, 62318, 62319)

62280 Injection/infusion of neurolytic substance (eg, alcohol, phenol, iced saline solutions), with or without other therapeutic substance; subarachnoid

➔ *CPT Assistant* Nov 99:32-34, Jan 00:2; *CPT Changes: An Insider's View* 2000

62281 epidural, cervical or thoracic

➔ *CPT Assistant* Apr 96:11, Nov 99:32-34, Jan 00:2; *CPT Changes: An Insider's View* 2000

62282 epidural, lumbar, sacral (caudal)

➔ *CPT Assistant* Apr 96:11, Nov 99:32-34, Jan 00:2; *CPT Changes: An Insider's View* 2000

▲ **62284** Injection procedure for myelography and/or computed tomography, spinal (other than C1-C2 and posterior fossa)

➔ *CPT Assistant* Fall 93:13, Sep 04:13; *CPT Changes: An Insider's View* 2003, 2008

➔ *Clinical Examples in Radiology* Fall 06:5-6, 11-12

(For injection procedure at C1-C2, use 61055)

(For radiological supervision and interpretation, see **Radiology**)

62287 Aspiration or decompression procedure, percutaneous, of nucleus pulposus of intervertebral disc, any method, single or multiple levels, lumbar (eg, manual or automated percutaneous discectomy, percutaneous laser discectomy)

➔ *CPT Assistant* Nov 99:34, Mar 02:11; *CPT Changes: An Insider's View* 2000

(For fluoroscopic guidance, use 77002)

(For injection of non-neurolytic diagnostic or therapeutic substance(s), see 62310, 62311)

62290   Injection procedure for discography, each level; lumbar

➔ *CPT Assistant* Nov 99:35, Apr 03:27; *CPT Changes: An Insider's View* 2000

62291   cervical or thoracic

➔ *CPT Assistant* Nov 99:35; *CPT Changes: An Insider's View* 2000

(For radiological supervision and interpretation, see 72285, 72295)

62292   Injection procedure for chemonucleolysis, including discography, intervertebral disc, single or multiple levels, lumbar

➔ *CPT Assistant* Oct 99:10

62294   Injection procedure, arterial, for occlusion of arteriovenous malformation, spinal

62310   Injection, single (not via indwelling catheter), not including neurolytic substances, with or without contrast (for either localization or epidurography), of diagnostic or therapeutic substance(s) (including anesthetic, antispasmodic, opioid, steroid, other solution), epidural or subarachnoid; cervical or thoracic

➔ *CPT Assistant* Nov 99:32-35, Jan 00:2, Dec 00:15, Sep 04:5; *CPT Changes: An Insider's View* 2000

62311   lumbar, sacral (caudal)

➔ *CPT Assistant* Nov 99:32-35, Jan 00:1, Dec 00:15, Sep 04:5; *CPT Changes: An Insider's View* 2000

62318   Injection, including catheter placement, continuous infusion or intermittent bolus, not including neurolytic substances, with or without contrast (for either localization or epidurography), of diagnostic or therapeutic substance(s) (including anesthetic, antispasmodic, opioid, steroid, other solution), epidural or subarachnoid; cervical or thoracic

➔ *CPT Assistant* Nov 99:32-35, Jan 00:2, Dec 00:15, Oct 01:9; *CPT Changes: An Insider's View* 2000

62319   lumbar, sacral (caudal)

➔ *CPT Assistant* Nov 99:32-35, Jan 00:2, Dec 00:15, Oct 01:9; *CPT Changes: An Insider's View* 2000

(For transforaminal epidural injection, see 64479-64484)

(Report 01996 for daily hospital management of continuous epidural or subarachnoid drug administration performed in conjunction with 62318-62319)

Catheter Implantation

(For percutaneous placement of intrathecal or epidural catheter, see codes 62270-62273, 62280-62284, 62310-62319)

62350   Implantation, revision or repositioning of tunneled intrathecal or epidural catheter, for long-term medication administration via an external pump or implantable reservoir/infusion pump; without laminectomy

➔ *CPT Assistant* Nov 99:36; *CPT Changes: An Insider's View* 2000, 2001

62351   with laminectomy

➔ *CPT Assistant* Nov 99:36; *CPT Changes: An Insider's View* 2000

(For refilling and maintenance of an implantable infusion pump for spinal or brain drug therapy, see 95990, 95991)

62355   Removal of previously implanted intrathecal or epidural catheter

Reservoir/Pump Implantation

62360   Implantation or replacement of device for intrathecal or epidural drug infusion; subcutaneous reservoir

62361   nonprogrammable pump

62362   programmable pump, including preparation of pump, with or without programming

➔ *CPT Assistant* Mar 97:11

Intrathecal or Epidural Drug Infusion Pump Implantation
62362

The reservoir is placed in the subcutaneous tissues and attached to a previously placed catheter for intrathecal or epidural drug infusion.

Catheter

Implanted infusion pump

62365   Removal of subcutaneous reservoir or pump, previously implanted for intrathecal or epidural infusion

62367 Electronic analysis of programmable, implanted pump for intrathecal or epidural drug infusion (includes evaluation of reservoir status, alarm status, drug prescription status); without reprogramming

62368 with reprogramming
→ *CPT Assistant* Nov 02:10, Jul 06:1

(For refilling and maintenance of an implantable infusion pump for spinal or brain drug therapy, use 95990-95991)

Posterior Extradural Laminotomy or Laminectomy for Exploration/ Decompression of Neural Elements or Excision of Herniated Intervertebral Discs

(When 63001-63048 are followed by arthrodesis, see 22590-22614)

63001 Laminectomy with exploration and/or decompression of spinal cord and/or cauda equina, without facetectomy, foraminotomy or discectomy (eg, spinal stenosis), 1 or 2 vertebral segments; cervical
→ *CPT Assistant* Jan 01:12

63003 thoracic
→ *CPT Assistant* Jan 01:12

63005 lumbar, except for spondylolisthesis
→ *CPT Assistant* Jan 01:12

Lumbar Laminectomy
63005

With the patient prone and under general anesthesia, the laminae and underlying ligamentum flavum are removed.

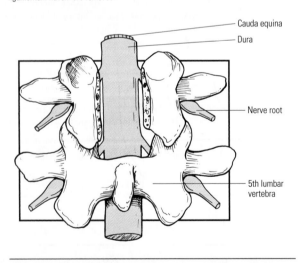

- Cauda equina
- Dura
- Nerve root
- 5th lumbar vertebra

63011 sacral
→ *CPT Assistant* Jan 01:12

63012 Laminectomy with removal of abnormal facets and/or pars inter-articularis with decompression of cauda equina and nerve roots for spondylolisthesis, lumbar (Gill type procedure)
→ *CPT Assistant* Jan 01:12

63015 Laminectomy with exploration and/or decompression of spinal cord and/or cauda equina, without facetectomy, foraminotomy or discectomy (eg, spinal stenosis), more than 2 vertebral segments; cervical
→ *CPT Assistant* Jan 01:12

63016 thoracic
→ *CPT Assistant* Jan 01:12

63017 lumbar
→ *CPT Assistant* Jan 01:12

63020 Laminotomy (hemilaminectomy), with decompression of nerve root(s), including partial facetectomy, foraminotomy and/or excision of herniated intervertebral disc; one interspace, cervical
→ *CPT Assistant* Nov 99:36, Jan 01:12; *CPT Changes: An Insider's View* 2000

(For bilateral procedure, report 63020 with modifier 50)

63030 one interspace, lumbar (including open or endoscopically-assisted approach)
→ *CPT Assistant* Mar 96:7, Nov 99:36, Jan 01:12, Feb 01:10, Sep 02:10, Oct 04:12; *CPT Changes: An Insider's View* 2000

(For bilateral procedure, report 63030 with modifier 50)

+ 63035 each additional interspace, cervical or lumbar (List separately in addition to code for primary procedure)
→ *CPT Assistant* Fall 91:8, Mar 96:7, Nov 99:36, Jan 01:12, Feb 01:10; *CPT Changes: An Insider's View* 2000

(Use 63035 in conjunction with 63020-63030)

(For bilateral procedure, report 63035 with modifier 50)

63040 Laminotomy (hemilaminectomy), with decompression of nerve root(s), including partial facetectomy, foraminotomy and/or excision of herniated intervertebral disc, reexploration, single interspace; cervical
→ *CPT Assistant* Jan 99:11, Jan 01:12; *CPT Changes: An Insider's View* 2001

(For bilateral procedure, report 63040 with modifier 50)

63042 lumbar
→ *CPT Assistant* Jan 99:11, Jan 01:12

(For bilateral procedure, report 63042 with modifier 50)

+ 63043 each additional cervical interspace (List separately in addition to code for primary procedure)
→ *CPT Changes: An Insider's View* 2001

(Use 63043 in conjunction with 63040)

(For bilateral procedure, report 63043 with modifier 50)

+ 63044 each additional lumbar interspace (List separately in addition to code for primary procedure)
→ *CPT Changes: An Insider's View* 2001

(Use 63044 in conjunction with 63042)

(For bilateral procedure, report 63044 with modifier 50)

63045   Laminectomy, facetectomy and foraminotomy (unilateral or bilateral with decompression of spinal cord, cauda equina and/or nerve root[s], [eg, spinal or lateral recess stenosis]), single vertebral segment; cervical
> *CPT Assistant* Jan 01:12

63046   thoracic
> *CPT Assistant* Jan 99:11, Jan 01:12

63047   lumbar
> *CPT Assistant* Jan 99:11, Jan 01:12, Feb 01:10, Nov 02:11

+ 63048   each additional segment, cervical, thoracic, or lumbar (List separately in addition to code for primary procedure)
> *CPT Assistant* Fall 91:8, Jan 99:11, Jan 01:12

(Use 63048 in conjunction with 63045-63047)

63050   Laminoplasty, cervical, with decompression of the spinal cord, two or more vertebral segments;
> *CPT Changes: An Insider's View* 2005

63051   with reconstruction of the posterior bony elements (including the application of bridging bone graft and non-segmental fixation devices (eg, wire, suture, mini-plates), when performed)
> *CPT Changes: An Insider's View* 2005

(Do not report 63050 or 63051 in conjunction with 22600, 22614, 22840-22842, 63001, 63015, 63045, 63048, 63295 for the same vertebral segment(s))

Transpedicular or Costovertebral Approach for Posterolateral Extradural Exploration/Decompression

63055   Transpedicular approach with decompression of spinal cord, equina and/or nerve root(s) (eg, herniated intervertebral disc), single segment; thoracic
> *CPT Assistant* Nov 99:36; *CPT Changes: An Insider's View* 2000

63056   lumbar (including transfacet, or lateral extraforaminal approach) (eg, far lateral herniated intervertebral disc)
> *CPT Assistant* Nov 99:36; *CPT Changes: An Insider's View* 2000

+ 63057   each additional segment, thoracic or lumbar (List separately in addition to code for primary procedure)
> *CPT Assistant* Nov 99:36; *CPT Changes: An Insider's View* 2000

(Use 63057 in conjunction with 63055, 63056)

63064   Costovertebral approach with decompression of spinal cord or nerve root(s) (eg, herniated intervertebral disc), thoracic; single segment
> *CPT Assistant* Fall 92:19

+ 63066   each additional segment (List separately in addition to code for primary procedure)

(Use 63066 in conjunction with 63064)

(For excision of thoracic intraspinal lesions by laminectomy, see 63266, 63271, 63276, 63281, 63286)

Anterior or Anterolateral Approach for Extradural Exploration/Decompression

For the following codes, when two surgeons work together as primary surgeons performing distinct part(s) of spinal cord exploration/decompression operation, each surgeon should report his/her distinct operative work by appending modifier 62 to the procedure code (and any associated add-on codes for that procedure code as long as both surgeons continue to work together as primary surgeons). In this situation, modifier 62 may be appended to the definitive procedure code(s) 63075, 63077, 63081, 63085, 63087, 63090 and, as appropriate, to associated additional interspace add-on code(s) 63076, 63078 or additional segment add-on code(s) 63082, 63086, 63088, 63091 as long as both surgeons continue to work together as primary surgeons.

63075   Discectomy, anterior, with decompression of spinal cord and/or nerve root(s), including osteophytectomy; cervical, single interspace
> *CPT Assistant* Nov 98:18, Jan 01:12, Feb 02:4; *CPT Changes: An Insider's View* 2002

+ 63076   cervical, each additional interspace (List separately in addition to code for primary procedure)
> *CPT Assistant* Nov 98:18, Jan 01:12, Feb 02:4; *CPT Changes: An Insider's View* 2002

(Use 63076 in conjunction with 63075)

63077   thoracic, single interspace
> *CPT Assistant* Nov 98:18, Jan 01:12, Feb 02:4; *CPT Changes: An Insider's View* 2002

+ 63078   thoracic, each additional interspace (List separately in addition to code for primary procedure)
> *CPT Assistant* Nov 98:18, Jan 01:12, Feb 02:4; *CPT Changes: An Insider's View* 2002

(Use 63078 in conjunction with 63077)

(Do not report code 69990 in addition to codes 63075-63078)

63081   Vertebral corpectomy (vertebral body resection), partial or complete, anterior approach with decompression of spinal cord and/or nerve root(s); cervical, single segment
> *CPT Assistant* Spring 93:37, Feb 02:4; *CPT Changes: An Insider's View* 2002

+ 63082   cervical, each additional segment (List separately in addition to code for primary procedure)
> *CPT Assistant* Spring 93:37, Feb 02:4; *CPT Changes: An Insider's View* 2002

(Use 63082 in conjunction with 63081)

(For transoral approach, see 61575, 61576)

63085 Vertebral corpectomy (vertebral body resection), partial or complete, transthoracic approach with decompression of spinal cord and/or nerve root(s); thoracic, single segment

➔ *CPT Assistant* Spring 93:37, Feb 02:4; *CPT Changes: An Insider's View* 2002

+ 63086 thoracic, each additional segment (List separately in addition to code for primary procedure)

➔ *CPT Assistant* Spring 93:37, Feb 02:4; *CPT Changes: An Insider's View* 2002

(Use 63086 in conjunction with 63085)

63087 Vertebral corpectomy (vertebral body resection), partial or complete, combined thoracolumbar approach with decompression of spinal cord, cauda equina or nerve root(s), lower thoracic or lumbar; single segment

➔ *CPT Assistant* Spring 93:37, Feb 02:4; *CPT Changes: An Insider's View* 2002

+ 63088 each additional segment (List separately in addition to code for primary procedure)

➔ *CPT Assistant* Spring 93:37, Feb 02:4; *CPT Changes: An Insider's View* 2002

(Use 63088 in conjunction with 63087)

63090 Vertebral corpectomy (vertebral body resection), partial or complete, transperitoneal or retroperitoneal approach with decompression of spinal cord, cauda equina or nerve root(s), lower thoracic, lumbar, or sacral; single segment

➔ *CPT Assistant* Spring 93:37, Mar 96:6, Feb 02:4; *CPT Changes: An Insider's View* 2002

+ 63091 each additional segment (List separately in addition to code for primary procedure)

➔ *CPT Assistant* Spring 93:37, Mar 96:6, Feb 02:4; *CPT Changes: An Insider's View* 2002

(Use 63091 in conjunction with 63090)

(Procedures 63081-63091 include discectomy above and/or below vertebral segment)

(If followed by arthrodesis, see 22548-22812)

(For reconstruction of spine, use appropriate vertebral corpectomy codes 63081-63091, bone graft codes 20930-20938, arthrodesis codes 22548-22812, and spinal instrumentation codes 22840-22855)

Lateral Extracavitary Approach for Extradural Exploration/Decompression

63101 Vertebral corpectomy (vertebral body resection), partial or complete, lateral extracavitary approach with decompression of spinal cord and/or nerve root(s) (eg, for tumor or retropulsed bone fragments); thoracic, single segment

➔ *CPT Changes: An Insider's View* 2004

63102 lumbar, single segment

➔ *CPT Changes: An Insider's View* 2004

+ 63103 thoracic or lumbar, each additional segment (List separately in addition to code for primary procedure)

➔ *CPT Changes: An Insider's View* 2004

(Use 63103 in conjunction with 63101 and 63102)

Incision

63170 Laminectomy with myelotomy (eg, Bischof or DREZ type), cervical, thoracic, or thoracolumbar

63172 Laminectomy with drainage of intramedullary cyst/syrinx; to subarachnoid space

63173 to peritoneal or pleural space

➔ *CPT Changes: An Insider's View* 2004

63180 Laminectomy and section of dentate ligaments, with or without dural graft, cervical; one or two segments

63182 more than two segments

63185 Laminectomy with rhizotomy; one or two segments

63190 more than two segments

63191 Laminectomy with section of spinal accessory nerve

(For bilateral procedure, report 63191 with modifier 50)

(For resection of sternocleidomastoid muscle, use 21720)

63194 Laminectomy with cordotomy, with section of one spinothalamic tract, one stage; cervical

63195 thoracic

63196 Laminectomy with cordotomy, with section of both spinothalamic tracts, one stage; cervical

63197 thoracic

63198 Laminectomy with cordotomy with section of both spinothalamic tracts, two stages within 14 days; cervical

63199 thoracic

63200 Laminectomy, with release of tethered spinal cord, lumbar

Excision by Laminectomy of Lesion Other Than Herniated Disc

63250 Laminectomy for excision or occlusion of arteriovenous malformation of spinal cord; cervical

63251 thoracic

63252 thoracolumbar

63265 Laminectomy for excision or evacuation of intraspinal lesion other than neoplasm, extradural; cervical

63266 thoracic

63267 lumbar

63268 sacral

63270 Laminectomy for excision of intraspinal lesion other than neoplasm, intradural; cervical

63271 thoracic

63272 lumbar

63273 sacral

63275   Laminectomy for biopsy/excision of intraspinal neoplasm; extradural, cervical

63276   extradural, thoracic

63277   extradural, lumbar

63278   extradural, sacral

63280   intradural, extramedullary, cervical

63281   intradural, extramedullary, thoracic

63282   intradural, extramedullary, lumbar

63283   intradural, sacral

63285   intradural, intramedullary, cervical

63286   intradural, intramedullary, thoracic

63287   intradural, intramedullary, thoracolumbar

63290   combined extradural-intradural lesion, any level

(For drainage of intramedullary cyst/syrinx, use 63172, 63173)

+ 63295   Osteoplastic reconstruction of dorsal spinal elements, following primary intraspinal procedure (List separately in addition to code for primary procedure)

➜ *CPT Changes: An Insider's View* 2005

(Use 63295 in conjunction with 63172, 63173, 63185, 63190, 63200-63290)

(Do not report 63295 in conjunction with 22590-22614, 22840-22844, 63050, 63051 for the same vertebral segment(s))

Excision, Anterior or Anterolateral Approach, Intraspinal Lesion

For the following codes, when two surgeons work together as primary surgeons performing distinct part(s) of an anterior approach for an intraspinal excision, each surgeon should report his/her distinct operative work by appending modifier 62 to the single definitive procedure code. In this situation, modifier 62 may be appended to the definitive procedure code(s) 63300-63307 and, as appropriate, to the associated additional segment add-on code 63308 as long as both surgeons continue to work together as primary surgeons.

(For arthrodesis, see 22548-22585)

(For reconstruction of spine, see 20930-20938)

63300   Vertebral corpectomy (vertebral body resection), partial or complete, for excision of intraspinal lesion, single segment; extradural, cervical

➜ *CPT Assistant* Feb 02:4

63301   extradural, thoracic by transthoracic approach

➜ *CPT Assistant* Feb 02:4

63302   extradural, thoracic by thoracolumbar approach

➜ *CPT Assistant* Feb 02:4

63303   extradural, lumbar or sacral by transperitoneal or retroperitoneal approach

➜ *CPT Assistant* Feb 02:4

63304   intradural, cervical

➜ *CPT Assistant* Feb 02:4

63305   intradural, thoracic by transthoracic approach

➜ *CPT Assistant* Feb 02:4

63306   intradural, thoracic by thoracolumbar approach

➜ *CPT Assistant* Feb 02:4

63307   intradural, lumbar or sacral by transperitoneal or retroperitoneal approach

➜ *CPT Assistant* Feb 02:4

+ 63308   each additional segment (List separately in addition to codes for single segment)

➜ *CPT Assistant* Feb 02:4

(Use 63308 in conjunction with 63300-63307)

Stereotaxis

63600   Creation of lesion of spinal cord by stereotactic method, percutaneous, any modality (including stimulation and/or recording)

63610   Stereotactic stimulation of spinal cord, percutaneous, separate procedure not followed by other surgery

63615   Stereotactic biopsy, aspiration, or excision of lesion, spinal cord

Neurostimulators (Spinal)

Codes 63650-63688 apply to both simple and complex neurostimulators. For initial or subsequent electronic analysis and programming of neurostimulator pulse generators, see codes 95970-95975.

Codes 63650, 63655, and 63660 describe the operative placement, revision, or removal of the spinal neurostimulator system components to provide spinal electrical stimulation. A neurostimulator system includes an implanted neurostimulator, external controller, extension, and collection of contacts. Multiple contacts or electrodes (4 or more) provide the actual electrical stimulation in the epidural space.

For percutaneously placed neurostimulator systems (63650, 63660), the contacts are on a catheter-like lead. An array defines the collection of contacts that are on one catheter.

For systems placed via an open surgical exposure (63655, 63660), the contacts are on a plate or paddle-shaped surface.

63650 Percutaneous implantation of neurostimulator electrode array, epidural

→ *CPT Assistant* Jun 98:3-4, Nov 98:18, Mar 99:11, Apr 99:10, Sep 99:3

Percutaneous Implantation of Neurostimulator Electrodes
63650

Single catheter electrode array is inserted percutaneously into the epidural space. A simple or complex receiver is subcutaneously implanted.

63655 Laminectomy for implantation of neurostimulator electrodes, plate/paddle, epidural

→ *CPT Assistant* Jun 98:3-4, Nov 98:18, Sep 99:3-4

Placement of Neurostimulator Electrodes Through Laminectomy
63655

The electrode plate or paddle is placed in the epidural space via open exposure through large laminotomy or small laminectomy. The simple or complex receiver is subcutaneously implanted.

63660 Revision or removal of spinal neurostimulator electrode percutaneous array(s) or plate/paddle(s)

→ *CPT Assistant* Jun 98:3-4, Jun 98:1, Nov 98:18

63685 Insertion or replacement of spinal neurostimulator pulse generator or receiver, direct or inductive coupling

→ *CPT Assistant* Jun 98:3-4, Sep 99:5; *CPT Changes: An Insider's View* 2005

(Do not report 63685 in conjunction with 63688 for the same pulse generator or receiver)

63688 Revision or removal of implanted spinal neurostimulator pulse generator or receiver

→ *CPT Assistant* Jun 98:3-4, Sep 99:5

(For electronic analysis of implanted neurostimulator pulse generator system, see 95970-95975)

Repair

63700 Repair of meningocele; less than 5 cm diameter

63702   larger than 5 cm diameter

(Do not use modifier 63 in conjunction with 63700, 63702)

63704 Repair of myelomeningocele; less than 5 cm diameter

63706   larger than 5 cm diameter

(Do not use modifier 63 in conjunction with 63704, 63706)

(For complex skin closure, see **Integumentary System**)

63707 Repair of dural/cerebrospinal fluid leak, not requiring laminectomy

→ *CPT Changes: An Insider's View* 2002

63709 Repair of dural/cerebrospinal fluid leak or pseudomeningocele, with laminectomy

→ *CPT Changes: An Insider's View* 2002

63710 Dural graft, spinal

(For laminectomy and section of dentate ligaments, with or without dural graft, cervical, see 63180, 63182)

Shunt, Spinal CSF

63740 Creation of shunt, lumbar, subarachnoid-peritoneal, -pleural, or other; including laminectomy

→ *CPT Assistant* Winter 90:8

63741   percutaneous, not requiring laminectomy

→ *CPT Assistant* Winter 90:8

63744 Replacement, irrigation or revision of lumbosubarachnoid shunt

63746 Removal of entire lumbosubarachnoid shunt system without replacement

(For insertion of subarachnoid catheter with reservoir and/or pump for intermittent or continuous infusion of drug including laminectomy, see 62351 and 62360, 62361 or 62362)

(For insertion or replacement of subarachnoid or epidural catheter, with reservoir and/or pump for drug infusion without laminectomy, see 62350 and 62360, 62361 or 62362)

Extracranial Nerves, Peripheral Nerves, and Autonomic Nervous System

(For intracranial surgery on cranial nerves, see 61450, 61460, 61790)

Introduction/Injection of Anesthetic Agent (Nerve Block), Diagnostic or Therapeutic

Somatic Nerves

64400   Injection, anesthetic agent; trigeminal nerve, any division or branch
➔ *CPT Assistant* Jul 98:10, May 99:8, Nov 99:36, Apr 05:13; *CPT Changes: An Insider's View* 2000

64402   facial nerve
➔ *CPT Assistant* Jul 98:10, Apr 05:13

64405   greater occipital nerve
➔ *CPT Assistant* Jul 98:10, Apr 05:13

64408   vagus nerve
➔ *CPT Assistant* Jul 98:10, Apr 05:13

64410   phrenic nerve
➔ *CPT Assistant* Jul 98:10, Apr 05:13

64412   spinal accessory nerve
➔ *CPT Assistant* Jul 98:10, Apr 05:13

64413   cervical plexus
➔ *CPT Assistant* Jul 98:10, Apr 05:13

64415   brachial plexus, single
➔ *CPT Assistant* Fall 92:17, Jul 98:10, May 99:8, Oct 01:9, Feb 04:7, Apr 05:13, Nov 06:23; *CPT Changes: An Insider's View* 2003

64416   brachial plexus, continuous infusion by catheter (including catheter placement) including daily management for anesthetic agent administration
➔ *CPT Assistant* Feb 04:7, Apr 05:13; *CPT Changes: An Insider's View* 2003

(Do not report 64416 in conjunction with 01996)

64417   axillary nerve
➔ *CPT Assistant* Jul 98:10, Apr 05:13

64418   suprascapular nerve
➔ *CPT Assistant* Jul 98:10, Apr 05:13

64420   intercostal nerve, single
➔ *CPT Assistant* Jul 98:10, Apr 05:13

64421   intercostal nerves, multiple, regional block
➔ *CPT Assistant* Jul 98:10, Apr 05:13

64425   ilioinguinal, iliohypogastric nerves
➔ *CPT Assistant* Jul 98:10, Apr 05:13

64430   pudendal nerve
➔ *CPT Assistant* Jul 98:10, Apr 05:13

64435   paracervical (uterine) nerve
➔ *CPT Assistant* Jul 98:10, Mar 03:22, Jul 03:15, Apr 05:13

64445   sciatic nerve, single
➔ *CPT Assistant* Jul 98:10, May 99:8, Feb 04:8, Apr 05:13; *CPT Changes: An Insider's View* 2003

64446   sciatic nerve, continuous infusion by catheter (including catheter placement), including daily management for anesthetic agent administration
➔ *CPT Assistant* Feb 04:9, Apr 05:13; *CPT Changes: An Insider's View* 2003

(Do not report 64446 in conjunction with 01996)

64447   femoral nerve, single
➔ *CPT Assistant* Feb 04:9, Apr 05:13; *CPT Changes: An Insider's View* 2003

(Do not report 64447 in conjunction with 01996)

64448   femoral nerve, continuous infusion by catheter (including catheter placement) including daily management for anesthetic agent administration
➔ *CPT Assistant* Feb 04:10, Apr 05:13; *CPT Changes: An Insider's View* 2003

(Do not report 64448 in conjunction with 01996)

64449   lumbar plexus, posterior approach, continuous infusion by catheter (including catheter placement) including daily management for anesthetic agent administration
➔ *CPT Assistant* Apr 05:13; *CPT Changes: An Insider's View* 2004

(Do not report 64449 in conjunction with 01996)

64450   other peripheral nerve or branch
➔ *CPT Assistant* Jul 98:10, Nov 99:37, Dec 99:7, Oct 01:9, Aug 03:6, Apr 05:13; *CPT Changes: An Insider's View* 2000

(For phenol destruction, see 64622-64627)

(For subarachnoid or subdural injection, see 62280, 62310-62319)

(For epidural or caudal injection, see 62273, 62281-62282, 62310-62319)

(Codes 64470-64484 are unilateral procedures. For bilateral procedures, use modifier 50)

(For fluoroscopic guidance and localization for needle placement and injection in conjunction with 64470-64484, use 77003)

64470   Injection, anesthetic agent and/or steroid, paravertebral facet joint or facet joint nerve; cervical or thoracic, single level
➔ *CPT Assistant* Nov 99:33, 37, Feb 00:4, Sep 04:3; *CPT Changes: An Insider's View* 2000

+ 64472 cervical or thoracic, each additional level (List separately in addition to code for primary procedure)

➡ *CPT Assistant* Nov 99:33, 37, Feb 00:4, Sep 04:3; *CPT Changes: An Insider's View* 2000

(Use 64472 in conjunction with 64470)

64475 lumbar or sacral, single level

➡ *CPT Assistant* Nov 99:33, 37, Feb 00:4, Mar 03:22, May 04:15, Sep 04:3; *CPT Changes: An Insider's View* 2000

+ 64476 lumbar or sacral, each additional level (List separately in addition to code for primary procedure)

➡ *CPT Assistant* Nov 99:33, 37, Feb 00:4, Sep 04:3; *CPT Changes: An Insider's View* 2000

(Use 64476 in conjunction with 64475)

64479 Injection, anesthetic agent and/or steroid, transforaminal epidural; cervical or thoracic, single level

➡ *CPT Assistant* Nov 99:33, 37, Feb 00:4; *CPT Changes: An Insider's View* 2000

+ 64480 cervical or thoracic, each additional level (List separately in addition to code for primary procedure)

➡ *CPT Assistant* Nov 99:33, 37, Feb 00:4, Feb 05:14; *CPT Changes: An Insider's View* 2000

(Use 64480 in conjunction with 64479)

64483 lumbar or sacral, single level

➡ *CPT Assistant* Nov 99:33, 37, Feb 00:4; *CPT Changes: An Insider's View* 2000

+ 64484 lumbar or sacral, each additional level (List separately in addition to code for primary procedure)

➡ *CPT Assistant* Nov 99:33, 37, Feb 00:4, Feb 05:14; *CPT Changes: An Insider's View* 2000

(Use 64484 in conjunction with 64483)

Sympathetic Nerves

64505 Injection, anesthetic agent; sphenopalatine ganglion

➡ *CPT Assistant* Jul 98:10, Apr 05:13

64508 carotid sinus (separate procedure)

➡ *CPT Assistant* Jul 98:10, Apr 05:13

64510 stellate ganglion (cervical sympathetic)

➡ *CPT Assistant* Jul 98:10, Apr 05:13

64517 superior hypogastric plexus

➡ *CPT Assistant* Oct 04:11, Apr 05:13; *CPT Changes: An Insider's View* 2004

64520 lumbar or thoracic (paravertebral sympathetic)

➡ *CPT Assistant* Jul 98:10, Apr 05:13

64530 celiac plexus, with or without radiologic monitoring

➡ *CPT Assistant* Jul 98:10, Apr 05:13

Neurostimulators (Peripheral Nerve)

Codes 64553-64595 apply to both simple and complex neurostimulators. For initial or subsequent electronic analysis and programming of neurostimulator pulse generators, see codes 95970-95975.

64550 Application of surface (transcutaneous) neurostimulator

➡ *CPT Assistant* Jan 02:11, Apr 02:18

64553 Percutaneous implantation of neurostimulator electrodes; cranial nerve

➡ *CPT Assistant* Nov 99:38, Apr 01:9; *CPT Changes: An Insider's View* 2000

(For open placement of cranial nerve (eg, vagal, trigeminal) neurostimulator pulse generator or receiver, see 61885, 61886, as appropriate)

64555 peripheral nerve (excludes sacral nerve)

➡ *CPT Changes: An Insider's View* 2002

64560 autonomic nerve

64561 sacral nerve (transforaminal placement)

➡ *CPT Changes: An Insider's View* 2002

64565 neuromuscular

➡ *CPT Assistant* Jul 00:11

64573 Incision for implantation of neurostimulator electrodes; cranial nerve

➡ *CPT Assistant* Sep 99:4, Nov 99:38, Apr 01:8; *CPT Changes: An Insider's View* 2000

(For open placement of cranial nerve (eg, vagal, trigeminal) neurostimulator pulse generator or receiver, see 61885, 61886, as appropriate)

(For revision or removal of cranial nerve (eg, vagal, trigeminal) neurostimulator pulse generator or receiver, use 61888)

Implantation Neurostimulator Electrodes, Cranial Nerve (Vagal Nerve Stimulation)
61885, 64573

Open incision for implantation of a neurostimulator electrode (64573) on the vagus nerve (a cranial nerve) with connection of the electrode to an implanted programmable pulse generator (61885) in the infraclavicular area

64575   peripheral nerve (excludes sacral nerve)

> *CPT Changes: An Insider's View* 2002

64577   autonomic nerve

64580   neuromuscular

64581   sacral nerve (transforaminal placement)

> *CPT Changes: An Insider's View* 2002

Incisional Implantation of Sacral Nerve Neurostimulator
64581

Posterior View

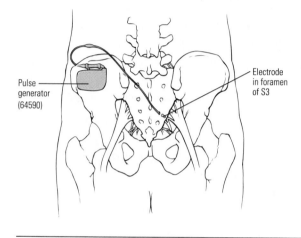

Pulse generator (64590)

Electrode in foramen of S3

64585   Revision or removal of peripheral neurostimulator electrodes

64590   Insertion or replacement of peripheral or gastric neurostimulator pulse generator or receiver, direct or inductive coupling

> *CPT Assistant* Sep 99:4, Apr 01:8, Mar 07:4, Apr 07:7;
> *CPT Changes: An Insider's View* 2002, 2005, 2007

(Do not report 64590 in conjunction with 64595)

64595   Revision or removal of peripheral or gastric neurostimulator pulse generator or receiver

> *CPT Assistant* Sep 99:3, Mar 07:4; *CPT Changes: An Insider's View* 2007

Destruction by Neurolytic Agent (eg, Chemical, Thermal, Electrical or Radiofrequency)

Codes 64600-64681 include the injection of other therapeutic agents (eg, corticosteroids).

Somatic Nerves

64600   Destruction by neurolytic agent, trigeminal nerve; supraorbital, infraorbital, mental, or inferior alveolar branch

> *CPT Assistant* Aug 05:13

64605   second and third division branches at foramen ovale

> *CPT Assistant* Aug 05:13

64610   second and third division branches at foramen ovale under radiologic monitoring

> *CPT Assistant* Aug 05:13

64612   Chemodenervation of muscle(s); muscle(s) innervated by facial nerve (eg, for blepharospasm, hemifacial spasm)

> *CPT Assistant* Oct 98:10, Apr 01:2, Aug 05:13, Sep 06:5;
> *CPT Changes: An Insider's View* 2000, 2001

Chemodenervation of Extremity
64612-64614

Flexor digitorum superficialis m. (cut)

Botulinum injection

Flexor digitorum profundus m.

Flexor carpi ulnaris m.

Cramped hand

Cramping relieved

64613   neck muscle(s) (eg, for spasmodic torticollis, spasmodic dysphonia)

> *CPT Assistant* Sep 00:10, Apr 01:2, Aug 05:13, Sep 06:5;
> *CPT Changes: An Insider's View* 2001, 2006

64614   extremity(s) and/or trunk muscle(s) (eg, for dystonia, cerebral palsy, multiple sclerosis)
CPT Assistant Apr 01:2, Feb 05:14, Aug 05:13, Sep 06:5; *CPT Changes: An Insider's View* 2001

(For chemodenervation guided by needle electromyography or muscle electrical stimulation, see 95873, 95874)

(For chemodenervation for strabismus involving the extraocular muscles, use 67345)

(For chemodenervation of internal anal sphincter, use 46505)

64620   Destruction by neurolytic agent, intercostal nerve
CPT Assistant Nov 99:38, Aug 05:13; *CPT Changes: An Insider's View* 2000

(For fluoroscopic guidance and localization for needle placement and neurolysis in conjunction with 64622-64627, use 77003)

64622   Destruction by neurolytic agent, paravertebral facet joint nerve; lumbar or sacral, single level
CPT Assistant Nov 99:33, 39, Dec 99:7, Mar 00:4, Sep 04:5, Aug 05:13; *CPT Changes: An Insider's View* 2000

(For bilateral procedure, report 64622 with modifier 50)

+ 64623   lumbar or sacral, each additional level (List separately in addition to code for primary procedure)
CPT Assistant Nov 99:33, 39, Mar 00:4, Sep 04:5, Aug 05:13; *CPT Changes: An Insider's View* 2000

(Use 64623 in conjunction with 64622)

(For bilateral procedure, report 64623 with modifier 50)

64626   cervical or thoracic, single level
CPT Assistant Nov 99:33, 39, Mar 00:4, Sep 04:5, Aug 05:13; *CPT Changes: An Insider's View* 2000

(For bilateral procedure, report 64626 with modifier 50)

+ 64627   cervical or thoracic, each additional level (List separately in addition to code for primary procedure)
CPT Assistant Nov 99:33, 39, Mar 00:4, Sep 04:5, Aug 05:13; *CPT Changes: An Insider's View* 2000

(Use 64627 in conjunction with 64626)

(For bilateral procedure, report 64627 with modifier 50)

64630   Destruction by neurolytic agent; pudendal nerve
CPT Assistant Aug 05:13; *CPT Changes: An Insider's View* 2001

64640   other peripheral nerve or branch
CPT Assistant Aug 05:13

Sympathetic Nerves

64650   Chemodenervation of eccrine glands; both axillae
CPT Changes: An Insider's View 2006

64653   other area(s) (eg, scalp, face, neck), per day
CPT Changes: An Insider's View 2006

(Report the specific service in conjunction with code(s) for the specific substance(s) or drug(s) provided)

(For chemodenervation of extremities (eg, hands or feet), use 64999)

64680   Destruction by neurolytic agent, with or without radiologic monitoring; celiac plexus
CPT Assistant Feb 99:10, Aug 05:13; *CPT Changes: An Insider's View* 2004

64681   superior hypogastric plexus
CPT Assistant Aug 05:13; *CPT Changes: An Insider's View* 2004

Neuroplasty (Exploration, Neurolysis or Nerve Decompression)

Neuroplasty is the decompression or freeing of intact nerve from scar tissue, including external neurolysis and/or transposition.

(For internal neurolysis requiring use of operating microscope, use 64727)

(For facial nerve decompression, use 69720)

▶(For neuroplasty with nerve wrapping, see 64702-64727, 64999)◄

64702   Neuroplasty; digital, one or both, same digit
CPT Assistant Jun 01:11

64704   nerve of hand or foot
CPT Assistant Jun 01:11

64708   Neuroplasty, major peripheral nerve, arm or leg; other than specified
CPT Assistant Jun 01:11

64712   sciatic nerve
CPT Assistant Jun 01:11

64713   brachial plexus
CPT Assistant Jun 01:11

64714   lumbar plexus
CPT Assistant Jun 97:11, Sep 98:16, Jun 01:11

64716   Neuroplasty and/or transposition; cranial nerve (specify)
CPT Assistant Jun 01:11

64718   ulnar nerve at elbow
CPT Assistant Jun 01:11

64719   ulnar nerve at wrist
CPT Assistant Jun 01:11

64721   median nerve at carpal tunnel
CPT Assistant Fall 92:17, Sep 97:10, Jun 01:11, Nov 06:23

(For arthroscopic procedure, use 29848)

64722   Decompression; unspecified nerve(s) (specify)
CPT Assistant Sep 98:16, May 99:11, Jun 01:11, Oct 04:12

64726   plantar digital nerve
CPT Assistant Jun 01:11

+ 64727   Internal neurolysis, requiring use of operating microscope (List separately in addition to code for neuroplasty) (Neuroplasty includes external neurolysis)
➔ *CPT Assistant* Nov 98:19, Jun 01:11

(Do not report code 69990 in addition to code 64727)

Transection or Avulsion

(For stereotactic lesion of gasserian ganglion, use 61790)

64732   Transection or avulsion of; supraorbital nerve
➔ *CPT Assistant* Nov 99:39; *CPT Changes: An Insider's View* 2000

64734   infraorbital nerve

64736   mental nerve

64738   inferior alveolar nerve by osteotomy

64740   lingual nerve

64742   facial nerve, differential or complete

64744   greater occipital nerve

64746   phrenic nerve

(For section of recurrent laryngeal nerve, use 31595)

64752   vagus nerve (vagotomy), transthoracic

64755   vagus nerves limited to proximal stomach (selective proximal vagotomy, proximal gastric vagotomy, parietal cell vagotomy, supra- or highly selective vagotomy)
➔ *CPT Assistant* Nov 99:39; *CPT Changes: An Insider's View* 2000, 2002

(For laparoscopic approach, use 43652)

64760   vagus nerve (vagotomy), abdominal
➔ *CPT Assistant* Nov 99:39; *CPT Changes: An Insider's View* 2000

(For laparoscopic approach, use 43651)

64761   pudendal nerve

(For bilateral procedure, report 64761 with modifier 50)

64763   Transection or avulsion of obturator nerve, extrapelvic, with or without adductor tenotomy

(For bilateral procedure, report 64763 with modifier 50)

64766   Transection or avulsion of obturator nerve, intrapelvic, with or without adductor tenotomy

(For bilateral procedure, report 64766 with modifier 50)

64771   Transection or avulsion of other cranial nerve, extradural

64772   Transection or avulsion of other spinal nerve, extradural

(For excision of tender scar, skin and subcutaneous tissue, with or without tiny neuroma, see 11400-11446, 13100-13153)

Excision

Somatic Nerves

(For Morton neurectomy, use 28080)

64774   Excision of neuroma; cutaneous nerve, surgically identifiable

64776   digital nerve, one or both, same digit

+ 64778   digital nerve, each additional digit (List separately in addition to code for primary procedure)

(Use 64778 in conjunction with 64776)

64782   hand or foot, except digital nerve

+ 64783   hand or foot, each additional nerve, except same digit (List separately in addition to code for primary procedure)

(Use 64783 in conjunction with 64782)

64784   major peripheral nerve, except sciatic

64786   sciatic nerve

+ 64787   Implantation of nerve end into bone or muscle (List separately in addition to neuroma excision)

(Use 64787 in conjunction with 64774-64786)

64788   Excision of neurofibroma or neurolemmoma; cutaneous nerve

64790   major peripheral nerve

64792   extensive (including malignant type)

64795   Biopsy of nerve

Sympathetic Nerves

64802   Sympathectomy, cervical

(For bilateral procedure, report 64802 with modifier 50)

64804   Sympathectomy, cervicothoracic

(For bilateral procedure, report 64804 with modifier 50)

64809   Sympathectomy, thoracolumbar

(For bilateral procedure, report 64809 with modifier 50)

64818   Sympathectomy, lumbar

(For bilateral procedure, report 64818 with modifier 50)

64820   Sympathectomy; digital arteries, each digit
➔ *CPT Assistant* Jan 04:27; *CPT Changes: An Insider's View* 2002

(Do not report 69990 in addition to code 64820)

64821   radial artery
➔ *CPT Changes: An Insider's View* 2002

(Do not report 69990 in addition to code 64821)

64822   ulnar artery
➔ *CPT Changes: An Insider's View* 2002

(Do not report 69990 in addition to code 64822)

64823   superficial palmar arch
> *CPT Changes: An Insider's View* 2002

(Do not report 69990 in addition to code 64823)

Neurorrhaphy

64831   Suture of digital nerve, hand or foot; one nerve
> *CPT Assistant* Apr 00:5

+ 64832   each additional digital nerve (List separately in addition to code for primary procedure)
> *CPT Assistant* Apr 00:5

(Use 64832 in conjunction with 64831)

▲ **64834**   Suture of one nerve; hand or foot, common sensory nerve
> *CPT Changes: An Insider's View* 2008

▲ **64835**   median motor thenar
> *CPT Changes: An Insider's View* 2008

▲ **64836**   ulnar motor
> *CPT Changes: An Insider's View* 2008

+ 64837   Suture of each additional nerve, hand or foot (List separately in addition to code for primary procedure)

(Use 64837 in conjunction with 64834-64836)

64840   Suture of posterior tibial nerve

64856   Suture of major peripheral nerve, arm or leg, except sciatic; including transposition

64857   without transposition

64858   Suture of sciatic nerve

+ 64859   Suture of each additional major peripheral nerve (List separately in addition to code for primary procedure)

(Use 64859 in conjunction with 64856, 64857)

64861   Suture of; brachial plexus

64862   lumbar plexus

64864   Suture of facial nerve; extracranial

64865   infratemporal, with or without grafting

64866   Anastomosis; facial-spinal accessory

64868   facial-hypoglossal

64870   facial-phrenic

+ 64872   Suture of nerve; requiring secondary or delayed suture (List separately in addition to code for primary neurorrhaphy)

(Use 64872 in conjunction with 64831-64865)

+ 64874   requiring extensive mobilization, or transposition of nerve (List separately in addition to code for nerve suture)

(Use 64874 in conjunction with 64831-64865)

+ 64876   requiring shortening of bone of extremity (List separately in addition to code for nerve suture)

(Use 64876 in conjunction with 64831-64865)

Neurorrhaphy With Nerve Graft, Vein Graft, or Conduit

64885   Nerve graft (includes obtaining graft), head or neck; up to 4 cm in length
> *CPT Assistant* Nov 00:11

64886   more than 4 cm length
> *CPT Assistant* Nov 00:11

64890   Nerve graft (includes obtaining graft), single strand, hand or foot; up to 4 cm length

64891   more than 4 cm length

64892   Nerve graft (includes obtaining graft), single strand, arm or leg; up to 4 cm length

64893   more than 4 cm length

64895   Nerve graft (includes obtaining graft), multiple strands (cable), hand or foot; up to 4 cm length
> *CPT Assistant* Nov 00:11

64896   more than 4 cm length
> *CPT Assistant* Nov 00:11

64897   Nerve graft (includes obtaining graft), multiple strands (cable), arm or leg; up to 4 cm length
> *CPT Assistant* Nov 00:11

64898   more than 4 cm length
> *CPT Assistant* Nov 00:11

+ 64901   Nerve graft, each additional nerve; single strand (List separately in addition to code for primary procedure)
> *CPT Assistant* Nov 00:11

(Use 64901 in conjunction with 64885-64893)

+ 64902   multiple strands (cable) (List separately in addition to code for primary procedure)
> *CPT Assistant* Nov 00:11

(Use 64902 in conjunction with 64885, 64886, 64895-64898)

64905   Nerve pedicle transfer; first stage

64907   second stage

64910   Nerve repair; with synthetic conduit or vein allograft (eg, nerve tube), each nerve
> *CPT Changes: An Insider's View* 2007

64911   with autogenous vein graft (includes harvest of vein graft), each nerve
> *CPT Changes: An Insider's View* 2007

(Do not report 69990 in addition to 64910, 64911)

Other Procedures

64999   Unlisted procedure, nervous system
> *CPT Assistant* Apr 96:11, Sep 98:16, Oct 98:10, Jan 00:10, Aug 00:7, Sep 00:10, Feb 02:10, Nov 03:5, Oct 04:11, Apr 05:13, Aug 05:13, Sep 05:9

Eye and Ocular Adnexa

(For diagnostic and treatment ophthalmological services, see **Medicine, Ophthalmology,** and 92002 et seq)

(Do not report code 69990 in addition to codes 65091-68850)

Eyeball

Removal of Eye

65091 Evisceration of ocular contents; without implant

65093   with implant

65101 Enucleation of eye; without implant

65103   with implant, muscles not attached to implant

65105   with implant, muscles attached to implant

(For conjunctivoplasty after enucleation, see 68320 et seq)

65110 Exenteration of orbit (does not include skin graft), removal of orbital contents; only

65112   with therapeutic removal of bone

65114   with muscle or myocutaneous flap

(For skin graft to orbit (split skin), see 15120, 15121; free, full thickness, see 15260, 15261)

(For eyelid repair involving more than skin, see 67930 et seq)

Secondary Implant(s) Procedures

An ocular implant is an implant inside muscular cone; an orbital implant is an implant outside muscular cone.

65125 Modification of ocular implant with placement or replacement of pegs (eg, drilling receptacle for prosthesis appendage) (separate procedure)

65130 Insertion of ocular implant secondary; after evisceration, in scleral shell

65135   after enucleation, muscles not attached to implant

65140   after enucleation, muscles attached to implant

65150 Reinsertion of ocular implant; with or without conjunctival graft

65155   with use of foreign material for reinforcement and/or attachment of muscles to implant

65175 Removal of ocular implant

(For orbital implant (implant outside muscle cone) insertion, use 67550; removal, use 67560)

Removal of Foreign Body

(For removal of implanted material: ocular implant, use 65175; anterior segment implant, use 65920; posterior segment implant, use 67120; orbital implant, use 67560)

(For diagnostic x-ray for foreign body, use 70030)

(For diagnostic echography for foreign body, use 76529)

(For removal of foreign body from orbit: frontal approach, use 67413; lateral approach, use 67430; transcranial approach, use 61334)

(For removal of foreign body from eyelid, embedded, use 67938)

(For removal of foreign body from lacrimal system, use 68530)

65205 Removal of foreign body, external eye; conjunctival superficial
> *CPT Assistant* Mar 05:17

65210   conjunctival embedded (includes concretions), subconjunctival, or scleral nonperforating

65220   corneal, without slit lamp

65222   corneal, with slit lamp

(For repair of corneal laceration with foreign body, use 65275)

65235 Removal of foreign body, intraocular; from anterior chamber of eye or lens
> *CPT Changes: An Insider's View* 2002

(For removal of implanted material from anterior segment, use 65920)

65260   from posterior segment, magnetic extraction, anterior or posterior route

65265   from posterior segment, nonmagnetic extraction

(For removal of implanted material from posterior segment, use 67120)

Repair of Laceration

(For fracture of orbit, see 21385 et seq)

(For repair of wound of eyelid, skin, linear, simple, see 12011-12018; intermediate, layered closure, see 12051-12057; linear, complex, see 13150-13160; other, see 67930, 67935)

(For repair of wound of lacrimal system, use 68700)

(For repair of operative wound, use 66250)

65270 Repair of laceration; conjunctiva, with or without nonperforating laceration sclera, direct closure

65272   conjunctiva, by mobilization and rearrangement, without hospitalization

65273   conjunctiva, by mobilization and rearrangement, with hospitalization

---

65275 cornea, nonperforating, with or without removal foreign body

65280 cornea and/or sclera, perforating, not involving uveal tissue

65285 cornea and/or sclera, perforating, with reposition or resection of uveal tissue

65286 application of tissue glue, wounds of cornea and/or sclera
➲ *CPT Assistant* May 99:11

(Repair of laceration includes use of conjunctival flap and restoration of anterior chamber, by air or saline injection when indicated)

(For repair of iris or ciliary body, use 66680)

65290 Repair of wound, extraocular muscle, tendon and/or Tenon's capsule

Anterior Segment

Cornea

Excision

65400 Excision of lesion, cornea (keratectomy, lamellar, partial), except pterygium

65410 Biopsy of cornea

65420 Excision or transposition of pterygium; without graft

65426 with graft

Removal or Destruction

65430 Scraping of cornea, diagnostic, for smear and/or culture

65435 Removal of corneal epithelium; with or without chemocauterization (abrasion, curettage)

65436 with application of chelating agent (eg, EDTA)

65450 Destruction of lesion of cornea by cryotherapy, photocoagulation or thermocauterization

---

Cryotherapy of Lesion on Cornea
65450

A freezing probe is applied directly to the corneal defect to destroy it.

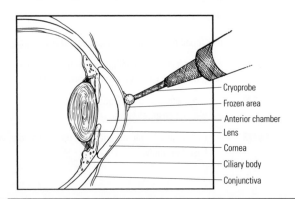

- Cryoprobe
- Frozen area
- Anterior chamber
- Lens
- Cornea
- Ciliary body
- Conjunctiva

65600 Multiple punctures of anterior cornea (eg, for corneal erosion, tattoo)

Keratoplasty

Corneal transplant includes use of fresh or preserved grafts, and preparation of donor material.

(Keratoplasty excludes refractive keratoplasty procedures, 65760, 65765, and 65767)

65710 Keratoplasty (corneal transplant); lamellar
➲ *CPT Assistant* Oct 02:8

65730 penetrating (except in aphakia)
➲ *CPT Assistant* Oct 02:8, Feb 06:1

65750 penetrating (in aphakia)
➲ *CPT Assistant* Oct 02:8

65755 penetrating (in pseudophakia)
➲ *CPT Assistant* Winter 90:8, Oct 02:9

Other Procedures

65760 Keratomileusis
➲ *CPT Assistant* Oct 02:9

65765 Keratophakia
➲ *CPT Assistant* Oct 02:10

65767 Epikeratoplasty
➲ *CPT Assistant* Winter 90:8, Oct 02:10

65770 Keratoprosthesis
➲ *CPT Assistant* Oct 02:10

65771 Radial keratotomy
➲ *CPT Assistant* Winter 90:8, Oct 02:10

65772 Corneal relaxing incision for correction of surgically induced astigmatism
➲ *CPT Assistant* Oct 02:10, 12

65775 Corneal wedge resection for correction of surgically induced astigmatism
➲ *CPT Assistant* Oct 02:10, 12

(For fitting of contact lens for treatment of disease, use 92070)

(For unlisted procedures on cornea, use 66999)

65780 Ocular surface reconstruction; amniotic membrane transplantation
➲ *CPT Assistant* May 04:10; *CPT Changes: An Insider's View* 2004

65781 limbal stem cell allograft (eg, cadaveric or living donor)
➲ *CPT Assistant* May 04:10; *CPT Changes: An Insider's View* 2004

65782 limbal conjunctival autograft (includes obtaining graft)
➲ *CPT Assistant* Feb 04:11, May 04:10, Feb 05:15-16; *CPT Changes: An Insider's View* 2004

(For harvesting conjunctival allograft, living donor, use 68371)

Anterior Chamber

Incision

65800 Paracentesis of anterior chamber of eye (separate procedure); with diagnostic aspiration of aqueous

65805 with therapeutic release of aqueous

65810 with removal of vitreous and/or discission of anterior hyaloid membrane, with or without air injection

65815 with removal of blood, with or without irrigation and/or air injection

(For injection, see 66020-66030)

(For removal of blood clot, use 65930)

65820 Goniotomy
➔ *CPT Assistant* Sep 05:12

(Do not report modifier 63 in conjunction with 65820)

(For use of ophthalmic endoscope with 65820, use 66990)

65850 Trabeculotomy ab externo

65855 Trabeculoplasty by laser surgery, one or more sessions (defined treatment series)
➔ *CPT Assistant* Mar 98:7, Mar 03:23

(If re-treatment is necessary after several months because of disease progression, a new treatment or treatment series should be reported with a modifier, if necessary, to indicate lesser or greater complexity)

(For trabeculectomy, use 66170)

65860 Severing adhesions of anterior segment, laser technique (separate procedure)

65865 Severing adhesions of anterior segment of eye, incisional technique (with or without injection of air or liquid) (separate procedure); goniosynechiae

(For trabeculoplasty by laser surgery, use 65855)

65870 anterior synechiae, except goniosynechiae

65875 posterior synechiae
➔ *CPT Assistant* Sep 05:12

(For use of ophthalmic endoscope with 65875, use 66990)

65880 corneovitreal adhesions

(For laser surgery, use 66821)

►Removal◄

65900 Removal of epithelial downgrowth, anterior chamber of eye
➔ *CPT Changes: An Insider's View* 2002

65920 Removal of implanted material, anterior segment of eye
➔ *CPT Assistant* Sep 05:12; *CPT Changes: An Insider's View* 2002

(For use of ophthalmic endoscope with 65920, use 66990)

65930 Removal of blood clot, anterior segment of eye
➔ *CPT Changes: An Insider's View* 2002

►Introduction◄

66020 Injection, anterior chamber of eye (separate procedure); air or liquid
➔ *CPT Changes: An Insider's View* 2002

66030 medication

(For unlisted procedures on anterior segment, use 66999)

Anterior Sclera

Excision

(For removal of intraocular foreign body, use 65235)

(For operations on posterior sclera, use 67250, 67255)

66130 Excision of lesion, sclera

66150 Fistulization of sclera for glaucoma; trephination with iridectomy

66155 thermocauterization with iridectomy

66160 sclerectomy with punch or scissors, with iridectomy

66165 iridencleisis or iridotasis

66170 trabeculectomy ab externo in absence of previous surgery
➔ *CPT Assistant* Jul 03:4, Nov 03:10

(For trabeculotomy ab externo, use 65850)

(For repair of operative wound, use 66250)

►(For dilation of Schlemm's Canal with or without retention of device, see 0176T, 0177T)◄

66172 trabeculectomy ab externo with scarring from previous ocular surgery or trauma (includes injection of antifibrotic agents)
➔ *CPT Assistant* Jul 03:4, Nov 03:10

(For transciliary body sclera fistulization, use Category III code 0123T)

Aqueous Shunt

66180 Aqueous shunt to extraocular reservoir (eg, Molteno, Schocket, Denver-Krupin)
➔ *CPT Assistant* Winter 90:8, Aug 03:9, Sep 03:2

66185 Revision of aqueous shunt to extraocular reservoir
➔ *CPT Assistant* Winter 90:8

(For removal of implanted shunt, use 67120)

Repair or Revision

(For scleral procedures in retinal surgery, see 67101 et seq)

66220   Repair of scleral staphyloma; without graft

66225   with graft

(For scleral reinforcement, see 67250, 67255)

66250   Revision or repair of operative wound of anterior segment, any type, early or late, major or minor procedure

(For unlisted procedures on anterior sclera, use 66999)

Iris, Ciliary Body

Incision

66500   Iridotomy by stab incision (separate procedure); except transfixion

66505   with transfixion as for iris bombe

(For iridotomy by photocoagulation, use 66761)

Excision

66600   Iridectomy, with corneoscleral or corneal section; for removal of lesion

66605   with cyclectomy

66625   peripheral for glaucoma (separate procedure)

66630   sector for glaucoma (separate procedure)

66635   optical (separate procedure)

(For coreoplasty by photocoagulation, use 66762)

Repair

66680   Repair of iris, ciliary body (as for iridodialysis)

(For reposition or resection of uveal tissue with perforating wound of cornea or sclera, use 65285)

66682   Suture of iris, ciliary body (separate procedure) with retrieval of suture through small incision (eg, McCannel suture)

Destruction

66700   Ciliary body destruction; diathermy

66710   cyclophotocoagulation, transscleral
  - ➥ *CPT Assistant* Mar 05:20, Sep 05:5; *CPT Changes: An Insider's View* 2005

66711   cyclophotocoagulation, endoscopic
  - ➥ *CPT Assistant* Mar 05:20, Sep 05:5, 12; *CPT Changes: An Insider's View* 2005

(Do not report 66711 in conjunction with 66990)

⊙ **66720**   cryotherapy

66740   cyclodialysis

66761   Iridotomy/iridectomy by laser surgery (eg, for glaucoma) (one or more sessions)
  - ➥ *CPT Assistant* Mar 98:7

66762   Iridoplasty by photocoagulation (one or more sessions) (eg, for improvement of vision, for widening of anterior chamber angle)
  - ➥ *CPT Assistant* Mar 98:7

66770   Destruction of cyst or lesion iris or ciliary body (nonexcisional procedure)

(For excision lesion iris, ciliary body, see 66600, 66605; for removal of epithelial downgrowth, use 65900)

(For unlisted procedures on iris, ciliary body, use 66999)

Lens

Incision

66820   Discission of secondary membranous cataract (opacified posterior lens capsule and/or anterior hyaloid); stab incision technique (Ziegler or Wheeler knife)

66821   laser surgery (eg, YAG laser) (one or more stages)

66825   Repositioning of intraocular lens prosthesis, requiring an incision (separate procedure)

►Removal◄

Lateral canthotomy, iridectomy, iridotomy, anterior capsulotomy, posterior capsulotomy, the use of viscoelastic agents, enzymatic zonulysis, use of other pharmacologic agents, and subconjunctival or sub-tenon injections are included as part of the code for the extraction of lens.

66830   Removal of secondary membranous cataract (opacified posterior lens capsule and/or anterior hyaloid) with corneo-scleral section, with or without iridectomy (iridocapsulotomy, iridocapsulectomy)

66840   Removal of lens material; aspiration technique, one or more stages
  - ➥ *CPT Assistant* Fall 92:4

66850   phacofragmentation technique (mechanical or ultrasonic) (eg, phacoemulsification), with aspiration
  - ➥ *CPT Assistant* Fall 92:6

66852   pars plana approach, with or without vitrectomy
  - ➥ *CPT Assistant* Fall 92:8

66920   intracapsular
  - ➥ *CPT Assistant* Fall 92:8

66930   intracapsular, for dislocated lens
  - ➥ *CPT Assistant* Fall 92:8

66940 extracapsular (other than 66840, 66850, 66852)
> *CPT Assistant* Fall 92:4

(For removal of intralenticular foreign body without lens extraction, use 65235)

(For repair of operative wound, use 66250)

▶Intraocular Lens Procedures◀

66982 Extracapsular cataract removal with insertion of intraocular lens prosthesis (one stage procedure), manual or mechanical technique (eg, irrigation and aspiration or phacoemulsification), complex, requiring devices or techniques not generally used in routine cataract surgery (eg, iris expansion device, suture support for intraocular lens, or primary posterior capsulorrhexis) or performed on patients in the amblyogenic developmental stage
> *CPT Assistant* Feb 01:7, Nov 03:10; *CPT Changes: An Insider's View* 2001, 2002

66983 Intracapsular cataract extraction with insertion of intraocular lens prosthesis (one stage procedure)
> *CPT Assistant* Fall 92:5, 8, Nov 03:10

66984 Extracapsular cataract removal with insertion of intraocular lens prosthesis (one stage procedure), manual or mechanical technique (eg, irrigation and aspiration or phacoemulsification)
> *CPT Assistant* Fall 92:5, 8, Feb 01:7, Nov 03:10, Mar 05:11

(For complex extracapsular cataract removal, use 66982)

66985 Insertion of intraocular lens prosthesis (secondary implant), not associated with concurrent cataract removal
> *CPT Assistant* Sep 05:12

(To code implant at time of concurrent cataract surgery, see 66982, 66983, 66984)

(For intraocular lens prosthesis supplied by physician, use 99070)

(For ultrasonic determination of intraocular lens power, use 76519)

(For removal of implanted material from anterior segment, use 65920)

(For secondary fixation (separate procedure), use 66682)

(For use of ophthalmic endoscope with 66985, use 66990)

66986 Exchange of intraocular lens
> *CPT Assistant* Sep 05:12

(For use of ophthalmic endoscope with 66986, use 66990)

▶Other Procedures◀

+ 66990 Use of ophthalmic endoscope (List separately in addition to code for primary procedure)
> *CPT Assistant* Sep 05:12; *CPT Changes: An Insider's View* 2003

▶(66990 may be used only with codes 65820, 65875, 65920, 66985, 66986, 67036, 67039, 67040, 67041, 67042, 67043, 67112)◀

66999 Unlisted procedure, anterior segment of eye

Posterior Segment

Vitreous

67005 Removal of vitreous, anterior approach (open sky technique or limbal incision); partial removal
> *CPT Assistant* Fall 92:4

67010 subtotal removal with mechanical vitrectomy
> *CPT Assistant* Fall 92:4

(For removal of vitreous by paracentesis of anterior chamber, use 65810)

(For removal of corneovitreal adhesions, use 65880)

67015 Aspiration or release of vitreous, subretinal or choroidal fluid, pars plana approach (posterior sclerotomy)

67025 Injection of vitreous substitute, pars plana or limbal approach (fluid-gas exchange), with or without aspiration (separate procedure)

67027 Implantation of intravitreal drug delivery system (eg, ganciclovir implant), includes concomitant removal of vitreous
> *CPT Assistant* Nov 97:23, Nov 98:1

Intravitreal Drug Delivery System
67027

A drug delivery system that releases medication into the vitreous is implanted into the vitreous by pars plana incision.

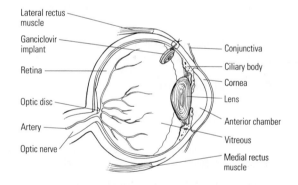

(For removal, use 67121)

67028 Intravitreal injection of a pharmacologic agent (separate procedure)
> *CPT Assistant* Winter 90:9

67030 Discission of vitreous strands (without removal), pars plana approach

67031 Severing of vitreous strands, vitreous face adhesions, sheets, membranes or opacities, laser surgery (one or more stages)

67036 Vitrectomy, mechanical, pars plana approach;

➔ *CPT Assistant* Fall 92:6

▶(67038 has been deleted. To report, see 67041, 67042, 67043)◀

67039 with focal endolaser photocoagulation

➔ *CPT Assistant* Winter 90:9, Sep 05:12

67040 with endolaser panretinal photocoagulation

➔ *CPT Assistant* Winter 90:9, Sep 05:12

●**67041** with removal of preretinal cellular membrane (eg, macular pucker)

➔ *CPT Changes: An Insider's View* 2008

●**67042** with removal of internal limiting membrane of retina (eg, for repair of macular hole, diabetic macular edema), includes, if performed, intraocular tamponade (ie, air, gas or silicone oil)

➔ *CPT Changes: An Insider's View* 2008

●**67043** with removal of subretinal membrane (eg, choroidal neovascularization), includes, if performed, intraocular tamponade (ie, air, gas or silicone oil) and laser photocoagulation

➔ *CPT Changes: An Insider's View* 2008

▶(For use of ophthalmic endoscope with 67036, 67039, 67040-67043, use 66990)◀

(For associated lensectomy, use 66850)

▶(For use of vitrectomy in retinal detachment surgery, see 67108, 67113)◀

(For associated removal of foreign body, see 65260, 65265)

(For unlisted procedures on vitreous, use 67299)

Retina or Choroid

Repair

(If diathermy, cryotherapy and/or photocoagulation are combined, report under principal modality used)

67101 Repair of retinal detachment, one or more sessions; cryotherapy or diathermy, with or without drainage of subretinal fluid

➔ *CPT Assistant* Mar 98:7

67105 photocoagulation, with or without drainage of subretinal fluid

➔ *CPT Assistant* Mar 98:7

67107 Repair of retinal detachment; scleral buckling (such as lamellar scleral dissection, imbrication or encircling procedure), with or without implant, with or without cryotherapy, photocoagulation, and drainage of subretinal fluid

Repair of Retinal Detachment
67107

The retinal tear is treated externally by placing a hot or cold probe over the sclera and then depressing it. The burn seals the choroid to the retina at the site of the tear. The healing scar is supported by the encircling band, which buckles the eye.

Clove hitch suture securing ends of buckle

Silicone sponge

Encircling silicone exoplant

67108 with vitrectomy, any method, with or without air or gas tamponade, focal endolaser photocoagulation, cryotherapy, drainage of subretinal fluid, scleral buckling, and/or removal of lens by same technique

➔ *CPT Assistant* Winter 90:9

67110 by injection of air or other gas (eg, pneumatic retinopexy)

➔ *CPT Assistant* Winter 90:9

67112 by scleral buckling or vitrectomy, on patient having previous ipsilateral retinal detachment repair(s) using scleral buckling or vitrectomy techniques

(For aspiration or drainage of subretinal or subchoroidal fluid, use 67015)

(For use of ophthalmic endoscope with 67112, use 66990)

●**67113** Repair of complex retinal detachment (eg, proliferative vitreoretinopathy, stage C-1 or greater, diabetic traction retinal detachment, retinopathy of prematurity, retinal tear of greater than 90 degrees), with vitrectomy and membrane peeling, may include air, gas, or silicone oil tamponade, cryotherapy, endolaser photocoagulation, drainage of subretinal fluid, scleral buckling, and/or removal of lens

➔ *CPT Changes: An Insider's View* 2008

▶(To report vitrectomy, pars plana approach, other than in retinal detachment surgery, see 67036-67043)◀

67115 Release of encircling material (posterior segment)

67120 Removal of implanted material, posterior segment; extraocular

67121 intraocular

➔ *CPT Assistant* Nov 97:23, Nov 98:19

(For removal from anterior segment, use 65920)

(For removal of foreign body, see 65260, 65265)

Prophylaxis

▶Codes 67141, 67145, 67208-67220, 67227, 67228, 67229 include treatment at one or more sessions that may occur at different encounters. These codes should be reported once during a defined treatment period.◀

Repetitive services. The services listed below are often performed in multiple sessions or groups of sessions. The methods of reporting vary.

The following descriptors are intended to include all sessions in a defined treatment period.

67141 Prophylaxis of retinal detachment (eg, retinal break, lattice degeneration) without drainage, one or more sessions; cryotherapy, diathermy

➔ *CPT Assistant* Mar 98:7

67145 photocoagulation (laser or xenon arc)

➔ *CPT Assistant* Fall 92:4, Mar 98:7

Destruction

67208 Destruction of localized lesion of retina (eg, macular edema, tumors), one or more sessions; cryotherapy, diathermy

➔ *CPT Assistant* Mar 98:7, Nov 98:19

67210 photocoagulation

➔ *CPT Assistant* Mar 98:7, Nov 98:19

67218 radiation by implantation of source (includes removal of source)

➔ *CPT Assistant* Mar 98:7

67220 Destruction of localized lesion of choroid (eg, choroidal neovascularization); photocoagulation (eg, laser), one or more sessions

➔ *CPT Assistant* Nov 98:19, Nov 99:39, Feb 01:8; *CPT Changes: An Insider's View* 2000, 2001

(For destruction of macular drusen, photocoagulation, use Category III code 0017T)

(For destruction of localized lesion of choroid by transpupillary thermotherapy, use Category III code 0016T)

67221 photodynamic therapy (includes intravenous infusion)

➔ *CPT Assistant* Feb 01:8, Sep 01:10, Jun 02:10; *CPT Changes: An Insider's View* 2001

+ 67225 photodynamic therapy, second eye, at single session (List separately in addition to code for primary eye treatment)

➔ *CPT Assistant* Jun 02:10; *CPT Changes: An Insider's View* 2002

(Use 67225 in conjunction with 67221)

▲ **67227** Destruction of extensive or progressive retinopathy (eg, diabetic retinopathy), one or more sessions, cryotherapy, diathermy

➔ *CPT Assistant* Mar 98:7; *CPT Changes: An Insider's View* 2008

▲ **67228** Treatment of extensive or progressive retinopathy, one or more sessions; (eg, diabetic retinopathy), photocoagulation

➔ *CPT Assistant* Mar 98:7; *CPT Changes: An Insider's View* 2008

● **67229** preterm infant (less than 37 weeks gestation at birth), performed from birth up to 1 year of age (eg, retinopathy of prematurity), photocoagulation or cryotherapy

➔ *CPT Changes: An Insider's View* 2008

▶(For bilateral procedure, use modifier 50)◀

(For unlisted procedures on retina, use 67299)

Posterior Sclera

Repair

(For excision lesion sclera, use 66130)

67250 Scleral reinforcement (separate procedure); without graft

67255 with graft

(For repair scleral staphyloma, see 66220, 66225)

Other Procedures

67299 Unlisted procedure, posterior segment

Ocular Adnexa

Extraocular Muscles of Right Eye

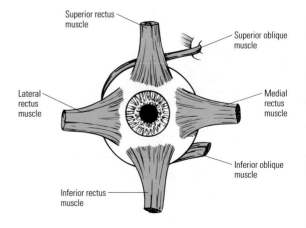

Superior rectus muscle

Superior oblique muscle

Lateral rectus muscle

Medial rectus muscle

Inferior oblique muscle

Inferior rectus muscle

Extraocular Muscles

67311   Strabismus surgery, recession or resection procedure; one horizontal muscle

➔ *CPT Assistant* Summer 93:20, Mar 97:5, Nov 98:19, Sep 02:10

Strabismus Surgery—Horizontal Muscles
67311-67312

In Figure A, the medial or lateral rectus muscle is made weaker by recession (retroplacement of the muscle attachment). In Figure B, it is made stronger by resection (removal of a segment). Use 67311 for one horizontal muscle and 67312 for two muscles of the same eye.

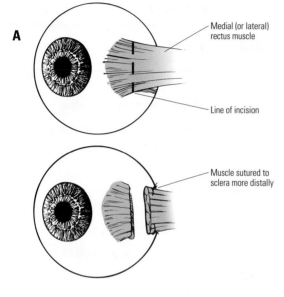

A

Medial (or lateral) rectus muscle

Line of incision

Muscle sutured to sclera more distally

B

Medial (or lateral) rectus muscle

Section of muscle to be removed to re-align eye

Muscle reattached

67312   two horizontal muscles

➔ *CPT Assistant* Summer 93:20, Mar 97:5

67314   one vertical muscle (excluding superior oblique)

➔ *CPT Assistant* Summer 93:20, Mar 97:5

67316   two or more vertical muscles (excluding superior oblique)

➔ *CPT Assistant* Summer 93:20, Mar 97:5

(For adjustable sutures, use 67335 in addition to codes 67311-67334 for primary procedure reflecting number of muscles operated on)

Strabismus Surgery—Vertical Muscles
67314-67316

Either the superior or inferior rectus muscle is strengthened or weakened. Use 67316 for two muscles of the same eye.

Inferior (or superior) rectus muscle

67318   Strabismus surgery, any procedure, superior oblique muscle

➔ *CPT Assistant* Summer 93:20, Mar 97:5, Nov 98:19

✛ 67320   Transposition procedure (eg, for paretic extraocular muscle), any extraocular muscle (specify) (List separately in addition to code for primary procedure)

➔ *CPT Assistant* Summer 93:20, Mar 97:5

(Use 67320 in conjunction with 67311-67318)

Transposition Procedure
67320

The extraocular muscles are transposed.

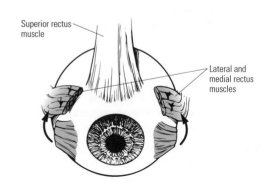

Superior rectus muscle

Lateral and medial rectus muscles

+ 67331   Strabismus surgery on patient with previous eye surgery or injury that did not involve the extraocular muscles (List separately in addition to code for primary procedure)

➔ *CPT Assistant* Summer 93:20, Mar 97:5

(Use 67331 in conjunction with 67311-67318)

+ 67332   Strabismus surgery on patient with scarring of extraocular muscles (eg, prior ocular injury, strabismus or retinal detachment surgery) or restrictive myopathy (eg, dysthyroid ophthalmopathy) (List separately in addition to code for primary procedure)

➔ *CPT Assistant* Summer 93:20, Mar 97:5

(Use 67332 in conjunction with 67311-67318)

+ 67334   Strabismus surgery by posterior fixation suture technique, with or without muscle recession (List separately in addition to code for primary procedure)

➔ *CPT Assistant* Summer 93:20, Mar 97:5

(Use 67334 in conjunction with 67311-67318)

+ 67335   Placement of adjustable suture(s) during strabismus surgery, including postoperative adjustment(s) of suture(s) (List separately in addition to code for specific strabismus surgery)

➔ *CPT Assistant* Summer 93:20, Mar 97:5

(Use 67335 in conjunction with 67311-67334)

Strabismus Surgery—Adjustable Sutures
67335

Sutures are tied in such a way as to allow the tension on the muscle to be adjusted after the anesthetic is not affecting the position of the globe.

Superior rectus muscle

Adjustable suture

+ 67340   Strabismus surgery involving exploration and/or repair of detached extraocular muscle(s) (List separately in addition to code for primary procedure)

➔ *CPT Assistant* Summer 93:20, Mar 97:5

(Use 67340 in conjunction with 67311-67334)

67343   Release of extensive scar tissue without detaching extraocular muscle (separate procedure)

➔ *CPT Assistant* Summer 93:20, Mar 97:5

(Use 67343 in conjunction with 67311-67340, when such procedures are performed other than on the affected muscle)

67345   Chemodenervation of extraocular muscle

➔ *CPT Assistant* Summer 93:20, Mar 97:5, Apr 00:2

(For chemodenervation for blepharospasm and other neurological disorders, see 64612 and 64613)

67346   Biopsy of extraocular muscle

➔ *CPT Changes: An Insider's View* 2007

(For repair of wound, extraocular muscle, tendon or Tenon's capsule, use 65290)

Other Procedures

(67350 has been deleted. To report, use 67346)

67399   Unlisted procedure, ocular muscle

Orbit

Exploration, Excision, Decompression

67400   Orbitotomy without bone flap (frontal or transconjunctival approach); for exploration, with or without biopsy

67405   with drainage only

67412   with removal of lesion

67413   with removal of foreign body

67414   with removal of bone for decompression

➔ *CPT Assistant* Jul 99:10

67415   Fine needle aspiration of orbital contents

(For exenteration, enucleation, and repair, see 65101 et seq; for optic nerve decompression, use 67570)

67420   Orbitotomy with bone flap or window, lateral approach (eg, Kroenlein); with removal of lesion

67430   with removal of foreign body

67440   with drainage

67445   with removal of bone for decompression

(For optic nerve sheath decompression, use 67570)

67450   for exploration, with or without biopsy

(For orbitotomy, transcranial approach, see 61330-61334)

(For orbital implant, see 67550, 67560)

(For removal of eyeball or for repair after removal, see 65091-65175)

Other Procedures

67500 Retrobulbar injection; medication (separate procedure, does not include supply of medication)

67505 alcohol

67515 Injection of medication or other substance into Tenon's capsule

➔ *CPT Changes: An Insider's View* 2002

(For subconjunctival injection, use 68200)

67550 Orbital implant (implant outside muscle cone); insertion

67560 removal or revision

(For ocular implant (implant inside muscle cone), see 65093-65105, 65130-65175)

(For treatment of fractures of malar area, orbit, see 21355 et seq)

67570 Optic nerve decompression (eg, incision or fenestration of optic nerve sheath)

67599 Unlisted procedure, orbit

Eyelids

Incision

67700 Blepharotomy, drainage of abscess, eyelid

67710 Severing of tarsorrhaphy

67715 Canthotomy (separate procedure)

(For canthoplasty, use 67950)

(For division of symblepharon, use 68340)

Excision, Destruction

Codes for removal of lesion include more than skin (ie, involving lid margin, tarsus, and/or palpebral conjunctiva).

(For removal of lesion, involving mainly skin of eyelid, see 11310-11313; 11440-11446, 11640-11646; 17000-17004)

(For repair of wounds, blepharoplasty, grafts, reconstructive surgery, see 67930-67975)

67800 Excision of chalazion; single

➔ *CPT Assistant* Sep 99:10

67801 multiple, same lid

67805 multiple, different lids

➔ *CPT Assistant* Sep 99:10

67808 under general anesthesia and/or requiring hospitalization, single or multiple

67810 Biopsy of eyelid

➔ *CPT Assistant* Dec 04:19

67820 Correction of trichiasis; epilation, by forceps only

➔ *CPT Assistant* Jul 98:10

Trichiasis
67820-67825

When the eyelashes are ingrown or misdirected (trichiasis), the physician uses a biomicroscope and forceps to remove the offending eyelashes. Report 67825 when cryosurgery or electrosurgery is used to destroy the follicles.

Forceps

Ingrown or misdirected eyelashes

67825 epilation by other than forceps (eg, by electrosurgery, cryotherapy, laser surgery)

➔ *CPT Assistant* Jul 98:10

67830 incision of lid margin

67835 incision of lid margin, with free mucous membrane graft

67840 Excision of lesion of eyelid (except chalazion) without closure or with simple direct closure

(For excision and repair of eyelid by reconstructive surgery, see 67961, 67966)

67850 Destruction of lesion of lid margin (up to 1 cm)

(For Mohs micrographic surgery, see 17311-17315)

(For initiation or follow-up care of topical chemotherapy (eg, 5-FU or similar agents), see appropriate office visits)

Tarsorrhaphy

67875 Temporary closure of eyelids by suture (eg, Frost suture)

➔ *CPT Assistant* Winter 90:9

67880 Construction of intermarginal adhesions, median tarsorrhaphy, or canthorrhaphy;

67882 with transposition of tarsal plate

(For severing of tarsorrhaphy, use 67710)

(For canthoplasty, reconstruction canthus, use 67950)

(For canthotomy, use 67715)

Repair (Brow Ptosis, Blepharoptosis, Lid Retraction, Ectropion, Entropion)

67900   Repair of brow ptosis (supraciliary, mid-forehead or coronal approach)

(For forehead rhytidectomy, use 15824)

67901   Repair of blepharoptosis; frontalis muscle technique with suture or other material (eg, banked fascia)

➔ *CPT Assistant* Sep 00:7, Oct 06:11; *CPT Changes: An Insider's View* 2006

67902   frontalis muscle technique with autologous fascial sling (includes obtaining fascia)

➔ *CPT Assistant* Sep 00:7, Oct 06:11; *CPT Changes: An Insider's View* 2006

67903   (tarso) levator resection or advancement, internal approach

➔ *CPT Assistant* Sep 00:7, Oct 06:11

67904   (tarso) levator resection or advancement, external approach

➔ *CPT Assistant* Sep 00:7, Oct 06:11

67906   superior rectus technique with fascial sling (includes obtaining fascia)

➔ *CPT Assistant* Sep 00:7, Oct 06:11

67908   conjunctivo-tarso-Muller's muscle-levator resection (eg, Fasanella-Servat type)

➔ *CPT Assistant* Sep 00:7, Oct 06:11

67909   Reduction of overcorrection of ptosis

67911   Correction of lid retraction

(For obtaining autogenous graft materials, see 20920, 20922 or 20926)

(For correction of trichiasis by mucous membrane graft, use 67835)

67912   Correction of lagophthalmos, with implantation of upper eyelid lid load (eg, gold weight)

➔ *CPT Assistant* May 04:12, Aug 04:10, Oct 06:11; *CPT Changes: An Insider's View* 2004

67914   Repair of ectropion; suture

67915   thermocauterization

67916   excision tarsal wedge

➔ *CPT Assistant* Feb 04:11, May 04:12, Feb 05:16, Oct 06:11; *CPT Changes: An Insider's View* 2004

67917   extensive (eg, tarsal strip operations)

➔ *CPT Assistant* Feb 04:11, May 04:12, Oct 06:11; *CPT Changes: An Insider's View* 2004

(For correction of everted punctum, use 68705)

67921   Repair of entropion; suture

67922   thermocauterization

67923   excision tarsal wedge

➔ *CPT Assistant* May 04:12, Oct 06:11; *CPT Changes: An Insider's View* 2004

67924   extensive (eg, tarsal strip or capsulopalpebral fascia repairs operation)

➔ *CPT Assistant* May 04:12, Oct 06:11; *CPT Changes: An Insider's View* 2004

(For repair of cicatricial ectropion or entropion requiring scar excision or skin graft, see also 67961 et seq)

Reconstruction

Codes for blepharoplasty involve more than skin (ie, involving lid margin, tarsus, and/or palpebral conjunctiva).

67930   Suture of recent wound, eyelid, involving lid margin, tarsus, and/or palpebral conjunctiva direct closure; partial thickness

67935   full thickness

67938   Removal of embedded foreign body, eyelid

(For repair of skin of eyelid, see 12011-12018; 12051-12057; 13150-13153)

(For tarsorrhaphy, canthorrhaphy, see 67880, 67882)

(For repair of blepharoptosis and lid retraction, see 67901-67911)

(For blepharoplasty for entropion, ectropion, see 67916, 67917, 67923, 67924)

(For correction of blepharochalasis (blepharorhytidectomy), see 15820-15823)

(For repair of skin of eyelid, adjacent tissue transfer, see 14060, 14061; preparation for graft, use 15004; free graft, see 15120, 15121, 15260, 15261)

(For excision of lesion of eyelid, use 67800 et seq)

(For repair of lacrimal canaliculi, use 68700)

67950   Canthoplasty (reconstruction of canthus)

67961   Excision and repair of eyelid, involving lid margin, tarsus, conjunctiva, canthus, or full thickness, may include preparation for skin graft or pedicle flap with adjacent tissue transfer or rearrangement; up to one-fourth of lid margin

67966   over one-fourth of lid margin

(For canthoplasty, use 67950)

(For free skin grafts, see 15120, 15121, 15260, 15261)

(For tubed pedicle flap preparation, use 15576; for delay, use 15630; for attachment, use 15650)

67971   Reconstruction of eyelid, full thickness by transfer of tarsoconjunctival flap from opposing eyelid; up to two-thirds of eyelid, one stage or first stage

67973   total eyelid, lower, one stage or first stage

67974   total eyelid, upper, one stage or first stage

67975   second stage

Other Procedures

67999 Unlisted procedure, eyelids

Conjunctiva

(For removal of foreign body, see 65205 et seq)

Incision and Drainage

68020 Incision of conjunctiva, drainage of cyst

68040 Expression of conjunctival follicles (eg, for trachoma)

Excision and/or Destruction

68100 Biopsy of conjunctiva

68110 Excision of lesion, conjunctiva; up to 1 cm

68115   over 1 cm

68130   with adjacent sclera

68135 Destruction of lesion, conjunctiva

Injection

(For injection into Tenon's capsule or retrobulbar injection, see 67500-67515)

68200 Subconjunctival injection
➔ *CPT Assistant* Aug 03:15

Conjunctivoplasty

(For wound repair, see 65270-65273)

68320 Conjunctivoplasty; with conjunctival graft or extensive rearrangement
➔ *CPT Assistant* Feb 04:11

68325   with buccal mucous membrane graft (includes obtaining graft)

68326 Conjunctivoplasty, reconstruction cul-de-sac; with conjunctival graft or extensive rearrangement

68328   with buccal mucous membrane graft (includes obtaining graft)

68330 Repair of symblepharon; conjunctivoplasty, without graft

68335   with free graft conjunctiva or buccal mucous membrane (includes obtaining graft)

68340   division of symblepharon, with or without insertion of conformer or contact lens

Other Procedures

68360 Conjunctival flap; bridge or partial (separate procedure)

68362   total (such as Gunderson thin flap or purse string flap)

(For conjunctival flap for perforating injury, see 65280, 65285)

(For repair of operative wound, use 66250)

(For removal of conjunctival foreign body, see 65205, 65210)

68371 Harvesting conjunctival allograft, living donor
➔ *CPT Assistant* May 04:10; *CPT Changes: An Insider's View* 2004

68399 Unlisted procedure, conjunctiva

Lacrimal System

Incision

68400 Incision, drainage of lacrimal gland

68420 Incision, drainage of lacrimal sac (dacryocystotomy or dacryocystostomy)

68440 Snip incision of lacrimal punctum

Excision

68500 Excision of lacrimal gland (dacryoadenectomy), except for tumor; total

68505   partial

68510 Biopsy of lacrimal gland

68520 Excision of lacrimal sac (dacryocystectomy)

68525 Biopsy of lacrimal sac

68530 Removal of foreign body or dacryolith, lacrimal passages

68540 Excision of lacrimal gland tumor; frontal approach

68550   involving osteotomy

Repair

68700 Plastic repair of canaliculi

68705 Correction of everted punctum, cautery

68720 Dacryocystorhinostomy (fistulization of lacrimal sac to nasal cavity)
➔ *CPT Assistant* Sep 01:10, Jul 03:15, Aug 03:14

68745 Conjunctivorhinostomy (fistulization of conjunctiva to nasal cavity); without tube

68750   with insertion of tube or stent

68760   Closure of the lacrimal punctum; by thermocauterization, ligation, or laser surgery

68761   by plug, each
              ➡ *CPT Assistant* Jun 96:10, Jan 07:28

Closure of Lacrimal Punctum by Plug
68761

The physician inserts a lacrimal duct implant into a lacrimal punctum.

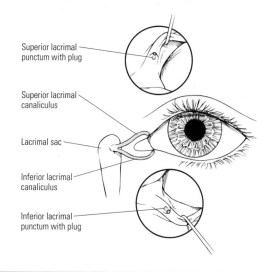

68770   Closure of lacrimal fistula (separate procedure)

Probing and/or Related Procedures

68801   Dilation of lacrimal punctum, with or without irrigation

            (To report a bilateral procedure, use 68801 with modifier 50)

68810   Probing of nasolacrimal duct, with or without irrigation;
            ➡ *CPT Assistant* Nov 02:11

            (For bilateral procedure, report 68810 with modifier 50)

68811   requiring general anesthesia
              ➡ *CPT Assistant* Nov 02:11

            (For bilateral procedure, report 68811 with modifier 50)

68815   with insertion of tube or stent
              ➡ *CPT Assistant* Nov 02:11

            (See also 92018)

            (For bilateral procedure, report 68815 with modifier 50)

● **68816**   with transluminal balloon catheter dilation
              ➡ *CPT Changes: An Insider's View* 2008

Probing of Nasolacrimal Duct
68816

A balloon catheter is in the nasolacrimal duct.

▶(Do not report 68816 in conjunction with 68810, 68811, 68815)◀

▶(For bilateral procedure, report 68816 with modifier 50)◀

68840   Probing of lacrimal canaliculi, with or without irrigation

68850   Injection of contrast medium for dacryocystography
            ➡ *CPT Assistant* Feb 01:9

            (For radiological supervision and interpretation, see 70170, 78660)

Other Procedures

68899   Unlisted procedure, lacrimal system

Notes

⊙=Moderate sedation ✚=Add-on code ✂=FDA approval pending ➜➜=See p xvii for details

Auditory System

(For diagnostic services (eg, audiometry, vestibular tests), see 92502 et seq)

External Ear

Incision

69000   Drainage external ear, abscess or hematoma; simple
➔ *CPT Assistant* Oct 97:11, Oct 99:10

69005   complicated

69020   Drainage external auditory canal, abscess
➔ *CPT Assistant* Oct 97:11

69090   Ear piercing

Excision

69100   Biopsy external ear

69105   Biopsy external auditory canal

69110   Excision external ear; partial, simple repair

69120   complete amputation

(For reconstruction of ear, see 15120 et seq)

69140   Excision exostosis(es), external auditory canal

69145   Excision soft tissue lesion, external auditory canal

69150   Radical excision external auditory canal lesion; without neck dissection

69155   with neck dissection

(For resection of temporal bone, use 69535)

(For skin grafting, see 15004-15261)

Removal

69200   Removal foreign body from external auditory canal; without general anesthesia

69205   with general anesthesia

69210   Removal impacted cerumen (separate procedure), one or both ears
➔ *CPT Assistant* Apr 03:9, Jul 05:14

69220   Debridement, mastoidectomy cavity, simple (eg, routine cleaning)

(For bilateral procedure, report 69220 with modifier 50)

69222   Debridement, mastoidectomy cavity, complex (eg, with anesthesia or more than routine cleaning)

(For bilateral procedure, report 69222 with modifier 50)

Repair

(For suture of wound or injury of external ear, see 12011-14300)

⊙ **69300**   Otoplasty, protruding ear, with or without size reduction

(For bilateral procedure, report 69300 with modifier 50)

69310   Reconstruction of external auditory canal (meatoplasty) (eg, for stenosis due to injury, infection) (separate procedure)
➔ *CPT Changes: An Insider's View* 2002

69320   Reconstruction external auditory canal for congenital atresia, single stage

(For combination with middle ear reconstruction, see 69631, 69641)

(For other reconstructive procedures with grafts (eg, skin, cartilage, bone), see 13150-15760, 21230-21235)

Other Procedures

(For otoscopy under general anesthesia, use 92502)

69399   Unlisted procedure, external ear

Middle Ear

Introduction

69400   Eustachian tube inflation, transnasal; with catheterization

69401   without catheterization

69405   Eustachian tube catheterization, transtympanic

(69410 has been deleted)

Incision

69420   Myringotomy including aspiration and/or eustachian tube inflation

69421   Myringotomy including aspiration and/or eustachian tube inflation requiring general anesthesia

69424   Ventilating tube removal requiring general anesthesia
➔ *CPT Assistant* Mar 05:17; *CPT Changes: An Insider's View* 2003

(For bilateral procedure, report 69424 with modifier 50)

(Do not report code 69424 in conjunction with 69205, 69210, 69420, 69421, 69433-69676, 69710-69745, 69801-69930)

69433   Tympanostomy (requiring insertion of ventilating tube), local or topical anesthesia

(For bilateral procedure, report 69433 with modifier 50)

Tympanostomy
69433-69436

A ventilating tube is inserted into the opening of the tympanum.

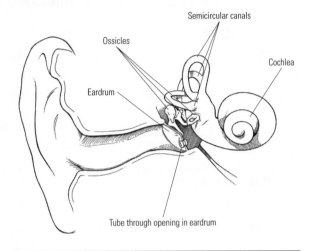

69436   Tympanostomy (requiring insertion of ventilating tube), general anesthesia

(For bilateral procedure, report 69436 with modifier 50)

69440   Middle ear exploration through postauricular or ear canal incision

(For atticotomy, see 69601 et seq)

69450   Tympanolysis, transcanal

Excision

69501   Transmastoid antrotomy (simple mastoidectomy)

69502   Mastoidectomy; complete

69505   modified radical

69511   radical

(For skin graft, see 15004 et seq)

(For mastoidectomy cavity debridement, see 69220, 69222)

69530   Petrous apicectomy including radical mastoidectomy

69535   Resection temporal bone, external approach

(For middle fossa approach, see 69950-69970)

69540   Excision aural polyp

69550   Excision aural glomus tumor; transcanal

69552   transmastoid

69554   extended (extratemporal)

Repair

69601   Revision mastoidectomy; resulting in complete mastoidectomy

69602   resulting in modified radical mastoidectomy

69603   resulting in radical mastoidectomy

69604   resulting in tympanoplasty

(For planned secondary tympanoplasty after mastoidectomy, see 69631, 69632)

69605   with apicectomy

(For skin graft, see 15120, 15121, 15260, 15261)

69610   Tympanic membrane repair, with or without site preparation of perforation for closure, with or without patch
➔ *CPT Assistant* Mar 01:10, Mar 03:21

69620   Myringoplasty (surgery confined to drumhead and donor area)
➔ *CPT Assistant* Mar 01:10

69631   Tympanoplasty without mastoidectomy (including canalplasty, atticotomy and/or middle ear surgery), initial or revision; without ossicular chain reconstruction
➔ *CPT Assistant* Jul 98:11, Mar 01:10, Mar 07:9

69632   with ossicular chain reconstruction (eg, postfenestration)

69633   with ossicular chain reconstruction and synthetic prosthesis (eg, partial ossicular replacement prosthesis (PORP), total ossicular replacement prosthesis (TORP))

69635   Tympanoplasty with antrotomy or mastoidotomy (including canalplasty, atticotomy, middle ear surgery, and/or tympanic membrane repair); without ossicular chain reconstruction

69636   with ossicular chain reconstruction

Tympanoplasty
69635-69646

A graft is used to repair the tympanic membrane perforation.

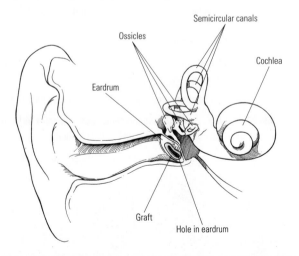

69637   with ossicular chain reconstruction and synthetic prosthesis (eg, partial ossicular replacement prosthesis (PORP), total ossicular replacement prosthesis (TORP))

69641   Tympanoplasty with mastoidectomy (including canalplasty, middle ear surgery, tympanic membrane repair); without ossicular chain reconstruction

69642   with ossicular chain reconstruction

69643   with intact or reconstructed wall, without ossicular chain reconstruction

69644   with intact or reconstructed canal wall, with ossicular chain reconstruction

69645   radical or complete, without ossicular chain reconstruction

69646   radical or complete, with ossicular chain reconstruction

69650   Stapes mobilization

69660   Stapedectomy or stapedotomy with reestablishment of ossicular continuity, with or without use of foreign material;

69661   with footplate drill out

69662   Revision of stapedectomy or stapedotomy

69666   Repair oval window fistula

69667   Repair round window fistula

69670   Mastoid obliteration (separate procedure)

69676   Tympanic neurectomy

(For bilateral procedure, report 69676 with modifier 50)

Other Procedures

69700   Closure postauricular fistula, mastoid (separate procedure)

69710   Implantation or replacement of electromagnetic bone conduction hearing device in temporal bone

(Replacement procedure includes removal of old device)

69711   Removal or repair of electromagnetic bone conduction hearing device in temporal bone

69714   Implantation, osseointegrated implant, temporal bone, with percutaneous attachment to external speech processor/cochlear stimulator; without mastoidectomy
➔ *CPT Changes: An Insider's View* 2001

69715   with mastoidectomy
➔ *CPT Changes: An Insider's View* 2001

69717   Replacement (including removal of existing device), osseointegrated implant, temporal bone, with percutaneous attachment to external speech processor/cochlear stimulator; without mastoidectomy
➔ *CPT Changes: An Insider's View* 2001

69718   with mastoidectomy
➔ *CPT Changes: An Insider's View* 2001

69720   Decompression facial nerve, intratemporal; lateral to geniculate ganglion

69725   including medial to geniculate ganglion

69740   Suture facial nerve, intratemporal, with or without graft or decompression; lateral to geniculate ganglion

69745   including medial to geniculate ganglion

(For extracranial suture of facial nerve, use 64864)

69799   Unlisted procedure, middle ear
➔ *CPT Assistant* Oct 99:10

Inner Ear

Incision and/or Destruction

69801   Labyrinthotomy, with or without cryosurgery including other nonexcisional destructive procedures or perfusion of vestibuloactive drugs (single or multiple perfusions); transcanal
➔ *CPT Assistant* Nov 96:12

(69801 includes all required infusions performed on initial and subsequent days of treatment)

69802   with mastoidectomy

69805   Endolymphatic sac operation; without shunt

69806   with shunt
➔ *CPT Assistant* Nov 96:12

69820   Fenestration semicircular canal

69840   Revision fenestration operation

Excision

69905   Labyrinthectomy; transcanal

69910   with mastoidectomy

69915   Vestibular nerve section, translabyrinthine approach

(For transcranial approach, use 69950)

Introduction

69930 Cochlear device implantation, with or without mastoidectomy

Cochlear Device Implantation
69930

An internal coil is attached to the temporal bone and the ground wire attached to the internal coil is connected to the temporalis muscle.

Other Procedures

69949 Unlisted procedure, inner ear

Temporal Bone, Middle Fossa Approach

(For external approach, use 69535)

69950 Vestibular nerve section, transcranial approach

69955 Total facial nerve decompression and/or repair (may include graft)

69960 Decompression internal auditory canal

69970 Removal of tumor, temporal bone

Other Procedures

69979 Unlisted procedure, temporal bone, middle fossa approach

Operating Microscope

The surgical microscope is employed when the surgical services are performed using the techniques of microsurgery. Code 69990 should be reported (without modifier 51 appended) in addition to the code for the primary procedure performed. Do not use 69990 for visualization with magnifying loupes or corrected vision. Do not report code 69990 in addition to procedures where use of the operating microscope is an inclusive component (15756-15758, 15842, 19364, 19368, 20955-20962, 20969-20973, 26551-26554, 26556, 31526, 31531, 31536, 31541, 31545, 31546, 31561, 31571, 43116, 43496, 49906, 61548, 63075-63078, 64727, 64820-64823, 65091-68850).

+ 69990 Microsurgical techniques, requiring use of operating microscope (List separately in addition to code for primary procedure)

➔ *CPT Assistant* Nov 98:20, Apr 99:11, Jun 99:11, Jul 99:11, Oct 99:10, Oct 00:3, Oct 02:8, Jan 04:28, Mar 05:11, Jul 05:14, Aug 05:1; *CPT Changes: An Insider's View* 2002

Operating Microscope
69990

A surgical operating microscope is used to obtain good visualization of the fine structures in the operating field. The lens system may be operated by hand or foot controls to adjust to working distance, with interchangeable oculars providing magnification as needed.

Radiology Guidelines (Including Nuclear Medicine and Diagnostic Ultrasound)

Items used by all physicians in reporting their services are presented in the **Introduction.** Some of the commonalities are repeated here for the convenience of those physicians referring to this section on **Radiology (Including Nuclear Medicine and Diagnostic Ultrasound).** Other definitions and items unique to Radiology are also listed.

Subject Listings

Subject listings apply when radiological services are performed by or under the responsible supervision of a physician.

Separate Procedures

Some of the procedures or services listed in the CPT codebook that are commonly carried out as an integral component of a total service or procedure have been identified by the inclusion of the term "separate procedure." The codes designated as "separate procedure" should not be reported in addition to the code for the total procedure or service of which it is considered an integral component.

However, when a procedure or service that is designated as a "separate procedure" is carried out independently or considered to be unrelated or distinct from other procedures/services provided at that time, it may be reported by itself, or in addition to other procedures/services by appending modifier 59 to the specific "separate procedure" code to indicate that the procedure is not considered to be a component of another procedure, but is a distinct, independent procedure. This may represent a different session or patient encounter, different procedure or surgery, different site or organ system, separate incision/excision, separate lesion, or separate injury (or area of injury in extensive injuries).

Subsection Information

Several of the subheadings or subsections have special needs or instructions unique to that section. Where these are indicated (eg, "Radiation Oncology") special **"Notes"** will be presented preceding those procedural terminology

listings, referring to that subsection specifically. If there is an "Unlisted Procedure" code number (see section below) for the individual subsection, it will be shown. Those subsections with **"Notes"** are as follows:

▶Functional MRI . . . . 70554-70555◀
Aorta and Arteries 75600-75790
Veins and Lymphatics 75801-75893
Transcatheter Procedures 75894-75989
Diagnostic Ultrasound 76506-76999
Abdomen and Retroperitoneum 76700-76776
Obstetrical 76801-76828
Non-Obstetrical 76830-76857
Radiation Oncology 77261-77799
Clinical Treatment Planning 77261-77299
Radiation Treatment Management 77427-77499
Proton Beam Treatment Delivery 77520-77525
Hyperthermia 77600-77620
Clinical Brachytherapy 77750-77799
Nuclear Medicine 78000-78299
Musculoskeletal System 78300-78399
Cardiovascular System 78414-78499
Therapeutic 79005-79999

Unlisted Service or Procedure

A service or procedure may be provided that is not listed in this edition of the CPT codebook. When reporting such a service, the appropriate "Unlisted Procedure" code may be used to indicate the service, identifying it by "Special Report" as discussed below. The "Unlisted Procedures" and accompanying codes for **Radiology (Including Nuclear Medicine and Diagnostic Ultrasound)** are as follows:

76496 Unlisted fluoroscopic procedure (eg, diagnostic, interventional)

76497 Unlisted computed tomography procedure (eg, diagnostic, interventional)

76498   Unlisted magnetic resonance procedure (eg, diagnostic, interventional)

76499   Unlisted diagnostic radiographic procedure

76999   Unlisted ultrasound procedure (eg, diagnostic, interventional)

77299   Unlisted procedure, therapeutic radiology clinical treatment planning

77399   Unlisted procedure, medical radiation physics, dosimetry and treatment devices, and special services

77499   Unlisted procedure, therapeutic radiology treatment management

77799   Unlisted procedure, clinical brachytherapy

78099   Unlisted endocrine procedure, diagnostic nuclear medicine

78199   Unlisted hematopoietic, reticuloendothelial and lymphatic procedure, diagnostic nuclear medicine

78299   Unlisted gastrointestinal procedure, diagnostic nuclear medicine

78399   Unlisted musculoskeletal procedure, diagnostic nuclear medicine

78499   Unlisted cardiovascular procedure, diagnostic nuclear medicine

78599   Unlisted respiratory procedure, diagnostic nuclear medicine

78699   Unlisted nervous system procedure, diagnostic nuclear medicine

78799   Unlisted genitourinary procedure, diagnostic nuclear medicine

78999   Unlisted miscellaneous procedure, diagnostic nuclear medicine

79999   Radiopharmaceutical therapy, unlisted procedure

Special Report

A service that is rarely provided, unusual, variable, or new may require a special report in determining medical appropriateness of the service. Pertinent information should include an adequate definition or description of the nature, extent, and need for the procedure; and the time, effort, and equipment necessary to provide the service. Additional items that may be included are:

- Complexity of symptoms
- Final diagnosis
- Pertinent physical findings
- Diagnostic and therapeutic procedures
- Concurrent problems
- Follow-up care

Supervision and Interpretation

When a procedure is performed by two physicians, the radiologic portion of the procedure is designated as "radiological supervision and interpretation." When a physician performs both the procedure and provides imaging supervision and interpretation, a combination of procedure codes outside the 70000 series and imaging supervision and interpretation codes are to be used.

(The Radiological Supervision and Interpretation codes are not applicable to the Radiation Oncology subsection.)

Administration of Contrast Material(s)

The phrase "with contrast" used in the codes for procedures performed using contrast for imaging enhancement represents contrast material administered intravascularly, intra-articularly or intrathecally.

For intra-articular injection, use the appropriate joint injection code. If radiographic arthrography is performed, also use the arthrography supervision and interpretation code for the appropriate joint (which includes fluoroscopy). If computed tomography (CT) or magnetic resonance (MR) arthrography are performed without radiographic arthrography, use the appropriate joint injection code, the appropriate CT or MR code ("with contrast" or "without followed by contrast"), and the appropriate imaging guidance code for needle placement for contrast injection.

For spine examinations using computed tomography, magnetic resonance imaging, magnetic resonance angiography, "with contrast" includes intrathecal or intravascular injection. For intrathecal injection, use also 61055 or 62284.

Injection of intravascular contrast material is part of the "with contrast" CT, computed tomographic angiography (CTA), magnetic resonance imaging (MRI), and magnetic resonance angiography (MRA) procedures.

Oral and/or rectal contrast administration alone does not qualify as a study "with contrast."

Written Report(s)

A written report, signed by the interpreting physician, should be considered an integral part of a radiologic procedure or interpretation.

Radiology

Diagnostic Radiology (Diagnostic Imaging)

Head and Neck

70010 Myelography, posterior fossa, radiological supervision and interpretation
➜ *CPT Assistant* Mar 05:11

70015 Cisternography, positive contrast, radiological supervision and interpretation

70030 Radiologic examination, eye, for detection of foreign body

70100 Radiologic examination, mandible; partial, less than four views

70110   complete, minimum of four views

70120 Radiologic examination, mastoids; less than three views per side

70130   complete, minimum of three views per side

70134 Radiologic examination, internal auditory meati, complete

70140 Radiologic examination, facial bones; less than three views

70150   complete, minimum of three views

70160 Radiologic examination, nasal bones, complete, minimum of three views

70170 Dacryocystography, nasolacrimal duct, radiological supervision and interpretation

70190 Radiologic examination; optic foramina

70200   orbits, complete, minimum of four views

70210 Radiologic examination, sinuses, paranasal, less than three views

70220 Radiologic examination, sinuses, paranasal, complete, minimum of three views

70240 Radiologic examination, sella turcica

70250 Radiologic examination, skull; less than four views
➜ *CPT Changes: An Insider's View* 2004

70260   complete, minimum of four views
➜ *CPT Changes: An Insider's View* 2004

70300 Radiologic examination, teeth; single view

70310   partial examination, less than full mouth

70320   complete, full mouth

70328 Radiologic examination, temporomandibular joint, open and closed mouth; unilateral

70330   bilateral

70332 Temporomandibular joint arthrography, radiological supervision and interpretation

(Do not report 70332 in conjunction with 77002)

70336 Magnetic resonance (eg, proton) imaging, temporomandibular joint(s)
➜ *CPT Assistant* Jul 99:11, Jul 01:7; *CPT Changes: An Insider's View* 2001

70350 Cephalogram, orthodontic

70355 Orthopantogram

70360 Radiologic examination; neck, soft tissue

70370   pharynx or larynx, including fluoroscopy and/or magnification technique

70371 Complex dynamic pharyngeal and speech evaluation by cine or video recording
➜ *CPT Assistant* Dec 04:17

70373 Laryngography, contrast, radiological supervision and interpretation

70380 Radiologic examination, salivary gland for calculus

70390 Sialography, radiological supervision and interpretation

70450 Computed tomography, head or brain; without contrast material
➜ *CPT Assistant* Apr 96:11; *CPT Changes: An Insider's View* 2003

70460   with contrast material(s)
➜ *CPT Assistant* Apr 96:11

70470   without contrast material, followed by contrast material(s) and further sections
➜ *CPT Assistant* Apr 96:11

(To report 3D rendering, see 76376, 76377)

70480 Computed tomography, orbit, sella, or posterior fossa or outer, middle, or inner ear; without contrast material
➜ *CPT Changes: An Insider's View* 2003

70481   with contrast material(s)

70482   without contrast material, followed by contrast material(s) and further sections

(To report 3D rendering, see 76376, 76377)

70486 Computed tomography, maxillofacial area; without contrast material
➜ *CPT Assistant* Mar 02:11; *CPT Changes: An Insider's View* 2003
➜ *Clinical Examples in Radiology* Winter 07:4-5, Spring 07:4

70487   with contrast material(s)

70488   without contrast material, followed by contrast material(s) and further sections

(To report 3D rendering, see 76376, 76377)

70490 Computed tomography, soft tissue neck; without contrast material

➔ *CPT Changes: An Insider's View* 2003

70491 with contrast material(s)

70492 without contrast material followed by contrast material(s) and further sections

(To report 3D rendering, see 76376, 76377)

(For cervical spine, see 72125, 72126)

▲ **70496** Computed tomographic angiography, head, with contrast material(s), including noncontrast images, if performed, and image postprocessing

➔ *CPT Assistant* Jul 01:4, Dec 05:7, Jan 07:31; *CPT Changes: An Insider's View* 2001, 2008

▲ **70498** Computed tomographic angiography, neck, with contrast material(s), including noncontrast images, if performed, and image postprocessing

➔ *CPT Assistant* Jul 01:4, Dec 05:7, Jan 07:31; *CPT Changes: An Insider's View* 2001, 2008

70540 Magnetic resonance (eg, proton) imaging, orbit, face, and/or neck; without contrast material(s)

➔ *CPT Assistant* Jul 01:6, Mar 07:7; *CPT Changes: An Insider's View* 2001, 2007

➔ *Clinical Examples in Radiology* Spring 05:3

(For head or neck magnetic resonance angiography studies, see 70544-70546, 70547-70549)

70542 with contrast material(s)

➔ *CPT Assistant* Jul 01:6; *CPT Changes: An Insider's View* 2001

➔ *Clinical Examples in Radiology* Spring 05:3

70543 without contrast material(s), followed by contrast material(s) and further sequences

➔ *CPT Assistant* Jul 01:6; *CPT Changes: An Insider's View* 2001

➔ *Clinical Examples in Radiology* Spring 05:2-3, Winter 07:7, 11

(Report 70540-70543 once per imaging session)

70544 Magnetic resonance angiography, head; without contrast material(s)

➔ *CPT Assistant* Sep 01:5, Dec 05:7, Jan 07:31; *CPT Changes: An Insider's View* 2001

70545 with contrast material(s)

➔ *CPT Assistant* Jul 01:5, Dec 05:7; *CPT Changes: An Insider's View* 2001

70546 without contrast material(s), followed by contrast material(s) and further sequences

➔ *CPT Assistant* Jul 01:5, Dec 05:7, Jan 07:31; *CPT Changes: An Insider's View* 2001

70547 Magnetic resonance angiography, neck; without contrast material(s)

➔ *CPT Assistant* Sep 01:5, Dec 05:7, Jan 07:31; *CPT Changes: An Insider's View* 2001

70548 with contrast material(s)

➔ *CPT Assistant* Sep 01:6, Dec 05:7, Jan 07:31; *CPT Changes: An Insider's View* 2001

70549 without contrast material(s), followed by contrast material(s) and further sequences

➔ *CPT Assistant* Sep 01:6, Dec 05:7, Jan 07:31; *CPT Changes: An Insider's View* 2001

70551 Magnetic resonance (eg, proton) imaging, brain (including brain stem); without contrast material

➔ *CPT Assistant* May 98:10, Mar 05:20, Feb 07:6

70552 with contrast material(s)

➔ *CPT Assistant* Jul 01:6, Mar 05:20, Feb 07:6

70553 without contrast material, followed by contrast material(s) and further sequences

➔ *CPT Assistant* Nov 97:24, Jul 01:6, Mar 05:20, Feb 07:6

➔ *Clinical Examples in Radiology* Spring 05:2, Spring 06:4-5

(For magnetic spectroscopy, use 76390)

Functional MRI involves identification and mapping of stimulation of brain function. When neurofunctional tests are administered by a technologist or other non-physician or non-psychologist, use 70554. When neurofunctional tests are entirely administered by a physician or psychologist, use 70555.

70554 Magnetic resonance imaging, brain, functional MRI; including test selection and administration of repetitive body part movement and/or visual stimulation, not requiring physician or psychologist administration

➔ *CPT Changes: An Insider's View* 2007

(Do not report 70554 in conjunction with 96020)

70555 requiring physician or psychologist administration of entire neurofunctional testing

➔ *CPT Changes: An Insider's View* 2007

(Do not report 70555 unless 96020 is performed)

(Do not report 70554, 70555 in conjunction with 70551-70553 unless a separate diagnostic MRI is performed)

70557 Magnetic resonance (eg, proton) imaging, brain (including brain stem and skull base), during open intracranial procedure (eg, to assess for residual tumor or residual vascular malformation); without contrast material

➔ *CPT Changes: An Insider's View* 2004

70558 with contrast material(s)

➔ *CPT Changes: An Insider's View* 2004

70559 without contrast material(s), followed by contrast material(s) and further sequences

➔ *CPT Changes: An Insider's View* 2004

(For stereotactic biopsy of intracranial lesion with magnetic resonance guidance, use 61751. 70557, 70558 or 70559 may be reported only if a separate report is generated. Report only one of the above codes once per operative session. Do not use these codes in conjunction with 61751, 77021, 77022)

Chest

(For fluoroscopic or ultrasonic guidance for needle placement procedures (eg, biopsy, aspiration, injection, localization device) of the thorax, see 76942, 77002)

71010   Radiologic examination, chest; single view, frontal

71015   stereo, frontal

71020   Radiologic examination, chest, two views, frontal and lateral;
> *CPT Assistant* Sep 03:3, Mar 05:11, Feb 07:10

71021   with apical lordotic procedure

71022   with oblique projections

71023   with fluoroscopy
> *CPT Assistant* Aug 03:14

71030   Radiologic examination, chest, complete, minimum of four views;

►(For concurrent computer-aided detection [CAD] performed in addition to codes 71010, 71020, 71021, 71022, and 71030, use 0174T. Do not report 71010, 71020, 71021, 71022, and 71030 in conjunction with 0175T for CAD performed remotely from the primary interpretation)◄

71034   with fluoroscopy
> *CPT Assistant* Aug 03:14

(For separate chest fluoroscopy, use 76000)

71035   Radiologic examination, chest, special views (eg, lateral decubitus, Bucky studies)

71040   Bronchography, unilateral, radiological supervision and interpretation

71060   Bronchography, bilateral, radiological supervision and interpretation

71090   Insertion pacemaker, fluoroscopy and radiography, radiological supervision and interpretation
> *CPT Assistant* Aug 02:11

(For procedure, see appropriate organ or site)

71100   Radiologic examination, ribs, unilateral; two views

71101   including posteroanterior chest, minimum of three views

71110   Radiologic examination, ribs, bilateral; three views

71111   including posteroanterior chest, minimum of four views

71120   Radiologic examination; sternum, minimum of two views

71130   sternoclavicular joint or joints, minimum of three views

71250   Computed tomography, thorax; without contrast material
> *CPT Changes: An Insider's View* 2003

71260   with contrast material(s)
> *CPT Assistant* Jul 01:4
> *Clinical Examples in Radiology* Summer 05:4

71270   without contrast material, followed by contrast material(s) and further sections
> *CPT Assistant* Jun 01:10

(For cardiac computed tomography of the heart, see Category III codes 0144T-0151T)

(To report 3D rendering, see 76376, 76377)

▲ **71275**   Computed tomographic angiography, chest (noncoronary), with contrast material(s), including noncontrast images, if performed, and image postprocessing
> *CPT Assistant* Jul 01:4, Jun 05:11, Dec 05:7, Jan 07:31, Mar 07:7; *CPT Changes: An Insider's View* 2001, 2007, 2008
> *Clinical Examples in Radiology* Spring 05:7

(For coronary artery computed tomographic angiography including calcification score and/or cardiac morphology, see Category III codes 0146T-0149T)

71550   Magnetic resonance (eg, proton) imaging, chest (eg, for evaluation of hilar and mediastinal lymphadenopathy); without contrast material(s)
> *CPT Assistant* Jul 01:7; *CPT Changes: An Insider's View* 2001

71551   with contrast material(s)
> *CPT Assistant* Jul 01:7; *CPT Changes: An Insider's View* 2001

71552   without contrast material(s), followed by contrast material(s) and further sequences
> *CPT Assistant* Jul 01:7; *CPT Changes: An Insider's View* 2001

(For breast MRI, see 77058, 77059)

71555   Magnetic resonance angiography, chest (excluding myocardium), with or without contrast material(s)
> *CPT Assistant* Fall 95:2, Dec 05:7, Jan 07:31

Spine and Pelvis

72010   Radiologic examination, spine, entire, survey study, anteroposterior and lateral
> *CPT Assistant* May 02:18, Jan 07:29

72020   Radiologic examination, spine, single view, specify level

72040   Radiologic examination, spine, cervical; two or three views
> *CPT Assistant* Sep 01:7; *CPT Changes: An Insider's View* 2001

72050   minimum of four views

72052   complete, including oblique and flexion and/or extension studies

72069   Radiologic examination, spine, thoracolumbar, standing (scoliosis)
> *CPT Assistant* Winter 90:9

72070   Radiologic examination, spine; thoracic, two views
> *CPT Assistant* Sep 01:7; *CPT Changes: An Insider's View* 2001

72072   thoracic, three views
> *CPT Assistant* Sep 01:7; *CPT Changes: An Insider's View* 2001

72074   thoracic, minimum of four views
> *CPT Assistant* Sep 01:7; *CPT Changes: An Insider's View* 2001

72080   thoracolumbar, two views
> *CPT Assistant* Sep 01:7; *CPT Changes: An Insider's View* 2001

72090   scoliosis study, including supine and erect studies

72100   Radiologic examination, spine, lumbosacral; two or three views
> *CPT Assistant* Sep 01:7; *CPT Changes: An Insider's View* 2001

72110   minimum of four views
> *CPT Assistant* Sep 01:7; *CPT Changes: An Insider's View* 2001

72114   complete, including bending views

72120   Radiologic examination, spine, lumbosacral, bending views only, minimum of four views

(Contrast material in CT of spine is either by intrathecal or intravenous injection. For intrathecal injection, use also 61055 or 62284. IV injection of contrast material is part of the CT procedure)

72125   Computed tomography, cervical spine; without contrast material
> *CPT Changes: An Insider's View* 2003

72126   with contrast material

72127   without contrast material, followed by contrast material(s) and further sections

(For intrathecal injection procedure, see 61055, 62284)

72128   Computed tomography, thoracic spine; without contrast material
> *CPT Changes: An Insider's View* 2003

72129   with contrast material

(For intrathecal injection procedure, see 61055, 62284)

72130   without contrast material, followed by contrast material(s) and further sections

(For intrathecal injection procedure, see 61055, 62284)

72131   Computed tomography, lumbar spine; without contrast material
> *CPT Changes: An Insider's View* 2003

72132   with contrast material
> *CPT Assistant* Fall 93:13
> *Clinical Examples in Radiology* Fall 06:5-6, 11-12

72133   without contrast material, followed by contrast material(s) and further sections

(For intrathecal injection procedure, see 61055, 62284)

(To report 3D rendering, see 76376, 76377)

72141   Magnetic resonance (eg, proton) imaging, spinal canal and contents, cervical; without contrast material

72142   with contrast material(s)

(For cervical spinal canal imaging without contrast material followed by contrast material, use 72156)

72146   Magnetic resonance (eg, proton) imaging, spinal canal and contents, thoracic; without contrast material
> *CPT Assistant* May 99:10

72147   with contrast material(s)
> *CPT Assistant* May 99:10

(For thoracic spinal canal imaging without contrast material followed by contrast material, use 72157)

72148   Magnetic resonance (eg, proton) imaging, spinal canal and contents, lumbar; without contrast material
> *CPT Assistant* Nov 05:15
> *Clinical Examples in Radiology* Spring 06:6, 11

72149   with contrast material(s)

(For lumbar spinal canal imaging without contrast material followed by contrast material, use 72158)

72156   Magnetic resonance (eg, proton) imaging, spinal canal and contents, without contrast material, followed by contrast material(s) and further sequences; cervical

72157   thoracic

72158   lumbar

72159   Magnetic resonance angiography, spinal canal and contents, with or without contrast material(s)
> *CPT Assistant* Dec 05:7, Jan 07:31

72170   Radiologic examination, pelvis; one or two views
> *CPT Assistant* Sep 01:7, Mar 03:23; *CPT Changes: An Insider's View* 2001
> *Clinical Examples in Radiology* Spring 05:12

72190   complete, minimum of three views

(For pelvimetry, use 74710)

▲ **72191**   Computed tomographic angiography, pelvis, with contrast material(s), including noncontrast images, if performed, and image postprocessing
> *CPT Assistant* Jul 01:4, 6, Dec 05:7, Jan 07:31; *CPT Changes: An Insider's View* 2001, 2008

(For CTA aorto-iliofemoral runoff, use 75635)

72192   Computed tomography, pelvis; without contrast material
> *CPT Assistant* Mar 05:1, 4, Mar 07:10; *CPT Changes: An Insider's View* 2003
> *Clinical Examples in Radiology* Winter 06:11, Spring 07:3, 11

72193   with contrast material(s)
> *CPT Assistant* Mar 05:1, 4, Mar 07:10
> *Clinical Examples in Radiology* Winter 05:1, 7, Spring 07:3, 11

72194   without contrast material, followed by contrast material(s) and further sections
> *CPT Assistant* Mar 05:1, 4, Mar 07:10
> *Clinical Examples in Radiology* Spring 07:3, 11

(To report 3D rendering, see 76376, 76377)

(For computed tomographic colonography, see Category III codes 0066T, 0067T. Do not report 72192-72194 in conjunction with 0066T, 0067T)

72195   Magnetic resonance (eg, proton) imaging, pelvis; without contrast material(s)

> *CPT Assistant* Jul 01:7, Jun 06:17; *CPT Changes: An Insider's View* 2001

> *Clinical Examples in Radiology* Spring 06:8-9, Fall 06:7-8

72196   with contrast material(s)

> *CPT Assistant* Jul 01:7, Jun 06:17; *CPT Changes: An Insider's View* 2001

> *Clinical Examples in Radiology* Spring 06:8-9, Fall 06:7-8

72197   without contrast material(s), followed by contrast material(s) and further sequences

> *CPT Assistant* Jul 01:7; *CPT Changes: An Insider's View* 2001

> *Clinical Examples in Radiology* Spring 06:8-9, Fall 06:2-3, 7-8

72198   Magnetic resonance angiography, pelvis, with or without contrast material(s)

> *CPT Assistant* Dec 05:7, Jan 07:31

72200   Radiologic examination, sacroiliac joints; less than three views

72202   three or more views

72220   Radiologic examination, sacrum and coccyx, minimum of two views

72240   Myelography, cervical, radiological supervision and interpretation

> *CPT Assistant* Fall 93:13

> *Clinical Examples in Radiology* Fall 06:5-6, 11-12

(For complete cervical myelography, see 61055, 62284, 72240)

72255   Myelography, thoracic, radiological supervision and interpretation

(For complete thoracic myelography, see 61055, 62284, 72255)

72265   Myelography, lumbosacral, radiological supervision and interpretation

> *CPT Assistant* Fall 93:13, Aug 00:7

(For complete lumbosacral myelography, see 61055, 62284, 72265)

72270   Myelography, two or more regions (eg, lumbar/thoracic, cervical/thoracic, lumbar/cervical, lumbar/thoracic/cervical), radiological supervision and interpretation

> *CPT Changes: An Insider's View* 2004

(For complete myelography of entire spinal canal, see 61055, 62284, 72270)

72275   Epidurography, radiological supervision and interpretation

> *CPT Assistant* Nov 99:40, Jan 00:2, Aug 00:7; *CPT Changes: An Insider's View* 2000

(72275 includes 77003)

(For injection procedure, see 62280-62282, 62310-62319, 64479-64484, 0027T)

(Use 72275 only when an epidurogram is performed, images documented, and a formal radiologic report is issued)

Epidurography
72275

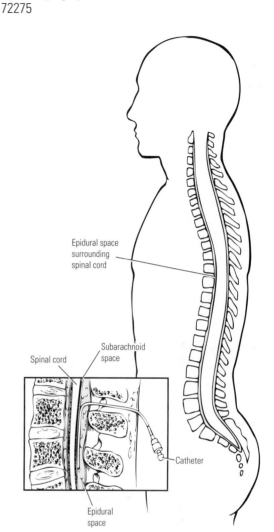

Epidural space surrounding spinal cord

Subarachnoid space

Spinal cord

Catheter

Epidural space

72285   Discography, cervical or thoracic, radiological supervision and interpretation

> *CPT Assistant* Nov 99:35, 40; *CPT Changes: An Insider's View* 2000

72291   Radiological supervision and interpretation, percutaneous vertebroplasty or vertebral augmentation including cavity creation, per vertebral body; under fluoroscopic guidance

> *CPT Changes: An Insider's View* 2007

72292   under CT guidance

> *CPT Changes: An Insider's View* 2007

(For procedure, see 22520-22525)

72295   Discography, lumbar, radiological supervision and interpretation

> *CPT Assistant* Apr 03:27

Upper Extremities

(For stress views, any joint, use 77071)

73000 Radiologic examination; clavicle, complete

73010   scapula, complete

73020 Radiologic examination, shoulder; one view

73030   complete, minimum of two views

73040 Radiologic examination, shoulder, arthrography, radiological supervision and interpretation
> *CPT Assistant* Jul 01:7, Feb 07:11
> *Clinical Examples in Radiology* Spring 05:6

(Do not report 77002 in conjunction with 73040)

73050 Radiologic examination; acromioclavicular joints, bilateral, with or without weighted distraction

73060   humerus, minimum of two views

73070 Radiologic examination, elbow; two views
> *CPT Assistant* Winter 90:9, Sep 01:8; *CPT Changes: An Insider's View* 2001

73080   complete, minimum of three views

73085 Radiologic examination, elbow, arthrography, radiological supervision and interpretation
> *Clinical Examples in Radiology* Spring 05:6

(Do not report 77002 in conjunction with 73085)

73090 Radiologic examination; forearm, two views
> *CPT Assistant* Sep 01:8, Apr 02:14; *CPT Changes: An Insider's View* 2001

73092   upper extremity, infant, minimum of two views

73100 Radiologic examination, wrist; two views
> *CPT Assistant* Winter 90:9, Sep 01:8; *CPT Changes: An Insider's View* 2001

73110   complete, minimum of three views
> *CPT Assistant* Mar 97:10, Nov 06:22

73115 Radiologic examination, wrist, arthrography, radiological supervision and interpretation
> *Clinical Examples in Radiology* Spring 05:6

(Do not report 77002 in conjunction with 73115)

73120 Radiologic examination, hand; two views
> *CPT Assistant* Winter 90:9

73130   minimum of three views
> *Clinical Examples in Radiology* Winter 05:9

73140 Radiologic examination, finger(s), minimum of two views

73200 Computed tomography, upper extremity; without contrast material
> *CPT Changes: An Insider's View* 2003

73201   with contrast material(s)

73202   without contrast material, followed by contrast material(s) and further sections

(To report 3D rendering, see 76376, 76377)

▲ **73206** Computed tomographic angiography, upper extremity, with contrast material(s), including noncontrast images, if performed, and image postprocessing
> *CPT Assistant* Jul 01:5, Dec 05:7, Jan 07:31; *CPT Changes: An Insider's View* 2001, 2008

73218 Magnetic resonance (eg, proton) imaging, upper extremity, other than joint; without contrast material(s)
> *CPT Assistant* Jul 01:7; *CPT Changes: An Insider's View* 2001

73219   with contrast material(s)
> *CPT Assistant* Jul 01:7; *CPT Changes: An Insider's View* 2001

73220   without contrast material(s), followed by contrast material(s) and further sequences
> *CPT Assistant* Jul 01:7; *CPT Changes: An Insider's View* 2001

73221 Magnetic resonance (eg, proton) imaging, any joint of upper extremity; without contrast material(s)
> *CPT Assistant* Jul 01:7; *CPT Changes: An Insider's View* 2001

73222   with contrast material(s)
> *CPT Assistant* Jul 01:7; *CPT Changes: An Insider's View* 2001
> *Clinical Examples in Radiology* Spring 05:5

73223   without contrast material(s), followed by contrast material(s) and further sequences
> *CPT Assistant* Jul 01:7; *CPT Changes: An Insider's View* 2001

73225 Magnetic resonance angiography, upper extremity, with or without contrast material(s)
> *CPT Assistant* Dec 05:7, Jan 07:31

Lower Extremities

(For stress views, any joint, use 77071)

73500 Radiologic examination, hip, unilateral; one view
> *Clinical Examples in Radiology* Spring 05:12

73510   complete, minimum of two views
> *CPT Assistant* Spring 92:9, May 99:10, Apr 02:19, Mar 03:23
> *Clinical Examples in Radiology* Spring 05:12

73520 Radiologic examination, hips, bilateral, minimum of two views of each hip, including anteroposterior view of pelvis
> *CPT Assistant* Apr 02:19
> *Clinical Examples in Radiology* Spring 05:12

73525 Radiologic examination, hip, arthrography, radiological supervision and interpretation
> *Clinical Examples in Radiology* Spring 05:6

(Do not report 73525 in conjunction with 77002)

73530 Radiologic examination, hip, during operative procedure

73540 Radiologic examination, pelvis and hips, infant or child, minimum of two views

73542 Radiological examination, sacroiliac joint arthrography, radiological supervision and interpretation
> *CPT Assistant* Nov 99:40-41; *CPT Changes: An Insider's View* 2000
> *Clinical Examples in Radiology* Spring 05:6

(Do not report 73542 in conjunction with 77002)

(For procedure, use 27096. If formal arthrography is not performed, recorded, and a formal radiologic report is not issued, use 77003 for fluoroscopic guidance for sacroiliac joint injections)

73550   Radiologic examination, femur, two views
➔ *CPT Assistant* Sep 01:8; *CPT Changes: An Insider's View* 2001

73560   Radiologic examination, knee; one or two views

73562   three views
➔ *CPT Assistant* Apr 02:15
➔ *Clinical Examples in Radiology* Fall 06:4

73564   complete, four or more views
➔ *CPT Assistant* Jun 98:11, Nov 98:21
➔ *Clinical Examples in Radiology* Fall 06:4

73565   both knees, standing, anteroposterior
➔ *CPT Assistant* Winter 90:9
➔ *Clinical Examples in Radiology* Fall 06:4

73580   Radiologic examination, knee, arthrography, radiological supervision and interpretation
➔ *Clinical Examples in Radiology* Spring 05:6

(Do not report 73580 in conjunction with 77002)

73590   Radiologic examination; tibia and fibula, two views
➔ *CPT Assistant* Sep 01:8; *CPT Changes: An Insider's View* 2001

73592   lower extremity, infant, minimum of two views

73600   Radiologic examination, ankle; two views
➔ *CPT Assistant* Sep 01:8, Apr 02:15, Mar 03:9; *CPT Changes: An Insider's View* 2001

73610   complete, minimum of three views
➔ *CPT Assistant* Apr 02:15, Mar 03:9

73615   Radiologic examination, ankle, arthrography, radiological supervision and interpretation

(Do not report 73615 in conjunction with 77002)

73620   Radiologic examination, foot; two views
➔ *CPT Assistant* Sep 01:8, Apr 02:15, Mar 03:9; *CPT Changes: An Insider's View* 2001

73630   complete, minimum of three views

73650   Radiologic examination; calcaneus, minimum of two views

73660   toe(s), minimum of two views

73700   Computed tomography, lower extremity; without contrast material
➔ *CPT Changes: An Insider's View* 2003

73701   with contrast material(s)

73702   without contrast material, followed by contrast material(s) and further sections

(To report 3D rendering, see 76376, 76377)

▲ **73706**   Computed tomographic angiography, lower extremity, with contrast material(s), including noncontrast images, if performed, and image postprocessing
➔ *CPT Assistant* Jul 01:5-6, Dec 05:7, Jan 07:31; *CPT Changes: An Insider's View* 2001, 2008

(For CTA aorto-iliofemoral runoff, use 75635)

73718   Magnetic resonance (eg, proton) imaging, lower extremity other than joint; without contrast material(s)
➔ *CPT Assistant* Jul 01:3; *CPT Changes: An Insider's View* 2001
➔ *Clinical Examples in Radiology* Spring 07:7-9, 12

73719   with contrast material(s)
➔ *CPT Assistant* Jul 01:3; *CPT Changes: An Insider's View* 2001
➔ *Clinical Examples in Radiology* Spring 07:7-9, 12

73720   without contrast material(s), followed by contrast material(s) and further sequences
➔ *CPT Assistant* Jul 01:3; *CPT Changes: An Insider's View* 2001
➔ *Clinical Examples in Radiology* Spring 07:7-9, 12

73721   Magnetic resonance (eg, proton) imaging, any joint of lower extremity; without contrast material
➔ *CPT Assistant* Jul 01:3, Jun 06:17; *CPT Changes: An Insider's View* 2001
➔ *Clinical Examples in Radiology* Spring 07:7-9, 12

73722   with contrast material(s)
➔ *CPT Assistant* Jul 01:3, Jun 06:17; *CPT Changes: An Insider's View* 2001
➔ *Clinical Examples in Radiology* Spring 07:7-9, 12

73723   without contrast material(s), followed by contrast material(s) and further sequences
➔ *CPT Assistant* Jul 01:3; *CPT Changes: An Insider's View* 2001
➔ *Clinical Examples in Radiology* Spring 07:7-9, 12

73725   Magnetic resonance angiography, lower extremity, with or without contrast material(s)
➔ *CPT Assistant* Dec 05:7, Jan 07:31
➔ *Clinical Examples in Radiology* Spring 06:1-3

Abdomen

74000   Radiologic examination, abdomen; single anteroposterior view
➔ *CPT Assistant* Nov 98:21
➔ *Clinical Examples in Radiology* Spring 07:4

74010   anteroposterior and additional oblique and cone views

74020   complete, including decubitus and/or erect views

74022   complete acute abdomen series, including supine, erect, and/or decubitus views, single view chest
➔ *CPT Changes: An Insider's View* 2003

74150   Computed tomography, abdomen; without contrast material
➔ *CPT Assistant* Oct 02:12, Mar 05:1, 4; *CPT Changes: An Insider's View* 2003
➔ *Clinical Examples in Radiology* Spring 07:3, 11

74160   with contrast material(s)
➔ *CPT Assistant* Mar 05:1, 4
➔ *Clinical Examples in Radiology* Spring 07:3, 11

74170   without contrast material, followed by contrast material(s) and further sections
> *CPT Assistant* Mar 05:4
> *Clinical Examples in Radiology* Winter 05:1, 7-8, 12, Spring 07:3, 11

(To report 3D rendering, see 76376, 76377)

(For computed tomographic colonography, see Category III codes 0066T, 0067T. Do not report 74150-74170 in conjunction with 0066T, 0067T)

▲ **74175**   Computed tomographic angiography, abdomen, with contrast material(s), including noncontrast images, if performed, and image postprocessing
> *CPT Assistant* Jul 01:6, Dec 05:7, Jan 07:31; *CPT Changes: An Insider's View* 2001, 2008

(For CTA aorto-iliofemoral runoff, use 75635)

74181   Magnetic resonance (eg, proton) imaging, abdomen; without contrast material(s)
> *CPT Assistant* Jul 01:3; *CPT Changes: An Insider's View* 2001

74182   with contrast material(s)
> *CPT Assistant* Jul 01:3; *CPT Changes: An Insider's View* 2001

74183   without contrast material(s), followed by with contrast material(s) and further sequences
> *CPT Assistant* Jul 01:3; *CPT Changes: An Insider's View* 2001

74185   Magnetic resonance angiography, abdomen, with or without contrast material(s)
> *CPT Assistant* Dec 05:7, Jan 07:31
> *Clinical Examples in Radiology* Spring 06:1-3

74190   Peritoneogram (eg, after injection of air or contrast), radiological supervision and interpretation

(For procedure, use 49400)

(For computed tomography, see 72192 or 74150)

Gastrointestinal Tract

▶(For percutaneous placement of gastrostomy tube, use 43246)◀

74210   Radiologic examination; pharynx and/or cervical esophagus

74220   esophagus

74230   Swallowing function, with cineradiography/videoradiography
> *CPT Assistant* Dec 04:17; *CPT Changes: An Insider's View* 2002
> *Clinical Examples in Radiology* Summer 06:4-5

74235   Removal of foreign body(s), esophageal, with use of balloon catheter, radiological supervision and interpretation

(For procedure, see 43215, 43247)

74240   Radiologic examination, gastrointestinal tract, upper; with or without delayed films, without KUB

74241   with or without delayed films, with KUB

74245   with small intestine, includes multiple serial films
> *CPT Changes: An Insider's View* 2002

74246   Radiological examination, gastrointestinal tract, upper, air contrast, with specific high density barium, effervescent agent, with or without glucagon; with or without delayed films, without KUB

74247   with or without delayed films, with KUB

74249   with small intestine follow-through
> *CPT Changes: An Insider's View* 2002

74250   Radiologic examination, small intestine, includes multiple serial films;
> *CPT Changes: An Insider's View* 2002

74251   via enteroclysis tube

74260   Duodenography, hypotonic

74270   Radiologic examination, colon; barium enema, with or without KUB
> *CPT Assistant* May 03:19

74280   air contrast with specific high density barium, with or without glucagon

74283   Therapeutic enema, contrast or air, for reduction of intussusception or other intraluminal obstruction (eg, meconium ileus)
> *CPT Assistant* Nov 97:24

74290   Cholecystography, oral contrast;

74291   additional or repeat examination or multiple day examination

74300   Cholangiography and/or pancreatography; intraoperative, radiological supervision and interpretation
> *CPT Assistant* Nov 99:41, Dec 00:14; *CPT Changes: An Insider's View* 2000

+ **74301**   additional set intraoperative, radiological supervision and interpretation (List separately in addition to code for primary procedure)

(Use 74301 in conjunction with 74300)

74305   through existing catheter, radiological supervision and interpretation
> *CPT Assistant* Nov 99:41; *CPT Changes: An Insider's View* 2000, 2002

(For procedure, see 47505, 48400, 47560-47561, 47563)

(For biliary duct stone extraction, percutaneous, see 47630, 74327)

74320   Cholangiography, percutaneous, transhepatic, radiological supervision and interpretation

74327   Postoperative biliary duct calculus removal, percutaneous via T-tube tract, basket, or snare (eg, Burhenne technique), radiological supervision and interpretation
> *CPT Changes: An Insider's View* 2002

(For procedure, use 47630)

74328   Endoscopic catheterization of the biliary ductal system, radiological supervision and interpretation

(For procedure, see 43260-43272 as appropriate)

74329   Endoscopic catheterization of the pancreatic ductal system, radiological supervision and interpretation

(For procedure, see 43260-43272 as appropriate)

74330   Combined endoscopic catheterization of the biliary and pancreatic ductal systems, radiological supervision and interpretation

(For procedure, see 43260-43272 as appropriate)

74340   Introduction of long gastrointestinal tube (eg, Miller-Abbott), including multiple fluoroscopies and films, radiological supervision and interpretation

(For tube placement, use 44500)

▶(74350 has been deleted. To report gastrostomy tube placement, use 49440)◀

74355   Percutaneous placement of enteroclysis tube, radiological supervision and interpretation

74360   Intraluminal dilation of strictures and/or obstructions (eg, esophagus), radiological supervision and interpretation
➔ *CPT Assistant* Spring 94:3

74363   Percutaneous transhepatic dilation of biliary duct stricture with or without placement of stent, radiological supervision and interpretation
➔ *CPT Changes: An Insider's View* 2002

(For procedure, see 47510, 47511, 47555, 47556)

Urinary Tract

74400   Urography (pyelography), intravenous, with or without KUB, with or without tomography

74410   Urography, infusion, drip technique and/or bolus technique;

74415   with nephrotomography

74420   Urography, retrograde, with or without KUB
➔ *CPT Assistant* Sep 00:11

74425   Urography, antegrade (pyelostogram, nephrostogram, loopogram), radiological supervision and interpretation
➔ *CPT Assistant* Fall 93:14, Dec 97:7, Oct 05:18
➔ *Clinical Examples in Radiology* Summer 06:1-3

74430   Cystography, minimum of 3 views, radiological supervision and interpretation

74440   Vasography, vesiculography, or epididymography, radiological supervision and interpretation

74445   Corpora cavernosography, radiological supervision and interpretation

74450   Urethrocystography, retrograde, radiological supervision and interpretation

74455   Urethrocystography, voiding, radiological supervision and interpretation

74470   Radiologic examination, renal cyst study, translumbar, contrast visualization, radiological supervision and interpretation
➔ *CPT Assistant* Oct 05:18, Feb 07:11

74475   Introduction of intracatheter or catheter into renal pelvis for drainage and/or injection, percutaneous, radiological supervision and interpretation
➔ *CPT Assistant* Dec 97:7, Oct 05:18, Feb 07:11

74480   Introduction of ureteral catheter or stent into ureter through renal pelvis for drainage and/or injection, percutaneous, radiological supervision and interpretation
➔ *CPT Assistant* Fall 93:14, Oct 05:18
➔ *Clinical Examples in Radiology* Summer 06:1-3

(For transurethral surgery [ureter and pelvis], see 52320-52355)

74485   Dilation of nephrostomy, ureters, or urethra, radiological supervision and interpretation
➔ *CPT Assistant* Oct 05:18
➔ *Clinical Examples in Radiology* Summer 06:1-3

(For dilation of ureter without radiologic guidance, use 52341, 52344)

(For change of nephrostomy or pyelostomy tube, use 50398)

Gynecological and Obstetrical

(For abdomen and pelvis, see 72170-72190, 74000-74170)

74710   Pelvimetry, with or without placental localization

74740   Hysterosalpingography, radiological supervision and interpretation
➔ *CPT Assistant* Nov 97:24, Jul 99:8

(For introduction of saline or contrast for hysterosalpingography, see 58340)

74742   Transcervical catheterization of fallopian tube, radiological supervision and interpretation

(For procedure, use 58345)

74775   Perineogram (eg, vaginogram, for sex determination or extent of anomalies)

Heart

▶Cardiac magnetic imaging differs from traditional magnetic resonance imaging (MRI) in its ability to provide a physiologic evaluation of cardiac function. Traditional MRI relies on static images to obtain clinical diagnoses based upon anatomic information. Improvement in spatial and temporal resolution has expanded the application from an anatomic test and includes physiologic evaluation of cardiac function. Flow and velocity assessment for valves and intracardiac shunts is performed in addition to a function and morphologic evaluation. Use 75559 and 75560 to report pharmacologic wall motion stress evaluation without contrast. Use 75563 and 75564 to report pharmacologic perfusion stress with contrast.

Listed procedures may be performed independently or in the course of overall medical care. If the physician providing these services is also responsible for diagnostic workup and/or follow-up care of the patient, see appropriate sections also. Only one procedure in the series 75557-75564 is appropriately reported per session.

Cardiac MRI studies may be performed at rest and/or during pharmacologic stress. Therefore, the appropriate stress testing code from the 93015-93018 series should be reported in addition to 75559, 75560, 75563, 75564.◄

> (For separate injection procedures for vascular radiology, see **Surgery** section, 36000-36299)

> (For cardiac catheterization procedures, see 93501-93556)

> ►(75552-75556 have been deleted. To report, see 75557-75564)◄

● **75557** Cardiac magnetic resonance imaging for morphology and function without contrast material;
➔ CPT Changes: An Insider's View 2008

● **75558**   with flow/velocity quantification
➔ CPT Changes: An Insider's View 2008

● **75559**   with stress imaging
➔ CPT Changes: An Insider's View 2008

● **75560**   with flow/velocity quantification and stress
➔ CPT Changes: An Insider's View 2008

● **75561** Cardiac magnetic resonance imaging for morphology and function without contrast material(s), followed by contrast material(s) and further sequences;
➔ CPT Changes: An Insider's View 2008

● **75562**   with flow/velocity quantification
➔ CPT Changes: An Insider's View 2008

● **75563**   with stress imaging
➔ CPT Changes: An Insider's View 2008

● **75564**   with flow/velocity quantification and stress
➔ CPT Changes: An Insider's View 2008

> ►(Do not report 75557-75564 in conjunction with 76376, 76377)◄

Vascular Procedures

Aorta and Arteries

Selective vascular catheterizations should be coded to include introduction and all lesser order selective catheterizations used in the approach (eg, the description for a selective right middle cerebral artery catheterization includes the introduction and placement catheterization of the right common and internal carotid arteries).

Additional second and/or third order arterial catheterizations within the same family of arteries supplied by a single first order artery should be expressed by 36218 or 36248. Additional first order or higher catheterizations in vascular families supplied by a first

order vessel different from a previously selected and coded family should be separately coded using the conventions described above.

For angiography performed in conjunction with therapeutic transcatheter radiological supervision and interpretation services, see the Radiology Transcatheter Procedures guidelines.

Diagnostic angiography (radiological supervision and interpretation) codes should NOT be used with interventional procedures for:

1. Contrast injections, angiography, roadmapping, and/or fluoroscopic guidance for the intervention,

2. Vessel measurement, and

3. Post-angioplasty/stent angiography,

as this work is captured in the radiological supervision and interpretation code(s).

Diagnostic angiography performed at the time of an interventional procedure is separately reportable if:

1. No prior catheter-based angiographic study is available and a full diagnostic study is performed, and the decision to intervene is based on the diagnostic study, OR

2. A prior study is available, but as documented in the medical record:

   a. The patient's condition with respect to the clinical indication has changed since the prior study, OR

   b. There is inadequate visualization of the anatomy and/or pathology, OR

   c. There is a clinical change during the procedure that requires new evaluation outside the target area of intervention.

Diagnostic angiography performed at a separate setting from an interventional procedure is separately reported.

Diagnostic angiography performed at the time of an interventional procedure is NOT separately reportable if it is specifically included in the interventional code descriptor.

> (For intravenous procedure, see 36000-36013, 36400-36425 and 36100-36248 for intra-arterial procedure)

> (For radiological supervision and interpretation, see 75600-75978)

75600 Aortography, thoracic, without serialography, radiological supervision and interpretation

> (For injection procedure, use 93544)

75605   Aortography, thoracic, by serialography, radiological supervision and interpretation

➜ *CPT Assistant* Spring 94:29, Dec 98:9

(For injection procedure, use 93544)

Aortography
75600-75630

A radiographic contrast study is performed on the abdominal or thoracic aorta.

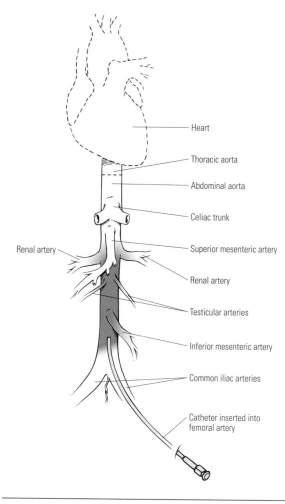

- Heart
- Thoracic aorta
- Abdominal aorta
- Celiac trunk
- Superior mesenteric artery
- Renal artery
- Renal artery
- Testicular arteries
- Inferior mesenteric artery
- Common iliac arteries
- Catheter inserted into femoral artery

75625   Aortography, abdominal, by serialography, radiological supervision and interpretation

➜ *CPT Assistant* Fall 93:16, Jan 01:14

(For injection procedure, use 93544)

75630   Aortography, abdominal plus bilateral iliofemoral lower extremity, catheter, by serialography, radiological supervision and interpretation

➜ *CPT Assistant* Fall 93:16, Jan 01:14

▲ **75635**   Computed tomographic angiography, abdominal aorta and bilateral iliofemoral lower extremity runoff, with contrast material(s), including noncontrast images, if performed, and image postprocessing

➜ *CPT Assistant* Jul 01:4-5, Dec 05:7, Jan 07:31; *CPT Changes: An Insider's View* 2001, 2008

➜ *Clinical Examples in Radiology* Spring 06:1-3

75650   Angiography, cervicocerebral, catheter, including vessel origin, radiological supervision and interpretation

➜ *CPT Assistant* Spring 94:29, Apr 98:9, Oct 00:6

75658   Angiography, brachial, retrograde, radiological supervision and interpretation

75660   Angiography, external carotid, unilateral, selective, radiological supervision and interpretation

Angiography, Carotid Artery
75660-75680

A radiographic contrast study is performed on the carotid artery vascular family.

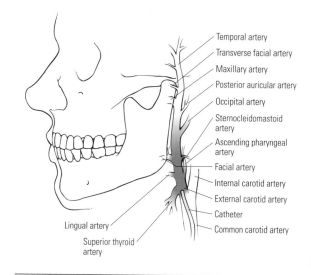

- Temporal artery
- Transverse facial artery
- Maxillary artery
- Posterior auricular artery
- Occipital artery
- Sternocleidomastoid artery
- Ascending pharyngeal artery
- Facial artery
- Internal carotid artery
- External carotid artery
- Catheter
- Common carotid artery
- Lingual artery
- Superior thyroid artery

75662   Angiography, external carotid, bilateral, selective, radiological supervision and interpretation

75665   Angiography, carotid, cerebral, unilateral, radiological supervision and interpretation

75671   Angiography, carotid, cerebral, bilateral, radiological supervision and interpretation

➜ *CPT Assistant* Oct 00:6

75676   Angiography, carotid, cervical, unilateral, radiological supervision and interpretation

75680   Angiography, carotid, cervical, bilateral, radiological supervision and interpretation

➜ *CPT Assistant* Oct 00:6

75685   Angiography, vertebral, cervical, and/or intracranial, radiological supervision and interpretation

➜ *CPT Assistant* Oct 00:6

75705   Angiography, spinal, selective, radiological supervision and interpretation

75710   Angiography, extremity, unilateral, radiological supervision and interpretation

➜ *CPT Assistant* Apr 99:11, Jan 01:14

75716   Angiography, extremity, bilateral, radiological supervision and interpretation

➜ *CPT Assistant* Fall 93:16, Jan 01:14

75722 Angiography, renal, unilateral, selective (including flush aortogram), radiological supervision and interpretation

75724 Angiography, renal, bilateral, selective (including flush aortogram), radiological supervision and interpretation

75726 Angiography, visceral, selective or supraselective (with or without flush aortogram), radiological supervision and interpretation

(For selective angiography, each additional visceral vessel studied after basic examination, use 75774)

75731 Angiography, adrenal, unilateral, selective, radiological supervision and interpretation

75733 Angiography, adrenal, bilateral, selective, radiological supervision and interpretation

75736 Angiography, pelvic, selective or supraselective, radiological supervision and interpretation
➔ *Clinical Examples in Radiology* Spring 05:14

75741 Angiography, pulmonary, unilateral, selective, radiological supervision and interpretation

(For injection procedure, use 93541)

75743 Angiography, pulmonary, bilateral, selective, radiological supervision and interpretation
➔ *CPT Assistant* Spring 94:29, Apr 98:7

(For injection procedure, use 93541)

75746 Angiography, pulmonary, by nonselective catheter or venous injection, radiological supervision and interpretation

(For injection procedure, use 93541)

(For introduction of catheter, injection procedure, see 93501-93533, 93539, 93540, 93545, 93556)

(For introduction of catheter, injection procedure, see 93501-93533, 93545, 93556)

(For introduction of catheter, injection procedure, see 93501-93533, 93539, 93540, 93545, 93556)

75756 Angiography, internal mammary, radiological supervision and interpretation

(For introduction of catheter, injection procedure, see 93501-93533, 93545, 93556)

+ 75774 Angiography, selective, each additional vessel studied after basic examination, radiological supervision and interpretation (List separately in addition to code for primary procedure)
➔ *CPT Assistant* Fall 93:17, Spring 94:29

(Use 75774 in addition to code for specific initial vessel studied)

(For angiography, see codes 75600-75790)

(For catheterizations, see codes 36215-36248)

(For introduction of catheter, injection procedure, see 93501-93533, 93545, 93555, 93556)

75790 Angiography, arteriovenous shunt (eg, dialysis patient), radiological supervision and interpretation
➔ *CPT Assistant* Feb 97:2, May 01:4
➔ *Clinical Examples in Radiology* Spring 05:8-10, Spring 07:1-3

(For introduction of catheter, use 36140, 36145, 36215-36217, 36245-36247)

Veins and Lymphatics

For venography performed in conjunction with therapeutic transcatheter radiological supervision and interpretation services, see the Radiology Transcatheter Procedures guidelines.

Diagnostic venography (radiological supervision and interpretation) codes should NOT be used with interventional procedures for:

1. Contrast injections, venography, roadmapping, and/or fluoroscopic guidance for the intervention,

2. Vessel measurement, and

3. Post-angioplasty/stent venography,

as this work is captured in the radiological supervision and interpretation code(s).

Diagnostic venography performed at the time of an interventional procedure is separately reportable if:

1. No prior catheter-based venographic study is available and a full diagnostic study is performed, and decision to intervene is based on the diagnostic study, OR

2. A prior study is available, but as documented in the medical record:

   a. The patient's condition with respect to the clinical indication has changed since the prior study, OR

   b. There is inadequate visualization of the anatomy and/or pathology, OR

   c. There is a clinical change during the procedure that requires new evaluation outside the target area of intervention.

Diagnostic venography performed at a separate setting from an interventional procedure is separately reported.

Diagnostic venography performed at the time of an interventional procedure is NOT separately reportable if it is specifically included in the interventional code descriptor.

(For injection procedure for venous system, see 36000-36015, 36400-36510)

(For injection procedure for lymphatic system, use 38790)

75801 Lymphangiography, extremity only, unilateral, radiological supervision and interpretation

75803 Lymphangiography, extremity only, bilateral, radiological supervision and interpretation

75805 Lymphangiography, pelvic/abdominal, unilateral, radiological supervision and interpretation

75807 Lymphangiography, pelvic/abdominal, bilateral, radiological supervision and interpretation

75809 Shuntogram for investigation of previously placed indwelling nonvascular shunt (eg, LeVeen shunt, ventriculoperitoneal shunt, indwelling infusion pump), radiological supervision and interpretation

➔ *CPT Changes: An Insider's View* 2001

(For procedure, see 49427 or 61070)

75810 Splenoportography, radiological supervision and interpretation

75820 Venography, extremity, unilateral, radiological supervision and interpretation

➔ *CPT Assistant* Oct 97:10

➔ *Clinical Examples in Radiology* Summer 06:8-9

Venography
75820-75822

A radiographic contrast study is performed on the veins of the lower extremities.

Inferior vena cava
Common iliac
Percutaneous catheter
Deep femoral vein
Femoral vein
Great saphenous vein
Popliteal vein
Anterior tibial vein
Small saphenous vein
Posterior tibial vein
Peroneal vein
Venous arch on dorsum of foot

75822 Venography, extremity, bilateral, radiological supervision and interpretation

75825 Venography, caval, inferior, with serialography, radiological supervision and interpretation

➔ *Clinical Examples in Radiology* Winter 05:5-6

75827 Venography, caval, superior, with serialography, radiological supervision and interpretation

➔ *CPT Assistant* Apr 98:12

75831 Venography, renal, unilateral, selective, radiological supervision and interpretation

➔ *CPT Assistant* Sep 98:7

75833 Venography, renal, bilateral, selective, radiological supervision and interpretation

➔ *CPT Assistant* Sep 98:7

75840 Venography, adrenal, unilateral, selective, radiological supervision and interpretation

75842 Venography, adrenal, bilateral, selective, radiological supervision and interpretation

75860 Venography, venous sinus (eg, petrosal and inferior sagittal) or jugular, catheter, radiological supervision and interpretation

➔ *CPT Changes: An Insider's View* 2004

75870 Venography, superior sagittal sinus, radiological supervision and interpretation

75872 Venography, epidural, radiological supervision and interpretation

75880 Venography, orbital, radiological supervision and interpretation

75885 Percutaneous transhepatic portography with hemodynamic evaluation, radiological supervision and interpretation

➔ *CPT Assistant* Oct 96:4, Mar 02:10, Dec 03:2, Feb 07:11

75887 Percutaneous transhepatic portography without hemodynamic evaluation, radiological supervision and interpretation

➔ *CPT Assistant* Mar 02:10, Dec 03:2, Feb 07:11

75889 Hepatic venography, wedged or free, with hemodynamic evaluation, radiological supervision and interpretation

75891 Hepatic venography, wedged or free, without hemodynamic evaluation, radiological supervision and interpretation

75893 Venous sampling through catheter, with or without angiography (eg, for parathyroid hormone, renin), radiological supervision and interpretation

(For procedure, use 36500)

Transcatheter Procedures

Therapeutic transcatheter radiological supervision and interpretation code(s) include the following services associated with that intervention:

1. Contrast injections, angiography/venography, roadmapping, and fluoroscopic guidance for the intervention,

2. Vessel measurement, and

3. Completion angiography/venography (except for those uses permitted by 75898).

Unless specifically included in the code descriptor, diagnostic angiography/venography performed at the time of transcatheter therapeutic radiological and interpretation service(s) is separately reportable (eg, no prior catheter-based diagnostic angiography/venography study of the target vessel is available, prior diagnostic study is inadequate, patient's condition with respect to the clinical indication has changed since the prior study or during the intervention). See 75600-75893.

Codes 75956 and 75957 include all angiography of the thoracic aorta and its branches for diagnostic imaging prior to deployment of the primary endovascular devices (including all routine components of modular devices), fluoroscopic guidance in the delivery of the endovascular components, and intraprocedural arterial angiography (eg, confirm position, detect endoleak, evaluate runoff).

Code 75958 includes the analogous services for placement of each proximal thoracic endovascular extension. Code 75959 includes the analogous services for placement of a distal thoracic endovascular extension(s) placed during a procedure after the primary repair.

75894 Transcatheter therapy, embolization, any method, radiological supervision and interpretation

➔ *CPT Assistant* Sep 98:7

➔ *Clinical Examples in Radiology* Winter 07:1-3

(For uterine fibroid embolization [uterine artery embolization performed to treat uterine fibroids], use 37210)

(For obstetrical and gynecologic embolization procedures other than uterine fibroid embolization [eg, embolization to treat obstetrical or postpartum hemorrhage], use 37204)

75896 Transcatheter therapy, infusion, any method (eg, thrombolysis other than coronary), radiological supervision and interpretation

➔ *CPT Assistant* May 01:4

(For infusion for coronary disease, see 92975, 92977)

75898 Angiography through existing catheter for follow-up study for transcatheter therapy, embolization or infusion

➔ *CPT Changes: An Insider's View* 2002

75900 Exchange of a previously placed intravascular catheter during thrombolytic therapy with contrast monitoring, radiological supervision and interpretation

➔ *CPT Changes: An Insider's View* 2006

➔ *Clinical Examples in Radiology* Winter 06:20

(For procedure, use 37209)

75901 Mechanical removal of pericatheter obstructive material (eg, fibrin sheath) from central venous device via separate venous access, radiologic supervision and interpretation

➔ *CPT Assistant* Jul 03:13, Dec 04:12; *CPT Changes: An Insider's View* 2003

(For procedure, use 36595)

(For venous catheterization, see 36010-36012)

75902 Mechanical removal of intraluminal (intracatheter) obstructive material from central venous device through device lumen, radiologic supervision and interpretation

➔ *CPT Assistant* Jul 03:13, Dec 04:12; *CPT Changes: An Insider's View* 2003

(For procedure, use 36596)

(For venous catheterization, see 36010-36012)

75940 Percutaneous placement of IVC filter, radiological supervision and interpretation

➔ *CPT Assistant* Nov 00:11

➔ *Clinical Examples in Radiology* Winter 05:5-6

75945 Intravascular ultrasound (non-coronary vessel), radiological supervision and interpretation; initial vessel

+ 75946 each additional non-coronary vessel (List separately in addition to code for primary procedure)

(Use 75946 in conjunction with 75945)

(For catheterizations, see codes 36215-36248)

(For transcatheter therapies, see codes 37200-37208, 61624, 61626)

(For procedure, see 37250, 37251)

75952 Endovascular repair of infrarenal abdominal aortic aneurysm or dissection, radiological supervision and interpretation

➔ *CPT Changes: An Insider's View* 2001

(For implantation of endovascular grafts, see 34800-34808)

(For radiologic supervision and interpretation of endovascular repair of abdominal aortic aneurysm involving visceral vessels, see Category III codes 0078T-0081T)

75953 Placement of proximal or distal extension prosthesis for endovascular repair of infrarenal aortic or iliac artery aneurysm, pseudoaneurysm, or dissection, radiological supervision and interpretation

➔ *CPT Assistant* Feb 03:3; *CPT Changes: An Insider's View* 2001, 2003

(For implantation of endovascular extension prostheses, see 34825, 34826)

75954 Endovascular repair of iliac artery aneurysm, pseudoaneurysm, arteriovenous malformation, or trauma, radiological supervision and interpretation

➔ *CPT Assistant* Feb 03:3; *CPT Changes: An Insider's View* 2003

(For implantation of endovascular graft, see 34900)

75956 Endovascular repair of descending thoracic aorta (eg, aneurysm, pseudoaneurysm, dissection, penetrating ulcer, intramural hematoma, or traumatic disruption); involving coverage of left subclavian artery origin, initial endoprosthesis plus descending thoracic aortic extension(s), if required, to level of celiac artery origin, radiological supervision and interpretation

➔ *CPT Changes: An Insider's View* 2006

➔ *Clinical Examples in Radiology* Winter 06:17

(For implantation of endovascular graft, use 33880)

75957　not involving coverage of left subclavian artery origin, initial endoprosthesis plus descending thoracic aortic extension(s), if required, to level of celiac artery origin, radiological supervision and interpretation

➔ *CPT Changes: An Insider's View* 2006

➔ *Clinical Examples in Radiology* Winter 06:17

(For implantation of endovascular graft, use 33881)

75958　Placement of proximal extension prosthesis for endovascular repair of descending thoracic aorta (eg, aneurysm, pseudoaneurysm, dissection, penetrating ulcer, intramural hematoma, or traumatic disruption), radiological supervision and interpretation

➔ *CPT Changes: An Insider's View* 2006

➔ *Clinical Examples in Radiology* Winter 06:17

(Report 75958 for each proximal extension)

(For implantation of proximal endovascular extension, see 33883, 33884)

75959　Placement of distal extension prosthesis(s) (delayed) after endovascular repair of descending thoracic aorta, as needed, to level of celiac origin, radiological supervision and interpretation

➔ *CPT Changes: An Insider's View* 2006

➔ *Clinical Examples in Radiology* Winter 06:17

(Do not report 75959 in conjunction with 75956, 75957)

(Report 75959 once, regardless of number of modules deployed)

(For implantation of distal endovascular extension, use 33886)

75960　Transcatheter introduction of intravascular stent(s) (except coronary, carotid, and vertebral vessel), percutaneous and/or open, radiological supervision and interpretation, each vessel

➔ *CPT Assistant* Fall 93:18, Oct 96:2, May 01:4, Dec 03:2; *CPT Changes: An Insider's View* 2005

(For procedure, see 37205-37208)

(For radiologic supervision and interpretation for transcatheter placement of extracranial vertebral or intrathoracic carotid artery stent(s), see Category III codes 0075T, 0076T)

75961　Transcatheter retrieval, percutaneous, of intravascular foreign body (eg, fractured venous or arterial catheter), radiological supervision and interpretation

(For procedure, use 37203)

75962　Transluminal balloon angioplasty, peripheral artery, radiological supervision and interpretation

➔ *CPT Assistant* Fall 93:18, May 01:4

➔ *Clinical Examples in Radiology* Spring 07:1-3

+ 75964　Transluminal balloon angioplasty, each additional peripheral artery, radiological supervision and interpretation (List separately in addition to code for primary procedure)

(Use 75964 in conjunction with 75962)

75966　Transluminal balloon angioplasty, renal or other visceral artery, radiological supervision and interpretation

+ 75968　Transluminal balloon angioplasty, each additional visceral artery, radiological supervision and interpretation (List separately in addition to code for primary procedure)

(Use 75968 in conjunction with 75966)

(For percutaneous transluminal coronary angioplasty, see 92982-92984)

75970　Transcatheter biopsy, radiological supervision and interpretation

(For injection procedure only for transcatheter therapy or biopsy, see 36100-36299)

(For transcatheter renal and ureteral biopsy, use 52007)

(For percutaneous needle biopsy of pancreas, use 48102; of retroperitoneal lymph node or mass, use 49180)

75978　Transluminal balloon angioplasty, venous (eg, subclavian stenosis), radiological supervision and interpretation

➔ *CPT Assistant* Oct 96:4, Feb 97:2, May 01:4, Dec 03:2

➔ *Clinical Examples in Radiology* Spring 05:8-10, Spring 07:1-3

75980　Percutaneous transhepatic biliary drainage with contrast monitoring, radiological supervision and interpretation

75982　Percutaneous placement of drainage catheter for combined internal and external biliary drainage or of a drainage stent for internal biliary drainage in patients with an inoperable mechanical biliary obstruction, radiological supervision and interpretation

▲ **75984**　Change of percutaneous tube or drainage catheter with contrast monitoring (eg, genitourinary system, abscess), radiological supervision and interpretation

➔ *CPT Assistant* Nov 97:24; *CPT Changes: An Insider's View* 2008

▶(For percutaneous replacement of gastrostomy, duodenostomy, jejunostomy, gastro-jejunostomy, or cecostomy [or other colonic] tube including fluoroscopic imaging guidance, see 49450-49452)◀

(For change of nephrostomy or pyelostomy tube only, use 50398)

(For introduction procedure only for percutaneous biliary drainage, see 47510, 47511)

(For percutaneous cholecystostomy, use 47490)

(For change of percutaneous biliary drainage catheter only, use 47525)

(For percutaneous nephrostolithotomy or pyelostolithotomy, see 50080, 50081)

▶(For removal and/or replacement of an internally dwelling ureteral stent via a transurethral approach, see 50385-50386)◀

75989　Radiological guidance (ie, fluoroscopy, ultrasound, or computed tomography), for percutaneous drainage (eg, abscess, specimen collection), with placement of catheter, radiological supervision and interpretation

➔ *CPT Assistant* Nov 97:24, Mar 98:8, Feb 07:11; *CPT Changes: An Insider's View* 2001, 2002

Transluminal Atherectomy

75992 Transluminal atherectomy, peripheral artery, radiological supervision and interpretation

(For procedure, see 35481-35485, 35491-35495)

+ 75993 Transluminal atherectomy, each additional peripheral artery, radiological supervision and interpretation (List separately in addition to code for primary procedure)

(Use 75993 in conjunction with 75992)

(For procedure, see 35481-35485, 35491-35495)

75994 Transluminal atherectomy, renal, radiological supervision and interpretation

(For procedure, see 35480, 35490)

75995 Transluminal atherectomy, visceral, radiological supervision and interpretation

(For procedure, see 35480, 35490)

+ 75996 Transluminal atherectomy, each additional visceral artery, radiological supervision and interpretation (List separately in addition to code for primary procedure)

(Use 75996 in conjunction with 75995)

(For procedure, see 35480, 35490)

Other Procedures

(For computed tomography cerebral perfusion analysis, see Category III code 0042T)

(For arthrography of shoulder, use 73040; elbow, use 73085; wrist, use 73115; hip, use 73525; knee, use 73580; ankle, use 73615)

(75998 has been deleted. To report, use 77001)

76000 Fluoroscopy (separate procedure), up to 1 hour physician time, other than 71023 or 71034 (eg, cardiac fluoroscopy)

→ *CPT Assistant* Apr 96:11, Nov 99:32, Dec 00:14, Apr 03:7, Jul 03:16, Aug 03:14; *CPT Changes: An Insider's View* 2000

76001 Fluoroscopy, physician time more than 1 hour, assisting a nonradiologic physician (eg, nephrostolithotomy, ERCP, bronchoscopy, transbronchial biopsy)

(76003 has been deleted. To report, use 77002)

(76005 has been deleted. To report, use 77003)

(76006 has been deleted. To report, use 77071)

76010 Radiologic examination from nose to rectum for foreign body, single view, child

→ *CPT Changes: An Insider's View* 2001

(76012, 76013 have been deleted. To report, see 72291, 72292)

(76020 has been deleted. To report, use 77072)

(76040 has been deleted. To report, use 77073)

(76061, 76062 have been deleted. To report, see 77074, 77075)

(76065 has been deleted. To report, use 77076)

(76066 has been deleted. To report, use 77077)

(76070, 76071 have been deleted. To report, see 77078, 77079)

(76075-76077 have been deleted. To report, see 77080-77082)

(76078 has been deleted. To report, use 77083)

76080 Radiologic examination, abscess, fistula or sinus tract study, radiological supervision and interpretation

→ *CPT Assistant* Nov 97:24, Mar 98:8, Nov 03:14, Dec 06:10

▶(For contrast injection[s] and radiological assessment of gastrostomy, duodenostomy, jejunostomy, gastro-jejunostomy, or cecostomy [or other colonic] tube including fluoroscopic imaging guidance, use 49465)◀

(76082, 76083 have been deleted. To report, see 77051, 77052)

(76085 has been deleted. To report, see 77051, 77052)

(76086 has been deleted. To report, use 77053)

(76088 has been deleted. To report, use 77054)

(76090, 76091 have been deleted. To report, see 77055, 77056)

(76092 has been deleted. To report, use 77057)

(76093, 76094 have been deleted. To report, see 77058, 77059)

(76095 has been deleted. To report, use 77031)

(76096 has been deleted. To report, use 77032)

76098 Radiological examination, surgical specimen

76100 Radiologic examination, single plane body section (eg, tomography), other than with urography

76101 Radiologic examination, complex motion (ie, hypercycloidal) body section (eg, mastoid polytomography), other than with urography; unilateral

76102   bilateral

(For nephrotomography, use 74415)

76120 Cineradiography/videoradiography, except where specifically included

→ *CPT Assistant* Sep 00:4, Apr 04:15; *CPT Changes: An Insider's View* 2002

+ 76125 Cineradiography/videoradiography to complement routine examination (List separately in addition to code for primary procedure)

→ *CPT Assistant* Oct 97:1, Sep 00:4; *CPT Changes: An Insider's View* 2002

76140 Consultation on X-ray examination made elsewhere, written report

→ *CPT Assistant* Summer 91:13, Oct 97:1

76150 Xeroradiography

(76150 is to be used for non-mammographic studies only)

76350   Subtraction in conjunction with contrast studies

(76355 has been deleted. To report, use 77011)

(76360 has been deleted. To report, use 77012)

(76362 has been deleted. To report, use 77013)

(76370 has been deleted. To report, use 77014)

(76375 has been deleted)

(2D reformatting is no longer separately reported. To report 3D rendering, see 76376, 76377)

(76376, 76377 require concurrent physician supervision of image postprocessing 3D manipulation of volumetric data set and image rendering)

76376   3D rendering with interpretation and reporting of computed tomography, magnetic resonance imaging, ultrasound, or other tomographic modality; not requiring image postprocessing on an independent workstation

➔ *CPT Assistant* Dec 05:1, 7, Jan 07:31; *CPT Changes: An Insider's View* 2006

➔ *Clinical Examples in Radiology* Winter 06:17, Spring 06:8-9, Fall 06:9-10, Winter 07:4-5

(Use 76376 in conjunction with code[s] for base imaging procedure[s])

▶(Do not report 76376 in conjunction with 70496, 70498, 70544-70549, 71275, 71555, 72159, 72191, 72198, 73206, 73225, 73706, 73725, 74175, 74185, 75635, 75557-75564, 76377, 78000-78999, 0066T, 0067T, 0144T-0151T, 0159T)◀

76377   requiring image postprocessing on an independent workstation

➔ *CPT Assistant* Dec 05:1, Jan 07:31; *CPT Changes: An Insider's View* 2006

➔ *Clinical Examples in Radiology* Winter 06:17, Spring 06:8-9, Fall 06:9-10, Winter 07:4-5

(Use 76377 in conjunction with code[s] for base imaging procedure[s])

▶(Do not report 76377 in conjunction with 70496, 70498, 70544-70549, 71275, 71555, 72159, 72191, 72198, 73206, 73225, 73706, 73725, 74175, 74185, 75557-75564, 75635, 76376, 78000-78999, 0066T, 0067T, 0144T-0151T, 0159T)◀

▶(To report computer-aided detection, including computer algorithm analysis of MRI data for lesion detection/characterization, pharmacokinetic analysis, breast MRI, use Category III code 0159T)◀

76380   Computed tomography, limited or localized follow-up study

➔ *CPT Changes: An Insider's View* 2002, 2003

76390   Magnetic resonance spectroscopy

➔ *CPT Assistant* Nov 97:25

(For magnetic resonance imaging, use appropriate MRI body site code)

(76393 has been deleted. To report, use 77021)

(76394 has been deleted. To report, use 77022)

(76400 has been deleted. To report, use 77084)

76496   Unlisted fluoroscopic procedure (eg, diagnostic, interventional)

➔ *CPT Changes: An Insider's View* 2003

76497   Unlisted computed tomography procedure (eg, diagnostic, interventional)

➔ *CPT Assistant* Jun 05:11; *CPT Changes: An Insider's View* 2003

➔ *Clinical Examples in Radiology* Spring 05:1, 7

76498   Unlisted magnetic resonance procedure (eg, diagnostic, interventional)

➔ *CPT Changes: An Insider's View* 2003

76499   Unlisted diagnostic radiographic procedure

➔ *CPT Assistant* Jul 99:10, Sep 00:4, Apr 04:15, Nov 06:22; *CPT Changes: An Insider's View* 2003

Diagnostic Ultrasound

All diagnostic ultrasound examinations require permanently recorded images with measurements, when such measurements are clinically indicated. For those codes whose sole diagnostic goal is a biometric measure (ie, 76514, 76516, and 76519), permanently recorded images are not required. A final, written report should be issued for inclusion in the patient's medical record. The prescription form for the intraocular lens satisfies the written report requirement for 76519. For those anatomic regions that have "complete" and "limited" ultrasound codes, note the elements that comprise a "complete" exam. The report should contain a description of these elements or the reason that an element could not be visualized (eg, obscured by bowel gas, surgically absent).

If less than the required elements for a "complete" exam are reported (eg, limited number of organs or limited portion of region evaluated), the "limited" code for that anatomic region should be used once per patient exam session. A "limited" exam of an anatomic region should not be reported for the same exam session as a "complete" exam of that same region.

▶Evaluation of vascular structures using both color and spectral Doppler is separately reportable. To report, see Noninvasive Vascular Diagnostic Studies (93875-93990). However, color Doppler alone, when performed for anatomic structure identification in conjunction with a real-time ultrasound examination, is not reported separately.◀

Ultrasound guidance procedures also require permanently recorded images of the site to be localized, as well as a documented description of the localization process, either separately or within the report of the procedure for which the guidance is utilized.

Use of ultrasound, without thorough evaluation of organ(s) or anatomic region, image documentation, and final, written report, is not separately reportable.

Definitions

A-mode implies a one-dimensional ultrasonic measurement procedure.

M-mode implies a one-dimensional ultrasonic measurement procedure with movement of the trace to record amplitude and velocity of moving echo-producing structures.

B-scan implies a two-dimensional ultrasonic scanning procedure with a two-dimensional display.

Real-time scan implies a two-dimensional ultrasonic scanning procedure with display of both two-dimensional structure and motion with time.

(To report diagnostic vascular ultrasound studies, see 93875-93990)

(For focused ultrasound ablation treatment of uterine leiomyomata, see Category III codes 0071T, 0072T)

Head and Neck

▲ **76506** Echoencephalography, real time with image documentation (gray scale) (for determination of ventricular size, delineation of cerebral contents, and detection of fluid masses or other intracranial abnormalities), including A-mode encephalography as secondary component where indicated
➔ *CPT Changes: An Insider's View* 2007, 2008

76510 Ophthalmic ultrasound, diagnostic; B-scan and quantitative A-scan performed during the same patient encounter
➔ *CPT Assistant* Dec 05:3; *CPT Changes: An Insider's View* 2005

76511 quantitative A-scan only
➔ *CPT Assistant* Winter 93:12, Oct 96:9, Nov 99:42, Jul 04:12, Dec 05:3; *CPT Changes: An Insider's View* 2005

76512 B-scan (with or without superimposed non-quantitative A-scan)
➔ *CPT Assistant* Winter 93:12, Oct 96:9, Dec 05:3; *CPT Changes: An Insider's View* 2005

76513 anterior segment ultrasound, immersion (water bath) B-scan or high resolution biomicroscopy
➔ *CPT Assistant* Winter 93:12, Nov 99:42; *CPT Changes: An Insider's View* 2000

76514 corneal pachymetry, unilateral or bilateral (determination of corneal thickness)
➔ *CPT Assistant* Jul 04:12, 15, Feb 05:13, Jun 05:11, Dec 05:3; *CPT Changes: An Insider's View* 2004

76516 Ophthalmic biometry by ultrasound echography, A-scan;
➔ *CPT Assistant* Oct 03:10, Dec 05:3

76519 with intraocular lens power calculation
➔ *CPT Assistant* Winter 93:12, Oct 03:10, Dec 05:3

(For partial coherence interferometry, use 92136)

76529 Ophthalmic ultrasonic foreign body localization
➔ *CPT Assistant* Winter 93:12

76536 Ultrasound, soft tissues of head and neck (eg, thyroid, parathyroid, parotid), real time with image documentation
➔ *CPT Changes: An Insider's View* 2002, 2007

Chest

76604 Ultrasound, chest (includes mediastinum), real time with image documentation
➔ *CPT Changes: An Insider's View* 2002, 2007

76645 Ultrasound, breast(s) (unilateral or bilateral), real time with image documentation
➔ *CPT Changes: An Insider's View* 2002, 2007
➔ *Clinical Examples in Radiology* Fall 05:8

Abdomen and Retroperitoneum

A complete ultrasound examination of the abdomen (76700) consists of real time scans of the liver, gall bladder, common bile duct, pancreas, spleen, kidneys, and the upper abdominal aorta and inferior vena cava including any demonstrated abdominal abnormality.

A complete ultrasound examination of the retroperitoneum (76770) consists of real time scans of the kidneys, abdominal aorta, common iliac artery origins, and inferior vena cava, including any demonstrated retroperitoneal abnormality. Alternatively, if clinical history suggests urinary tract pathology, complete evaluation of the kidneys and urinary bladder also comprises a complete retroperitoneal ultrasound.

Use of ultrasound, without thorough evaluation of organ(s) or anatomic region, image documentation and final, written report, is not separately reportable.

76700 Ultrasound, abdominal, real time with image documentation; complete
➔ *CPT Assistant* Fall 93:13, Oct 01:3, Dec 05:3, Mar 07:7; *CPT Changes: An Insider's View* 2002, 2007
➔ *Clinical Examples in Radiology* Winter 05:9, 11

76705 limited (eg, single organ, quadrant, follow-up)
➔ *CPT Assistant* Fall 93:13, Oct 01:3, Apr 03:27, Dec 05:3
➔ *Clinical Examples in Radiology* Winter 05:9, 11

76770 Ultrasound, retroperitoneal (eg, renal, aorta, nodes), real time with image documentation; complete
➔ *CPT Assistant* May 99:10, Jun 99:10; *CPT Changes: An Insider's View* 2002, 2007
➔ *Clinical Examples in Radiology* Winter 05:9, 11

76775 limited
➔ *CPT Assistant* May 99:10, Jun 99:10, Dec 05:3
➔ *Clinical Examples in Radiology* Winter 05:9, 11, Winter 07:8-10, Spring 07:5-6

76776 Ultrasound, transplanted kidney, real time and duplex Doppler with image documentation
➔ *CPT Changes: An Insider's View* 2007

(For ultrasound of transplanted kidney without duplex Doppler, use 76775)

(Do not report 76776 in conjunction with 93975, 93976)

(76778 has been deleted. To report, see 76775, 76776)

Spinal Canal

76800   Ultrasound, spinal canal and contents

> *CPT Assistant* Apr 98:15; *CPT Changes: An Insider's View* 2002

Pelvis

Obstetrical

Codes 76801 and 76802 include determination of the number of gestational sacs and fetuses, gestational sac/fetal measurements appropriate for gestation (younger than 14 weeks 0 days), survey of visible fetal and placental anatomic structure, qualitative assessment of amniotic fluid volume/gestational sac shape and examination of the maternal uterus and adnexa.

Codes 76805 and 76810 include determination of number of fetuses and amniotic/chorionic sacs, measurements appropriate for gestational age (older than or equal to 14 weeks 0 days), survey of intracranial/spinal/abdominal anatomy, 4 chambered heart, umbilical cord insertion site, placenta location and amniotic fluid assessment and, when visible, examination of maternal adnexa.

Codes 76811 and 76812 include all elements of codes 76805 and 76810 plus detailed anatomic evaluation of the fetal brain/ventricles, face, heart/outflow tracts and chest anatomy, abdominal organ specific anatomy, number/length/architecture of limbs and detailed evaluation of the umbilical cord and placenta and other fetal anatomy as clinically indicated.

Report should document the results of the evaluation of each element described above or the reason for non-visualization.

Code 76815 represents a focused "quick look" exam limited to the assessment of one or more of the elements listed in code 76815.

Code 76816 describes an examination designed to reassess fetal size and interval growth or reevaluate one or more anatomic abnormalities of a fetus previously demonstrated on ultrasound, and should be coded once for each fetus requiring reevaluation using modifier 59 for each fetus after the first.

Code 76817 describes a transvaginal obstetric ultrasound performed separately or in addition to one of the transabdominal examinations described above. For transvaginal examinations performed for non-obstetrical purposes, use code 76830.

76801   Ultrasound, pregnant uterus, real time with image documentation, fetal and maternal evaluation, first trimester (< 14 weeks 0 days), transabdominal approach; single or first gestation

> *CPT Assistant* Mar 03:7, Nov 05:15; *CPT Changes: An Insider's View* 2003

> *Clinical Examples in Radiology* Winter 07:6-7

(To report first trimester fetal nuchal translucency measurement, use 76813)

+ 76802   each additional gestation (List separately in addition to code for primary procedure)

> *CPT Assistant* Mar 03:7, Nov 05:15; *CPT Changes: An Insider's View* 2003

> *Clinical Examples in Radiology* Winter 07:6-7

(Use 76802 in conjunction with 76801)

(To report first trimester fetal nuchal translucency measurement, use 76814)

76805   Ultrasound, pregnant uterus, real time with image documentation, fetal and maternal evaluation, after first trimester (> or = 14 weeks 0 days), transabdominal approach; single or first gestation

> *CPT Assistant* Apr 97:2, Nov 97:25, Oct 01:3, Aug 02:2, Mar 03:7; *CPT Changes: An Insider's View* 2002, 2003

> *Clinical Examples in Radiology* Winter 05:3-4

+ 76810   each additional gestation (List separately in addition to code for primary procedure)

> *CPT Assistant* Apr 97:2, Oct 01:3, Aug 02:2, Mar 03:7; *CPT Changes: An Insider's View* 2003

> *Clinical Examples in Radiology* Winter 05:4

(Use 76810 in conjunction with 76805)

76811   Ultrasound, pregnant uterus, real time with image documentation, fetal and maternal evaluation plus detailed fetal anatomic examination, transabdominal approach; single or first gestation

> *CPT Assistant* Mar 03:7; *CPT Changes: An Insider's View* 2003

> *Clinical Examples in Radiology* Winter 05:4

+ 76812   each additional gestation (List separately in addition to code for primary procedure)

> *CPT Assistant* Mar 03:7; *CPT Changes: An Insider's View* 2003

(Use 76812 in conjunction with 76811)

76813   Ultrasound, pregnant uterus, real time with image documentation, first trimester fetal nuchal translucency measurement, transabdominal or transvaginal approach; single or first gestation

> *CPT Changes: An Insider's View* 2007

+ 76814   each additional gestation (List separately in addition to code for primary procedure)

> *CPT Changes: An Insider's View* 2007

(Use 76814 in conjunction with 76813)

76815   Ultrasound, pregnant uterus, real time with image documentation, limited (eg, fetal heart beat, placental location, fetal position and/or qualitative amniotic fluid volume), one or more fetuses

> *CPT Assistant* Apr 97:2, Nov 97:25, Oct 01:3, Dec 01:6, Aug 02:2, Mar 03:7, Nov 03:14; *CPT Changes: An Insider's View* 2003

> *Clinical Examples in Radiology* Winter 07:6-7

(Use 76815 only once per exam and not per element)

(To report first trimester fetal nuchal translucency measurement, see 76813, 76814)

76816 Ultrasound, pregnant uterus, real time with image documentation, follow-up (eg, re-evaluation of fetal size by measuring standard growth parameters and amniotic fluid volume, re-evaluation of organ system(s) suspected or confirmed to be abnormal on a previous scan), transabdominal approach, per fetus

➜ *CPT Assistant* Apr 97:2, Oct 01:3, Aug 02:2, Mar 03:7; *CPT Changes: An Insider's View* 2003

(Report 76816 with modifier 59 for each additional fetus examined in a multiple pregnancy)

76817 Ultrasound, pregnant uterus, real time with image documentation, transvaginal

➜ *CPT Assistant* Mar 03:7; *CPT Changes: An Insider's View* 2003

(For non-obstetrical transvaginal ultrasound, use 76830)

(If transvaginal examination is done in addition to transabdominal obstetrical ultrasound exam, use 76817 in addition to appropriate transabdominal exam code)

76818 Fetal biophysical profile; with non-stress testing

➜ *CPT Assistant* Apr 97:2, May 98:10, Sep 01:4, Oct 01:3, Dec 01:6, Oct 04:10; *CPT Changes: An Insider's View* 2001

76819 without non-stress testing

➜ *CPT Assistant* Sep 01:8, Dec 01:6; *CPT Changes: An Insider's View* 2001, 2002

(Fetal biophysical profile assessments for the second and any additional fetuses, should be reported separately by code 76818 or 76819 with the modifier 59 appended)

(For amniotic fluid index without non-stress test, use 76815)

76820 Doppler velocimetry, fetal; umbilical artery

➜ *CPT Assistant* Dec 05:3; *CPT Changes: An Insider's View* 2005

76821 middle cerebral artery

➜ *CPT Assistant* Dec 05:3; *CPT Changes: An Insider's View* 2005

76825 Echocardiography, fetal, cardiovascular system, real time with image documentation (2D), with or without M-mode recording;

➜ *CPT Assistant* Apr 97:2, Aug 02:2

76826 follow-up or repeat study

➜ *CPT Assistant* Apr 97:2, Aug 02:2

76827 Doppler echocardiography, fetal, pulsed wave and/or continuous wave with spectral display; complete

➜ *CPT Assistant* Apr 97:2, Aug 02:2, Dec 05:3; *CPT Changes: An Insider's View* 2005

76828 follow-up or repeat study

➜ *CPT Assistant* Apr 97:2, Aug 02:2, Dec 05:3

(To report the use of color mapping, use 93325)

Nonobstetrical

Code 76856 includes the complete evaluation of the female pelvic anatomy. Elements of this examination include a description and measurements of the uterus and adnexal structures, measurement of the endometrium, measurement of the bladder (when applicable), and a description of any pelvic pathology (eg, ovarian cysts, uterine leiomyomata, free pelvic fluid).

Code 76856 is also applicable to a complete evaluation of the male pelvis. Elements of the examination include evaluation and measurement (when applicable) of the urinary bladder, evaluation of the prostate and seminal vesicles to the extent that they are visualized transabdominally, and any pelvic pathology (eg, bladder tumor, enlarged prostate, free pelvic fluid, pelvic abscess).

Code 76857 represents a focused examination limited to the assessment of one or more elements listed in code 76856 and/or the reevaluation of one or more pelvic abnormalities previously demonstrated on ultrasound. Code 76857, rather than 76770, should be utilized if the urinary bladder alone (ie, not including the kidneys) is imaged, whereas code 51798 should be utilized if a bladder volume or post-void residual measurement is obtained without imaging the bladder.

Use of ultrasound, without thorough evaluation of organ(s) or anatomic region, image documentation, and final, written report, is not separately reportable.

76830 Ultrasound, transvaginal

➜ *CPT Assistant* Aug 96:10, Jul 99:8, Aug 02:2, Mar 03:7, Dec 05:3; *CPT Changes: An Insider's View* 2002

➜ *Clinical Examples in Radiology* Inaugural 04:6-7

(For obstetrical transvaginal ultrasound, use 76817)

(If transvaginal examination is done in addition to transabdominal non-obstetrical ultrasound exam, use 76830 in addition to appropriate transabdominal exam code)

76831 Saline infusion sonohysterography (SIS), including color flow Doppler, when performed

➜ *CPT Assistant* Nov 97:25, Jul 99:8, Dec 05:3; *CPT Changes: An Insider's View* 2004

(For introduction of saline for saline infusion sonohysterography, use 58340)

76856 Ultrasound, pelvic (nonobstetric), real time with image documentation; complete

➜ *CPT Assistant* Oct 01:3, Dec 05:3, Jan 06:47, Mar 07:7; *CPT Changes: An Insider's View* 2002, 2007

➜ *Clinical Examples in Radiology* Inaugural 04:6-7

76857 limited or follow-up (eg, for follicles)

➜ *CPT Assistant* Jun 97:10, Oct 01:3, Dec 05:3

Genitalia

76870   Ultrasound, scrotum and contents
> *CPT Assistant* May 05:3; *CPT Changes: An Insider's View* 2002

76872   Ultrasound, transrectal;
> *CPT Assistant* May 96:3, Nov 99:42; *CPT Changes: An Insider's View* 2000, 2004

76873   prostate volume study for brachytherapy treatment planning (separate procedure)
> *CPT Assistant* Nov 99:42; *CPT Changes: An Insider's View* 2000

Extremities

76880   Ultrasound, extremity, nonvascular, real time with image documentation
> *CPT Changes: An Insider's View* 2002, 2007

76885   Ultrasound, infant hips, real time with imaging documentation; dynamic (requiring physician manipulation)
> *CPT Assistant* Nov 97:25; *CPT Changes: An Insider's View* 2002

76886   limited, static (not requiring physician manipulation)
> *CPT Assistant* Nov 97:25; *CPT Changes: An Insider's View* 2002

Ultrasonic Guidance Procedures

76930   Ultrasonic guidance for pericardiocentesis, imaging supervision and interpretation
> *CPT Changes: An Insider's View* 2001

76932   Ultrasonic guidance for endomyocardial biopsy, imaging supervision and interpretation
> *CPT Changes: An Insider's View* 2001

76936   Ultrasound guided compression repair of arterial pseudoaneurysm or arteriovenous fistulae (includes diagnostic ultrasound evaluation, compression of lesion and imaging)

+ 76937   Ultrasound guidance for vascular access requiring ultrasound evaluation of potential access sites, documentation of selected vessel patency, concurrent realtime ultrasound visualization of vascular needle entry, with permanent recording and reporting (List separately in addition to code for primary procedure)
> *CPT Assistant* Dec 04:13; *CPT Changes: An Insider's View* 2004
> *Clinical Examples in Radiology* Inaugural 04:1-2, Winter 05:5-6, Summer 06:8-9

(Do not use 76937 in conjunction with 76942)

(If extremity venous non-invasive vascular diagnostic study is performed separate from venous access guidance, use 93965, 93970 or 93971)

76940   Ultrasound guidance for, and monitoring of, parenchymal tissue ablation
> *CPT Assistant* Oct 02:2, Mar 07:7; *CPT Changes: An Insider's View* 2004, 2007

(Do not report 76940 in conjunction with 76998)

►(For ablation, see 32998, 47370-47382, 50592, 50593)◄

76941   Ultrasonic guidance for intrauterine fetal transfusion or cordocentesis, imaging supervision and interpretation
> *CPT Changes: An Insider's View* 2001

(For procedure, see 36460, 59012)

76942   Ultrasonic guidance for needle placement (eg, biopsy, aspiration, injection, localization device), imaging supervision and interpretation
> *CPT Assistant* Fall 93:12, Fall 94:2, May 96:3, Jun 97:5, Oct 01:2, May 04:7, Dec 04:12, Apr 05:15-16; *CPT Changes: An Insider's View* 2001
> *Clinical Examples in Radiology* Summer 05:1, 2, 6, Fall 05:1

(Do not report 76942 in conjunction with 43232, 43237, 43242, 45341, 45342, or 76975)

(For microwave thermotherapy of the breast, use Category III code 0061T)

76945   Ultrasonic guidance for chorionic villus sampling, imaging supervision and interpretation
> *CPT Changes: An Insider's View* 2001

(For procedure, use 59015)

76946   Ultrasonic guidance for amniocentesis, imaging supervision and interpretation
> *CPT Changes: An Insider's View* 2001

76948   Ultrasonic guidance for aspiration of ova, imaging supervision and interpretation
> *CPT Changes: An Insider's View* 2001

76950   Ultrasonic guidance for placement of radiation therapy fields
> *CPT Changes: An Insider's View* 2001

76965   Ultrasonic guidance for interstitial radioelement application

Other Procedures

76970   Ultrasound study follow-up (specify)

76975   Gastrointestinal endoscopic ultrasound, supervision and interpretation
> *CPT Assistant* Spring 94:5, May 04:7; *CPT Changes: An Insider's View* 2001

(Do not report 76975 in conjunction with 43231, 43232, 43237, 43238, 43242, 43259, 45341, 45342, or 76942)

76977   Ultrasound bone density measurement and interpretation, peripheral site(s), any method
> *CPT Assistant* Nov 98:21

(76986 has been deleted. To report, use 76998)

76998   Ultrasonic guidance, intraoperative
> *CPT Changes: An Insider's View* 2007

(Do not report 76998 in conjunction with 47370-47382)

(For ultrasound guidance for open and laparoscopic radiofrequency tissue ablation, use 76940)

76999 Unlisted ultrasound procedure (eg, diagnostic, interventional)

→ *CPT Changes: An Insider's View* 2003

Radiologic Guidance

Fluoroscopic Guidance

+ **77001** Fluoroscopic guidance for central venous access device placement, replacement (catheter only or complete), or removal (includes fluoroscopic guidance for vascular access and catheter manipulation, any necessary contrast injections through access site or catheter with related venography radiologic supervision and interpretation, and radiographic documentation of final catheter position) (List separately in addition to code for primary procedure)

→ *CPT Changes: An Insider's View* 2007

(Do not use 77001 in conjunction with 77002)

(If formal extremity venography is performed from separate venous access and separately interpreted, use 36005 and 75820, 75822, 75825, or 75827)

77002 Fluoroscopic guidance for needle placement (eg, biopsy, aspiration, injection, localization device)

→ *CPT Changes: An Insider's View* 2007

(See appropriate surgical code for procedure and anatomic location)

(77002 includes all radiographic arthrography with the exception of supervision and interpretation for CT and MR arthrography)

(Do not report 77002 in addition to 70332, 73040, 73085, 73115, 73525, 73580, 73615)

▶(77002 is included in the organ/anatomic specific radiological supervision and interpretation procedures 49440, 74320, 74355, 74445, 74470, 74475, 75809, 75810, 75885, 75887, 75980, 75982, 75989)◀

77003 Fluoroscopic guidance and localization of needle or catheter tip for spine or paraspinous diagnostic or therapeutic injection procedures (epidural, transforaminal epidural, subarachnoid, paravertebral facet joint, paravertebral facet joint nerve, or sacroiliac joint), including neurolytic agent destruction

→ *CPT Changes: An Insider's View* 2007

(Injection of contrast during fluoroscopic guidance and localization [77003] is included in 22526, 22527, 62263, 62264, 62270-62282, 62310-62319, 0027T)

(Fluoroscopic guidance for subarachnoid puncture for diagnostic radiographic myelography is included in supervision and interpretation codes 72240-72270)

(For epidural or subarachnoid needle or catheter placement and injection, see 62270-62282, 62310-62319)

(For sacroiliac joint arthrography, see 27096, 73542. If formal arthrography is not performed and recorded, and a formal radiographic report is not issued, use 77003 for fluoroscopic guidance for sacroiliac joint injections)

(For paravertebral facet joint injection, see 64470-64476. For transforaminal epidural needle placement and injection, see 64479-64484)

(For destruction by neurolytic agent, see 64600-64680)

(For percutaneous or endoscopic lysis of epidural adhesions, 62263, 62264, 0027T include fluoroscopic guidance and localization)

Computed Tomography Guidance

77011 Computed tomography guidance for stereotactic localization

→ *CPT Changes: An Insider's View* 2007

77012 Computed tomography guidance for needle placement (eg, biopsy, aspiration, injection, localization device), radiological supervision and interpretation

→ *CPT Changes: An Insider's View* 2007

77013 Computed tomography guidance for, and monitoring of, parenchymal tissue ablation

→ *CPT Changes: An Insider's View* 2007

(Do not report 77013 in conjunction with 20982)

▶(For percutaneous radiofrequency ablation, see 32998, 47382, 50592, 50593)◀

77014 Computed tomography guidance for placement of radiation therapy fields

→ *CPT Changes: An Insider's View* 2007

▶(For placement of interstitial device[s] for radiation therapy guidance, prostate, use 55876)◀

Magnetic Resonance Guidance

77021 Magnetic resonance guidance for needle placement (eg, for biopsy, needle aspiration, injection, or placement of localization device) radiological supervision and interpretation

→ *CPT Changes: An Insider's View* 2007

(For procedure, see appropriate organ or site)

77022 Magnetic resonance guidance for, and monitoring of, parenchymal tissue ablation

→ *CPT Changes: An Insider's View* 2007

▶(For percutaneous radiofrequency ablation, see 32998, 47382, 50592, 50593)◀

(For focused ultrasound ablation treatment of uterine leiomyomata, see Category III codes 0071T, 0072T)

Other Radiologic Guidance

77031   Stereotactic localization guidance for breast biopsy or needle placement (eg, for wire localization or for injection), each lesion, radiological supervision and interpretation

➲ *CPT Changes: An Insider's View* 2007

(For procedure, see 10022, 19000-19103, 19290, 19291)

(For injection for sentinel node localization without lymphoscintigraphy, use 38792)

77032   Mammographic guidance for needle placement, breast (eg, for wire localization or for injection), each lesion, radiological supervision and interpretation

➲ *CPT Changes: An Insider's View* 2007

(For procedure, see 10022, 19000, 19102, 19103, 19290, 19291)

(For injection for sentinel node localization without lymphoscintigraphy, use 38792)

Breast, Mammography

(For mammographic guidance for needle placement of breast lesion, use 77032)

+ 77051   Computer-aided detection (computer algorithm analysis of digital image data for lesion detection) with further physician review for interpretation, with or without digitization of film radiographic images; diagnostic mammography (List separately in addition to code for primary procedure)

➲ *CPT Changes: An Insider's View* 2007

(Use 77051 in conjunction with 77055, 77056)

+ 77052   screening mammography (List separately in addition to code for primary procedure)

➲ *CPT Changes: An Insider's View* 2007

(Use 77052 in conjunction with 77057)

77053   Mammary ductogram or galactogram, single duct, radiological supervision and interpretation

➲ *CPT Changes: An Insider's View* 2007

(For mammary ductogram or galactogram injection, use 19030)

77054   Mammary ductogram or galactogram, multiple ducts, radiological supervision and interpretation

➲ *CPT Changes: An Insider's View* 2007

77055   Mammography; unilateral

➲ *CPT Changes: An Insider's View* 2007

77056   bilateral

➲ *CPT Changes: An Insider's View* 2007

(Use 77055, 77056 in conjunction with 77051 for computer-aided detection applied to a diagnostic mammogram)

77057   Screening mammography, bilateral (2-view film study of each breast)

➲ *CPT Changes: An Insider's View* 2007

(Use 77057 in conjunction with 77052 for computer-aided detection applied to a screening mammogram)

(To report electrical impedance scan of the breast, bilateral, use Category III code 0060T)

Screening Mammography
77057

Mammogram

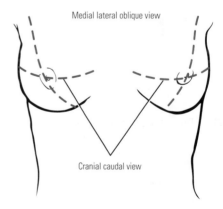

Medial lateral oblique view

Cranial caudal view

77058   Magnetic resonance imaging, breast, without and/or with contrast material(s); unilateral

➲ *CPT Changes: An Insider's View* 2007

77059   bilateral

➲ *CPT Changes: An Insider's View* 2007

Bone/Joint Studies

77071 Manual application of stress performed by physician for joint radiography, including contralateral joint if indicated

→ *CPT Changes: An Insider's View* 2007

(For radiographic interpretation of stressed images, see appropriate anatomic site and number of views)

77072 Bone age studies

→ *CPT Changes: An Insider's View* 2007

77073 Bone length studies (orthoroentgenogram, scanogram)

→ *CPT Changes: An Insider's View* 2007

77074 Radiologic examination, osseous survey; limited (eg, for metastases)

→ *CPT Changes: An Insider's View* 2007

77075   complete (axial and appendicular skeleton)

→ *CPT Changes: An Insider's View* 2007

77076 Radiologic examination, osseous survey, infant

→ *CPT Changes: An Insider's View* 2007

77077 Joint survey, single view, 2 or more joints (specify)

→ *CPT Changes: An Insider's View* 2007

77078 Computed tomography, bone mineral density study, 1 or more sites; axial skeleton (eg, hips, pelvis, spine)

→ *CPT Changes: An Insider's View* 2007

77079   appendicular skeleton (peripheral) (eg, radius, wrist, heel)

→ *CPT Changes: An Insider's View* 2007

77080 Dual-energy X-ray absorptiometry (DXA), bone density study, 1 or more sites; axial skeleton (eg, hips, pelvis, spine)

→ *CPT Changes: An Insider's View* 2007

77081   appendicular skeleton (peripheral) (eg, radius, wrist, heel)

→ *CPT Changes: An Insider's View* 2007

77082   vertebral fracture assessment

→ *CPT Changes: An Insider's View* 2007

(To report dual-energy X-ray absorptiometry [DXA] body composition study, 1 or more sites, use Category III code 0028T)

77083 Radiographic absorptiometry (eg, photodensitometry, radiogrammetry), 1 or more sites

→ *CPT Changes: An Insider's View* 2007

77084 Magnetic resonance (eg, proton) imaging, bone marrow blood supply

→ *CPT Changes: An Insider's View* 2007

Radiation Oncology

Listings for Radiation Oncology provide for teletherapy and brachytherapy to include initial consultation, clinical treatment planning, simulation, medical radiation physics, dosimetry, treatment devices, special services, and clinical treatment management procedures. They include normal follow-up care during course of treatment and for three months following its completion.

When a service or procedure is provided that is not listed in this edition of the CPT codebook it should be identified by a Special Report (see page 300) and one of the following unlisted procedure codes:

77299 Unlisted procedure, therapeutic radiology clinical treatment planning

77399 Unlisted procedure, medical radiation physics, dosimetry and treatment devices, and special services

77499 Unlisted procedure, therapeutic radiology treatment management

77799 Unlisted procedure, clinical brachytherapy

For treatment by injectable or ingestible isotopes, see subsection **Nuclear Medicine.**

Consultation: Clinical Management

Preliminary consultation, evaluation of patient prior to decision to treat, or full medical care (in addition to treatment management) when provided by the therapeutic radiologist may be identified by the appropriate procedure codes from **Evaluation and Management, Medicine,** or **Surgery** sections.

Clinical Treatment Planning (External and Internal Sources)

The clinical treatment planning process is a complex service including interpretation of special testing, tumor localization, treatment volume determination, treatment time/dosage determination, choice of treatment modality, determination of number and size of treatment ports, selection of appropriate treatment devices, and other procedures.

Definitions

Simple planning requires a single treatment area of interest encompassed in a single port or simple parallel opposed ports with simple or no blocking.

Intermediate planning requires three or more converging ports, two separate treatment areas, multiple blocks, or special time dose constraints.

Complex planning requires highly complex blocking, custom shielding blocks, tangential ports, special wedges or compensators, three or more separate treatment areas, rotational or special beam considerations, combination of therapeutic modalities.

77261 Therapeutic radiology treatment planning; simple

→ *CPT Assistant* Fall 91:12, 15, Oct 97:2

77262   intermediate

→ *CPT Assistant* Fall 91:12, 15, Oct 97:2

77263   complex

→ *CPT Assistant* Fall 91:15, Oct 97:2

Definitions

Simple simulation of a single treatment area with either a single port or parallel opposed ports. Simple or no blocking.

Intermediate simulation of three or more converging ports, two separate treatment areas, multiple blocks.

Complex simulation of tangential portals, three or more treatment areas, rotation or arc therapy, complex blocking, custom shielding blocks, brachytherapy source verification, hyperthermia probe verification, any use of contrast materials.

Three-dimensional (3D) computer-generated 3D reconstruction of tumor volume and surrounding critical normal tissue structures from direct CT scans and/or MRI data in preparation for non-coplanar or coplanar therapy. The simulation uses documented 3D beam's eye view volume-dose displays of multiple or moving beams. Documentation with 3D volume reconstruction and dose distribution is required.

Simulation may be carried out on a dedicated simulator, a radiation therapy treatment unit, or diagnostic X-ray machine.

77280   Therapeutic radiology simulation-aided field setting; simple
> *CPT Assistant* Fall 91:15, Oct 97:2, Nov 97:26

77285   intermediate
> *CPT Assistant* Fall 91:15, Oct 97:3

77290   complex
> *CPT Assistant* Fall 91:12, 15, Oct 97:3

77295   3-dimensional
> *CPT Assistant* Fall 91:15, Oct 97:3, Nov 97:26, May 05:7

77299   Unlisted procedure, therapeutic radiology clinical treatment planning

Medical Radiation Physics, Dosimetry, Treatment Devices, and Special Services

77300   Basic radiation dosimetry calculation, central axis depth dose calculation, TDF, NSD, gap calculation, off axis factor, tissue inhomogeneity factors, calculation of non-ionizing radiation surface and depth dose, as required during course of treatment, only when prescribed by the treating physician
> *CPT Assistant* Fall 91:14, Oct 97:3; *CPT Changes: An Insider's View* 2002

77301   Intensity modulated radiotherapy plan, including dose-volume histograms for target and critical structure partial tolerance specifications
> *CPT Assistant* Mar 05:1, 6, May 05:7; *CPT Changes: An Insider's View* 2002

(Dose plan is optimized using inverse or forward planning technique for modulated beam delivery (eg, binary, dynamic MLC) to create highly conformal dose distribution. Computer plan distribution must be verified for positional accuracy based on dosimetric verification of the intensity map with verification of treatment set-up and interpretation of verification methodology)

77305   Teletherapy, isodose plan (whether hand or computer calculated); simple (one or two parallel opposed unmodified ports directed to a single area of interest)
> *CPT Assistant* Fall 91:15, Oct 97:3

77310   intermediate (three or more treatment ports directed to a single area of interest)
> *CPT Assistant* Fall 91:15, Oct 97:3

77315   complex (mantle or inverted Y, tangential ports, the use of wedges, compensators, complex blocking, rotational beam, or special beam considerations)
> *CPT Assistant* Fall 91:15, Oct 97:3

(Only one teletherapy isodose plan may be reported for a given course of therapy to a specific treatment area)

77321   Special teletherapy port plan, particles, hemibody, total body
> *CPT Assistant* Fall 91:14, Oct 97:4

77326   Brachytherapy isodose plan; simple (calculation made from single plane, one to four sources/ribbon application, remote afterloading brachytherapy, 1 to 8 sources)
> *CPT Assistant* Winter 91:17; *CPT Changes: An Insider's View* 2003

(For definition of source/ribbon, see page 328)

77327   intermediate (multiplane dosage calculations, application involving 5 to 10 sources/ribbons, remote afterloading brachytherapy, 9 to 12 sources)
> *CPT Assistant* Winter 91:17

77328   complex (multiplane isodose plan, volume implant calculations, over 10 sources/ribbons used, special spatial reconstruction, remote afterloading brachytherapy, over 12 sources)
> *CPT Assistant* Winter 91:17

77331   Special dosimetry (eg, TLD, microdosimetry) (specify), only when prescribed by the treating physician
> *CPT Assistant* Fall 91:13, Oct 97:4

77332   Treatment devices, design and construction; simple (simple block, simple bolus)
> *CPT Assistant* Oct 97:4

77333   intermediate (multiple blocks, stents, bite blocks, special bolus)
> *CPT Assistant* Oct 97:3

77334   complex (irregular blocks, special shields, compensators, wedges, molds or casts)
> *CPT Assistant* Fall 91:14, Oct 97:4

77336   Continuing medical physics consultation, including assessment of treatment parameters, quality assurance of dose delivery, and review of patient treatment documentation in support of the radiation oncologist, reported per week of therapy
➔ *CPT Assistant* Fall 91:15, Oct 97:4, Nov 98:21

77370   Special medical radiation physics consultation
➔ *CPT Assistant* Fall 91:14, Oct 97:4

Stereotactic Radiation Treatment Delivery

▲ **77371**   Radiation treatment delivery, stereotactic radiosurgery (SRS), complete course of treatment of cranial lesion(s) consisting of 1 session; multi-source Cobalt 60 based
➔ *CPT Changes: An Insider's View* 2007, 2008

▲ **77372**   linear accelerator based
➔ *CPT Changes: An Insider's View* 2007, 2008

(For radiation treatment management, use 77432)

77373   Stereotactic body radiation therapy, treatment delivery, per fraction to 1 or more lesions, including image guidance, entire course not to exceed 5 fractions
➔ *CPT Changes: An Insider's View* 2007

(Do not report 77373 in conjunction with 77401-77416, 77418)

(For single fraction cranial lesion[s], see 77371, 77372)

Other Procedures

77399   Unlisted procedure, medical radiation physics, dosimetry and treatment devices, and special services
➔ *CPT Assistant* Nov 98:21

Radiation Treatment Delivery

(Radiation treatment delivery [77401-77416] recognizes the technical component and the various energy levels)

77401   Radiation treatment delivery, superficial and/or ortho voltage
➔ *CPT Assistant* Apr 03:14, Aug 03:10

77402   Radiation treatment delivery, single treatment area, single port or parallel opposed ports, simple blocks or no blocks; up to 5 MeV
➔ *CPT Assistant* Apr 03:14, Aug 03:10
➔ *Clinical Examples in Radiology* Spring 07:7-9, 12

77403   6-10 MeV
➔ *CPT Assistant* Apr 03:14
➔ *Clinical Examples in Radiology* Spring 07:7-9, 12

77404   11-19 MeV
➔ *CPT Assistant* Apr 03:14
➔ *Clinical Examples in Radiology* Spring 07:7-9, 12

77406   20 MeV or greater
➔ *CPT Assistant* Apr 03:14, Aug 03:10
➔ *Clinical Examples in Radiology* Spring 07:7-9, 12

77407   Radiation treatment delivery, two separate treatment areas, three or more ports on a single treatment area, use of multiple blocks; up to 5 MeV
➔ *CPT Assistant* Apr 03:14, Aug 03:10
➔ *Clinical Examples in Radiology* Spring 07:7-9, 12

77408   6-10 MeV
➔ *CPT Assistant* Apr 03:14
➔ *Clinical Examples in Radiology* Spring 07:7-9, 12

77409   11-19 MeV
➔ *CPT Assistant* Apr 03:14

77411   20 MeV or greater
➔ *CPT Assistant* Apr 03:14, Aug 03:10
➔ *Clinical Examples in Radiology* Spring 07:7-9, 12

77412   Radiation treatment delivery, three or more separate treatment areas, custom blocking, tangential ports, wedges, rotational beam, compensators, electron beam; up to 5 MeV
➔ *CPT Assistant* Apr 03:14, Aug 03:10; *CPT Changes: An Insider's View* 2006
➔ *Clinical Examples in Radiology* Winter 06:20, Spring 07:7-9, 12

77413   6-10 MeV
➔ *CPT Assistant* Fall 91:14, Apr 03:14
➔ *Clinical Examples in Radiology* Spring 07:7-9, 12

77414   11-19 MeV
➔ *CPT Assistant* Apr 03:14
➔ *Clinical Examples in Radiology* Spring 07:7-9, 12

77416   20 MeV or greater
➔ *CPT Assistant* Aug 03:10
➔ *Clinical Examples in Radiology* Spring 07:7-9, 12

77417   Therapeutic radiology port film(s)
➔ *CPT Assistant* Fall 91:14, Dec 97:11, Feb 06:14

77418   Intensity modulated treatment delivery, single or multiple fields/arcs, via narrow spatially and temporally modulated beams, binary, dynamic MLC, per treatment session
➔ *CPT Assistant* Mar 05:1, 6, May 05:7; *CPT Changes: An Insider's View* 2002, 2005

(For intensity modulated treatment planning, use 77301)

(For compensator-based beam modulation treatment delivery, use Category III code 0073T)

77421   Stereoscopic X-ray guidance for localization of target volume for the delivery of radiation therapy
➔ *CPT Changes: An Insider's View* 2006
➔ *Clinical Examples in Radiology* Winter 06:18

(Do not report 77421 in conjunction with 77432, 77435)

▶(For placement of interstitial device[s] for radiation therapy guidance, prostate, use 55876)◀

Neutron Beam Treatment Delivery

77422   High energy neutron radiation treatment delivery; single treatment area using a single port or parallel-opposed ports with no blocks or simple blocking

> *CPT Changes: An Insider's View* 2006

> *Clinical Examples in Radiology* Winter 06:18

77423   1 or more isocenter(s) with coplanar or non-coplanar geometry with blocking and/or wedge, and/or compensator(s)

> *CPT Changes: An Insider's View* 2006

> *Clinical Examples in Radiology* Winter 06:18

Radiation Treatment Management

Radiation treatment management is reported in units of five fractions or treatment sessions, regardless of the actual time period in which the services are furnished. The services need not be furnished on consecutive days. Multiple fractions representing two or more treatment sessions furnished on the same day may be counted separately as long as there has been a distinct break in therapy sessions, and the fractions are of the character usually furnished on different days. Code 77427 is also reported if there are three or four fractions beyond a multiple of five at the end of a course of treatment; one or two fractions beyond a multiple of five at the end of a course of treatment are not reported separately. The professional services furnished during treatment management typically consist of:

■ Review of port films;

■ Review of dosimetry, dose delivery, and treatment parameters;

■ Review of patient treatment set-up;

■ Examination of patient for medical evaluation and management (eg, assessment of the patient's response to treatment, coordination of care and treatment, review of imaging and/or lab test results).

77427   Radiation treatment management, five treatments

> *CPT Assistant* Nov 99:42, Feb 00:7; *CPT Changes: An Insider's View* 2000

77431   Radiation therapy management with complete course of therapy consisting of one or two fractions only

> *CPT Assistant* Winter 90:10, Oct 97:4

(77431 is not to be used to fill in the last week of a long course of therapy)

▲ **77432**   Stereotactic radiation treatment management of cranial lesion(s) (complete course of treatment consisting of one session)

> *CPT Assistant* Oct 97:4; *CPT Changes: An Insider's View* 2008

▶(Single fraction cranial stereotactic radiation treatment is performed jointly by a surgeon and a radiation oncologist. The surgeon reports radiosurgery with 61793)◀

▶(For stereotactic body radiation therapy treatment, use 77435)◀

77435   Stereotactic body radiation therapy, treatment management, per treatment course, to one or more lesions, including image guidance, entire course not to exceed 5 fractions

> *CPT Changes: An Insider's View* 2007

(Do not report 77435 in conjunction with 77427-77432)

▶(When stereotactic radiation therapy is performed jointly by a surgeon and a radiation oncologist [ie, spinal or cranial], the surgeon reports radiosurgery with 61793)◀

77470   Special treatment procedure (eg, total body irradiation, hemibody radiation, per oral, endocavitary or intraoperative cone irradiation)

> *CPT Assistant* Winter 91:22, Oct 97:1; *CPT Changes: An Insider's View* 2001

(77470 assumes that the procedure is performed one or more times during the course of therapy, in addition to daily or weekly patient management)

77499   Unlisted procedure, therapeutic radiology treatment management

> *CPT Assistant* Nov 99:42, Feb 00:7; *CPT Changes: An Insider's View* 2000

Proton Beam Treatment Delivery

Definitions

Simple proton treatment delivery to a single treatment area utilizing a single non-tangential/oblique port, custom block with compensation (77522) and without compensation (77520).

Intermediate proton treatment delivery to one or more treatment areas utilizing two or more ports or one or more tangential/oblique ports, with custom blocks and compensators.

Complex proton treatment delivery to one or more treatment areas utilizing two or more ports per treatment area with matching or patching fields and/or multiple isocenters, with custom blocks and compensators.

77520   Proton treatment delivery; simple, without compensation

> *CPT Assistant* Nov 99:43; *CPT Changes: An Insider's View* 2000, 2001

77522   simple, with compensation

> *CPT Changes: An Insider's View* 2001

77523   intermediate

> *CPT Assistant* Nov 99:43; *CPT Changes: An Insider's View* 2000, 2001

77525   complex

> *CPT Changes: An Insider's View* 2001

Hyperthermia

Hyperthermia treatments as listed in this section include external (superficial and deep), interstitial, and intracavitary.

Radiation therapy when given concurrently is listed separately.

Hyperthermia is used only as an adjunct to radiation therapy or chemotherapy. It may be induced by a variety of sources (eg, microwave, ultrasound, low energy radio-frequency conduction, or by probes).

The listed treatments include management during the course of therapy and follow-up care for three months after completion.

Preliminary consultation is not included (see **Evaluation and Management** 99241-99255).

Physics planning and interstitial insertion of temperature sensors, and use of external or interstitial heat generating sources are included.

The following descriptors are included in the treatment schedule:

⊙ **77600** Hyperthermia, externally generated; superficial (ie, heating to a depth of 4 cm or less)
➔ *CPT Assistant* Winter 91:22

⊙ **77605** deep (ie, heating to depths greater than 4 cm)
➔ *CPT Assistant* Winter 91:22

⊙ **77610** Hyperthermia generated by interstitial probe(s); 5 or fewer interstitial applicators
➔ *CPT Assistant* Winter 91:22

⊙ **77615** more than 5 interstitial applicators
➔ *CPT Assistant* Winter 91:22

Clinical Intracavitary Hyperthermia

77620 Hyperthermia generated by intracavitary probe(s)
➔ *CPT Assistant* Winter 91:22

Clinical Brachytherapy

Clinical brachytherapy requires the use of either natural or man-made radioelements applied into or around a treatment field of interest. The supervision of radioelements and dose interpretation are performed solely by the therapeutic radiologist.

Services 77750-77799 include admission to the hospital and daily visits.

For insertion of ovoids and tandems, use 57155.

For insertion of Heyman capsules, use 58346.

Definitions

(Sources refer to intracavitary placement or permanent interstitial placement; ribbons refer to temporary interstitial placement)

A simple application has one to four sources/ribbons.

An intermediate application has five to 10 sources/ribbons.

A complex application has greater than 10 sources/ribbons.

▶(For high dose rate electronic brachytherapy, per fraction, use Category III code 0182T)◀

77750 Infusion or instillation of radioelement solution (includes 3 months follow-up care)
➔ *CPT Assistant* Sep 05:1; *CPT Changes: An Insider's View* 2005

(For administration of radiolabeled monoclonal antibodies, use 79403)

(For non-antibody radiopharmaceutical therapy by intravenous administration only, not including 3-month follow-up care, use 79101)

77761 Intracavitary radiation source application; simple
➔ *CPT Assistant* Winter 91:23, Jan 96:7, Mar 99:3, Feb 02:7, Sep 05:1; *CPT Changes: An Insider's View* 2001

77762 intermediate
➔ *CPT Assistant* Winter 91:23, Feb 02:7, Sep 05:1

77763 complex
➔ *CPT Assistant* Winter 91:23, Mar 99:3, Feb 02:7, Sep 05:1

▶(Do not report 77761-77763 in conjunction with Category III code 0182T)◀

77776 Interstitial radiation source application; simple
➔ *CPT Assistant* Winter 91:23, Sep 05:1; *CPT Changes: An Insider's View* 2001

77777 intermediate
➔ *CPT Assistant* Winter 91:23, Sep 05:1

77778 complex
➔ *CPT Assistant* Winter 91:23, Apr 04:6, Sep 05:1

▶(Do not report 77776-77778 in conjunction with Category III code 0182T)◀

77781 Remote afterloading high intensity brachytherapy; 1-4 source positions or catheters
➔ *CPT Assistant* Winter 90:10, Winter 91:23, Mar 99:3, Feb 02:7, Mar 02:2, Sep 05:1, Nov 05:15

77782 5-8 source positions or catheters
➔ *CPT Assistant* Winter 90:10, Winter 91:23, Mar 99:3, Feb 02:7, Mar 02:2, Sep 05:1, Nov 05:15

77783 9-12 source positions or catheters
➔ *CPT Assistant* Winter 90:10, Winter 91:23, Mar 99:3, Feb 02:7, Mar 02:2, Sep 05:1, Nov 05:15

77784 over 12 source positions or catheters
➔ *CPT Assistant* Winter 90:10, Winter 91:23, Mar 99:3, Feb 02:7, Mar 02:2, Sep 05:1, Nov 05:15

▶(Do not report 77781-77784 in conjunction with Category III code 0182T)◀

77789   Surface application of radiation source
    ➲ *CPT Assistant* Sep 05:1; *CPT Changes: An Insider's View* 2001

    ▶(Do not report 77789 in conjunction with Category III code 0182T)◄

77790   Supervision, handling, loading of radiation source
    ➲ *CPT Assistant* Sep 05:1; *CPT Changes: An Insider's View* 2001

77799   Unlisted procedure, clinical brachytherapy
    ➲ *CPT Assistant* Sep 05:1

Nuclear Medicine

Listed procedures may be performed independently or in the course of overall medical care. If the physician providing these services is also responsible for diagnostic work-up and/or follow-up care of patient, see appropriate sections also.

Radioimmunoassay tests are found in the **Clinical Pathology** section (codes 82000-84999). These codes can be appropriately used by any specialist performing such tests in a laboratory licensed and/or certified for radioimmunoassays. The reporting of these tests is not confined to clinical pathology laboratories alone.

The services listed do not include the radiopharmaceutical or drug. Diagnostic and therapeutic radiopharmaceuticals and drugs supplied by the physician should be reported separately using the appropriate supply code(s), in addition to the procedure code.

Diagnostic

Endocrine System

78000   Thyroid uptake; single determination
    ➲ *CPT Assistant* Dec 05:7, 9, Jan 07:31

78001   multiple determinations

78003   stimulation, suppression or discharge (not including initial uptake studies)

78006   Thyroid imaging, with uptake; single determination

78007   multiple determinations

78010   Thyroid imaging; only

78011   with vascular flow

78015   Thyroid carcinoma metastases imaging; limited area (eg, neck and chest only)
    ➲ *CPT Assistant* Nov 98:21, Jan 07:31

78016   with additional studies (eg, urinary recovery)

78018   whole body
    ➲ *CPT Assistant* Apr 99:4, Jan 07:31

+ 78020   Thyroid carcinoma metastases uptake (List separately in addition to code for primary procedure)
    ➲ *CPT Assistant* Nov 98:21, Apr 99:4, Jan 07:31

(Use 78020 in conjunction with 78018 only)

78070   Parathyroid imaging

78075   Adrenal imaging, cortex and/or medulla

78099   Unlisted endocrine procedure, diagnostic nuclear medicine
    ➲ *CPT Assistant* Dec 05:7, Jan 07:31

(For chemical analysis, see **Chemistry** section)

Hematopoietic, Reticuloendothelial and Lymphatic System

78102   Bone marrow imaging; limited area
    ➲ *CPT Assistant* Dec 05:7

78103   multiple areas

78104   whole body

78110   Plasma volume, radiopharmaceutical volume-dilution technique (separate procedure); single sampling

78111   multiple samplings

78120   Red cell volume determination (separate procedure); single sampling

78121   multiple samplings

78122   Whole blood volume determination, including separate measurement of plasma volume and red cell volume (radiopharmaceutical volume-dilution technique)

78130   Red cell survival study;

78135   differential organ/tissue kinetics (eg, splenic and/or hepatic sequestration)

78140   Labeled red cell sequestration, differential organ/tissue (eg, splenic and/or hepatic)

(78160, 78162, 78170, 78172 have been deleted)

78185   Spleen imaging only, with or without vascular flow

(If combined with liver study, use procedures 78215 and 78216)

78190   Kinetics, study of platelet survival, with or without differential organ/tissue localization

78191   Platelet survival study

78195   Lymphatics and lymph nodes imaging
    ➲ *CPT Assistant* Nov 98:22, Jul 99:6, Nov 99:43, Dec 99:8; *CPT Changes: An Insider's View* 2000, 2002

(For sentinel node identification without scintigraphy imaging, use 38792)

(For sentinal node excision, see 38500-38542)

78199   Unlisted hematopoietic, reticuloendothelial and lymphatic procedure, diagnostic nuclear medicine
    ➲ *CPT Assistant* Dec 05:7

(For chemical analysis, see **Chemistry** section)

Gastrointestinal System

78201 Liver imaging; static only
➔ *CPT Assistant* Dec 05:7

78202   with vascular flow

(For spleen imaging only, use 78185)

78205 Liver imaging (SPECT);
➔ *CPT Assistant* Nov 98:22

78206   with vascular flow
➔ *CPT Assistant* Nov 98:22

78215 Liver and spleen imaging; static only

78216   with vascular flow

78220 Liver function study with hepatobiliary agents, with serial images

78223 Hepatobiliary ductal system imaging, including gallbladder, with or without pharmacologic intervention, with or without quantitative measurement of gallbladder function

78230 Salivary gland imaging;

78231   with serial images

78232 Salivary gland function study

78258 Esophageal motility

78261 Gastric mucosa imaging

78262 Gastroesophageal reflux study

78264 Gastric emptying study

78267 Urea breath test, C-14 (isotopic); acquisition for analysis
➔ *CPT Assistant* Nov 99:43; *CPT Changes: An Insider's View* 2000, 2005

78268   analysis
➔ *CPT Assistant* Nov 99:43; *CPT Changes: An Insider's View* 2000

78270 Vitamin B-12 absorption study (eg, Schilling test); without intrinsic factor

78271   with intrinsic factor

78272 Vitamin B-12 absorption studies combined, with and without intrinsic factor

78278 Acute gastrointestinal blood loss imaging

78282 Gastrointestinal protein loss

78290 Intestine imaging (eg, ectopic gastric mucosa, Meckel's localization, volvulus)
➔ *CPT Changes: An Insider's View* 2002

78291 Peritoneal-venous shunt patency test (eg, for LeVeen, Denver shunt)

(For injection procedure, use 49427)

78299 Unlisted gastrointestinal procedure, diagnostic nuclear medicine
➔ *CPT Assistant* Dec 05:7

Musculoskeletal System

Bone and joint imaging can be used in the diagnosis of a variety of inflammatory processes (eg, osteomyelitis), as well as for localization of primary and/or metastatic neoplasms.

78300 Bone and/or joint imaging; limited area
➔ *CPT Assistant* Mar 97:11, Dec 05:7

78305   multiple areas
➔ *CPT Assistant* Mar 97:11

78306   whole body
➔ *CPT Assistant* Mar 97:11, Jan 02:10, Jun 03:11
➔ *Clinical Examples in Radiology* Summer 06:7, 12

78315   three phase study
➔ *CPT Assistant* Jan 02:10
➔ *Clinical Examples in Radiology* Summer 06:7, 12

78320   tomographic (SPECT)
➔ *CPT Assistant* Mar 97:11, Jun 03:11

78350 Bone density (bone mineral content) study, one or more sites; single photon absorptiometry
➔ *CPT Assistant* Nov 97:26

78351   dual photon absorptiometry, one or more sites
➔ *CPT Assistant* Nov 97:26

(For radiographic bone density [photodensitometry], use 77083)

78399 Unlisted musculoskeletal procedure, diagnostic nuclear medicine
➔ *CPT Assistant* Dec 05:7

Cardiovascular System

Myocardial perfusion and cardiac blood pool imaging studies may be performed at rest and/or during stress. When performed during exercise and/or pharmacologic stress, the appropriate stress testing code from the 93015-93018 series should be reported in addition to 78460-78465, 78472-78492.

78414 Determination of central c-v hemodynamics (non-imaging) (eg, ejection fraction with probe technique) with or without pharmacologic intervention or exercise, single or multiple determinations
➔ *CPT Assistant* Dec 05:7

78428 Cardiac shunt detection

78445 Non-cardiac vascular flow imaging (ie, angiography, venography)

(78455 has been deleted)

78456 Acute venous thrombosis imaging, peptide
➔ *CPT Assistant* Nov 99:43; *CPT Changes: An Insider's View* 2000

78457 Venous thrombosis imaging, venogram; unilateral
➔ *CPT Assistant* Nov 99:43; *CPT Changes: An Insider's View* 2000

78458   bilateral
➔ *CPT Assistant* Nov 99:43; *CPT Changes: An Insider's View* 2000

78459 Myocardial imaging, positron emission tomography (PET), metabolic evaluation
➜ *CPT Assistant* Jun 96:5, Nov 97:26

(For myocardial perfusion study, see 78491-78492)

78460 Myocardial perfusion imaging; (planar) single study, at rest or stress (exercise and/or pharmacologic), with or without quantification
➜ *CPT Assistant* Mar 99:10, Apr 00:1

78461 multiple studies (planar), at rest and/or stress (exercise and/or pharmacologic), and redistribution and/or rest injection, with or without quantification
➜ *CPT Assistant* Mar 99:10

78464 tomographic (SPECT), single study (including attenuation correction when performed), at rest or stress (exercise and/or pharmacologic), with or without quantification
➜ *CPT Assistant* Mar 99:10; *CPT Changes: An Insider's View* 2005

78465 tomographic (SPECT), multiple studies (including attenuation correction when performed), at rest and/or stress (exercise and/or pharmacologic) and redistribution and/or rest injection, with or without quantification
➜ *CPT Assistant* Aug 98:11, Mar 99:10, Oct 04:10, Mar 05:11; *CPT Changes: An Insider's View* 2005
➜ *Clinical Examples in Radiology* Inaugural 04:3-5

78466 Myocardial imaging, infarct avid, planar; qualitative or quantitative

78468 with ejection fraction by first pass technique

78469 tomographic SPECT with or without quantification

78472 Cardiac blood pool imaging, gated equilibrium; planar, single study at rest or stress (exercise and/or pharmacologic), wall motion study plus ejection fraction, with or without additional quantitative processing
➜ *CPT Assistant* Nov 98:22, Jun 99:8, Nov 99:44; *CPT Changes: An Insider's View* 2000

(For assessment of right ventricular ejection fraction by first pass technique, use 78496)

78473 multiple studies, wall motion study plus ejection fraction, at rest and stress (exercise and/or pharmacologic), with or without additional quantification
➜ *CPT Assistant* Jun 99:11

+ 78478 Myocardial perfusion study with wall motion, qualitative or quantitative study (List separately in addition to code for primary procedure)
➜ *CPT Assistant* Mar 99:10, Oct 04:10, Apr 07:1
➜ *Clinical Examples in Radiology* Inaugural 04:3-5

(Use 78478 in conjunction with 78460, 78461, 78464, 78465)

+ 78480 Myocardial perfusion study with ejection fraction (List separately in addition to code for primary procedure)
➜ *CPT Assistant* Mar 97:10, Oct 04:10, Apr 07:1
➜ *Clinical Examples in Radiology* Inaugural 04:3-5

(Use 78480 in conjunction with 78460, 78461, 78464, 78465)

78481 Cardiac blood pool imaging (planar), first pass technique; single study, at rest or with stress (exercise and/or pharmacologic), wall motion study plus ejection fraction, with or without quantification

78483 multiple studies, at rest and with stress (exercise and/ or pharmacologic), wall motion study plus ejection fraction, with or without quantification

▶(For cerebral blood flow study, use 78610)◀

78491 Myocardial imaging, positron emission tomography (PET), perfusion; single study at rest or stress
➜ *CPT Assistant* Nov 97:27

78492 multiple studies at rest and/or stress
➜ *CPT Assistant* Nov 97:27

78494 Cardiac blood pool imaging, gated equilibrium, SPECT, at rest, wall motion study plus ejection fraction, with or without quantitative processing
➜ *CPT Assistant* Nov 98:22, Jun 99:3

+ 78496 Cardiac blood pool imaging, gated equilibrium, single study, at rest, with right ventricular ejection fraction by first pass technique (List separately in addition to code for primary procedure)
➜ *CPT Assistant* Nov 98:22, Jun 99:3, 11

(Use 78496 in conjunction with 78472)

78499 Unlisted cardiovascular procedure, diagnostic nuclear medicine
➜ *CPT Assistant* Dec 05:7

Respiratory System

78580 Pulmonary perfusion imaging, particulate
➜ *CPT Assistant* Mar 99:4, Dec 05:7

78584 Pulmonary perfusion imaging, particulate, with ventilation; single breath
➜ *CPT Assistant* Mar 99:4

78585 rebreathing and washout, with or without single breath
➜ *CPT Assistant* Mar 99:4

78586 Pulmonary ventilation imaging, aerosol; single projection
➜ *CPT Assistant* Mar 99:4

78587 multiple projections (eg, anterior, posterior, lateral views)
➜ *CPT Assistant* Mar 99:4

78588 Pulmonary perfusion imaging, particulate, with ventilation imaging, aerosol, one or multiple projections
➜ *CPT Assistant* Nov 98:22, Mar 99:4

78591 Pulmonary ventilation imaging, gaseous, single breath, single projection
➜ *CPT Assistant* Mar 99:4

78593 Pulmonary ventilation imaging, gaseous, with rebreathing and washout with or without single breath; single projection
➜ *CPT Assistant* Mar 99:4

78594 multiple projections (eg, anterior, posterior, lateral views)

78596 Pulmonary quantitative differential function (ventilation/perfusion) study
➜ *CPT Assistant* Winter 90:10

78599 Unlisted respiratory procedure, diagnostic nuclear medicine
➜ *CPT Assistant* Dec 05:7

Nervous System

▲ **78600** Brain imaging, less than 4 static views;
➜ *CPT Assistant* Dec 05:7; *CPT Changes: An Insider's View* 2008

▲ **78601** with vascular flow
➜ *CPT Changes: An Insider's View* 2008

▲ **78605** Brain imaging, minimum 4 static views;
➜ *CPT Changes: An Insider's View* 2008

▲ **78606** with vascular flow
➜ *CPT Changes: An Insider's View* 2008

▲ **78607** Brain imaging, tomographic (SPECT)
➜ *CPT Changes: An Insider's View* 2008

78608 Brain imaging, positron emission tomography (PET); metabolic evaluation

78609 perfusion evaluation

78610 Brain imaging, vascular flow only

▶(78615 has been deleted. To report, use 78610)◀

78630 Cerebrospinal fluid flow, imaging (not including introduction of material); cisternography

(For injection procedure, see 61000-61070, 62270-62319)

78635 ventriculography

(For injection procedure, see 61000-61070, 62270-62294)

78645 shunt evaluation

(For injection procedure, see 61000-61070, 62270-62294)

78647 tomographic (SPECT)

78650 Cerebrospinal fluid leakage detection and localization
➜ *CPT Changes: An Insider's View* 2002

(For injection procedure, see 61000-61070, 62270-62294)

78660 Radiopharmaceutical dacryocystography

78699 Unlisted nervous system procedure, diagnostic nuclear medicine
➜ *CPT Assistant* Dec 05:7

Genitourinary System

78700 Kidney imaging morphology;
➜ *CPT Assistant* Dec 05:7, Mar 07:7; *CPT Changes: An Insider's View* 2007

78701 with vascular flow

(78704 has been deleted. To report, see 78707-78709)

78707 with vascular flow and function, single study without pharmacological intervention
➜ *CPT Assistant* Nov 97:27, Mar 07:7; *CPT Changes: An Insider's View* 2007

78708 with vascular flow and function, single study, with pharmacological intervention (eg, angiotensin converting enzyme inhibitor and/or diuretic)
➜ *CPT Assistant* Nov 97:27, Mar 07:7; *CPT Changes: An Insider's View* 2007

78709 with vascular flow and function, multiple studies, with and without pharmacological intervention (eg, angiotensin converting enzyme inhibitor and/or diuretic)
➜ *CPT Assistant* Nov 97:27, Mar 07:7; *CPT Changes: An Insider's View* 2007

(For introduction of radioactive substance in association with renal endoscopy, see 77776-77778)

78710 tomographic (SPECT)
➜ *CPT Assistant* Nov 97:27, Mar 07:7; *CPT Changes: An Insider's View* 2007

(78715 has been deleted. To report, see 78701-78709)

78725 Kidney function study, non-imaging radioisotopic study
➜ *CPT Assistant* Nov 98:22

+ **78730** Urinary bladder residual study (List separately in addition to code for primary procedure)
➜ *CPT Changes: An Insider's View* 2007

(Use 78730 in conjunction with 78740)

(For measurement of postvoid residual urine and/or bladder capacity by ultrasound, nonimaging, use 51798)

(For ultrasound imaging of the bladder only, with measurement of postvoid residual urine when performed, use 76857)

78740 Ureteral reflux study (radiopharmaceutical voiding cystogram)

(Use 78740 in conjunction with 78730 for urinary bladder residual study)

(For catheterization, see 51701, 51702, 51703)

(78760 has been deleted. To report, use 78761)

78761 Testicular imaging with vascular flow
➜ *CPT Changes: An Insider's View* 2007

78799 Unlisted genitourinary procedure, diagnostic nuclear medicine
➜ *CPT Assistant* Dec 05:7

(For chemical analysis, see **Chemistry** section)

Other Procedures

(For specific organ, see appropriate heading)

(For radiophosphorus tumor identification, ocular, see 78800)

78800   Radiopharmaceutical localization of tumor or distribution of radiopharmaceutical agent(s); limited area

➔ *CPT Assistant* Dec 05:7; *CPT Changes: An Insider's View* 2004

➔ *Clinical Examples in Radiology* Summer 06:6, 10-11

(For specific organ, see appropriate heading)

78801   multiple areas

78802   whole body, single day imaging

➔ *CPT Assistant* Jun 03:11; *CPT Changes: An Insider's View* 2004

➔ *Clinical Examples in Radiology* Summer 06:6, 10-11

78803   tomographic (SPECT)

➔ *CPT Assistant* Jun 03:11

➔ *Clinical Examples in Radiology* Summer 06:6, 10-11

78804   whole body, requiring two or more days imaging

➔ *CPT Changes: An Insider's View* 2004

78805   Radiopharmaceutical localization of inflammatory process; limited area

➔ *CPT Assistant* Nov 99:44; *CPT Changes: An Insider's View* 2001

78806   whole body

➔ *CPT Assistant* Nov 99:44, Jun 03:11; *CPT Changes: An Insider's View* 2000

78807   tomographic (SPECT)

➔ *CPT Assistant* Jun 03:11

(For imaging bone infectious or inflammatory disease with a bone imaging radiopharmaceutical, see 78300, 78305, 78306)

(For PET of brain, see 78608, 78609)

(For PET myocardial imaging, see 78459, 78491, 78492)

▲ **78811**   Positron emission tomography (PET) imaging; limited area (eg, chest, head/neck)

➔ *CPT Assistant* Dec 05:7; *CPT Changes: An Insider's View* 2005, 2008

➔ *Clinical Examples in Radiology* Spring 05:13, 15

▲ **78812**   skull base to mid-thigh

➔ *CPT Assistant* Dec 05:7; *CPT Changes: An Insider's View* 2005, 2008

➔ *Clinical Examples in Radiology* Spring 05:13, 15

▲ **78813**   whole body

➔ *CPT Assistant* Dec 05:7; *CPT Changes: An Insider's View* 2005, 2008

➔ *Clinical Examples in Radiology* Spring 05:13, 15

▲ **78814**   Positron emission tomography (PET) with concurrently acquired computed tomography (CT) for attenuation correction and anatomical localization imaging; limited area (eg, chest, head/neck)

➔ *CPT Assistant* Feb 05:13, Jun 05:10, Dec 05:7; *CPT Changes: An Insider's View* 2005, 2008

➔ *Clinical Examples in Radiology* Spring 05:13, 15

▲ **78815**   skull base to mid-thigh

➔ *CPT Assistant* Feb 05:13, Jun 05:10, Dec 05:7; *CPT Changes: An Insider's View* 2005, 2008

➔ *Clinical Examples in Radiology* Spring 05:13, 15

▲ **78816**   whole body

➔ *CPT Assistant* Feb 05:13, Jun 05:10, Dec 05:7; *CPT Changes: An Insider's View* 2005, 2008

➔ *Clinical Examples in Radiology* Spring 05:13, 15

(Report 78811-78816 only once per imaging session)

(Computed tomography (CT) performed for other than attenuation correction and anatomical localization is reported using the appropriate site specific CT code with modifier 59)

78890   Generation of automated data: interactive process involving nuclear physician and/or allied health professional personnel; simple manipulations and interpretation, not to exceed 30 minutes

78891   complex manipulations and interpretation, exceeding 30 minutes

(Use 78890 or 78891 in addition to primary procedure)

78999   Unlisted miscellaneous procedure, diagnostic nuclear medicine

➔ *CPT Assistant* Dec 05:7

Therapeutic

The oral and intravenous administration codes in this section are inclusive of the mode of administration. For intra-arterial, intra-cavitary, and intra-articular administration, also use the appropriate injection and/or procedure codes, as well as imaging guidance and radiological supervision and interpretation codes, when appropriate.

79005   Radiopharmaceutical therapy, by oral administration

➔ *CPT Assistant* Sep 05:1; *CPT Changes: An Insider's View* 2005

➔ *Clinical Examples in Radiology* Spring 05:14

(For monoclonal antibody therapy, use 79403)

79101   Radiopharmaceutical therapy, by intravenous administration

➔ *CPT Assistant* Sep 05:1; *CPT Changes: An Insider's View* 2005

(Do not report 79101 in conjunction with 36400, 36410, 79403, 90760, 90774 or 90775, 96409)

(For radiolabeled monoclonal antibody by intravenous infusion, use 79403)

(For infusion or instillation of non-antibody radioelement solution that includes 3 months follow-up care, use 77750)

79200   Radiopharmaceutical therapy, by intracavitary administration

➔ *CPT Assistant* Sep 05:1; *CPT Changes: An Insider's View* 2005

79300   Radiopharmaceutical therapy, by interstitial radioactive colloid administration

➔ *CPT Assistant* Sep 05:1; *CPT Changes: An Insider's View* 2005

79403 Radiopharmaceutical therapy, radiolabeled monoclonal antibody by intravenous infusion

➔ *CPT Assistant* Sep 05:1; *CPT Changes: An Insider's View* 2004

(For pre-treatment imaging, see 78802, 78804)

(Do not report 79403 in conjunction with 79101)

79440 Radiopharmaceutical therapy, by intra-articular administration

➔ *CPT Assistant* Sep 05:1; *CPT Changes: An Insider's View* 2005

79445 Radiopharmaceutical therapy, by intra-arterial particulate administration

➔ *CPT Assistant* Sep 05:1, Dec 06:10; *CPT Changes: An Insider's View* 2005

▶(Do not report 79445 in conjunction with 90773, 96420)◀

(Use appropriate procedural and radiological supervision and interpretation codes for the angiographic and interventional procedures provided prerequisite to intra-arterial radiopharmaceutical therapy)

79999 Radiopharmaceutical therapy, unlisted procedure

➔ *CPT Assistant* Mar 05:11, Sep 05:1, Jan 07:30; *CPT Changes: An Insider's View* 2005

Pathology and Laboratory Guidelines

Items used by all physicians in reporting their services are presented in the **Introduction.** Some of the commonalities are repeated here for the convenience of those physicians referring to this section on **Pathology and Laboratory.** Other definitions and items unique to Pathology and Laboratory are also listed.

Services in Pathology and Laboratory

Services in Pathology and Laboratory are provided by a physician or by technologists under responsible supervision of a physician.

Separate or Multiple Procedures

It is appropriate to designate multiple procedures that are rendered on the same date by separate entries.

Subsection Information

Several of the subheadings or subsections have special needs or instructions unique to that section. Where these are indicated (eg, "Panel Tests"), special **"Notes"** will be presented preceding those procedural terminology listings referring to that subsection specifically. If there is an "Unlisted Procedure" code number (see the following section) for the individual subsection, it will be shown. Those subsections with **"Notes"** are as follows:

Organ or Disease Panels	80048-80076
Drug Testing	80100-80103
Therapeutic Drug Assays	80150-80299
Evocative/Suppression Testing	80400-80440
Consultations (Clinical Pathology)	80500-80502
Urinalysis	81000-81099
Chemistry	82000-84999
Molecular Diagnostics	83890-83912
Infectious Agent: Detection of Antibodies	86602-86804
Microbiology	87001-87255
Infectious Agent Detection	87260-87999
Anatomic Pathology	88000-88099

Cytopathology	88104-88199
Cytogenetic Studies	88230-88299
Surgical Pathology	88300-88399

Unlisted Service or Procedure

A service or procedure may be provided that is not listed in this edition of the CPT codebook. When reporting such a service, the appropriate "Unlisted Procedure" code may be used to indicate the service, identifying it by "Special Report" as discussed below. The "Unlisted Procedures" and accompanying codes for **Pathology and Laboratory** are as follows:

81099	Unlisted urinalysis procedure
84999	Unlisted chemistry procedure
85999	Unlisted hematology and coagulation procedure
86849	Unlisted immunology procedure
86999	Unlisted transfusion medicine procedure
87999	Unlisted microbiology procedure
88099	Unlisted necropsy (autopsy) procedure
88199	Unlisted cytopathology procedure
88299	Unlisted cytogenetic study
88399	Unlisted surgical pathology procedure
89240	Unlisted miscellaneous pathology test

Special Report

A service that is rarely provided, unusual, variable, or new may require a special report in determining medical appropriateness of the service. Pertinent information should include an adequate definition or description of the nature, extent, and need for the procedure; and the time, effort, and equipment necessary to provide the service. Additional items that may be included are:

- Complexity of symptoms
- Final diagnosis
- Pertinent physical findings
- Diagnostic and therapeutic procedures
- Concurrent problems
- Follow-up care

Notes

⊙=Moderate sedation   ✚=Add-on code   ✗=FDA approval pending   ➲➲=See p xvii for details

Pathology and Laboratory

Organ or Disease-Oriented Panels

These panels were developed for coding purposes only and should not be interpreted as clinical parameters. The tests listed with each panel identify the defined components of that panel.

These panel components are not intended to limit the performance of other tests. If one performs tests in addition to those specifically indicated for a particular panel, those tests should be reported separately in addition to the panel code.

● **80047**   Basic metabolic panel (Calcium, ionized)

This panel must include the following:

Calcium, ionized (82330)

Carbon dioxide (82374)

Chloride (82435)

Creatinine (82565)

Glucose (82947)

Potassium (84132)

Sodium (84295)

Urea Nitrogen (BUN) (84520)

➔ *CPT Changes: An Insider's View* 2008

▶(Do not report 80047 in conjunction with 80053)◀

▲ **80048**   Basic metabolic panel (Calcium, total)

This panel must include the following:

Calcium (82310)

Carbon dioxide (82374)

Chloride (82435)

Creatinine (82565)

Glucose (82947)

Potassium (84132)

Sodium (84295)

Urea nitrogen (BUN) (84520)

➔ *CPT Assistant* Jan 98:6, Sep 99:11, Nov 99:44, Jan 00:7, Aug 05:9; *CPT Changes: An Insider's View* 2000, 2008

(Do not use 80048 in addition to 80053)

80050   General health panel

This panel must include the following:

Comprehensive metabolic panel (80053)

Blood count, complete (CBC), automated and automated differential WBC count (85025 or 85027 and 85004)

OR

Blood count, complete (CBC), automated (85027) and appropriate manual differential WBC count (85007 or 85009)

Thyroid stimulating hormone (TSH) (84443)

➔ *CPT Assistant* Winter 92:14, Summer 93:14, Jun 97:10, Nov 97:28, Jan 98:6, Sep 99:11; *CPT Changes: An Insider's View* 2001, 2004

80051   Electrolyte panel

This panel must include the following:

Carbon dioxide (82374)

Chloride (82435)

Potassium (84132)

Sodium (84295)

➔ *CPT Assistant* Nov 97:28, Jan 98:7, Sep 99:11

80053   Comprehensive metabolic panel

This panel must include the following:

Albumin (82040)

Bilirubin, total (82247)

Calcium (82310)

Carbon dioxide (bicarbonate) (82374)

Chloride (82435)

Creatinine (82565)

Glucose (82947)

Phosphatase, alkaline (84075)

Potassium (84132)

Protein, total (84155)

Sodium (84295)

Transferase, alanine amino (ALT) (SGPT) (84460)

Transferase, aspartate amino (AST) (SGOT) (84450)

Urea nitrogen (BUN) (84520)

➔ *CPT Assistant* Jan 98:6, Nov 98:23, Sep 99:11, Nov 99:44, May 00:11; *CPT Changes: An Insider's View* 2000

▶(Do not use 80053 in addition to 80047, 80048, 80076)◀

▲=Revised code   ●=New code   ▶◀=Contains new or revised text   ⊘=Modifier 51 exempt

80055   Obstetric panel

This panel must include the following:

Blood count, complete (CBC), automated and automated differential WBC count (85025 or 85027 and 85004)

OR

Blood count, complete (CBC), automated (85027) and appropriate manual differential WBC count (85007 or 85009)

Hepatitis B surface antigen (HBsAg) (87340)

Antibody, rubella (86762)

Syphilis test, qualitative (eg, VDRL, RPR, ART) (86592)

Antibody screen, RBC, each serum technique (86850)

Blood typing, ABO (86900) AND

Blood typing, Rh (D) (86901)

➲ *CPT Assistant* Winter 92:14, Summer 93:14, Jun 97:10, Apr 99:6, Sep 99:11; *CPT Changes: An Insider's View* 2004

80061   Lipid panel

This panel must include the following:

Cholesterol, serum, total (82465)

Lipoprotein, direct measurement, high density cholesterol (HDL cholesterol) (83718)

Triglycerides (84478)

➲ *CPT Assistant* Winter 92:14, Summer 93:14, Jun 97:10, Sep 99:11, Mar 00:11, Feb 05:9

80069   Renal function panel

This panel must include the following:

Albumin (82040)

Calcium (82310)

Carbon dioxide (bicarbonate) (82374)

Chloride (82435)

Creatinine (82565)

Glucose (82947)

Phosphorus inorganic (phosphate) (84100)

Potassium (84132)

Sodium (84295)

Urea nitrogen (BUN) (84520)

➲ *CPT Assistant* Sep 99:11, Nov 99:44; *CPT Changes: An Insider's View* 2000

80074   Acute hepatitis panel

This panel must include the following:

Hepatitis A antibody (HAAb), IgM antibody (86709)

Hepatitis B core antibody (HBcAb), IgM antibody (86705)

Hepatitis B surface antigen (HBsAg) (87340)

Hepatitis C antibody (86803)

➲ *CPT Assistant* Sep 99:11, Nov 99:45; *CPT Changes: An Insider's View* 2000

80076   Hepatic function panel

This panel must include the following:

Albumin (82040)

Bilirubin, total (82247)

Bilirubin, direct (82248)

Phosphatase, alkaline (84075)

Protein, total (84155)

Transferase, alanine amino (ALT) (SGPT) (84460)

Transferase, aspartate amino (AST) (SGOT) (84450)

➲ *CPT Assistant* Winter 92:14, Summer 93:14, Jun 97:10, Jan 98:6, Apr 99:6, Sep 99:11, Nov 99:45, Jan 00:7, Aug 05:9; *CPT Changes: An Insider's View* 2000

(Do not use 80076 in addition to 80053)

Drug Testing

The following list contains examples of drugs or classes of drugs that are commonly assayed by qualitative screen, followed by confirmation with a second method:

- Alcohols
- Amphetamines
- Barbiturates
- Benzodiazepines
- Cocaine and metabolites
- Methadones
- Methaqualones
- Opiates
- Phencyclidines
- Phenothiazines
- Propoxyphenes
- Tetrahydrocannabinoids
- Tricyclic antidepressants

Confirmed drugs may also be quantitated.

Use 80100 for each multiple drug class chromatographic procedure. Use 80102 for each procedure necessary for confirmation. For chromatography, each combination of stationary and mobile phase is to be counted as one procedure. For example, if detection of three drugs by chromatography requires one stationary phase with three mobile phases, use 80100 three times. However, if multiple drugs can be detected using a single analysis (eg, one stationary phase with one mobile phase), use 80100 only once.

For quantitation of drugs screened, use appropriate code in **Chemistry** section (82000-84999) or **Therapeutic Drug Assay** section (80150-80299).

80100 Drug screen, qualitative; multiple drug classes chromatographic method, each procedure
➔ *CPT Assistant* Fall 93:26, Mar 00:2, Aug 05:9; *CPT Changes: An Insider's View* 2001

80101 single drug class method (eg, immunoassay, enzyme assay), each drug class
➔ *CPT Assistant* Fall 93:26, Mar 00:2, Nov 06:22; *CPT Changes: An Insider's View* 2001

80102 Drug confirmation, each procedure
➔ *CPT Assistant* Fall 93:26, Mar 00:2; *CPT Changes: An Insider's View* 2001

80103 Tissue preparation for drug analysis
➔ *CPT Assistant* Aug 05:9

Therapeutic Drug Assays

The material for examination may be from any source. Examination is quantitative. For nonquantitative testing, see Drug Testing (80100-80103).
➔ *CPT Assistant* (80150-80299) Winter 92:14, Fall 93:26, Mar 00:1

80150 Amikacin
➔ *CPT Assistant* Aug 05:9

80152 Amitriptyline

80154 Benzodiazepines

80156 Carbamazepine; total
➔ *CPT Changes: An Insider's View* 2001

80157 free
➔ *CPT Changes: An Insider's View* 2001

80158 Cyclosporine

80160 Desipramine

80162 Digoxin

80164 Dipropylacetic acid (valproic acid)

80166 Doxepin

80168 Ethosuximide

80170 Gentamicin

80172 Gold

80173 Haloperidol
➔ *CPT Changes: An Insider's View* 2001

80174 Imipramine

80176 Lidocaine

80178 Lithium

80182 Nortriptyline

80184 Phenobarbital

80185 Phenytoin; total

80186 free

80188 Primidone

80190 Procainamide;

80192 with metabolites (eg, n-acetyl procainamide)

80194 Quinidine

80195 Sirolimus
➔ *CPT Assistant* Mar 06:6; *CPT Changes: An Insider's View* 2006

80196 Salicylate

80197 Tacrolimus

80198 Theophylline

80200 Tobramycin

80201 Topiramate
➔ *CPT Assistant* Nov 97:28

80202 Vancomycin

80299 Quantitation of drug, not elsewhere specified
➔ *CPT Assistant* Mar 00:3, Oct 04:14, Aug 05:9

Evocative/Suppression Testing

The following test panels involve the administration of evocative or suppressive agents, and the baseline and subsequent measurement of their effects on chemical constituents. These codes are to be used for the reporting of the laboratory component of the overall testing protocol. For the physician's administration of the evocative or suppressive agents, see 90760, 90761, 90772-90774, 90775; for the supplies and drugs, see 99070. To report physician attendance and monitoring during the testing, use the appropriate evaluation and management code, including the prolonged physician care codes if required. Prolonged physician care codes are not separately reported when evocative/suppression testing involves prolonged infusions reported with 90760-90761. In the code descriptors where reference is made to a particular analyte (eg, Cortisol: 82533 x 2) the "x 2" refers to the number of times the test for that particular analyte is performed.

80400 ACTH stimulation panel; for adrenal insufficiency

This panel must include the following:

Cortisol (82533 x 2)
➔ *CPT Assistant* Summer 94:1, Fall 94:10, Aug 05:9

80402 for 21 hydroxylase deficiency

This panel must include the following:

Cortisol (82533 x 2)

17 hydroxyprogesterone (83498 x 2)
➔ *CPT Assistant* Summer 94:1, Fall 94:10

80406   for 3 beta-hydroxydehydrogenase deficiency

This panel must include the following:

Cortisol (82533 x 2)

17 hydroxypregnenolone (84143 x 2)
➔ *CPT Assistant* Summer 94:1, Fall 94:10

80408 Aldosterone suppression evaluation panel (eg, saline infusion)

This panel must include the following:

Aldosterone (82088 x 2)

Renin (84244 x 2)
➔ *CPT Assistant* Summer 94:1, Fall 94:10

80410 Calcitonin stimulation panel (eg, calcium, pentagastrin)

This panel must include the following:

Calcitonin (82308 x 3)
➔ *CPT Assistant* Summer 94:1, Fall 94:11

80412 Corticotropic releasing hormone (CRH) stimulation panel

This panel must include the following:

Cortisol (82533 x 6)

Adrenocorticotropic hormone (ACTH) (82024 x 6)
➔ *CPT Assistant* Summer 94:1, Fall 94:11

80414 Chorionic gonadotropin stimulation panel; testosterone response

This panel must include the following:

Testosterone (84403 x 2 on three pooled blood samples)
➔ *CPT Assistant* Summer 94:1, Fall 94:11

80415   estradiol response

This panel must include the following:

Estradiol (82670 x 2 on three pooled blood samples)
➔ *CPT Assistant* Summer 94:1, Fall 94:11

80416 Renal vein renin stimulation panel (eg, captopril)

This panel must include the following:

Renin (84244 x 6)
➔ *CPT Assistant* Summer 94:1

80417 Peripheral vein renin stimulation panel (eg, captopril)

This panel must include the following:

Renin (84244 x 2)

80418 Combined rapid anterior pituitary evaluation panel

This panel must include the following:

Adrenocorticotropic hormone (ACTH) (82024 x 4)

Luteinizing hormone (LH) (83002 x 4)

Follicle stimulating hormone (FSH) (83001 x 4)

Prolactin (84146 x 4)

Human growth hormone (HGH) (83003 x 4)

Cortisol (82533 x 4)

Thyroid stimulating hormone (TSH) (84443 x 4)
➔ *CPT Assistant* Summer 94:1, Fall 94:13

80420 Dexamethasone suppression panel, 48 hour

This panel must include the following:

Free cortisol, urine (82530 x 2)

Cortisol (82533 x 2)

Volume measurement for timed collection (81050 x 2)
➔ *CPT Assistant* Fall 94:13

(For single dose dexamethasone, use 82533)
➔ *CPT Assistant* Summer 94:1

80422 Glucagon tolerance panel; for insulinoma

This panel must include the following:

Glucose (82947 x 3)

Insulin (83525 x 3)
➔ *CPT Assistant* Summer 94:1, Fall 94:13

80424   for pheochromocytoma

This panel must include the following:

Catecholamines, fractionated (82384 x 2)
➔ *CPT Assistant* Summer 94:1, Fall 94:14

80426 Gonadotropin releasing hormone stimulation panel

This panel must include the following:

Follicle stimulating hormone (FSH) (83001 x 4)

Luteinizing hormone (LH) (83002 x 4)
➔ *CPT Assistant* Summer 94:1, Fall 94:14

80428 Growth hormone stimulation panel (eg, arginine infusion, l-dopa administration)

This panel must include the following:

Human growth hormone (HGH) (83003 x 4)
➔ *CPT Assistant* Summer 94:1, Fall 94:14

80430 Growth hormone suppression panel (glucose administration)

This panel must include the following:

Glucose (82947 x 3)

Human growth hormone (HGH) (83003 x 4)
➔ *CPT Assistant* Summer 94:1, Fall 94:14

80432 Insulin-induced C-peptide suppression panel

This panel must include the following:

Insulin (83525)

C-peptide (84681 x 5)

Glucose (82947 x 5)
➔ *CPT Assistant* Summer 94:1, Fall 94:15

80434   Insulin tolerance panel; for ACTH insufficiency

This panel must include the following:

Cortisol (82533 x 5)

Glucose (82947 x 5)

➔ *CPT Assistant* Summer 94:1, Fall 94:15

80435   for growth hormone deficiency

This panel must include the following:

Glucose (82947 x 5)

Human growth hormone (HGH) (83003 x 5)

➔ *CPT Assistant* Summer 94:1, Fall 94:15

80436   Metyrapone panel

This panel must include the following:

Cortisol (82533 x 2)

11 deoxycortisol (82634 x 2)

➔ *CPT Assistant* Summer 94:1, Fall 94:16

80438   Thyrotropin releasing hormone (TRH) stimulation panel; one hour

This panel must include the following:

Thyroid stimulating hormone (TSH) (84443 x 3)

➔ *CPT Assistant* Summer 94:1, Fall 94:16

80439   two hour

This panel must include the following:

Thyroid stimulating hormone (TSH) (84443 x 4)

➔ *CPT Assistant* Summer 94:1, Fall 94:16

80440   for hyperprolactinemia

This panel must include the following:

Prolactin (84146 x 3)

➔ *CPT Assistant* Summer 94:1, Fall 94:16, Aug 05:9

Consultations (Clinical Pathology)

A clinical pathology consultation is a service, including a written report, rendered by the pathologist in response to a request from an attending physician in relation to a test result(s) requiring additional medical interpretive judgment.

Reporting of a test result(s) without medical interpretive judgment is not considered a clinical pathology consultation.

80500   Clinical pathology consultation; limited, without review of patient's history and medical records

➔ *CPT Assistant* Apr 97:9, Nov 02:9, Aug 05:9

80502   comprehensive, for a complex diagnostic problem, with review of patient's history and medical records

➔ *CPT Assistant* Apr 97:9, Nov 02:9, Aug 05:9

(These codes may also be used for pharmacokinetic consultations)

(For consultations involving the examination and evaluation of the patient, see 99241-99255)

Urinalysis

For specific analyses, see appropriate section.

(For urinalysis, infectious agent detection, semi-quantitative analysis of volatile compounds, use Category III code 0041T)

81000   Urinalysis, by dip stick or tablet reagent for bilirubin, glucose, hemoglobin, ketones, leukocytes, nitrite, pH, protein, specific gravity, urobilinogen, any number of these constituents; non-automated, with microscopy

➔ *CPT Assistant* Winter 90, Winter 91:10, Fall 93:25, Aug 05:9

81001   automated, with microscopy

81002   non-automated, without microscopy

➔ *CPT Assistant* Mar 98:3, Apr 07:1

81003   automated, without microscopy

81005   Urinalysis; qualitative or semiquantitative, except immunoassays

➔ *CPT Assistant* Winter 90, Winter 91:10, Fall 93:25

(For non-immunoassay reagent strip urinalysis, see 81000, 81002)

(For immunoassay, qualitative or semiquantitative, use 83518)

(For microalbumin, see 82043, 82044)

81007   bacteriuria screen, except by culture or dipstick

➔ *CPT Changes: An Insider's View* 2001

(For culture, see 87086-87088)

(For dipstick, use 81000 or 81002)

81015   microscopic only

▶(For sperm evaluation for retrograde ejaculation, use 89331)◀

81020   two or three glass test

➔ *CPT Assistant* Winter 90, Winter 91:10

81025   Urine pregnancy test, by visual color comparison methods

➔ *CPT Assistant* Mar 98:3

81050   Volume measurement for timed collection, each

81099   Unlisted urinalysis procedure

➔ *CPT Assistant* Aug 05:9

Chemistry

The material for examination may be from any source unless otherwise specified in the code descriptor. When an analyte is measured in multiple specimens from different sources, or in specimens that are obtained at different times, the analyte is reported separately for each source and for each specimen. The examination is quantitative unless specified. To report an organ or disease oriented panel, see codes 80048-80076.

When a code describes a method where measurement of multiple analytes may require one or several procedures, each procedure is coded separately (eg, 82491-82492, 82541-82544). For example, if two analytes are measured using column chromatography using a single stationary or mobile phase, use 82492. If the same two analytes are measured using different stationary or mobile phase conditions, 82491 would be used twice. If a total of four analytes are measured where two analytes are measured with a single stationary and mobile phase, and the other two analytes are measured using a different stationary and mobile phase, use 82492 twice. If a total of three analytes are measured where two analytes are measured using a single stationary or mobile phase condition, and the third analyte is measured separately using a different stationary or mobile phase procedure, use 82492 once for the two analytes measured under the same condition, and use 82491 once for the third analyte measured separately.

Clinical information derived from the results of laboratory data that is mathematically calculated (eg, free thyroxine index [T7]) is considered part of the test procedure and therefore is not a separately reportable service.

82000 Acetaldehyde, blood
➲ *CPT Assistant* Aug 05:9

82003 Acetaminophen

82009 Acetone or other ketone bodies, serum; qualitative

82010   quantitative

82013 Acetylcholinesterase

(Acid, gastric, see gastric acid, 82926, 82928)

(Acid phosphatase, see 84060-84066)

82016 Acylcarnitines; qualitative, each specimen
➲ *CPT Assistant* Nov 98:23

82017   quantitative, each specimen
➲ *CPT Assistant* Nov 98:23; *CPT Changes: An Insider's View* 2000

(For carnitine, use 82379)

82024 Adrenocorticotropic hormone (ACTH)

82030 Adenosine, 5-monophosphate, cyclic (cyclic AMP)

82040 Albumin; serum
➲ *CPT Assistant* Dec 99:2

82042   urine or other source, quantitative, each specimen
➲ *CPT Changes: An Insider's View* 2001

82043   urine, microalbumin, quantitative
➲ *CPT Assistant* Summer 94:2

82044   urine, microalbumin, semiquantitative (eg, reagent strip assay)
➲ *CPT Assistant* Summer 94:2, Mar 98:3, Sep 02:10

(For prealbumin, use 84134)

82045   ischemia modified
➲ *CPT Changes: An Insider's View* 2005

82055 Alcohol (ethanol); any specimen except breath

(For other volatiles, alcohol, use 84600)

82075   breath

82085 Aldolase

82088 Aldosterone

(Alkaline phosphatase, see 84075, 84080)

82101 Alkaloids, urine, quantitative
➲ *CPT Assistant* Aug 05:9

(Alphaketoglutarate, see 82009, 82010)

(Alpha tocopherol (Vitamin E), use 84446)

82103 Alpha-1-antitrypsin; total

82104   phenotype

82105 Alpha-fetoprotein (AFP); serum

82106   amniotic fluid

82107   AFP-L3 fraction isoform and total AFP (including ratio)
➲ *CPT Changes: An Insider's View* 2007

82108 Aluminum

82120 Amines, vaginal fluid, qualitative
➲ *CPT Assistant* Nov 99:45; *CPT Changes: An Insider's View* 2000

(For combined pH and amines test for vaginitis, use 82120 and 83986)

82127 Amino acids; single, qualitative, each specimen
➲ *CPT Assistant* Nov 98:24

82128   multiple, qualitative, each specimen
➲ *CPT Assistant* Nov 98:24

82131   single, quantitative, each specimen
➲ *CPT Assistant* May 98:11, Nov 98:24

82135 Aminolevulinic acid, delta (ALA)

82136 Amino acids, 2 to 5 amino acids, quantitative, each specimen
➲ *CPT Assistant* Nov 98:24

82139 Amino acids, 6 or more amino acids, quantitative, each specimen
➲ *CPT Assistant* Nov 98:24

82140   Ammonia

82143   Amniotic fluid scan (spectrophotometric)

(For L/S ratio, use 83661)

(Amobarbital, see 80100-80103 for qualitative analysis, 82205 for quantitative analysis)

82145   Amphetamine or methamphetamine

(For qualitative analysis, see 80100-80103)

82150   Amylase

82154   Androstanediol glucuronide
➔ *CPT Assistant* Summer 94:5

82157   Androstenedione

82160   Androsterone

82163   Angiotensin II

82164   Angiotensin I - converting enzyme (ACE)

(Antidiuretic hormone (ADH), use 84588)

(Antimony, use 83015)

(Antitrypsin, alpha-1-, see 82103, 82104)

82172   Apolipoprotein, each

82175   Arsenic

(For heavy metal screening, use 83015)

82180   Ascorbic acid (Vitamin C), blood

(Aspirin, see acetylsalicylic acid, 80196)

(Atherogenic index, blood, ultracentrifugation, quantitative, use 83701)

82190   Atomic absorption spectroscopy, each analyte

82205   Barbiturates, not elsewhere specified
➔ *CPT Assistant* Jul 03:7, Aug 05:9

(For qualitative analysis, see 80100-80103)

(For B-Natriuretic peptide, use 83880)

82232   Beta-2 microglobulin

(Bicarbonate, use 82374)

82239   Bile acids; total

82240   cholylglycine

(For bile pigments, urine, see 81000-81005)

82247   Bilirubin; total
➔ *CPT Assistant* Nov 98:24, Apr 99:6, Dec 99:1, Jan 00:7

82248   direct
➔ *CPT Assistant* Nov 98:24, Apr 99:6, Dec 99:1

82252   feces, qualitative

82261   Biotinidase, each specimen
➔ *CPT Assistant* Nov 98:24

82270   Blood, occult, by peroxidase activity (eg, guaiac), qualitative; feces, consecutive collected specimens with single determination, for colorectal neoplasm screening (ie, patient was provided 3 cards or single triple card for consecutive collection)
➔ *CPT Assistant* Sep 03:15, Feb 06:7; *CPT Changes: An Insider's View* 2002, 2006

82271   other sources
➔ *CPT Assistant* Feb 06:7; *CPT Changes: An Insider's View* 2006

▲ **82272**   Blood, occult, by peroxidase activity (eg, guaiac), qualitative, feces, 1-3 simultaneous determinations, performed for other than colorectal neoplasm screening
➔ *CPT Assistant* Feb 06:7; *CPT Changes: An Insider's View* 2006, 2008

(82273 has been deleted. To report, use 82271)

(Blood urea nitrogen (BUN), see 84520, 84525)

82274   Blood, occult, by fecal hemoglobin determination by immunoassay, qualitative, feces, 1-3 simultaneous determinations
➔ *CPT Changes: An Insider's View* 2002

82286   Bradykinin

82300   Cadmium
➔ *CPT Assistant* Aug 05:9

82306   Calcifediol (25-OH Vitamin D-3)

82307   Calciferol (Vitamin D)

(For 1,25-Dihydroxyvitamin D, use 82652)

82308   Calcitonin

82310   Calcium; total
➔ *CPT Assistant* Dec 99:2

82330   ionized

82331   after calcium infusion test

82340   urine quantitative, timed specimen

82355   Calculus; qualitative analysis
➔ *CPT Changes: An Insider's View* 2002

82360   quantitative analysis, chemical

82365   infrared spectroscopy

82370   X-ray diffraction
➔ *CPT Changes: An Insider's View* 2001

(Carbamates, see individual listings)

82373   Carbohydrate deficient transferrin
➔ *CPT Changes: An Insider's View* 2001

82374   Carbon dioxide (bicarbonate)
➔ *CPT Assistant* Dec 99:2

(See also 82803)

82375   Carbon monoxide (carboxyhemoglobin); quantitative

82376   qualitative

(To report end-tidal carbon monoxide, use Category III code 0043T)

82378 Carcinoembryonic antigen (CEA)
➲ *CPT Assistant* Fall 93:25, Aug 96:11

82379 Carnitine (total and free), quantitative, each specimen
➲ *CPT Assistant* Nov 98:24

(For acylcarnitine, see 82016, 82017)

82380 Carotene

82382 Catecholamines; total urine

82383 blood

82384 fractionated

(For urine metabolites, see 83835, 84585)

82387 Cathepsin-D

82390 Ceruloplasmin

82397 Chemiluminescent assay
➲ *CPT Assistant* Fall 93:25

82415 Chloramphenicol
➲ *CPT Assistant* Aug 05:9

82435 Chloride; blood
➲ *CPT Assistant* Dec 99:2

82436 urine

82438 other source
➲ *CPT Assistant* Jul 03:7

(For sweat collection by iontophoresis, use 89230)

82441 Chlorinated hydrocarbons, screen

(Chlorpromazine, use 84022)

(Cholecalciferol (Vitamin D), use 82307)

82465 Cholesterol, serum or whole blood, total
➲ *CPT Assistant* Dec 99:2, Mar 00:11, Feb 05:9; *CPT Changes: An Insider's View* 2001

(For high density lipoprotein (HDL), use 83718)

82480 Cholinesterase; serum

82482 RBC

82485 Chondroitin B sulfate, quantitative

(Chorionic gonadotropin, see gonadotropin, 84702, 84703)

82486 Chromatography, qualitative; column (eg, gas liquid or HPLC), analyte not elsewhere specified
➲ *CPT Assistant* Nov 98:24-25

82487 paper, 1-dimensional, analyte not elsewhere specified

82488 paper, 2-dimensional, analyte not elsewhere specified

82489 thin layer, analyte not elsewhere specified

82491 Chromatography, quantitative, column (eg, gas liquid or HPLC); single analyte not elsewhere specified, single stationary and mobile phase
➲ *CPT Assistant* Fall 93:25, Nov 98:24-25, Mar 00:3

82492 multiple analytes, single stationary and mobile phase
➲ *CPT Assistant* Nov 98:24-25, Mar 00:3

82495 Chromium

82507 Citrate
➲ *CPT Assistant* Aug 05:9

82520 Cocaine or metabolite

(Cocaine, qualitative analysis, see 80100-80103)

(Codeine, qualitative analysis, see 80100-80103)

(Codeine, quantitative analysis, see 82101)

(Complement, see 86160-86162)

82523 Collagen cross links, any method

82525 Copper

(Coproporphyrin, see 84119, 84120)

(Corticosteroids, use 83491)

82528 Corticosterone

82530 Cortisol; free
➲ *CPT Assistant* Summer 94:3

82533 total
➲ *CPT Assistant* Summer 94:3

(C-peptide, use 84681)

82540 Creatine

82541 Column chromatography/mass spectrometry (eg, GC/MS, or HPLC/MS), analyte not elsewhere specified; qualitative, single stationary and mobile phase
➲ *CPT Assistant* Nov 98:24-25

82542 quantitative, single stationary and mobile phase
➲ *CPT Assistant* Nov 98:24-25

82543 stable isotope dilution, single analyte, quantitative, single stationary and mobile phase
➲ *CPT Assistant* Nov 98:24-25

82544 stable isotope dilution, multiple analytes, quantitative, single stationary and mobile phase
➲ *CPT Assistant* Nov 98:24-25, Dec 99:7

82550 Creatine kinase (CK), (CPK); total
➲ *CPT Assistant* Feb 98:1, Dec 99:2

82552 isoenzymes
➲ *CPT Assistant* Feb 98:1

82553 MB fraction only
➲ *CPT Assistant* Feb 98:1

82554 isoforms
➲ *CPT Assistant* Feb 98:1

82565 Creatinine; blood
➲ *CPT Assistant* Dec 99:2

82570 other source

82575 clearance

82585 Cryofibrinogen

82595 Cryoglobulin, qualitative or semi-quantitative (eg, cryocrit)
➔ *CPT Changes: An Insider's View* 2001

(For quantitative, cryoglobulin, see 82784, 82785)

(Crystals, pyrophosphate vs urate, use 89060)

82600 Cyanide
➔ *CPT Assistant* Aug 05:9

82607 Cyanocobalamin (Vitamin B-12);

82608 unsaturated binding capacity

(Cyclic AMP, use 82030)

(Cyclic GMP, use 83008)

(Cyclosporine, use 80158)

● **82610** Cystatin C
➔ *CPT Changes: An Insider's View* 2008

82615 Cystine and homocystine, urine, qualitative

82626 Dehydroepiandrosterone (DHEA)
➔ *CPT Assistant* Summer 94:4

82627 Dehydroepiandrosterone-sulfate (DHEA-S)
➔ *CPT Assistant* Summer 94:4

(Delta-aminolevulinic acid (ALA), use 82135)

82633 Desoxycorticosterone, 11-

82634 Deoxycortisol, 11-

(Dexamethasone suppression test, use 80420)

(Diastase, urine, use 82150)

82638 Dibucaine number

(Dichloroethane, use 84600)

(Dichloromethane, use 84600)

(Diethylether, use 84600)

82646 Dihydrocodeinone

(For qualitative analysis, see 80100-80103)

82649 Dihydromorphinone

(For qualitative analysis, see 80100-80103)

82651 Dihydrotestosterone (DHT)

82652 Dihydroxyvitamin D, 1,25-

82654 Dimethadione

(For qualitative analysis, see 80100-80103)

(Diphenylhydantoin, use 80185)

(Dipropylacetic acid, use 80164)

(Dopamine, see 82382-82384)

(Duodenal contents, see individual enzymes; for intubation and collection, use 89100)

82656 Elastase, pancreatic (EL-1), fecal, qualitative or semi-quantitative
➔ *CPT Assistant* Sep 05:9; *CPT Changes: An Insider's View* 2005

82657 Enzyme activity in blood cells, cultured cells, or tissue, not elsewhere specified; nonradioactive substrate, each specimen
➔ *CPT Assistant* Nov 98:25

82658 radioactive substrate, each specimen
➔ *CPT Assistant* Nov 98:25

82664 Electrophoretic technique, not elsewhere specified

(Endocrine receptor assays, see 84233-84235)

82666 Epiandrosterone

(Epinephrine, see 82382-82384)

82668 Erythropoietin

82670 Estradiol

82671 Estrogens; fractionated

82672 total

(Estrogen receptor assay, use 84233)

82677 Estriol

82679 Estrone

(Ethanol, see 82055 and 82075)

82690 Ethchlorvynol

(Ethyl alcohol, see 82055 and 82075)

82693 Ethylene glycol

82696 Etiocholanolone

(For fractionation of ketosteroids, use 83593)

82705 Fat or lipids, feces; qualitative
➔ *CPT Assistant* Aug 05:9

82710 quantitative

82715 Fat differential, feces, quantitative

82725 Fatty acids, nonesterified

82726 Very long chain fatty acids
➔ *CPT Assistant* Nov 98:25

(For long-chain (C20-22) omega-3 fatty acids in red blood cell (RBC) membranes, use Category III code 0111T)

82728 Ferritin

(Fetal hemoglobin, see hemoglobin 83030, 83033, and 85460)

(Fetoprotein, alpha-1, see 82105, 82106)

82731 Fetal fibronectin, cervicovaginal secretions, semi-quantitative
➔ *CPT Assistant* Nov 98:25

82735 Fluoride

82742 Flurazepam

(For qualitative analysis, see 80100-80103)

(Foam stability test, use 83662)

82746	Folic acid; serum
82747	RBC

(Follicle stimulating hormone (FSH), use 83001)

82757 Fructose, semen

(Fructosamine, use 82985)

(Fructose, TLC screen, use 84375)

82759 Galactokinase, RBC

82760 Galactose

82775 Galactose-1-phosphate uridyl transferase; quantitative

82776 screen

82784 Gammaglobulin; IgA, IgD, IgG, IgM, each
➔ *CPT Assistant* Spring 94:31, Aug 00:11

82785 IgE
➔ *CPT Assistant* Spring 94:31

(For allergen specific IgE, see 86003, 86005)

82787 immunoglobulin subclasses (IgG1, 2, 3, or 4), each
➔ *CPT Changes: An Insider's View* 2001

(Gamma-glutamyltransferase [GGT], use 82977)

82800 Gases, blood, pH only
➔ *CPT Assistant* Aug 05:9

82803 Gases, blood, any combination of pH, pCO_2, pO_2, CO_2, HCO_3 (including calculated O_2 saturation);

(Use 82803 for 2 or more of the above listed analytes)

82805 with O_2 saturation, by direct measurement, except pulse oximetry

82810 Gases, blood, O_2 saturation only, by direct measurement, except pulse oximetry

(For pulse oximetry, use 94760)

82820 Hemoglobin-oxygen affinity (pO_2 for 50% hemoglobin saturation with oxygen)

82926 Gastric acid, free and total, each specimen

82928 Gastric acid, free or total, each specimen

82938 Gastrin after secretin stimulation

82941 Gastrin
➔ *CPT Assistant* Aug 05:9

(Gentamicin, use 80170)

(GGT, use 82977)

(GLC, gas liquid chromatography, use 82486)

82943 Glucagon

82945 Glucose, body fluid, other than blood
➔ *CPT Changes: An Insider's View* 2001

82946 Glucagon tolerance test

82947 Glucose; quantitative, blood (except reagent strip)
➔ *CPT Assistant* Summer 93:14, Summer 94:5, Sep 99:10, Dec 99:2, Jun 02:3, Feb 05:9; *CPT Changes: An Insider's View* 2001

82948 blood, reagent strip
➔ *CPT Assistant* Summer 94:5, Jan 99:10

82950 post glucose dose (includes glucose)
➔ *CPT Assistant* Sep 99:10, Jun 02:3, Feb 05:9

82951 tolerance test (GTT), three specimens (includes glucose)
➔ *CPT Assistant* Feb 01:10, Feb 05:9

82952 tolerance test, each additional beyond three specimens
➔ *CPT Assistant* Feb 01:10

82953 tolbutamide tolerance test

(For insulin tolerance test, see 80434, 80435)

(For leucine tolerance test, use 80428)

(For semiquantitative urine glucose, see 81000, 81002, 81005, 81099)

82955 Glucose-6-phosphate dehydrogenase (G6PD); quantitative

82960 screen

(For glucose tolerance test with medication, use 90774 in addition)

82962 Glucose, blood by glucose monitoring device(s) cleared by the FDA specifically for home use
➔ *CPT Assistant* Summer 94:4, Jan 99:10

82963 Glucosidase, beta

82965 Glutamate dehydrogenase

82975 Glutamine (glutamic acid amide)

82977 Glutamyltransferase, gamma (GGT)
➔ *CPT Assistant* Dec 99:1

82978 Glutathione

82979 Glutathione reductase, RBC

82980 Glutethimide

(Glycohemoglobin, use 83036)

82985 Glycated protein
➔ *CPT Assistant* Summer 94:2

(Gonadotropin, chorionic, see 84702, 84703)

83001 Gonadotropin; follicle stimulating hormone (FSH)
➔ *CPT Assistant* Aug 05:9

83002 luteinizing hormone (LH)

(For luteinizing releasing factor (LRH), use 83727)

83003 Growth hormone, human (HGH) (somatotropin)

(For antibody to human growth hormone, use 86277)

83008 Guanosine monophosphate (GMP), cyclic

83009 Helicobacter pylori, blood test analysis for urease activity, non-radioactive isotope (eg, C-13)
➔ *CPT Changes: An Insider's View* 2005

(For H. pylori, breath test analysis for urease activity, see 83013, 83014)

83010 Haptoglobin; quantitative

83012 phenotypes

83013 Helicobacter pylori; breath test analysis for urease activity, non-radioactive isotope (eg, C-13)
> *CPT Assistant* Nov 98:25, Feb 99:8, Nov 99:45; *CPT Changes: An Insider's View* 2001, 2002, 2005

83014 drug administration
> *CPT Assistant* Nov 98:25, Feb 99:8, Nov 99:45; *CPT Changes: An Insider's View* 2005

(For H. pylori, stool, use 87338. For H. pylori, liquid scintillation counter, see 78267, 78268. For H. pylori, enzyme immunoassay, use 87339)

(For H. pylori, blood test analysis for urease activity, use 83009)

83015 Heavy metal (eg, arsenic, barium, beryllium, bismuth, antimony, mercury); screen

83018 quantitative, each

83020 Hemoglobin fractionation and quantitation; electrophoresis (eg, A2, S, C, and/or F)
> *CPT Assistant* Nov 98:25

83021 chromatography (eg, A2, S, C, and/or F)
> *CPT Assistant* Nov 98:25, Dec 99:7

►(For glycosylated [A1c] hemoglobin analysis, by chromatography, in the absence of an identified hemoglobin variant, use 83036)◄

83026 Hemoglobin; by copper sulfate method, non-automated

83030 F (fetal), chemical

83033 F (fetal), qualitative
> *CPT Changes: An Insider's View* 2001

83036 glycosylated (A1C)
> *CPT Assistant* Summer 94:2, Feb 06:7, Oct 06:15; *CPT Changes: An Insider's View* 2006

►(For glycosylated [A1c] hemoglobin analysis, by chromatography, in the setting of an identified hemoglobin variant, use 83021)◄

(For fecal hemoglobin detection by immunoassay, use 82274)

83037 glycosylated (A1C) by device cleared by FDA for home use
> *CPT Assistant* Feb 06:7, Oct 06:15; *CPT Changes: An Insider's View* 2006

83045 methemoglobin, qualitative

83050 methemoglobin, quantitative

83051 plasma

83055 sulfhemoglobin, qualitative

83060 sulfhemoglobin, quantitative

83065 thermolabile

83068 unstable, screen

83069 urine

83070 Hemosiderin; qualitative

83071 quantitative

(Heroin, see 80100-80103)

(HIAA, use 83497)

(High performance liquid chromatography (HPLC), use 82486)

83080 b-Hexosaminidase, each assay
> *CPT Assistant* Nov 98:25

83088 Histamine

(Hollander test, use 91052)

83090 Homocysteine
> *CPT Assistant* Jan 01:13; *CPT Changes: An Insider's View* 2001

83150 Homovanillic acid (HVA)
> *CPT Assistant* Aug 05:9

(Hormones, see individual alphabetic listings in **Chemistry** section)

(Hydrogen breath test, use 91065)

83491 Hydroxycorticosteroids, 17- (17-OHCS)
> *CPT Assistant* Aug 05:9

(For cortisol, see 82530, 82533. For deoxycortisol, use 82634)

83497 Hydroxyindolacetic acid, 5-(HIAA)

(For urine qualitative test, use 81005)

(5-Hydroxytryptamine, use 84260)

83498 Hydroxyprogesterone, 17-d

83499 Hydroxyprogesterone, 20-

83500 Hydroxyproline; free
> *CPT Assistant* Aug 05:9

83505 total

83516 Immunoassay for analyte other than infectious agent antibody or infectious agent antigen, qualitative or semiquantitative; multiple step method
> *CPT Assistant* Nov 98:25

83518 single step method (eg, reagent strip)
> *CPT Assistant* Fall 93:26

83519 Immunoassay, analyte, quantitative; by radiopharmaceutical technique (eg, RIA)
> *CPT Assistant* Fall 93:26, Summer 94:2

83520 not otherwise specified
> *CPT Assistant* Fall 93:26

(For immunoassays for antibodies to infectious agent antigens, see analyte and method specific codes in the **Immunology** section)

(For immunoassay of tumor antigen not elsewhere specified, use 86316)

(Immunoglobulins, see 82784, 82785)

83525	Insulin; total
	(For proinsulin, use 84206)
83527	free
	➡ *CPT Assistant* Summer 94:5
83528	Intrinsic factor
	(For intrinsic factor antibodies, use 86340)
83540	Iron
	➡ *CPT Assistant* Fall 93:25
83550	Iron binding capacity
83570	Isocitric dehydrogenase (IDH)
	(Isonicotinic acid hydrazide, INH, see code for specific method)
	(Isopropyl alcohol, use 84600)
83582	Ketogenic steroids, fractionation
	(Ketone bodies, for serum, see 82009, 82010; for urine, see 81000-81003)
83586	Ketosteroids, 17- (17-KS); total
83593	fractionation
83605	Lactate (lactic acid)
	➡ *CPT Assistant* Aug 05:9
83615	Lactate dehydrogenase (LD), (LDH);
	➡ *CPT Assistant* Fall 93:25, Feb 98:1, Dec 99:2
83625	isoenzymes, separation and quantitation
	➡ *CPT Assistant* Fall 93:25, Feb 98:1
83630	Lactoferrin, fecal; qualitative
	➡ *CPT Assistant* Feb 06:7; *CPT Changes: An Insider's View* 2005, 2006
83631	quantitative
	➡ *CPT Assistant* Feb 06:7, Jan 07:29; *CPT Changes: An Insider's View* 2006
83632	Lactogen, human placental (HPL) human chorionic somatomammotropin
83633	Lactose, urine; qualitative
83634	quantitative
	(For tolerance, see 82951, 82952)
	(For breath hydrogen test for lactase deficiency, use 91065)
83655	Lead
83661	Fetal lung maturity assessment; lecithin sphingomyelin (L/S) ratio
	➡ *CPT Changes: An Insider's View* 2001
83662	foam stability test
83663	fluorescence polarization
	➡ *CPT Changes: An Insider's View* 2001
83664	lamellar body density
	➡ *CPT Changes: An Insider's View* 2001
	(For phosphatidylglycerol, use 84081)

83670	Leucine aminopeptidase (LAP)
83690	Lipase
83695	Lipoprotein (a)
	➡ *CPT Assistant* Feb 06:7; *CPT Changes: An Insider's View* 2006
83698	Lipoprotein-associated phospholipase A_2 (Lp-PLA$_2$)
	➡ *CPT Changes: An Insider's View* 2007
83700	Lipoprotein, blood; electrophoretic separation and quantitation
	➡ *CPT Assistant* Feb 06:7; *CPT Changes: An Insider's View* 2006
83701	high resolution fractionation and quantitation of lipoproteins including lipoprotein subclasses when performed (eg, electrophoresis, ultracentrifugation)
	➡ *CPT Assistant* Feb 06:7; *CPT Changes: An Insider's View* 2006
83704	quantitation of lipoprotein particle numbers and lipoprotein particle subclasses (eg, by nuclear magnetic resonance spectroscopy)
	➡ *CPT Assistant* Feb 06:7; *CPT Changes: An Insider's View* 2006
	(83715, 83716 have been deleted. To report, use 83700, 83701)
83718	Lipoprotein, direct measurement; high density cholesterol (HDL cholesterol)
	➡ *CPT Assistant* Oct 99:11, Mar 00:11, Feb 05:9
83719	VLDL cholesterol
	➡ *CPT Assistant* Oct 99:11
83721	LDL cholesterol
	➡ *CPT Assistant* Nov 98:25, Oct 99:11
	(For fractionation by high resolution electrophoresis or ultracentrifugation, use 83701)
	(For lipoprotein particle numbers and subclasses analysis by nuclear magnetic resonance spectroscopy, use 83704)
	(To report direct measurement, intermediate density lipoproteins [remnant lipoproteins], use Category III code 0026T)
83727	Luteinizing releasing factor (LRH)
	(Luteinizing hormone (LH), use 83002)
	(For qualitative analysis, see 80100-80103)
	(Macroglobulins, alpha-2, use 86329)
83735	Magnesium
83775	Malate dehydrogenase
	(Maltose tolerance, see 82951, 82952)
	(Mammotropin, use 84146)
83785	Manganese
	(Marijuana, see 80100-80103)
83788	Mass spectrometry and tandem mass spectrometry (MS, MS/MS), analyte not elsewhere specified; qualitative, each specimen
	➡ *CPT Assistant* Nov 98:26

83789   quantitative, each specimen
> *CPT Assistant* Nov 98:26

83805   Meprobamate
> *CPT Assistant* Aug 05:9

(For qualitative analysis, see 80100-80103)

83825   Mercury, quantitative

(Mercury screen, use 83015)

83835   Metanephrines

(For catecholamines, see 82382-82384)

83840   Methadone

(For methadone qualitative analysis, see 80100-80103)

(Methamphetamine, see 80100-80103, 82145)

(Methanol, use 84600)

83857   Methemalbumin

(Methemoglobin, see hemoglobin 83045, 83050)

83858   Methsuximide

(Methyl alcohol, use 84600)

(Microalbumin, see 82043 for quantitative, see 82044 for semiquantitative)

(Microglobulin, beta-2, use 82232)

83864   Mucopolysaccharides, acid; quantitative

83866   screen

83872   Mucin, synovial fluid (Ropes test)

83873   Myelin basic protein, cerebrospinal fluid
> *CPT Changes: An Insider's View* 2002

(For oligoclonal bands, use 83916)

83874   Myoglobin
> *CPT Assistant* Feb 98:1

(Nalorphine, use 83925)

83880   Natriuretic peptide
> *CPT Assistant* Jul 03:7; *CPT Changes: An Insider's View* 2003

83883   Nephelometry, each analyte not elsewhere specified

83885   Nickel

83887   Nicotine

Codes 83890-83914 are intended for use with molecular diagnostic techniques for analysis of nucleic acids.

Codes 83890-83914 are coded by procedure rather than analyte.

Code separately for each procedure used in an analysis. For example, a procedure requiring isolation of DNA, restriction endonuclease digestion, electrophoresis, and nucleic acid probe amplification would be coded 83890, 83892, 83894, and 83898.

When molecular diagnostic procedures are performed to test for oncology, hematology, neurology or inherited disorder, use the appropriate modifier to specify probe type or condition tested. (See **Appendix I** for a listing of appropriate modifiers to report with molecular diagnostic and cytogenetic procedures.)

(For microbial identification, see 87470-87801)

(For array technology using more than 10 probes, see 88384-88386)

83890   Molecular diagnostics; molecular isolation or extraction
> *CPT Assistant* Fall 93:26, Nov 98:26, Jul 05:1, Jan 06:5

83891   isolation or extraction of highly purified nucleic acid
> *CPT Assistant* Nov 98:26, Jul 05:1, Jan 06:5

83892   enzymatic digestion
> *CPT Assistant* Fall 93:26, Jul 05:1, Jan 06:5

83893   dot/slot blot production
> *CPT Assistant* Nov 98:26, Jul 05:1, Jan 06:5

83894   separation by gel electrophoresis (eg, agarose, polyacrylamide)
> *CPT Assistant* Fall 93:25, Nov 98:26, Jul 05:1, Jan 06:5

83896   nucleic acid probe, each
> *CPT Assistant* Fall 93:26, Aug 02:10, Jul 05:1, Jan 06:5

83897   nucleic acid transfer (eg, Southern, Northern)
> *CPT Assistant* Nov 98:26, Jul 05:1, Jan 06:5

▲ **83898**   amplification, target, each nucleic acid sequence
> *CPT Assistant* Fall 93:26, Nov 98:26, Jul 05:1, Jan 06:5, Feb 06:7; *CPT Changes: An Insider's View* 2001, 2006, 2008

▶(For multiplex target amplification, see 83900, 83901)◀

▶(For signal amplification, use 83908)◀

▲ **83900**   amplification, target, multiplex, first two nucleic acid sequences
> *CPT Assistant* Jan 06:5, Feb 06:7; *CPT Changes: An Insider's View* 2006, 2008

+▲ **83901**   amplification, target, multiplex, each additional nucleic acid sequence beyond 2 (List separately in addition to code for primary procedure)
> *CPT Assistant* Nov 98:26, Jul 05:1, Aug 05:9, Jan 06:5, Feb 06:7; *CPT Changes: An Insider's View* 2006, 2008

(Use 83901 in conjunction with 83900)

83902   reverse transcription
> *CPT Assistant* Jul 05:1, Jan 06:5; *CPT Changes: An Insider's View* 2001

83903   mutation scanning, by physical properties (eg, single strand conformational polymorphisms (SSCP), heteroduplex, denaturing gradient gel electrophoresis (DGGE), RNA'ase A), single segment, each
> *CPT Assistant* Nov 98:26, Jul 05:1, Jan 06:5

83904   mutation identification by sequencing, single segment, each segment
> *CPT Assistant* Nov 98:26, Jul 05:1, Jan 06:5

83905　mutation identification by allele specific transcription, single segment, each segment
➔ *CPT Assistant* Nov 98:26, Jul 05:1, Jan 06:5

83906　mutation identification by allele specific translation, single segment, each segment
➔ *CPT Assistant* Nov 98:26, Jul 05:1, Jan 06:5

83907　lysis of cells prior to nucleic acid extraction (eg, stool specimens, paraffin embedded tissue)
➔ *CPT Assistant* Jan 06:5, Feb 06:7; *CPT Changes: An Insider's View* 2006

▲ **83908**　amplification, signal, each nucleic acid sequence
➔ *CPT Assistant* Jan 06:5, Feb 06:7; *CPT Changes: An Insider's View* 2006, 2008

▶(For target amplification, see 83898, 83900, 83901)◀

83909　separation and identification by high resolution technique (eg, capillary electrophoresis)
➔ *CPT Assistant* Jan 06:5, Feb 06:7; *CPT Changes: An Insider's View* 2006

83912　interpretation and report
➔ *CPT Assistant* Jul 05:1, Jan 06:5

83913　RNA stabilization
➔ *CPT Changes: An Insider's View* 2007

83914　Mutation identification by enzymatic ligation or primer extension, single segment, each segment (eg, oligonucleotide ligation assay (OLA), single base chain extension (SBCE), or allele-specific primer extension (ASPE))
➔ *CPT Assistant* Feb 06:7; *CPT Changes: An Insider's View* 2006

83915　Nucleotidase 5'-

83916　Oligoclonal immune (oligoclonal bands)
➔ *CPT Changes: An Insider's View* 2002

83918　Organic acids; total, quantitative, each specimen
➔ *CPT Assistant* Mar 96:11, Nov 98:26; *CPT Changes: An Insider's View* 2001

83919　qualitative, each specimen
➔ *CPT Assistant* Nov 98:26

83921　Organic acid, single, quantitative
➔ *CPT Changes: An Insider's View* 2001

83925　Opiates (eg, morphine, meperidine)

83930　Osmolality; blood

83935　urine

83937　Osteocalcin (bone g1a protein)
➔ *CPT Assistant* Summer 94:5

83945　Oxalate

83950　Oncoprotein, HER-2/neu
➔ *CPT Changes: An Insider's View* 2002

(For tissue, see 88342, 88365)

83970　Parathormone (parathyroid hormone)

(Pesticide, quantitative, see code for specific method. For screen for chlorinated hydrocarbons, use 82441)

83986　pH, body fluid, except blood

(For blood pH, see 82800, 82803)

83992　Phencyclidine (PCP)

(For qualitative analysis, see 80100-80103)

(Phenobarbital, use 80184)

● **83993**　Calprotectin, fecal
➔ *CPT Changes: An Insider's View* 2008

84022　Phenothiazine
➔ *CPT Assistant* Aug 05:9

(For qualitative analysis, see 80100, 80101)

84030　Phenylalanine (PKU), blood

(Phenylalanine-tyrosine ratio, see 84030, 84510)

84035　Phenylketones, qualitative

84060　Phosphatase, acid; total

84061　　forensic examination

84066　　prostatic

84075　Phosphatase, alkaline;
➔ *CPT Assistant* Dec 99:2

84078　　heat stable (total not included)

84080　　isoenzymes

84081　Phosphatidylglycerol

(Phosphates inorganic, use 84100)

(Phosphates, organic, see code for specific method. For cholinesterase, see 82480, 82482)

84085　Phosphogluconate, 6-, dehydrogenase, RBC

84087　Phosphohexose isomerase

84100　Phosphorus inorganic (phosphate);
➔ *CPT Assistant* Dec 99:2, Aug 05:9

84105　　urine

(Pituitary gonadotropins, see 83001-83002)

(PKU, see 84030, 84035)

84106　Porphobilinogen, urine; qualitative

84110　　quantitative

84119　Porphyrins, urine; qualitative

84120　　quantitation and fractionation

84126　Porphyrins, feces; quantitative

84127　　qualitative

(Porphyrin precursors, see 82135, 84106, 84110)

(For protoporphyrin, RBC, see 84202, 84203)

84132　Potassium; serum
➔ *CPT Assistant* Dec 99:2, Jun 02:3

84133　　urine

84134	Prealbumin
	(For microalbumin, see 82043, 82044)
84135	Pregnanediol
84138	Pregnanetriol
84140	Pregnenolone
	➔ *CPT Assistant* Summer 94:6
84143	17-hydroxypregnenolone
	➔ *CPT Assistant* Summer 94:6
84144	Progesterone
	(Progesterone receptor assay, use 84234)
	(For proinsulin, use 84206)
84146	Prolactin
84150	Prostaglandin, each
84152	Prostate specific antigen (PSA); complexed (direct measurement)
	➔ *CPT Changes: An Insider's View* 2001
84153	total
	➔ *CPT Assistant* Fall 93:26, May 96:10, Aug 96:10, Jan 97:10, Nov 98:26, Aug 99:5, Dec 99:10
84154	free
	➔ *CPT Assistant* Nov 98:26, Aug 99:5, Dec 99:10
84155	Protein, total, except by refractometry; serum
	➔ *CPT Assistant* Dec 99:2, Jan 00:7; *CPT Changes: An Insider's View* 2004
84156	urine
	➔ *CPT Changes: An Insider's View* 2004
84157	other source (eg, synovial fluid, cerebrospinal fluid)
	➔ *CPT Changes: An Insider's View* 2004
84160	Protein, total, by refractometry, any source
	➔ *CPT Changes: An Insider's View* 2004
	(For urine total protein by dipstick method, use 81000-81003)
84163	Pregnancy-associated plasma protein-A (PAPP-A)
	➔ *CPT Changes: An Insider's View* 2005
84165	Protein; electrophoretic fractionation and quantitation, serum
	➔ *CPT Changes: An Insider's View* 2004, 2005
84166	electrophoretic fractionation and quantitation, other fluids with concentration (eg, urine, CSF)
	➔ *CPT Changes: An Insider's View* 2005
84181	Western Blot, with interpretation and report, blood or other body fluid
84182	Western Blot, with interpretation and report, blood or other body fluid, immunological probe for band identification, each
	(For Western Blot tissue analysis, use 88371)

84202	Protoporphyrin, RBC; quantitative
	➔ *CPT Assistant* Aug 05:9
84203	screen
84206	Proinsulin
	(Pseudocholinesterase, use 82480)
84207	Pyridoxal phosphate (Vitamin B-6)
84210	Pyruvate
84220	Pyruvate kinase
84228	Quinine
84233	Receptor assay; estrogen
84234	progesterone
84235	endocrine, other than estrogen or progesterone (specify hormone)
84238	non-endocrine (specify receptor)
	➔ *CPT Assistant* Nov 05:14; *CPT Changes: An Insider's View* 2006
84244	Renin
84252	Riboflavin (Vitamin B-2)
	(Salicylates, use 80196)
	(Secretin test, see 99070, 89100 and appropriate analyses)
84255	Selenium
84260	Serotonin
	(For urine metabolites (HIAA), use 83497)
84270	Sex hormone binding globulin (SHBG)
	➔ *CPT Assistant* Summer 94:4
84275	Sialic acid
	(Sickle hemoglobin, use 85660)
84285	Silica
84295	Sodium; serum
	➔ *CPT Assistant* Dec 99:2
84300	urine
	➔ *CPT Assistant* Aug 05:9
84302	other source
	➔ *CPT Assistant* Jul 03:7; *CPT Changes: An Insider's View* 2003
	(Somatomammotropin, use 83632)
	(Somatotropin, use 83003)
84305	Somatomedin
	➔ *CPT Assistant* Summer 94:4
84307	Somatostatin
	➔ *CPT Assistant* Summer 94:4
84311	Spectrophotometry, analyte not elsewhere specified
84315	Specific gravity (except urine)
	(For specific gravity, urine, see 81000-81003)
	(Stone analysis, see 82355-82370)

84375 Sugars, chromatographic, TLC or paper chromatography

84376 Sugars (mono-, di-, and oligosaccharides); single qualitative, each specimen
➜ *CPT Assistant* Nov 98:26-27, Dec 99:7

84377 multiple qualitative, each specimen
➜ *CPT Assistant* Nov 98:26-27, Jul 03:7

84378 single quantitative, each specimen
➜ *CPT Assistant* Nov 98:26-27

84379 multiple quantitative, each specimen
➜ *CPT Assistant* Nov 98:26-27, Dec 99:7, Jul 03:7

84392 Sulfate, urine

(Sulfhemoglobin, see hemoglobin, 83055, 83060)

(T-3, see 84479-84481)

(T-4, see 84436-84439)

84402 Testosterone; free
➜ *CPT Assistant* Aug 05:9

84403 total

84425 Thiamine (Vitamin B-1)

84430 Thiocyanate

84432 Thyroglobulin
➜ *CPT Assistant* Summer 94:2

(Thyroglobulin, antibody, use 86800)

(Thyrotropin releasing hormone (TRH) test, see 80438, 80439)

84436 Thyroxine; total
➜ *CPT Assistant* Fall 93:25, Summer 94:3

84437 requiring elution (eg, neonatal)

84439 free

84442 Thyroxine binding globulin (TBG)

84443 Thyroid stimulating hormone (TSH)
➜ *CPT Assistant* Summer 94:3

84445 Thyroid stimulating immune globulins (TSI)
➜ *CPT Assistant* Summer 94:3; *CPT Changes: An Insider's View* 2002

(Tobramycin, use 80200)

84446 Tocopherol alpha (Vitamin E)

(Tolbutamide tolerance, use 82953)

84449 Transcortin (cortisol binding globulin)
➜ *CPT Assistant* Summer 94:6

84450 Transferase; aspartate amino (AST) (SGOT)
➜ *CPT Assistant* Dec 99:2

84460 alanine amino (ALT) (SGPT)
➜ *CPT Assistant* Dec 99:2

84466 Transferrin
➜ *CPT Assistant* Summer 94:4

(Iron binding capacity, use 83550)

84478 Triglycerides
➜ *CPT Assistant* Dec 99:2, Mar 00:11, Feb 05:9

84479 Thyroid hormone (T3 or T4) uptake or thyroid hormone binding ratio (THBR)
➜ *CPT Assistant* Fall 93:25, Summer 94:3

84480 Triiodothyronine T3; total (TT-3)

84481 free

84482 reverse
➜ *CPT Assistant* Summer 94:2

84484 Troponin, quantitative
➜ *CPT Assistant* Nov 97:29, Jan 98:6, Feb 98:1

(For troponin, qualitative assay, use 84512)

84485 Trypsin; duodenal fluid

84488 feces, qualitative

84490 feces, quantitative, 24-hour collection

84510 Tyrosine

(Urate crystal identification, use 89060)

84512 Troponin, qualitative
➜ *CPT Assistant* Nov 97:29, Jan 98:6, Feb 98:1

(For troponin, quantitative assay, use 84484)

84520 Urea nitrogen; quantitative
➜ *CPT Assistant* Dec 99:2

84525 semiquantitative (eg, reagent strip test)
➜ *CPT Assistant* Mar 98:3

84540 Urea nitrogen, urine

84545 Urea nitrogen, clearance

84550 Uric acid; blood
➜ *CPT Assistant* Dec 99:2

84560 other source

84577 Urobilinogen, feces, quantitative

84578 Urobilinogen, urine; qualitative

84580 quantitative, timed specimen

84583 semiquantitative

(Uroporphyrins, use 84120)

(Valproic acid (dipropylacetic acid), use 80164)

84585 Vanillylmandelic acid (VMA), urine

84586 Vasoactive intestinal peptide (VIP)
➜ *CPT Assistant* Summer 94:6

84588 Vasopressin (antidiuretic hormone, ADH)

84590 Vitamin A
➜ *CPT Assistant* Aug 05:9

(Vitamin B-1, use 84425)

(Vitamin B-2, use 84252)

(Vitamin B-6, use 84207)

(Vitamin B-12, use 82607)

(Vitamin B-12, absorption (Schilling), see 78270, 78271)

(Vitamin C, use 82180)

(Vitamin D, see 82306, 82307, 82652)

(Vitamin E, use 84446)

84591   Vitamin, not otherwise specified
> *CPT Changes: An Insider's View* 2001

84597   Vitamin K

(VMA, use 84585)

84600   Volatiles (eg, acetic anhydride, carbon tetrachloride, dichloroethane, dichloromethane, diethylether, isopropyl alcohol, methanol)
> *CPT Assistant* Aug 05:9

(For acetaldehyde, use 82000)

(Volume, blood, RISA or Cr-51, see 78110, 78111)

84620   Xylose absorption test, blood and/or urine

(For administration, use 99070)

84630   Zinc

84681   C-peptide

84702   Gonadotropin, chorionic (hCG); quantitative

84703   qualitative

(For urine pregnancy test by visual color comparison, use 81025)

● **84704**   free beta chain
> *CPT Changes: An Insider's View* 2008

84830   Ovulation tests, by visual color comparison methods for human luteinizing hormone

84999   Unlisted chemistry procedure
> *CPT Assistant* Oct 00:24, Aug 05:9

Hematology and Coagulation

(For blood banking procedures, see **Transfusion Medicine**)

(Agglutinins, see **Immunology**)

(Antiplasmin, use 85410)

(Antithrombin III, see 85300, 85301)

85002   Bleeding time
> *CPT Assistant* Aug 05:9

85004   Blood count; automated differential WBC count
> *CPT Assistant* Jan 04:26; *CPT Changes: An Insider's View* 2003

85007   blood smear, microscopic examination with manual differential WBC count
> *CPT Assistant* Jul 03:7, Jan 04:26; *CPT Changes: An Insider's View* 2003

85008   blood smear, microscopic examination without manual differential WBC count
> *CPT Assistant* Jul 03:8, Jan 04:26; *CPT Changes: An Insider's View* 2003

(For other fluids (eg, CSF), see 89050, 89051)

85009   manual differential WBC count, buffy coat
> *CPT Assistant* Jul 03:7, Jan 04:26; *CPT Changes: An Insider's View* 2003

(Eosinophils, nasal smear, use 89190)

85013   spun microhematocrit

85014   hematocrit (Hct)
> *CPT Assistant* Jul 03:7; *CPT Changes: An Insider's View* 2003

85018   hemoglobin (Hgb)
> *CPT Assistant* Jul 03:8; *CPT Changes: An Insider's View* 2003

(For other hemoglobin determination, see 83020-83069)

(For immunoassay, hemoglobin, fecal, use 82274)

85025   complete (CBC), automated (Hgb, Hct, RBC, WBC and platelet count) and automated differential WBC count
> *CPT Assistant* Jul 00:11, Jul 03:7, Jan 04:26; *CPT Changes: An Insider's View* 2003

85027   complete (CBC), automated (Hgb, Hct, RBC, WBC and platelet count)
> *CPT Assistant* Jul 03:8, Jan 04:26; *CPT Changes: An Insider's View* 2003

85032   manual cell count (erythrocyte, leukocyte, or platelet) each
> *CPT Assistant* Jul 03:8, Nov 03:15; *CPT Changes: An Insider's View* 2003

85041   red blood cell (RBC), automated
> *CPT Assistant* Jul 03:8; *CPT Changes: An Insider's View* 2003

(Do not report code 85041 in conjunction with 85025 or 85027)

85044   reticulocyte, manual
> *CPT Assistant* Jul 03:8; *CPT Changes: An Insider's View* 2003

85045   reticulocyte, automated
> *CPT Assistant* Jul 03:8; *CPT Changes: An Insider's View* 2003

85046   reticulocytes, automated, including one or more cellular parameters (eg, reticulocyte hemoglobin content (CHr), immature reticulocyte fraction (IRF), reticulocyte volume (MRV), RNA content), direct measurement
> *CPT Assistant* Nov 98:27; *CPT Changes: An Insider's View* 2005

85048   leukocyte (WBC), automated
> *CPT Assistant* Jul 03:8; *CPT Changes: An Insider's View* 2003

85049   platelet, automated
> *CPT Changes: An Insider's View* 2003

85055   Reticulated platelet assay
> *CPT Changes: An Insider's View* 2004

85060	Blood smear, peripheral, interpretation by physician with written report
85097	Bone marrow, smear interpretation

➔ *CPT Assistant* Winter 92:17, Jul 98:4, Mar 03:22; *CPT Changes: An Insider's View* 2002

(For special stains, see 88312, 88313)

(For bone biopsy, see 20220, 20225, 20240, 20245, 20250, 20251)

85130	Chromogenic substrate assay

➔ *CPT Assistant* Aug 05:9

(Circulating anti-coagulant screen (mixing studies), see 85611, 85732)

85170	Clot retraction
85175	Clot lysis time, whole blood dilution

(Clotting factor I (fibrinogen), see 85384, 85385)

85210	Clotting; factor II, prothrombin, specific

➔ *CPT Assistant* Aug 05:9

(See also 85610-85613)

85220	factor V (AcG or proaccelerin), labile factor
85230	factor VII (proconvertin, stable factor)
85240	factor VIII (AHG), one stage
85244	factor VIII related antigen
85245	factor VIII, VW factor, ristocetin cofactor
85246	factor VIII, VW factor antigen
85247	factor VIII, von Willebrand factor, multimetric analysis
85250	factor IX (PTC or Christmas)
85260	factor X (Stuart-Prower)
85270	factor XI (PTA)
85280	factor XII (Hageman)
85290	factor XIII (fibrin stabilizing)
85291	factor XIII (fibrin stabilizing), screen solubility
85292	prekallikrein assay (Fletcher factor assay)
85293	high molecular weight kininogen assay (Fitzgerald factor assay)
85300	Clotting inhibitors or anticoagulants; antithrombin III, activity

➔ *CPT Assistant* Aug 05:9

85301	antithrombin III, antigen assay
85302	protein C, antigen
85303	protein C, activity
85305	protein S, total
85306	protein S, free
85307	Activated Protein C (APC) resistance assay

➔ *CPT Changes: An Insider's View* 2001

85335	Factor inhibitor test
85337	Thrombomodulin

(For mixing studies for inhibitors, use 85732)

85345	Coagulation time; Lee and White
85347	activated
85348	other methods

(Differential count, see 85007 et seq)

(Duke bleeding time, use 85002)

(Eosinophils, nasal smear, use 89190)

85360	Euglobulin lysis

(Fetal hemoglobin, see 83030, 83033, 85460)

85362	Fibrin(ogen) degradation (split) products (FDP) (FSP); agglutination slide, semiquantitative

(Immunoelectrophoresis, use 86320)

85366	paracoagulation
85370	quantitative
85378	Fibrin degradation products, D-dimer; qualitative or semiquantitative

➔ *CPT Assistant* Jul 03:8; *CPT Changes: An Insider's View* 2003

85379	quantitative

(For ultrasensitive and standard sensitivity quantitative D-dimer, use 85379)

85380	ultrasensitive (eg, for evaluation for venous thromboembolism), qualitative or semiquantitative

➔ *CPT Assistant* Jul 03:8; *CPT Changes: An Insider's View* 2003

85384	Fibrinogen; activity
85385	antigen
85390	Fibrinolysins or coagulopathy screen, interpretation and report
85396	Coagulation/fibrinolysis assay, whole blood (eg, viscoelastic clot assessment), including use of any pharmacologic additive(s), as indicated, including interpretation and written report, per day

➔ *CPT Changes: An Insider's View* 2004

85400	Fibrinolytic factors and inhibitors; plasmin

➔ *CPT Assistant* Aug 05:9

85410	alpha-2 antiplasmin
85415	plasminogen activator
85420	plasminogen, except antigenic assay
85421	plasminogen, antigenic assay

(Fragility, red blood cell, see 85547, 85555-85557)

85441	Heinz bodies; direct
85445	induced, acetyl phenylhydrazine

(Hematocrit (PCV), see 85014, 85025, 85027)

(Hemoglobin, see 83020-83068, 85018, 85025, 85027)

85460   Hemoglobin or RBCs, fetal, for fetomaternal hemorrhage; differential lysis (Kleihauer-Betke)
→ *CPT Assistant* Fall 93:25

(See also 83030, 83033)

(Hemolysins, see 86940, 86941)

85461   rosette

85475   Hemolysin, acid

(See also 86940, 86941)

85520   Heparin assay
→ *CPT Assistant* Aug 05:9

85525   Heparin neutralization

85530   Heparin-protamine tolerance test

85536   Iron stain, peripheral blood
→ *CPT Changes: An Insider's View* 2001

(For iron stains on bone marrow or other tissues with physician evaluation, use 88313)

85540   Leukocyte alkaline phosphatase with count

85547   Mechanical fragility, RBC

85549   Muramidase

(Nitroblue tetrazolium dye test, use 86384)

85555   Osmotic fragility, RBC; unincubated

85557   incubated

(Packed cell volume, use 85013)

(Partial thromboplastin time, see 85730, 85732)

(Parasites, blood (eg, malaria smears), use 87207)

(Plasmin, use 85400)

(Plasminogen, use 85420)

(Plasminogen activator, use 85415)

85576   Platelet, aggregation (in vitro), each agent
→ *CPT Assistant* Jul 96:10; *CPT Changes: An Insider's View* 2003

85597   Platelet neutralization

85610   Prothrombin time;
→ *CPT Assistant* Aug 05:9

85611   substitution, plasma fractions, each

85612   Russell viper venom time (includes venom); undiluted

85613   diluted

(Red blood cell count, see 85025, 85027, 85041)

85635   Reptilase test

(Reticulocyte count, see 85044, 85045)

85651   Sedimentation rate, erythrocyte; non-automated

85652   automated

85660   Sickling of RBC, reduction

(Hemoglobin electrophoresis, use 83020)

(Smears [eg, for parasites, malaria], use 87207)

85670   Thrombin time; plasma

85675   titer

85705   Thromboplastin inhibition, tissue
→ *CPT Assistant* Aug 05:9

(For individual clotting factors, see 85245-85247)

85730   Thromboplastin time, partial (PTT); plasma or whole blood

85732   substitution, plasma fractions, each

85810   Viscosity

(von Willebrand factor assay, see 85245-85247)

(WBC count, see 85025, 85027, 85048, 89050)

85999   Unlisted hematology and coagulation procedure
→ *CPT Assistant* Aug 05:9

Immunology

(Acetylcholine receptor antibody, see 83519, 86255, 86256)

(Actinomyces, antibodies to, use 86602)

(Adrenal cortex antibodies, see 86255, 86256)

86000   Agglutinins, febrile (eg, Brucella, Francisella, Murine typhus, Q fever, Rocky Mountain spotted fever, scrub typhus), each antigen
→ *CPT Assistant* Aug 05:9

(For antibodies to infectious agents, see 86602-86804)

86001   Allergen specific IgG quantitative or semiquantitative, each allergen
→ *CPT Changes: An Insider's View* 2001

(Agglutinins and autohemolysins, see 86940, 86941)

86003   Allergen specific IgE; quantitative or semiquantitative, each allergen
→ *CPT Assistant* Spring 94:31

(For total quantitative IgE, use 82785)

86005   qualitative, multiallergen screen (dipstick, paddle, or disk)
→ *CPT Assistant* Spring 94:31

(For total qualitative IgE, use 83518)

(Alpha-1 antitrypsin, see 82103, 82104)

(Alpha-1 feto-protein, see 82105, 82106)

(Anti-AChR [acetylcholine receptor] antibody titer, see 86255, 86256)

(Anticardiolipin antibody, use 86147)

(Anti-DNA, use 86225)

(Anti-deoxyribonuclease titer, use 86215)

86021   Antibody identification; leukocyte antibodies

86022   platelet antibodies

86023   platelet associated immunoglobulin assay

86038   Antinuclear antibodies (ANA);

86039   titer

(Antistreptococcal antibody, ie, anti-DNAse, use 86215)

(Antistreptokinase titer, use 86590)

86060   Antistreptolysin O; titer

(For antibodies to infectious agents, see 86602-86804)

86063   screen

(For antibodies to infectious agents, see 86602-86804)

(Blastomyces, antibodies to, use 86612)

(86064 has been deleted. For B cells, total count, use 86355)

86077   Blood bank physician services; difficult cross match and/or evaluation of irregular antibody(s), interpretation and written report

86078   investigation of transfusion reaction including suspicion of transmissible disease, interpretation and written report

86079   authorization for deviation from standard blood banking procedures (eg, use of outdated blood, transfusion of Rh incompatible units), with written report

(Brucella, antibodies to, use 86622)

(Candida, antibodies to, use 86628. For skin testing, use 86485)

86140   C-reactive protein;
   CPT Assistant Aug 05:9; *CPT Changes: An Insider's View* 2002

(Candidiasis, use 86628)

86141   high sensitivity (hsCRP)
   CPT Changes: An Insider's View 2002

86146   Beta 2 Glycoprotein I antibody, each
   CPT Changes: An Insider's View 2001

86147   Cardiolipin (phospholipid) antibody, each Ig class
   CPT Changes: An Insider's View 2001

86148   Anti-phosphatidylserine (phospholipid) antibody
   CPT Assistant Nov 97:30, Jul 03:8, Nov 03:5

(To report antiprothrombin [phospholipid cofactor] antibody, use Category III code 0030T)

86155   Chemotaxis assay, specify method

(Clostridium difficile toxin, use 87230)

(Coccidioides, antibodies to, see 86635. For skin testing, use 86490)

86156   Cold agglutinin; screen

86157   titer

86160   Complement; antigen, each component

86161   functional activity, each component

86162   total hemolytic (CH50)

86171   Complement fixation tests, each antigen

(Coombs test, see 86880-86886)

86185   Counterimmunoelectrophoresis, each antigen

(Cryptococcus, antibodies to, use 86641)

86200   Cyclic citrullinated peptide (CCP), antibody
   CPT Assistant Mar 06:6; *CPT Changes: An Insider's View* 2006

86215   Deoxyribonuclease, antibody
   CPT Assistant Aug 05:9

86225   Deoxyribonucleic acid (DNA) antibody; native or double stranded

(Echinococcus, antibodies to, see code for specific method)

(For HIV antibody tests, see 86701-86703)

86226   single stranded

(Anti D.S., DNA, IFA, eg, using C.Lucilae, see 86255 and 86256)

86235   Extractable nuclear antigen, antibody to, any method (eg, nRNP, SS-A, SS-B, Sm, RNP, Sc170, J01), each antibody

86243   Fc receptor

(Filaria, antibodies to, see code for specific method)

86255   Fluorescent noninfectious agent antibody; screen, each antibody
   CPT Assistant Nov 98:27

86256   titer, each antibody

(Fluorescent technique for antigen identification in tissue, use 88346; for indirect fluorescence, use 88347)

(FTA, see 86781)

(Gel [agar] diffusion tests, use 86331)

86277   Growth hormone, human (HGH), antibody

86280   Hemagglutination inhibition test (HAI)

(For rubella, use 86762)

(For antibodies to infectious agents, see 86602-86804)

86294   Immunoassay for tumor antigen, qualitative or semiquantitative (eg, bladder tumor antigen)
   CPT Changes: An Insider's View 2001

86300   Immunoassay for tumor antigen, quantitative; CA 15-3 (27.29)
   CPT Assistant Aug 05:9; *CPT Changes: An Insider's View* 2001

86301   CA 19-9
   CPT Changes: An Insider's View 2001

86304   CA 125
➔ *CPT Changes: An Insider's View* 2001

(For measurement of serum HER-2/neu oncoprotein, see 83950)

(For hepatitis delta agent, antibody, use 86692)

86308   Heterophile antibodies; screening

(For antibodies to infectious agents, see 86602-86804)

86309   titer

(For antibodies to infectious agents, see 86602-86804)

86310   titers after absorption with beef cells and guinea pig kidney

(Histoplasma, antibodies to, use 86698. For skin testing, use 86510)

(For antibodies to infectious agents, see 86602-86804)

(Human growth hormone antibody, use 86277)

86316   Immunoassay for tumor antigen, other antigen, quantitative (eg, CA 50, 72-4, 549), each
➔ *CPT Assistant* May 96:11, Aug 96:11, Apr 98:15, Aug 99:5, Dec 99:10; *CPT Changes: An Insider's View* 2001

86317   Immunoassay for infectious agent antibody, quantitative, not otherwise specified
➔ *CPT Assistant* Nov 97:30-31

(For immunoassay techniques for antigens, see 83516, 83518, 83519, 83520, 87301-87450, 87810-87899)

(For particle agglutination procedures, use 86403)

86318   Immunoassay for infectious agent antibody, qualitative or semiquantitative, single step method (eg, reagent strip)

86320   Immunoelectrophoresis; serum

86325   other fluids (eg, urine, cerebrospinal fluid) with concentration
➔ *CPT Changes: An Insider's View* 2002

86327   crossed (2-dimensional assay)

86329   Immunodiffusion; not elsewhere specified
➔ *CPT Assistant* Aug 00:11

86331   gel diffusion, qualitative (Ouchterlony), each antigen or antibody

86332   Immune complex assay

86334   Immunofixation electrophoresis; serum
➔ *CPT Changes: An Insider's View* 2005

86335   other fluids with concentration (eg, urine, CSF)
➔ *CPT Changes: An Insider's View* 2005

86336   Inhibin A
➔ *CPT Changes: An Insider's View* 2002

86337   Insulin antibodies

86340   Intrinsic factor antibodies

(Leptospira, antibodies to, use 86720)

(Leukoagglutinins, use 86021)

86341   Islet cell antibody
➔ *CPT Assistant* Summer 94:6

86343   Leukocyte histamine release test (LHR)

86344   Leukocyte phagocytosis

86353   Lymphocyte transformation, mitogen (phytomitogen) or antigen induced blastogenesis

(Malaria antibodies, use 86750)

86355   B cells, total count
➔ *CPT Assistant* Mar 06:6; *CPT Changes: An Insider's View* 2006

● **86356**   Mononuclear cell antigen, quantitative (eg, flow cytometry), not otherwise specified, each antigen
➔ *CPT Changes: An Insider's View* 2008

►(Do not report 88187-88189 for interpretation of 86355, 86356, 86357, 86359, 86360, 86361, 86367)◄

86357   Natural killer (NK) cells, total count
➔ *CPT Assistant* Mar 06:6; *CPT Changes: An Insider's View* 2006

86359   T cells; total count
➔ *CPT Assistant* Nov 97:30

86360   absolute CD4 and CD8 count, including ratio
➔ *CPT Assistant* Nov 97:30, Jan 07:29

86361   absolute CD4 count
➔ *CPT Assistant* Nov 97:30

86367   Stem cells (ie, CD34), total count
➔ *CPT Assistant* Mar 06:6; *CPT Changes: An Insider's View* 2006

(For flow cytometric immunophenotyping for the assessment of potential hematolymphoid neoplasia, see 88184-88189)

86376   Microsomal antibodies (eg, thyroid or liver-kidney), each

86378   Migration inhibitory factor test (MIF)

(Mitochondrial antibody, liver, see 86255, 86256)

(Mononucleosis, see 86308-86310)

(86379 has been deleted. For natural killer cells, total count, use 86357)

86382   Neutralization test, viral

86384   Nitroblue tetrazolium dye test (NTD)

(Ouchterlony diffusion, use 86331)

(Platelet antibodies, see 86022, 86023)

86403   Particle agglutination; screen, each antibody
➔ *CPT Assistant* Aug 05:9

86406   titer, each antibody

(Pregnancy test, see 84702, 84703)

(Rapid plasma reagin test (RPR), see 86592, 86593)

86430   Rheumatoid factor; qualitative

86431   quantitative

(Serologic test for syphilis, see 86592, 86593)

86480 Tuberculosis test, cell mediated immunity measurement of gamma interferon antigen response

> *CPT Assistant* Mar 06:6; *CPT Changes: An Insider's View* 2006

86485 Skin test; candida

(For antibody, candida, use 86628)

● **86486** unlisted antigen, each

> *CPT Changes: An Insider's View* 2008

86490 coccidioidomycosis

86510 histoplasmosis

> *CPT Assistant* Aug 05:9

(For histoplasma, antibody, use 86698)

86580 tuberculosis, intradermal

(For tuberculosis test, cell mediated immunity measurement of gamma interferon antigen response, use 86480)

(86585 has been deleted. To report tuberculosis testing by intradermal (Mantoux) test, use 86580)

(For skin tests for allergy, see 95010-95199)

(Smooth muscle antibody, see 86255, 86256)

(Sporothrix, antibodies to, see code for specific method)

▶(86586 has been deleted. For skin testing, unlisted antigen, use 86486. For flow cytometry, quantitative, not otherwise specified, use 86356)◀

(86587 has been deleted. For stem cells, total count, use 86367)

86590 Streptokinase, antibody

(For antibodies to infectious agents, see 86602-86804)

(Streptolysin O antibody, see antistreptolysin O, 86060, 86063)

86592 Syphilis test; qualitative (eg, VDRL, RPR, ART)

(For antibodies to infectious agents, see 86602-86804)

86593 quantitative

(For antibodies to infectious agents, see 86602-86804)

(Tetanus antibody, use 86774)

(Thyroglobulin antibody, use 86800)

(Thyroglobulin, use 84432)

(Thyroid microsomal antibody, use 86376)

(For toxoplasma antibody, see 86777-86778)

The following codes (86602-86804) are qualitative or semiquantitative immunoassays performed by multiple-step methods for the detection of antibodies to infectious agents. For immunoassays by single-step method (eg, reagent strips), use code 86318. Procedures for the identification of antibodies should be coded as precisely as possible. For example, an antibody to a virus could be coded with increasing specificity for virus, family, genus, species, or type. In some cases, further precision may be added to codes by specifying the class of immunoglobulin being detected. When multiple tests are done to detect antibodies to organisms classified more precisely than the specificity allowed by available codes, it is appropriate to code each as a separate service. For example, a test for antibody to an enterovirus is coded as 86658. Coxsackie viruses are enteroviruses, but there are no codes for the individual species of enterovirus. If assays are performed for antibodies to coxsackie A and B species, each assay should be separately coded. Similarly, if multiple assays are performed for antibodies of different immuno-globulin classes, each assay should be coded separately. When a coding option exists for reporting IgM specific antibodies (eg, 86632), the corresponding nonspecific code (eg, 86631) may be reported for performance of either an antibody analysis not specific for a particular immunoglobulin class or for an IgG analysis.

(For the detection of antibodies other than those to infectious agents, see specific antibody [eg, 86021-86023, 86376, 86800, 86850-86870] or specific method [eg, 83516, 86255, 86256]).

(For infectious agent/antigen detection, see 87260-87899)

> *CPT Assistant* Fall 93:26

86602 Antibody; actinomyces

> *CPT Assistant* Aug 05:9

86603 adenovirus

86606 Aspergillus

86609 bacterium, not elsewhere specified

86611 Bartonella

> *CPT Changes: An Insider's View* 2001

86612 Blastomyces

86615 Bordetella

86617 Borrelia burgdorferi (Lyme disease) confirmatory test (eg, Western Blot or immunoblot)

86618 Borrelia burgdorferi (Lyme disease)

86619 Borrelia (relapsing fever)

86622 Brucella

86625 Campylobacter

86628 Candida

(For skin test, candida, use 86485)

86631 Chlamydia

86632 Chlamydia, IgM

> *CPT Assistant* Nov 97:31

(For chlamydia antigen, see 87270, 87320. For fluorescent antibody technique, see 86255, 86256)

86635 Coccidioides

86638 Coxiella burnetii (Q fever)

86641	Cryptococcus
86644	cytomegalovirus (CMV)
86645	cytomegalovirus (CMV), IgM
	➲ *CPT Assistant* Jul 03:7
86648	Diphtheria
86651	encephalitis, California (La Crosse)
86652	encephalitis, Eastern equine
86653	encephalitis, St. Louis
86654	encephalitis, Western equine
86658	enterovirus (eg, coxsackie, echo, polio)

(Trichinella, antibodies to, use 86784)

(Trypanosoma, antibodies to, see code for specific method)

(Tuberculosis, use 86580 for skin testing)

(Viral antibodies, see code for specific method)

86663	Epstein-Barr (EB) virus, early antigen (EA)
86664	Epstein-Barr (EB) virus, nuclear antigen (EBNA)
86665	Epstein-Barr (EB) virus, viral capsid (VCA)
86666	Ehrlichia
	➲ *CPT Changes: An Insider's View* 2001
86668	Francisella tularensis
86671	fungus, not elsewhere specified
86674	Giardia lamblia
86677	Helicobacter pylori
	➲ *CPT Assistant* Jan 98:6
86682	helminth, not elsewhere specified
86684	Haemophilus influenza
86687	HTLV-I
86688	HTLV-II
86689	HTLV or HIV antibody, confirmatory test (eg, Western Blot)
86692	hepatitis, delta agent
	➲ *CPT Assistant* Nov 97:31

(For hepatitis delta agent, antigen, use 87380)

86694	herpes simplex, non-specific type test
86695	herpes simplex, type 1
86696	herpes simplex, type 2
	➲ *CPT Changes: An Insider's View* 2001
86698	histoplasma
86701	HIV-1
	➲ *CPT Assistant* Aug 05:9
86702	HIV-2

86703	HIV-1 and HIV-2, single assay
	➲ *CPT Assistant* Nov 97:31

►(When HIV antibody immunoassay [HIV testing 86701-86703] is performed using a kit or transportable instrument that wholly or in part consists of a single use, disposable analytical chamber, the service may be identified by adding modifier 92 to the usual code)◄

(For HIV-1 antigen, use 87390)

(For HIV-2 antigen, use 87391)

(For confirmatory test for HIV antibody (eg, Western Blot), use 86689)

86704	Hepatitis B core antibody (HBcAb); total
	➲ *CPT Assistant* Nov 97:31-32; *CPT Changes: An Insider's View* 2001
86705	IgM antibody
	➲ *CPT Assistant* Nov 97:31-32
86706	Hepatitis B surface antibody (HBsAb)
	➲ *CPT Assistant* Nov 97:31-32
86707	Hepatitis Be antibody (HBeAb)
	➲ *CPT Assistant* Nov 97:31-32
86708	Hepatitis A antibody (HAAb); total
	➲ *CPT Assistant* Nov 97:31-32, Jun 00:11; *CPT Changes: An Insider's View* 2001
86709	IgM antibody
	➲ *CPT Assistant* Nov 97:31-32, Jun 00:11
86710	Antibody; influenza virus
86713	Legionella
86717	Leishmania
86720	Leptospira
86723	Listeria monocytogenes
86727	lymphocytic choriomeningitis
86729	lymphogranuloma venereum
86732	mucormycosis
86735	mumps
86738	mycoplasma
86741	Neisseria meningitidis
86744	Nocardia
86747	parvovirus
86750	Plasmodium (malaria)
86753	protozoa, not elsewhere specified
86756	respiratory syncytial virus
86757	Rickettsia
	➲ *CPT Changes: An Insider's View* 2001
86759	rotavirus
86762	rubella
86765	rubeola

86768	Salmonella
86771	Shigella
86774	tetanus
86777	Toxoplasma
86778	Toxoplasma, IgM
86781	Treponema pallidum, confirmatory test (eg, FTA-abs)
86784	Trichinella
86787	varicella-zoster
86788	West Nile virus, IgM

➔ *CPT Changes: An Insider's View* 2007

86789	West Nile virus

➔ *CPT Changes: An Insider's View* 2007

86790	virus, not elsewhere specified
86793	Yersinia
86800	Thyroglobulin antibody

➔ *CPT Assistant* Aug 05:9

(For thyroglobulin, use 84432)

86803	Hepatitis C antibody;

➔ *CPT Assistant* Nov 97:31-32

86804	confirmatory test (eg, immunoblot)

➔ *CPT Assistant* Nov 97:31-32

Tissue Typing

(For pretransplant cross-match, see appropriate code or codes)

86805	Lymphocytotoxicity assay, visual crossmatch; with titration
86806	without titration
86807	Serum screening for cytotoxic percent reactive antibody (PRA); standard method

➔ *CPT Assistant* Jun 01:11

86808	quick method

➔ *CPT Assistant* Jun 01:11

86812	HLA typing; A, B, or C (eg, A10, B7, B27), single antigen

➔ *CPT Assistant* Mar 03:23, Jun 06:17

86813	A, B, or C, multiple antigens

➔ *CPT Assistant* Mar 03:23, Jun 06:17

86816	DR/DQ, single antigen

➔ *CPT Assistant* Mar 03:23

86817	DR/DQ, multiple antigens

➔ *CPT Assistant* Mar 03:23

86821	lymphocyte culture, mixed (MLC)

➔ *CPT Assistant* Mar 03:23

86822	lymphocyte culture, primed (PLC)

➔ *CPT Assistant* Mar 03:23

86849	Unlisted immunology procedure

➔ *CPT Assistant* Mar 98:10

Transfusion Medicine

(For apheresis, use 36511, 36512)

(For therapeutic phlebotomy, use 99195)

86850	Antibody screen, RBC, each serum technique

➔ *CPT Assistant* Fall 93:25

86860	Antibody elution (RBC), each elution
86870	Antibody identification, RBC antibodies, each panel for each serum technique

➔ *CPT Assistant* Fall 93:25, Mar 01:10

86880	Antihuman globulin test (Coombs test); direct, each antiserum
▲ 86885	indirect, qualitative, each reagent red cell

➔ *CPT Changes: An Insider's View* 2008

▲ 86886	indirect, each antibody titer

➔ *CPT Changes: An Insider's View* 2008

▶(For indirect antihuman globulin [Coombs] test for RBC antibody screening, use 86850)◀

▶(For indirect antihuman globulin [Coombs] test for RBC antibody identification using reagent red cell panels, use 86870)◀

86890	Autologous blood or component, collection processing and storage; predeposited

➔ *CPT Assistant* Apr 96:2

86891	intra- or postoperative salvage

(For physician services to autologous donors, see 99201-99204)

86900	Blood typing; ABO

➔ *CPT Assistant* Aug 05:9

86901	Rh (D)

➔ *CPT Assistant* Fall 93:25

86903	antigen screening for compatible blood unit using reagent serum, per unit screened
86904	antigen screening for compatible unit using patient serum, per unit screened
86905	RBC antigens, other than ABO or Rh (D), each
86906	Rh phenotyping, complete
86910	Blood typing, for paternity testing, per individual; ABO, Rh and MN
86911	each additional antigen system
86920	Compatibility test each unit; immediate spin technique

➔ *CPT Assistant* Mar 06:6

86921	incubation technique

➔ *CPT Assistant* Mar 06:6

86922	antiglobulin technique

➔ *CPT Assistant* Mar 06:6

86923   electronic
> *CPT Assistant* Mar 06:6; *CPT Changes: An Insider's View* 2006

(Do not use 86923 in conjunction with 86920-86922 for same unit crossmatch)

86927   Fresh frozen plasma, thawing, each unit

86930   Frozen blood, each unit; freezing (includes preparation)
> *CPT Assistant* Apr 96:2, Jul 03:8; *CPT Changes: An Insider's View* 2003

86931   thawing
> *CPT Assistant* Jul 03:8; *CPT Changes: An Insider's View* 2003

86932   freezing (includes preparation) and thawing
> *CPT Assistant* Jul 03:8; *CPT Changes: An Insider's View* 2003

86940   Hemolysins and agglutinins; auto, screen, each

86941   incubated

86945   Irradiation of blood product, each unit

86950   Leukocyte transfusion

(For leukapheresis, use 36511)

86960   Volume reduction of blood or blood product (eg, red blood cells or platelets), each unit
> *CPT Assistant* Mar 06:6; *CPT Changes: An Insider's View* 2006

86965   Pooling of platelets or other blood products

86970   Pretreatment of RBCs for use in RBC antibody detection, identification, and/or compatibility testing; incubation with chemical agents or drugs, each

86971   incubation with enzymes, each

86972   by density gradient separation

86975   Pretreatment of serum for use in RBC antibody identification; incubation with drugs, each

86976   by dilution

86977   incubation with inhibitors, each

86978   by differential red cell absorption using patient RBCs or RBCs of known phenotype, each absorption

86985   Splitting of blood or blood products, each unit
> *CPT Assistant* Apr 96:2

86999   Unlisted transfusion medicine procedure
> *CPT Assistant* Aug 05:9, Nov 05:14

Microbiology

Includes bacteriology, mycology, parasitology, and virology.

Presumptive identification of microorganisms is defined as identification by colony morphology, growth on selective media, Gram stains, or up to three tests (eg, catalase, oxidase, indole, urease). Definitive identification of microorganisms is defined as an identification to the genus or species level that requires additional tests (eg, biochemical panels, slide cultures). If additional studies involve molecular probes, chromatography, or immunologic techniques, these should be separately coded in addition to definitive identification codes (87140-87158). For multiple specimens/sites use modifier 59. For repeat laboratory tests performed on the same day, use modifier 91.

87001   Animal inoculation, small animal; with observation
> *CPT Assistant* Aug 05:9

87003   with observation and dissection

87015   Concentration (any type), for infectious agents
> *CPT Changes: An Insider's View* 2001

(Do not report 87015 in conjunction with 87177)

87040   Culture, bacterial; blood, aerobic, with isolation and presumptive identification of isolates (includes anaerobic culture, if appropriate)
> *CPT Assistant* Aug 97:18, Jun 02:2; *CPT Changes: An Insider's View* 2001, 2004

87045   stool, aerobic, with isolation and preliminary examination (eg, KIA, LIA), Salmonella and Shigella species
> *CPT Changes: An Insider's View* 2001, 2002, 2004

87046   stool, aerobic, additional pathogens, isolation and presumptive identification of isolates, each plate
> *CPT Changes: An Insider's View* 2001, 2002, 2004, 2005

87070   any other source except urine, blood or stool, aerobic, with isolation and presumptive identification of isolates
> *CPT Assistant* Aug 97:18, Nov 01:10, Oct 03:10; *CPT Changes: An Insider's View* 2001, 2004

(For urine, use 87088)

87071   quantitative, aerobic with isolation and presumptive identification of isolates, any source except urine, blood or stool
> *CPT Assistant* Jun 02:3, Sep 03:3; *CPT Changes: An Insider's View* 2001

(For urine, use 87088)

87073   quantitative, anaerobic with isolation and presumptive identification of isolates, any source except urine, blood or stool
> *CPT Assistant* Jun 02:3; *CPT Changes: An Insider's View* 2001

(For definitive identification of isolates, use 87076 or 87077. For typing of isolates see 87140-87158)

87075   any source, except blood, anaerobic with isolation and presumptive identification of isolates
> *CPT Changes: An Insider's View* 2001, 2004

87076   anaerobic isolate, additional methods required for definitive identification, each isolate
> *CPT Changes: An Insider's View* 2001

(For gas liquid chromatography (GLC) or high pressure liquid chromatography (HPLC), use 87143)

87077 aerobic isolate, additional methods required for definitive identification, each isolate

➔ *CPT Assistant* Nov 01:10; *CPT Changes: An Insider's View* 2001

(For gas liquid chromatography (GLC) or high pressure liquid chromatography (HPLC), use 87143)

87081 Culture, presumptive, pathogenic organisms, screening only;

➔ *CPT Assistant* Nov 01:10; *CPT Changes: An Insider's View* 2001

87084 with colony estimation from density chart

87086 Culture, bacterial; quantitative colony count, urine

➔ *CPT Changes: An Insider's View* 2001

87088 with isolation and presumptive identification of each isolate, urine

➔ *CPT Changes: An Insider's View* 2001, 2007

87101 Culture, fungi (mold or yeast) isolation, with presumptive identification of isolates; skin, hair, or nail

➔ *CPT Assistant* Sep 99:10, Aug 05:9; *CPT Changes: An Insider's View* 2001

87102 other source (except blood)

87103 blood

87106 Culture, fungi, definitive identification, each organism; yeast

➔ *CPT Changes: An Insider's View* 2001

(Use 87106 in addition to codes 87101, 87102, or 87103 when appropriate)

87107 mold

➔ *CPT Changes: An Insider's View* 2001

87109 Culture, mycoplasma, any source

87110 Culture, chlamydia, any source

➔ *CPT Changes: An Insider's View* 2001

(For immunofluorescence staining of shell vials, use 87140)

87116 Culture, tubercle or other acid-fast bacilli (eg, TB, AFB, mycobacteria) any source, with isolation and presumptive identification of isolates

➔ *CPT Changes: An Insider's View* 2001

(For concentration, use 87015)

87118 Culture, mycobacterial, definitive identification, each isolate

➔ *CPT Changes: An Insider's View* 2001

(For nucleic acid probe identification, use 87149)

(For GLC or HPLC identification, use 87143)

87140 Culture, typing; immunofluorescent method, each antiserum

➔ *CPT Assistant* Nov 01:10, Sep 03:3; *CPT Changes: An Insider's View* 2001

87143 gas liquid chromatography (GLC) or high pressure liquid chromatography (HPLC) method

➔ *CPT Changes: An Insider's View* 2001

87147 immunologic method, other than immunofluoresence (eg, agglutination grouping), per antiserum

➔ *CPT Assistant* Apr 02:18, Oct 03:10; *CPT Changes: An Insider's View* 2001

87149 identification by nucleic acid probe

➔ *CPT Assistant* Nov 01:10; *CPT Changes: An Insider's View* 2001

87152 identification by pulse field gel typing

➔ *CPT Changes: An Insider's View* 2001

87158 other methods

➔ *CPT Assistant* Nov 01:10, Sep 03:3

87164 Dark field examination, any source (eg, penile, vaginal, oral, skin); includes specimen collection

87166 without collection

87168 Macroscopic examination; arthropod

➔ *CPT Changes: An Insider's View* 2001

87169 parasite

➔ *CPT Changes: An Insider's View* 2001

87172 Pinworm exam (eg, cellophane tape prep)

➔ *CPT Changes: An Insider's View* 2001

87176 Homogenization, tissue, for culture

➔ *CPT Changes: An Insider's View* 2001

87177 Ova and parasites, direct smears, concentration and identification

➔ *CPT Assistant* Jul 03:8, Nov 03:15, Mar 06:6

(Do not report 87177 in conjunction with 87015)

(For direct smears from a primary source, use 87207)

(For coccidia or microsporidia exam, use 87207)

(For complex special stain (trichrome, iron hematoxylin), use 87209)

(For nucleic acid probes in cytologic material, use 88365)

(For molecular diagnostics, see 83890-83898, 87470-87799)

87181 Susceptibility studies, antimicrobial agent; agar dilution method, per agent (eg, antibiotic gradient strip)

➔ *CPT Assistant* Nov 01:10; *CPT Changes: An Insider's View* 2001

87184 disk method, per plate (12 or fewer agents)

➔ *CPT Assistant* Nov 01:10; *CPT Changes: An Insider's View* 2001

87185 enzyme detection (eg, beta lactamase), per enzyme

➔ *CPT Assistant* Nov 01:10; *CPT Changes: An Insider's View* 2001

87186 microdilution or agar dilution (minimum inhibitory concentration (MIC) or breakpoint), each multi-antimicrobial, per plate

➔ *CPT Assistant* Nov 01:10; *CPT Changes: An Insider's View* 2001

+ 87187   microdilution or agar dilution, minimum lethal
              concentration (MLC), each plate (List separately in
              addition to code for primary procedure)
              ➔ *CPT Assistant* Nov 01:10; *CPT Changes: An Insider's View*
                 2001

(Use 87187 in conjunction with 87186 or 87188)

87188   macrobroth dilution method, each agent
              ➔ *CPT Assistant* Nov 01:10; *CPT Changes: An Insider's View*
                 2001

87190   mycobacteria, proportion method, each agent
              ➔ *CPT Changes: An Insider's View* 2001

(For other mycobacterial susceptibility studies, see
87181, 87184, 87186, or 87188)

87197   Serum bactericidal titer (Schlicter test)

87205   Smear, primary source with interpretation; Gram or
              Giemsa stain for bacteria, fungi, or cell types
              ➔ *CPT Assistant* Aug 05:9; *CPT Changes: An Insider's View* 2001

87206   fluorescent and/or acid fast stain for bacteria, fungi,
              parasites, viruses or cell types
              ➔ *CPT Changes: An Insider's View* 2001

87207   special stain for inclusion bodies or parasites (eg,
              malaria, coccidia, microsporidia, trypanosomes,
              herpes viruses)
              ➔ *CPT Assistant* Jul 03:8, Mar 06:6; *CPT Changes: An Insider's*
                 View 2001, 2003

(For direct smears with concentration and identification,
use 87177)

(For thick smear preparation, use 87015)

(For fat, meat, fibers, nasal eosinophils, and starch, see
miscellaneous section)

87209   complex special stain (eg, trichrome, iron
              hemotoxylin) for ova and parasites
              ➔ *CPT Assistant* Mar 06:6; *CPT Changes: An Insider's View*
                 2006

87210   wet mount for infectious agents (eg, saline, India ink,
              KOH preps)
              ➔ *CPT Changes: An Insider's View* 2001

(For KOH examination of skin, hair or nails, see 87220)

87220   Tissue examination by KOH slide of samples from skin,
              hair, or nails for fungi or ectoparasite ova or mites (eg,
              scabies)
              ➔ *CPT Changes: An Insider's View* 2001

87230   Toxin or antitoxin assay, tissue culture (eg, Clostridium
              difficile toxin)

87250   Virus isolation; inoculation of embryonated eggs, or small
              animal, includes observation and dissection
              ➔ *CPT Changes: An Insider's View* 2001

87252   tissue culture inoculation, observation, and
              presumptive identification by cytopathic effect
              ➔ *CPT Changes: An Insider's View* 2001

87253   tissue culture, additional studies or definitive
              identification (eg, hemabsorption, neutralization,
              immunofluoresence stain), each isolate
              ➔ *CPT Changes: An Insider's View* 2001

(Electron microscopy, use 88348)

(Inclusion bodies in tissue sections, see 88304-88309; in
smears, see 87207-87210; in fluids, use 88106)

87254   centrifuge enhanced (shell vial) technique, includes
              identification with immunofluorescence stain, each
              virus
              ➔ *CPT Assistant* Jul 03:8; *CPT Changes: An Insider's View*
                 2001, 2003

(Report 87254 in addition to 87252 as appropriate)

87255   including identification by non-immunologic method,
              other than by cytopathic effect (eg, virus specific
              enzymatic activity)
              ➔ *CPT Assistant* Jul 03:9; *CPT Changes: An Insider's View* 2003

▶These codes are intended for primary source only. For
similar studies on culture material, refer to codes 87140-
87158. Infectious agents by antigen detection,
immunofluorescence microscopy, or nucleic acid probe
techniques should be reported as precisely as possible.
The most specific code possible should be reported. If
there is no specific agent code, the general methodology
code (eg, 87299, 87449, 87450, 87797, 87798, 87799,
87899) should be used. For identification of antibodies to
many of the listed infectious agents, see 86602-86804.
When separate results are reported for different species or
strain of organisms, each result should be coded
separately.◀

87260   Infectious agent antigen detection by immunofluorescent
              technique; adenovirus
              ➔ *CPT Assistant* Nov 97:32; *CPT Changes: An Insider's View* 2001

87265   Bordetella pertussis/parapertussis
              ➔ *CPT Assistant* Nov 97:32

87267   Enterovirus, direct fluorescent antibody (DFA)
              ➔ *CPT Assistant* Jul 03:8

87269   giardia
              ➔ *CPT Changes: An Insider's View* 2004

87270   Chlamydia trachomatis
              ➔ *CPT Assistant* Nov 97:32

87271   Cytomegalovirus, direct fluorescent antibody (DFA)
              ➔ *CPT Assistant* Jul 03:7

87272   cryptosporidium
              ➔ *CPT Assistant* Nov 97:32; *CPT Changes: An Insider's View*
                 2004

87273   Herpes simplex virus type 2
              ➔ *CPT Changes: An Insider's View* 2001

87274   Herpes simplex virus type 1
              ➔ *CPT Assistant* Nov 97:32; *CPT Changes: An Insider's View*
                 2001

▲=Revised code   ●=New code   ▶◀=Contains new or revised text   ⊘=Modifier 51 exempt

87275   influenza B virus
➤ *CPT Changes: An Insider's View* 2001

87276   influenza A virus
➤ *CPT Assistant* Nov 97:32

87277   Legionella micdadei
➤ *CPT Changes: An Insider's View* 2001

87278   Legionella pneumophila
➤ *CPT Assistant* Nov 97:32

87279   Parainfluenza virus, each type
➤ *CPT Changes: An Insider's View* 2001

87280   respiratory syncytial virus
➤ *CPT Assistant* Nov 97:32

87281   Pneumocystis carinii
➤ *CPT Changes: An Insider's View* 2001

87283   Rubeola
➤ *CPT Changes: An Insider's View* 2001

87285   Treponema pallidum
➤ *CPT Assistant* Nov 97:32

87290   Varicella zoster virus
➤ *CPT Assistant* Nov 97:32

87299   not otherwise specified, each organism
➤ *CPT Assistant* Nov 97:32, Nov 01:10; *CPT Changes: An Insider's View* 2001

87300   Infectious agent antigen detection by immunofluorescent technique, polyvalent for multiple organisms, each polyvalent antiserum
➤ *CPT Assistant* Aug 05:9; *CPT Changes: An Insider's View* 2001

(For physician evaluation of infectious disease agents by immunofluorescence, use 88346)

87301   Infectious agent antigen detection by enzyme immunoassay technique, qualitative or semiquantitative, multiple-step method; adenovirus enteric types 40/41
➤ *CPT Assistant* Nov 97:32, Nov 99:46

87305   Aspergillus
➤ *CPT Changes: An Insider's View* 2007

87320   Chlamydia trachomatis
➤ *CPT Assistant* Nov 97:32

87324   Clostridium difficile toxin(s)
➤ *CPT Assistant* Nov 97:32; *CPT Changes: An Insider's View* 2001

87327   Cryptococcus neoformans
➤ *CPT Changes: An Insider's View* 2001

(For Cryptococcus latex agglutination, use 86403)

87328   cryptosporidium
➤ *CPT Assistant* Nov 97:32; *CPT Changes: An Insider's View* 2004

87329   giardia
➤ *CPT Changes: An Insider's View* 2004

87332   cytomegalovirus
➤ *CPT Assistant* Nov 97:32

87335   Escherichia coli 0157
➤ *CPT Assistant* Nov 97:32

(For giardia antigen, use 87329)

87336   Entamoeba histolytica dispar group
➤ *CPT Changes: An Insider's View* 2001

87337   Entamoeba histolytica group
➤ *CPT Changes: An Insider's View* 2001

87338   Helicobacter pylori, stool
➤ *CPT Assistant* Nov 99:46; *CPT Changes: An Insider's View* 2000

87339   Helicobacter pylori
➤ *CPT Changes: An Insider's View* 2001

(For H. pylori, stool, use 87338. For H. pylori, breath and blood by mass spectrometry, see 83013, 83014. For H. pylori, liquid scintillation counter, see 78267, 78268)

87340   hepatitis B surface antigen (HBsAg)
➤ *CPT Assistant* Nov 97:32, Jan 00:11

87341   hepatitis B surface antigen (HBsAg) neutralization
➤ *CPT Changes: An Insider's View* 2001

87350   hepatitis Be antigen (HBeAg)
➤ *CPT Assistant* Nov 97:32

87380   hepatitis, delta agent
➤ *CPT Assistant* Nov 97:32

87385   Histoplasma capsulatum
➤ *CPT Assistant* Nov 97:32

87390   HIV-1
➤ *CPT Assistant* Nov 97:32

87391   HIV-2
➤ *CPT Assistant* Nov 97:32

87400   Influenza, A or B, each
➤ *CPT Assistant* Jun 01:11, Dec 01:6, Aug 05:9; *CPT Changes: An Insider's View* 2001

87420   respiratory syncytial virus
➤ *CPT Assistant* Nov 97:32

87425   rotavirus
➤ *CPT Assistant* Nov 97:32

87427   Shiga-like toxin
➤ *CPT Changes: An Insider's View* 2001

87430   Streptococcus, group A
➤ *CPT Assistant* Nov 97:32

87449   Infectious agent antigen detection by enzyme immunoassay technique qualitative or semiquantitative; multiple step method, not otherwise specified, each organism
➤ *CPT Assistant* Nov 97:32, Jan 00:11, Nov 01:10; *CPT Changes: An Insider's View* 2001

87450   single step method, not otherwise specified, each organism
➤ *CPT Assistant* Nov 97:33; *CPT Changes: An Insider's View* 2001

87451	multiple step method, polyvalent for multiple organisms, each polyvalent antiserum
	➔ *CPT Changes: An Insider's View* 2001
87470	Infectious agent detection by nucleic acid (DNA or RNA); Bartonella henselae and Bartonella quintana, direct probe technique
	➔ *CPT Assistant* Nov 97:33-34
87471	Bartonella henselae and Bartonella quintana, amplified probe technique
87472	Bartonella henselae and Bartonella quintana, quantification
87475	Borrelia burgdorferi, direct probe technique
87476	Borrelia burgdorferi, amplified probe technique
87477	Borrelia burgdorferi, quantification
87480	Candida species, direct probe technique
87481	Candida species, amplified probe technique
87482	Candida species, quantification
87485	Chlamydia pneumoniae, direct probe technique
87486	Chlamydia pneumoniae, amplified probe technique
87487	Chlamydia pneumoniae, quantification
87490	Chlamydia trachomatis, direct probe technique
87491	Chlamydia trachomatis, amplified probe technique
87492	Chlamydia trachomatis, quantification
87495	cytomegalovirus, direct probe technique
87496	cytomegalovirus, amplified probe technique
87497	cytomegalovirus, quantification
87498	enterovirus, amplified probe technique
	➔ *CPT Changes: An Insider's View* 2007
● **87500**	vancomycin resistance (eg, enterococcus species van A, van B), amplified probe technique
	➔ *CPT Changes: An Insider's View* 2008
87510	Gardnerella vaginalis, direct probe technique
	➔ *CPT Assistant* Aug 05:9
87511	Gardnerella vaginalis, amplified probe technique
87512	Gardnerella vaginalis, quantification
87515	hepatitis B virus, direct probe technique
87516	hepatitis B virus, amplified probe technique
87517	hepatitis B virus, quantification
87520	hepatitis C, direct probe technique
87521	hepatitis C, amplified probe technique
87522	hepatitis C, quantification
87525	hepatitis G, direct probe technique
87526	hepatitis G, amplified probe technique
87527	hepatitis G, quantification

87528	Herpes simplex virus, direct probe technique
87529	Herpes simplex virus, amplified probe technique
87530	Herpes simplex virus, quantification
87531	Herpes virus-6, direct probe technique
87532	Herpes virus-6, amplified probe technique
87533	Herpes virus-6, quantification
87534	HIV-1, direct probe technique
87535	HIV-1, amplified probe technique
87536	HIV-1, quantification
87537	HIV-2, direct probe technique
87538	HIV-2, amplified probe technique
87539	HIV-2, quantification
87540	Legionella pneumophila, direct probe technique
87541	Legionella pneumophila, amplified probe technique
87542	Legionella pneumophila, quantification
87550	Mycobacteria species, direct probe technique
87551	Mycobacteria species, amplified probe technique
87552	Mycobacteria species, quantification
87555	Mycobacteria tuberculosis, direct probe technique
87556	Mycobacteria tuberculosis, amplified probe technique
87557	Mycobacteria tuberculosis, quantification
87560	Mycobacteria avium-intracellulare, direct probe technique
87561	Mycobacteria avium-intracellulare, amplified probe technique
87562	Mycobacteria avium-intracellulare, quantification
87580	Mycoplasma pneumoniae, direct probe technique
87581	Mycoplasma pneumoniae, amplified probe technique
87582	Mycoplasma pneumoniae, quantification
87590	Neisseria gonorrhoeae, direct probe technique
87591	Neisseria gonorrhoeae, amplified probe technique
87592	Neisseria gonorrhoeae, quantification
87620	papillomavirus, human, direct probe technique
	➔ *CPT Assistant* Feb 02:10, Aug 05:9
87621	papillomavirus, human, amplified probe technique
87622	papillomavirus, human, quantification
87640	Staphylococcus aureus, amplified probe technique
	➔ *CPT Changes: An Insider's View* 2007
87641	Staphylococcus aureus, methicillin resistant, amplified probe technique
	➔ *CPT Changes: An Insider's View* 2007

(For assays that detect methicillin resistance and identify Staphylococcus aureus using a single nucleic acid sequence, use 87641)

▲=Revised code   ●=New code   ►◄=Contains new or revised text   ⊘=Modifier 51 exempt

87650 Streptococcus, group A, direct probe technique

87651 Streptococcus, group A, amplified probe technique

87652 Streptococcus, group A, quantification

87653 Streptococcus, group B, amplified probe technique
> *CPT Changes: An Insider's View* 2007

87660 Trichomonas vaginalis, direct probe technique
> *CPT Changes: An Insider's View* 2004

87797 Infectious agent detection by nucleic acid (DNA or RNA), not otherwise specified; direct probe technique, each organism
> *CPT Assistant* Nov 97:34, Nov 01:10, Aug 05:9; *CPT Changes: An Insider's View* 2001

87798 amplified probe technique, each organism
> *CPT Assistant* Nov 97:34, Nov 01:10; *CPT Changes: An Insider's View* 2001

87799 quantification, each organism
> *CPT Assistant* Nov 97:34; *CPT Changes: An Insider's View* 2001

87800 Infectious agent detection by nucleic acid (DNA or RNA), multiple organisms; direct probe(s) technique
> *CPT Assistant* Aug 05:9; *CPT Changes: An Insider's View* 2001

87801 amplified probe(s) technique
> *CPT Changes: An Insider's View* 2001

(For each specific organism nucleic acid detection from a primary source, see 87470-87660. For detection of specific infectious agents not otherwise specified, see 87797, 87798, or 87799 one time for each agent)

87802 Infectious agent antigen detection by immunoassay with direct optical observation; Streptococcus, group B
> *CPT Assistant* Jun 03:12; *CPT Changes: An Insider's View* 2002

87803 Clostridium difficile toxin A
> *CPT Assistant* Jun 03:12; *CPT Changes: An Insider's View* 2002

87804 Influenza
> *CPT Assistant* Jun 03:11-12; *CPT Changes: An Insider's View* 2002

87807 respiratory syncytial virus
> *CPT Changes: An Insider's View* 2005

87808 Trichomonas vaginalis
> *CPT Changes: An Insider's View* 2007

● **87809** adenovirus
> *CPT Changes: An Insider's View* 2008

87810 Infectious agent detection by immunoassay with direct optical observation; Chlamydia trachomatis
> *CPT Assistant* Nov 97:34, Jan 98:6

87850 Neisseria gonorrhoeae
> *CPT Assistant* Nov 97:34, Jan 98:6

87880 Streptococcus, group A
> *CPT Assistant* Nov 97:34, Jan 98:6, Dec 98:8

87899 not otherwise specified
> *CPT Assistant* Jan 98:6, Jun 01:11

87900 Infectious agent drug susceptibility phenotype prediction using regularly updated genotypic bioinformatics
> *CPT Assistant* Mar 06:6; *CPT Changes: An Insider's View* 2006

87901 Infectious agent genotype analysis by nucleic acid (DNA or RNA); HIV 1, reverse transcriptase and protease
> *CPT Assistant* Aug 05:9, Mar 06:6; *CPT Changes: An Insider's View* 2001, 2002

(For infectious agent drug susceptibility phenotype prediction for HIV-1, use 87900)

87902 Hepatitis C virus
> *CPT Changes: An Insider's View* 2002

87903 Infectious agent phenotype analysis by nucleic acid (DNA or RNA) with drug resistance tissue culture analysis, HIV 1; first through 10 drugs tested
> *CPT Assistant* Apr 04:15, Mar 06:6; *CPT Changes: An Insider's View* 2001, 2002

+ **87904** each additional drug tested (List separately in addition to code for primary procedure)
> *CPT Assistant* Apr 04:15, Mar 06:6; *CPT Changes: An Insider's View* 2001, 2002, 2006

(Use 87904 in conjunction with 87903)

87999 Unlisted microbiology procedure
> *CPT Assistant* Aug 05:9

Anatomic Pathology

Postmortem Examination

Procedures 88000 through 88099 represent physician services only. Use modifier 90 for outside laboratory services.
> *CPT Assistant* Fall 93:26

88000 Necropsy (autopsy), gross examination only; without CNS
> *CPT Assistant* Aug 05:9

88005 with brain

88007 with brain and spinal cord

88012 infant with brain

88014 stillborn or newborn with brain

88016 macerated stillborn

88020 Necropsy (autopsy), gross and microscopic; without CNS

88025 with brain

88027 with brain and spinal cord

88028 infant with brain

88029 stillborn or newborn with brain

88036 Necropsy (autopsy), limited, gross and/or microscopic; regional

88037 single organ

88040	Necropsy (autopsy); forensic examination
88045	coroner's call
88099	Unlisted necropsy (autopsy) procedure

Cytopathology

(For cervicography, see Category III code 0003T)

(For collection of cytology specimens via mammary duct catheter lavage, report 0046T-0047T)

88104 Cytopathology, fluids, washings or brushings, except cervical or vaginal; smears with interpretation

➔ *CPT Assistant* Spring 91:6, Fall 94:3, Aug 05:9

88106 simple filter method with interpretation

➔ *CPT Assistant* Fall 94:3; *CPT Changes: An Insider's View* 2007

88107 smears and simple filter preparation with interpretation

➔ *CPT Assistant* Fall 94:3; *CPT Changes: An Insider's View* 2007

(For nongynecological selective cellular enhancement including filter transfer techniques, use 88112)

88108 Cytopathology, concentration technique, smears and interpretation (eg, Saccomanno technique)

➔ *CPT Assistant* Fall 94:3, Nov 97:34, Jan 98:6

(For cervical or vaginal smears, see 88150-88155)

(For gastric intubation with lavage, see 89130-89141, 91055)

(For x-ray localization, use 74340)

88112 Cytopathology, selective cellular enhancement technique with interpretation (eg, liquid based slide preparation method), except cervical or vaginal

➔ *CPT Changes: An Insider's View* 2004

(Do not report 88112 with 88108)

88125 Cytopathology, forensic (eg, sperm)

88130 Sex chromatin identification; Barr bodies

88140 peripheral blood smear, polymorphonuclear drumsticks

➔ *CPT Assistant* Nov 98:27-28, Mar 06:6

(For Guard stain, use 88313)

Codes 88141-88155, 88164-88167, 88174-88175 are used to report cervical or vaginal screening by various methods and to report physician interpretation services. Use codes 88150-88154 to report conventional Pap smears that are examined using non-Bethesda reporting. Use codes 88164-88167 to report conventional Pap smears that are examined using the Bethesda System of reporting. Use codes 88142-88143 to report liquid-based specimens processed as thin-layer preparations that are examined using any system of reporting (Bethesda or non-Bethesda). Use codes 88174-88175 to report

automated screening of liquid-based specimens that are examined using any system of reporting (Bethesda or non-Bethesda). Within each of these three code families choose the one code that describes the screening method(s) used. Codes 88141 and 88155 should be reported in addition to the screening code chosen when the additional services are provided. Manual rescreening requires a complete visual reassessment of the entire slide initially screened by either an automated or manual process. Manual review represents an assessment of selected cells or regions of a slide identified by initial automated review.

88141 Cytopathology, cervical or vaginal (any reporting system), requiring interpretation by physician

➔ *CPT Assistant* Nov 97:35, Jan 98:6, Jan 99:11, May 99:6, Nov 99:46, Mar 04:6, Mar 05:16

(Use 88141 in conjunction with 88142-88154, 88164-88167, 88174-88175)

88142 Cytopathology, cervical or vaginal (any reporting system), collected in preservative fluid, automated thin layer preparation; manual screening under physician supervision

➔ *CPT Assistant* Nov 97:34-35, Jan 98:6, Nov 98:28, May 99:6, Jul 03:7, Mar 04:4

88143 with manual screening and rescreening under physician supervision

➔ *CPT Assistant* Nov 97:34-35, Nov 98:28, May 99:6, Jul 03:7, Mar 04:4, Mar 05:16

(For automated screening of automated thin layer preparation, see 88174, 88175)

88147 Cytopathology smears, cervical or vaginal; screening by automated system under physician supervision

➔ *CPT Assistant* Nov 97:35, Nov 98:28, Jan 99:11, May 99:6, Nov 99:46, Mar 04:6

88148 screening by automated system with manual rescreening under physician supervision

➔ *CPT Assistant* Jan 99:1, May 99:6, Nov 99:46, Mar 04:6; *CPT Changes: An Insider's View* 2000

88150 Cytopathology, slides, cervical or vaginal; manual screening under physician supervision

➔ *CPT Assistant* Winter 91:19, Nov 97:34-35, Nov 98:28, May 99:6, Mar 04:5

88152 with manual screening and computer-assisted rescreening under physician supervision

➔ *CPT Assistant* Nov 97:35, Jan 98:6, May 99:6, Mar 04:5

88153 with manual screening and rescreening under physician supervision

➔ *CPT Assistant* Nov 97:34-35, Nov 98:28, May 99:6, Mar 04:5, Mar 05:16

88154 with manual screening and computer-assisted rescreening using cell selection and review under physician supervision

➔ *CPT Assistant* Nov 97:34-35, Nov 98:28, May 99:6, Mar 04:5

+ **88155** Cytopathology, slides, cervical or vaginal, definitive hormonal evaluation (eg, maturation index, karyopyknotic index, estrogenic index) (List separately in addition to code(s) for other technical and interpretation services)

➔ *CPT Assistant* Nov 97:35, Nov 98:28, May 99:6, Nov 99:46, Mar 04:5

(Use 88155 in conjunction with 88142-88154, 88164-88167, 88174-88175)

88160 Cytopathology, smears, any other source; screening and interpretation

➔ *CPT Assistant* Jan 98:6

88161 preparation, screening and interpretation

➔ *CPT Assistant* Aug 97:18, Jan 98:6

88162 extended study involving over 5 slides and/or multiple stains

(For aerosol collection of sputum, use 89220)

(For special stains, see 88312-88314)

88164 Cytopathology, slides, cervical or vaginal (the Bethesda System); manual screening under physician supervision

➔ *CPT Assistant* Nov 98:28, May 99:6, Mar 04:5

88165 with manual screening and rescreening under physician supervision

➔ *CPT Assistant* Nov 98:28, May 99:6, Mar 04:5, Mar 05:16

88166 with manual screening and computer-assisted rescreening under physician supervision

➔ *CPT Assistant* Nov 98:28, May 99:6, Mar 04:5

88167 with manual screening and computer-assisted rescreening using cell selection and review under physician supervision

➔ *CPT Assistant* Nov 98:28, May 99:6, Jul 03:7, Mar 04:5

(88170, 88171 have been deleted)

(To report collection of specimen via fine needle aspiration, see 10021, 10022)

88172 Cytopathology, evaluation of fine needle aspirate; immediate cytohistologic study to determine adequacy of specimen(s)

➔ *CPT Assistant* Fall 93:26, Fall 94:2, Dec 98:8; *CPT Changes: An Insider's View* 2001

88173 interpretation and report

➔ *CPT Assistant* Fall 93:26, Fall 94:2, Dec 98:8

(For fine needle aspirate, see 10021, 10022)

(Do not report 88172, 88173 in conjunction with 88333 and 88334 for the same specimen)

88174 Cytopathology, cervical or vaginal (any reporting system), collected in preservative fluid, automated thin layer preparation; screening by automated system, under physician supervision

➔ *CPT Assistant* Jul 03:9, Mar 04:4; *CPT Changes: An Insider's View* 2003

88175 with screening by automated system and manual rescreening or review, under physician supervision

➔ *CPT Assistant* Jul 03:9, Mar 04:4, Mar 06:6; *CPT Changes: An Insider's View* 2003, 2006

(For manual screening, see 88142, 88143)

88182 Flow cytometry, cell cycle or DNA analysis

(For DNA ploidy analysis by morphometric technique, use 88358)

88184 Flow cytometry, cell surface, cytoplasmic, or nuclear marker, technical component only; first marker

➔ *CPT Changes: An Insider's View* 2005

+ **88185** each additional marker (List separately in addition to code for first marker)

➔ *CPT Changes: An Insider's View* 2005

(Report 88185 in conjunction with 88184)

88187 Flow cytometry, interpretation; 2 to 8 markers

➔ *CPT Assistant* Apr 05:14; *CPT Changes: An Insider's View* 2005

88188 9 to 15 markers

➔ *CPT Assistant* Apr 05:14; *CPT Changes: An Insider's View* 2005

88189 16 or more markers

➔ *CPT Assistant* Apr 05:14; *CPT Changes: An Insider's View* 2005

►(Do not report 88187-88189 for interpretation of 86355, 86356, 86357, 86359, 86360, 86361, 86367)◄

88199 Unlisted cytopathology procedure

(For electron microscopy, see 88348, 88349)

Cytogenetic Studies

When molecular diagnostic procedures are performed to test for oncologic or inherited disorder, use the appropriate modifier to specify probe type or condition tested. (See **Appendix I** for a listing of appropriate modifiers to report with molecular diagnostic and cytogenetic procedures.)

(For acetylcholinesterase, use 82013)

(For alpha-fetoprotein, serum or amniotic fluid, see 82105, 82106)

(For laser microdissection of cells from tissue sample, see 88380)

88230 Tissue culture for non-neoplastic disorders; lymphocyte

➔ *CPT Assistant* Nov 98:29, Oct 99:2, Aug 05:9

88233 skin or other solid tissue biopsy

➔ *CPT Assistant* Nov 98:29, Oct 99:2

88235 amniotic fluid or chorionic villus cells

➔ *CPT Assistant* Nov 98:29, Oct 99:2

88237   Tissue culture for neoplastic disorders; bone marrow, blood cells
> *CPT Assistant* Nov 98:29, Oct 99:2

88239   solid tumor
> *CPT Assistant* Nov 98:29, Oct 99:2

88240   Cryopreservation, freezing and storage of cells, each cell line
> *CPT Assistant* Nov 98:29, Oct 99:2, Jul 03:9

(For therapeutic cryopreservation and storage, use 38207)

88241   Thawing and expansion of frozen cells, each aliquot
> *CPT Assistant* Nov 98:29, Oct 99:2, Jul 03:9

(For therapeutic thawing of previous harvest, use 38208)

88245   Chromosome analysis for breakage syndromes; baseline Sister Chromatid Exchange (SCE), 20-25 cells
> *CPT Assistant* Nov 98:29, Oct 99:2, Jul 05:1

88248   baseline breakage, score 50-100 cells, count 20 cells, 2 karyotypes (eg, for ataxia telangiectasia, Fanconi anemia, fragile X)
> *CPT Assistant* Nov 98:29, Oct 99:2, Jul 05:1

88249   score 100 cells, clastogen stress (eg, diepoxybutane, mitomycin C, ionizing radiation, UV radiation)
> *CPT Assistant* Nov 98:29, Oct 99:2, Jul 05:1

88261   Chromosome analysis; count 5 cells, 1 karyotype, with banding
> *CPT Assistant* Nov 98:29, Oct 99:2, Jul 05:1

88262   count 15-20 cells, 2 karyotypes, with banding
> *CPT Assistant* Nov 98:29, Oct 99:2

88263   count 45 cells for mosaicism, 2 karyotypes, with banding
> *CPT Assistant* Nov 98:29, Oct 99:2, Jul 05:1

88264   analyze 20-25 cells
> *CPT Assistant* Nov 98:29, Oct 99:2, Jul 05:1

88267   Chromosome analysis, amniotic fluid or chorionic villus, count 15 cells, 1 karyotype, with banding
> *CPT Assistant* Jul 05:1

88269   Chromosome analysis, in situ for amniotic fluid cells, count cells from 6-12 colonies, 1 karyotype, with banding
> *CPT Assistant* Jul 05:1

88271   Molecular cytogenetics; DNA probe, each (eg, FISH)
> *CPT Assistant* Nov 98:29, Mar 99:10, Oct 99:3, Jun 02:11, Jul 05:1

88272   chromosomal in situ hybridization, analyze 3-5 cells (eg, for derivatives and markers)
> *CPT Assistant* Nov 98:29, Mar 99:10, Oct 99:3, Jun 02:11, Jul 05:1

88273   chromosomal in situ hybridization, analyze 10-30 cells (eg, for microdeletions)
> *CPT Assistant* Nov 98:29, Mar 99:10, Oct 99:3, Jun 02:11, Jul 05:1

88274   interphase in situ hybridization, analyze 25-99 cells
> *CPT Assistant* Nov 98:29, Mar 99:10, Oct 99:3, Jun 02:11, Jul 05:1

88275   interphase in situ hybridization, analyze 100-300 cells
> *CPT Assistant* Nov 98:29, Mar 99:10, Oct 99:3, Jun 02:11, Jul 05:1

88280   Chromosome analysis; additional karyotypes, each study
> *CPT Assistant* Jul 05:1

88283   additional specialized banding technique (eg, NOR, C-banding)
> *CPT Assistant* Jul 05:1

88285   additional cells counted, each study
> *CPT Assistant* Jul 05:1

88289   additional high resolution study
> *CPT Assistant* Oct 99:3, Jul 05:1

88291   Cytogenetics and molecular cytogenetics, interpretation and report
> *CPT Assistant* Nov 98:29, Oct 99:3, Jul 05:1

88299   Unlisted cytogenetic study
> *CPT Assistant* Oct 99:3

Surgical Pathology

Services 88300 through 88309 include accession, examination, and reporting. They do not include the services designated in codes 88311 through 88365 and 88399, which are coded in addition when provided.

The unit of service for codes 88300 through 88309 is the specimen.

A specimen is defined as tissue or tissues that is (are) submitted for individual and separate attention, requiring individual examination and pathologic diagnosis. Two or more such specimens from the same patient (eg, separately identified endoscopic biopsies, skin lesions) are each appropriately assigned an individual code reflective of its proper level of service.

Service code 88300 is used for any specimen that in the opinion of the examining pathologist can be accurately diagnosed without microscopic examination. Service code 88302 is used when gross and microscopic examination is performed on a specimen to confirm identification and the absence of disease. Service codes 88304 through 88309 describe all other specimens requiring gross and microscopic examination, and represent additional ascending levels of physician work. Levels 88302 through 88309 are specifically defined by the assigned specimens.

Any unlisted specimen should be assigned to the code which most closely reflects the physician work involved when compared to other specimens assigned to that code.

(Do not report 88302-88309 on the same specimen as part of Mohs surgery)

88300   **Level I** - Surgical pathology, gross examination only
> *CPT Assistant* Winter 91:18, Sep 00:10, Aug 05:9

88302 **Level II** - Surgical pathology, gross and microscopic examination

Appendix, incidental

Fallopian tube, sterilization

Fingers/toes, amputation, traumatic

Foreskin, newborn

Hernia sac, any location

Hydrocele sac

Nerve

Skin, plastic repair

Sympathetic ganglion

Testis, castration

Vaginal mucosa, incidental

Vas deferens, sterilization

➔ *CPT Assistant* Winter 91:18, Sep 00:10, Nov 06:1, Jan 07:29

88304 **Level III** - Surgical pathology, gross and microscopic examination

Abortion, induced

Abscess

Aneurysm - arterial/ventricular

Anus, tag

Appendix, other than incidental

Artery, atheromatous plaque

Bartholin's gland cyst

Bone fragment(s), other than pathologic fracture

Bursa/synovial cyst

Carpal tunnel tissue

Cartilage, shavings

Cholesteatoma

Colon, colostomy stoma

Conjunctiva - biopsy/pterygium

Cornea

Diverticulum - esophagus/small intestine

Dupuytren's contracture tissue

Femoral head, other than fracture

Fissure/fistula

Foreskin, other than newborn

Gallbladder

Ganglion cyst

Hematoma

Hemorrhoids

Hydatid of Morgagni

Intervertebral disc

Joint, loose body

Meniscus

Mucocele, salivary

Neuroma - Morton's/traumatic

Pilonidal cyst/sinus

Polyps, inflammatory - nasal/sinusoidal

Skin - cyst/tag/debridement

Soft tissue, debridement

Soft tissue, lipoma

Spermatocele

Tendon/tendon sheath

Testicular appendage

Thrombus or embolus

Tonsil and/or adenoids

Varicocele

Vas deferens, other than sterilization

Vein, varicosity

➔ *CPT Assistant* Winter 91:18, Spring 91:2, Aug 97:18, Sep 00:10, Jan 07:29; *CPT Changes: An Insider's View* 2002

88305 **Level IV** - Surgical pathology, gross and microscopic examination

Abortion - spontaneous/missed

Artery, biopsy

Bone marrow, biopsy

Bone exostosis

Brain/meninges, other than for tumor resection

Breast, biopsy, not requiring microscopic evaluation of surgical margins

Breast, reduction mammoplasty

Bronchus, biopsy

Cell block, any source

Cervix, biopsy

Colon, biopsy

Duodenum, biopsy

Endocervix, curettings/biopsy

Endometrium, curettings/biopsy

Esophagus, biopsy

Extremity, amputation, traumatic

Fallopian tube, biopsy

Fallopian tube, ectopic pregnancy

Femoral head, fracture

Fingers/toes, amputation, non-traumatic

Gingiva/oral mucosa, biopsy

Heart valve

Joint, resection

Kidney, biopsy

Larynx, biopsy

Leiomyoma(s), uterine myomectomy - without uterus

Lip, biopsy/wedge resection

Lung, transbronchial biopsy

Lymph node, biopsy

Muscle, biopsy

Nasal mucosa, biopsy

Nasopharynx/oropharynx, biopsy

Nerve, biopsy

Odontogenic/dental cyst

Omentum, biopsy

Ovary with or without tube, non-neoplastic

Ovary, biopsy/wedge resection

Parathyroid gland

Peritoneum, biopsy

Pituitary tumor

Placenta, other than third trimester

Pleura/pericardium - biopsy/tissue

Polyp, cervical/endometrial

Polyp, colorectal

Polyp, stomach/small intestine

Prostate, needle biopsy

Prostate, TUR

Salivary gland, biopsy

Sinus, paranasal biopsy

Skin, other than cyst/tag/debridement/plastic repair

Small intestine, biopsy

Soft tissue, other than tumor/mass/lipoma/debridement

Spleen

Stomach, biopsy

Synovium

Testis, other than tumor/biopsy/castration

Thyroglossal duct/brachial cleft cyst

Tongue, biopsy

Tonsil, biopsy

Trachea, biopsy

Ureter, biopsy

Urethra, biopsy

Urinary bladder, biopsy

Uterus, with or without tubes and ovaries, for prolapse

Vagina, biopsy

Vulva/labia, biopsy

→ *CPT Assistant* Winter 90:2, Winter 91:18, Spring 91:6, Winter 92:17, Aug 97:18, Jul 98:4, Nov 98:29-30, Jul 00:4, Sep 00:10, Dec 00:15, Jul 05:13, Nov 06:1, Jan 07:29; *CPT Changes: An Insider's View* 2002

88307 **Level V** - Surgical pathology, gross and microscopic examination

Adrenal, resection

Bone - biopsy/curettings

Bone fragment(s), pathologic fracture

Brain, biopsy

Brain/meninges, tumor resection

Breast, excision of lesion, requiring microscopic evaluation of surgical margins

Breast, mastectomy - partial/simple

Cervix, conization

Colon, segmental resection, other than for tumor

Extremity, amputation, non-traumatic

Eye, enucleation

Kidney, partial/total nephrectomy

Larynx, partial/total resection

Liver, biopsy - needle/wedge

Liver, partial resection

Lung, wedge biopsy

Lymph nodes, regional resection

Mediastinum, mass

Myocardium, biopsy

Odontogenic tumor

Ovary with or without tube, neoplastic

Pancreas, biopsy

Placenta, third trimester

Prostate, except radical resection

Salivary gland

Sentinel lymph node

Small intestine, resection, other than for tumor

Soft tissue mass (except lipoma) - biopsy/simple excision

Stomach - subtotal/total resection, other than for tumor

Testis, biopsy

Thymus, tumor

Thyroid, total/lobe

Ureter, resection

Urinary bladder, TUR

Uterus, with or without tubes and ovaries, other than neoplastic/prolapse

⮕ *CPT Assistant* Winter 91:18, Winter 92:18, Jul 98:4, Nov 98:29-30, Jul 99:10, Jul 00:4, Sep 00:10, Dec 00:15, Dec 03:11, Nov 06:1, Jan 07:29; *CPT Changes: An Insider's View* 2001

88309 **Level VI** - Surgical pathology, gross and microscopic examination

Bone resection

Breast, mastectomy - with regional lymph nodes

Colon, segmental resection for tumor

Colon, total resection

Esophagus, partial/total resection

Extremity, disarticulation

Fetus, with dissection

Larynx, partial/total resection - with regional lymph nodes

Lung - total/lobe/segment resection

Pancreas, total/subtotal resection

Prostate, radical resection

Small intestine, resection for tumor

Soft tissue tumor, extensive resection

Stomach - subtotal/total resection for tumor

Testis, tumor

Tongue/tonsil -resection for tumor

Urinary bladder, partial/total resection

Uterus, with or without tubes and ovaries, neoplastic

Vulva, total/subtotal resection

⮕ *CPT Assistant* Winter 91:18, Spring 91:2, Fall 93:2, 26, Jul 00:4, Sep 00:10, Dec 03:11, Nov 06:1, Jan 07:29

(For fine needle aspiration, see 10021, 10022)

(For evaluation of fine needle aspirate, see 88172-88173)

(Do not report 88302-88309 on the same specimen as part of Mohs surgery)

✚ **88311** Decalcification procedure (List separately in addition to code for surgical pathology examination)

⮕ *CPT Assistant* Winter 92:18, Jul 98:4, Jun 02:11, Nov 02:7, Nov 06:1

✚ **88312** Special stains (List separately in addition to code for primary service); Group I for microorganisms (eg, Gridley, acid fast, methenamine silver), each

⮕ *CPT Assistant* Winter 91:19, Jun 02:11, Nov 02:7, Nov 06:1; *CPT Changes: An Insider's View* 2004

✚ **88313** Group II, all other (eg, iron, trichrome), except immunocytochemistry and immunoperoxidase stains, each

⮕ *CPT Assistant* Jun 02:11, Nov 02:7, Mar 03:22, Nov 03:15, Jun 06:17, Nov 06:1

(For immunocytochemistry and immunoperoxidase tissue studies, use 88342)

✚ **88314** histochemical staining with frozen section(s)

⮕ *CPT Assistant* Nov 02:7, Nov 06:1

(Do not report 88314 with 17311-17315 for routine frozen section stain (eg, hematoxylin and eosin, toluidine blue), performed during Mohs surgery. When a nonroutine histochemical stain on frozen tissue is utilized, report 88314 with modifier 59)

88318 Determinative histochemistry to identify chemical components (eg, copper, zinc)

88319 Determinative histochemistry or cytochemistry to identify enzyme constituents, each

88321 Consultation and report on referred slides prepared elsewhere

⮕ *CPT Assistant* Winter 91:19, Apr 97:9, Oct 00:7, Dec 02:10

88323 Consultation and report on referred material requiring preparation of slides

⮕ *CPT Assistant* Winter 91:19, Apr 97:9, Oct 00:7, Dec 02:10

88325 Consultation, comprehensive, with review of records and specimens, with report on referred material

⮕ *CPT Assistant* Winter 91:19, Apr 97:9, Dec 02:10

88329 Pathology consultation during surgery;

⮕ *CPT Assistant* Winter 91:19, Apr 97:12, Aug 97:18, Jan 07:29

88331 first tissue block, with frozen section(s), single specimen

⮕ *CPT Assistant* Winter 91:19, Spring 91:2, Apr 97:12, Aug 97:18, Jul 00:4, Nov 02:7, Mar 06:6, Nov 06:1, Jan 07:29; *CPT Changes: An Insider's View* 2001

88332 each additional tissue block with frozen section(s)

⮕ *CPT Assistant* Winter 91:19, Apr 97:12, Aug 97:18, Jul 00:4, Mar 06:6, Jan 07:29

88333 cytologic examination (eg, touch prep, squash prep), initial site

⮕ *CPT Assistant* Mar 06:6, Jan 07:29; *CPT Changes: An Insider's View* 2006

88334 cytologic examination (eg, touch prep, squash prep), each additional site

⮕ *CPT Assistant* Mar 06:6, Jan 07:29; *CPT Changes: An Insider's View* 2006

(For intraoperative consultation on a specimen requiring both frozen section and cytologic evaluation, use 88331 and 88334)

(For percutaneous needle biopsy requiring intraprocedural cytologic examination, use 88333)

(Do not report 88333 and 88334 for non-intraoperative cytologic examination, see 88160-88162)

(Do not report 88333 and 88334 for intraprocedural cytologic evaluation of fine needle aspirate, see 88172)

88342   Immunohistochemistry (including tissue immunoperoxidase), each antibody
→ *CPT Assistant* Winter 91:17, Jul 00:10, Nov 02:6-7, Nov 06:1; *CPT Changes: An Insider's View* 2004

(Do not report 88342 in conjunction with 88360 or 88361 for the same antibody)

(For quantitative or semiquantitative immunohistochemistry, see 88360, 88361)

88346   Immunofluorescent study, each antibody; direct method

88347   indirect method

88348   Electron microscopy; diagnostic

88349   scanning

88355   Morphometric analysis; skeletal muscle

88356   nerve

88358   tumor (eg, DNA ploidy)
→ *CPT Assistant* Jul 98:4, Jul 99:11, Jun 02:11, Jun 06:17; *CPT Changes: An Insider's View* 2004

(Do not report 88358 with 88313 unless each procedure is for a different special stain)

88360   Morphometric analysis, tumor immunohistochemistry (eg, Her-2/neu, estrogen receptor/progesterone receptor), quantitative or semiquantitative, each antibody; manual
→ *CPT Changes: An Insider's View* 2005

88361   using computer-assisted technology
→ *CPT Changes: An Insider's View* 2004, 2005

(Do not report 88360, 88361 with 88342 unless each procedure is for a different antibody)

(For morphometric analysis using in situ hybridization techniques, see 88367, 88368)

(When semi-thin plastic-embedded sections are performed in conjunction with morphometric analysis, only the morphometric analysis should be reported; if performed as an independent procedure, see codes 88300-88309 for surgical pathology.)

88362   Nerve teasing preparations

88365   In situ hybridization (eg, FISH), each probe
→ *CPT Assistant* Jun 02:11, Mar 05:16; *CPT Changes: An Insider's View* 2005

(Do not report 88365 in conjunction with 88367, 88368 for the same probe)

88367   Morphometric analysis, in situ hybridization (quantitative or semi-quantitative) each probe; using computer-assisted technology
→ *CPT Assistant* Mar 05:16; *CPT Changes: An Insider's View* 2005

88368   manual
→ *CPT Assistant* Mar 05:16; *CPT Changes: An Insider's View* 2005

88371   Protein analysis of tissue by Western Blot, with interpretation and report;

88372   immunological probe for band identification, each

▲ **88380**   Microdissection (ie, sample preparation of microscopically identified target); laser capture
→ *CPT Assistant* Apr 02:17; *CPT Changes: An Insider's View* 2002, 2008

● **88381**   manual
→ *CPT Changes: An Insider's View* 2008

►(Do not report 88380 in conjunction with 88381)◄

88384   Array-based evaluation of multiple molecular probes; 11 through 50 probes
→ *CPT Assistant* Jan 06:5, Mar 06:6; *CPT Changes: An Insider's View* 2006

88385   51 through 250 probes
→ *CPT Assistant* Jan 06:5, Mar 06:6; *CPT Changes: An Insider's View* 2006

88386   251 through 500 probes
→ *CPT Assistant* Jan 06:5, Mar 06:6; *CPT Changes: An Insider's View* 2006

(For preparation of array-based evaluation, see 83890-83892, 83898-83901)

(For preparation and analyses of less than 11 probes, see 83890-83914)

88399   Unlisted surgical pathology procedure

Transcutaneous Procedures

88400   Bilirubin, total, transcutaneous
→ *CPT Assistant* Aug 05:9

Other Procedures

89049   Caffeine halothane contracture test (CHCT) for malignant hyperthermia susceptibility, including interpretation and report
→ *CPT Assistant* Mar 06:6, May 06:19; *CPT Changes: An Insider's View* 2006

89050   Cell count, miscellaneous body fluids (eg, cerebrospinal fluid, joint fluid), except blood;
→ *CPT Assistant* Aug 05:9; *CPT Changes: An Insider's View* 2002

89051   with differential count

89055   Leukocyte assessment, fecal, qualitative or semiquantitative
→ *CPT Assistant* Jul 03:9; *CPT Changes: An Insider's View* 2003, 2004

89060   Crystal identification by light microscopy with or without polarizing lens analysis, tissue or any body fluid (except urine)
→ *CPT Changes: An Insider's View* 2007

(Do not report 89060 for crystal identification on paraffin-embedded tissue)

89100 Duodenal intubation and aspiration; single specimen (eg, simple bile study or afferent loop culture) plus appropriate test procedure

89105 collection of multiple fractional specimens with pancreatic or gallbladder stimulation, single or double lumen tube
➡ *CPT Assistant* Aug 05:9

(For radiological localization, use 74340)

(For chemical analyses, see **Chemistry,** this section)

(Electrocardiogram, see 93000-93268)

(Esophagus acid perfusion test (Bernstein), see 91030)

89125 Fat stain, feces, urine, or respiratory secretions
➡ *CPT Changes: An Insider's View* 2001

89130 Gastric intubation and aspiration, diagnostic, each specimen, for chemical analyses or cytopathology;

89132 after stimulation

89135 Gastric intubation, aspiration, and fractional collections (eg, gastric secretory study); one hour

89136 2 hours

89140 2 hours including gastric stimulation (eg, histalog, pentagastrin)

89141 3 hours, including gastric stimulation

(For gastric lavage, therapeutic, use 91105)

(For radiologic localization of gastric tube, use 74340)

(For chemical analyses, see 82926, 82928)

(Joint fluid chemistry, see **Chemistry,** this section)

89160 Meat fibers, feces

89190 Nasal smear for eosinophils

(Occult blood, feces, use 82270)

(Paternity tests, use 86910)

89220 Sputum, obtaining specimen, aerosol induced technique (separate procedure)
➡ *CPT Assistant* Aug 05:9; *CPT Changes: An Insider's View* 2004

89225 Starch granules, feces
➡ *CPT Changes: An Insider's View* 2004

89230 Sweat collection by iontophoresis
➡ *CPT Changes: An Insider's View* 2004

89235 Water load test
➡ *CPT Changes: An Insider's View* 2004

89240 Unlisted miscellaneous pathology test
➡ *CPT Assistant* Nov 05:14, Jan 07:30; *CPT Changes: An Insider's View* 2004

Reproductive Medicine Procedures

89250 Culture of oocyte(s)/embryo(s), less than 4 days;
➡ *CPT Assistant* Nov 97:35-36, Jan 98:6, Oct 98:1, Apr 04:2, May 04:16, Jun 04:9; *CPT Changes: An Insider's View* 2004

89251 with co-culture of oocyte(s)/embryos
➡ *CPT Assistant* Nov 97:35-36, Jan 98:6, Oct 98:1, Apr 04:2; *CPT Changes: An Insider's View* 2004

(For extended culture of oocyte(s)/embryo(s), see 89272)

89253 Assisted embryo hatching, microtechniques (any method)
➡ *CPT Assistant* Nov 97:35-36, Jan 98:6, Oct 98:1, Apr 04:2, May 04:16, Jun 04:9

89254 Oocyte identification from follicular fluid
➡ *CPT Assistant* Nov 97:35-36, Jan 98:6, Oct 98:1, Apr 04:2, May 04:16, Jun 04:9

89255 Preparation of embryo for transfer (any method)
➡ *CPT Assistant* Nov 97:35-36, Jan 98:6, Oct 98:1, Apr 04:2, May 04:16, Jun 04:9

89257 Sperm identification from aspiration (other than seminal fluid)
➡ *CPT Assistant* Nov 97:35-36, Jan 98:6, Oct 98:1, Nov 98:30, Apr 04:2

(For semen analysis, see 89300-89320)

(For sperm identification from testis tissue, use 89264)

89258 Cryopreservation; embryo(s)
➡ *CPT Assistant* Nov 97:36, Jan 98:6, Oct 98:1, Apr 04:2, 4; *CPT Changes: An Insider's View* 2004

89259 sperm
➡ *CPT Assistant* Nov 97:36, Jan 98:6, Oct 98:1, Apr 04:2, 4

(For cryopreservation of reproductive tissue, testicular, use 89335)

(For cryopreservation of reproductive tissue, ovarian, use Category III code 0058T)

(For cryopreservation of oocyte(s), use Category III code 0059T)

89260 Sperm isolation; simple prep (eg, sperm wash and swim-up) for insemination or diagnosis with semen analysis
➡ *CPT Assistant* Nov 97:36, Jan 98:6, Oct 98:1, Apr 04:3-4

89261 complex prep (eg, Percoll gradient, albumin gradient) for insemination or diagnosis with semen analysis
➡ *CPT Assistant* Nov 97:36, Jan 98:6, Oct 98:1, Apr 04:3-4

(For semen analysis without sperm wash or swim-up, use 89320)

89264 Sperm identification from testis tissue, fresh or cryopreserved
➡ *CPT Assistant* Nov 98:30, Apr 04:3-4

(For biopsy of testis, see 54500, 54505)

(For sperm identification from aspiration, use 89257)

(For semen analysis, see 89300-89320)

89268 Insemination of oocytes
➔ *CPT Assistant* Apr 04:3-4; *CPT Changes: An Insider's View* 2004

89272 Extended culture of oocyte(s)/embryo(s), 4-7 days
➔ *CPT Assistant* Apr 04:3-4; *CPT Changes: An Insider's View* 2004

89280 Assisted oocyte fertilization, microtechnique; less than or equal to 10 oocytes
➔ *CPT Assistant* Apr 04:3-4; *CPT Changes: An Insider's View* 2004

89281 greater than 10 oocytes
➔ *CPT Assistant* Apr 04:3-4; *CPT Changes: An Insider's View* 2004

89290 Biopsy, oocyte polar body or embryo blastomere, microtechnique (for pre-implantation genetic diagnosis); less than or equal to 5 embryos
➔ *CPT Assistant* Apr 04:5; *CPT Changes: An Insider's View* 2004

89291 greater than 5 embryos
➔ *CPT Assistant* Apr 04:3, 5; *CPT Changes: An Insider's View* 2004

89300 Semen analysis; presence and/or motility of sperm including Huhner test (post coital)
➔ *CPT Assistant* Nov 97:36, Jul 98:10, Oct 98:4, Apr 04:3, Aug 05:9

89310 motility and count (not including Huhner test)
➔ *CPT Assistant* Jul 03:9, Apr 04:3; *CPT Changes: An Insider's View* 2003

▲ **89320** volume, count, motility, and differential
➔ *CPT Assistant* Apr 04:3; *CPT Changes: An Insider's View* 2008

(Skin tests, see 86485-86580 and 95010-95199)

▲ **89321** sperm presence and motility of sperm, if performed
➔ *CPT Changes: An Insider's View* 2001, 2008

(To report Hyaluronan binding assay (HBA), use Category III code 0087T)

● **89322** volume, count, motility, and differential using strict morphologic criteria (eg, Kruger)
➔ *CPT Changes: An Insider's View* 2008

89325 Sperm antibodies

(For medicolegal identification of sperm, use 88125)

89329 Sperm evaluation; hamster penetration test

89330 cervical mucus penetration test, with or without spinnbarkeit test
➔ *CPT Assistant* Nov 05:14

● **89331** Sperm evaluation, for retrograde ejaculation, urine (sperm concentration, motility, and morphology, as indicated)
➔ *CPT Changes: An Insider's View* 2008

▶(For semen analysis on concurrent semen specimen, see 89300-89322 in conjunction with 89331)◀

▶(For detection of sperm in urine, use 81015)◀

89335 Cryopreservation, reproductive tissue, testicular
➔ *CPT Assistant* Apr 04:5; *CPT Changes: An Insider's View* 2004

(For cryopreservation of embryo(s), use 89258. For cryopreservation of sperm, use 89259)

(For cryopreservation of reproductive tissue, ovarian, use Category III code 0058T)

(For cryopreservation of oocyte, use Category III code 0059T)

89342 Storage (per year); embryo(s)
➔ *CPT Assistant* Apr 04:5; *CPT Changes: An Insider's View* 2004

89343 sperm/semen
➔ *CPT Assistant* Apr 04:5; *CPT Changes: An Insider's View* 2004

89344 reproductive tissue, testicular/ovarian
➔ *CPT Assistant* Apr 04:5; *CPT Changes: An Insider's View* 2004

89346 oocyte(s)
➔ *CPT Assistant* Apr 04:5; *CPT Changes: An Insider's View* 2004, 2005

89352 Thawing of cryopreserved; embryo(s)
➔ *CPT Assistant* Apr 04:5; *CPT Changes: An Insider's View* 2004

89353 sperm/semen, each aliquot
➔ *CPT Assistant* Apr 04:5; *CPT Changes: An Insider's View* 2004

89354 reproductive tissue, testicular/ovarian
➔ *CPT Assistant* Apr 04:5; *CPT Changes: An Insider's View* 2004

89356 oocytes, each aliquot
➔ *CPT Assistant* Apr 04:5, Aug 05:9; *CPT Changes: An Insider's View* 2004

Notes

⊙=Moderate sedation ✚=Add-on code ✗=FDA approval pending ➔➔=See p xvii for details

Medicine Guidelines

In addition to the definitions and commonly used terms presented in the **Introduction**, several other items unique to this section on **Medicine** are defined or identified here.

Multiple Procedures

It is appropriate to designate multiple procedures that are rendered on the same date by separate entries. For example: If individual medical psychotherapy (90829) is rendered in addition to subsequent hospital care (eg, 99231), the psychotherapy would be reported separately from the hospital visit. In this instance, both 99231 and 90829 would be reported.

Add-on Codes

Some of the listed procedures are commonly carried out in addition to the primary procedure performed. All add-on codes found in the CPT codebook are exempt from the multiple procedure concept. They are exempt from the use of modifier 51, as these procedures are not reported as stand-alone codes. These additional or supplemental procedures are designated as "add-on" codes. Add-on codes in the CPT codebook can be readily identified by specific descriptor nomenclature which includes phrases such as "each additional" or "(List separately in addition to primary procedure)."

Separate Procedures

Some of the procedures or services listed in the CPT codebook that are commonly carried out as an integral component of a total service or procedure have been identified by the inclusion of the term "separate procedure." The codes designated as "separate procedure" should not be reported in addition to the code for the total procedure or service of which it is considered an integral component.

However, when a procedure or service that is designated as a "separate procedure" is carried out independently or considered to be unrelated or distinct from other procedures/services provided at that time, it may be reported by itself, or in addition to other procedures/services by appending modifier 59 to the specific "separate procedure" code to indicate that the procedure is not considered to be a component of another procedure, but is a distinct, independent procedure. This may represent a different session or patient encounter, different procedure or surgery, different site or organ system, separate incision/excision, separate lesion, or separate injury (or area of injury in extensive injuries).

Subsection Information

Several of the subheadings or subsections have special instructions unique to that section. These special instructions will be presented preceding those procedural terminology listings, referring to that subsection specifically. If there is an "Unlisted Procedure" code number (see section below) for the individual subsection, it will also be shown. Those subsections within the **Medicine** section that have special instructions are as follows:

Immune Globulins 90281-90399
Immunization Administration for
   Vaccines/Toxoids 90465-90474
Vaccines, Toxoids 90476-90749
Hydration, Therapeutic, Prophylactic,
   and Diagnostic Injections and
   Infusions 90760-90779
   Hydration 90760-90761
   Therapeutic, Prophylactic, and Diagnostic
   Injections and Infusions 90765-90779
Psychiatry 90801-90899
Dialysis 90918-90999
   Hemodialysis 90935-90940
   Miscellaneous Dialysis
   Procedures 90945-90999
Ophthalmology 92002-92499
   General Ophthalmological
   Services 92002-92014
   Ophthalmoscopy 92225-92260
   Contact Lens Services 92310-92326
   Spectacle Services 92340-92371
Special Otorhinolaryngologic
   Services 92502-92700
   Audiologic Function Tests 92551-92597
   Evaluative and Therapeutic
   Services 92601-92633
►Cardiography . . . . 93000-93278◄
Echocardiography 93303-93350
Cardiac Catheterization 93501-93533
►Injection Procedures . . . . 93539-93572◄
Intracardiac Electrophysiological
   Procedures/Studies 93600-93662
Peripheral Arterial Disease
   Rehabilitation 93668
Noninvasive Vascular
   Diagnostic Studies 93875-93990
Cerebrovascular Arterial Studies 93875-93893
Pulmonary 94002-94799
Allergy and Clinical Immunology . . . 95004-95199
Neurology and Neuromuscular 95805-95999
   Sleep Testing 95805-95811
Routine Electroencephalography (EEG) . . . 95812-95830

Special Report

A service that is rarely provided, unusual, variable, or new may require a special report in determining medical appropriateness of the service. Pertinent information should include an adequate definition or description of the nature, extent, and need for the procedure; and the time, effort, and equipment necessary to provide the service. Additional items that may be included are:

- Complexity of symptoms
- Final diagnosis
- Pertinent physical findings
- Diagnostic and therapeutic procedures
- Concurrent problems
- Follow-up care

Unlisted Service or Procedure

A service or procedure may be provided that is not listed in this edition of the CPT codebook. When reporting such a service, the appropriate "Unlisted Procedure" code may be used to indicate the service, identifying it by "Special Report" as discussed on this page. The "Unlisted Procedures" and accompanying codes for **Medicine** are as follows:

▲ **90399**	Unlisted immune globulin
▲ **90749**	Unlisted vaccine/toxoid
90779	Unlisted therapeutic, prophylactic or diagnostic intravenous or intra-arterial injection or infusion
90899	Unlisted psychiatric service or procedure

Materials Supplied by Physician

Supplies and materials provided by the physician (eg, sterile trays/drugs), over and above those usually included with the procedure(s) rendered are reported separately. List drugs, trays, supplies, and materials provided. Identify as 99070 or specific supply code.

Medicine

Immune Globulins

►Codes 90281-90399 identify the immune globulin product only and are reported in addition to the administration codes 90765-90768, 90772, 90774, 90775 as appropriate. Modifier 51 should not be reported with the immune globulin codes when performed with another procedure. Immune globulin products listed here include broad-spectrum and anti-infective immune globulins, antitoxins, and various isoantibodies.◄

▲ **90281** Immune globulin (Ig), human, for intramuscular use
→ *CPT Assistant* Nov 98:30, Jan 99:3, Sep 99:10; *CPT Changes: An Insider's View* 2008

▲ **90283** Immune globulin (IgIV), human, for intravenous use
→ *CPT Assistant* Nov 98:30, Jan 99:3; *CPT Changes: An Insider's View* 2008

● **90284** Immune globulin (SCIg), human, for use in subcutaneous infusions, 100 mg, each
→ *CPT Changes: An Insider's View* 2008

▲ **90287** Botulinum antitoxin, equine, any route
→ *CPT Assistant* Nov 98:30, Jan 99:3; *CPT Changes: An Insider's View* 2008

▲ **90288** Botulism immune globulin, human, for intravenous use
→ *CPT Assistant* Nov 98:30, Jan 99:3; *CPT Changes: An Insider's View* 2008

▲ **90291** Cytomegalovirus immune globulin (CMV-IgIV), human, for intravenous use
→ *CPT Assistant* Nov 98:30, Jan 99:3; *CPT Changes: An Insider's View* 2008

▲ **90296** Diphtheria antitoxin, equine, any route
→ *CPT Assistant* Nov 98:30, Jan 99:3; *CPT Changes: An Insider's View* 2008

▲ **90371** Hepatitis B immune globulin (HBIg), human, for intramuscular use
→ *CPT Assistant* Nov 98:30, Jan 99:3; *CPT Changes: An Insider's View* 2008

▲ **90375** Rabies immune globulin (RIg), human, for intramuscular and/or subcutaneous use
→ *CPT Assistant* Nov 98:30, Jan 99:3; *CPT Changes: An Insider's View* 2008

▲ **90376** Rabies immune globulin, heat-treated (RIg-HT), human, for intramuscular and/or subcutaneous use
→ *CPT Assistant* Nov 98:30, Jan 99:3; *CPT Changes: An Insider's View* 2008

▲ **90378** Respiratory syncytial virus immune globulin (RSV-IgIM), for intramuscular use, 50 mg, each
→ *CPT Assistant* Jan 99:3, Nov 99:47, Jun 00:10; *CPT Changes: An Insider's View* 2000, 2001, 2008

▲ **90379** Respiratory syncytial virus immune globulin (RSV-IgIV), human, for intravenous use
→ *CPT Assistant* Nov 98:30, Jan 99:3; *CPT Changes: An Insider's View* 2008

▲ **90384** Rho(D) immune globulin (RhIg), human, full-dose, for intramuscular use
→ *CPT Assistant* Nov 98:30, Jan 99:3; *CPT Changes: An Insider's View* 2008

▲ **90385** Rho(D) immune globulin (RhIg), human, mini-dose, for intramuscular use
→ *CPT Assistant* Nov 98:30, Jan 99:3; *CPT Changes: An Insider's View* 2008

▲ **90386** Rho(D) immune globulin (RhIgIV), human, for intravenous use
→ *CPT Assistant* Nov 98:30, Jan 99:3; *CPT Changes: An Insider's View* 2008

▲ **90389** Tetanus immune globulin (TIg), human, for intramuscular use
→ *CPT Assistant* Nov 98:30, Jan 99:3; *CPT Changes: An Insider's View* 2008

▲ **90393** Vaccinia immune globulin, human, for intramuscular use
→ *CPT Assistant* Nov 98:30, Jan 99:3; *CPT Changes: An Insider's View* 2008

▲ **90396** Varicella-zoster immune globulin, human, for intramuscular use
→ *CPT Assistant* Nov 98:30, Jan 99:3; *CPT Changes: An Insider's View* 2008

▲ **90399** Unlisted immune globulin
→ *CPT Assistant* Nov 98:30, Jan 99:3, Feb 99:11, Sep 99:10; *CPT Changes: An Insider's View* 2008

Immunization Administration for Vaccines/Toxoids

Codes 90465-90474 must be reported in addition to the vaccine and toxoid code(s) 90476-90749.

Report codes 90465-90468 only when the physician provides face-to-face counseling of the patient and family during the administration of a vaccine. For immunization administration of any vaccine that is not accompanied by face-to-face physician counseling to the patient/family, report codes 90471-90474.

If a significant separately identifiable Evaluation and Management service (eg, office or other outpatient services, preventive medicine services) is performed, the appropriate E/M service code should be reported in addition to the vaccine and toxoid administration codes.

(For allergy testing, see 95004 et seq)

▲=Revised code   ●=New code   ►◄=Contains new or revised text   ⊘=Modifier 51 exempt   American Medical Association   **379**

▶(For skin testing of bacterial, viral, fungal extracts, see 86485-86580)◀

(For therapeutic or diagnostic injections, see 90772-90779)

90465 Immunization administration younger than 8 years of age (includes percutaneous, intradermal, subcutaneous, or intramuscular injections) when the physician counsels the patient/family; first injection (single or combination vaccine/toxoid), per day

➔ *CPT Assistant* Apr 05:1-3, Aug 05:15, Nov 05:1; *CPT Changes: An Insider's View* 2005

(Do not report 90465 in conjunction with 90467)

+ 90466 each additional injection (single or combination vaccine/toxoid), per day (List separately in addition to code for primary procedure)

➔ *CPT Assistant* Apr 05:1-3, Aug 05:15, Nov 05:1; *CPT Changes: An Insider's View* 2005

(Use 90466 in conjunction with 90465 or 90467)

90467 Immunization administration younger than age 8 years (includes intranasal or oral routes of administration) when the physician counsels the patient/family; first administration (single or combination vaccine/toxoid), per day

➔ *CPT Assistant* Apr 05:1-3, Aug 05:15; *CPT Changes: An Insider's View* 2005

(Do not report 90467 in conjunction with 90465)

+ 90468 each additional administration (single or combination vaccine/toxoid), per day (List separately in addition to code for primary procedure)

➔ *CPT Assistant* Apr 05:1-3, Aug 05:15; *CPT Changes: An Insider's View* 2005

(Use 90468 in conjunction with 90465 or 90467)

90471 Immunization administration (includes percutaneous, intradermal, subcutaneous, or intramuscular injections); one vaccine (single or combination vaccine/toxoid)

➔ *CPT Assistant* Nov 98:31, Jan 99:2, Apr 99:10, Oct 99:9, Nov 99:47-48, Nov 00:10, Feb 01:5, Jul 01:2, Nov 02:11, Mar 04:11, Apr 04:14, Apr 05:1-3, 5, Nov 05:1; *CPT Changes: An Insider's View* 2002, 2005

(Do not report 90471 in conjunction with 90473)

+ 90472 each additional vaccine (single or combination vaccine/toxoid) (List separately in addition to code for primary procedure)

➔ *CPT Assistant* Nov 98:31, Jan 99:2, Apr 99:10, Oct 99:9, Nov 99:47-48, Nov 00:10, Feb 01:5, Jul 01:2, Nov 02:11, Mar 04:11, Apr 04:14, Apr 05:1-3, Nov 05:1; *CPT Changes: An Insider's View* 2000

(Use 90472 in conjunction with 90471 or 90473)

(For administration of immune globulins, see 90281-90399, 90760, 90761, 90765-90768, 90774)

(For intravesical administration of BCG vaccine, see 51720, 90586)

90473 Immunization administration by intranasal or oral route; one vaccine (single or combination vaccine/toxoid)

➔ *CPT Assistant* Feb 01:5, Nov 02:11, Apr 04:14, Apr 05:1-3; *CPT Changes: An Insider's View* 2002

(Do not report 90473 in conjunction with 90471)

+ 90474 each additional vaccine (single or combination vaccine/toxoid) (List separately in addition to code for primary procedure)

➔ *CPT Assistant* Feb 01:5, Nov 02:11, Apr 04:14, Apr 05:1-3; *CPT Changes: An Insider's View* 2002

(Use 90474 in conjunction with 90471 or 90473)

Vaccines, Toxoids

To assist users to report the most recent new or revised vaccine product codes, the American Medical Association (AMA) currently uses the CPT Website, which features updates of CPT Editorial Panel actions regarding these products. Once approved by the CPT Editorial Panel, these codes will be made available for release on a semi-annual (twice a year: July 1 and January 1) basis. As part of the electronic distribution, there is a six-month implementation period from the initial release date (ie, codes released on January 1 are eligible for use on July 1 and codes released on July 1 are eligible for use January 1).

The CPT Editorial Panel, in recognition of the public health interest in vaccine products, has chosen to publish new vaccine product codes prior to approval by the Food and Drug Administration (FDA). These codes are indicated with the ⁄ symbol and will be tracked by the AMA to monitor FDA approval status. Once the FDA status changes to approval, the ⁄ symbol will be removed. CPT users should refer to the AMA Internet site (www.ama-assn.org/ama/pub/category/10902.html) for the most up-to-date information on codes with the ⁄ symbol.

▶Codes 90476-90748 identify the vaccine product **only.** To report the administration of a vaccine/toxoid, the vaccine/toxoid product codes 90476-90749 must be used in addition to an immunization administration code(s) 90465-90474. Modifier 51 should not be reported for the vaccines, toxoids when performed with these administration procedures.◀

If a significantly separately identifiable Evaluation and Management (E/M) service (eg, office or other outpatient services, preventive medicine services) is performed, the appropriate E/M service code should be reported in addition to the vaccine and toxoid administration codes.

To meet the reporting requirements of immunization registries, vaccine distribution programs, and reporting systems (eg, Vaccine Adverse Event Reporting System) the exact vaccine product administered needs to be reported. Multiple codes for a particular vaccine are provided in the CPT codebook when the schedule (number of doses or timing) differs for two or more products of the same vaccine type (eg, hepatitis A, Hib) or the vaccine product is available in more than one chemical formulation, dosage, or route of administration.

▶The "age" descriptions included in CPT vaccine codes (eg, 90655-90660, 90714, 90715, 90718, 90732) are not intended to identify a product's licensed age indication. Refer to the product's prescribing information (PI) for the FDA approved age indication before administering vaccine to a patient.◀

Separate codes are available for combination vaccines (eg, DTP-Hib, DtaP-Hib, HepB-Hib). It is inappropriate to code each component of a combination vaccine separately. If a specific vaccine code is not available, the unlisted procedure code should be reported, until a new code becomes available.

(For immune globulins, see codes 90281-90399, 90765-90768, 90772-90775 for administration of immune globulins)

➔ *CPT Assistant* Nov 99:48

▲ **90476**   Adenovirus vaccine, type 4, live, for oral use
    ➔ *CPT Assistant* Nov 98:31-33, Jan 99:2, Sep 99:10, Oct 99:9; *CPT Changes: An Insider's View* 2008

▲ **90477**   Adenovirus vaccine, type 7, live, for oral use
    ➔ *CPT Assistant* Nov 98:31-33, Jan 99:2, Oct 99:9; *CPT Changes: An Insider's View* 2008

▲ **90581**   Anthrax vaccine, for subcutaneous use
    ➔ *CPT Assistant* Nov 98:31-33, Jan 99:2, Oct 99:9; *CPT Changes: An Insider's View* 2008

▲ **90585**   Bacillus Calmette-Guerin vaccine (BCG) for tuberculosis, live, for percutaneous use
    ➔ *CPT Assistant* Nov 98:31-33, Jan 99:2, Oct 99:9; *CPT Changes: An Insider's View* 2008

▲ **90586**   Bacillus Calmette-Guerin vaccine (BCG) for bladder cancer, live, for intravesical use
    ➔ *CPT Assistant* Nov 98:31-33, Jan 99:2, Oct 99:9, Nov 02:11; *CPT Changes: An Insider's View* 2008

▲ **90632**   Hepatitis A vaccine, adult dosage, for intramuscular use
    ➔ *CPT Assistant* Nov 98:31-33, Jan 99:2, Oct 99:9; *CPT Changes: An Insider's View* 2008

▲ **90633**   Hepatitis A vaccine, pediatric/adolescent dosage-2 dose schedule, for intramuscular use
    ➔ *CPT Assistant* Nov 98:31-33, Jan 99:2, Oct 99:9; *CPT Changes: An Insider's View* 2008

▲ **90634**   Hepatitis A vaccine, pediatric/adolescent dosage-3 dose schedule, for intramuscular use
    ➔ *CPT Assistant* Nov 98:31-33, Jan 99:2, Oct 99:9; *CPT Changes: An Insider's View* 2008

▲ **90636**   Hepatitis A and hepatitis B vaccine (HepA-HepB), adult dosage, for intramuscular use
    ➔ *CPT Assistant* Nov 98:31-33, Jan 99:2, Oct 99:9; *CPT Changes: An Insider's View* 2008

▲ **90645**   Hemophilus influenza b vaccine (Hib), HbOC conjugate (4 dose schedule), for intramuscular use
    ➔ *CPT Assistant* Nov 98:31-33, Jan 99:2, Oct 99:9; *CPT Changes: An Insider's View* 2008

▲ **90646**   Hemophilus influenza b vaccine (Hib), PRP-D conjugate, for booster use only, intramuscular use
    ➔ *CPT Assistant* Nov 98:31-33, Jan 99:2, Oct 99:9; *CPT Changes: An Insider's View* 2008

▲ **90647**   Hemophilus influenza b vaccine (Hib), PRP-OMP conjugate (3 dose schedule), for intramuscular use
    ➔ *CPT Assistant* Nov 98:31-33, Jan 99:2, Oct 99:9; *CPT Changes: An Insider's View* 2008

▲ **90648**   Hemophilus influenza b vaccine (Hib), PRP-T conjugate (4 dose schedule), for intramuscular use
    ➔ *CPT Assistant* Nov 98:31-33, Jan 99:2, Oct 99:9; *CPT Changes: An Insider's View* 2008

▲ **90649**   Human Papilloma virus (HPV) vaccine, types 6, 11, 16, 18 (quadrivalent), 3 dose schedule, for intramuscular use
    ➔ *CPT Assistant* Dec 05:9, Jun 06:8, Sep 06:14; *CPT Changes: An Insider's View* 2006, 2008

▲ **90655**   Influenza virus vaccine, split virus, preservative free, when administered to children 6-35 months of age, for intramuscular use
    ➔ *CPT Assistant* Oct 99:9, Feb 04:2, Apr 07:12; *CPT Changes: An Insider's View* 2004, 2007, 2008

▲ **90656**   Influenza virus vaccine, split virus, preservative free, when administered to individuals 3 years and older, for intramuscular use
    ➔ *CPT Changes: An Insider's View* 2005, 2007, 2008

▲ **90657**   Influenza virus vaccine, split virus, when administered to children 6-35 months of age, for intramuscular use
    ➔ *CPT Assistant* Nov 98:31-33, Jan 99:2, Oct 99:9, Feb 02:10, Feb 04:2, Apr 05:5; *CPT Changes: An Insider's View* 2004, 2007, 2008

▲ **90658**   Influenza virus vaccine, split virus, when administered to individuals 3 years of age and older, for intramuscular use
    ➔ *CPT Assistant* Nov 98:31-33, Jan 99:2, Oct 99:9, Feb 04:2, Apr 07:12; *CPT Changes: An Insider's View* 2004, 2007, 2008

▲ **90660**   Influenza virus vaccine, live, for intranasal use
    ➔ *CPT Assistant* Nov 98:31-33, Jan 99:2, Oct 99:9, Mar 04:11, Apr 04:14; *CPT Changes: An Insider's View* 2008

✎● **90661**   Influenza virus vaccine, derived from cell cultures, subunit, preservative and antibiotic free, for intramuscular use
    ➔ *CPT Changes: An Insider's View* 2008

✎● **90662**   Influenza virus vaccine, split virus, preservative free, enhanced immunogenicity via increased antigen content, for intramuscular use
    ➔ *CPT Changes: An Insider's View* 2008

✎● **90663**   Influenza virus vaccine, pandemic formulation
    ➔ *CPT Changes: An Insider's View* 2008

▲ **90665**   Lyme disease vaccine, adult dosage, for intramuscular use
    ➔ *CPT Assistant* Nov 98:31-33, Jan 99:2, Oct 99:9; *CPT Changes: An Insider's View* 2008

▲ **90669**　Pneumococcal conjugate vaccine, polyvalent, when administered to children younger than 5 years, for intramuscular use

　　➜ *CPT Assistant* Nov 98:31-33, Jan 99:2, Oct 99:9, Jun 00:10; *CPT Changes: An Insider's View* 2001, 2007, 2008

▲ **90675**　Rabies vaccine, for intramuscular use

　　➜ *CPT Assistant* Nov 98:31-33, Jan 99:2, Oct 99:9; *CPT Changes: An Insider's View* 2008

▲ **90676**　Rabies vaccine, for intradermal use

　　➜ *CPT Assistant* Nov 98:31-33, Jan 99:2, Oct 99:9; *CPT Changes: An Insider's View* 2008

▲ **90680**　Rotavirus vaccine, pentavalent, 3 dose schedule, live, for oral use

　　➜ *CPT Assistant* Nov 98:31-33, Jan 99:2, Oct 99:9, Jun 05:6, Dec 05:9, Jun 06:8; *CPT Changes: An Insider's View* 2006, 2008

▲ **90690**　Typhoid vaccine, live, oral

　　➜ *CPT Assistant* Nov 98:31-33, Jan 99:2, Oct 99:9; *CPT Changes: An Insider's View* 2008

▲ **90691**　Typhoid vaccine, Vi capsular polysaccharide (ViCPs), for intramuscular use

　　➜ *CPT Assistant* Nov 98:31-33, Jan 99:2, Oct 99:9; *CPT Changes: An Insider's View* 2008

▲ **90692**　Typhoid vaccine, heat- and phenol-inactivated (H-P), for subcutaneous or intradermal use

　　➜ *CPT Assistant* Nov 98:31-33, Jan 99:2, Oct 99:9; *CPT Changes: An Insider's View* 2008

▲ **90693**　Typhoid vaccine, acetone-killed, dried (AKD), for subcutaneous use (U.S. military)

　　➜ *CPT Assistant* Nov 98:31-33, Jan 99:2, Oct 99:9; *CPT Changes: An Insider's View* 2004, 2008

✎ ▲ **90698**　Diphtheria, tetanus toxoids, acellular pertussis vaccine, haemophilus influenza Type B, and poliovirus vaccine, inactivated (DTaP - Hib - IPV), for intramuscular use

　　➜ *CPT Assistant* Oct 99:9, Dec 05:9, Jun 06:8; *CPT Changes: An Insider's View* 2008

▲ **90700**　Diphtheria, tetanus toxoids, and acellular pertussis vaccine (DTaP), when administered to individuals younger than 7 years, for intramuscular use

　　➜ *CPT Assistant* Jan 96:5, Apr 97:10, Nov 98:31-33, Jan 99:2, Oct 99:9, Nov 03:13; *CPT Changes: An Insider's View* 2005, 2007, 2008

▲ **90701**　Diphtheria, tetanus toxoids, and whole cell pertussis vaccine (DTP), for intramuscular use

　　➜ *CPT Assistant* Jan 96:6, Apr 97:10, Nov 98:31-33, Jan 99:2, Oct 99:9; *CPT Changes: An Insider's View* 2008

▲ **90702**　Diphtheria and tetanus toxoids (DT) adsorbed when administered to individuals younger than 7 years, for intramuscular use

　　➜ *CPT Assistant* Jan 96:6, Aug 96:10, Apr 97:10, Nov 98:31-33, Jan 99:2, Sep 99:10, Oct 99:9, Jun 00:10, Feb 07:11; *CPT Changes: An Insider's View* 2001, 2007, 2008

▲ **90703**　Tetanus toxoid adsorbed, for intramuscular use

　　➜ *CPT Assistant* Jan 96:6, Apr 97:10, Nov 98:31-33, Jan 99:2, Sep 99:10, Oct 99:9; *CPT Changes: An Insider's View* 2004, 2008

▲ **90704**　Mumps virus vaccine, live, for subcutaneous use

　　➜ *CPT Assistant* Apr 97:10, Nov 98:31-33, Jan 99:2, Oct 99:9; *CPT Changes: An Insider's View* 2004, 2008

▲ **90705**　Measles virus vaccine, live, for subcutaneous use

　　➜ *CPT Assistant* Apr 97:10, Nov 98:31-33, Jan 99:2, Oct 99:9; *CPT Changes: An Insider's View* 2004, 2008

▲ **90706**　Rubella virus vaccine, live, for subcutaneous use

　　➜ *CPT Assistant* Apr 97:10, Nov 98:31-33, Jan 99:2, Oct 99:9; *CPT Changes: An Insider's View* 2004, 2008

▲ **90707**　Measles, mumps and rubella virus vaccine (MMR), live, for subcutaneous use

　　➜ *CPT Assistant* Jan 96:6, May 96:10, Apr 97:10, Nov 98:31-33, Jan 99:2, Oct 99:9, Apr 05:1, 5; *CPT Changes: An Insider's View* 2004, 2008

▲ **90708**　Measles and rubella virus vaccine, live, for subcutaneous use

　　➜ *CPT Assistant* Apr 97:10, Nov 98:31-33, Jan 99:2, Oct 99:9; *CPT Changes: An Insider's View* 2004, 2008

▲ **90710**　Measles, mumps, rubella, and varicella vaccine (MMRV), live, for subcutaneous use

　　➜ *CPT Assistant* May 96:10, Apr 97:10, Nov 98:31-33, Jan 99:2, Oct 99:9, Dec 05:9, Jun 06:8; *CPT Changes: An Insider's View* 2008

▲ **90712**　Poliovirus vaccine, (any type[s]) (OPV), live, for oral use

　　➜ *CPT Assistant* Jan 96:6, Apr 97:10, Nov 98:31-33, Jan 99:2, Oct 99:9; *CPT Changes: An Insider's View* 2008

▲ **90713**　Poliovirus vaccine, inactivated (IPV), for subcutaneous or intramuscular use

　　➜ *CPT Assistant* Apr 97:10, Nov 98:31-33, Jan 99:2, Oct 99:9, Jun 05:6; *CPT Changes: An Insider's View* 2006, 2008

▲ **90714**　Tetanus and diphtheria toxoids (Td) adsorbed, preservative free, when administered to individuals 7 years or older, for intramuscular use

　　➜ *CPT Assistant* Jun 05:6; *CPT Changes: An Insider's View* 2006, 2007, 2008

▲ **90715**　Tetanus, diphtheria toxoids and acellular pertussis vaccine (Tdap), when administered to individuals 7 years or older, for intramuscular use

　　➜ *CPT Assistant* Oct 99:9, Jun 05:6, Dec 05:9, Jun 06:8; *CPT Changes: An Insider's View* 2006, 2007, 2008

▲ **90716**　Varicella virus vaccine, live, for subcutaneous use

　　➜ *CPT Assistant* Jan 96:6, May 96:10, Apr 97:10, Nov 98:31-33, Jan 99:2, Oct 99:9; *CPT Changes: An Insider's View* 2008

▲ **90717**　Yellow fever vaccine, live, for subcutaneous use

　　➜ *CPT Assistant* Apr 97:10, Nov 98:31-33, Jan 99:2, Oct 99:9; *CPT Changes: An Insider's View* 2008

▲ **90718**　Tetanus and diphtheria toxoids (Td) adsorbed when administered to individuals 7 years or older, for intramuscular use

　　➜ *CPT Assistant* Aug 96:10, Apr 97:10, Nov 98:31-33, Jan 99:2, Oct 99:9, Jun 00:10, Feb 07:11; *CPT Changes: An Insider's View* 2001, 2004, 2007, 2008

▲ **90719**　Diphtheria toxoid, for intramuscular use

　　➜ *CPT Assistant* Apr 97:10, Nov 98:31-33, Jan 99:2, Sep 99:10, Oct 99:9; *CPT Changes: An Insider's View* 2008

▲ **90720**　Diphtheria, tetanus toxoids, and whole cell pertussis vaccine and Hemophilus influenza B vaccine (DTP-Hib), for intramuscular use

　　➜ *CPT Assistant* Jan 96:5, Apr 97:10, Nov 98:31-33, Jan 99:2, Oct 99:9; *CPT Changes: An Insider's View* 2008

▲ **90721**   Diphtheria, tetanus toxoids, and acellular pertussis vaccine and Hemophilus influenza B vaccine (DtaP-Hib), for intramuscular use

➡ *CPT Assistant* Jan 96:5, Apr 97:10, Nov 98:31-33, Jan 99:2, Oct 99:9; *CPT Changes: An Insider's View* 2000, 2008

▲ **90723**   Diphtheria, tetanus toxoids, acellular pertussis vaccine, Hepatitis B, and poliovirus vaccine, inactivated (DtaP-HepB-IPV), for intramuscular use

➡ *CPT Assistant* Apr 97:10, Oct 99:9; *CPT Changes: An Insider's View* 2001, 2008

▲ **90725**   Cholera vaccine for injectable use

➡ *CPT Assistant* Apr 97:10, Nov 98:31-33, Jan 99:2, Oct 99:9; *CPT Changes: An Insider's View* 2008

▲ **90727**   Plague vaccine, for intramuscular use

➡ *CPT Assistant* Apr 97:10, Nov 98:31-33, Jan 99:2, Oct 99:9; *CPT Changes: An Insider's View* 2004, 2008

▲ **90732**   Pneumococcal polysaccharide vaccine, 23-valent, adult or immunosuppressed patient dosage, when administered to individuals 2 years or older, for subcutaneous or intramuscular use

➡ *CPT Assistant* Apr 97:10, Nov 98:31-33, Jan 99:2, Oct 99:9; *CPT Changes: An Insider's View* 2002, 2007, 2008

▲ **90733**   Meningococcal polysaccharide vaccine (any group(s)), for subcutaneous use

➡ *CPT Assistant* Apr 97:10, Nov 98:31-33, Jan 99:2, Oct 99:9, Dec 99:7; *CPT Changes: An Insider's View* 2001, 2004, 2008

▲ **90734**   Meningococcal conjugate vaccine, serogroups A, C, Y and W-135 (tetravalent), for intramuscular use

➡ *CPT Assistant* Oct 99:9; *CPT Changes: An Insider's View* 2008

▲ **90735**   Japanese encephalitis virus vaccine, for subcutaneous use

➡ *CPT Assistant* Apr 97:10, Nov 98:31-33, Jan 99:2, Oct 99:9; *CPT Changes: An Insider's View* 2008

▲ **90736**   Zoster (shingles) vaccine, live, for subcutaneous injection

➡ *CPT Assistant* Dec 05:9, Jun 06:8; *CPT Changes: An Insider's View* 2006, 2008

▲ **90740**   Hepatitis B vaccine, dialysis or immunosuppressed patient dosage (3 dose schedule), for intramuscular use

➡ *CPT Assistant* Apr 97:10, Oct 99:9, Apr 01:10; *CPT Changes: An Insider's View* 2001, 2008

▲ **90743**   Hepatitis B vaccine, adolescent (2 dose schedule), for intramuscular use

➡ *CPT Assistant* Apr 97:10, Oct 99:9; *CPT Changes: An Insider's View* 2001, 2008

▲ **90744**   Hepatitis B vaccine, pediatric/adolescent dosage (3 dose schedule), for intramuscular use

➡ *CPT Assistant* Jan 96:5, Apr 97:10, Jun 97:10, Nov 98:31-33, Jan 99:2, Oct 99:9, Nov 99:48-49, Jun 00:10; *CPT Changes: An Insider's View* 2000, 2001, 2008

▲ **90746**   Hepatitis B vaccine, adult dosage, for intramuscular use

➡ *CPT Assistant* Jan 96:5, Apr 97:10, Nov 98:31-33, Jan 99:2, Oct 99:9; *CPT Changes: An Insider's View* 2008

▲ **90747**   Hepatitis B vaccine, dialysis or immunosuppressed patient dosage (4 dose schedule), for intramuscular use

➡ *CPT Assistant* Jan 96:5, Apr 97:10, Jun 97:10, Nov 98:31-33, Jan 99:2, Oct 99:9, Jun 00:10, Apr 01:10; *CPT Changes: An Insider's View* 2001, 2008

▲ **90748**   Hepatitis B and Hemophilus influenza b vaccine (HepB-Hib), for intramuscular use

➡ *CPT Assistant* Apr 97:10, Nov 97:37, Nov 98:31-33, Jan 99:2, Sep 99:10, Oct 99:9; *CPT Changes: An Insider's View* 2008

▲ **90749**   Unlisted vaccine/toxoid

➡ *CPT Assistant* Jan 96:6, Apr 97:10, Jun 97:10, Nov 98:31-33, Jan 99:2, Oct 99:9, Nov 02:11; *CPT Changes: An Insider's View* 2008

Hydration, Therapeutic, Prophylactic, and Diagnostic Injections and Infusions (Excludes Chemotherapy)

▶Physician work related to hydration, injection, and infusion services predominantly involves affirmation of treatment plan and direct supervision of staff. These codes are not intended to be reported by the physician in the facility setting.

When these codes are reported *by the facility*, the following instructions apply. The initial code should be selected using a hierarchy whereby chemotherapy services are primary to therapeutic, prophylactic, and diagnostic services which are primary to hydration services. Infusions are primary to pushes, which are primary to injections. This hierarchy does not apply to physician reporting.◀

If a significant separately identifiable Evaluation and Management service is performed, the appropriate E/M service code should be reported using modifier 25 in addition to 90760-90779. For same day E/M service a different diagnosis is not required.

If performed to facilitate the infusion or injection, the following services are included and are not reported separately:

a. Use of local anesthesia

b. IV start

c. Access to indwelling IV, subcutaneous catheter or port

d. Flush at conclusion of infusion

e. Standard tubing, syringes, and supplies

▶(For declotting a catheter or port, see 36593)◀

When multiple drugs are administered, report the service(s) and the specific materials or drugs for each.

When administering multiple infusions, injections or combinations, only one "initial" service code should be reported, unless protocol requires that two separate IV sites must be used. The "initial" code that best describes the key or primary reason for the encounter should always be reported irrespective of the order in which the infusions or injections occur. If an injection or infusion is of a subsequent or concurrent nature, even if it is the first such service within that group of services, then a subsequent or concurrent code from the appropriate section should be reported (eg, the first IV push given subsequent to an initial one-hour infusion is reported using a subsequent IV push code).

When reporting codes for which infusion time is a factor, use the actual time over which the infusion is administered.

Hydration *can/list w/ chemo*

Codes 90760-90761 are intended to report a hydration IV infusion to consist of a pre-packaged fluid and electrolytes (eg, normal saline, D5-1/2 normal saline+30mEq KCl/liter), but are not used to report infusion of drugs or other substances. Hydration IV infusions typically require direct physician supervision for purposes of consent, safety oversight, or intraservice supervision of staff. Typically such infusions require little special handling to prepare or dispose of, and staff that administer these do not typically require advanced practice training. After initial set-up, infusion typically entails little patient risk and thus little monitoring.

▲ **90760** Intravenous infusion, hydration; initial, 31 minutes to 1 hour

➔ *CPT Assistant* Nov 05:1, Jul 06:4, Sep 06:14, Dec 06:14; *CPT Changes: An Insider's View* 2006, 2008

(Do not report 90760 if performed as a concurrent infusion service)

+ **90761** each additional hour (List separately in addition to code for primary procedure)

➔ *CPT Assistant* Nov 05:1, Jul 06:4, Sep 06:14, Dec 06:14, Mar 07:10; *CPT Changes: An Insider's View* 2006, 2007

(Use 90761 in conjunction with 90760)

(Report 90761 for hydration infusion intervals of greater than 30 minutes beyond 1 hour increments)

►(Report 90761 to identify hydration if provided as a secondary or subsequent service after a different initial service [90760, 90765, 90774, 96409, 96413] is administered through the same IV access)◄

►(Do not report intravenous infusion for hydration of 30 minutes or less)◄

Therapeutic, Prophylactic, and Diagnostic Injections and Infusions

A therapeutic, prophylactic, or diagnostic IV infusion or injection (90765-90779) (other than hydration) is for the administration of substances/drugs. When fluids are used to administer the drug(s), the administration of the fluid is considered incidental hydration and is not separately reportable. These services typically require direct physician supervision for any or all purposes of patient assessment, provision of consent, safety oversight, and intra-service supervision of staff. Typically, such infusions require special consideration to prepare, dose or dispose

of, require practice training and competency for staff who administer the infusions, and require periodic patient assessment with vital sign monitoring during the infusion.

Intravenous or intra-arterial push is defined as: a) an injection in which the health care professional who administers the substance/drug is continuously present to administer the injection and observe the patient, or b) an infusion of 15 minutes or less.

(Do not report 90765-90779 with codes for which IV push or infusion is an inherent part of the procedure (eg, administration of contrast material for a diagnostic imaging study))

90765 Intravenous infusion, for therapy, prophylaxis, or diagnosis (specify substance or drug); initial, up to 1 hour

➔ *CPT Assistant* Nov 05:1, Sep 06:14, Nov 06:22, Dec 06:14; *CPT Changes: An Insider's View* 2006

+ **90766** each additional hour (List separately in addition to code for primary procedure)

➔ *CPT Assistant* Nov 05:1, Sep 06:14, Dec 06:14, Mar 07:10; *CPT Changes: An Insider's View* 2006, 2007

(Report 90766 in conjunction with 90765, 90767)

(Report 90766 for additional hour(s) of sequential infusion)

(Report 90766 for infusion intervals of greater than 30 minutes beyond 1 hour increments)

+ **90767** additional sequential infusion, up to 1 hour (List separately in addition to code for primary procedure)

➔ *CPT Assistant* Nov 05:1, Sep 06:14, Nov 06:22, Dec 06:14; *CPT Changes: An Insider's View* 2006

►(Report 90767 in conjunction with 90765, 90774, 96409, 96413 if provided as a secondary or subsequent service after a different initial service is administered through the same IV access. Report 90767 only once per sequential infusion of same infusate mix)◄

+ **90768** concurrent infusion (List separately in addition to code for primary procedure)

➔ *CPT Assistant* Nov 05:1, Aug 06:11, Sep 06:14, Nov 06:22, Dec 06:14; *CPT Changes: An Insider's View* 2006

(Report 90768 only once per encounter)

►(Report 90768 in conjunction with 90765, 90766, 96413, 96415, 96416)◄

● **90769** Subcutaneous infusion for therapy or prophylaxis (specify substance or drug); initial, up to one hour, including pump set-up and establishment of subcutaneous infusion site(s)

➔ *CPT Changes: An Insider's View* 2008

►(For infusions of 15 minutes or less, use 90772)◄

+● **90770** each additional hour (List separately in addition to code for primary procedure)

➔ *CPT Changes: An Insider's View* 2008

►(Use 90770 in conjunction with 90769)◄

►(Use 90770 for infusion intervals of greater than 30 minutes beyond one hour increments)◄

+● **90771**   additional pump set-up with establishment of new subcutaneous infusion site(s) (List separately in addition to code for primary procedure)

→ *CPT Changes: An Insider's View* 2008

►(Use 90771 in conjunction with 90769)◄

►(Use 90769 and 90771 only once per encounter)◄

90772   Therapeutic, prophylactic or diagnostic injection (specify substance or drug); subcutaneous or intramuscular

→ *CPT Assistant* Nov 05:1, Sep 06:14, Dec 06:14; *CPT Changes: An Insider's View* 2006

(For administration of vaccines/toxoids, see 90465-90466, 90471-90472)

(Report 90772 for non-antineoplastic hormonal therapy injections)

(Report 96401 for anti-neoplastic nonhormonal injection therapy)

(Report 96402 for anti-neoplastic hormonal injection therapy)

►(Physicians do not report 90772 for injections given without direct physician supervision. To report, use 99211. Hospitals may report 90772 when the physician is not present)◄

(90772 does not include injections for allergen immunotherapy. For allergen immunotherapy injections, see 95115-95117)

90773   intra-arterial

→ *CPT Assistant* Nov 05:1, Sep 06:14, Dec 06:14; *CPT Changes: An Insider's View* 2006

90774   intravenous push, single or initial substance/drug

→ *CPT Assistant* Nov 05:1, Sep 06:14, Dec 06:14; *CPT Changes: An Insider's View* 2006

+ **90775**   each additional sequential intravenous push of a new substance/drug (List separately in addition to code for primary procedure)

→ *CPT Assistant* Nov 05:1, Sep 06:14, Dec 06:14; *CPT Changes: An Insider's View* 2006

(Use 90775 in conjunction with 90765, 90774, 96409, 96413)

►(Report 90775 to identify intravenous push of a new substance/drug if provided as a secondary or subsequent service after a different initial service is administered through the same IV access)◄

+● **90776**   each additional sequential intravenous push of the same substance/drug provided in a facility (List separately in addition to code for primary procedure)

→ *CPT Changes: An Insider's View* 2008

►(Do not report 90776 for a push performed within 30 minutes of a reported push of the same substance or drug)◄

►(90776 may be reported by facilities only)◄

90779   Unlisted therapeutic, prophylactic or diagnostic intravenous or intra-arterial injection or infusion

→ *CPT Assistant* Nov 05:1, Sep 06:14, Dec 06:14; *CPT Changes: An Insider's View* 2006

(For allergy immunizations, see 95004 et seq)

(90780 and 90781 have been deleted. To report, see 90760, 90761, 90765-90768)

(90782 has been deleted. To report, use 90772)

(90783 has been deleted. To report, use 90773)

(90784 has been deleted. To report, use 90774)

(90788 has been deleted. To report, use 90772)

(90799 has been deleted. To report, use 90779)

Psychiatry

Hospital care by the attending physician in treating a psychiatric inpatient or partial hospitalization may be initial or subsequent in nature (see 99221-99233) and may include exchanges with nursing and ancillary personnel. Hospital care services involve a variety of responsibilities unique to the medical management of inpatients, such as physician hospital orders, interpretation of laboratory or other medical diagnostic studies and observations.

Some patients receive hospital evaluation and management services only and others receive evaluation and management services and other procedures. If other procedures such as electroconvulsive therapy or psychotherapy are rendered in addition to hospital evaluation and management services, these should be listed separately (ie, hospital care service plus electroconvulsive therapy or when psychotherapy is done, an appropriate code defining psychotherapy with medical evaluation and management services). Modifier 22 may be used to indicate a more extensive service. Modifier 52 may be used to signify a service that is reduced or less extensive than the usual procedure.

Other evaluation and management services, such as office medical service or other patient encounters, may be described as listed in the section on **Evaluation and Management,** if appropriate.

The evaluation and management services should not be reported separately, when reporting codes 90805, 90807, 90809, 90811, 90813, 90815, 90817, 90819, 90822, 90824, 90827, 90829.

Consultation for psychiatric evaluation of a patient includes examination of a patient and exchange of information with the primary physician and other informants such as nurses or family members, and preparation of a report. These consultation services (99241-99255) are limited to initial or follow-up evaluation and do not involve psychiatric treatment.

→ *CPT Assistant* Nov 97:37

Psychiatric Diagnostic or Evaluative Interview Procedures

Psychiatric diagnostic interview examination includes a history, mental status, and a disposition, and may include communication with family or other sources, ordering and medical interpretation of laboratory or other medical diagnostic studies. In certain circumstances other informants will be seen in lieu of the patient.

Interactive psychiatric diagnostic interview examination is typically furnished to children. It involves the use of physical aids and non-verbal communication to overcome barriers to therapeutic interaction between the clinician and a patient who has not yet developed, or has lost, either the expressive language communication skills to explain his/her symptoms and response to treatment, or the receptive communication skills to understand the clinician if he/she were to use ordinary adult language for communication.

➔ *CPT Assistant* Nov 97:37-38

90801   Psychiatric diagnostic interview examination
➔ *CPT Assistant* Summer 92:12, Nov 97:39-40, Mar 01:5, Mar 02:4, May 05:1

90802   Interactive psychiatric diagnostic interview examination using play equipment, physical devices, language interpreter, or other mechanisms of communication
➔ *CPT Assistant* Nov 97:39-40, Mar 01:5, Mar 02:4, May 05:1

Psychiatric Therapeutic Procedures

Psychotherapy is the treatment for mental illness and behavioral disturbances in which the clinician establishes a professional contract with the patient and, through definitive therapeutic communication, attempts to alleviate the emotional disturbances, reverse or change maladaptive patterns of behavior, and encourage personality growth and development. The codes for reporting psychotherapy are divided into two broad categories: Interactive Psychotherapy; and Insight Oriented, Behavior Modifying and/or Supportive Psychotherapy.

Interactive psychotherapy is typically furnished to children. It involves the use of physical aids and non-verbal communication to overcome barriers to therapeutic interaction between the clinician and a patient who has not yet developed, or has lost, either the expressive language communication skills to explain his/her symptoms and response to treatment, or the receptive communication skills to understand the clinician if he/she were to use ordinary adult language for communication.

Insight oriented, behavior modifying and/or supportive psychotherapy refers to the development of insight or affective understanding, the use of behavior modification techniques, the use of supportive interactions, the use of cognitive discussion of reality, or any combination of the above to provide therapeutic change.

Some patients receive psychotherapy only and others receive psychotherapy and medical evaluation and management services. These evaluation and management services involve a variety of responsibilities unique to the medical management of psychiatric patients, such as medical diagnostic evaluation (eg, evaluation of comorbid medical conditions, drug interactions, and physical examinations), drug management when indicated, physician orders, interpretation of laboratory or other medical diagnostic studies and observations.

In reporting psychotherapy, the appropriate code is chosen on the basis of the type of psychotherapy (interactive using non-verbal techniques versus insight oriented, behavior modifying and/or supportive using verbal techniques), the place of service (office versus inpatient), the face-to-face time spent with the patient during psychotherapy, and whether evaluation and management services are furnished on the same date of service as psychotherapy.

To report medical evaluation and management services furnished on a day when psychotherapy is not provided, select the appropriate code from the **Evaluation and Management Services Guidelines.**

➔ *CPT Assistant* Nov 97:38

Office or Other Outpatient Facility

Insight Oriented, Behavior Modifying and/or Supportive Psychotherapy

90804   Individual psychotherapy, insight oriented, behavior modifying and/or supportive, in an office or outpatient facility, approximately 20 to 30 minutes face-to-face with the patient;
➔ *CPT Assistant* Nov 97:39, Jul 99:10, Mar 01:5, Mar 02:4, Oct 02:11, May 05:1

90805   with medical evaluation and management services
➔ *CPT Assistant* Nov 97:39, Jul 99:10, Mar 01:5, Mar 02:4, May 05:1

90806   Individual psychotherapy, insight oriented, behavior modifying and/or supportive, in an office or outpatient facility, approximately 45 to 50 minutes face-to-face with the patient;
➔ *CPT Assistant* Nov 97:39, Jul 99:10, Mar 01:6, Mar 02:4, Sep 03:3, Sep 04:13, Mar 05:16, May 05:1

90807   with medical evaluation and management services
➔ *CPT Assistant* Nov 97:39, Jul 99:10, Mar 01:6, May 05:1

90808   Individual psychotherapy, insight oriented, behavior modifying and/or supportive, in an office or outpatient facility, approximately 75 to 80 minutes face-to-face with the patient;
➔ *CPT Assistant* Nov 97:39, Jul 99:10, Mar 01:5, Mar 02:4, May 05:1

90809   with medical evaluation and management services
➔ *CPT Assistant* Nov 97:39, Jul 99:10, Mar 01:5, May 05:1

Interactive Psychotherapy

90810 Individual psychotherapy, interactive, using play equipment, physical devices, language interpreter, or other mechanisms of non-verbal communication, in an office or outpatient facility, approximately 20 to 30 minutes face-to-face with the patient;
➔ *CPT Assistant* Nov 97:39, Mar 01:5, Mar 02:4, May 05:1

90811 with medical evaluation and management services
➔ *CPT Assistant* Nov 97:39, Mar 01:5, May 05:1

90812 Individual psychotherapy, interactive, using play equipment, physical devices, language interpreter, or other mechanisms of non-verbal communication, in an office or outpatient facility, approximately 45 to 50 minutes face-to-face with the patient;
➔ *CPT Assistant* Nov 97:39, Mar 01:5, Mar 02:4, May 05:1

90813 with medical evaluation and management services
➔ *CPT Assistant* Nov 97:39, Mar 01:5, Mar 02:4, May 05:1

90814 Individual psychotherapy, interactive, using play equipment, physical devices, language interpreter, or other mechanisms of non-verbal communication, in an office or outpatient facility, approximately 75 to 80 minutes face-to-face with the patient;
➔ *CPT Assistant* Nov 97:39, Mar 01:5, Mar 02:4, May 05:1

90815 with medical evaluation and management services
➔ *CPT Assistant* Nov 97:39, Mar 01:5, Mar 02:4, May 05:1

Inpatient Hospital, Partial Hospital or Residential Care Facility

Insight Oriented, Behavior Modifying and/or Supportive Psychotherapy

90816 Individual psychotherapy, insight oriented, behavior modifying and/or supportive, in an inpatient hospital, partial hospital or residential care setting, approximately 20 to 30 minutes face-to-face with the patient;
➔ *CPT Assistant* Nov 97:39-40, Mar 01:6-7, Mar 02:4, May 05:1

90817 with medical evaluation and management services
➔ *CPT Assistant* Nov 97:39-40, Mar 01:6-7, Mar 02:4, May 05:1

90818 Individual psychotherapy, insight oriented, behavior modifying and/or supportive, in an inpatient hospital, partial hospital or residential care setting, approximately 45 to 50 minutes face-to-face with the patient;
➔ *CPT Assistant* Nov 97:39-40, Mar 01:6-7, Mar 02:4, May 05:1

90819 with medical evaluation and management services
➔ *CPT Assistant* Summer 92:24, Nov 97:39-40, Mar 01:6-7, Mar 02:4, May 05:1

90821 Individual psychotherapy, insight oriented, behavior modifying and/or supportive, in an inpatient hospital, partial hospital or residential care setting, approximately 75 to 80 minutes face-to-face with the patient;
➔ *CPT Assistant* Nov 97:39-40, Mar 01:6-7, Mar 02:4, May 05:1

90822 with medical evaluation and management services
➔ *CPT Assistant* Nov 97:39-40, Mar 01:6-7, Mar 02:4, May 05:1

Interactive Psychotherapy

90823 Individual psychotherapy, interactive, using play equipment, physical devices, language interpreter, or other mechanisms of non-verbal communication, in an inpatient hospital, partial hospital or residential care setting, approximately 20 to 30 minutes face-to-face with the patient;
➔ *CPT Assistant* Nov 97:40, Mar 01:6-7, Mar 02:4, May 05:1

90824 with medical evaluation and management services
➔ *CPT Assistant* Nov 97:40, Mar 01:6-7, Mar 02:4, May 05:1

90826 Individual psychotherapy, interactive, using play equipment, physical devices, language interpreter, or other mechanisms of non-verbal communication, in an inpatient hospital, partial hospital or residential care setting, approximately 45 to 50 minutes face-to-face with the patient;
➔ *CPT Assistant* Nov 97:40, Mar 01:6-7, Mar 02:4, May 05:1

90827 with medical evaluation and management services
➔ *CPT Assistant* Nov 97:40, Mar 01:6-7, Mar 02:4, May 05:1

90828 Individual psychotherapy, interactive, using play equipment, physical devices, language interpreter, or other mechanisms of non-verbal communication, in an inpatient hospital, partial hospital or residential care setting, approximately 75 to 80 minutes face-to-face with the patient;
➔ *CPT Assistant* Nov 97:40, Mar 01:6-7, Mar 02:4, May 05:1

90829 with medical evaluation and management services
➔ *CPT Assistant* Summer 92:13, Nov 97:40, Mar 01:6-7, Mar 02:4, May 05:1

Other Psychotherapy

90845 Psychoanalysis
➔ *CPT Assistant* Summer 92:15, Nov 97:40-41, Mar 01:8, Mar 02:4, May 05:1, Feb 06:15

90846 Family psychotherapy (without the patient present)
➔ *CPT Assistant* Summer 92:15, Nov 97:40-41, Mar 01:8, Mar 02:4, May 05:1

90847 Family psychotherapy (conjoint psychotherapy) (with patient present)
➔ *CPT Assistant* Summer 92:15, Nov 97:40-41, Mar 01:5, Mar 02:4, May 05:1

90849 Multiple-family group psychotherapy
➔ *CPT Assistant* Summer 92:15, Nov 97:40-41, Mar 01:5, Mar 02:4, May 05:1

90853 Group psychotherapy (other than of a multiple-family group)
➔ *CPT Assistant* Summer 92:15, Nov 97:40-41, Mar 01:8, Mar 02:4, May 05:1

90857 Interactive group psychotherapy
➔ *CPT Assistant* Summer 92:15, Nov 97:40-41, Mar 01:8, Mar 02:4, May 05:1

Other Psychiatric Services or Procedures

(For repetitive transcranial magnetic stimulation for treatment of clinical depression, see Category III codes 0160T, 0161T)

►(For analysis/programming of neurostimulators used for vagus nerve stimulation therapy, see 95970, 95974, 95975)◄

90862 Pharmacologic management, including prescription, use, and review of medication with no more than minimal medical psychotherapy

⊃ *CPT Assistant* Summer 92:16, Nov 97:40-41, Mar 01:5, Mar 02:4, May 05:1, Dec 06:10

90865 Narcosynthesis for psychiatric diagnostic and therapeutic purposes (eg, sodium amobarbital (Amytal) interview)

⊃ *CPT Assistant* Nov 97:41, Mar 01:5, Mar 02:4, May 05:1

90870 Electroconvulsive therapy (includes necessary monitoring)

⊃ *CPT Assistant* Summer 92:16, Mar 01:5, Mar 02:4, May 05:1; *CPT Changes: An Insider's View* 2006

(90871 has been deleted)

90875 Individual psychophysiological therapy incorporating biofeedback training by any modality (face-to-face with the patient), with psychotherapy (eg, insight oriented, behavior modifying or supportive psychotherapy); approximately 20-30 minutes

⊃ *CPT Assistant* Nov 96:15, Sep 97:11, Nov 97:41, Apr 98:14, Jun 99:5, Mar 01:5, Mar 02:4, Mar 05:16, May 05:1

90876 approximately 45-50 minutes

⊃ *CPT Assistant* Nov 96:15, Sep 97:11, Nov 97:41, Jun 99:5, Mar 01:5, Mar 05:16, May 05:1

90880 Hypnotherapy

⊃ *CPT Assistant* Summer 92:16, Nov 97:41, Mar 01:5, Mar 02:4, May 05:1

90882 Environmental intervention for medical management purposes on a psychiatric patient's behalf with agencies, employers, or institutions

⊃ *CPT Assistant* Summer 92:16, Mar 01:5, Mar 02:4, May 05:1

90885 Psychiatric evaluation of hospital records, other psychiatric reports, psychometric and/or projective tests, and other accumulated data for medical diagnostic purposes

⊃ *CPT Assistant* Nov 97:41, Mar 01:5, Mar 02:4, Oct 04:10, May 05:1

90887 Interpretation or explanation of results of psychiatric, other medical examinations and procedures, or other accumulated data to family or other responsible persons, or advising them how to assist patient

⊃ *CPT Assistant* Summer 92:17, Mar 01:5, Mar 02:4, Oct 02:11, May 05:1

90889 Preparation of report of patient's psychiatric status, history, treatment, or progress (other than for legal or consultative purposes) for other physicians, agencies, or insurance carriers

⊃ *CPT Assistant* Summer 92:17, Mar 01:5, Mar 02:4, May 05:1

90899 Unlisted psychiatric service or procedure

⊃ *CPT Assistant* Mar 01:5, Mar 02:4, May 05:1

Biofeedback

(For psychophysiological therapy incorporating biofeedback training, see 90875, 90876)

90901 Biofeedback training by any modality

⊃ *CPT Assistant* Sep 97:11, Apr 98:14, Jun 98:10, Jun 99:5, May 02:18, Sep 04:13, Mar 05:16

90911 Biofeedback training, perineal muscles, anorectal or urethral sphincter, including EMG and/or manometry

⊃ *CPT Assistant* Sep 97:11, Nov 97:41, Jun 98:10, Jun 99:5

(For incontinence treatment by pulsed magnetic neuromodulation, use Category III code 0029T)

(For testing of rectal sensation, tone and compliance, use 91120)

Dialysis

Codes 90918-90921 are reported ONCE per month to distinguish age-specific services related to the patient's end-stage renal disease (ESRD) performed in an outpatient setting. ESRD-related physician services include establishment of a dialyzing cycle, outpatient evaluation and management of the dialysis visits, telephone calls, and patient management during the dialysis, provided during a full month. These codes are not used if the physician also submits hospitalization codes during the month.

Codes 90918-90921 describe a full month of ESRD-related services provided in an outpatient setting. For ESRD and non-ESRD dialysis services performed in an inpatient setting, and for non-ESRD dialysis services performed in an outpatient setting, see 90935-90937 and 90945-90947.

Evaluation and management services unrelated to ESRD services that cannot be performed during the dialysis session may be reported separately.

Codes 90922-90925 are reported when outpatient ESRD-related services are not performed consecutively during an entire full month (eg, when the patient spends part of the month as a hospital inpatient, or when the outpatient ESRD-related services are initiated after the first of the month). The appropriate age-related code from this series (90922-90925) is reported daily less the days of hospitalization. For reporting purposes, each month is considered 30 days.

Example:

Outpatient ESRD-related services are initiated on July 1 for a 57-year-old male. On July 11, he is admitted to the hospital as an inpatient and is discharged on July 27.

In this example, code 90925 should be reported for each day outside of the inpatient hospitalization (30 days/month less 17 days/hospitalization = 13 days). Report inpatient E/M services as appropriate. Dialysis procedures rendered during the hospitalization (July 11-27) should be reported as appropriate (90935-90937, 90945-90947).

End-Stage Renal Disease Services

90918 End-stage renal disease (ESRD) related services per full month; for patients younger than two years of age to include monitoring for the adequacy of nutrition, assessment of growth and development, and counseling of parents

→ *CPT Assistant* Fall 93:5, May 96:4, May 02:17, Jan 03:22

90919 for patients between two and eleven years of age to include monitoring for the adequacy of nutrition, assessment of growth and development, and counseling of parents

→ *CPT Assistant* Fall 93:5, May 96:5, May 02:17, Jan 03:22

90920 for patients between twelve and nineteen years of age to include monitoring for the adequacy of nutrition, assessment of growth and development, and counseling of parents

→ *CPT Assistant* Fall 93:5, May 96:5, May 02:17, Jan 03:22

90921 for patients twenty years of age and older

→ *CPT Assistant* Fall 93:5, May 96:5, May 02:17, Jan 03:22

90922 End-stage renal disease (ESRD) related services (less than full month), per day; for patients younger than two years of age

→ *CPT Assistant* Fall 93:5, May 96:5, May 02:17, Jan 03:22

90923 for patients between two and eleven years of age

→ *CPT Assistant* May 96:5, May 02:17, Jan 03:22

90924 for patients between twelve and nineteen years of age

→ *CPT Assistant* May 96:5, May 02:17, Jan 03:22

90925 for patients twenty years of age and older

→ *CPT Assistant* May 96:5, May 02:17, Jan 03:22

Hemodialysis

Codes 90935, 90937 are reported to describe the hemodialysis procedure with all evaluation and management services related to the patient's renal disease on the day of the hemodialysis procedure. These codes are used for inpatient ESRD and non-ESRD procedures or for outpatient non-ESRD dialysis services. Code 90935 is reported if only one evaluation of the patient is required related to that hemodialysis procedure. Code 90937 is reported when patient re-evaluation(s) is required during a hemodialysis procedure. Use modifier 25 with Evaluation and Management codes for separately identifiable services unrelated to the dialysis procedure or renal failure which cannot be rendered during the dialysis session.

(For home visit hemodialysis services performed by a non-physician health care professional, use 99512)

(For cannula declotting, see 36831, 36833, 36860, 36861)

▶(For declotting of implanted vascular access device or catheter by thrombolytic agent, use 36593)◀

→ *CPT Assistant* Nov 99:49

▶(For collection of blood specimen from a partially or completely implantable venous access device, use 36591)◀

(For prolonged physician attendance, see 99354-99360)

90935 Hemodialysis procedure with single physician evaluation

→ *CPT Assistant* Fall 93:2, May 02:17, Jan 03:22

90937 Hemodialysis procedure requiring repeated evaluation(s) with or without substantial revision of dialysis prescription

→ *CPT Assistant* Fall 93:2, May 02:17, Jan 03:22

(90939 has been deleted. To report, use 90940)

90940 Hemodialysis access flow study to determine blood flow in grafts and arteriovenous fistulae by an indicator method

→ *CPT Assistant* Jan 03:22, May 06:18; *CPT Changes: An Insider's View* 2001, 2006

→ *Clinical Examples in Radiology* Summer 06:7, 12

(For duplex scan of hemodialysis access, use 93990)

Miscellaneous Dialysis Procedures

Codes 90945, 90947 describe dialysis procedures other than hemodialysis (eg, peritoneal dialysis, hemofiltration or continuous renal replacement therapies), and all evaluation and management services related to the patient's renal disease on the day of the procedure. Code 90945 is reported if only one evaluation of the patient is required related to that procedure. Code 90947 is reported when patient re-evaluation(s) is required during a procedure. Utilize modifier 25 with Evaluation and Management codes for separately identifiable services unrelated to the procedure or the renal failure which cannot be rendered during the dialysis session.

(For insertion of intraperitoneal cannula or catheter, see 49420, 49421)

(For prolonged physician attendance, see 99354-99360)

90945 Dialysis procedure other than hemodialysis (eg, peritoneal dialysis, hemofiltration, or other continuous renal replacement therapies), with single physician evaluation

→ *CPT Assistant* Fall 93:2, Nov 97:41, Jul 98:10, Oct 01:11, Jan 03:22; *CPT Changes: An Insider's View* 2001

(For home infusion of peritoneal dialysis, use 99601, 99602)

90947 Dialysis procedure other than hemodialysis (eg, peritoneal dialysis, hemofiltration, or other continuous renal replacement therapies) requiring repeated physician evaluations, with or without substantial revision of dialysis prescription

> *CPT Assistant* Fall 93:2, Nov 97:41, Jul 98:10, Oct 01:11, Jan 03:22; *CPT Changes: An Insider's View* 2001

90989 Dialysis training, patient, including helper where applicable, any mode, completed course

> *CPT Assistant* Fall 93:5, Jun 01:10

90993 Dialysis training, patient, including helper where applicable, any mode, course not completed, per training session

> *CPT Assistant* Winter 90:11, Fall 93:5, Jun 01:10

90997 Hemoperfusion (eg, with activated charcoal or resin)

90999 Unlisted dialysis procedure, inpatient or outpatient

Gastroenterology

(For duodenal intubation and aspiration, see 89100-89105)

(For gastrointestinal radiologic procedures, see 74210-74363)

(For esophagoscopy procedures, see 43200-43228; upper GI endoscopy 43234-43259; endoscopy, small intestine and stomal 44360-44393; proctosigmoidoscopy 45300-45321; sigmoidoscopy 45330-45339; colonoscopy 45355-45385; anoscopy 46600-46615)

91000 Esophageal intubation and collection of washings for cytology, including preparation of specimens (separate procedure)

91010 Esophageal motility (manometric study of the esophagus and/or gastroesophageal junction) study;

> *CPT Assistant* Nov 97:42

91011 with mecholyl or similar stimulant

91012 with acid perfusion studies

91020 Gastric motility (manometric) studies

> *CPT Assistant* Nov 97:42

91022 Duodenal motility (manometric) study

> *CPT Changes: An Insider's View* 2006

(If gastrointestinal endoscopy is performed, use 43235)

(If fluoroscopy is performed, use 76000)

(If gastric motility study is performed, use 91020)

91030 Esophagus, acid perfusion (Bernstein) test for esophagitis

91034 Esophagus, gastroesophageal reflux test; with nasal catheter pH electrode(s) placement, recording, analysis and interpretation

> *CPT Assistant* May 05:3; *CPT Changes: An Insider's View* 2005

Esophageal Acid Reflux Test
91034

A catheter with a pH electrode is placed into the esophagus, either through the nares or swallowed, to measure intraesophageal pH (an indicator of gastric reflux).

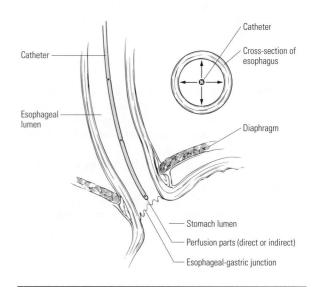

91035 with mucosal attached telemetry pH electrode placement, recording, analysis and interpretation

> *CPT Assistant* May 05:3; *CPT Changes: An Insider's View* 2005

91037 Esophageal function test, gastroesophageal reflux test with nasal catheter intraluminal impedance electrode(s) placement, recording, analysis and interpretation;

> *CPT Assistant* May 05:3; *CPT Changes: An Insider's View* 2005

91038 prolonged (greater than 1 hour, up to 24 hours)

> *CPT Assistant* May 05:3; *CPT Changes: An Insider's View* 2005

91040 Esophageal balloon distension provocation study

> *CPT Assistant* May 05:3; *CPT Changes: An Insider's View* 2005

(For balloon dilatation with endoscopy, see 43220, 43249, 43456, or 43458)

91052 Gastric analysis test with injection of stimulant of gastric secretion (eg, histamine, insulin, pentagastrin, calcium and secretin)

(For gastric biopsy by capsule, peroral, via tube, one or more specimens, use 43600)

(For gastric laboratory procedures, see also 89130-89141)

91055 Gastric intubation, washings, and preparing slides for cytology (separate procedure)

(For gastric lavage, therapeutic, use 91105)

(91060 has been deleted)

(For biopsy by capsule, small intestine, per oral, via tube [one or more specimens], use 44100)

91065 Breath hydrogen test (eg, for detection of lactase deficiency, fructose intolerance, bacterial overgrowth, or oro-cecal gastrointestinal transit)

➜ *CPT Assistant* May 05:3; *CPT Changes: An Insider's View* 2005

(For H. pylori breath test analysis, use 83013 for non-radioactive (C-13) isotope or 78268 for radioactive (C-14) isotope)

91100 Intestinal bleeding tube, passage, positioning and monitoring

91105 Gastric intubation, and aspiration or lavage for treatment (eg, for ingested poisons)

➜ *CPT Assistant* Winter 91:7, Spring 93:34, Sep 96:10, Nov 99:49, Aug 00:2, Feb 07:10

Gastric Intubation
91105

A large-bore gastric lavage tube is inserted orally through the esophagus into the stomach for expedient lavage and evacuation of stomach contents (eg, poisonings, hemorrhage).

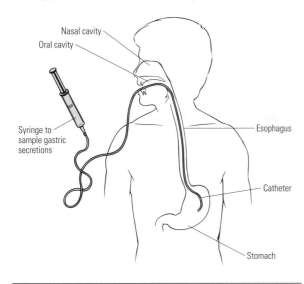

Nasal cavity
Oral cavity
Syringe to sample gastric secretions
Esophagus
Catheter
Stomach

(For cholangiography, see 47500, 74320)

(For abdominal paracentesis, see 49080, 49081; with instillation of medication, see 96440, 96445)

(For peritoneoscopy, use 49320; with biopsy, use 49321)

(For peritoneoscopy and guided transhepatic cholangiography, use 47560; with biopsy, use 47561)

(For splenoportography, see 38200, 75810)

91110 Gastrointestinal tract imaging, intraluminal (eg, capsule endoscopy), esophagus through ileum, with physician interpretation and report

➜ *CPT Assistant* Oct 04:15, Aug 05:14; *CPT Changes: An Insider's View* 2004

(Visualization of the colon is not reported separately)

(Append modifier 52 if the ileum is not visualized)

91111 Gastrointestinal tract imaging, intraluminal (eg, capsule endoscopy), esophagus with physician interpretation and report

➜ *CPT Changes: An Insider's View* 2007

(Do not report 91111 in conjunction with 91110)

91120 Rectal sensation, tone, and compliance test (ie, response to graded balloon distention)

➜ *CPT Assistant* May 05:3; *CPT Changes: An Insider's View* 2005

(For biofeedback training, use 90911)

(For anorectal manometry, use 91122)

91122 Anorectal manometry

91123 Pulsed irrigation of fecal impaction

➜ *CPT Changes: An Insider's View* 2002

Gastric Physiology

91132 Electrogastrography, diagnostic, transcutaneous;

➜ *CPT Changes: An Insider's View* 2001

91133 with provocative testing

➜ *CPT Changes: An Insider's View* 2001

Other Procedures

91299 Unlisted diagnostic gastroenterology procedure

➜ *CPT Assistant* Aug 05:14

Ophthalmology

(For surgical procedures, see **Surgery,** Eye and Ocular Adnexa, 65091 et seq)

Definitions

Intermediate ophthalmological services describes an evaluation of a new or existing condition complicated with a new diagnostic or management problem not necessarily relating to the primary diagnosis, including history, general medical observation, external ocular and adnexal examination and other diagnostic procedures as indicated; may include the use of mydriasis for ophthalmoscopy.

For example:

a. Review of history, external examination, ophthalmoscopy, biomicroscopy for an acute complicated condition (eg, iritis) not requiring comprehensive ophthalmological services.

b. Review of interval history, external examination, ophthalmoscopy, biomicroscopy and tonometry in established patient with known cataract not requiring comprehensive ophthalmological services.

Comprehensive ophthalmological services describes a general evaluation of the complete visual system. The comprehensive services constitute a single service entity but need not be performed at one session. The service includes history, general medical observation, external

---

and ophthalmoscopic examinations, gross visual fields and basic sensorimotor examination. It often includes, as indicated: biomicroscopy, examination with cycloplegia or mydriasis and tonometry. It always includes initiation of diagnostic and treatment programs.

Intermediate and comprehensive ophthalmological services constitute integrated services in which medical decision making cannot be separated from the examining techniques used. Itemization of service components, such as slit lamp examination, keratometry, routine ophthalmoscopy, retinoscopy, tonometry, or motor evaluation is not applicable.

For example:

The comprehensive services required for diagnosis and treatment of a patient with symptoms indicating possible disease of the visual system, such as glaucoma, cataract or retinal disease, or to rule out disease of the visual system, new or established patient.

Initiation of diagnostic and treatment program includes the prescription of medication, and arranging for special ophthalmological diagnostic or treatment services, consultations, laboratory procedures and radiological services.

Special ophthalmological services describes services in which a special evaluation of part of the visual system is made, which goes beyond the services included under general ophthalmological services, or in which special treatment is given. Special ophthalmological services may be reported in addition to the general ophthalmological services or evaluation and management services.

For example:

Fluorescein angioscopy, quantitative visual field examination, refraction or extended color vision examination (such as Nagel's anomaloscope) should be separately reported.

Prescription of lenses, when required, is included in 92015. It includes specification of lens type (monofocal, bifocal, other), lens power, axis, prism, absorptive factor, impact resistance, and other factors.

Interpretation and report by the physician is an integral part of special ophthalmological services where indicated. Technical procedures (which may or may not be performed by the physician personally) are often part of the service, but should not be mistaken to constitute the service itself.

➔ *CPT Assistant* Nov 97:42-43

General Ophthalmological Services

New Patient

Solely for the purposes of distinguishing between new and established patients, **professional services** are those face-to-face services rendered by a physician and reported by a specific code(s). A new patient is one who has not

received any professional services from the physician or another physician of the same specialty who belongs to the same group practice within the past three years.

92002 Ophthalmological services: medical examination and evaluation with initiation of diagnostic and treatment program; intermediate, new patient
➔ *CPT Assistant* Feb 97:6, Aug 98:3, Jun 05:11, Dec 05:10, Jan 07:30

92004 comprehensive, new patient, one or more visits
➔ *CPT Assistant* Feb 97:6, Aug 98:3, Jun 05:11, Dec 05:10, Jan 07:30

Established Patient

Solely for the purposes of distinguishing between new and established patients, **professional services** are those face-to-face services rendered by a physician and reported by a specific code(s). An established patient is one who has received professional services from the physician or another physician of the same specialty who belongs to the same group practice within the past three years.

92012 Ophthalmological services: medical examination and evaluation, with initiation or continuation of diagnostic and treatment program; intermediate, established patient
➔ *CPT Assistant* Feb 97:6, Aug 98:3, Jun 05:11, Dec 05:10, Jan 07:30

92014 comprehensive, established patient, one or more visits
➔ *CPT Assistant* Feb 97:6, Aug 98:3, Dec 99:10, Jun 05:11, Dec 05:10, Jan 07:30

(For surgical procedures, see **Surgery,** Eye and Ocular Adnexa, 65091 et seq)

Special Ophthalmological Services

92015 Determination of refractive state
➔ *CPT Assistant* Mar 96:11, Feb 97:6, Aug 98:3, Aug 06:11

92018 Ophthalmological examination and evaluation, under general anesthesia, with or without manipulation of globe for passive range of motion or other manipulation to facilitate diagnostic examination; complete
➔ *CPT Assistant* Feb 97:6, Aug 98:3

92019 limited
➔ *CPT Assistant* Feb 97:6, Aug 98:3

92020 Gonioscopy (separate procedure)
➔ *CPT Assistant* Feb 97:6, Aug 98:3

(For gonioscopy under general anesthesia, use 92018)

92025 Computerized corneal topography, unilateral or bilateral, with interpretation and report
➔ *CPT Changes: An Insider's View* 2007

(Do not report 92025 in conjunction with 65710-65755)

(92025 is not used for manual keratoscopy, which is part of a single system Evaluation and Management or ophthalmological service)

92060   Sensorimotor examination with multiple measurements of ocular deviation (eg, restrictive or paretic muscle with diplopia) with interpretation and report (separate procedure)
> *CPT Assistant* Feb 97:6, Aug 98:3

92065   Orthoptic and/or pleoptic training, with continuing medical direction and evaluation
> *CPT Assistant* Feb 97:6, Jun 98:10, Aug 98:3

92070   Fitting of contact lens for treatment of disease, including supply of lens
> *CPT Assistant* Feb 97:6, Aug 98:3

92081   Visual field examination, unilateral or bilateral, with interpretation and report; limited examination (eg, tangent screen, Autoplot, arc perimeter, or single stimulus level automated test, such as Octopus 3 or 7 equivalent)
> *CPT Assistant* Feb 97:6, Aug 98:3

92082   intermediate examination (eg, at least 2 isopters on Goldmann perimeter, or semiquantitative, automated suprathreshold screening program, Humphrey suprathreshold automatic diagnostic test, Octopus program 33)
> *CPT Assistant* Feb 97:6, Aug 98:3

92083   extended examination (eg, Goldmann visual fields with at least 3 isopters plotted and static determination within the central 30°, or quantitative, automated threshold perimetry, Octopus program G-1, 32 or 42, Humphrey visual field analyzer full threshold programs 30-2, 24-2, or 30/60-2)
> *CPT Assistant* Feb 97:6, Aug 98:3

(Gross visual field testing (eg, confrontation testing) is a part of general ophthalmological services and is not reported separately)

92100   Serial tonometry (separate procedure) with multiple measurements of intraocular pressure over an extended time period with interpretation and report, same day (eg, diurnal curve or medical treatment of acute elevation of intraocular pressure)
> *CPT Assistant* Feb 97:6, Jun 98:10, Aug 98:3

92120   Tonography with interpretation and report, recording indentation tonometer method or perilimbal suction method
> *CPT Assistant* Feb 97:6, Aug 98:3

92130   Tonography with water provocation
> *CPT Assistant* Feb 97:6, Aug 98:3

▲ **92135**   Scanning computerized ophthalmic diagnostic imaging, posterior segment, (eg, scanning laser) with interpretation and report, unilateral
> *CPT Assistant* Aug 98:3, Nov 98:33, Mar 99:10, Apr 99:10; *CPT Changes: An Insider's View* 2008

92136   Ophthalmic biometry by partial coherence interferometry with intraocular lens power calculation
> *CPT Assistant* Aug 98:3, Apr 02:18; *CPT Changes: An Insider's View* 2002

92140   Provocative tests for glaucoma, with interpretation and report, without tonography
> *CPT Assistant* Feb 97:6, Aug 98:3

Ophthalmoscopy

Routine ophthalmoscopy is part of general and special ophthalmologic services whenever indicated. It is a non-itemized service and is not reported separately.

92225   Ophthalmoscopy, extended, with retinal drawing (eg, for retinal detachment, melanoma), with interpretation and report; initial
> *CPT Assistant* Feb 97:6, Aug 98:2, Dec 99:10

Extended Ophthalmoscopy
92225, 92226

Illustration of retinal structures to document for comparison with future examinations

Indirect ophthalmoscope

Indirect lens

Optic disc

Fovea

Vein

Artery

Ophthalmoscopic appearance of retina

92226   subsequent
> *CPT Assistant* Feb 97:6, Aug 98:2

92230 Fluorescein angioscopy with interpretation and report
➔ *CPT Assistant* Feb 97:6

92235 Fluorescein angiography (includes multiframe imaging) with interpretation and report
➔ *CPT Assistant* Feb 97:6

Fluorescein Angiography
92235

Fluorescein dye is injected in a peripheral vein to enhance imaging. Serial multiframe angiography is performed to evaluate choroidal and retinal circulation. In this illustration, arteries display an even fluorescence, while veins appear striped from the laminar dye flow.

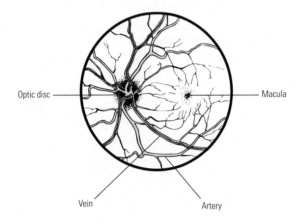

92240 Indocyanine-green angiography (includes multiframe imaging) with interpretation and report

92250 Fundus photography with interpretation and report
➔ *CPT Assistant* Feb 97:6, Apr 99:10

92260 Ophthalmodynamometry
➔ *CPT Assistant* Feb 97:6

(For ophthalmoscopy under general anesthesia, use 92018)

Other Specialized Services

92265 Needle oculoelectromyography, one or more extraocular muscles, one or both eyes, with interpretation and report
➔ *CPT Assistant* Feb 97:6

92270 Electro-oculography with interpretation and report
➔ *CPT Assistant* Feb 97:6

92275 Electroretinography with interpretation and report
➔ *CPT Assistant* Feb 97:6

(For electronystagmography for vestibular function studies, see 92541 et seq)

(For ophthalmic echography (diagnostic ultrasound), see 76511-76529)

92283 Color vision examination, extended, eg, anomaloscope or equivalent
➔ *CPT Assistant* Feb 97:6

(Color vision testing with pseudoisochromatic plates (such as HRR or Ishihara) is not reported separately. It is included in the appropriate general or ophthalmological service, or 99172)

92284 Dark adaptation examination with interpretation and report
➔ *CPT Assistant* Feb 97:6

92285 External ocular photography with interpretation and report for documentation of medical progress (eg, close-up photography, slit lamp photography, goniophotography, stereo-photography)
➔ *CPT Assistant* Feb 97:6, Sep 97:10

92286 Special anterior segment photography with interpretation and report; with specular endothelial microscopy and cell count
➔ *CPT Assistant* Feb 97:6

92287 with fluorescein angiography
➔ *CPT Assistant* Feb 97:6

Contact Lens Services

The prescription of contact lens includes specification of optical and physical characteristics (such as power, size, curvature, flexibility, gas-permeability). It is NOT a part of the general ophthalmological services.

The fitting of contact lens includes instruction and training of the wearer and incidental revision of the lens during the training period.

Follow-up of successfully fitted extended wear lenses is reported as part of a general ophthalmological service (92012 et seq).

The supply of contact lenses may be reported as part of the service of fitting. It may also be reported separately by using the appropriate supply codes.

(For therapeutic or surgical use of contact lens, see 68340, 92070)

92310 Prescription of optical and physical characteristics of and fitting of contact lens, with medical supervision of adaptation; corneal lens, both eyes, except for aphakia
➔ *CPT Assistant* Feb 97:6

(For prescription and fitting of one eye, add modifier 52)

92311 corneal lens for aphakia, one eye
➔ *CPT Assistant* Feb 97:6

92312 corneal lens for aphakia, both eyes
➔ *CPT Assistant* Feb 97:6

92313 corneoscleral lens
➔ *CPT Assistant* Feb 97:7, Mar 03:1

92314   Prescription of optical and physical characteristics of contact lens, with medical supervision of adaptation and direction of fitting by independent technician; corneal lens, both eyes except for aphakia
➔ *CPT Assistant* Feb 97:7

(For prescription and fitting of one eye, add modifier 52)

92315   corneal lens for aphakia, one eye
➔ *CPT Assistant* Feb 97:7

92316   corneal lens for aphakia, both eyes
➔ *CPT Assistant* Feb 97:7

92317   corneoscleral lens
➔ *CPT Assistant* Feb 97:7

92325   Modification of contact lens (separate procedure), with medical supervision of adaptation
➔ *CPT Assistant* Feb 97:7

92326   Replacement of contact lens
➔ *CPT Assistant* Feb 97:7

(92330, 92335 have been deleted)

(For prescription, fitting, and/or medical supervision of ocular prosthetic adaptation by a physician, see Evaluation and Management services or General Ophthalmological service codes 92002-92014)

Spectacle Services (Including Prosthesis for Aphakia)

Prescription of lenses, when required, is included in 92015 Determination of refractive state. It includes specification of lens type (monofocal, bifocal, other), lens power, axis, prism, absorptive factor, impact resistance, and other factors.

Fitting of spectacles is a separate service; when provided by the physician, it is reported as indicated by 92340-92371.

Fitting includes measurement of anatomical facial characteristics, the writing of laboratory specifications, and the final adjustment of the spectacles to the visual axes and anatomical topography. Presence of physician is not required.

Supply of materials is a separate service component; it is not part of the service of fitting spectacles.
➔ *CPT Assistant* Nov 97:43

92340   Fitting of spectacles, except for aphakia; monofocal
➔ *CPT Assistant* Feb 97:7, Aug 98:4

92341   bifocal
➔ *CPT Assistant* Feb 97:7, Aug 98:4

92342   multifocal, other than bifocal
➔ *CPT Assistant* Feb 97:7, Aug 98:4

92352   Fitting of spectacle prosthesis for aphakia; monofocal
➔ *CPT Assistant* Feb 97:7, Aug 98:4

92353   multifocal
➔ *CPT Assistant* Feb 97:7, Aug 98:4

92354   Fitting of spectacle mounted low vision aid; single element system
➔ *CPT Assistant* Feb 97:7, Aug 98:4

92355   telescopic or other compound lens system
➔ *CPT Assistant* Feb 97:7, Aug 98:4

92358   Prosthesis service for aphakia, temporary (disposable or loan, including materials)
➔ *CPT Assistant* Feb 97:7, Aug 98:4

92370   Repair and refitting spectacles; except for aphakia
➔ *CPT Assistant* Feb 97:7

92371   spectacle prosthesis for aphakia
➔ *CPT Assistant* Feb 97:7, Aug 98:4

(Codes 92390-92396 have been deleted. For supply of spectacles or contact lenses, use the appropriate supply codes)

Other Procedures

92499   Unlisted ophthalmological service or procedure
➔ *CPT Assistant* Feb 97:7

Special Otorhinolaryngologic Services

Diagnostic or treatment procedures usually included in a comprehensive otorhinolaryngologic evaluation or office visit, are reported as an integrated medical service, using appropriate descriptors from the 99201 series. Itemization of component procedures (eg, otoscopy, rhinoscopy, tuning fork test) does not apply.

Special otorhinolaryngologic services are those diagnostic and treatment services not usually included in a comprehensive otorhinolaryngologic evaluation or office visit. These services are reported separately, using codes 92502-92700.

All services include medical diagnostic evaluation. Technical procedures (which may or may not be performed by the physician personally) are often part of the service, but should not be mistaken to constitute the service itself.

Code 92506 is used to report evaluation of speech production, receptive language, and expressive language abilities. Tests may examine speech sound production, articulatory movements of oral musculature, the patient's ability to understand the meaning and intent of written and verbal expressions, and the appropriate formulation and utterance of expressive thought. In contrast, 92626 and 92627 are reported for an evaluation of auditory rehabilitation status determining the patient's ability to use residual hearing in order to identify the acoustic characteristics of sounds associated with speech communication.

(For laryngoscopy with stroboscopy, use 31579)

92502 Otolaryngologic examination under general anesthesia

92504 Binocular microscopy (separate diagnostic procedure)
➔ *CPT Assistant* Jul 05:14

92506 Evaluation of speech, language, voice, communication, and/or auditory processing
➔ *CPT Assistant* Sep 04:13, Dec 04:14, Mar 05:7, Jan 06:7; *CPT Changes: An Insider's View* 2006

92507 Treatment of speech, language, voice, communication, and/or auditory processing disorder; individual
➔ *CPT Assistant* Dec 04:14, Jan 06:7; *CPT Changes: An Insider's View* 2006

92508 group, 2 or more individuals
➔ *CPT Assistant* Dec 04:14

(92510 has been deleted)

(For auditory rehabilitation, prelingual hearing loss, use 92630)

(For auditory rehabilitation, postlingual hearing loss, use 92633)

(For cochlear implant programming, see 92601-92604)

92511 Nasopharyngoscopy with endoscope (separate procedure)

92512 Nasal function studies (eg, rhinomanometry)

92516 Facial nerve function studies (eg, electroneuronography)

92520 Laryngeal function studies (ie, aerodynamic testing and acoustic testing)
➔ *CPT Assistant* Dec 04:17, Jan 06:7; *CPT Changes: An Insider's View* 2006

(For performance of a single test, use modifier 52)

(To report flexible fiberoptic laryngeal evaluation of swallowing and laryngeal sensory testing, see 92611-92617)

(To report other testing of laryngeal function (eg, electroglottography), use 92700)

92526 Treatment of swallowing dysfunction and/or oral function for feeding

Vestibular Function Tests, With Observation and Evaluation by Physician, Without Electrical Recording

92531 Spontaneous nystagmus, including gaze

92532 Positional nystagmus test
➔ *CPT Changes: An Insider's View* 2002

92533 Caloric vestibular test, each irrigation (binaural, bithermal stimulation constitutes four tests)
➔ *CPT Assistant* May 96:5

92534 Optokinetic nystagmus test
➔ *CPT Changes: An Insider's View* 2002

Vestibular Function Tests, With Recording (eg, ENG, PENG), and Medical Diagnostic Evaluation

92541 Spontaneous nystagmus test, including gaze and fixation nystagmus, with recording
➔ *CPT Assistant* Feb 05:13

92542 Positional nystagmus test, minimum of 4 positions, with recording
➔ *CPT Assistant* Feb 05:13

92543 Caloric vestibular test, each irrigation (binaural, bithermal stimulation constitutes four tests), with recording
➔ *CPT Assistant* May 96:5, Oct 04:10, Feb 05:13, Sep 06:13

92544 Optokinetic nystagmus test, bidirectional, foveal or peripheral stimulation, with recording
➔ *CPT Assistant* Feb 05:13

92545 Oscillating tracking test, with recording
➔ *CPT Assistant* Feb 05:13

92546 Sinusoidal vertical axis rotational testing
➔ *CPT Assistant* Sep 04:13, Feb 05:13

+ 92547 Use of vertical electrodes (List separately in addition to code for primary procedure)
➔ *CPT Assistant* May 04:14, Feb 05:13

(Use 92547 in conjunction with 92541-92546)

(For unlisted vestibular tests, use 92700)

92548 Computerized dynamic posturography

Audiologic Function Tests With Medical Diagnostic Evaluation

The audiometric tests listed below imply the use of calibrated electronic equipment. Other hearing tests (such as whispered voice, tuning fork) are considered part of the general otorhinolaryngologic services and are not reported separately. All services include testing of both ears. Use modifier 52 if a test is applied to one ear instead of to two ears. All codes (except 92559) apply to testing of individuals; for testing of groups, use 92559 and specify test(s) used.

(For evaluation of speech, language and/or hearing problems through observation and assessment of performance, use 92506)

92551 Screening test, pure tone, air only

92552   Pure tone audiometry (threshold); air only

92553   air and bone

92555   Speech audiometry threshold;

92556   with speech recognition

92557   Comprehensive audiometry threshold evaluation and speech recognition (92553 and 92556 combined)

(For hearing aid evaluation and selection, see 92590-92595)

92559   Audiometric testing of groups

92560   Bekesy audiometry; screening

92561   diagnostic

92562   Loudness balance test, alternate binaural or monaural
→ *CPT Assistant* Mar 05:7, 9

92563   Tone decay test

92564   Short increment sensitivity index (SISI)
→ *CPT Assistant* Oct 96:9

92565   Stenger test, pure tone

92567   Tympanometry (impedance testing)
→ *CPT Assistant* Winter 90:11

92568   Acoustic reflex testing; threshold
→ *CPT Assistant* Jan 06:7; *CPT Changes: An Insider's View* 2006

92569   decay
→ *CPT Assistant* Jan 06:7; *CPT Changes: An Insider's View* 2006

92571   Filtered speech test
→ *CPT Assistant* Mar 05:7

92572   Staggered spondaic word test
→ *CPT Assistant* Mar 05:7

(92573 has been deleted. To report the Lombard test, use 92700)

92575   Sensorineural acuity level test

92576   Synthetic sentence identification test
→ *CPT Assistant* Mar 05:7

92577   Stenger test, speech

92579   Visual reinforcement audiometry (VRA)

92582   Conditioning play audiometry

92583   Select picture audiometry

92584   Electrocochleography

92585   Auditory evoked potentials for evoked response audiometry and/or testing of the central nervous system; comprehensive
→ *CPT Assistant* Winter 90:11; *CPT Changes: An Insider's View* 2001

92586   limited
→ *CPT Changes: An Insider's View* 2001

92587   Evoked otoacoustic emissions; limited (single stimulus level, either transient or distortion products)

92588   comprehensive or diagnostic evaluation (comparison of transient and/or distortion product otoacoustic emissions at multiple levels and frequencies)

(For central auditory function evaluation, see 92620, 92621)

92590   Hearing aid examination and selection; monaural

92591   binaural

92592   Hearing aid check; monaural

92593   binaural

92594   Electroacoustic evaluation for hearing aid; monaural

92595   binaural

92596   Ear protector attenuation measurements

92597   Evaluation for use and/or fitting of voice prosthetic device to supplement oral speech

(To report augmentative and alternative communication device services, see 92605, 92607, 92608)

Evaluative and Therapeutic Services

Codes 92601 and 92603 describe post-operative analysis and fitting of previously placed external devices, connection to the cochlear implant, and programming of the stimulator. Codes 92602 and 92604 describe subsequent sessions for measurements and adjustment of the external transmitter and re-programming of the internal stimulator.

(For placement of cochlear implant, use 69930)

92601   Diagnostic analysis of cochlear implant, patient younger than 7 years of age; with programming
→ *CPT Assistant* Mar 03:1, Jan 06:7; *CPT Changes: An Insider's View* 2003

92602   subsequent reprogramming
→ *CPT Assistant* Mar 03:1, 21, Jan 06:7; *CPT Changes: An Insider's View* 2003

(Do not report 92602 in addition to 92601)

(For aural rehabilitation services following cochlear implant, including evaluation of rehabilitation status, see 92626-92627, 92630-92633)

92603 Diagnostic analysis of cochlear implant, age 7 years or older; with programming

➲ *CPT Assistant* Mar 03:2, 4, Jan 06:7; *CPT Changes: An Insider's View* 2003

92604 subsequent reprogramming

➲ *CPT Assistant* Mar 03:2, 21, Jan 06:7; *CPT Changes: An Insider's View* 2003

(Do not report 92604 in addition to 92603)

A View of the Outer Cochlear Implant
92601-92604

An example of the elements that are addressed in the diagnostic analysis and reprogramming of the cochlear implant

Transmitting coil

Headset with microphone

Cord to speech processor

92605 Evaluation for prescription of non-speech-generating augmentative and alternative communication device

➲ *CPT Assistant* Mar 03:2, 4; *CPT Changes: An Insider's View* 2003

92606 Therapeutic service(s) for the use of non-speech-generating device, including programming and modification

➲ *CPT Assistant* Mar 03:2, 4; *CPT Changes: An Insider's View* 2003

92607 Evaluation for prescription for speech-generating augmentative and alternative communication device, face-to-face with the patient; first hour

➲ *CPT Assistant* Mar 03:2, 4, Dec 04:16; *CPT Changes: An Insider's View* 2003

(For evaluation for prescription of a non-speech-generating device, use 92605)

+ 92608 each additional 30 minutes (List separately in addition to code for primary procedure)

➲ *CPT Assistant* Mar 03:2, 5, Dec 04:16; *CPT Changes: An Insider's View* 2003

(Use 92608 in conjunction with 92607)

92609 Therapeutic services for the use of speech-generating device, including programming and modification

➲ *CPT Assistant* Mar 03:2, 4, Dec 04:16; *CPT Changes: An Insider's View* 2003

(For therapeutic service(s) for the use of a non-speech-generating device, use 92606)

92610 Evaluation of oral and pharyngeal swallowing function

➲ *CPT Assistant* Mar 03:2, 5, Dec 04:17; *CPT Changes: An Insider's View* 2003

(For motion fluoroscopic evaluation of swallowing function, use 92611)

(For flexible endoscopic examination, use 92612-92617)

92611 Motion fluoroscopic evaluation of swallowing function by cine or video recording

➲ *CPT Assistant* Mar 03:2, 5, Dec 04:17, Jan 06:7; *CPT Changes: An Insider's View* 2003

➲ *Clinical Examples in Radiology* Summer 06:4-5

(For radiological supervision and interpretation, use 74230)

(For evaluation of oral and pharyngeal swallowing function, use 92610)

(For flexible fiberoptic diagnostic laryngoscopy, use 31575. Do not report 31575 in conjunction with 92612-92617)

92612 Flexible fiberoptic endoscopic evaluation of swallowing by cine or video recording;

➲ *CPT Assistant* Mar 03:6, Jan 06:7; *CPT Changes: An Insider's View* 2003

(If flexible fiberoptic or endoscopic evaluation of swallowing is performed without cine or video recording, use 92700)

92613 physician interpretation and report only

➲ *CPT Assistant* Jan 06:7; *CPT Changes: An Insider's View* 2003

(To report an evaluation of oral and pharyngeal swallowing function, use 92610)

(To report motion fluoroscopic evaluation of swallowing function, use 92611)

92614 Flexible fiberoptic endoscopic evaluation, laryngeal sensory testing by cine or video recording;

➲ *CPT Assistant* Mar 03:6, Jan 06:7; *CPT Changes: An Insider's View* 2003

(If flexible fiberoptic or endoscopic evaluation of swallowing is performed without cine or video recording, use 92700)

92615 physician interpretation and report only

➲ *CPT Assistant* Mar 03:6, Jan 06:7; *CPT Changes: An Insider's View* 2003

92616   Flexible fiberoptic endoscopic evaluation of swallowing and laryngeal sensory testing by cine or video recording;
→ *CPT Assistant* Mar 03:6, Jan 06:7; *CPT Changes: An Insider's View* 2003

(If flexible fiberoptic or endoscopic evaluation of swallowing is performed without cine or video recording, use 92700)

92617   physician interpretation and report only
→ *CPT Assistant* Mar 03:6, Jan 06:7; *CPT Changes: An Insider's View* 2003

92620   Evaluation of central auditory function, with report; initial 60 minutes
→ *CPT Assistant* Mar 05:7-8; *CPT Changes: An Insider's View* 2005

92621   each additional 15 minutes
→ *CPT Assistant* Mar 05:7; *CPT Changes: An Insider's View* 2005

(Do not report 92620, 92621 in conjunction with 92506)

92625   Assessment of tinnitus (includes pitch, loudness matching, and masking)
→ *CPT Assistant* Mar 05:7-10; *CPT Changes: An Insider's View* 2005

(Do not report 92625 in conjunction with 92562)

(For unilateral assessment, use modifier 52)

92626   Evaluation of auditory rehabilitation status; first hour
→ *CPT Assistant* Jan 06:7; *CPT Changes: An Insider's View* 2006

+ 92627   each additional 15 minutes (List separately in addition to code for primary procedure)
→ *CPT Assistant* Jan 06:7; *CPT Changes: An Insider's View* 2006

(Use 92627 in conjunction with 92626)

(When reporting 92626, 92627, use the face-to-face time with the patient or family)

92630   Auditory rehabilitation; prelingual hearing loss
→ *CPT Assistant* Jan 06:7; *CPT Changes: An Insider's View* 2006

92633   postlingual hearing loss
→ *CPT Assistant* Jan 06:7; *CPT Changes: An Insider's View* 2006

Special Diagnostic Procedures

92640   Diagnostic analysis with programming of auditory brainstem implant, per hour
→ *CPT Changes: An Insider's View* 2007

(Report nonprogramming services separately [eg, cardiac monitoring])

Other Procedures

92700   Unlisted otorhinolaryngological service or procedure
→ *CPT Assistant* Sep 04:14, Oct 04:10, Jan 06:7, Sep 06:13; *CPT Changes: An Insider's View* 2003

Cardiovascular

Therapeutic Services and Procedures

(For nonsurgical septal reduction therapy [eg, alcohol ablation], use Category III code 0024T)

92950   Cardiopulmonary resuscitation (eg, in cardiac arrest)
→ *CPT Assistant* Jan 96:7

(See also critical care services, 99291, 99292)

⊙ **92953**   Temporary transcutaneous pacing
→ *CPT Assistant* Nov 99:49, Feb 07:10

(For physician direction of ambulance or rescue personnel outside the hospital, use 99288)

⊙ **92960**   Cardioversion, elective, electrical conversion of arrhythmia; external
→ *CPT Assistant* Summer 93:13, Nov 99:49, Jun 00:5, Nov 00:9, Jul 01:11; *CPT Changes: An Insider's View* 2000

⊙ **92961**   internal (separate procedure)
→ *CPT Assistant* Summer 93:13, Nov 99:49, Jun 00:5, Jul 00:5, Nov 00:9; *CPT Changes: An Insider's View* 2000

(Do not report 92961 in addition to codes 93662, 93618-93624, 93631, 93640-93642, 93650-93652, 93741-93744)

92970   Cardioassist-method of circulatory assist; internal

92971   external

(For balloon atrial-septostomy, use 92992)

(For placement of catheters for use in circulatory assist devices such as intra-aortic balloon pump, use 33970)

⊙**+ 92973**   Percutaneous transluminal coronary thrombectomy (List separately in addition to code for primary procedure)
→ *CPT Assistant* Mar 02:2, 10, Mar 04:10; *CPT Changes: An Insider's View* 2002

(Use 92973 in conjunction with 92980, 92982)

⊙**+ 92974**   Transcatheter placement of radiation delivery device for subsequent coronary intravascular brachytherapy (List separately in addition to code for primary procedure)
→ *CPT Assistant* Mar 02:2; *CPT Changes: An Insider's View* 2002

(Use 92974 in conjunction with 92980, 92982, 92995, 93508)

(For intravascular radioelement application, see 77781-77784)

⊙ **92975**   Thrombolysis, coronary; by intracoronary infusion, including selective coronary angiography

92977   by intravenous infusion

(For thrombolysis of vessels other than coronary, see 37201, 75896)

(For cerebral thrombolysis, use 37195)

⊙✚ **92978**   Intravascular ultrasound (coronary vessel or graft) during diagnostic evaluation and/or therapeutic intervention including imaging supervision, interpretation and report; initial vessel (List separately in addition to code for primary procedure)

➔ *CPT Assistant* Nov 97:43-44, Nov 99:49, Mar 02:2, Jan 07:28; *CPT Changes: An Insider's View* 2000

Intravascular Ultrasound (Coronary Vessel or Graft)
92978

A catheter with a transducer at its tip is inserted and threaded through a selected coronary artery(s) or coronary bypass graft(s).

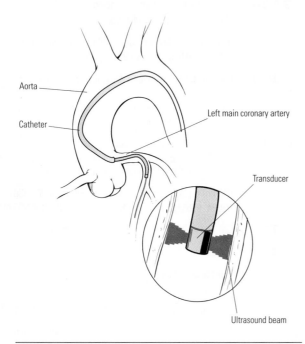

⊙✚ **92979**   each additional vessel (List separately in addition to code for primary procedure)

➔ *CPT Assistant* Nov 97:43-44, Nov 99:49; *CPT Changes: An Insider's View* 2000

(Use 92979 in conjunction with 92978)

(Intravascular ultrasound services include all transducer manipulations and repositioning within the specific vessel being examined, both before and after therapeutic intervention (eg, stent placement))

⊙ **92980**   Transcatheter placement of an intracoronary stent(s), percutaneous, with or without other therapeutic intervention, any method; single vessel

➔ *CPT Assistant* Aug 96:2, Dec 96:11, Apr 98:9, Aug 98:3, Aug 00:11, Mar 01:11, Apr 01:10, Mar 02:2, Aug 03:10, Apr 05:14

⊙✚ **92981**   each additional vessel (List separately in addition to code for primary procedure)

➔ *CPT Assistant* Mar 01:11, Apr 01:10, Aug 03:10

(Use 92981 in conjunction with 92980)

(Codes 92980, 92981 are used to report coronary artery stenting. Coronary angioplasty (92982, 92984) or atherectomy (92995, 92996), in the same artery, is considered part of the stenting procedure and is not reported separately. Codes 92973 (percutaneous transluminal coronary thombectomy), 92974 (coronary brachytherapy) and 92978, 92979 (intravascular ultrasound) are add-on codes for reporting procedures performed in addition to coronary stenting, atherectomy, and angioplasty and are not included in the "therapeutic interventions" in 92980)

(To report additional vessels treated by angioplasty or atherectomy only during the same session, see 92984, 92996)

(To report transcatheter placement of radiation delivery device for coronary intravascular brachytherapy, use 92974)

(For intravascular radioelement application, see 77781-77784)

⊙ **92982**   Percutaneous transluminal coronary balloon angioplasty; single vessel

➔ *CPT Assistant* Winter 92:15, Aug 96:2, Apr 97:10, Mar 02:2, Apr 05:14

Percutaneous Transluminal Coronary Angioplasty (PTCA)
92982

PTCA of a single coronary vessel

⊙✛ **92984**   each additional vessel (List separately in addition to code for primary procedure)

> *CPT Assistant* Winter 92:15, Aug 96:2, Dec 96:11, Apr 97:10, Apr 05:14

(Use 92984 in conjunction with 92980, 92982, 92995)

(For stent placement following completion of angioplasty or atherectomy, see 92980, 92981)

(To report transcatheter placement of radiation delivery device for coronary intravascular brachytherapy, use 92974)

(For intravascular radioelement application, see 77781-77784)

⊙ **92986**   Percutaneous balloon valvuloplasty; aortic valve

⊙ **92987**   mitral valve

92990   pulmonary valve

> *CPT Assistant* Winter 91:3

92992   Atrial septectomy or septostomy; transvenous method, balloon (eg, Rashkind type) (includes cardiac catheterization)

> *CPT Assistant* Nov 97:44, Apr 98:3, 10

92993   blade method (Park septostomy) (includes cardiac catheterization)

> *CPT Assistant* Apr 98:10

⊙ **92995**   Percutaneous transluminal coronary atherectomy, by mechanical or other method, with or without balloon angioplasty; single vessel

> *CPT Assistant* Winter 92:15

⊙✛ **92996**   each additional vessel (List separately in addition to code for primary procedure)

> *CPT Assistant* Winter 92:15, Apr 98:3

(Use 92996 in conjunction with 92980, 92982, 92995)

(For stent placement following completion of angioplasty or atherectomy, see 92980, 92981)

(To report additional vessels treated by angioplasty only during the same session, use 92984)

92997   Percutaneous transluminal pulmonary artery balloon angioplasty; single vessel

> *CPT Assistant* Nov 97:44

✛ **92998**   each additional vessel (List separately in addition to code for primary procedure)

> *CPT Assistant* Nov 97:44

(Use 92998 in conjunction with 92997)

Cardiography

▶Codes 93040-93042 are appropriate when an order for the test is triggered by an event, the rhythm strip is used to help diagnose the presence or absence of an arrhythmia, and a report is generated. There must be a specific order for an electrocardiogram or rhythm strip followed by a separate, signed, written, and retrievable report. It is not appropriate to use these codes for reviewing the telemetry monitor strips taken from a monitoring system. The need for an electrocardiogram or rhythm strip should be supported by documentation in the patient medical record.◀

(For echocardiography, see 93303-93350)

▶(For electrocardiogram, 64 leads or greater, with graphic presentation and analysis, see 0178T-0180T)◀

93000   Electrocardiogram, routine ECG with at least 12 leads; with interpretation and report

> *CPT Assistant* Aug 97:9, Feb 05:9, Mar 05:1, 11

93005   tracing only, without interpretation and report

> *CPT Assistant* Aug 97:9, Mar 05:1

93010   interpretation and report only

> *CPT Assistant* Aug 97:9, Mar 05:1, Apr 07:1

▶(For acoustic heart sound recording, see Category III codes 0068T-0070T)◀

(For ECG monitoring, see 99354-99360)

93012   Telephonic transmission of post-symptom electrocardiogram rhythm strip(s), 24-hour attended monitoring, per 30 day period of time; tracing only

> *CPT Assistant* Jun 96:2, Oct 05:14; *CPT Changes: An Insider's View* 2003

93014   physician review with interpretation and report only

> *CPT Assistant* Jun 96:2, Oct 05:14

93015   Cardiovascular stress test using maximal or submaximal treadmill or bicycle exercise, continuous electrocardiographic monitoring, and/or pharmacological stress; with physician supervision, with interpretation and report

> *CPT Assistant* Apr 96:11, Jun 96:10, Aug 02:10

93016   physician supervision only, without interpretation and report

> *CPT Assistant* Apr 96:11, Aug 02:10

93017   tracing only, without interpretation and report

> *CPT Assistant* Aug 02:10

93018   interpretation and report only

> *CPT Assistant* Apr 96:11, Jun 96:10

(For inert gas rebreathing measurement, see Category III codes 0104T, 0105T)

93024   Ergonovine provocation test

93025 Microvolt T-wave alternans for assessment of ventricular arrhythmias

> *CPT Assistant* Mar 02:3; *CPT Changes: An Insider's View* 2002

93040 Rhythm ECG, one to three leads; with interpretation and report

> *CPT Assistant* Apr 04:8

93041 tracing only without interpretation and report

> *CPT Assistant* Apr 04:8

93042 interpretation and report only

> *CPT Assistant* Apr 04:8

93224 Electrocardiographic monitoring for 24 hours by continuous original ECG waveform recording and storage, with visual superimposition scanning; includes recording, scanning analysis with report, physician review and interpretation

> *CPT Assistant* Oct 05:14, Apr 07:3

93225 recording (includes hook-up, recording, and disconnection)

> *CPT Assistant* Oct 05:14, Apr 07:3

93226 scanning analysis with report

> *CPT Assistant* Oct 05:14, Apr 07:3

93227 physician review and interpretation

93230 Electrocardiographic monitoring for 24 hours by continuous original ECG waveform recording and storage without superimposition scanning utilizing a device capable of producing a full miniaturized printout; includes recording, microprocessor-based analysis with report, physician review and interpretation

> *CPT Assistant* Oct 05:14, Apr 07:3

93231 recording (includes hook-up, recording, and disconnection)

> *CPT Assistant* Oct 05:14, Apr 07:3

93232 microprocessor-based analysis with report

> *CPT Assistant* Oct 05:14, Apr 07:3

93233 physician review and interpretation

> *CPT Assistant* Oct 05:14, Apr 07:3

93235 Electrocardiographic monitoring for 24 hours by continuous computerized monitoring and non-continuous recording, and real-time data analysis utilizing a device capable of producing intermittent full-sized waveform tracings, possibly patient activated; includes monitoring and real-time data analysis with report, physician review and interpretation

> *CPT Assistant* Oct 05:14, Apr 07:3

93236 monitoring and real-time data analysis with report

> *CPT Assistant* Oct 05:14, Apr 07:3

93237 physician review and interpretation

> *CPT Assistant* Oct 05:14, Apr 07:3

93268 Patient demand single or multiple event recording with presymptom memory loop, 24-hour attended monitoring, per 30 day period of time; includes transmission, physician review and interpretation

> *CPT Assistant* Jun 96:2, Nov 99:49-50, Oct 05:14, Apr 07:3; *CPT Changes: An Insider's View* 2003

93270 recording (includes hook-up, recording, and disconnection)

> *CPT Assistant* Jun 96:2, Oct 05:14, Apr 07:3

93271 monitoring, receipt of transmissions, and analysis

> *CPT Assistant* Jun 96:2, Oct 05:14, Apr 07:3

93272 physician review and interpretation only

> *CPT Assistant* Jun 96:2, Apr 98:14, Nov 99:49-50, Oct 05:14, Apr 07:3

(For postsymptom recording, see 93012, 93014)

(For implanted patient activated cardiac event recording, see 33282, 93727)

93278 Signal-averaged electrocardiography (SAECG), with or without ECG

(For interpretation and report only, use 93278 with modifier 26)

(For unlisted cardiographic procedure, use 93799)

Echocardiography

Echocardiography includes obtaining ultrasonic signals from the heart and great arteries, with two-dimensional image and/or Doppler ultrasonic signal documentation, and interpretation and report. When interpretation is performed separately use modifier 26.

Echocardiography is an ultrasound examination of the cardiac chambers and valves, the adjacent great vessels, and the pericardium. A complete transthoracic echocardiogram (93307) is a comprehensive procedure that includes 2-dimensional and selected M-mode examination of the left and right atria, left and right ventricles, the aortic, mitral, and tricuspid valves, the pericardium, and adjacent portions of the aorta. These structures are assessed using multiple views as required to obtain a complete functional and anatomic evaluation, and appropriate measurements are obtained and recorded. Despite significant effort, identification and measurement of some structures may not always be possible. In such instances, the reason that an element could not be visualized must be documented. Additional structures that may be visualized (eg, pulmonary veins, pulmonary artery, pulmonic valve, inferior vena cava) would be included as part of the service.

A follow-up or limited echocardiographic study (93308) is an examination that does not evaluate or document the attempt to evaluate all the structures that comprise the complete echocardiographic exam. This is typically performed in follow-up of a complete echocardiographic examination when a repeat complete exam is unnecessary due to the more focused clinical concern. In some emergent clinical situations, a limited echocardiographic study may be performed primarily.

Report of an echocardiographic study, whether complete or limited, includes an interpretation of all obtained information, documentation of all clinically relevant findings including quantitative measurements obtained, plus a description of any recognized abnormalities. Pertinent images, videotape, and/or digital data are archived for permanent storage and are available for subsequent review. Use of echocardiography not meeting these criteria is not separately reportable.

Use of ultrasound, without thorough evaluation of organ(s) or anatomic region, image documentation and final, written report, is not separately reportable.

(For fetal echocardiography, see 76825-76828)

93303   Transthoracic echocardiography for congenital cardiac anomalies; complete
> *CPT Assistant* Nov 97:44, Dec 97:5, Sep 05:10-11
> *Clinical Examples in Radiology* Fall 06:9-10

93304   follow-up or limited study
> *CPT Assistant* Nov 97:44, Dec 97:5
> *Clinical Examples in Radiology* Fall 06:9-10

93307   Echocardiography, transthoracic, real-time with image documentation (2D) with or without M-mode recording; complete
> *CPT Assistant* Dec 97:5, Sep 05:11
> *Clinical Examples in Radiology* Fall 06:9-10

93308   follow-up or limited study
> *CPT Assistant* Dec 97:5, Sep 05:11
> *Clinical Examples in Radiology* Fall 06:9-10

⊙ **93312**   Echocardiography, transesophageal, real time with image documentation (2D) (with or without M-mode recording); including probe placement, image acquisition, interpretation and report
> *CPT Assistant* Dec 97:5, Jan 00:10

Transesophageal Echocardiography (TEE)
93312-93318

An endoscopic ultrasound transducer is passed through the mouth into the esophagus and 2-dimensional images are obtained from the posterior aspect of the heart.

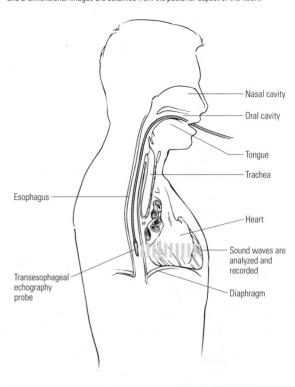

⊙ **93313**   placement of transesophageal probe only
> *CPT Assistant* Dec 97:5

⊙ **93314**   image acquisition, interpretation and report only
> *CPT Assistant* Dec 97:5, Jan 00:10

⊙ **93315**   Transesophageal echocardiography for congenital cardiac anomalies; including probe placement, image acquisition, interpretation and report
> *CPT Assistant* Nov 97:44, Dec 97:5

⊙ **93316**   placement of transesophageal probe only
> *CPT Assistant* Nov 97:44, Dec 97:5

⊙ **93317**   image acquisition, interpretation and report only
> *CPT Assistant* Nov 97:44, Dec 97:5

⊙ **93318**   Echocardiography, transesophageal (TEE) for monitoring purposes, including probe placement, real time 2-dimensional image acquisition and interpretation leading to ongoing (continuous) assessment of (dynamically changing) cardiac pumping function and to therapeutic measures on an immediate time basis
> *CPT Changes: An Insider's View* 2001

+ **93320**   Doppler echocardiography, pulsed wave and/or continuous wave with spectral display (List separately in addition to codes for echocardiographic imaging); complete
> *CPT Assistant* Nov 97:44, Dec 97:5
> *Clinical Examples in Radiology* Fall 06:9-10

(Use 93320 in conjunction with 93303, 93304, 93307, 93308, 93312, 93314, 93315, 93317, 93350)

+ **93321**   follow-up or limited study (List separately in addition to codes for echocardiographic imaging)
> *CPT Assistant* Nov 97:44, Dec 97:5
> *Clinical Examples in Radiology* Fall 06:9-10

(Use 93321 in conjunction with 93303, 93304, 93307, 93308, 93312, 93314, 93315, 93317, 93350)

+ **93325**   Doppler echocardiography color flow velocity mapping (List separately in addition to codes for echocardiography)
> *CPT Assistant* Nov 97:44, Dec 97:5
> *Clinical Examples in Radiology* Fall 06:9-10

(Use 93325 in conjunction with 76825, 76826, 76827, 76828, 93303, 93304, 93307, 93308, 93312, 93314, 93315, 93317, 93320, 93321, 93350)

93350   Echocardiography, transthoracic, real-time with image documentation (2D), with or without M-mode recording, during rest and cardiovascular stress test using treadmill, bicycle exercise and/or pharmacologically induced stress, with interpretation and report
> *CPT Assistant* Aug 02:11

(The appropriate stress testing code from the 93015-93018 series should be reported in addition to 93350 to capture the exercise stress portion of the study)

Cardiac Catheterization

Cardiac catheterization is a diagnostic medical procedure which includes introduction, positioning and repositioning of catheter(s), when necessary, recording of intracardiac and intravascular pressure, obtaining blood samples for measurement of blood gases or dilution curves and cardiac output measurements (Fick or other method, with or without rest and exercise and/or studies) with or without electrode catheter placement, final evaluation and report of procedure. When selective injection procedures are performed without a preceding cardiac catheterization, these services should be reported using codes in the Vascular Injection Procedures section, 36011-36015 and 36215-36218.

When coronary artery, arterial coronary conduit or venous bypass graft angiography is performed without concomitant left heart cardiac catheterization, use 93508. Injection procedures 93539, 93540, 93544, and 93545 represent separate identifiable services and may be reported in conjunction with one another in addition to 93508, as appropriate. To report imaging supervision, interpretation and report in conjunction with 93508, use 93556.

Modifier 51 should not be appended to 93501-93533, 93539-93556.
> *CPT Assistant* Nov 98:33

⊙▲ **93501**   Right heart catheterization
> *CPT Assistant* Spring 94:24, Jan 98:11, Apr 98:2, Apr 00:10;
> *CPT Changes: An Insider's View* 2008

Right Heart Catheterization
93501

The physician introduces a cardiac catheter into the venous system. The catheter is directed into the right atrium, right ventricle, and pulmonary artery.

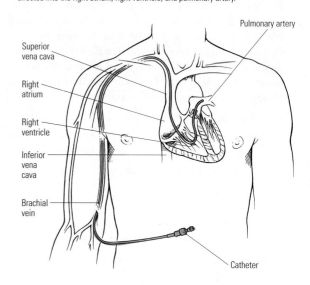

Catheter is advanced retrograde through the arterial system to the ascending aorta; pressures are measured in the aortic root; the catheter is manipulated using fluoroscopic guidance into the ostium of a coronary artery, arterial bypass conduit, or venous coronary bypass graft.

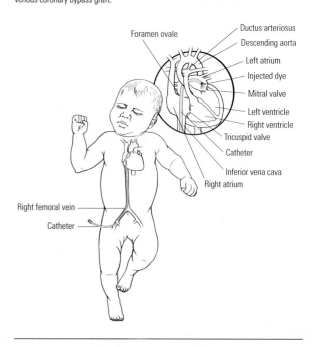

(For bundle of His recording, use 93600)

⊘ **93503** Insertion and placement of flow directed catheter (eg, Swan-Ganz) for monitoring purposes

→ *CPT Assistant* Winter 91:3, Fall 95:8, Feb 97:5, Apr 98:2

(For subsequent monitoring, see 99356-99357)

⊙▲ **93505** Endomyocardial biopsy

→ *CPT Assistant* Apr 98:2, Apr 00:10; *CPT Changes: An Insider's View* 2008

⊙▲ **93508** Catheter placement in coronary artery(s), arterial coronary conduit(s), and/or venous coronary bypass graft(s) for coronary angiography without concomitant left heart catheterization

→ *CPT Assistant* Nov 97:44-45, Jan 98:11, Apr 98:2, Apr 00:10, Aug 00:11; *CPT Changes: An Insider's View* 2008

(93508 is to be used only when left heart catheterization 93510, 93511, 93524, 93526 is not performed)

(93508 is to be used only once per procedure)

Coronary Angiography Without Concomitant Left Heart Catheterization
93508

Cardiac catheterization procedure performed wherein the catheter does not cross the aortic valve into the left ventricle (left heart catheterization).

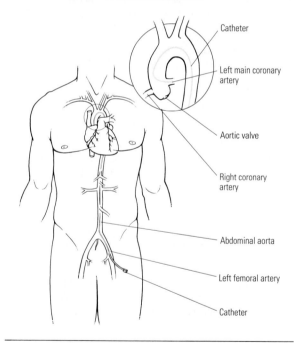

(To report transcatheter placement of radiation delivery device for coronary intravascular brachytherapy, use 92974)

(For intravascular radioelement application, see 77781-77784)

⊙▲ **93510** Left heart catheterization, retrograde, from the brachial artery, axillary artery or femoral artery; percutaneous

→ *CPT Assistant* Spring 94:26, Nov 97:44-45, Jan 98:11, Apr 98:2; *CPT Changes: An Insider's View* 2008

Left Heart Catheterization
93510

A catheter is inserted into the arterial system and then into the left ventricle.

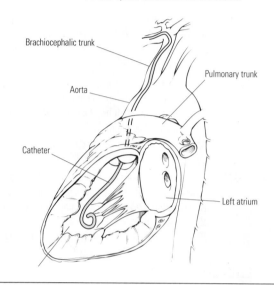

⊙▲ **93511** by cutdown

→ *CPT Assistant* Spring 94:24, Nov 97:44-45, Jan 98:11, Apr 98:2; *CPT Changes: An Insider's View* 2008

⊙▲ **93514** Left heart catheterization by left ventricular puncture

→ *CPT Assistant* Spring 94:24, Jan 98:11, Apr 98:2; *CPT Changes: An Insider's View* 2008

⊙▲ **93524** Combined transseptal and retrograde left heart catheterization

→ *CPT Assistant* Spring 94:24, Nov 97:44-45, Jan 98:11, Apr 98:2; *CPT Changes: An Insider's View* 2008

⊙▲ **93526** Combined right heart catheterization and retrograde left heart catheterization

→ *CPT Assistant* Spring 94:28, Nov 97:44-45, Jan 98:11, Apr 98:2; *CPT Changes: An Insider's View* 2008

⊙▲ **93527** Combined right heart catheterization and transseptal left heart catheterization through intact septum (with or without retrograde left heart catheterization)

→ *CPT Assistant* Jan 98:11, Apr 98:2; *CPT Changes: An Insider's View* 2008

⊙▲ **93528** Combined right heart catheterization with left ventricular puncture (with or without retrograde left heart catheterization)

→ *CPT Assistant* Jan 98:11, Apr 98:2; *CPT Changes: An Insider's View* 2008

⊙▲ **93529**   Combined right heart catheterization and left heart catheterization through existing septal opening (with or without retrograde left heart catheterization)

➔ *CPT Assistant* Jan 98:11, Apr 98:2; *CPT Changes: An Insider's View* 2008

⊙▲ **93530**   Right heart catheterization, for congenital cardiac anomalies

➔ *CPT Assistant* Nov 97:45, Jan 98:11, Mar 98:11, Apr 98:3, 6-7; *CPT Changes: An Insider's View* 2008

▲ **93531**   Combined right heart catheterization and retrograde left heart catheterization, for congenital cardiac anomalies

➔ *CPT Assistant* Nov 97:45, Jan 98:11, Mar 98:11, Apr 98:8, 10-11; *CPT Changes: An Insider's View* 2008

▲ **93532**   Combined right heart catheterization and transseptal left heart catheterization through intact septum with or without retrograde left heart catheterization, for congenital cardiac anomalies

➔ *CPT Assistant* Nov 97:45, Jan 98:11, Mar 98:11, Apr 98:10-11; *CPT Changes: An Insider's View* 2008

▲ **93533**   Combined right heart catheterization and transseptal left heart catheterization through existing septal opening, with or without retrograde left heart catheterization, for congenital cardiac anomalies

➔ *CPT Assistant* Nov 97:45, Jan 98:11, Mar 98:11, Apr 98:12-13; *CPT Changes: An Insider's View* 2008

►Injection Procedures◄

►When injection procedures are performed in conjunction with cardiac catheterization, these services do not include introduction of catheters but do include repositioning of catheters when necessary and use of automatic power injectors. Injection procedures 93539-93545 represent separate identifiable services and may be coded in conjunction with one another when appropriate. The technical details of angiography, supervision of filming and processing, interpretation, and report are not included. To report radiological supervision, interpretation, and report for 93542 or 93543, use 93555. To report radiological supervision, interpretation, and report for 93539, 93540, 93541, 93544, or 93545, use 93556. Modifier 51 should not be appended to 93539-93556.◄

⊙⊘ **93539**   Injection procedure during cardiac catheterization; for selective opacification of arterial conduits (eg, internal mammary), whether native or used for bypass

➔ *CPT Assistant* Spring 94:27, Nov 97:44-45, Apr 98:3, Oct 01:11

⊙⊘ **93540**   for selective opacification of aortocoronary venous bypass grafts, one or more coronary arteries

➔ *CPT Assistant* Spring 94:27, Nov 97:44-45, Apr 98:3

⊙▲ **93541**   for pulmonary angiography

➔ *CPT Assistant* Spring 94:28, Nov 97:44-45, Apr 98:3, Jan 01:16; *CPT Changes: An Insider's View* 2008

⊙▲ **93542**   for selective right ventricular or right atrial angiography

➔ *CPT Assistant* Spring 94:24, Nov 97:44-45, Apr 98:3, Jan 01:16; *CPT Changes: An Insider's View* 2008

⊙▲ **93543**   for selective left ventricular or left atrial angiography

➔ *CPT Assistant* Spring 94:28, Nov 97:44-45, Apr 98:3, Jan 01:16; *CPT Changes: An Insider's View* 2008

⊙⊘ **93544**   for aortography

➔ *CPT Assistant* Spring 94:28, Nov 97:44-45, Apr 98:3, Jan 01:16

⊙⊘ **93545**   for selective coronary angiography (injection of radiopaque material may be by hand)

➔ *CPT Assistant* Spring 94:28, Nov 97:44-45, Apr 98:3, Jan 01:16, Nov 02:10

⊙⊘ **93555**   Imaging supervision, interpretation and report for injection procedure(s) during cardiac catheterization; ventricular and/or atrial angiography

➔ *CPT Assistant* Spring 94:28, Oct 97:10, Nov 97:44-45, Apr 98:3, 11-12

⊙⊘ **93556**   pulmonary angiography, aortography, and/or selective coronary angiography including venous bypass grafts and arterial conduits (whether native or used in bypass)

➔ *CPT Assistant* Spring 94:28, Oct 97:10, Nov 97:44-45, Apr 98:3, 11-12

⊙ **93561**   Indicator dilution studies such as dye or thermal dilution, including arterial and/or venous catheterization; with cardiac output measurement (separate procedure)

➔ *CPT Assistant* Winter 91:25, Summer 95:2, Aug 00:2, Feb 07:10

⊙ **93562**   subsequent measurement of cardiac output

➔ *CPT Assistant* Winter 91:25, Summer 95:2, Aug 00:2, Feb 07:10

►(93561, 93562 are not to be used with cardiac catheterization codes)◄

(For radioisotope method of cardiac output, see 78472, 78473, or 78481)

⊙+ **93571**   Intravascular Doppler velocity and/or pressure derived coronary flow reserve measurement (coronary vessel or graft) during coronary angiography including pharmacologically induced stress; initial vessel (List separately in addition to code for primary procedure)

➔ *CPT Assistant* Nov 98:33, Apr 00:2

Intravascular Distal Blood Flow Velocity
93571

A Doppler guidewire is positioned in a proximal coronary artery with the transducer beam parallel to blood flow to measure blood flow velocity.

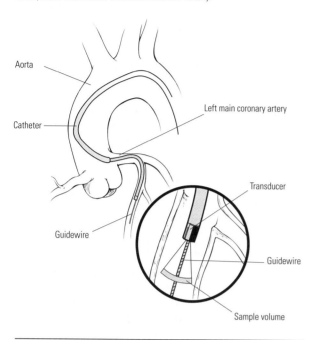

Aorta

Left main coronary artery

Catheter

Guidewire

Transducer

Guidewire

Sample volume

⊙**+ 93572**   each additional vessel (List separately in addition to code for primary procedure)

➔ *CPT Assistant* Nov 98:34, Apr 00:2

(Intravascular distal coronary blood flow velocity measurements include all Doppler transducer manipulations and repositioning within the specific vessel being examined, during coronary angiography or therapeutic intervention (eg, angioplasty))

(For unlisted cardiac catheterization procedure, use 93799)

Repair of Septal Defect

93580   Percutaneous transcatheter closure of congenital interatrial communication (ie, Fontan fenestration, atrial septal defect) with implant

➔ *CPT Assistant* Mar 03:23; *CPT Changes: An Insider's View* 2003

(Percutaneous transcatheter closure of atrial septal defect includes a right heart catheterization procedure. Code 93580 includes injection of contrast for atrial and ventricular angiograms. Codes 93501, 93529-93533, 93539, 93543, 93555 should not be reported separately in addition to code 93580)

93581   Percutaneous transcatheter closure of a congenital ventricular septal defect with implant

➔ *CPT Assistant* Mar 03:23; *CPT Changes: An Insider's View* 2003

(Percutaneous transcatheter closure of ventricular septal defect includes a right heart catheterization procedure. Code 93581 includes injection of contrast for atrial and ventricular angiograms. Codes 93501, 93529-93533, 93539, 93543, 93555 should not be reported separately in addition to code 93581)

(For ventricular septal defect closure via transmyocardial implant delivery, see 0166T, 0167T)

(For echocardiographic services performed in addition to 93580, 93581, see 93303-93317, 93662 as appropriate)

Intracardiac Electrophysiological Procedures/Studies

Intracardiac electrophysiologic studies (EPS) are an invasive diagnostic medical procedure which include the insertion and repositioning of electrode catheters, recording of electrograms before and during pacing or programmed stimulation of multiple locations in the heart, analysis of recorded information, and report of the procedure. Electrophysiologic studies are most often performed with two or more electrode catheters. In many circumstances, patients with arrhythmias are evaluated and treated at the same encounter. In this situation, a diagnostic *electrophysiologic study* is performed, induced tachycardia(s) are *mapped*, and on the basis of the diagnostic and mapping information, the tissue is *ablated*. Electrophysiologic study(ies), mapping, and ablation represent distinctly different procedures, requiring individual reporting whether performed on the same or subsequent dates.

Definitions

Arrhythmia Induction: In most electrophysiologic studies, an attempt is made to induce arrhythmia(s) from single or multiple sites within the heart. Arrhythmia induction is achieved by performing pacing at different rates, programmed stimulation (introduction of critically timed electrical impulses), and other techniques. Because arrhythmia induction occurs via the same catheter(s) inserted for the electrophysiologic study(ies), catheter insertion and temporary pacemaker codes are not additionally reported. Codes 93600-93603, 93610-93612 and 93618 are used to describe unusual situations where there may be recording, pacing or an attempt at arrhythmia induction from only one site in the heart. Code 93619 describes only evaluation of the sinus node, atrioventricular node and His-Purkinje conduction system, without arrhythmia induction. Codes 93620-93624 and 93640-93642 all include recording, pacing and attempted arrhythmia induction from one or more site(s) in the heart.

Mapping: Mapping is a distinct procedure performed in addition to a diagnostic electrophysiologic procedure and should be separately reported using 93609 or 93613. Do not report standard mapping (93609) in addition to 3-D mapping (93613). When a tachycardia is induced, the site of tachycardia origination or its electrical path through the heart is often defined by mapping. Mapping creates a multidimensional depiction of a tachycardia by recording multiple electrograms obtained sequentially or simultaneously from multiple catheter sites in the heart. Depending upon the technique, certain types of mapping catheters may be repositioned from point-to-point within the heart, allowing sequential recording from the various sites to construct maps. Other types of mapping catheters allow mapping without a point-to-point technique by allowing simultaneous recording from many electrodes on the same catheter and computer-assisted three dimensional reconstruction of the tachycardia activation sequence.

Ablation: Once the part of the heart involved in the tachycardia is localized, the tachycardia may be treated by ablation (the delivery of a radiofrequency energy to the area to selectively destroy cardiac tissue). Ablation procedures (93651-93652) may be performed: independently on a date subsequent to a diagnostic electrophysiologic study and mapping; or, at the time a diagnostic electrophysiologic study, tachycardia(s) induction and mapping is performed. When an electrophysiologic study, mapping, and ablation are performed on the same date, each procedure should be separately reported. In reporting catheter ablation, 93651 and/or 93652 should be reported once to describe ablation of cardiac arrhythmias, regardless of the number of arrhythmias ablated.

Modifier 51 should not be appended to 93600-93660.

⊘ **93600** Bundle of His recording
➔ *CPT Assistant* Summer 94:12, Aug 97:9, Apr 04:9, Jul 04:13, Aug 05:13

⊘ **93602** Intra-atrial recording
➔ *CPT Assistant* Summer 94:12, Aug 97:9, Apr 04:9, Jul 04:13, Aug 05:13

⊘ **93603** Right ventricular recording
➔ *CPT Assistant* Summer 94:12, Aug 97:9, Apr 04:9, Jul 04:13, Aug 05:13

⊙✚ **93609** Intraventricular and/or intra-atrial mapping of tachycardia site(s) with catheter manipulation to record from multiple sites to identify origin of tachycardia (List separately in addition to code for primary procedure)
➔ *CPT Assistant* Summer 94:12, Aug 97:9, Apr 04:9, Aug 05:13; *CPT Changes: An Insider's View* 2002

(Use 93609 in conjunction with 93620, 93651, 93652)

(Do not report 93609 in addition to 93613)

⊘ **93610** Intra-atrial pacing
➔ *CPT Assistant* Summer 94:12, Aug 97:9, Apr 04:9, Jul 04:13

⊘ **93612** Intraventricular pacing
➔ *CPT Assistant* Summer 94:12, Aug 97:9, Apr 04:9, Jul 04:13

(Do not report 93612 in conjunction with 93620-93622)

⊙✚ **93613** Intracardiac electrophysiologic 3-dimensional mapping (List separately in addition to code for primary procedure)
➔ *CPT Assistant* Apr 04:8, Aug 05:13; *CPT Changes: An Insider's View* 2002

(Use 93613 in conjunction with 93620, 93651, 93652)

(Do not report 93613 in addition to 93609)

⊙⊘ **93615** Esophageal recording of atrial electrogram with or without ventricular electrogram(s);
➔ *CPT Assistant* Summer 94:12, Aug 97:9, Apr 04:9, Aug 05:13

⊙⊘ **93616** with pacing
➔ *CPT Assistant* Summer 94:12, Aug 97:9, Apr 04:9, Aug 05:13

⊙⊘ **93618** Induction of arrhythmia by electrical pacing
➔ *CPT Assistant* Summer 94:12, Aug 97:9, Oct 97:10, Apr 99:10, Jun 00:5, Nov 00:9, Apr 04:9, Jul 04:13, Aug 05:13

(For intracardiac phonocardiogram, use 93799)

⊙▲ **93619** Comprehensive electrophysiologic evaluation with right atrial pacing and recording, right ventricular pacing and recording, His bundle recording, including insertion and repositioning of multiple electrode catheters, without induction or attempted induction of arrhythmia
➔ *CPT Assistant* Aug 97:9, Oct 97:10, Nov 00:9, Apr 04:9, Jul 04:13, Aug 05:13; *CPT Changes: An Insider's View* 2002, 2008

(Do not report 93619 in conjunction with 93600, 93602, 93610, 93612, 93618, or 93620-93622)

⊙▲ **93620** Comprehensive electrophysiologic evaluation including insertion and repositioning of multiple electrode catheters with induction or attempted induction of arrhythmia; with right atrial pacing and recording, right ventricular pacing and recording, His bundle recording
➔ *CPT Assistant* Summer 94:12, Aug 97:9, Oct 97:10, Jul 98:10, Aug 98:7, Nov 00:9, Apr 04:9, Jul 04:13, Aug 05:13; *CPT Changes: An Insider's View* 2002, 2003, 2008

(Do not report 93620 in conjunction with 93600, 93602, 93610, 93612, 93618 or 93619)

⊙✚ **93621** with left atrial pacing and recording from coronary sinus or left atrium (List separately in addition to code for primary procedure)
➔ *CPT Assistant* Summer 94:12, Aug 97:9, Oct 97:10, Jul 98:10, Aug 98:7, Nov 98:34, Nov 00:9, Apr 04:9, Jul 04:13, Aug 05:13; *CPT Changes: An Insider's View* 2002

(Use 93621 in conjunction with 93620)

⊙✚ **93622** with left ventricular pacing and recording (List separately in addition to code for primary procedure)
➔ *CPT Assistant* Summer 94:14, Aug 97:9, Oct 97:10, Jul 98:10, Aug 98:7, Nov 98:34, Nov 00:9, Apr 04:9, Jul 04:13, Aug 05:13; *CPT Changes: An Insider's View* 2002

(Use 93622 in conjunction with 93620)

+ 93623 Programmed stimulation and pacing after intravenous drug infusion (List separately in addition to code for primary procedure)

➔ *CPT Assistant* Summer 94:14, Aug 97:9, Nov 00:9, Aug 05:13

(Use 93623 in conjunction with 93619, 93620)

⊙▲ 93624 Electrophysiologic follow-up study with pacing and recording to test effectiveness of therapy, including induction or attempted induction of arrhythmia

➔ *CPT Assistant* Summer 94:14, Aug 97:9, Nov 00:9, Aug 05:13; *CPT Changes: An Insider's View* 2008

⊘ 93631 Intra-operative epicardial and endocardial pacing and mapping to localize the site of tachycardia or zone of slow conduction for surgical correction

➔ *CPT Assistant* Summer 94:14, Aug 97:9, Nov 00:9, Aug 05:13

⊙▲ 93640 Electrophysiologic evaluation of single or dual chamber pacing cardioverter-defibrillator leads including defibrillation threshold evaluation (induction of arrhythmia, evaluation of sensing and pacing for arrhythmia termination) at time of initial implantation or replacement;

➔ *CPT Assistant* Summer 94:14, Aug 97:9, Apr 99:10, Nov 99:50, Nov 00:9, Aug 05:13; *CPT Changes: An Insider's View* 2000, 2008

⊙▲ 93641 with testing of single or dual chamber pacing cardioverter-defibrillator pulse generator

➔ *CPT Assistant* Summer 94:14, Aug 97:9, Apr 99:10, Nov 99:50, Jun 00:5, Jul 00:5, Nov 00:9, Aug 05:13; *CPT Changes: An Insider's View* 2000, 2008

(For subsequent or periodic electronic analysis and/or reprogramming of single or dual chamber pacing cardioverter-defibrillators, see 93642, 93741-93744)

⊙▲ 93642 Electrophysiologic evaluation of single or dual chamber pacing cardioverter-defibrillator (includes defibrillation threshold evaluation, induction of arrhythmia, evaluation of sensing and pacing for arrhythmia termination, and programming or reprogramming of sensing or therapeutic parameters)

➔ *CPT Assistant* Summer 94:14, Aug 97:9, Nov 99:50, Jun 00:5, Nov 00:9, Aug 05:13; *CPT Changes: An Insider's View* 2000, 2008

⊙▲ 93650 Intracardiac catheter ablation of atrioventricular node function, atrioventricular conduction for creation of complete heart block, with or without temporary pacemaker placement

➔ *CPT Assistant* Summer 94:15, Aug 97:9, Nov 00:9, Aug 05:13; *CPT Changes: An Insider's View* 2008

⊙▲ 93651 Intracardiac catheter ablation of arrhythmogenic focus; for treatment of supraventricular tachycardia by ablation of fast or slow atrioventricular pathways, accessory atrioventricular connections or other atrial foci, singly or in combination

➔ *CPT Assistant* Summer 94:15, Aug 97:9, Nov 00:9, Aug 05:13; *CPT Changes: An Insider's View* 2008

⊙▲ 93652 for treatment of ventricular tachycardia

➔ *CPT Assistant* Summer 94:15, Aug 97:9, Nov 00:9, Aug 05:13; *CPT Changes: An Insider's View* 2008

▲ 93660 Evaluation of cardiovascular function with tilt table evaluation, with continuous ECG monitoring and intermittent blood pressure monitoring, with or without pharmacological intervention

➔ *CPT Changes: An Insider's View* 2008

(For testing of autonomic nervous system function, see 95921-95923)

+ 93662 Intracardiac echocardiography during therapeutic/diagnostic intervention, including imaging supervision and interpretation (List separately in addition to code for primary procedure)

➔ *CPT Assistant* Mar 03:23; *CPT Changes: An Insider's View* 2001

(Use 93662 in conjunction with 92987, 93527, 93532, 93580, 93581, 93621, 93622, 93651, or 93652, as appropriate)

(Do not report 92961 in addition to 93662)

Peripheral Arterial Disease Rehabilitation

Peripheral arterial disease (PAD) rehabilitative physical exercise consists of a series of sessions, lasting 45-60 minutes per session, involving use of either a motorized treadmill or a track to permit each patient to achieve symptom-limited claudication. Each session is supervised by an exercise physiologist or nurse. The supervising provider monitors the individual patient's claudication threshold and other cardiovascular limitations for adjustment of workload. During this supervised rehabilitation program, the development of new arrhythmias, symptoms that might suggest angina or the continued inability of the patient to progress to an adequate level of exercise may require physician review and examination of the patient. These physician services would be separately reported with an appropriate level E/M service code.

93668 Peripheral arterial disease (PAD) rehabilitation, per session

➔ *CPT Changes: An Insider's View* 2001

Noninvasive Physiologic Studies and Procedures

(For arterial cannulization and recording of direct arterial pressure, use 36620)

(For radiographic injection procedures, see 36000-36299)

(For vascular cannulization for hemodialysis, see 36800-36821)

(For chemotherapy for malignant disease, see 96409-96549)

(For penile plethysmography, use 54240)

93701 Bioimpedance, thoracic, electrical

➔ *CPT Assistant* Mar 02:3; *CPT Changes: An Insider's View* 2002

93720   Plethysmography, total body; with interpretation and report

➔ *CPT Assistant* Mar 99:10, Sep 03:15

93721   tracing only, without interpretation and report

➔ *CPT Assistant* Mar 99:10

93722   interpretation and report only

➔ *CPT Assistant* Mar 99:10

(For regional plethysmography, see 93875-93931)

93724   Electronic analysis of antitachycardia pacemaker system (includes electrocardiographic recording, programming of device, induction and termination of tachycardia via implanted pacemaker, and interpretation of recordings)

➔ *CPT Assistant* Summer 94:23

93727   Electronic analysis of implantable loop recorder (ILR) system (includes retrieval of recorded and stored ECG data, physician review and interpretation of retrieved ECG data and reprogramming)

➔ *CPT Assistant* Nov 99:50, Jul 00:5; *CPT Changes: An Insider's View* 2000

93731   Electronic analysis of dual-chamber pacemaker system (includes evaluation of programmable parameters at rest and during activity where applicable, using electrocardiographic recording and interpretation of recordings at rest and during exercise, analysis of event markers and device response); without reprogramming

➔ *CPT Assistant* Summer 94:23, Feb 98:11

93732   with reprogramming

➔ *CPT Assistant* Summer 94:23, Feb 98:11, Mar 00:10

93733   Electronic analysis of dual chamber internal pacemaker system (may include rate, pulse amplitude and duration, configuration of wave form, and/or testing of sensory function of pacemaker), telephonic analysis

➔ *CPT Assistant* Summer 94:23

93734   Electronic analysis of single chamber pacemaker system (includes evaluation of programmable parameters at rest and during activity where applicable, using electrocardiographic recording and interpretation of recordings at rest and during exercise, analysis of event markers and device response); without reprogramming

➔ *CPT Assistant* Summer 94:23, Feb 98:11

93735   with reprogramming

➔ *CPT Assistant* Summer 94:23, Feb 98:11

93736   Electronic analysis of single chamber internal pacemaker system (may include rate, pulse amplitude and duration, configuration of wave form, and/or testing of sensory function of pacemaker), telephonic analysis

➔ *CPT Assistant* Summer 94:23

93740   Temperature gradient studies

93741   Electronic analysis of pacing cardioverter-defibrillator (includes interrogation, evaluation of pulse generator status, evaluation of programmable parameters at rest and during activity where applicable, using electrocardiographic recording and interpretation of recordings at rest and during exercise, analysis of event markers and device response); single chamber or wearable cardioverter-defibrillator system, without reprogramming

➔ *CPT Assistant* Nov 99:50-51, Jul 00:5, Nov 00:9, Sep 05:8; *CPT Changes: An Insider's View* 2000, 2005

(Do not report 93741 in conjunction with 93745)

93742   single chamber or wearable cardioverter-defibrillator system, with reprogramming

➔ *CPT Assistant* Nov 99:50-51, Jul 00:5, Nov 00:9; *CPT Changes: An Insider's View* 2000, 2005

(Do not report 93742 in conjunction with 93745)

93743   dual chamber, without reprogramming

➔ *CPT Assistant* Nov 99:50-51, Jul 00:5, Nov 00:9, Sep 05:8; *CPT Changes: An Insider's View* 2000

93744   dual chamber, with reprogramming

➔ *CPT Assistant* Nov 99:50-51, Jul 00:5, Nov 00:9; *CPT Changes: An Insider's View* 2000

93745   Initial set-up and programming by a physician of wearable cardioverter-defibrillator includes initial programming of system, establishing baseline electronic ECG, transmission of data to data repository, patient instruction in wearing system and patient reporting of problems or events

➔ *CPT Changes: An Insider's View* 2005

(Do not report 93745 in conjunction with 93741, 93742)

93760   Thermogram; cephalic

93762   peripheral

93770   Determination of venous pressure

(For central venous cannulization see 36555-36556, 36500)

93784   Ambulatory blood pressure monitoring, utilizing a system such as magnetic tape and/or computer disk, for 24 hours or longer; including recording, scanning analysis, interpretation and report

93786   recording only

93788   scanning analysis with report

93790   physician review with interpretation and report

Other Procedures

93797   Physician services for outpatient cardiac rehabilitation; without continuous ECG monitoring (per session)

93798   with continuous ECG monitoring (per session)

93799   Unlisted cardiovascular service or procedure

➔ *CPT Assistant* Mar 98:11, Mar 02:10, Nov 05:15

Noninvasive Vascular Diagnostic Studies

Vascular studies include patient care required to perform the studies, supervision of the studies and interpretation of study results with copies for patient records of hard copy output with analysis of all data, including bidirectional vascular flow or imaging when provided.

The use of a simple hand-held or other Doppler device that does not produce hard copy output, or that produces a record that does not permit analysis of bidirectional vascular flow, is considered to be part of the physical examination of the vascular system and is not separately reported.

▶*Duplex scan* (eg, 93880, 93882) describes an ultrasonic scanning procedure for characterizing the pattern and direction of blood flow in arteries or veins with the production of real-time images integrating B-mode two-dimensional vascular structure, Doppler spectral analysis, and color flow Doppler imaging.◀

Noninvasive physiologic studies are performed using equipment separate and distinct from the duplex scanner. Codes 93875, 93965, 93922, 93923, and 93924 describe the evaluation of non-imaging physiologic recordings of pressures, Doppler analysis of bi-directional blood flow, plethysmography, and/or oxygen tension measurements appropriate for the anatomic area studied.

Cerebrovascular Arterial Studies

A complete transcranial Doppler (TCD) study (93886) includes ultrasound evaluation of the right and left anterior circulation territories and the posterior circulation territory (to include vertebral arteries and basilar artery). In a limited TCD study (93888) there is ultrasound evaluation of two or fewer of these territories. For TCD, ultrasound evaluation is a reasonable and concerted attempt to identify arterial signals through an acoustic window.

93875   Noninvasive physiologic studies of extracranial arteries, complete bilateral study (eg, periorbital flow direction with arterial compression, ocular pneumoplethysmography, Doppler ultrasound spectral analysis)
> *CPT Assistant* Jun 96:9, Dec 97:10, Dec 05:3
> *Clinical Examples in Radiology* Spring 07:5-6

93880   Duplex scan of extracranial arteries; complete bilateral study
> *CPT Assistant* Jun 96:9, Dec 05:3

93882   unilateral or limited study
> *CPT Assistant* Jun 96:9, Dec 05:3

(To report common carotid intima-media thickness (IMT) study for evaluation of atherosclerotic burden or coronary heart disease risk factor assessment, use Category III code 0126T)

93886   Transcranial Doppler study of the intracranial arteries; complete study
> *CPT Assistant* Jun 96:9, Dec 05:3

93888   limited study
> *CPT Assistant* Jun 96:9, Dec 05:3

93890   vasoreactivity study
> *CPT Assistant* Dec 05:3; *CPT Changes: An Insider's View* 2005

93892   emboli detection without intravenous microbubble injection
> *CPT Assistant* Dec 05:3; *CPT Changes: An Insider's View* 2005

93893   emboli detection with intravenous microbubble injection
> *CPT Assistant* Dec 05:3; *CPT Changes: An Insider's View* 2005

(Do not report 93890-93893 in conjunction with 93888)

Extremity Arterial Studies (Including Digits)

93922   Noninvasive physiologic studies of upper or lower extremity arteries, single level, bilateral (eg, ankle/brachial indices, Doppler waveform analysis, volume plethysmography, transcutaneous oxygen tension measurement)
> *CPT Assistant* Jun 96:9, Dec 05:3

93923   Noninvasive physiologic studies of upper or lower extremity arteries, multiple levels or with provocative functional maneuvers, complete bilateral study (eg, segmental blood pressure measurements, segmental Doppler waveform analysis, segmental volume plethysmography, segmental transcutaneous oxygen tension measurements, measurements with postural provocative tests, measurements with reactive hyperemia)
> *CPT Assistant* Jun 96:9, Jun 01:10, Dec 05:3

93924   Noninvasive physiologic studies of lower extremity arteries, at rest and following treadmill stress testing, complete bilateral study
> *CPT Assistant* Jun 96:9, Dec 05:3

93925   Duplex scan of lower extremity arteries or arterial bypass grafts; complete bilateral study
> *CPT Assistant* Jun 96:9, Dec 05:3

93926   unilateral or limited study
> *CPT Assistant* Jun 96:9, Oct 01:2, Dec 05:3

93930   Duplex scan of upper extremity arteries or arterial bypass grafts; complete bilateral study
> *CPT Assistant* Jun 96:9, Dec 05:3

93931   unilateral or limited study
> *CPT Assistant* Jun 96:9, Oct 01:2, Dec 05:3

Extremity Venous Studies (Including Digits)

93965 Noninvasive physiologic studies of extremity veins, complete bilateral study (eg, Doppler waveform analysis with responses to compression and other maneuvers, phleborheography, impedance plethysmography)
➔ *CPT Assistant* Jun 96:9, Dec 05:3; *CPT Changes: An Insider's View* 2007

93970 Duplex scan of extremity veins including responses to compression and other maneuvers; complete bilateral study
➔ *CPT Assistant* Jun 96:9, Dec 05:3

93971 unilateral or limited study
➔ *CPT Assistant* Jun 96:9, Oct 01:2, Mar 03:21, Dec 05:3

Visceral and Penile Vascular Studies

93975 Duplex scan of arterial inflow and venous outflow of abdominal, pelvic, scrotal contents and/or retroperitoneal organs; complete study
➔ *CPT Assistant* Apr 96:11, Jun 96:9, Dec 05:3

93976 limited study
➔ *CPT Assistant* Apr 96:11, Jun 96:9, Dec 05:3

93978 Duplex scan of aorta, inferior vena cava, iliac vasculature, or bypass grafts; complete study
➔ *CPT Assistant* Jun 96:9, Dec 05:3
➔ *Clinical Examples in Radiology* Spring 07:5-6

93979 unilateral or limited study
➔ *CPT Assistant* Jun 96:9, Dec 05:3

93980 Duplex scan of arterial inflow and venous outflow of penile vessels; complete study
➔ *CPT Assistant* Jun 96:9, Dec 05:3

93981 follow-up or limited study
➔ *CPT Assistant* Jun 96:9, Dec 05:3

● **93982** Noninvasive physiologic study of implanted wireless pressure sensor in aneurysmal sac following endovascular repair, complete study including recording, analysis of pressure and waveform tracings, interpretation and report
➔ *CPT Changes: An Insider's View* 2008

▶(Do not report 93982 in conjunction with 34806)◀

Extremity Arterial-Venous Studies

93990 Duplex scan of hemodialysis access (including arterial inflow, body of access and venous outflow)
➔ *CPT Assistant* Jun 96:9, Dec 05:3
➔ *Clinical Examples in Radiology* Spring 07:5-6

(For measurement of hemodialysis access flow using indicator dilution methods, use 90940)

Pulmonary

Ventilator Management

94002 Ventilation assist and management, initiation of pressure or volume preset ventilators for assisted or controlled breathing; hospital inpatient/observation, initial day
➔ *CPT Changes: An Insider's View* 2007

94003 hospital inpatient/observation, each subsequent day
➔ *CPT Changes: An Insider's View* 2007

94004 nursing facility, per day
➔ *CPT Changes: An Insider's View* 2007

(Do not report 94002-94004 in conjunction with Evaluation and Management services 99201-99499)

94005 Home ventilator management care plan oversight of a patient (patient not present) in home, domiciliary or rest home (eg, assisted living) requiring review of status, review of laboratories and other studies and revision of orders and respiratory care plan (as appropriate), within a calendar month, 30 minutes or more
➔ *CPT Changes: An Insider's View* 2007

(Do not report 94005 in conjunction with 99339, 99340, 99374-99378)

(Ventilator management care plan oversight is reported separately from home or domiciliary, rest home [eg, assisted living] services. A physician may report 94005, when performed, including when a different physician reports 99339, 99340, 99374-99378 for the same 30 days)

Other Procedures

Codes 94010-94799 include laboratory procedure(s) and interpretation of test results. If a separate identifiable Evaluation and Management service is performed, the appropriate E/M service code should be reported in addition to 94010-94799.
➔ *CPT Assistant* Summer 95:4, Feb 96:9, Mar 96:10, Jan 99:8, Feb 99:9

94010 Spirometry, including graphic record, total and timed vital capacity, expiratory flow rate measurement(s), with or without maximal voluntary ventilation
➔ *CPT Assistant* Summer 91:16, Summer 95:4, Feb 96:9, Nov 97:45, Nov 98:35, Feb 99:9, Aug 03:15, Jul 05:11

94014 Patient-initiated spirometric recording per 30-day period of time; includes reinforced education, transmission of spirometric tracing, data capture, analysis of transmitted data, periodic recalibration and physician review and interpretation
➔ *CPT Assistant* Summer 95:4, Nov 98:34, Jan 99:8, Jul 05:11; *CPT Changes: An Insider's View* 2000

94015 recording (includes hook-up, reinforced education, data transmission, data capture, trend analysis, and periodic recalibration)
➔ *CPT Assistant* Summer 95:4, Nov 98:34, Jan 99:8, Jul 05:11

94016 physician review and interpretation only
➔ *CPT Assistant* Summer 95:4, Nov 98:34, Jan 99:8, Jul 05:11

94060 Bronchodilation responsiveness, spirometry as in 94010, pre- and post-bronchodilator administration

➔ *CPT Assistant* Summer 95:4, Feb 96:9, Feb 97:10, Nov 98:34, Jan 99:8, Feb 99:9, Jul 05:11; *CPT Changes: An Insider's View* 2005

(Report bronchodilator supply separately with 99070 or appropriate supply code)

(For prolonged exercise test for bronchospasm with pre- and post-spirometry, use 94620)

94070 Bronchospasm provocation evaluation, multiple spirometric determinations as in 94010, with administered agents (eg, antigen[s], cold air, methacholine)

➔ *CPT Assistant* Summer 91:16, Summer 95:4, Feb 96:9, Nov 97:45, Jan 99:8, Jul 05:11; *CPT Changes: An Insider's View* 2005

(Report antigen[s] administration separately with 99070 or appropriate supply code)

94150 Vital capacity, total (separate procedure)

➔ *CPT Assistant* Summer 95:4, Feb 96:9, Jul 05:11

94200 Maximum breathing capacity, maximal voluntary ventilation

➔ *CPT Assistant* Summer 95:4, Feb 96:9, Aug 03:15, Jul 05:11

94240 Functional residual capacity or residual volume: helium method, nitrogen open circuit method, or other method

➔ *CPT Assistant* Summer 95:4, Feb 96:9, Jul 05:11

94250 Expired gas collection, quantitative, single procedure (separate procedure)

➔ *CPT Assistant* Summer 95:4, Feb 96:9, Jul 05:11

94260 Thoracic gas volume

➔ *CPT Assistant* Summer 95:4, Feb 96:9, Jul 05:11

(For plethysmography, see 93720-93722)

94350 Determination of maldistribution of inspired gas: multiple breath nitrogen washout curve including alveolar nitrogen or helium equilibration time

➔ *CPT Assistant* Summer 95:4, Feb 96:9, Jul 05:11

94360 Determination of resistance to airflow, oscillatory or plethysmographic methods

➔ *CPT Assistant* Summer 95:4, Feb 96:9, Jul 05:11

94370 Determination of airway closing volume, single breath tests

➔ *CPT Assistant* Summer 95:4, Feb 96:9, Jul 05:11

94375 Respiratory flow volume loop

➔ *CPT Assistant* Summer 95:4, Feb 96:9, Oct 03:2, Jul 05:11, Jul 06:4

94400 Breathing response to CO_2 (CO_2 response curve)

➔ *CPT Assistant* Summer 95:4, Feb 96:9, Jul 05:11

94450 Breathing response to hypoxia (hypoxia response curve)

➔ *CPT Assistant* Summer 95:4, Feb 96:9, Jul 05:11

(For high altitude simulation test [HAST], see 94452, 94453)

94452 High altitude simulation test (HAST), with physician interpretation and report;

➔ *CPT Assistant* Jul 05:11; *CPT Changes: An Insider's View* 2005

(For obtaining arterial blood gases, use 36600)

(Do not report 94452 in conjunction with 94453, 94760, 94761)

94453 with supplemental oxygen titration

➔ *CPT Assistant* Jul 05:11; *CPT Changes: An Insider's View* 2005

(For obtaining arterial blood gases, use 36600)

(Do not report 94453 in conjunction with 94452, 94760, 94761)

⊘ **94610** Intrapulmonary surfactant administration by a physician through endotracheal tube

➔ *CPT Changes: An Insider's View* 2007

(Do not report 94610 in conjunction with 99293-99296)

(For endotracheal intubation, use 31500)

(Report 94610 once per dosing episode)

94620 Pulmonary stress testing; simple (eg, 6-minute walk test, prolonged exercise test for bronchospasm with pre- and post-spirometry and oximetry)

➔ *CPT Assistant* Summer 95:4, Feb 96:9, Nov 98:35, Jan 99:8, Mar 04:10, Jul 05:11, 13, Apr 07:3; *CPT Changes: An Insider's View* 2007

94621 complex (including measurements of CO_2 production, O_2 uptake, and electrocardiographic recordings)

➔ *CPT Assistant* Summer 95:4, Nov 98:35, Jan 99:8, Aug 02:10, Jul 05:11

94640 Pressurized or nonpressurized inhalation treatment for acute airway obstruction or for sputum induction for diagnostic purposes (eg, with an aerosol generator, nebulizer, metered dose inhaler or intermittent positive pressure breathing [IPPB] device)

➔ *CPT Assistant* Summer 95:4, Feb 96:9, May 98:10, Apr 00:11, Jul 05:11, Apr 07:3; *CPT Changes: An Insider's View* 2003

(For more than 1 inhalation treatment performed on the same date, append modifier 76)

(For continuous inhalation treatment of 1 hour or more, see 94644, 94645)

94642 Aerosol inhalation of pentamidine for pneumocystis carinii pneumonia treatment or prophylaxis

➔ *CPT Assistant* Summer 95:4, Feb 96:9, Jul 05:11

94644 Continuous inhalation treatment with aerosol medication for acute airway obstruction; first hour

➔ *CPT Changes: An Insider's View* 2007

(For services of less than 1 hour, use 94640)

+ **94645** each additional hour (List separately in addition to code for primary procedure)

➔ *CPT Changes: An Insider's View* 2007

(Use 94645 in conjunction with 94644)

(94656, 94657 have been deleted. To report, see 94002-94005)

94660 Continuous positive airway pressure ventilation (CPAP), initiation and management
➔ *CPT Assistant* Fall 92:30, Spring 95:4, Summer 95:4, Feb 96:9, Jan 99:10, Aug 00:2, Oct 03:2, Jul 05:11, Jul 06:4, Feb 07:10

94662 Continuous negative pressure ventilation (CNP), initiation and management
➔ *CPT Assistant* Fall 92:30, Spring 94:4, Summer 95:4, Feb 96:9, Aug 00:2, Jul 05:11, Feb 07:10

94664 Demonstration and/or evaluation of patient utilization of an aerosol generator, nebulizer, metered dose inhaler or IPPB device
➔ *CPT Assistant* Summer 95:4, Feb 96:9, May 98:10, Apr 00:11, Jul 05:11; *CPT Changes: An Insider's View* 2003

(94664 can be reported one time only per day of service)

94667 Manipulation chest wall, such as cupping, percussing, and vibration to facilitate lung function; initial demonstration and/or evaluation
➔ *CPT Assistant* Summer 95:4, Feb 96:9, Jul 05:11

94668 subsequent
➔ *CPT Assistant* Summer 95:4, Feb 96:9, Jul 05:11

94680 Oxygen uptake, expired gas analysis; rest and exercise, direct, simple
➔ *CPT Assistant* Summer 95:4, Feb 96:9, Jul 05:11

94681 including CO_2 output, percentage oxygen extracted
➔ *CPT Assistant* Summer 95:4, Feb 96:9, Jul 05:11

94690 rest, indirect (separate procedure)
➔ *CPT Assistant* Summer 95:4, Feb 96:9, Jul 05:11

(For single arterial puncture, use 36600)

94720 Carbon monoxide diffusing capacity (eg, single breath, steady state)
➔ *CPT Assistant* Summer 95:4, Feb 96:9, Jul 05:11; *CPT Changes: An Insider's View* 2002

94725 Membrane diffusion capacity
➔ *CPT Assistant* Summer 95:4, Feb 96:9, Jul 05:11

94750 Pulmonary compliance study (eg, plethysmography, volume and pressure measurements)
➔ *CPT Assistant* Summer 95:4, Feb 96:9, Jul 05:11; *CPT Changes: An Insider's View* 2002

94760 Noninvasive ear or pulse oximetry for oxygen saturation; single determination
➔ *CPT Assistant* Summer 95:4, Feb 96:9, Feb 97:10, Jul 98:2, Oct 03:2, Jul 05:11, Feb 06:9, Jul 06:4, Feb 07:10, Apr 07:1

(For blood gases, see 82803-82810)

94761 multiple determinations (eg, during exercise)
➔ *CPT Assistant* Summer 95:4, Feb 96:9, Jul 98:2, Jun 99:10, Jul 05:11, Feb 06:9, Jul 06:4, Feb 07:10, Apr 07:1

94762 by continuous overnight monitoring (separate procedure)
➔ *CPT Assistant* Summer 95:4, Feb 96:9, Jul 98:2, Oct 03:2, Jul 05:11, Feb 06:9, Jul 06:4, Feb 07:10, Apr 07:1

94770 Carbon dioxide, expired gas determination by infrared analyzer
➔ *CPT Assistant* Summer 95:4, Feb 96:9, Jul 05:11

(For bronchoscopy, see 31622-31656)

(For placement of flow directed catheter, use 93503)

(For venipuncture, use 36410)

(For central venous catheter placement, see 36555-36556)

(For arterial puncture, use 36600)

(For arterial catheterization, use 36620)

▶(For thoracentesis, use 32421)◀

(For phlebotomy, therapeutic, use 99195)

(For lung biopsy, needle, use 32405)

(For intubation, orotracheal or nasotracheal, use 31500)

94772 Circadian respiratory pattern recording (pediatric pneumogram), 12-24 hour continuous recording, infant
➔ *CPT Assistant* Summer 95:4, Feb 96:9, Jul 05:11

(Separate procedure codes for electromyograms, EEG, ECG, and recordings of respiration are excluded when 94772 is reported)

94774 Pediatric home apnea monitoring event recording including respiratory rate, pattern and heart rate per 30-day period of time; includes monitor attachment, download of data, physician review, interpretation, and preparation of a report
➔ *CPT Changes: An Insider's View* 2007

(Do not report 94774 in conjunction with 94775-94777 during the same reporting period)

94775 monitor attachment only (includes hook-up, initiation of recording and disconnection)
➔ *CPT Changes: An Insider's View* 2007

94776 monitoring, download of information, receipt of transmission(s) and analyses by computer only
➔ *CPT Changes: An Insider's View* 2007

94777 physician review, interpretation and preparation of report only
➔ *CPT Changes: An Insider's View* 2007

(When oxygen saturation monitoring is used in addition to heart rate and respiratory monitoring, it is not reported separately)

(Do not report 94774-94777 in conjunction with 93224-93272)

(Do not report apnea recording device separately)

(For sleep study, see 95805-95811)

94799 Unlisted pulmonary service or procedure
➔ *CPT Assistant* Summer 95:4, Feb 96:9, Mar 96:10, Jul 05:11

Allergy and Clinical Immunology

Definitions

Immunotherapy (desensitization, hyposensitization) is the parenteral administration of allergenic extracts as antigens at periodic intervals, usually on an increasing dosage scale to a dosage which is maintained as maintenance therapy. Indications for immunotherapy are determined by appropriate diagnostic procedures coordinated with clinical judgment and knowledge of the natural history of allergic diseases.

Other therapy: for medical conferences on the use of mechanical and electronic devices (precipitators, air conditioners, air filters, humidifiers, dehumidifiers), climatotherapy, physical therapy, occupational and recreational therapy, see **Evaluation and Management** section.

▶Do not report Evaluation and Management (E/M) services for test interpretation and report. If a significant separately identifiable E/M service is performed, the appropriate E/M service code should be reported using modifier 25.◀

Allergy Testing

(For allergy laboratory tests, see 86000-86999)

(For therapy for severe or intractable allergic disease, see 90765-90768, 90772, 90774, 90775)

▲ **95004** Percutaneous tests (scratch, puncture, prick) with allergenic extracts, immediate type reaction, including test interpretation and report by a physician, specify number of tests
➔ *CPT Assistant* Summer 91:15; *CPT Changes: An Insider's View* 2007, 2008

95010 Percutaneous tests (scratch, puncture, prick) sequential and incremental, with drugs, biologicals or venoms, immediate type reaction, specify number of tests
➔ *CPT Assistant* Summer 91:15

95012 Nitric oxide expired gas determination
➔ *CPT Changes: An Insider's View* 2007

(For nitric oxide determination by spectroscopy, use Category III code 0064T)

95015 Intracutaneous (intradermal) tests, sequential and incremental, with drugs, biologicals, or venoms, immediate type reaction, specify number of tests
➔ *CPT Assistant* Summer 91:15; *CPT Changes: An Insider's View* 2003

▲ **95024** Intracutaneous (intradermal) tests with allergenic extracts, immediate type reaction, including test interpretation and report by a physician, specify number of tests
➔ *CPT Assistant* Summer 91:15; *CPT Changes: An Insider's View* 2003, 2008

▲ **95027** Intracutaneous (intradermal) tests, sequential and incremental, with allergenic extracts for airborne allergens, immediate type reaction, including test interpretation and report by a physician, specify number of tests
➔ *CPT Assistant* Summer 91:15, Jun 97:10; *CPT Changes: An Insider's View* 2003, 2008

95028 Intracutaneous (intradermal) tests with allergenic extracts, delayed type reaction, including reading, specify number of tests
➔ *CPT Assistant* Summer 91:14; *CPT Changes: An Insider's View* 2003

95044 Patch or application test(s) (specify number of tests)
➔ *CPT Assistant* Summer 91:15, Spring 94:31

95052 Photo patch test(s) (specify number of tests)
➔ *CPT Assistant* Spring 94:31

95056 Photo tests
➔ *CPT Assistant* Summer 91:16

95060 Ophthalmic mucous membrane tests
➔ *CPT Assistant* Summer 91:16

95065 Direct nasal mucous membrane test
➔ *CPT Assistant* Summer 91:15

95070 Inhalation bronchial challenge testing (not including necessary pulmonary function tests); with histamine, methacholine, or similar compounds
➔ *CPT Assistant* Summer 91:16

95071 with antigens or gases, specify
➔ *CPT Assistant* Summer 91:16

(For pulmonary function tests, see 94060, 94070)

95075 Ingestion challenge test (sequential and incremental ingestion of test items, eg, food, drug or other substance such as metabisulfite)
➔ *CPT Assistant* Summer 91:16, Sep 01:10, Oct 02:11

(95078 has been deleted)

Allergen Immunotherapy

Codes 95115-95199 include the professional services necessary for allergen immunotherapy. Office visit codes may be used in addition to allergen immunotherapy if other identifiable services are provided at that time.

95115 Professional services for allergen immunotherapy not including provision of allergenic extracts; single injection
➔ *CPT Assistant* Fall 91:19, Spring 94:30, Summer 95:4, Summer 95:4, May 96:1, Nov 98:35, Apr 00:4, Feb 05:10-12, Nov 05:1, Nov 06:23

95117 two or more injections
➔ *CPT Assistant* Fall 91:19, Spring 94:30, Summer 95:4, May 96:1, Aug 96:10, Nov 98:35, Apr 00:4, Feb 05:10-12, Nov 05:1, Nov 06:23

95120   Professional services for allergen immunotherapy in prescribing physicians office or institution, including provision of allergenic extract; single injection

➜ *CPT Assistant* Fall 91:19, Spring 94:30, Summer 95:4, May 96:2, Nov 98:35, Feb 05:10-12

95125   two or more injections

➜ *CPT Assistant* Fall 91:19, Spring 94:30, Summer 95:4, May 96:2, Aug 96:10, Nov 98:35, Feb 05:10, 12

95130   single stinging insect venom

➜ *CPT Assistant* Fall 91:19, Summer 95:4, May 96:2, Jun 96:10, Nov 98:35, Sep 99:10, Feb 05:10, 12

95131   two stinging insect venoms

➜ *CPT Assistant* Fall 91:19, Summer 95:4, May 96:2, Jun 96:10, Nov 98:35, Sep 99:10, Feb 05:10, 12

95132   three stinging insect venoms

➜ *CPT Assistant* Fall 91:19, Summer 95:4, May 96:2, Nov 98:35, Sep 99:11, Feb 05:10, 12

95133   four stinging insect venoms

➜ *CPT Assistant* Fall 91:19, Summer 95:4, May 96:2, Nov 98:35, Sep 99:11, Feb 05:10, 12

95134   five stinging insect venoms

➜ *CPT Assistant* Fall 91:19, Summer 95:4, May 96:2, Nov 98:35, Sep 99:11, Feb 05:10, 12

95144   Professional services for the supervision of preparation and provision of antigens for allergen immunotherapy, single dose vial(s) (specify number of vials)

➜ *CPT Assistant* Fall 91:19, Spring 94:30, Summer 95:4, May 96:11, Nov 98:35, Feb 05:10-11; *CPT Changes: An Insider's View* 2002

(A single dose vial contains a single dose of antigen administered in one injection)

95145   Professional services for the supervision of preparation and provision of antigens for allergen immunotherapy (specify number of doses); single stinging insect venom

➜ *CPT Assistant* Fall 91:19, Summer 95:4, May 96:11, Nov 98:35, Feb 05:10-12; *CPT Changes: An Insider's View* 2002

95146   two single stinging insect venoms

➜ *CPT Assistant* Fall 91:19, Summer 95:4, May 96:11, Nov 98:35, Feb 05:10-12

95147   three single stinging insect venoms

➜ *CPT Assistant* Fall 91:19, Summer 95:4, May 96:11, Nov 98:35, Feb 05:10-12

95148   four single stinging insect venoms

➜ *CPT Assistant* Fall 91:19, Summer 95:4, May 96:11, Nov 98:35, Feb 05:10-12

95149   five single stinging insect venoms

➜ *CPT Assistant* Fall 91:19, Summer 95:4, May 96:11, Nov 98:35, Feb 05:10-12

95165   Professional services for the supervision of preparation and provision of antigens for allergen immunotherapy; single or multiple antigens (specify number of doses)

➜ *CPT Assistant* Fall 91:19, Spring 94:30, Summer 95:4, May 96:11, Nov 98:35, Apr 00:4, Apr 01:11, Feb 05:10-12, Jun 05:9; *CPT Changes: An Insider's View* 2002

95170   whole body extract of biting insect or other arthropod (specify number of doses)

➜ *CPT Assistant* Fall 91:19, Spring 94:30, Summer 95:4, May 96:12, Apr 01:11, Feb 05:10-12, Jun 05:9

(For allergy immunotherapy reporting, a dose is the amount of antigen(s) administered in a single injection from a multiple dose vial)

95180   Rapid desensitization procedure, each hour (eg, insulin, penicillin, equine serum)

➜ *CPT Assistant* Summer 95:4; *CPT Changes: An Insider's View* 2002

95199   Unlisted allergy/clinical immunologic service or procedure

➜ *CPT Assistant* Summer 95:4, Summer 95:4, Nov 98:35

►(For skin testing of bacterial, viral, fungal extracts, see 86485-86580, 95028)◄

(For special reports on allergy patients, use 99080)

(For testing procedures such as radioallergosorbent testing (RAST), rat mast cell technique (RMCT), mast cell degranulation test (MCDT), lymphocytic transformation test (LTT), leukocyte histamine release (LHR), migration inhibitory factor test (MIF), transfer factor test (TFT), nitroblue tetrazolium dye test (NTD), see Immunology section in **Pathology** or use 95199)

Endocrinology

95250   Ambulatory continuous glucose monitoring of interstitial tissue fluid via a subcutaneous sensor for up to 72 hours; sensor placement, hook-up, calibration of monitor, patient training, removal of sensor, and printout of recording

➜ *CPT Changes: An Insider's View* 2002, 2006

(Do not report 95250 in conjunction with 99091)

95251   physician interpretation and report

➜ *CPT Changes: An Insider's View* 2006

(Do not report 95250, 95251 in conjunction with 99091)

Neurology and Neuromuscular Procedures

Neurologic services are typically consultative, and any of the levels of consultation (99241-99255) may be appropriate.

In addition, services and skills outlined under **Evaluation and Management** levels of service appropriate to neurologic illnesses should be reported similarly.

The EEG, autonomic function, evoked potential, reflex tests, EMG, NCV, and MEG services (95812-95829 and 95860-95967) include recording, interpretation by a physician, and report. For interpretation only, use modifier 26. For EMG guidance, see 95873, 95874.

(For repetitive transcranial magnetic stimulation for treatment of clinical depression, see Category III codes 0160T, 0161T)

(Do not report codes 95860-95875 in addition to 96000-96004)

Sleep Testing

Sleep studies and polysomnography refer to the continuous and simultaneous monitoring and recording of various physiological and pathophysiological parameters of sleep for 6 or more hours with physician review, interpretation and report. The studies are performed to diagnose a variety of sleep disorders and to evaluate a patient's response to therapies such as nasal continuous positive airway pressure (NCPAP). Polysomnography is distinguished from sleep studies by the inclusion of sleep staging which is defined to include a 1-4 lead electroencephalogram (EEG), an electro-oculogram (EOG), and a submental electromyogram (EMG). Additional parameters of sleep include (1) ECG; (2) airflow; (3) ventilation and respiratory effort; (4) gas exchange by oximetry, transcutaneous monitoring, or end tidal gas analysis; (5) extremity muscle activity, motor activity-movement; (6) extended EEG monitoring; (7) penile tumescence; (8) gastro-esophageal reflux; (9) continuous blood pressure monitoring; (10) snoring; (11) body positions; etc.

The sleep services (95805-95811) include recording, interpretation and report. For interpretation only, use modifier 26.

For a study to be reported as polysomnography, sleep must be recorded and staged.

(Report with modifier 52 if less than 6 hours of recording or in other cases of reduced services as appropriate)

(For unattended sleep study, use 95806)

95805 Multiple sleep latency or maintenance of wakefulness testing, recording, analysis and interpretation of physiological measurements of sleep during multiple trials to assess sleepiness
➔ *CPT Assistant* Nov 97:45-46, Nov 98:35, Dec 01:3, Sep 02:2-3

95806 Sleep study, simultaneous recording of ventilation, respiratory effort, ECG or heart rate, and oxygen saturation, unattended by a technologist
➔ *CPT Assistant* Nov 97:45-46, Aug 98:10, Nov 98:35

95807 Sleep study, simultaneous recording of ventilation, respiratory effort, ECG or heart rate, and oxygen saturation, attended by a technologist
➔ *CPT Assistant* Nov 97:46, Nov 98:35

95808 Polysomnography; sleep staging with 1-3 additional parameters of sleep, attended by a technologist
➔ *CPT Assistant* Sep 96:11, Nov 97:46, Feb 98:6, Nov 98:35, Sep 02:2-3

95810 sleep staging with 4 or more additional parameters of sleep, attended by a technologist
➔ *CPT Assistant* Feb 98:6, Nov 98:35, Sep 02:2-3

95811 sleep staging with 4 or more additional parameters of sleep, with initiation of continuous positive airway pressure therapy or bilevel ventilation, attended by a technologist
➔ *CPT Assistant* Nov 97:46, Feb 98:6, Nov 98:35, Sep 02:2-3

Routine Electroencephalography (EEG)

EEG codes 95812-95822 include hyperventilation and/or photic stimulation when appropriate. Routine EEG codes 95816-95822 include 20 to 40 minutes of recording. Extended EEG codes 95812-95813 include reporting times longer than 40 minutes.

95812 Electroencephalogram (EEG) extended monitoring; 41-60 minutes
➔ *CPT Assistant* Winter 94:18, Nov 98:35; *CPT Changes: An Insider's View* 2003

95813 greater than one hour
➔ *CPT Assistant* Winter 94:18, Nov 98:35

95816 Electroencephalogram (EEG); including recording awake and drowsy
➔ *CPT Assistant* Sep 96:11, Nov 98:35, Nov 99:51, Jul 00:1; *CPT Changes: An Insider's View* 2000, 2003

95819 including recording awake and asleep
➔ *CPT Assistant* Nov 98:35, Nov 99:51, Jul 00:1; *CPT Changes: An Insider's View* 2000, 2003

95822 recording in coma or sleep only
➔ *CPT Assistant* Nov 98:35; *CPT Changes: An Insider's View* 2003

95824 cerebral death evaluation only
➔ *CPT Assistant* Nov 98:35

95827 all night recording
➔ *CPT Assistant* Nov 98:35; *CPT Changes: An Insider's View* 2003

(For 24-hour EEG monitoring, see 95950-95953 or 95956)

(For EEG during nonintracranial surgery, use 95955)

(For Wada test, use 95958)

(For digital analysis of EEG, use 95957)

95829 Electrocorticogram at surgery (separate procedure)
➔ *CPT Assistant* Nov 98:35

95830 Insertion by physician of sphenoidal electrodes for electroencephalographic (EEG) recording

Muscle and Range of Motion Testing

95831 Muscle testing, manual (separate procedure) with report; extremity (excluding hand) or trunk

> *CPT Assistant* Nov 99:51, Dec 99:10, Mar 00:11, Jul 00:2, Nov 01:5, Apr 03:28, Dec 03:7, Feb 04:5; *CPT Changes: An Insider's View* 2000

95832 hand, with or without comparison with normal side

> *CPT Assistant* Nov 99:51, Dec 99:10, Mar 00:11, Jul 00:2, Nov 01:5, Apr 03:28, Dec 03:7, Feb 04:5

95833 total evaluation of body, excluding hands

> *CPT Assistant* Nov 99:51, Dec 99:10, Jul 00:2, Nov 01:5, Jul 02:2, Apr 03:28, Dec 03:7, Feb 04:5

95834 total evaluation of body, including hands

> *CPT Assistant* Nov 99:51, Dec 99:10, Jul 00:2, Nov 01:5, Apr 03:28, Dec 03:7, Feb 04:5

95851 Range of motion measurements and report (separate procedure); each extremity (excluding hand) or each trunk section (spine)

> *CPT Assistant* Sep 99:10, Nov 01:5, Apr 03:28, Dec 03:7, Feb 04:5

95852 hand, with or without comparison with normal side

> *CPT Assistant* Nov 01:5, Apr 03:28, Dec 03:7

95857 Tensilon test for myasthenia gravis

(95858 has been deleted)

Electromyography and Nerve Conduction Tests

Needle electromyographic procedures include the interpretation of electrical waveforms measured by equipment that produces both visible and audible components of electrical signals recorded from the muscle(s) studied by the needle electrode.

95860 Needle electromyography; one extremity with or without related paraspinal areas

> *CPT Assistant* Nov 97:46, Jul 00:2, Apr 02:2, May 03:20, Jun 03:3, Feb 04:4, Jul 04:6, Oct 04:15, Jun 06:8, Sep 06:5; *CPT Changes: An Insider's View* 2003

95861 two extremities with or without related paraspinal areas

> *CPT Assistant* Nov 97:46, Jul 00:2, Apr 02:2, May 03:20, Jun 03:3, Feb 04:4, Jul 04:6, Oct 04:15, Jun 05:9, Jun 06:8, Sep 06:5; *CPT Changes: An Insider's View* 2003

(For dynamic electromyography performed during motion analysis studies, see 96002-96003)

95863 three extremities with or without related paraspinal areas

> *CPT Assistant* Nov 97:46, Jul 00:2, Apr 02:2, May 03:20, Jun 03:3, Feb 04:4, Jul 04:6, Oct 04:15, Jun 06:8, Sep 06:5; *CPT Changes: An Insider's View* 2003

95864 four extremities with or without related paraspinal areas

> *CPT Assistant* Nov 97:46, Jul 00:2, Jan 02:11, Apr 02:2, May 03:20, Jun 03:3, Feb 04:4, Jul 04:6, Oct 04:15, Jun 06:8, Sep 06:5; *CPT Changes: An Insider's View* 2003

95865 larynx

> *CPT Changes: An Insider's View* 2006

(Do not report modifier 50 in conjunction with 95865)

(For unilateral procedure, report modifier 52 in conjunction with 95865)

95866 hemidiaphragm

> *CPT Changes: An Insider's View* 2006

95867 cranial nerve supplied muscle(s), unilateral

> *CPT Assistant* Apr 02:2, May 03:20, Jun 03:3, Jun 06:8, Sep 06:5; *CPT Changes: An Insider's View* 2003

95868 cranial nerve supplied muscles, bilateral

> *CPT Assistant* Apr 02:2, May 03:20, Jun 03:3, Jun 06:8, Sep 06:5; *CPT Changes: An Insider's View* 2003

95869 thoracic paraspinal muscles (excluding T1 or T12)

> *CPT Assistant* Nov 97:46, Apr 02:2, May 03:20, Jun 03:3, Feb 04:4, Jun 06:8, Sep 06:5; *CPT Changes: An Insider's View* 2003

95870 limited study of muscles in one extremity or non-limb (axial) muscles (unilateral or bilateral), other than thoracic paraspinal, cranial nerve supplied muscles, or sphincters

> *CPT Assistant* Nov 97:46, Nov 99:51, Jul 00:2, Apr 02:2, May 03:20, Jun 03:3, Feb 04:4, Jul 04:6, Jun 05:9, Jun 06:8, Sep 06:5; *CPT Changes: An Insider's View* 2000

(To report a complete study of the extremities, see 95860-95864)

(For anal or urethral sphincter, detrusor, urethra, perineum musculature, see 51785-51792)

(For eye muscles, use 92265)

95872 Needle electromyography using single fiber electrode, with quantitative measurement of jitter, blocking and/or fiber density, any/all sites of each muscle studied

> *CPT Assistant* Apr 02:2, May 03:20, Jun 03:3, Sep 06:5

+ 95873 Electrical stimulation for guidance in conjunction with chemodenervation (List separately in addition to code for primary procedure)

> *CPT Changes: An Insider's View* 2006

+ 95874 Needle electromyography for guidance in conjunction with chemodenervation (List separately in addition to code for primary procedure)

> *CPT Changes: An Insider's View* 2006

(Use 95873, 95874 in conjunction with 64612-64614)

(Do not report 95874 in conjunction with 95873)

(Do not report 95873, 95874 in conjunction with 95860-95870)

95875 Ischemic limb exercise test with serial specimen(s) acquisition for muscle(s) metabolite(s)

> *CPT Assistant* Jun 03:3; *CPT Changes: An Insider's View* 2002, 2003

(For listing of nerves considered for separate study, see Appendix J)

⊘ **95900**   Nerve conduction, amplitude and latency/velocity study, each nerve; motor, without F-wave study

→ *CPT Assistant* Jan 96:2, Nov 99:51-52, Jan 00:10, Jul 00:3, Apr 02:2, Apr 03:4, May 03:20, Jul 04:13, Mar 05:17, Dec 05:9, Jun 06:8; *CPT Changes: An Insider's View* 2000

⊘ **95903**   motor, with F-wave study

→ *CPT Assistant* Jan 96:2, Nov 99:51-52, Jan 00:10, Jul 00:3, 12, Apr 02:2, Apr 03:4, May 03:20, Mar 05:17, Dec 05:9, Jun 06:8

⊘ **95904**   sensory

→ *CPT Assistant* Jan 96:2, Sep 99:11, Nov 99:51-52, Jul 00:12, Apr 02:2, Apr 03:4, May 03:20, Mar 05:17, Dec 05:9, Jun 06:8; *CPT Changes: An Insider's View* 2002

(Report 95900, 95903, and/or 95904 only once when multiple sites on the same nerve are stimulated or recorded)

Intraoperative Neurophysiology

+ **95920**   Intraoperative neurophysiology testing, per hour (List separately in addition to code for primary procedure)

→ *CPT Assistant* Winter 90:14, Nov 98:35-36, Nov 99:52, Jun 05:9

(Use 95920 in conjunction with the study performed, 92585, 95822, 95860, 95861, 95867, 95868, 95870, 95900, 95904, 95925-95937)

(Code 95920 describes ongoing electrophysiologic testing and monitoring performed during surgical procedures. Code 95920 is reported per hour of service, and includes only the ongoing electrophysiologic monitoring time distinct from performance of specific type(s) of baseline electrophysiologic study(s) (95860, 95861, 95867, 95868, 95870, 95900, 95904, 95928, 95929, 95933-95937) or interpretation of specific type(s) of baseline electrophysiologic study(s) (92585, 95822, 95870, 95925-95928, 95929, 95930). The time spent performing or interpreting the baseline electrophysiologic study(s) should not be counted as intraoperative monitoring, but represents separately reportable procedures. Code 95920 should be used once per hour even if multiple electrophysiologic studies are performed. The baseline electrophysiologic study(s) should be used once per operative session.)

(For electrocorticography, use 95829)

(For intraoperative EEG during nonintracranial surgery, use 95955)

(For intraoperative functional cortical or subcortical mapping, see 95961-95962)

(For intraoperative neurostimulator programming and analysis, see 95970-95975)

Autonomic Function Tests

95921   Testing of autonomic nervous system function; cardiovagal innervation (parasympathetic function), including two or more of the following: heart rate response to deep breathing with recorded R-R interval, Valsalva ratio, and 30:15 ratio

→ *CPT Assistant* Nov 98:35-36, Apr 02:2, Oct 03:11, Feb 06:15

95922   vasomotor adrenergic innervation (sympathetic adrenergic function), including beat-to-beat blood pressure and R-R interval changes during Valsalva maneuver and at least five minutes of passive tilt

→ *CPT Assistant* Nov 98:35-36, Apr 02:2, Jun 03:11, Feb 06:15, Nov 06:23

95923   sudomotor, including one or more of the following: quantitative sudomotor axon reflex test (QSART), silastic sweat imprint, thermoregulatory sweat test, and changes in sympathetic skin potential

→ *CPT Assistant* Nov 98:35-36, Apr 02:2, Feb 06:15

Evoked Potentials and Reflex Tests

95925   Short-latency somatosensory evoked potential study, stimulation of any/all peripheral nerves or skin sites, recording from the central nervous system; in upper limbs

→ *CPT Assistant* Nov 98:35-36, Apr 02:2

95926   in lower limbs

→ *CPT Assistant* May 01:11, Apr 02:2

95927   in the trunk or head

→ *CPT Assistant* Apr 02:2

(To report a unilateral study, use modifier 52)

(For auditory evoked potentials, use 92585)

95928   Central motor evoked potential study (transcranial motor stimulation); upper limbs

→ *CPT Changes: An Insider's View* 2005

95929   lower limbs

→ *CPT Changes: An Insider's View* 2005

95930   Visual evoked potential (VEP) testing central nervous system, checkerboard or flash

95933   Orbicularis oculi (blink) reflex, by electrodiagnostic testing

→ *CPT Assistant* Nov 98:35-36

95934   H-reflex, amplitude and latency study; record gastrocnemius/soleus muscle

→ *CPT Assistant* Jan 96:3, Nov 98:35-36, Jul 01:11, Apr 02:2, Jun 06:8

95936   record muscle other than gastrocnemius/soleus muscle

→ *CPT Assistant* Jan 96:3, Apr 02:2, Jun 06:8

(To report a bilateral study, use modifier 50)

95937   Neuromuscular junction testing (repetitive stimulation, paired stimuli), each nerve, any one method

→ *CPT Assistant* Nov 98:35-36, Apr 02:2, Jun 06:8

Special EEG Tests

95950 Monitoring for identification and lateralization of cerebral seizure focus, electroencephalographic (eg, 8 channel EEG) recording and interpretation, each 24 hours

→ *CPT Assistant* Nov 98:35

95951 Monitoring for localization of cerebral seizure focus by cable or radio, 16 or more channel telemetry, combined electroencephalographic (EEG) and video recording and interpretation (eg, for presurgical localization), each 24 hours

→ *CPT Assistant* Nov 98:35, Mar 03:21, Dec 04:18

Electroencephalographic (EEG) Monitoring and Video Recording
95951

Video-EEG monitoring

95953 Monitoring for localization of cerebral seizure focus by computerized portable 16 or more channel EEG, electroencephalographic (EEG) recording and interpretation, each 24 hours

→ *CPT Assistant* Nov 98:35

95954 Pharmacological or physical activation requiring physician attendance during EEG recording of activation phase (eg, thiopental activation test)

→ *CPT Assistant* Winter 94:18, Nov 98:35

95955 Electroencephalogram (EEG) during nonintracranial surgery (eg, carotid surgery)

→ *CPT Assistant* Nov 98:35

95956 Monitoring for localization of cerebral seizure focus by cable or radio, 16 or more channel telemetry, electroencephalographic (EEG) recording and interpretation, each 24 hours

→ *CPT Assistant* Nov 98:35

95957 Digital analysis of electroencephalogram (EEG) (eg, for epileptic spike analysis)

→ *CPT Assistant* Winter 94:18, Nov 98:35

95958 Wada activation test for hemispheric function, including electroencephalographic (EEG) monitoring

→ *CPT Assistant* Nov 98:35

95961 Functional cortical and subcortical mapping by stimulation and/or recording of electrodes on brain surface, or of depth electrodes, to provoke seizures or identify vital brain structures; initial hour of physician attendance

→ *CPT Assistant* Winter 94:18, Nov 98:35, Nov 99:52-53; *CPT Changes: An Insider's View* 2000

+ 95962 each additional hour of physician attendance (List separately in addition to code for primary procedure)

→ *CPT Assistant* Winter 94:18, Nov 98:35, Nov 99:52-53

(Use 95962 in conjunction with 95961)

95965 Magnetoencephalography (MEG), recording and analysis; for spontaneous brain magnetic activity (eg, epileptic cerebral cortex localization)

→ *CPT Changes: An Insider's View* 2002

95966 for evoked magnetic fields, single modality (eg, sensory, motor, language, or visual cortex localization)

→ *CPT Changes: An Insider's View* 2002

+ 95967 for evoked magnetic fields, each additional modality (eg, sensory, motor, language, or visual cortex localization) (List separately in addition to code for primary procedure)

→ *CPT Changes: An Insider's View* 2002

(Use 95967 in conjunction with 95966)

(For electroencephalography performed in addition to magnetoencephalography, see 95812-95827)

(For somatosensory evoked potentials, auditory evoked potentials, and visual evoked potentials performed in addition to magnetic evoked field responses, see 92585, 95925, 95926, and/or 95930)

(For computerized tomography performed in addition to magnetoencephalography, see 70450-70470, 70496)

(For magnetic resonance imaging performed in addition to magnetoencephalography, see 70551-70553)

Neurostimulators, Analysis-Programming

▶A simple neurostimulator pulse generator/transmitter (95970, 95971) is one capable of affecting three or fewer of the following: pulse amplitude, pulse duration, pulse frequency, eight or more electrode contacts, cycling, stimulation train duration, train spacing, number of programs, number of channels, alternating electrode polarities, dose time (stimulation parameters changing in time periods of minutes including dose lockout times), more than one clinical feature (eg, rigidity, dyskinesia, tremor). A complex neurostimulator pulse generator/ transmitter (95970, 95972- 95975) is one capable of affecting more than three of the above.◄

Code 95970 describes subsequent electronic analysis of a previously-implanted simple or complex brain, spinal cord, or peripheral neurostimulator pulse generator system, without reprogramming. Code 95971 describes intraoperative or subsequent electronic analysis of an implanted simple spinal cord, or peripheral (i.e., peripheral nerve, autonomic nerve, neuromuscular) neurostimulator pulse generator system, with programming. Codes 95972 and 95973 describe intraoperative (at initial insertion/revision) or subsequent electronic analysis of an implanted complex spinal cord or peripheral (except cranial nerve) neurostimulator pulse generator system, with programming. Codes 95974 and 95975 describe intraoperative (at initial insertion/revision) or subsequent electronic analysis of an implanted complex cranial nerve neurostimulator pulse generator system, with programming. Codes 95978 and 95979 describe initial or subsequent electronic analysis of an implanted brain neurostimulator pulse generator system, with programming.

►Code 95980 describes intraoperative electronic analysis of an implanted gastric neurostimulator pulse generator system, with programming; code 95981 describes subsequent analysis of the device; code 95982 describes subsequent analysis and reprogramming. For electronic analysis and reprogramming of gastric neurostimulator, lesser curvature, , use 0162T.◄

(For insertion of neurostimulator pulse generator, see 61885, 63685, 64590)

(For revision or removal of neurostimulator pulse generator or receiver, see 61888, 63688, 64595)

(For implantation of neurostimulator electrodes, see 43647, 43881, 61850-61875, 63650-63655, 64553-64580, 0155T, 0157T. For revision or removal of neurostimulator electrodes, see 43648, 43882, 61880, 63660, 64585, 0156T, 0158T)

95970 Electronic analysis of implanted neurostimulator pulse generator system (eg, rate, pulse amplitude and duration, configuration of wave form, battery status, electrode selectability, output modulation, cycling, impedance and patient compliance measurements); simple or complex brain, spinal cord, or peripheral (ie, cranial nerve, peripheral nerve, autonomic nerve, neuromuscular) neurostimulator pulse generator/transmitter, without reprogramming

➜ *CPT Assistant* Nov 98:36-37, Sep 99:1, Nov 99:53-54, Aug 05:7, Sep 05:10; *CPT Changes: An Insider's View* 2000

95971 simple spinal cord, or peripheral (ie, peripheral nerve, autonomic nerve, neuromuscular) neurostimulator pulse generator/transmitter, with intraoperative or subsequent programming

➜ *CPT Assistant* Nov 98:36-37, Sep 99:1, Nov 99:53-54, Aug 05:7; *CPT Changes: An Insider's View* 2000, 2005

95972 complex spinal cord, or peripheral (except cranial nerve) neurostimulator pulse generator/transmitter, with intraoperative or subsequent programming, first hour

➜ *CPT Assistant* Nov 98:36-37, Sep 99:1, Nov 99:53-54, Aug 05:7; *CPT Changes: An Insider's View* 2000, 2005

+ 95973 complex spinal cord, or peripheral (except cranial nerve) neurostimulator pulse generator/transmitter, with intraoperative or subsequent programming, each additional 30 minutes after first hour (List separately in addition to code for primary procedure)

➜ *CPT Assistant* Nov 98:36-37, Sep 99:1, Nov 99:53-54, Aug 05:7; *CPT Changes: An Insider's View* 2000, 2005

(Use 95973 in conjunction with 95972)

95974 complex cranial nerve neurostimulator pulse generator/transmitter, with intraoperative or subsequent programming, with or without nerve interface testing, first hour

➜ *CPT Assistant* Nov 98:36-37, Sep 99:1, Nov 99:53-54, Sep 05:10

+ 95975 complex cranial nerve neurostimulator pulse generator/transmitter, with intraoperative or subsequent programming, each additional 30 minutes after first hour (List separately in addition to code for primary procedure)

➜ *CPT Assistant* Nov 98:36-37, Sep 99:1, Nov 99:53-54, Sep 05:10

(Use 95975 in conjunction with 95974)

(For electronic analysis programming of gastric neurostimulator, lesser curvature, use Category III code 0162T)

95978 Electronic analysis of implanted neurostimulator pulse generator system (eg, rate, pulse amplitude and duration, battery status, electrode selectability and polarity, impedance and patient compliance measurements), complex deep brain neurostimulator pulse generator/transmitter, with initial or subsequent programming; first hour

➜ *CPT Assistant* Aug 05:7; *CPT Changes: An Insider's View* 2005

+ 95979 each additional 30 minutes after first hour (List separately in addition to code for primary procedure)

➜ *CPT Assistant* Aug 05:7; *CPT Changes: An Insider's View* 2005

(Use 95979 in conjunction with 95978)

● **95980** Electronic analysis of implanted neurostimulator pulse generator system (eg, rate, pulse amplitude and duration, configuration of wave form, battery status, electrode selectability, output modulation, cycling, impedance and patient measurements) gastric neurostimulator pulse generator/transmitter; intraoperative, with programming

➔ *CPT Changes: An Insider's View* 2008

● **95981** subsequent, without reprogramming

➔ *CPT Changes: An Insider's View* 2008

● **95982** subsequent, with reprogramming

➔ *CPT Changes: An Insider's View* 2008

Other Procedures

95990 Refilling and maintenance of implantable pump or reservoir for drug delivery, spinal (intrathecal, epidural) or brain (intraventricular);

➔ *CPT Assistant* Nov 02:4, Nov 05:1, Jul 06:1; *CPT Changes: An Insider's View* 2003

(For analysis and/or reprogramming of implantable infusion pump, see 62367-62368)

(For refill and maintenance of implanted infusion pump or reservoir for systemic drug therapy [eg, chemotherapy or insulin], use 96522)

95991 administered by physician

➔ *CPT Assistant* Nov 05:1, Jul 06:1; *CPT Changes: An Insider's View* 2004

95999 Unlisted neurological or neuromuscular diagnostic procedure

➔ *CPT Assistant* Feb 99:11, Jan 02:11, Mar 07:4, Apr 07:7

Motion Analysis

Codes 96000-96004 describe services performed as part of a major therapeutic or diagnostic decision making process. Motion analysis is performed in a dedicated motion analysis laboratory (ie, a facility capable of performing videotaping from the front, back and both sides, computerized 3-D kinematics, 3-D kinetics, and dynamic electromyography). Code 96000 may include 3-D kinetics and stride characteristics. Codes 96002-96003 describe dynamic electromyography.

Code 96004 should only be reported once regardless of the number of study(ies) reviewed/interpreted.

(For performance of needle electromyography procedures, see 95860-95875)

(For gait training, use 97116)

96000 Comprehensive computer-based motion analysis by video-taping and 3-D kinematics;

➔ *CPT Assistant* Aug 02:5, Jun 03:2; *CPT Changes: An Insider's View* 2002

96001 with dynamic plantar pressure measurements during walking

➔ *CPT Assistant* Aug 02:5, Jun 03:2; *CPT Changes: An Insider's View* 2002

96002 Dynamic surface electromyography, during walking or other functional activities, 1-12 muscles

➔ *CPT Assistant* Aug 02:5, Jun 03:3; *CPT Changes: An Insider's View* 2002

96003 Dynamic fine wire electromyography, during walking or other functional activities, 1 muscle

➔ *CPT Assistant* Aug 02:5, Jun 03:3; *CPT Changes: An Insider's View* 2002

(Do not report 96002, 96003 in conjunction with 95860-95864, 95869-95872)

96004 Physician review and interpretation of comprehensive computer-based motion analysis, dynamic plantar pressure measurements, dynamic surface electromyography during walking or other functional activities, and dynamic fine wire electromyography, with written report

➔ *CPT Assistant* Aug 02:5, Jun 03:3; *CPT Changes: An Insider's View* 2002

Functional Brain Mapping

Code 96020 includes selection and administration of testing of language, memory, cognition, movement, sensation, and other neurological functions when conducted in association with functional neuroimaging, monitoring of performance of this testing, and determination of validity of neurofunctional testing relative to separately interpreted functional magnetic resonance images.

96020 Neurofunctional testing selection and administration during noninvasive imaging functional brain mapping, with test administered entirely by a physician or psychologist, with review of test results and report

➔ *CPT Changes: An Insider's View* 2007

(For functional magnetic resonance imaging [fMRI], brain, use 70555)

(Do not report 96020 in conjunction with 96101-96103, 96116-96120)

(Do not report 96020 in conjunction with 70554)

(Evaluation and Management services codes should not be reported on the same day as 96020)

Medical Genetics and Genetic Counseling Services

These services are provided by trained genetic counselors and may include obtaining a structured family genetic history, pedigree construction, analysis for genetic risk assessment, and counseling of the patient and family. These activities may be provided during one or more sessions and may include review of medical data and family information, face-to-face interviews, and counseling services.

96040   Medical genetics and genetic counseling services, each 30 minutes face-to-face with patient/family

➔ *CPT Changes: An Insider's View* 2007

(For genetic counseling and education provided by a physician to an individual, see the appropriate Evaluation and Management codes)

(For genetic counseling and education provided by a physician to a group, use 99078)

(For education regarding genetic risks by a nonphysician to a group, see 98961, 98962)

(For genetic counseling and/or risk factor reduction intervention provided by a physician to patient(s) without symptoms or established disease, see 99401-99412)

Central Nervous System Assessments/Tests (eg, Neuro-Cognitive, Mental Status, Speech Testing)

The following codes are used to report the services provided during testing of the cognitive function of the central nervous system. The testing of cognitive processes, visual motor responses, and abstractive abilities is accomplished by the combination of several types of testing procedures. It is expected that the administration of these tests will generate material that will be formulated into a report.

(96100 has been deleted. To report, see 96101, 96102, 96103)

(For development of cognitive skills, see 97532, 97533)

(For mini-mental status examination performed by a physician, see **Evaluation and Management** services codes)

▲ **96101**   Psychological testing (includes psychodiagnostic assessment of emotionality, intellectual abilities, personality and psychopathology, eg, MMPI, Rorschach, WAIS), per hour of the psychologist's or physician's time, both face-to-face time administering tests to the patient and time interpreting these test results and preparing the report

➔ *CPT Changes: An Insider's View* 2006, 2008

►(96101 is also used in those circumstances when additional time is necessary to integrate other sources of clinical data, including previously completed and reported technician- and computer-administered tests)◄

►(Do not report 96101 for the interpretation and report of 96102, 96103)◄

96102   Psychological testing (includes psychodiagnostic assessment of emotionality, intellectual abilities, personality and psychopathology, eg, MMPI and WAIS), with qualified health care professional interpretation and report, administered by technician, per hour of technician time, face-to-face

➔ *CPT Changes: An Insider's View* 2006

96103   Psychological testing (includes psychodiagnostic assessment of emotionality, intellectual abilities, personality and psychopathology, eg, MMPI), administered by a computer, with qualified health care professional interpretation and report

➔ *CPT Changes: An Insider's View* 2006

96105   Assessment of aphasia (includes assessment of expressive and receptive speech and language function, language comprehension, speech production ability, reading, spelling, writing, eg, by Boston Diagnostic Aphasia Examination) with interpretation and report, per hour

➔ *CPT Assistant* Jul 96:8, May 05:1

96110   Developmental testing; limited (eg, Developmental Screening Test II, Early Language Milestone Screen), with interpretation and report

➔ *CPT Assistant* Jul 96:9, May 05:1

96111   extended (includes assessment of motor, language, social, adaptive and/or cognitive functioning by standardized developmental instruments) with interpretation and report

➔ *CPT Assistant* Jul 96:9, May 05:1; *CPT Changes: An Insider's View* 2005

(96115 has been deleted. To report, use 96116)

96116   Neurobehavioral status exam (clinical assessment of thinking, reasoning and judgment, eg, acquired knowledge, attention, language, memory, planning and problem solving, and visual spatial abilities), per hour of the psychologist's or physician's time, both face-to-face time with the patient and time interpreting test results and preparing the report

➔ *CPT Changes: An Insider's View* 2006

(96117 has been deleted. To report, see 96118, 96119, 96120)

▲ **96118**   Neuropsychological testing (eg, Halstead-Reitan Neuropsychological Battery, Wechsler Memory Scales and Wisconsin Card Sorting Test), per hour of the psychologist's or physician's time, both face-to-face time administering tests to the patient and time interpreting these test results and preparing the report

➔ *CPT Changes: An Insider's View* 2006, 2008

►(96118 is also used in those circumstances when additional time is necessary to integrate other sources of clinical data, including previously completed and reported technician- and computer-administered tests)◄

►(Do not report 96118 for the interpretation and report of 96119 or 96120)◄

96119   Neuropsychological testing (eg, Halstead-Reitan Neuropsychological Battery, Wechsler Memory Scales and Wisconsin Card Sorting Test), with qualified health care professional interpretation and report, administered by technician, per hour of technician time, face-to-face

➔ *CPT Changes: An Insider's View* 2006

96120   Neuropsychological testing (eg, Wisconsin Card Sorting Test), administered by a computer, with qualified health care professional interpretation and report

➔ *CPT Changes: An Insider's View* 2006

● **96125**   Standardized cognitive performance testing (eg, Ross Information Processing Assessment) per hour of a qualified health care professional's time, both face-to-face time administering tests to the patient and time interpreting these test results and preparing the report

➔ *CPT Changes: An Insider's View* 2008

▶(For psychological and neuropsychological testing by a physician or psychologist, see 96101-96103, 96118-96120)◀

Health and Behavior Assessment/Intervention

Health and behavior assessment procedures are used to identify the psychological, behavioral, emotional, cognitive, and social factors important to the prevention, treatment, or management of physical health problems.

The focus of the assessment is not on mental health but on the biopsychosocial factors important to physical health problems and treatments. The focus of the intervention is to improve the patient's health and well-being utilizing cognitive, behavioral, social, and/or psychophysiological procedures designed to ameliorate specific disease-related problems.

Codes 96150-96155 describe services offered to patients who present with primary physical illnesses, diagnoses, or symptoms and may benefit from assessments and interventions that focus on the biopsychosocial factors related to the patient's health status. These services do not represent preventive medicine counseling and risk factor reduction interventions.

For patients that require psychiatric services (90801-90899) as well as health and behavior assessment/intervention (96150-96155), report the predominant service performed. Do not report 96150-96155 in conjunction with 90801-90899 on the same date.

Evaluation and Management services codes (including **Preventive Medicine, Individual Counseling** codes 99401-99404, and **Preventive Medicine, Group Counseling** codes 99411-99412), should not be reported on the same day.

(For health and behavior assessment and/or intervention performed by a physician, see **Evaluation and Management** or **Preventive Medicine** services codes)

96150   Health and behavior assessment (eg, health-focused clinical interview, behavioral observations, psychophysiological monitoring, health-oriented questionnaires), each 15 minutes face-to-face with the patient; initial assessment

➔ *CPT Assistant* Mar 02:4, Feb 04:11, Mar 04:10, May 05:1, Jun 05:10; *CPT Changes: An Insider's View* 2002

96151   re-assessment

➔ *CPT Assistant* Mar 02:4, Feb 04:11, Mar 04:10, May 05:1, Jun 05:10; *CPT Changes: An Insider's View* 2002

96152   Health and behavior intervention, each 15 minutes, face-to-face; individual

➔ *CPT Assistant* Mar 02:4, Feb 04:11, Mar 04:10, May 05:1, Jun 05:10; *CPT Changes: An Insider's View* 2002

96153   group (2 or more patients)

➔ *CPT Assistant* Mar 02:4, Feb 04:11, Mar 04:10, May 05:1, Jun 05:10; *CPT Changes: An Insider's View* 2002

96154   family (with the patient present)

➔ *CPT Assistant* Mar 02:4, Feb 04:11, Mar 04:10, May 05:1, Jun 05:10; *CPT Changes: An Insider's View* 2002

96155   family (without the patient present)

➔ *CPT Assistant* Mar 02:4, 12, Feb 04:11, Mar 04:10, May 05:1, Jun 05:10; *CPT Changes: An Insider's View* 2002

Chemotherapy Administration

▶Chemotherapy administration codes 96401-96549 apply to parenteral administration of non-radionuclide anti-neoplastic drugs; and also to anti-neoplastic agents provided for treatment of noncancer diagnoses (eg, cyclophosphamide for auto-immune conditions) or to substances such as certain monoclonal antibody agents, and other biologic response modifiers. The infusion of chemotherapy drug agents requires physician work and/or clinical staff monitoring well beyond that of therapeutic drug agents (90760-90779) because the incidence of severe adverse patient reactions are typically greater. These services can be provided by any physician. Chemotherapy services are typically highly complex and require direct physician supervision for any or all purposes of patient assessment, provision of consent, safety oversight, and intraservice supervision of staff. Typically, such chemotherapy services require advanced practice training and competency for staff who provide these services; special considerations for preparation, dosage, or disposal; and commonly, these services entail significant patient risk and frequent monitoring. Examples are frequent changes in the infusion rate, prolonged presence of the nurse administering the solution for patient monitoring and infusion adjustments, and frequent conferring with the physician about these issues. These codes are not intended to be reported by the physician in the facility setting.◀

15 min or less considered a push

If performed to facilitate the infusion or injection, the following services are included and are not reported separately:

a. Use of local anesthesia

b. IV start

c. Access to indwelling IV, subcutaneous catheter or port

d. Flush at conclusion of infusion

e. Standard tubing, syringes and supplies

f. Preparation of chemotherapy agent(s)

▶(For declotting a catheter or port, use 36593)◀

Report separate codes for each parenteral method of administration employed when chemotherapy is administered by different techniques. The administration of medications (eg, antibiotics, steroidal agents, antiemetics, narcotics, analgesics) administered independently or sequentially as supportive management of chemotherapy administration, should be separately reported using 90760, 90761, 90765, 90779 as appropriate.

Report both the specific service as well as code(s) for the specific substance(s) or drug(s) provided. The fluid used to administer the drug(s) is considered incidental hydration and is not separately reportable.

When administering multiple infusions, injections or combinations, only one "initial" service code should be reported, unless protocol requires that two separate IV sites must be used. The "initial" code that best describes the key or primary reason for the encounter should always be reported irrespective of the order in which the infusions or injections occur. If an injection or infusion is of a subsequent or concurrent nature, even if it is the first such service within that group of services, then a subsequent or concurrent code from the appropriate section should be reported (eg, the first IV push given subsequent to an initial one-hour infusion is reported using a subsequent IV push code).

When reporting codes for which infusion time is a factor, use the actual time over which the infusion is administered.

If a significant separately identifiable Evaluation and Management service is performed, the appropriate E/M service code should be reported using modifier 25 in addition to 96401-96549. For same day E/M service, a different diagnosis is not required.

Regional (isolation) chemotherapy perfusion should be reported using the codes for arterial infusion (96420-96425). Placement of the intra-arterial catheter should be reported using the appropriate code from the **Cardiovascular Surgery** section. Placement of arterial and venous cannula(s) for extracorporeal circulation via a membrane oxygenator perfusion pump should be reported using 36823. Code 36823 includes dose

calculation and administration of the chemotherapy agent by injection into the perfusate. Do not report 96409-96425 in conjunction with 36823.

(For home infusion services, see 99601-99602)

Injection and Intravenous Infusion Chemotherapy

Intravenous or intra-arterial push is defined as: a) an injection in which the healthcare professional who administers the substance/drug is continuously present to administer the injection and observe the patient, or b) an infusion of 15 minutes or less.

(96400 has been deleted. To report, see 96401, 96402)

96401　Chemotherapy administration, subcutaneous or intramuscular; non-hormonal anti-neoplastic
➔ *CPT Assistant* Nov 05:1, Jan 06:47, Jan 07:30; *CPT Changes: An Insider's View* 2006

96402　　hormonal anti-neoplastic
➔ *CPT Assistant* Nov 05:1, Jan 07:30; *CPT Changes: An Insider's View* 2006

96405　Chemotherapy administration; intralesional, up to and including 7 lesions
➔ *CPT Assistant* Sep 96:5, Aug 97:19, Feb 01:10, Jul 01:2, Nov 05:1, Jan 07:30; *CPT Changes: An Insider's View* 2006

96406　　intralesional, more than 7 lesions
➔ *CPT Assistant* Sep 96:5, Aug 97:19, Feb 01:10, Jul 01:2, Nov 05:1, Jan 07:30; *CPT Changes: An Insider's View* 2006

(96408 has been deleted. To report, use 96409)

96409　　intravenous, push technique, single or initial substance/drug
➔ *CPT Assistant* Nov 05:1, Jan 07:30; *CPT Changes: An Insider's View* 2006

(96410 has been deleted. To report, use 96413)

+ 96411　　intravenous, push technique, each additional substance/drug (List separately in addition to code for primary procedure)
➔ *CPT Assistant* Nov 05:1, Jan 07:30; *CPT Changes: An Insider's View* 2006

(Use 96411 in conjunction with 96409, 96413)

(96412 has been deleted. To report, use 96415)

96413　Chemotherapy administration, intravenous infusion technique; up to 1 hour, single or initial substance/drug
➔ *CPT Assistant* Nov 05:1, Jan 07:30; *CPT Changes: An Insider's View* 2006

(96414 has been deleted. To report, use 96416)

▶(Report 90761 to identify hydration if administered as a secondary or subsequent service in association with 96413 through the same IV access)◀

▶(Report 90766, 90767, 90775 to identify therapeutic, prophylactic, or diagnostic drug infusion or injection, if administered as a secondary or subsequent service in association with 96413 through the same IV access)◀

+ 96415   each additional hour (List separately in addition to code for primary procedure)

> *CPT Assistant* Nov 05:1, Jan 07:30; *CPT Changes: An Insider's View* 2006, 2007

(handwritten: use only if over 30 min additional time)

(Use 96415 in conjunction with 96413)

(handwritten arrow) (Report 96415 for infusion intervals of greater than 30 minutes beyond 1-hour increments)

96416   initiation of prolonged chemotherapy infusion (more than 8 hours), requiring use of a portable or implantable pump

> *CPT Assistant* Nov 05:1, Jan 07:30; *CPT Changes: An Insider's View* 2006

(For refilling and maintenance of a portable pump or an implantable infusion pump or reservoir for drug delivery, see 96521-96523)

+ 96417   each additional sequential infusion (different substance/drug), up to 1 hour (List separately in addition to code for primary procedure)

(handwritten: add on)

> *CPT Assistant* Nov 05:1, Jan 07:30; *CPT Changes: An Insider's View* 2006

(Use 96417 in conjunction with 96413)

(handwritten arrow) (Report only once per sequential infusion. Report 96415 for additional hour(s) of sequential infusion)

Intra-Arterial Chemotherapy

96420   Chemotherapy administration, intra-arterial; push technique

> *CPT Assistant* Aug 97:19, Nov 98:37, Nov 99:54, Feb 01:10, Jul 01:2, Nov 05:1, Jan 07:30

96422   infusion technique, up to one hour

> *CPT Assistant* Dec 96:10, Aug 97:19, Nov 98:37, Feb 01:10, Jul 01:2, Nov 05:1, Jan 07:30

+ 96423   infusion technique, each additional hour (List separately in addition to code for primary procedure)

> *CPT Assistant* Dec 96:10, Nov 98:37, Feb 01:10, Jul 01:2, Nov 05:1, Jan 07:30; *CPT Changes: An Insider's View* 2006, 2007

(Use 96423 in conjunction with 96422)

(Report 96423 for infusion intervals of greater than 30 minutes beyond 1-hour increments)

(For regional chemotherapy perfusion via membrane oxygenator perfusion pump to an extremity, use 36823)

96425   infusion technique, initiation of prolonged infusion (more than 8 hours), requiring the use of a portable or implantable pump

> *CPT Assistant* Nov 99:54, Feb 01:10, Jul 01:2, Nov 05:1, Jan 07:30

(For refilling and maintenance of a portable pump or an implantable infusion pump or reservoir for drug delivery, see 96521-96523)

Other Chemotherapy

Code 96523 does not require direct physician supervision. Codes 96521-96523 may be reported when these devices are used for therapeutic drugs other than chemotherapy.

> ▶(For collection of blood specimen from a completely implantable venous access device, use 36591)◀

96440   Chemotherapy administration into pleural cavity, requiring and including thoracentesis

> *CPT Assistant* Feb 01:10, Jul 01:2, Nov 05:1, Jan 07:30

96445   Chemotherapy administration into peritoneal cavity, requiring and including peritoneocentesis

> *CPT Assistant* Feb 01:10, Jul 01:2, Nov 05:1, Jan 07:30

96450   Chemotherapy administration, into CNS (eg, intrathecal), requiring and including spinal puncture

> *CPT Assistant* Feb 01:10, Jul 01:2, Nov 05:1, Jan 07:30; *CPT Changes: An Insider's View* 2002

(For intravesical (bladder) chemotherapy administration, use 51720)

(For insertion of subarachnoid catheter and reservoir for infusion of drug, see 62350, 62351, 62360-62362; for insertion of intraventricular catheter and reservoir, see 61210, 61215)

(96520 has been deleted. To report, use 96521)

96521   Refilling and maintenance of portable pump

> *CPT Assistant* Nov 05:1, Jan 07:30; *CPT Changes: An Insider's View* 2006

96522   Refilling and maintenance of implantable pump or reservoir for drug delivery, systemic (eg, intravenous, intra-arterial)

> *CPT Changes: An Insider's View* 2006

(For refilling and maintenance of an implantable infusion pump for spinal or brain drug infusion, use 95990-95991)

96523   Irrigation of implanted venous access device for drug delivery systems

> *CPT Changes: An Insider's View* 2006

> ▶(Do not report 96523 if any other services are provided on the same day)◀

(96530 has been deleted. To report, use 96522)

96542   Chemotherapy injection, subarachnoid or intraventricular via subcutaneous reservoir, single or multiple agents

> *CPT Assistant* Aug 97:19, Jul 01:2, Nov 05:1, Jan 07:30

(96545 has been deleted)

(For radioactive isotope therapy, use 79005)

96549   Unlisted chemotherapy procedure

> *CPT Assistant* Aug 97:19, Jul 01:2, Nov 05:1, Jan 07:30

(handwritten: Use for concurrent infusion)

Photodynamic Therapy

(To report ocular photodynamic therapy, use 67221)

96567 Photodynamic therapy by external application of light to destroy premalignant and/or malignant lesions of the skin and adjacent mucosa (eg, lip) by activation of photosensitive drug(s), each phototherapy exposure session

➔ *CPT Assistant* Aug 03:15; *CPT Changes: An Insider's View* 2002

+ 96570 Photodynamic therapy by endoscopic application of light to ablate abnormal tissue via activation of photosensitive drug(s); first 30 minutes (List separately in addition to code for endoscopy or bronchoscopy procedures of lung and esophagus)

➔ *CPT Assistant* Nov 99:54, Sep 00:5; *CPT Changes: An Insider's View* 2000

+ 96571 each additional 15 minutes (List separately in addition to code for endoscopy or bronchoscopy procedures of lung and esophagus)

➔ *CPT Assistant* Nov 99:54, Sep 00:5; *CPT Changes: An Insider's View* 2000

(96570, 96571 are to be used in addition to bronchoscopy, endoscopy codes)

(Use 96570, 96571 in conjunction with 31641, 43228 as appropriate)

Special Dermatological Procedures

Dermatologic services are typically consultative, and any of the five levels of consultation (99241-99255) may be appropriate.

In addition, services and skills outlined under **Evaluation and Management** levels of service appropriate to dermatologic illnesses should be coded similarly.

(For intralesional injections, see 11900, 11901)

(For Tzanck smear, see 88160-88161)

96900 Actinotherapy (ultraviolet light)

96902 Microscopic examination of hairs plucked or clipped by the examiner (excluding hair collected by the patient) to determine telogen and anagen counts, or structural hair shaft abnormality

➔ *CPT Assistant* Nov 97:46-47

96904 Whole body integumentary photography, for monitoring of high risk patients with dysplastic nevus syndrome or a history of dysplastic nevi, or patients with a personal or familial history of melanoma

➔ *CPT Changes: An Insider's View* 2007

96910 Photochemotherapy; tar and ultraviolet B (Goeckerman treatment) or petrolatum and ultraviolet B

96912 psoralens and ultraviolet A (PUVA)

96913 Photochemotherapy (Goeckerman and/or PUVA) for severe photoresponsive dermatoses requiring at least four to eight hours of care under direct supervision of the physician (includes application of medication and dressings)

96920 Laser treatment for inflammatory skin disease (psoriasis); total area less than 250 sq cm

➔ *CPT Changes: An Insider's View* 2003

96921 250 sq cm to 500 sq cm

➔ *CPT Changes: An Insider's View* 2003

96922 over 500 sq cm

➔ *CPT Changes: An Insider's View* 2003

96999 Unlisted special dermatological service or procedure

Physical Medicine and Rehabilitation

Codes 97001-97755 should be used to report each distinct procedure performed. Do not append modifier 51 to 97001-97755.

(For muscle testing, range of joint motion, electromyography, see 95831 et seq)

(For biofeedback training by EMG, use 90901)

(For transcutaneous nerve stimulation (TNS), use 64550)

97001 Physical therapy evaluation

➔ *CPT Assistant* Nov 97:47, Feb 00:11, Sep 01:10, Oct 02:11, Dec 03:4, Feb 04:5, Apr 05:13, Aug 06:11

97002 Physical therapy re-evaluation

➔ *CPT Assistant* Nov 97:47, Feb 00:11, Sep 01:10, Oct 02:11, Dec 03:4, Feb 04:5

97003 Occupational therapy evaluation

➔ *CPT Assistant* Nov 97:47, Oct 02:11, Feb 04:5, Aug 06:11

97004 Occupational therapy re-evaluation

➔ *CPT Assistant* Nov 97:47, Oct 02:11, Feb 04:5

97005 Athletic training evaluation

➔ *CPT Assistant* Jun 02:9, Feb 04:5; *CPT Changes: An Insider's View* 2002

97006 Athletic training re-evaluation

➔ *CPT Assistant* Jun 02:9, Feb 04:5; *CPT Changes: An Insider's View* 2002

Modalities

Any physical agent applied to produce therapeutic changes to biologic tissue; includes but not limited to thermal, acoustic, light, mechanical, or electric energy.

Supervised

The application of a modality that does not require direct (one-on-one) patient contact by the provider.

97010 Application of a modality to one or more areas; hot or cold packs
> *CPT Assistant* Summer 95:5, Apr 96:11, Nov 97:47, Dec 98:1, Nov 01:5, Aug 02:11, Aug 06:11

97012 traction, mechanical
> *CPT Assistant* Summer 95:5, Apr 96:11, Nov 97:47, Dec 98:1, May 99:11, Nov 01:5, Aug 02:11, Dec 03:4, Oct 04:9

97014 electrical stimulation (unattended)
> *CPT Assistant* Summer 95:5, Apr 96:11, Nov 97:47, May 98:10, Nov 01:5, Jan 02:11, Apr 02:18, Aug 02:11, Dec 03:4

(For acupuncture with electrical stimulation, see 97813, 97814)

97016 vasopneumatic devices
> *CPT Assistant* Summer 95:6, Apr 96:11, Dec 98:1, Nov 01:5, Aug 02:11, May 05:14

97018 paraffin bath
> *CPT Assistant* Summer 95:6, Apr 96:11, Dec 98:1, Nov 01:5, Aug 02:11

(97020 has been deleted. To report, use 97024)

97022 whirlpool
> *CPT Assistant* Summer 95:6, Apr 96:11, May 98:10, Dec 98:1, Nov 01:5, Aug 02:11

97024 diathermy (eg, microwave)
> *CPT Assistant* Summer 95:6, Apr 96:11, Dec 98:1, Nov 01:5, Aug 02:11; *CPT Changes: An Insider's View* 2006

97026 infrared
> *CPT Assistant* Summer 95:6, Apr 96:11, Dec 98:1, Nov 01:5, Aug 02:11

97028 ultraviolet
> *CPT Assistant* Summer 95:6, Apr 96:11, Dec 98:1, Nov 01:5, Aug 02:11

Constant Attendance

The application of a modality that requires direct (one-on-one) patient contact by the provider.

97032 Application of a modality to one or more areas; electrical stimulation (manual), each 15 minutes
> *CPT Assistant* Summer 95:6, Dec 98:1, Nov 01:5, Apr 02:18, Jul 04:14

97033 iontophoresis, each 15 minutes
> *CPT Assistant* Summer 95:7, Dec 98:1, Nov 01:5

97034 contrast baths, each 15 minutes
> *CPT Assistant* Summer 95:7, Dec 98:1, Nov 01:5

97035 ultrasound, each 15 minutes
> *CPT Assistant* Summer 95:7, Sep 96:10, Dec 98:1, Nov 01:5

97036 Hubbard tank, each 15 minutes
> *CPT Assistant* Summer 95:7, Dec 98:1, Nov 01:5

97039 Unlisted modality (specify type and time if constant attendance)
> *CPT Assistant* Summer 95:7, May 98:10, Dec 98:1, Jan 00:10, Nov 01:5, May 05:14

Therapeutic Procedures

A manner of effecting change through the application of clinical skills and/or services that attempt to improve function.

Physician or therapist required to have direct (one-on-one) patient contact.

97110 Therapeutic procedure, one or more areas, each 15 minutes; therapeutic exercises to develop strength and endurance, range of motion and flexibility
> *CPT Assistant* Summer 95:7, Feb 97:10, Nov 98:37, Dec 99:11, Mar 05:11, Apr 05:14, Aug 05:11, Dec 05:8, Mar 06:15, Aug 06:11

97112 neuromuscular reeducation of movement, balance, coordination, kinesthetic sense, posture, and/or proprioception for sitting and/or standing activities
> *CPT Assistant* Summer 95:7, Feb 97:10, Apr 05:14, Aug 05:11, Mar 06:15, Aug 06:11; *CPT Changes: An Insider's View* 2002

97113 aquatic therapy with therapeutic exercises
> *CPT Assistant* Summer 95:7, Feb 97:10, Apr 05:14, Mar 06:15, Aug 06:11

97116 gait training (includes stair climbing)
> *CPT Assistant* Summer 95:8, Sep 96:7, Feb 97:10, Jun 03:3, Apr 05:14, Mar 06:15, Aug 06:11

(Use 96000-96003 to report comprehensive gait and motion analysis procedures)

97124 massage, including effleurage, petrissage and/or tapotement (stroking, compression, percussion)
> *CPT Assistant* Summer 95:8, May 96:10, Feb 97:10, Dec 99:7, Apr 05:14, May 05:14, Mar 06:15, Aug 06:11

(For myofascial release, use 97140)

97139 Unlisted therapeutic procedure (specify)
> *CPT Assistant* Summer 95:8, Feb 97:10, Apr 05:14, Aug 06:11

97140 Manual therapy techniques (eg, mobilization/manipulation, manual lymphatic drainage, manual traction), one or more regions, each 15 minutes
> *CPT Assistant* Nov 98:37, Feb 99:10, Mar 99:1, Jul 99:11, Aug 01:10, Dec 03:5

97150 Therapeutic procedure(s), group (2 or more individuals)
> *CPT Assistant* Summer 95:8, Dec 96:10, Feb 97:10, Oct 99:10, Nov 99:54-55, Dec 99:11, Apr 05:14, Aug 06:11

(Report 97150 for each member of group)

(Group therapy procedures involve constant attendance of the physician or therapist, but by definition do not require one-on-one patient contact by the physician or therapist)

(For manipulation under general anesthesia, see appropriate anatomic section in **Musculoskeletal System**)

(For osteopathic manipulative treatment (OMT), see 98925-98929)

(97504 has been deleted. To report, use 97760)

(97520 has been deleted. To report, use 97761)

97530 Therapeutic activities, direct (one-on-one) patient contact by the provider (use of dynamic activities to improve functional performance), each 15 minutes
➔ *CPT Assistant* Summer 95:9, Dec 01:6, Apr 03:26, Jul 03:15, Aug 05:11

97532 Development of cognitive skills to improve attention, memory, problem solving (includes compensatory training), direct (one-on-one) patient contact by the provider, each 15 minutes
➔ *CPT Assistant* Dec 01:1; *CPT Changes: An Insider's View* 2001

97533 Sensory integrative techniques to enhance sensory processing and promote adaptive responses to environmental demands, direct (one-on-one) patient contact by the provider, each 15 minutes
➔ *CPT Assistant* Dec 01:1; *CPT Changes: An Insider's View* 2001

97535 Self-care/home management training (eg, activities of daily living (ADL) and compensatory training, meal preparation, safety procedures, and instructions in use of assistive technology devices/adaptive equipment) direct one-on-one contact by provider, each 15 minutes
➔ *CPT Assistant* Sep 96:7, Apr 00:11, Dec 03:6; *CPT Changes: An Insider's View* 2002

97537 Community/work reintegration training (eg, shopping, transportation, money management, avocational activities and/or work environment/modification analysis, work task analysis, use of assistive technology device/adaptive equipment), direct one-on-one contact by provider, each 15 minutes
➔ *CPT Assistant* Sep 96:7, Dec 03:6; *CPT Changes: An Insider's View* 2004

(For wheelchair management/propulsion training, use 97542)

97542 Wheelchair management (eg, assessment, fitting, training), each 15 minutes
➔ *CPT Assistant* Sep 96:8; *CPT Changes: An Insider's View* 2006

97545 Work hardening/conditioning; initial 2 hours
➔ *CPT Assistant* Apr 03:26, Jul 03:15

+ 97546 each additional hour (List separately in addition to code for primary procedure)

(Use 97546 in conjunction with 97545)

Active Wound Care Management

Active wound care procedures are performed to remove devitalized and/or necrotic tissue and promote healing. Provider is required to have direct (one-on-one) patient contact.

(Do not report 97597-97602 in conjunction with 11040-11044)

97597 Removal of devitalized tissue from wound(s), selective debridement, without anesthesia (eg, high pressure waterjet with/without suction, sharp selective debridement with scissors, scalpel and forceps), with or without topical application(s), wound assessment, and instruction(s) for ongoing care, may include use of a whirlpool, per session; total wound(s) surface area less than or equal to 20 square centimeters
➔ *CPT Assistant* Jun 05:1, 0; *CPT Changes: An Insider's View* 2005

97598 total wound(s) surface area greater than 20 square centimeters
➔ *CPT Assistant* Jun 05:1, 0; *CPT Changes: An Insider's View* 2005

97602 Removal of devitalized tissue from wound(s), non-selective debridement, without anesthesia (eg, wet-to-moist dressings, enzymatic, abrasion), including topical application(s), wound assessment, and instruction(s) for ongoing care, per session
➔ *CPT Assistant* May 02:5, Jun 05:1, 0; *CPT Changes: An Insider's View* 2001

97605 Negative pressure wound therapy (eg, vacuum assisted drainage collection), including topical application(s), wound assessment, and instruction(s) for ongoing care, per session; total wound(s) surface area less than or equal to 50 square centimeters
➔ *CPT Assistant* Apr 05:13, Jun 05:1, 0; *CPT Changes: An Insider's View* 2005

97606 total wound(s) surface area greater than 50 square centimeters
➔ *CPT Assistant* Apr 05:13, Jun 05:1, 0; *CPT Changes: An Insider's View* 2005

Tests and Measurements

Requires direct one-on-one patient contact.

(For muscle testing, manual or electrical, joint range of motion, electromyography or nerve velocity determination, see 95831-95904)

(97703 has been deleted. To report, use 97762)

97750 Physical performance test or measurement (eg, musculoskeletal, functional capacity), with written report, each 15 minutes
➔ *CPT Assistant* Summer 95:5, Feb 97:10, Aug 98:11, Mar 00:11, Nov 01:5, May 02:18, Apr 03:28, Dec 03:7, Feb 04:5, Feb 07:12

97755 Assistive technology assessment (eg, to restore, augment or compensate for existing function, optimize functional tasks and/or maximize environmental accessibility), direct one-on-one contact by provider, with written report, each 15 minutes

➡ *CPT Changes: An Insider's View* 2004

(To report augmentative and alternative communication devices, see 92605, 92607)

Orthotic Management and Prosthetic Management

97760 Orthotic(s) management and training (including assessment and fitting when not otherwise reported), upper extremity(s), lower extremity(s) and/or trunk, each 15 minutes

➡ *CPT Assistant* Dec 05:8, 11, Feb 07:8; *CPT Changes: An Insider's View* 2006

(Code 97760 should not be reported with 97116 for the same extremity)

97761 Prosthetic training, upper and/or lower extremity(s), each 15 minutes

➡ *CPT Assistant* Dec 05:8, 11, Feb 07:8; *CPT Changes: An Insider's View* 2006

97762 Checkout for orthotic/prosthetic use, established patient, each 15 minutes

➡ *CPT Assistant* Dec 05:8, 11, Feb 07:8; *CPT Changes: An Insider's View* 2006

Other Procedures

(For extracorporeal shock wave musculoskeletal therapy, see Category III codes 0019T, 0101T, 0102T)

97799 Unlisted physical medicine/rehabilitation service or procedure

➡ *CPT Assistant* Summer 95:5, Oct 99:10

Medical Nutrition Therapy

97802 Medical nutrition therapy; initial assessment and intervention, individual, face-to-face with the patient, each 15 minutes

➡ *CPT Assistant* Apr 03:10, Nov 03:1; *CPT Changes: An Insider's View* 2001

97803 re-assessment and intervention, individual, face-to-face with the patient, each 15 minutes

➡ *CPT Assistant* Apr 03:10, Nov 03:1; *CPT Changes: An Insider's View* 2001

97804 group (2 or more individual(s)), each 30 minutes

➡ *CPT Assistant* Apr 03:10, Nov 03:1; *CPT Changes: An Insider's View* 2001

(For medical nutrition therapy assessment and/or intervention performed by a physician, see **Evaluation and Management** or **Preventive Medicine** service codes)

Acupuncture

Acupuncture is reported based on 15-minute increments of personal (face-to-face) contact with the patient, not the duration of acupuncture needle(s) placement.

If no electrical stimulation is used during a 15-minute increment, use 97810, 97811. If electrical stimulation of any needle is used during a 15-minute increment, use 97813, 97814.

Only one code may be reported for each 15-minute increment. Use either 97810 or 97813 for the initial 15-minute increment. Only one initial code is reported per day.

Evaluation and Management services may be reported separately, using modifier 25, if the patient's condition requires a significant separately identifiable E/M service, above and beyond the usual preservice and postservice work associated with the acupuncture services. The time of the E/M service is not included in the time of the acupuncture service.

97810 Acupuncture, 1 or more needles; without electrical stimulation, initial 15 minutes of personal one-on-one contact with the patient

➡ *CPT Assistant* Jan 05:16-17, Jun 05:5, Jun 06:20, Aug 06:4; *CPT Changes: An Insider's View* 2005

(Do not report 97810 in conjunction with 97813)

+ 97811 without electrical stimulation, each additional 15 minutes of personal one-on-one contact with the patient, with re-insertion of needle(s) (List separately in addition to code for primary procedure)

➡ *CPT Assistant* Jan 05:16, Jun 05:5, Aug 06:4; *CPT Changes: An Insider's View* 2005, 2006

(Use 97811 in conjunction with 97810, 97813)

Acupuncture, Needle
97810-97811

Acupuncture needle

97813   with electrical stimulation, initial 15 minutes of personal one-on-one contact with the patient

> ➔ *CPT Assistant* Jan 05:16-18, Jun 05:5, Jun 06:20, Aug 06:4; *CPT Changes: An Insider's View* 2005, 2006

(Do not report 97813 in conjunction with 97810)

+ 97814   with electrical stimulation, each additional 15 minutes of personal one-on-one contact with the patient, with re-insertion of needle(s) (List separately in addition to code for primary procedure)

> ➔ *CPT Assistant* Jan 05:16, Jun 05:5, Aug 06:4; *CPT Changes: An Insider's View* 2005, 2006

(Use 97814 in conjunction with 97810, 97813)

Osteopathic Manipulative Treatment

Osteopathic manipulative treatment (OMT) is a form of manual treatment applied by a physician to eliminate or alleviate somatic dysfunction and related disorders. This treatment may be accomplished by a variety of techniques.

Evaluation and Management services may be reported separately if, using modifier 25, the patient's condition requires a significant separately identifiable E/M service, above and beyond the usual preservice and postservice work associated with the procedure. The E/M service may be caused or prompted by the same symptoms or condition for which the OMT service was provided. As such, different diagnoses are not required for the reporting of the OMT and E/M service on the same date.

Body regions referred to are: head region; cervical region; thoracic region; lumbar region; sacral region; pelvic region; lower extremities; upper extremities; rib cage region; abdomen and viscera region.

> ➔ *CPT Assistant* Nov 98:37-38

98925   Osteopathic manipulative treatment (OMT); one to two body regions involved

> ➔ *CPT Assistant* May 96:10, Jan 97:8, 10, Jul 98:10, Aug 00:11, Dec 00:15

98926   three to four body regions involved

> ➔ *CPT Assistant* May 96:10, Jan 97:8, Aug 00:11, Dec 00:15

98927   five to six body regions involved

> ➔ *CPT Assistant* May 96:10, Jan 97:8, Aug 00:11, Dec 00:15

98928   seven to eight body regions involved

> ➔ *CPT Assistant* May 96:10, Jan 97:8, Aug 00:11, Dec 00:15

98929   nine to ten body regions involved

> ➔ *CPT Assistant* May 96:10, Jan 97:8, 10, Aug 00:11

Chiropractic Manipulative Treatment

Chiropractic manipulative treatment (CMT) is a form of manual treatment to influence joint and neurophysiological function. This treatment may be accomplished using a variety of techniques.

The chiropractic manipulative treatment codes include a pre-manipulation patient assessment. Additional Evaluation and Management services may be reported separately using modifier 25, if the patient's condition requires a significant separately identifiable E/M service, above and beyond the usual preservice and postservice work associated with the procedure. The E/M service may be caused or prompted by the same symptoms or condition for which the CMT service was provided. As such, different diagnoses are not required for the reporting of the CMT and E/M service on the same date.

For purposes of CMT, the five spinal regions referred to are: cervical region (includes atlanto-occipital joint); thoracic region (includes costovertebral and costotransverse joints); lumbar region; sacral region; and pelvic (sacro-iliac joint) region. The five extraspinal regions referred to are: head (including temporomandibular joint, excluding atlanto-occipital) region; lower extremities; upper extremities; rib cage (excluding costotransverse and costovertebral joints) and abdomen.

> ➔ *CPT Assistant* Nov 98:38

98940   Chiropractic manipulative treatment (CMT); spinal, one to two regions

> ➔ *CPT Assistant* Jan 97:7, 11, Feb 99:10, Dec 00:15, Mar 06:15

98941   spinal, three to four regions

> ➔ *CPT Assistant* Jan 97:7, 11, Mar 97:10, Feb 99:10, Dec 00:15, Mar 06:15

98942   spinal, five regions

> ➔ *CPT Assistant* Jan 97:7, 11, Feb 99:10, Dec 00:15, Mar 06:15

98943   extraspinal, one or more regions

> ➔ *CPT Assistant* Jan 97:7, 11, Mar 97:10, Feb 99:10, Dec 00:15, Mar 06:15

Education and Training for Patient Self-Management

The following codes are used to report educational and training services prescribed by a physician and provided by a qualified, nonphysician healthcare professional using a standardized curriculum to an individual or a group of patients for the treatment of established illness(s)/disease(s) or to delay comorbidity(s). Education and training for patient self-management may be

---

reported with these codes only when using a standardized curriculum as described below. This curriculum may be modified as necessary for the clinical needs, cultural norms and health literacy of the individual patient(s).

The purpose of the educational and training services is to teach the patient (may include caregiver(s)) how to effectively self-manage the patient's illness(s)/disease(s) or delay disease comorbidity(s) in conjunction with the patient's professional healthcare team. Education and training related to subsequent reinforcement or due to changes in the patient's condition or treatment plan are reported in the same manner as the original education and training. The type of education and training provided for the patient's clinical condition will be identified by the appropriate diagnosis code(s) reported.

The qualifications of the nonphysician healthcare professionals and the content of the educational and training program must be consistent with guidelines or standards established or recognized by a physician society, nonphysician healthcare professional society/association, or other appropriate source.

(For counseling and education provided by a physician to an individual, see the appropriate Evaluation and Management codes)

(For counseling and education provided by a physician to a group, use 99078)

(For counseling and/or risk factor reduction intervention provided by a physician to patient(s) without symptoms or established disease, see 99401-99412)

(For medical nutrition therapy, see 97802-97804)

(For health and behavior assessment/intervention that is not part of a standardized curriculum, see 96150-96155)

(For education provided as genetic counseling services, use 96040. For education to a group regarding genetic risks, see 98961, 98962)

98960 Education and training for patient self-management by a qualified, nonphysician health care professional using a standardized curriculum, face-to-face with the patient (could include caregiver/family) each 30 minutes; individual patient
➔ *CPT Changes: An Insider's View* 2006

98961 2-4 patients
➔ *CPT Changes: An Insider's View* 2006

98962 5-8 patients
➔ *CPT Changes: An Insider's View* 2006

▶Non-Face-to-Face Nonphysician Services◀

▶Telephone Services◀

▶Telephone services are non-face-to-face assessment and management services provided by a qualified health care professional to a patient using the telephone. These codes are used to report episodes of care by the qualified health care professional initiated by an established patient or guardian of an established patient. If the telephone service ends with a decision to see the patient within 24 hours or the next available urgent visit appointment, the code is not reported; rather the encounter is considered part of the preservice work of the subsequent assessment and management service, procedure and visit. Likewise, if the telephone call refers to a service performed and reported by the qualified health care professional within the previous seven days (either qualified health care professional requested or unsolicited patient follow-up) or within the postoperative period of the previously completed procedure, then the service(s) are considered part of that previous service or procedure. (Do not report 98966-98969 if reporting 98966-98969 performed in the previous seven days.)◀

▶(For telephone services provided by a physician, see 99441-99443)◀

● **98966** Telephone assessment and management service provided by a qualified nonphysician health care professional to an established patient, parent, or guardian not originating from a related assessment and management service provided within the previous seven days nor leading to an assessment and management service or procedure within the next 24 hours or soonest available appointment; 5-10 minutes of medical discussion
➔ *CPT Changes: An Insider's View* 2008

● **98967** 11-20 minutes of medical discussion
➔ *CPT Changes: An Insider's View* 2008

● **98968** 21-30 minutes of medical discussion
➔ *CPT Changes: An Insider's View* 2008

▶On-line Medical Evaluation◀

▶An on-line electronic medical evaluation is a non-face-to-face assessment and management service by a qualified health care professional to a patient using Internet resources in response to a patient's on-line inquiry. Reportable services involve the qualified health care professional's personal timely response to the patient's inquiry and must involve permanent storage (electronic or hard copy) of the encounter. This service is reported only once for the same episode of care during a seven-day period, although multiple qualified healthcare professionals could report their exchange with the same patient. If the on-line medical evaluation refers to an assessment and management service previously performed and reported by the qualified health care professional within the previous seven days (either qualified health care professional requested or unsolicited patient follow-up) or within the postoperative period of the previously completed procedure, then the service(s) are considered covered by the previous assessment and management office service or procedure. A reportable service encompasses the sum of communication (eg, related telephone calls, prescription provision, laboratory orders) pertaining to the on-line patient encounter.◄

▶(For an on-line medical evaluation provided by a physician, use 99444)◄

● **98969**   On-line assessment and management service provided by a qualified nonphysician health care professional to an established patient, guardian, or health care provider not originating from a related assessment and management service provided within the previous 7 days, using the Internet or similar electronic communications network

➔ *CPT Changes: An Insider's View* 2008

▶(Do not report 98969 when using 99339-99340, 99374-99380 for the same communication[s])◄

▶(Do not report 98969 for anticoagulation management when reporting 99363, 99364)◄

Special Services, Procedures and Reports

The procedures with code numbers 99000 through 99091 provide the reporting physician or other qualified healthcare professional with the means of identifying the completion of special reports and services that are an adjunct to the basic services rendered. The specific number assigned indicates the special circumstances under which a basic procedure is performed.

Code 99091 should be reported no more than once in a 30-day period to include the physician or health care provider time involved with data accession, review and interpretation, modification of care plan as necessary (including communication to patient and/or caregiver), and associated documentation.

If the services described by 99091 are provided on the same day the patient presents for an E/M service, these services should be considered part of the E/M service and not separately reported.

Do not report 99091 if it occurs within 30 days of care plan oversight services 99374-99380. Do not report 99091 if other more specific CPT codes exist (eg, 93014, 93227, 93233, 93272 for cardiographic services; 95250 for continuous glucose monitoring). Do not report 99091 for transfer and interpretation of data from hospital or clinical laboratory computers.

Codes 99050-99060 are reported in addition to an associated basic service. Typically only a single adjunct code from among 99050-99060 would be reported per patient encounter. However, there may be circumstances in which reporting multiple adjunct codes per patient encounter may be appropriate.

Miscellaneous Services

99000   Handling and/or conveyance of specimen for transfer from the physician's office to a laboratory

➔ *CPT Assistant* Winter 94:26, Feb 99:10, Oct 99:11, May 02:19, Aug 06:6, Sep 06:15, Jan 07:30

99001   Handling and/or conveyance of specimen for transfer from the patient in other than a physician's office to a laboratory (distance may be indicated)

➔ *CPT Assistant* Winter 94:26, May 02:19, Aug 06:6, Sep 06:15, Jan 07:30

99002   Handling, conveyance, and/or any other service in connection with the implementation of an order involving devices (eg, designing, fitting, packaging, handling, delivery or mailing) when devices such as orthotics, protectives, prosthetics are fabricated by an outside laboratory or shop but which items have been designed, and are to be fitted and adjusted by the attending physician

➔ *CPT Assistant* Winter 94:26, May 02:19, Aug 06:6, Sep 06:15, Jan 07:30

(For routine collection of venous blood, use 36415)

99024   Postoperative follow-up visit, normally included in the surgical package, to indicate that an evaluation and management service was performed during a postoperative period for a reason(s) related to the original procedure

➔ *CPT Assistant* Winter 94:26, Sep 97:10, Aug 98:5, May 02:19, Nov 03:13, Aug 06:6, Sep 06:15, Jan 07:30; *CPT Changes: An Insider's View* 2004

(As a component of a surgical "package," see **Surgery Guidelines**)

99026   Hospital mandated on call service; in-hospital, each hour

➔ *CPT Assistant* Jun 03:10, Aug 06:6, Sep 06:15, Jan 07:30; *CPT Changes: An Insider's View* 2003

99027   out-of-hospital, each hour

➔ *CPT Assistant* Jun 03:10, Aug 06:6, Sep 06:15, Jan 07:30; *CPT Changes: An Insider's View* 2003

(For physician standby services requiring prolonged physician attendance, use 99360, as appropriate. Time spent performing separately reportable procedure(s) or service(s) should not be included in the time reported as mandated on call service)

99050   Services provided in the office at times other than regularly scheduled office hours, or days when the office is normally closed (eg, holidays, Saturday or Sunday), in addition to basic service

➔ *CPT Assistant* Winter 94:27, May 02:19, Jun 03:10, May 06:18, Aug 06:6, Sep 06:15, Jan 07:30; *CPT Changes: An Insider's View* 2004, 2006

99051 Service(s) provided in the office during regularly scheduled evening, weekend, or holiday office hours, in addition to basic service

➔ *CPT Changes: An Insider's View* 2006

(99052 has been deleted)

99053 Service(s) provided between 10:00 PM and 8:00 AM at 24-hour facility, in addition to basic service

➔ *CPT Changes: An Insider's View* 2006

(99054 has been deleted)

99056 Service(s) typically provided in the office, provided out of the office at request of patient, in addition to basic service

➔ *CPT Assistant* Winter 94:27, May 02:19, May 06:18, Aug 06:6, Sep 06:15, Jan 07:30; *CPT Changes: An Insider's View* 2006

99058 Service(s) provided on an emergency basis in the office, which disrupts other scheduled office services, in addition to basic service

➔ *CPT Assistant* Winter 94:27, May 02:19, May 06:18, Aug 06:6, Sep 06:15, Jan 07:30; *CPT Changes: An Insider's View* 2006

99060 Service(s) provided on an emergency basis, out of the office, which disrupts other scheduled office services, in addition to basic service

➔ *CPT Changes: An Insider's View* 2006

99070 Supplies and materials (except spectacles), provided by the physician over and above those usually included with the office visit or other services rendered (list drugs, trays, supplies, or materials provided)

➔ *CPT Assistant* Winter 94:28, May 98:10, Jun 99:10, Jun 00:11, Jul 01:2, May 02:19, Aug 02:11, Jun 05:1, Jul 06:1, Aug 06:6, Sep 06:15, Jan 07:30, 31, Feb 07:8

(For supply of spectacles, use the appropriate supply codes)

99071 Educational supplies, such as books, tapes, and pamphlets, provided by the physician for the patient's education at cost to physician

➔ *CPT Assistant* Winter 94:28, May 02:19, Aug 06:6, Sep 06:15, Jan 07:30

99075 Medical testimony

➔ *CPT Assistant* Winter 94:28, May 02:19, Aug 06:6, Sep 06:15, Jan 07:30

99078 Physician educational services rendered to patients in a group setting (eg, prenatal, obesity, or diabetic instructions)

➔ *CPT Assistant* Winter 94:28, Jan 98:12, May 02:19, Aug 06:6, Sep 06:15, Jan 07:30

99080 Special reports such as insurance forms, more than the information conveyed in the usual medical communications or standard reporting form

➔ *CPT Assistant* Winter 94:28, May 02:19, Aug 06:6, Sep 06:15, Jan 07:30

(Do not report 99080 in conjunction with 99455, 99456 for the completion of Workmen's Compensation forms)

99082 Unusual travel (eg, transportation and escort of patient)

➔ *CPT Assistant* May 02:19, Jan 03:24, Nov 03:14, Aug 06:6, Sep 06:15, Jan 07:30

99090 Analysis of clinical data stored in computers (eg, ECGs, blood pressures, hematologic data)

➔ *CPT Assistant* Winter 94:28, May 02:19, Jun 03:10, Aug 06:6, Sep 06:15, Jan 07:30, Feb 07:10; *CPT Changes: An Insider's View* 2002

(For physician/health care professional collection and interpretation of physiologic data stored/transmitted by patient/caregiver, see 99091)

▶(Do not report 99090 if other more specific CPT codes exist, eg, 93227, 93233, 93272 for cardiographic services; 95250 for continuous glucose monitoring, 97750 for musculoskeletal function testing)◄

99091 Collection and interpretation of physiologic data (eg, ECG, blood pressure, glucose monitoring) digitally stored and/or transmitted by the patient and/or caregiver to the physician or other qualified health care professional, requiring a minimum of 30 minutes of time

➔ *CPT Assistant* May 02:19, Jun 03:10, Aug 06:6, Sep 06:15, Jan 07:30; *CPT Changes: An Insider's View* 2002

Qualifying Circumstances for Anesthesia

(For explanation of these services, see **Anesthesia Guidelines**)

+ 99100 Anesthesia for patient of extreme age, younger than 1 year and older than 70 (List separately in addition to code for primary anesthesia procedure)

(For procedure performed on infants younger than 1 year of age at time of surgery, see 00326, 00561, 00834, 00836)

+ 99116 Anesthesia complicated by utilization of total body hypothermia (List separately in addition to code for primary anesthesia procedure)

+ 99135 Anesthesia complicated by utilization of controlled hypotension (List separately in addition to code for primary anesthesia procedure)

+ 99140 Anesthesia complicated by emergency conditions (specify) (List separately in addition to code for primary anesthesia procedure)

➔ *CPT Assistant* Mar 01:10

(An emergency is defined as existing when delay in treatment of the patient would lead to a significant increase in the threat to life or body part.)

Moderate (Conscious) Sedation

Moderate (conscious) sedation is a drug induced depression of consciousness during which patients respond purposefully to verbal commands, either alone or accompanied by light tactile stimulation. No interventions are required to maintain a patent airway, and spontaneous ventilation is adequate. Cardiovascular function is usually maintained.

Moderate sedation does not include minimal sedation (anxiolysis), deep sedation or monitored anesthesia care (00100-01999).

When providing moderate sedation, the following services are included and NOT reported separately:

- Assessment of the patient (not included in intraservice time);

- Establishment of IV access and fluids to maintain patency, when performed;

- Administration of agent(s);

- Maintenance of sedation;

- Monitoring of oxygen saturation, heart rate and blood pressure; and

- Recovery (not included in intraservice time).

Intraservice time starts with the administration of the sedation agent(s), requires continuous face-to-face attendance, and ends at the conclusion of personal contact by the physician providing the sedation.

Do not report 99143-99150 in conjunction with 94760-94762.

Do not report 99143-99145 in conjunction with codes listed in Appendix G. Do not report 99148-99150 in conjunction with codes listed in Appendix G when performed in the nonfacility setting.

When a second physician other than the healthcare professional performing the diagnostic or therapeutic services provides moderate sedation in the facility setting (eg, hospital, outpatient hospital/ambulatory surgery center, skilled nursing facility) for the procedures listed in Appendix G, the second physician reports 99148-99150. However, for the circumstance in which these services are performed by the second physician in the nonfacility setting (eg, physician office, freestanding imaging center), codes 99148-99150 are not reported.

(99141, 99142 have been deleted. To report, see 99143-99145)

⊘ **99143**   Moderate sedation services (other than those services described by codes 00100-01999) provided by the same physician performing the diagnostic or therapeutic service that the sedation supports, requiring the presence of an independent trained observer to assist in the monitoring of the patient's level of consciousness and physiological status; younger than 5 years of age, first 30 minutes intra-service time

➲ *CPT Assistant* Feb 06:9, May 06:19, 20; *CPT Changes: An Insider's View* 2006

➲ *Clinical Examples in Radiology* Winter 06:18

⊘ **99144**   age 5 years or older, first 30 minutes intra-service time

➲ *CPT Assistant* Feb 06:9, May 06:19, 20; *CPT Changes: An Insider's View* 2006

➲ *Clinical Examples in Radiology* Winter 06:18, Summer 06:1-3

+ **99145**   each additional 15 minutes intra-service time (List separately in addition to code for primary service)

➲ *CPT Assistant* Feb 06:9, May 06:19, 20; *CPT Changes: An Insider's View* 2006

➲ *Clinical Examples in Radiology* Winter 06:18, Summer 06:1-3

(Use 99145 in conjunction with 99143, 99144)

▲ **99148**   Moderate sedation services (other than those services described by codes 00100-01999), provided by a physician other than the health care professional performing the diagnostic or therapeutic service that the sedation supports; younger than 5 years of age, first 30 minutes intra-service time

➲ *CPT Assistant* Feb 06:9, May 06:19, 20; *CPT Changes: An Insider's View* 2006, 2008

➲ *Clinical Examples in Radiology* Winter 06:18

▲ **99149**   age 5 years or older, first 30 minutes intra-service time

➲ *CPT Assistant* Feb 06:9, May 06:19, 20; *CPT Changes: An Insider's View* 2006, 2008

➲ *Clinical Examples in Radiology* Winter 06:18

+ **99150**   each additional 15 minutes intra-service time (List separately in addition to code for primary service)

➲ *CPT Assistant* Feb 06:9, May 06:19, 20; *CPT Changes: An Insider's View* 2006

➲ *Clinical Examples in Radiology* Winter 06:18

(Use 99150 in conjunction with 99148, 99149)

Other Services and Procedures

99170   Anogenital examination with colposcopic magnification in childhood for suspected trauma

➲ *CPT Assistant* Nov 99:55, Apr 06:1

(For conscious sedation, use 99143-99150)

99172 Visual function screening, automated or semi-automated bilateral quantitative determination of visual acuity, ocular alignment, color vision by pseudoisochromatic plates, and field of vision (may include all or some screening of the determination[s] for contrast sensitivity, vision under glare)

➔ *CPT Assistant* Feb 01:7, Mar 05:1, 3; *CPT Changes: An Insider's View* 2001

(This service must employ graduated visual acuity stimuli that allow a quantitative determination of visual acuity [eg, Snellen chart]. This service may not be used in addition to a general ophthalmological service or an E/M service)

(Do not report 99172 in conjunction with 99173)

99173 Screening test of visual acuity, quantitative, bilateral

➔ *CPT Assistant* Nov 99:55, May 02:2, Mar 05:1, 3; *CPT Changes: An Insider's View* 2000

(The screening test used must employ graduated visual acuity stimuli that allow a quantitative estimate of visual acuity [eg, Snellen chart]. Other identifiable services unrelated to this screening test provided at the same time may be reported separately [eg, preventive medicine services]. When acuity is measured as part of a general ophthalmological service or of an E/M service of the eye, it is a diagnostic examination and not a screening test.)

(Do not report 99173 in conjunction with 99172)

● **99174** Ocular photoscreening with interpretation and report, bilateral

➔ *CPT Changes: An Insider's View* 2008

►(Do not report 99174 in conjunction with 92002-92014, 99172, 99173)◄

99175 Ipecac or similar administration for individual emesis and continued observation until stomach adequately emptied of poison

(For diagnostic intubation, see 82926-82928, 89130-89141)

(For gastric lavage for diagnostic purposes, see 91055)

99183 Physician attendance and supervision of hyperbaric oxygen therapy, per session

➔ *CPT Assistant* Jan 03:23

(Evaluation and Management services and/or procedures [eg, wound debridement] provided in a hyperbaric oxygen treatment facility in conjunction with a hyperbaric oxygen therapy session should be reported separately)

99185 Hypothermia; regional

99186 total body

99190 Assembly and operation of pump with oxygenator or heat exchanger (with or without ECG and/or pressure monitoring); each hour

99191 45 minutes

99192 30 minutes

99195 Phlebotomy, therapeutic (separate procedure)

➔ *CPT Assistant* Apr 96:3, Jun 96:10

99199 Unlisted special service, procedure or report

➔ *CPT Assistant* Nov 99:55; *CPT Changes: An Insider's View* 2000

Home Health Procedures/Services

These codes are used by non-physician health care professionals. Physicians should utilize the home visit codes 99341-99350 and utilize CPT codes other than 99500-99600 for any additional procedure/service provided to a patient living in a residence.

The following codes are used to report services provided in a patient's residence (including assisted living apartments, group homes, nontraditional private homes, custodial care facilities, or schools).

Health care professionals who are authorized to use Evaluation and Management (E/M) Home Visit codes (99341-99350) may report 99500-99600 in addition to 99341-99350 if both services are performed. E/M services may be reported separately, using modifier 25, if the patient's condition requires a significant separately identifiable E/M service, above and beyond the home health service(s)/procedure(s) codes 99500-99600.

99500 Home visit for prenatal monitoring and assessment to include fetal heart rate, non-stress test, uterine monitoring, and gestational diabetes monitoring

➔ *CPT Assistant* Oct 03:7, Jan 07:30; *CPT Changes: An Insider's View* 2002

99501 Home visit for postnatal assessment and follow-up care

➔ *CPT Assistant* Oct 03:7, Jan 07:30; *CPT Changes: An Insider's View* 2002

99502 Home visit for newborn care and assessment

➔ *CPT Assistant* Oct 03:7, Jan 07:30; *CPT Changes: An Insider's View* 2002

99503 Home visit for respiratory therapy care (eg, bronchodilator, oxygen therapy, respiratory assessment, apnea evaluation)

➔ *CPT Assistant* Oct 03:7, Jan 07:30; *CPT Changes: An Insider's View* 2002

99504 Home visit for mechanical ventilation care

➔ *CPT Assistant* Oct 03:7, Jan 07:30; *CPT Changes: An Insider's View* 2002, 2003

99505 Home visit for stoma care and maintenance including colostomy and cystostomy

➔ *CPT Assistant* Oct 03:7, Jan 07:30; *CPT Changes: An Insider's View* 2002

99506 Home visit for intramuscular injections

➔ *CPT Assistant* Oct 03:7, Jan 07:30; *CPT Changes: An Insider's View* 2002

99507   Home visit for care and maintenance of catheter(s) (eg, urinary, drainage, and enteral)

➔ *CPT Assistant* Oct 03:7, Jan 07:30; *CPT Changes: An Insider's View* 2002

99509   Home visit for assistance with activities of daily living and personal care

➔ *CPT Assistant* Oct 03:7, Jan 07:30; *CPT Changes: An Insider's View* 2002

(To report self-care/home management training, see 97535)

(To report home medical nutrition assessment and intervention services, see 97802-97804)

(To report home speech therapy services, see 92507-92508)

99510   Home visit for individual, family, or marriage counseling

➔ *CPT Assistant* Oct 03:7, Jan 07:30; *CPT Changes: An Insider's View* 2002

99511   Home visit for fecal impaction management and enema administration

➔ *CPT Assistant* Oct 03:7, Jan 07:30; *CPT Changes: An Insider's View* 2002

99512   Home visit for hemodialysis

➔ *CPT Assistant* Oct 03:7, Jan 07:30; *CPT Changes: An Insider's View* 2002, 2004

(For home infusion of peritoneal dialysis, use 99601, 99602)

99600   Unlisted home visit service or procedure

➔ *CPT Assistant* Oct 03:7, Jan 07:30; *CPT Changes: An Insider's View* 2003

Home Infusion Procedures/Services

99601   Home infusion/specialty drug administration, per visit (up to 2 hours);

➔ *CPT Assistant* Nov 05:1; *CPT Changes: An Insider's View* 2004

+ 99602   each additional hour (List separately in addition to code for primary procedure)

➔ *CPT Assistant* Nov 05:1; *CPT Changes: An Insider's View* 2004

(Use 99602 in conjunction with 99601)

►Medication Therapy Management Services◄

►Medication therapy management service(s) (MTMS) describe face-to-face patient assessment and intervention as appropriate, by a pharmacist, upon request. MTMS is provided to optimize the response to medications or to manage treatment-related medication interactions or complications.

MTMS includes the following documented elements: review of the pertinent patient history, medication profile (prescription and nonprescription), and recommendations for improving health outcomes and treatment compliance. These codes are not to be used to describe the provision of product-specific information at the point of dispensing or any other routine dispensing-related activities.◄

● **99605**   Medication therapy management service(s) provided by a pharmacist, individual, face-to-face with patient, with assessment and intervention if provided; initial 15 minutes, new patient

➔ *CPT Changes: An Insider's View* 2008

● **99606**   initial 15 minutes, established patient

➔ *CPT Changes: An Insider's View* 2008

+● **99607**   each additional 15 minutes (List separately in addition to code for primary service)

➔ *CPT Changes: An Insider's View* 2008

►(Use 99607 in conjunction with 99605, 99606)◄

Notes

⊙=Moderate sedation　✛=Add-on code　✗=FDA approval pending　➲➲=See p xvii for details

Category II Codes

The following section of *Current Procedural Terminology (CPT)* contains a set of supplemental tracking codes that can be used for performance measurement. It is anticipated that the use of Category II codes for performance measurement will decrease the need for record abstraction and chart review, and thereby minimize administrative burden on physicians, other health care professionals, hospitals, and entities seeking to measure the quality of patient care. These codes are intended to facilitate data collection about the quality of care rendered by coding certain services and test results that support nationally established performance measures and that have an evidence base as contributing to quality patient care.

The use of these codes is optional. The codes are not required for correct coding and may not be used as a substitute for Category I codes.

These codes describe clinical components that may be typically included in evaluation and management services or clinical services and, therefore, do not have a relative value associated with them. Category II codes may also describe results from clinical laboratory or radiology tests and other procedures, identified processes intended to address patient safety practices, or services reflecting compliance with state or federal law.

Category II codes described in this section make use of alphabetical characters as the 5th character in the string (ie, 4 digits followed by the letter **F**). These digits are not intended to reflect the placement of the code in the regular (Category I) part of the CPT codebook. To promote understanding of these codes and their associated measures, users are referred to Appendix H, which contains information about performance measurement exclusion modifiers, measures, and the measure's source.

CPT Category II codes are arranged according to the following categories derived from standard clinical documentation format:

▶Composite Measures . . . . 0001F-0012F◀

▶Patient Management . . . . 0500F-0509F◀

▶Patient History . . . . 1000F-1111F◀

▶Physical Examination. . . . . 2000F-2031F◀

▶Diagnostic/Screening Processes
or Results . . . . 3006F-3210F◀

▶Therapeutic, Preventive or Other
Interventions . . . . 4000F-4124F◀

▶Follow-up or Other Outcomes
. . . . 5005F-5015F◀

▶Patient Safety . . . . 6005F-6020F◀

Cross-references to the measures associated with each Category II code and their source are included for reference in Appendix H. In addition, acronyms for the related diseases or clinical condition(s) have been added at the end of each code descriptor to identify the topic or clinical category in which that code is included. A complete listing of the diseases/clinical conditions, and their acronyms are provided in alphabetical order in Appendix H. Users should review the complete measure(s) associated with each code prior to implementation.

Category II codes are reviewed by the Performance Measures Advisory Group (PMAG), an advisory body to the CPT Editorial Panel and the CPT/HCPAC Advisory Committee. The PMAG is comprised of performance measurement experts representing the Agency for Healthcare Research and Quality (AHRQ), the American Medical Association (AMA), the Centers for Medicare and Medicaid Services (CMS), the Joint Commission on Accreditation of Healthcare Organizations (JCAHO), the National Committee for Quality Assurance (NCQA), and the Physician Consortium for Performance Improvement (PCPI). The PMAG may seek additional expertise and/or input from other national health care organizations, as necessary, for the development of tracking codes. These may include national medical specialty societies, other national health care professional associations, accrediting bodies, and federal regulatory agencies.

The most current listing of Category II codes, including guidelines, Code Change Proposal forms, and release and implementation dates for Category II codes may be accessed at http://www.ama-assn.org/go/cpt.

(For blood pressure measured, use 2000F)

(0003F has been deleted. To report, see 1034F-1036F)

(For tobacco use cessation intervention, pharmacologic therapy, use 4001F)

Modifiers

The following performance measurement modifiers may be used for Category II codes to indicate that a service specified in the associated measure(s) was considered but, due to either medical, patient, or system circumstance(s) documented in the medical record, the service was not provided. These modifiers serve as denominator exclusions from the performance measure. The user should note that not all listed measures provide for exclusions (see Appendix H for more discussion regarding exclusion criteria).

Category II modifiers should only be reported with Category II codes—they should not be reported with Category I or Category III codes. In addition, the modifiers in the Category II section should only be used where specified in the guidelines, reporting instructions, parenthetic notes, or code descriptor language listed in the Category II section (code listing and Appendix H).

1P Performance Measure Exclusion Modifier due to Medical Reasons

Reasons include:

- Not indicated (absence of organ/limb, already received/performed, other)

- Contraindicated (patient allergic history, potential adverse drug interaction, other)

▶Other medical reasons◀

2P Performance Measure Exclusion Modifier due to Patient Reasons

Reasons include:

- Patient declined

- Economic, social, or religious reasons

- Other patient reasons

3P Performance Measure Exclusion Modifier due to System Reasons

Reasons include:

- Resources to perform the services not available

- Insurance coverage/payor-related limitations

- Other reasons attributable to health care delivery system

▶Modifier 8P is intended to be used as a "reporting modifier" to allow the reporting of circumstances when an action described in a measure's numerator is not performed and the reason is not otherwise specified.◀

8P Performance measure reporting modifier—action not performed, reason not otherwise specified

Composite Codes

Composite codes combine several measures grouped within a single code descriptor to facilitate reporting for a clinical condition when all components are met. If only some of the components are met or if services are provided in addition to those included in the composite code, they may be reported individually using the corresponding CPT Category II codes for those services.

0001F Heart failure assessed (includes assessment of all the following components) (CAD, HF)[1]:

Blood pressure measured (2000F)[1]

Level of activity assessed (1003F)[1]

Clinical symptoms of volume overload (excess) assessed (1004F)[1]

Weight, recorded (2001F)[1]

Clinical signs of volume overload (excess) assessed (2002F)[1]

➜ *CPT Assistant* Oct 05:1; *CPT Changes: An Insider's View* 2006, 2007

(To report blood pressure measured, use 2000F)

0005F Osteoarthritis assessed (OA)[1]

Includes assessment of all the following components:

Osteoarthritis symptoms and functional status assessed (1006F)[1]

Use of anti-inflammatory or over-the-counter (OTC) analgesic medications assessed (1007F)[1]

Initial examination of the involved joint(s) (includes visual inspection, palpation, range of motion) (2004F)[1]

➜ *CPT Assistant* Oct 05:1, 6; *CPT Changes: An Insider's View* 2006, 2007

(To report tobacco use cessation intervention, use 4001F)

Footnotes
[1] Physician Consortium for Performance Improvement, www.physicianconsortium.org
[2] National Committee on Quality Assurance (NCQA), Health Employer Data Information Set (HEDIS®), www.ncqa.org
[3] Joint Commission on Accreditation of Healthcare Organizations (JCAHO), ORYX Initiative Performance Measures, www.jcaho.org/pms
[4] National Diabetes Quality Improvement Alliance (NDQIA), www.nationaldiabetesalliance.org
[5] Joint measure from the Physician Consortium for Performance Improvement, www.physicianconsortium.org and National Committee on Quality Assurance (NCQA), www.ncqa.org
[6] The Society of Thoracic Surgeons, www.sts.org, National Quality Forum, www.qualityforum.org

0012F   Community-acquired bacterial pneumonia assessment (includes all of the following components) (CAP)[1]:

Co-morbid conditions assessed (1026F)[1]

Vital signs recorded (2010F)[1]

Mental status assessed (2014F)[1]

Hydration status assessed (2018F)[1]

➔ *CPT Changes: An Insider's View* 2007

Patient Management

Patient management codes describe utilization measures or measures of patient care provided for specific clinical purposes (eg, prenatal care, pre- and post-surgical care).

0500F   Initial prenatal care visit (report at first prenatal encounter with health care professional providing obstetrical care. Report also date of visit and, in a separate field, the date of the last menstrual period - LMP) (Prenatal)[2]

➔ *CPT Assistant* Oct 05:1, 6; *CPT Changes: An Insider's View* 2005

0501F   Prenatal flow sheet documented in medical record by first prenatal visit (documentation includes at minimum blood pressure, weight, urine protein, uterine size, fetal heart tones, and estimated date of delivery). Report also: date of visit and, in a separate field, the date of the last menstrual period - LMP (Note: If reporting 0501F Prenatal flow sheet, it is not necessary to report 0500F Initial prenatal care visit) (Prenatal)[1]

➔ *CPT Assistant* Oct 05:6; *CPT Changes: An Insider's View* 2005

0502F   Subsequent prenatal care visit (Prenatal)[2]

[Excludes: patients who are seen for a condition unrelated to pregnancy or prenatal care (eg, an upper respiratory infection; patients seen for consultation only, not for continuing care)]

➔ *CPT Assistant* Oct 05:6; *CPT Changes: An Insider's View* 2005, 2007

0503F   Postpartum care visit (Prenatal)[2]

➔ *CPT Assistant* Oct 05:6; *CPT Changes: An Insider's View* 2005

● **0505F**   Hemodialysis plan of care documented (ESRD)[1]

➔ *CPT Changes: An Insider's View* 2008

● **0507F**   Peritoneal dialysis plan of care documented (ESRD)[1]

➔ *CPT Changes: An Insider's View* 2008

● **0509F**   Urinary incontinence plan of care documented (GER)[5]

➔ *CPT Changes: An Insider's View* 2008

Patient History

Patient history codes describe measures for select aspects of patient history or review of systems.

1000F   Tobacco use assessed (CAD, CAP, COPD, PV)[1] (DM)[4]

➔ *CPT Assistant* Oct 05:1, 6; *CPT Changes: An Insider's View* 2005, 2007

(1001F has been deleted. To report smoking use, tobacco use, or non-use of tobacco products, see 1034F-1036F)

1002F   Anginal symptoms and level of activity assessed (CAD)[1]

➔ *CPT Assistant* Oct 05:6; *CPT Changes: An Insider's View* 2005

1003F   Level of activity assessed (HF)[1]

➔ *CPT Assistant* Oct 05:6; *CPT Changes: An Insider's View* 2006

1004F   Clinical symptoms of volume overload (excess) assessed (HF)[1]

➔ *CPT Assistant* Oct 05:6; *CPT Changes: An Insider's View* 2006

1005F   Asthma symptoms evaluated (includes physician documentation of numeric frequency of symptoms or patient completion of an asthma assessment tool/survey/questionnaire) (Asthma)[1]

➔ *CPT Assistant* Oct 05:6; *CPT Changes: An Insider's View* 2006

1006F   Osteoarthritis symptoms and functional status assessed (may include the use of a standardized scale or the completion of an assessment questionnaire, such as the SF-36, AAOS Hip & Knee Questionnaire) (OA)[1]

[Instructions: Report when osteoarthritis is addressed during the patient encounter]

➔ *CPT Assistant* Oct 05:6; *CPT Changes: An Insider's View* 2006

1007F   Use of anti-inflammatory or analgesic over-the-counter (OTC) medications for symptom relief assessed (OA)[1]

➔ *CPT Assistant* Oct 05:6; *CPT Changes: An Insider's View* 2006

1008F   Gastrointestinal and renal risk factors assessed for patients on prescribed or OTC non-steroidal anti-inflammatory drug (NSAID) (OA)[1]

➔ *CPT Assistant* Oct 05:6; *CPT Changes: An Insider's View* 2006

Footnotes

[1] Physician Consortium for Performance Improvement, www.physicianconsortium.org

[2] National Committee on Quality Assurance (NCQA), Health Employer Data Information Set (HEDIS®), www.ncqa.org

[3] Joint Commission on Accreditation of Healthcare Organizations (JCAHO), ORYX Initiative Performance Measures, www.jcaho.org/pms

[4] National Diabetes Quality Improvement Alliance (NDQIA), www.nationaldiabetesalliance.org

[5] Joint measure from the Physician Consortium for Performance Improvement, www.physicianconsortium.org and National Committee on Quality Assurance (NCQA), www.ncqa.org

[6] The Society of Thoracic Surgeons, www.sts.org, National Quality Forum, www.qualityforum.org

---

1015F   Chronic obstructive pulmonary disease (COPD) symptoms assessed (Includes assessment of at least one of the following: dyspnea, cough/sputum, wheezing), or respiratory symptom assessment tool completed (COPD)[1]

➔ *CPT Changes: An Insider's View 2007*

1018F   Dyspnea assessed, not present (COPD)[1]

➔ *CPT Changes: An Insider's View 2007*

1019F   Dyspnea assessed, present (COPD)[1]

➔ *CPT Changes: An Insider's View 2007*

1022F   Pneumococcus immunization status assessed (CAP, COPD)[1]

➔ *CPT Changes: An Insider's View 2007*

1026F   Co-morbid conditions assessed (eg, includes assessment for presence or absence of: malignancy, liver disease, congestive heart failure, cerebrovascular disease, renal disease, chronic obstructive pulmonary disease, asthma, diabetes, other co-morbid conditions) (CAP)[1]

➔ *CPT Changes: An Insider's View 2007*

1030F   Influenza immunization status assessed (CAP)[1]

➔ *CPT Changes: An Insider's View 2007*

1034F   Current tobacco smoker (CAD, CAP, COPD, PV)[1] (DM)[4]

➔ *CPT Changes: An Insider's View 2007*

1035F   Current smokeless tobacco user (eg, chew, snuff) (PV)[1]

➔ *CPT Changes: An Insider's View 2007*

1036F   Current tobacco non-user (CAD, CAP, COPD, PV)[1] (DM)[4]

➔ *CPT Changes: An Insider's View 2007*

1038F   Persistent asthma (mild, moderate or severe) (Asthma)[1]

➔ *CPT Changes: An Insider's View 2007*

1039F   Intermittent asthma (Asthma)[1]

➔ *CPT Changes: An Insider's View 2007*

● **1040F**   DSM-IV™ criteria for major depressive disorder documented (MDD)[1]

➔ *CPT Changes: An Insider's View 2008*

● **1050F**   History obtained regarding new or changing moles (ML)[5]

➔ *CPT Changes: An Insider's View 2008*

● **1055F**   Visual functional status assessed (EC)[5]

➔ *CPT Changes: An Insider's View 2008*

● **1060F**   Documentation of permanent OR persistent OR paroxysmal atrial fibrillation (STR)[5]

➔ *CPT Changes: An Insider's View 2008*

● **1061F**   Documentation of absence of permanent AND persistent AND paroxysmal atrial fibrillation (STR)[5]

➔ *CPT Changes: An Insider's View 2008*

● **1065F**   Ischemic stroke symptom onset of less than 3 hours prior to arrival (STR)[5]

➔ *CPT Changes: An Insider's View 2008*

● **1066F**   Ischemic stroke symptom onset greater than or equal to 3 hours prior to arrival (STR)[5]

➔ *CPT Changes: An Insider's View 2008*

● **1070F**   Alarm symptoms (involuntary weight loss, dysphagia, or gastrointestinal bleeding) assessed; none present (GERD)[5]

➔ *CPT Changes: An Insider's View 2008*

● **1071F**   Alarm symptoms (involuntary weight loss, dysphagia, or gastrointestinal bleeding) assessed; one or more present (GERD)[5]

➔ *CPT Changes: An Insider's View 2008*

● **1080F**   Surrogate decision maker or advance care plan documented in the medical record (GER)[5]

➔ *CPT Changes: An Insider's View 2008*

● **1090F**   Presence or absence of urinary incontinence assessed (GER)[5]

➔ *CPT Changes: An Insider's View 2008*

● **1091F**   Urinary incontinence characterized (eg frequency, volume, timing, type of symptoms, how bothersome) (GER)[5]

➔ *CPT Changes: An Insider's View 2008*

● **1100F**   Patient screened for future fall risk; documentation of two or more falls in the past year or any fall with injury in the past year (GER)[5]

➔ *CPT Changes: An Insider's View 2008*

● **1101F**   Patient screened for future fall risk; documentation of no falls in the past year or only one fall without injury in the past year (GER)[5]

➔ *CPT Changes: An Insider's View 2008*

● **1110F**   Patient discharged from an inpatient facility (eg hospital, skilled nursing facility, or rehabilitation facility) within the last 60 days (GER)[5]

➔ *CPT Changes: An Insider's View 2008*

● **1111F**   Discharge medications reconciled with the current medication list in outpatient medical record (GER)[5]

➔ *CPT Changes: An Insider's View 2008*

Footnotes

[1] Physician Consortium for Performance Improvement, www.physicianconsortium.org

[2] National Committee on Quality Assurance (NCQA), Health Employer Data Information Set (HEDIS®), www.ncqa.org

[3] Joint Commission on Accreditation of Healthcare Organizations (JCAHO), ORYX Initiative Performance Measures, www.jcaho.org/pms

[4] National Diabetes Quality Improvement Alliance (NDQIA), www.nationaldiabetesalliance.org

[5] Joint measure from the Physician Consortium for Performance Improvement, www.physicianconsortium.org and National Committee on Quality Assurance (NCQA), www.ncqa.org

[6] The Society of Thoracic Surgeons, www.sts.org, National Quality Forum, www.qualityforum.org

Physical Examination

Physical examination codes describe aspects of physical examination or clinical assessment.

2000F Blood pressure measured (CAD, HF, HTN)[1]
    ➔ *CPT Assistant* Oct 05:1, 6; *CPT Changes: An Insider's View* 2005

2001F Weight recorded (HF, PAG)[1]
    ➔ *CPT Assistant* Oct 05:6; *CPT Changes: An Insider's View* 2006

2002F Clinical signs of volume overload (excess) assessed (HF)[1]
    ➔ *CPT Assistant* Oct 05:6; *CPT Changes: An Insider's View* 2006

    (Code 2003F has been deleted. For performance measurement coding information regarding heart failure, see the Heart Failure Clinical Topic listing in Appendix H)

2004F Initial examination of the involved joint(s) (includes visual inspection, palpation, range of motion) (OA)[1]

    [Instructions: Report only for initial osteoarthritis visit or for visits for new joint involvement]
    ➔ *CPT Assistant* Oct 05:6; *CPT Changes: An Insider's View* 2006

▲ **2010F** Vital signs (temperature, pulse, respiratory rate, and blood pressure) documented and reviewed (CAP)[2] (EM)[5]
    ➔ *CPT Changes: An Insider's View* 2007, 2008

▲ **2014F** Mental status assessed (CAP)[1] (EM)[5]
    ➔ *CPT Changes: An Insider's View* 2007

2018F Hydration status assessed (normal/mildly dehydrated/severely dehydrated) (CAP)[1]
    ➔ *CPT Changes: An Insider's View* 2007

● **2019F** Dilated macular exam performed, including documentation of the presence or absence of macular thickening or hemorrhage AND the level of macular degeneration severity (EC)[5]
    ➔ *CPT Changes: An Insider's View* 2008

● **2020F** Dilated fundus evaluation performed within six months prior to cataract surgery (EC)[5]
    ➔ *CPT Changes: An Insider's View* 2008

● **2021F** Dilated macular or fundus exam performed, including documentation of the presence or absence of macular edema AND level of severity of retinopathy (EC)[5]
    ➔ *CPT Changes: An Insider's View* 2008

2022F Dilated retinal eye exam with interpretation by an ophthalmologist or optometrist documented and reviewed (DM)[4]
    ➔ *CPT Changes: An Insider's View* 2007

2024F Seven standard field stereoscopic photos with interpretation by an ophthalmologist or optometrist documented and reviewed (DM)[4]
    ➔ *CPT Changes: An Insider's View* 2007

2026F Eye imaging validated to match diagnosis from seven standard field stereoscopic photos results documented and reviewed (DM)[4]
    ➔ *CPT Changes: An Insider's View* 2007

● **2027F** Optic nerve head evaluation performed (EC)[5]
    ➔ *CPT Changes: An Insider's View* 2008

2028F Foot examination performed (includes examination through visual inspection, sensory exam with monofilament, and pulse exam – report when any of the three components are completed) (DM)[4]
    ➔ *CPT Changes: An Insider's View* 2007

● **2029F** Complete physical skin exam performed (ML)[5]
    ➔ *CPT Changes: An Insider's View* 2008

● **2030F** Hydration status documented, normally hydrated (PAG)[1]
    ➔ *CPT Changes: An Insider's View* 2008

● **2031F** Hydration status documented, dehydrated (PAG)[1]
    ➔ *CPT Changes: An Insider's View* 2008

Diagnostic/Screening Processes or Results

Diagnostic/screening processes or results codes describe results of tests ordered (clinical laboratory tests, radiological or other procedural examinations).

    ▶(Code 3000F has been deleted. To report blood pressure use the corresponding systolic codes (3074F, 3075F, 3077F) and diastolic codes (3078F, 3079F, 3080F)◀

    ▶(Code 3002F has been deleted. To report blood pressure use the corresponding systolic codes (3074F, 3075F, 3077F) and diastolic codes (3078F, 3079F, 3080F)◀

3006F Chest X-ray results documented and reviewed (CAP)[1]
    ➔ *CPT Changes: An Insider's View* 2007

3011F Lipid panel results documented and reviewed (must include total cholesterol, HDL-C, triglycerides and calculated LDL-C) (CAD)[1]
    ➔ *CPT Changes: An Insider's View* 2007

Footnotes

[1] Physician Consortium for Performance Improvement, www.physicianconsortium.org

[2] National Committee on Quality Assurance (NCQA), Health Employer Data Information Set (HEDIS®), www.ncqa.org

[3] Joint Commission on Accreditation of Healthcare Organizations (JCAHO), ORYX Initiative Performance Measures, www.jcaho.org/pms

[4] National Diabetes Quality Improvement Alliance (NDQIA), www.nationaldiabetesalliance.org

[5] Joint measure from the Physician Consortium for Performance Improvement, www.physicianconsortium.org and National Committee on Quality Assurance (NCQA), www.ncqa.org

[6] The Society of Thoracic Surgeons, www.sts.org, National Quality Forum, www.qualityforum.org

3014F   Screening mammography results documented and reviewed (PV)[1]

➔ *CPT Changes: An Insider's View* 2007

▲ **3017F**   Colorectal cancer screening results documented and reviewed (PV)[1] (Includes: fecal occult blood testing annually, flexible sigmoidoscopy every 5 years, annual fecal occult blood testing plus flexible sigmoidoscopy every 5 years, double-contrast barium enema every 5 years, or colonoscopy every 10 years)

3020F   Left ventricular function (LVF) assessment (eg, echocardiography, nuclear test, or ventriculography) documented in the medical record (Includes quantitative or qualitative assessment results) (HF)[1]

➔ *CPT Changes: An Insider's View* 2007

3021F   Left ventricular ejection fraction (LVEF) <40% or documentation of moderately or severely depressed left ventricular systolic function (CAD, HF)[1]

➔ *CPT Changes: An Insider's View* 2007

3022F   Left ventricular ejection fraction (LVEF) ≥40% or documentation as normal or mildly depressed left ventricular systolic function (CAD, HF)[1]

➔ *CPT Changes: An Insider's View* 2007

3023F   Spirometry results documented and reviewed (COPD)[1]

➔ *CPT Changes: An Insider's View* 2007

3025F   Spirometry test results demonstrate $FEV_1/FVC<70\%$ with COPD symptoms (eg, dyspnea, cough/sputum, wheezing) (CAP, COPD)[1]

➔ *CPT Changes: An Insider's View* 2007

3027F   Spirometry test results demonstrate $FEV_1/FVC≥70\%$ or patient does not have COPD symptoms (COPD)[1]

➔ *CPT Changes: An Insider's View* 2007

3028F   Oxygen saturation results documented and reviewed (includes assessment through pulse oximetry or arterial blood gas measurement) (CAP, COPD)[1] (EM)[5]

➔ *CPT Changes: An Insider's View* 2007

3035F   Oxygen saturation ≤ 88 % or a PaO_2 ≤ 55 mm Hg (COPD)[1]

➔ *CPT Changes: An Insider's View* 2007

3037F   Oxygen saturation > 88% or PaO_2 > 55 mmHg (COPD)[1]

➔ *CPT Changes: An Insider's View* 2007

3040F   Functional expiratory volume (FEV_1) < 40% of predicted value (COPD)[1]

➔ *CPT Changes: An Insider's View* 2007

3042F   Functional expiratory volume (FEV_1) ≥ 40% of predicted value (COPD)[1]

➔ *CPT Changes: An Insider's View* 2007

● **3044F**   Most recent hemoglobin A1c (HbA1c) level < 7.0% (DM)[2,4]

➔ *CPT Changes: An Insider's View* 2008

● **3045F**   Most recent hemoglobin A1c (HbA1c) level 7.0 – 9.0 % (DM)[2,4]

➔ *CPT Changes: An Insider's View* 2008

3046F   Most recent hemoglobin A1c level > 9.0% (DM)[4]

➔ *CPT Changes: An Insider's View* 2007

▶(Code 3047F has been deleted. To report most recent hemoglobin A1c level ≤ 9.0%, see codes 3044F-3045F)◀

3048F   Most recent LDL-C < 100 mg/dL (DM)[4]

➔ *CPT Changes: An Insider's View* 2007

3049F   Most recent LDL-C 100-129 mg/dL (DM)[4]

➔ *CPT Changes: An Insider's View* 2007

3050F   Most recent LDL-C ≥ 130 mg/dL (DM)[4]

➔ *CPT Changes: An Insider's View* 2007

3060F   Positive microalbuminuria test result documented and reviewed (DM)[4]

➔ *CPT Changes: An Insider's View* 2007

3061F   Negative microalbuminuria test result documented and reviewed (DM)[4]

➔ *CPT Changes: An Insider's View* 2007

3062F   Positive macroalbuminuria test result documented and reviewed (DM)[4]

➔ *CPT Changes: An Insider's View* 2007

3066F   Documentation of treatment for nephropathy (eg, patient receiving dialysis, patient being treated for ESRD, CRF, ARF, or renal insufficiency, any visit to a nephrologist) (DM)[4]

➔ *CPT Changes: An Insider's View* 2007

3072F   Low risk for retinopathy (no evidence of retinopathy in the prior year) (DM)[4]

➔ *CPT Changes: An Insider's View* 2007

● **3073F**   Pre-surgical (cataract) axial length, corneal power measurement and method of intraocular lens power calculation documented within six months prior to surgery (EC)[5]

➔ *CPT Changes: An Insider's View* 2008

● **3074F**   Most recent systolic blood pressure < 130 mm Hg (DM)[2,4] (HTN)[1]

➔ *CPT Changes: An Insider's View* 2008

Footnotes

[1] Physician Consortium for Performance Improvement, www.physicianconsortium.org

[2] National Committee on Quality Assurance (NCQA), Health Employer Data Information Set (HEDIS®), www.ncqa.org

[3] Joint Commission on Accreditation of Healthcare Organizations (JCAHO), ORYX Initiative Performance Measures, www.jcaho.org/pms

[4] National Diabetes Quality Improvement Alliance (NDQIA), www.nationaldiabetesalliance.org

[5] Joint measure from the Physician Consortium for Performance Improvement, www.physicianconsortium.org and National Committee on Quality Assurance (NCQA), www.ncqa.org

[6] The Society of Thoracic Surgeons, www.sts.org, National Quality Forum, www.qualityforum.org

● **3075F**   Most recent systolic blood pressure 130 - 139 mm Hg (DM)[2,4] (HTN)[1]

→ *CPT Changes: An Insider's View* 2008

▶(Code 3076F has been deleted. To report most recent systolic blood pressure < 140 mm Hg, see codes 3074F-3075F)◀

3077F   Most recent systolic blood pressure ≥ 140 mm Hg (HTN)[1] (DM)[4]

→ *CPT Changes: An Insider's View* 2007

3078F   Most recent diastolic blood pressure < 80 mm Hg (HTN)[1] (DM)[4]

→ *CPT Changes: An Insider's View* 2007

3079F   Most recent diastolic blood pressure 80-89 mm Hg (HTN)[1] (DM)[4]

→ *CPT Changes: An Insider's View* 2007

3080F   Most recent diastolic blood pressure ≥ 90 mm Hg (HTN)[1] (DM)[4]

→ *CPT Changes: An Insider's View* 2007

● **3082F**   Kt/V < 1.2 (Clearance of urea (Kt)/volume (V)) (ESRD)[1]

→ *CPT Changes: An Insider's View* 2008

● **3083F**   Kt/V equal to or greater than 1.2 and less than 1.7 (Clearance of urea (Kt)/volume (V)) (ESRD)[1]

→ *CPT Changes: An Insider's View* 2008

● **3084F**   Kt/V ≥ 1.7 (Clearance of urea Kt)/volume (V)) (ESRD)[1]

→ *CPT Changes: An Insider's View* 2008

● **3085F**   Suicide risk assessed (MDD)[1]

→ *CPT Changes: An Insider's View* 2008

● **3088F**   Major depressive disorder, mild (MDD)[1]

→ *CPT Changes: An Insider's View* 2008

● **3089F**   Major depressive disorder, moderate (MDD)[1]

→ *CPT Changes: An Insider's View* 2008

● **3090F**   Major depressive disorder, severe without psychotic features (MDD)[1]

→ *CPT Changes: An Insider's View* 2008

● **3091F**   Major depressive disorder, severe with psychotic features (MDD)[1]

→ *CPT Changes: An Insider's View* 2008

● **3092F**   Major depressive disorder, in remission (MDD)[1]

→ *CPT Changes: An Insider's View* 2008

● **3093F**   Documentation of new diagnosis of initial or recurrent episode of major depressive disorder (MDD)[1]

→ *CPT Changes: An Insider's View* 2008

● **3095F**   Central Dual-energy X-Ray Absorptiometry (DXA) results documented (OP)[5]

→ *CPT Changes: An Insider's View* 2008

● **3096F**   Central Dual-energy X-Ray Absorptiometry (DXA) ordered (OP)[5]

→ *CPT Changes: An Insider's View* 2008

● **3100F**   Carotid imaging study report (includes direct or indirect reference to measurements of distal internal carotid diameter as the denominator for stenosis measurement) (STR)[5]

→ *CPT Changes: An Insider's View* 2008

▶(Code 3101F has been deleted)◀

▶(Code 3102F has been deleted)◀

● **3110F**   Presence or absence of hemorrhage and mass lesion and acute infarction documented in final CT or MRI report (STR)[5]

→ *CPT Changes: An Insider's View* 2008

● **3111F**   CT or MRI of the brain performed within 24 hours of arrival to the hospital (STR)[5]

→ *CPT Changes: An Insider's View* 2008

● **3112F**   CT or MRI of the brain performed greater than 24 hours after arrival to the hospital (STR)[5]

→ *CPT Changes: An Insider's View* 2008

● **3120F**   12-Lead ECG Performed (EM)[5]

→ *CPT Changes: An Insider's View* 2008

● **3130F**   Upper gastrointestinal endoscopy performed (GERD)[5]

→ *CPT Changes: An Insider's View* 2008

● **3132F**   Documentation of referral for upper gastrointestinal endoscopy (GERD)[5]

→ *CPT Changes: An Insider's View* 2008

● **3140F**   Upper gastrointestinal endoscopy report indicates suspicion of Barrett's esophagus (GERD)[5]

→ *CPT Changes: An Insider's View* 2008

● **3141F**   Upper gastrointestinal endoscopy report indicates no suspicion of Barrett's esophagus (GERD)[5]

→ *CPT Changes: An Insider's View* 2008

● **3142F**   Barium swallow test ordered (GERD)[1]

→ *CPT Changes: An Insider's View* 2008

▶(Code 3143F has been deleted. To report documentation of barium swallow study, use code 3142F)◀

● **3150F**   Forceps esophageal biopsy performed (GERD)[5]

→ *CPT Changes: An Insider's View* 2008

Footnotes

[1] Physician Consortium for Performance Improvement, www.physicianconsortium.org

[2] National Committee on Quality Assurance (NCQA), Health Employer Data Information Set (HEDIS®), www.ncqa.org

[3] Joint Commission on Accreditation of Healthcare Organizations (JCAHO), ORYX Initiative Performance Measures, www.jcaho.org/pms

[4] National Diabetes Quality Improvement Alliance (NDQIA), www.nationaldiabetesalliance.org

[5] Joint measure from the Physician Consortium for Performance Improvement, www.physicianconsortium.org and National Committee on Quality Assurance (NCQA), www.ncqa.org

[6] The Society of Thoracic Surgeons, www.sts.org, National Quality Forum, www.qualityforum.org

● **3155F**   Cytogenetic testing performed on bone marrow at time of diagnosis or prior to initiating treatment (HEM)[1]
➔ *CPT Changes: An Insider's View* 2008

● **3160F**   Documentation of iron stores prior to initiating erythropoietin therapy (HEM)[1]
➔ *CPT Changes: An Insider's View* 2008

● **3170F**   Flow cytometry studies performed at time of diagnosis or prior to initiating treatment (HEM)[1]
➔ *CPT Changes: An Insider's View* 2008

● **3200F**   Barium swallow test not ordered (GERD)[5]
➔ *CPT Changes: An Insider's View* 2008

● **3210F**   Group A Strep Test Performed (PHAR)[2]
➔ *CPT Changes: An Insider's View* 2008

Therapeutic, Preventive, or Other Interventions

Therapeutic, preventive, or other interventions codes describe pharmacologic, procedural, or behavioral therapies, including preventive services such as patient education and counseling.

4000F   Tobacco use cessation intervention, counseling (COPD, CAP, CAD)[1]
➔ *CPT Assistant* Oct 05:1; *CPT Changes: An Insider's View* 2005

4001F   Tobacco use cessation intervention, pharmacologic therapy (COPD, CAD, CAP, PV)[1] (DM)[4]
➔ *CPT Assistant* Oct 05:6; *CPT Changes: An Insider's View* 2005

4002F   Statin therapy, prescribed (CAD)[1]
➔ *CPT Assistant* Oct 05:6; *CPT Changes: An Insider's View* 2005

4003F   Patient education, written/oral, appropriate for patients with heart failure, performed (HF)[1]
➔ *CPT Assistant* Oct 05:6; *CPT Changes: An Insider's View* 2006

● **4005F**   Pharmacologic therapy (other than minerals/vitamins) for osteoporosis prescribed (OP)[5]
➔ *CPT Changes: An Insider's View* 2008

4006F   Beta-blocker therapy, prescribed[2]
➔ *CPT Assistant* Oct 05:6; *CPT Changes: An Insider's View* 2005

● **4007F**   Age-Related Eye Disease Study (AREDS) formulation prescribed or recommended (EC)[5]
➔ *CPT Changes: An Insider's View* 2008

4009F   Angiotensin converting enzyme (ACE) inhibitor or Angiotensin Receptor Blocker (ARB) therapy, prescribed (HF, CAD)[1]
➔ *CPT Assistant* Oct 05:6; *CPT Changes: An Insider's View* 2005, 2007

4011F   Oral antiplatelet therapy prescribed (eg, aspirin, clopidogrel/Plavix, or combination of aspirin and dipyridamole/Aggrenox) (CAD)[1]
➔ *CPT Assistant* Oct 05:6; *CPT Changes: An Insider's View* 2005

4012F   Warfarin therapy prescribed (CHF)[1]
➔ *CPT Assistant* Oct 05:6; *CPT Changes: An Insider's View* 2006

4014F   Written discharge instructions provided to heart failure patients discharged home. (Instructions include all of the following components: activity level, diet, discharge medications, follow-up appointment, weight monitoring, what to do if symptoms worsen)[3]

(Excludes patients < 18 years of age)
➔ *CPT Changes: An Insider's View* 2006, 2007

4015F   Persistent asthma, preferred long term control medication or an acceptable alternative treatment, prescribed (Asthma)[1]

(Note: There are no medical exclusion criteria)
➔ *CPT Changes: An Insider's View* 2006, 2007

(Do not report modifier 1P with 4015F)

(To report patient reasons for not prescribing, use modifier 2P)

4016F   Anti-inflammatory/analgesic agent prescribed (OA)[1]

(Use for prescribed or continued medication[s], including over-the-counter medication[s])
➔ *CPT Assistant* Oct 05:6; *CPT Changes: An Insider's View* 2006

4017F   Gastrointestinal prophylaxis for NSAID use prescribed (OA)[1]
➔ *CPT Assistant* Oct 05:6; *CPT Changes: An Insider's View* 2006

4018F   Therapeutic exercise for the involved joint(s) instructed or physical or occupational therapy prescribed (OA)[1]
➔ *CPT Assistant* Oct 05:6; *CPT Changes: An Insider's View* 2006

● **4019F**   Documentation of receipt of counseling on exercise AND either both calcium and vitamin D use or counseling regarding both calcium and vitamin D use (OP)[5]
➔ *CPT Changes: An Insider's View* 2008

4025F   Inhaled bronchodilator prescribed (COPD)[1]
➔ *CPT Changes: An Insider's View* 2007

Footnotes
[1] Physician Consortium for Performance Improvement, www.physicianconsortium.org
[2] National Committee on Quality Assurance (NCQA), Health Employer Data Information Set (HEDIS®), www.ncqa.org
[3] Joint Commission on Accreditation of Healthcare Organizations (JCAHO), ORYX Initiative Performance Measures, www.jcaho.org/pms
[4] National Diabetes Quality Improvement Alliance (NDQIA), www.nationaldiabetesalliance.org
[5] Joint measure from the Physician Consortium for Performance Improvement, www.physicianconsortium.org and National Committee on Quality Assurance (NCQA), www.ncqa.org
[6] The Society of Thoracic Surgeons, www.sts.org, National Quality Forum, www.qualityforum.org

4030F Long-term oxygen therapy prescribed (more than 15 hours per day) (COPD)[1]

→ *CPT Changes: An Insider's View* 2007

4033F Pulmonary rehabilitation exercise training recommended (COPD)[1]

→ *CPT Changes: An Insider's View* 2007

(Report 4033F with 1019F)

4035F Influenza immunization recommended (COPD)[1]

→ *CPT Changes: An Insider's View* 2007

4037F Influenza immunization ordered or administered (COPD, PV)[1]

→ *CPT Changes: An Insider's View* 2007

4040F Pneumococcal immunization ordered or administered (COPD)[1]

→ *CPT Changes: An Insider's View* 2007

● **4041F** Documentation of order for cefazolin OR cefuroxime for antimicrobial prophylaxis (PERI 2)[5]

→ *CPT Changes: An Insider's View* 2008

● **4042F** Documentation that prophylactic antibiotics were neither given within 4 hours prior to surgical incision nor given intraoperatively (PERI 2)[5]

→ *CPT Changes: An Insider's View* 2008

● **4043F** Documentation that an order was given to discontinue prophylactic antibiotics within 48 hours of surgical end time, cardiac procedures (PERI 2)[5]

→ *CPT Changes: An Insider's View* 2008

● **4044F** Documentation that an order was given for venous thromboembolism (VTE) prophylaxis to be given within 24 hrs prior to incision time or 24 hours after surgery end time (PERI 2)[5]

→ *CPT Changes: An Insider's View* 2008

▲ **4045F** Appropriate empiric antibiotic prescribed (CAP)[1], (EM)[5]

→ *CPT Changes: An Insider's View* 2007, 2008

● **4046F** Documentation that prophylactic antibiotics were given within 4 hours prior to surgical incision or given intraoperatively (PERI 2)[5]

→ *CPT Changes: An Insider's View* 2008

● **4047F** Documentation of order for prophylactic antibiotics to be given within one hour (if fluoroquinolone or vancomycin, two hours) prior to surgical incision (or start of procedure when no incision is required) (PERI 2)[5]

→ *CPT Changes: An Insider's View* 2008

● **4048F** Documentation that prophylactic antibiotic was given within one hour (if fluoroquinolone or vancomycin, two hours) prior to surgical incision (or start of procedure when no incision is required) (PERI 2)[5]

→ *CPT Changes: An Insider's View* 2008

● **4049F** Documentation that order was given to discontinue prophylactic antibiotics within 24 hours of surgical end time, non-cardiac procedure (PERI 2)[5]

→ *CPT Changes: An Insider's View* 2008

4050F Hypertension plan of care documented as appropriate (HTN)[1]

→ *CPT Changes: An Insider's View* 2007

● **4051F** Referred for an arterio-venous (AV) fistula (ESRD)[1]

→ *CPT Changes: An Insider's View* 2008

● **4052F** Hemodialysis via functioning arterio-venous (AV) fistula (ESRD)[1]

→ *CPT Changes: An Insider's View* 2008

● **4053F** Hemodialysis via functioning arterio-venous (AV) graft (ESRD)[1]

→ *CPT Changes: An Insider's View* 2008

● **4054F** Hemodialysis via catheter (ESRD)[1]

→ *CPT Changes: An Insider's View* 2008

● **4055F** Patient receiving peritoneal dialysis (ESRD)[1]

→ *CPT Changes: An Insider's View* 2008

● **4056F** Appropriate oral rehydration solution recommended (PAG)[1]

→ *CPT Changes: An Insider's View* 2008

● **4058F** Pediatric Gastroenteritis Education provided to caregiver (PAG)[1]

→ *CPT Changes: An Insider's View* 2008

● **4060F** Psychotherapy services provided (MDD)[1]

→ *CPT Changes: An Insider's View* 2008

● **4062F** Patient referral for psychotherapy documented (MDD)[1]

→ *CPT Changes: An Insider's View* 2008

● **4064F** Antidepressant pharmacotherapy prescribed (MDD)[1]

→ *CPT Changes: An Insider's View* 2008

● **4065F** Antipsychotic pharmacotherapy prescribed (MDD)[1]

→ *CPT Changes: An Insider's View* 2008

● **4066F** Electroconvulsive Therapy (ECT) provided (MDD)[1]

→ *CPT Changes: An Insider's View* 2008

● **4067F** Patient referral for electroconvulsive therapy (ECT) documented (MDD)[1]

→ *CPT Changes: An Insider's View* 2008

● **4070F** Deep Vein Thrombosis (DVT) prophylaxis received by end of hospital day 2 (STR)[5]

→ *CPT Changes: An Insider's View* 2008

Footnotes

[1] Physician Consortium for Performance Improvement, www.physicianconsortium.org

[2] National Committee on Quality Assurance (NCQA), Health Employer Data Information Set (HEDIS®), www.ncqa.org

[3] Joint Commission on Accreditation of Healthcare Organizations (JCAHO), ORYX Initiative Performance Measures, www.jcaho.org/pms

[4] National Diabetes Quality Improvement Alliance (NDQIA), www.nationaldiabetesalliance.org

[5] Joint measure from the Physician Consortium for Performance Improvement, www.physicianconsortium.org and National Committee on Quality Assurance (NCQA), www.ncqa.org

[6] The Society of Thoracic Surgeons, www.sts.org, National Quality Forum, www.qualityforum.org

● **4073F** Oral antiplatelet therapy prescribed at discharge (STR)[5]
➔ *CPT Changes: An Insider's View* 2008

● **4075F** Anticoagulant therapy prescribed at discharge (STR)[5]
➔ *CPT Changes: An Insider's View* 2008

● **4077F** Documentation that tissue plasminogen activator (t-PA) administration was considered (STR)[5]
➔ *CPT Changes: An Insider's View* 2008

● **4079F** Documentation that rehabilitation services were considered (STR)[5]
➔ *CPT Changes: An Insider's View* 2008

● **4084F** Aspirin received within 24 hours before emergency department arrival or during emergency department stay (EM)[5]
➔ *CPT Changes: An Insider's View* 2008

● **4090F** Patient receiving erythropoietin therapy (HEM)[1]
➔ *CPT Changes: An Insider's View* 2008

● **4095F** Patient not receiving erythropoietin therapy (HEM)[1]
➔ *CPT Changes: An Insider's View* 2008

● **4100F** Bisphosphonate therapy, intravenous, ordered or received (HEM)[1]
➔ *CPT Changes: An Insider's View* 2008

● **4110F** Internal mammary artery graft performed for primary, isolated coronary artery bypass graft procedure (CABG)[6]
➔ *CPT Changes: An Insider's View* 2008

● **4115F** Beta blocker administered within 24 hours prior to surgical incision (CABG)[6]
➔ *CPT Changes: An Insider's View* 2008

● **4120F** Antibiotic prescribed or dispensed (URI, PHAR)[2]
➔ *CPT Changes: An Insider's View* 2008

● **4124F** Antibiotic neither prescribed nor dispensed (URI, PHAR)[2]
➔ *CPT Changes: An Insider's View* 2008

Follow-up or Other Outcomes

Follow-up or other outcomes codes describe review and communication of test results to patients, patient satisfaction or experience with care, patient functional status, and patient morbidity and mortality.

● **5005F** Patient counseled on self-examination for new or changing moles (ML)[5]
➔ *CPT Changes: An Insider's View* 2008

● **5010F** Findings of dilated macular or fundus exam communicated to the physician managing the diabetes care (EC)[5]
➔ *CPT Changes: An Insider's View* 2008

● **5015F** Documentation of communication that a fracture occurred and that the patient was or should be tested or treated for osteoporosis (OP)[5]
➔ *CPT Changes: An Insider's View* 2008

Patient Safety

Patient safety codes that describe patient safety practices.

6005F Rationale (eg, severity of illness and safety) for level of care (eg, home, hospital) documented (CAP)[1]
➔ *CPT Changes: An Insider's View* 2007

● **6010F** Dysphagia screening conducted prior to order for or receipt of any foods, fluids or medication by mouth (STR)[5]
➔ *CPT Changes: An Insider's View* 2008

● **6015F** Patient receiving or eligible to receive foods, fluids or medication by mouth (STR)[5]
➔ *CPT Changes: An Insider's View* 2008

● **6020F** NPO (nothing by mouth) ordered (STR)[5]
➔ *CPT Changes: An Insider's View* 2008

Footnotes

[1] Physician Consortium for Performance Improvement, www.physicianconsortium.org

[2] National Committee on Quality Assurance (NCQA), Health Employer Data Information Set (HEDIS®), www.ncqa.org

[3] Joint Commission on Accreditation of Healthcare Organizations (JCAHO), ORYX Initiative Performance Measures, www.jcaho.org/pms

[4] National Diabetes Quality Improvement Alliance (NDQIA), www.nationaldiabetesalliance.org

[5] Joint measure from the Physician Consortium for Performance Improvement, www.physicianconsortium.org and National Committee on Quality Assurance (NCQA), www.ncqa.org

[6] The Society of Thoracic Surgeons, www.sts.org, National Quality Forum, www.qualityforum.org

Category III Codes

The following section contains a set of temporary codes for emerging technology, services, and procedures. Category III codes allow data collection for these services/procedures. Use of unlisted codes does not offer the opportunity for the collection of specific data. If a Category III code is available, this code must be reported instead of a Category I unlisted code. This is an activity that is critically important in the evaluation of health care delivery and the formation of public and private policy. The use of the codes in this section allow physicians and other qualified health care professionals, insurers, health services researchers, and health policy experts to identify emerging technology, services, and procedures for clinical efficacy, utilization and outcomes.

The inclusion of a service or procedure in this section neither implies nor endorses clinical efficacy, safety or the applicability to clinical practice. The codes in this section may not conform to the usual requirements for CPT Category I codes established by the Editorial Panel. For Category I codes, the Panel requires that the service/procedure be performed by many health care professionals in clinical practice in multiple locations and that FDA approval, as appropriate, has already been received. The nature of emerging technology, services, and procedures is such that these requirements may not be met. For these reasons, temporary codes for emerging technology, services, and procedures have been placed in a separate section of the CPT codebook and the codes are differentiated from Category I CPT codes by the use of alphanumeric characters.

Services/procedures described in this section make use of alphanumeric characters. These codes have an alpha character as the 5th character in the string, preceded by four digits. The digits are not intended to reflect the placement of the code in the Category I section of CPT nomenclature. Codes in this section may or may not eventually receive a Category I CPT code. In either case, a given Category III code will be archived five years from its date of publication or revision in the CPT code book unless it is demonstrated that a temporary code is still needed. New codes in this section are released semi-annually via the AMA/CPT internet site, to expedite dissemination for reporting. The full set of temporary codes for emerging technology, services, and procedures are published annually in the CPT codebook. Go to www.ama-assn.org/go/cpt for the most current listing.

(0003T has been deleted)

(0008T has been deleted)

(0010T has been deleted. To report, use 86480)

0016T   Destruction of localized lesion of choroid (eg, choroidal neovascularization), transpupillary thermotherapy
➔ *CPT Changes: An Insider's View* 2002

0017T   Destruction of macular drusen, photocoagulation
➔ *CPT Changes: An Insider's View* 2002

(0018T has been deleted. To report, see 0160T, 0161T)

0019T   Extracorporeal shock wave involving musculoskeletal system, not otherwise specified, low energy
➔ *CPT Assistant* Jun 05:6, Mar 06:1; *CPT Changes: An Insider's View* 2002, 2006

(For application of high energy extracorporeal shock wave involving musculoskeletal system not otherwise specified, use 0101T)

(For application of high energy extracorporeal shock wave involving lateral humeral epicondyle, use 0102T)

(0020T has been deleted. To report, use 28890)

(0021T has been deleted)

(0023T has been deleted. To report, use 87900)

▶(0024T has been deleted. To report, use 93799)◀

0026T   Lipoprotein, direct measurement, intermediate density lipoproteins (IDL) (remnant lipoproteins)
➔ *CPT Changes: An Insider's View* 2002

0027T   Endoscopic lysis of epidural adhesions with direct visualization using mechanical means (eg, spinal endoscopic catheter system) or solution injection (eg, normal saline) including radiologic localization and epidurography
➔ *CPT Assistant* Jan 02:9; *CPT Changes: An Insider's View* 2003

(For diagnostic epidurography, use 64999)

0028T   Dual energy x-ray absorptiometry (DEXA) body composition study, one or more sites
➔ *CPT Assistant* Jan 02:9; *CPT Changes: An Insider's View* 2003

0029T   Treatment(s) for incontinence, pulsed magnetic neuromodulation, per day
➔ *CPT Changes: An Insider's View* 2003

0030T Antiprothrombin (phospholipid cofactor) antibody, each Ig class
> *CPT Changes: An Insider's View* 2003

0031T Speculoscopy;
> *CPT Changes: An Insider's View* 2003

0032T with directed sampling
> *CPT Changes: An Insider's View* 2003

(0033T has been deleted. For endovascular repair of descending thoracic aorta, involving coverage of left subclavian artery origin, use 33880)

(0034T has been deleted. For endovascular repair of descending thoracic aorta, not involving coverage of left subclavian artery origin, use 33881)

(0035T has been deleted. For proximal extension during endovascular repair of descending thoracic aorta, use 33883. Distal extensions are included in 33880, 33881. Distal extensions performed after endovascular repair of descending thoracic aorta are reported with 33886)

(0036T has been deleted. For additional proximal extensions use 33884. Additional distal extensions during endovascular repair of descending thoracic aorta are included in 33880, 33881. Additional distal extensions placed after endovascular repair of thoracic aorta are included in 33886)

(0037T has been deleted. For open subclavian to carotid artery transposition performed in conjunction with endovascular thoracic aortic repair by neck incision, use 33889)

(0038T has been deleted. For endovascular repair of descending thoracic aorta, involving coverage of left subclavian artery origin, radiological supervision and interpretation, use 75956)

(0039T has been deleted. For endovascular repair of descending thoracic aorta, not involving coverage of left subclavian artery origin, radiological supervision and interpretation, use 75957)

(0040T has been deleted. For placement of proximal extension prosthesis for endovascular repair of descending thoracic aorta, radiological supervision and interpretation, use 75958. For placement of distal extension prosthesis after thoracic endovascular repair of descending thoracic aorta, radiological supervision and interpretation, use 75959)

0041T Urinalysis infectious agent detection, semi-quantitative analysis of volatile compounds
> *CPT Changes: An Insider's View* 2003

0042T Cerebral perfusion analysis using computed tomography with contrast administration, including post-processing of parametric maps with determination of cerebral blood flow, cerebral blood volume, and mean transit time
> *CPT Changes: An Insider's View* 2003

0043T Carbon monoxide, expired gas analysis (eg, $ETCO_c$/hemolysis breath test)
> *CPT Changes: An Insider's View* 2003

(0044T and 0045T have been deleted. To report, use 96904)

0046T Catheter lavage of a mammary duct(s) for collection of cytology specimen(s), in high risk individuals (GAIL risk scoring or prior personal history of breast cancer), each breast; single duct
> *CPT Assistant* Jul 04:7; *CPT Changes: An Insider's View* 2004

0047T each additional duct
> *CPT Assistant* Jul 04:7; *CPT Changes: An Insider's View* 2004

0048T Implantation of a ventricular assist device, extracorporeal, percutaneous transseptal access, single or dual cannulation
> *CPT Assistant* Jul 04:7-8; *CPT Changes: An Insider's View* 2004

+ 0049T Prolonged extracorporeal percutaneous transseptal ventricular assist device, greater than 24 hours, each subsequent 24 hour period (List separately in addition to code for primary procedure)
> *CPT Assistant* Jul 04:7; *CPT Changes: An Insider's View* 2004

(Use 0049T in conjunction with 0048T)

0050T Removal of a ventricular assist device, extracorporeal, percutaneous transseptal access, single or dual cannulation
> *CPT Assistant* Jul 04:7; *CPT Changes: An Insider's View* 2004

0051T Implantation of a total replacement heart system (artificial heart) with recipient cardiectomy
> *CPT Assistant* Jun 04:7; *CPT Changes: An Insider's View* 2004

(For implantation of heart assist or ventricular assist device, see 33975, 33976)

0052T Replacement or repair of thoracic unit of a total replacement heart system (artificial heart)
> *CPT Assistant* Jun 04:7; *CPT Changes: An Insider's View* 2004

(For replacement or repair of other implantable components in a total replacement heart system (artificial heart), use 0053T)

0053T Replacement or repair of implantable component or components of total replacement heart system (artificial heart), excluding thoracic unit
> *CPT Assistant* Jun 04:7; *CPT Changes: An Insider's View* 2004

(For replacement or repair of a thoracic unit of a total replacement heart system (artificial heart), use 0052T)

▶(0054T-0056T have been deleted. To report, see 20985-20987)◄

(0057T has been deleted. To report, use 43257)

0058T Cryopreservation; reproductive tissue, ovarian
> *CPT Assistant* Jun 04:8; *CPT Changes: An Insider's View* 2004

0059T oocyte(s)
> *CPT Changes: An Insider's View* 2004

(For cryopreservation of embryo(s), sperm and testicular reproductive tissue, see 89258, 89259, 89335)

0060T   Electrical impedance scan of the breast, bilateral (risk assessment device for breast cancer)

➔ *CPT Assistant* Jul 04:11; *CPT Changes: An Insider's View* 2004

0061T   Destruction/reduction of malignant breast tumor including breast carcinoma cells in the margins, microwave phased array thermotherapy, disposable catheter with combined temperature monitoring probe and microwave sensor, externally applied microwave energy, including interstitial placement of sensor

➔ *CPT Assistant* Jul 04:11; *CPT Changes: An Insider's View* 2004

(For imaging guidance performed in conjunction with 0061T, see 76942, 76998)

0062T   Percutaneous intradiscal annuloplasty, any method except electrothermal, unilateral or bilateral including fluoroscopic guidance; single level

➔ *CPT Assistant* Mar 05:1-3, Apr 05:14-16; *CPT Changes: An Insider's View* 2005, 2007

+ 0063T   1 or more additional levels (List separately in addition to 0062T for primary procedure)

➔ *CPT Assistant* Mar 05:1-2; *CPT Changes: An Insider's View* 2005

(For CT or MRI guidance and localization for needle placement and annuloplasty in conjunction with 0062T, 0063T, see 77012, 77021)

(For intradiscal electrothermal annuloplasty, see 22526-22527)

0064T   Spectroscopy, expired gas analysis (eg, nitric oxide/carbon dioxide test)

➔ *CPT Assistant* Mar 05:1, 3, Mar 07:11; *CPT Changes: An Insider's View* 2005

▶(0065T has been deleted. To report, use 99174)◀

0066T   Computed tomographic (CT) colonography (ie, virtual colonoscopy); screening

➔ *CPT Assistant* Mar 05:1, 4, Dec 05:7, Jan 07:31; *CPT Changes: An Insider's View* 2005

➔ *Clinical Examples in Radiology* Winter 05:8, 12

0067T   diagnostic

➔ *CPT Assistant* Mar 05:1, 4, Dec 05:7, Jan 07:31; *CPT Changes: An Insider's View* 2005

➔ *Clinical Examples in Radiology* Winter 05:8

(Do not report 0066T or 0067T in conjunction with 72192-72194, 74150-74170)

▲ **0068T**   Acoustic heart sound recording and computer analysis; with interpretation and report

➔ *CPT Assistant* Mar 05:1, 4-5, Dec 06:8; *CPT Changes: An Insider's View* 2005, 2008

▲ **0069T**   acoustic heart sound recording and computer analysis only

➔ *CPT Assistant* Mar 05:1, 4-5, Dec 06:8; *CPT Changes: An Insider's View* 2005, 2008

▲ **0070T**   interpretation and report only

➔ *CPT Assistant* Mar 05:1, 5, Dec 06:8; *CPT Changes: An Insider's View* 2005, 2008

0071T   Focused ultrasound ablation of uterine leiomyomata, including MR guidance; total leiomyomata volume less than 200 cc of tissue

➔ *CPT Assistant* Mar 05:1, 5, Dec 05:3; *CPT Changes: An Insider's View* 2005

0072T   total leiomyomata volume greater or equal to 200 cc of tissue

➔ *CPT Assistant* Mar 05:1, 5, Dec 05:3; *CPT Changes: An Insider's View* 2005

(Do not report 0071T, 0072T in conjunction with 51702 or 77022)

0073T   Compensator-based beam modulation treatment delivery of inverse planned treatment using three or more high resolution (milled or cast) compensator convergent beam modulated fields, per treatment session

➔ *CPT Assistant* Mar 05:1, 6, May 05:7; *CPT Changes: An Insider's View* 2005

(For treatment planning, use 77301)

(Do not report 0073T in conjunction with 77401-77416, 77418)

▶(0074T has been deleted. To report, see 98969, 99444)◀

0075T   Transcatheter placement of extracranial vertebral or intrathoracic carotid artery stent(s), including radiologic supervision and interpretation, percutaneous; initial vessel

➔ *CPT Assistant* May 05:7; *CPT Changes: An Insider's View* 2005

+ 0076T   each additional vessel (List separately in addition to code for primary procedure)

➔ *CPT Assistant* May 05:7; *CPT Changes: An Insider's View* 2005

(Use 0076T in conjunction with 0075T)

(When the ipsilateral extracranial vertebral or intrathoracic carotid arteriogram (including imaging and selective catheterization) confirms the need for stenting, then 0075T and 0076T include all ipsilateral extracranial vertebral or intrathoracic selective carotid catheterization, all diagnostic imaging for ipsilateral extracranial vertebral or intrathoracic carotid artery stenting, and all related radiologic supervision and interpretation. If stenting is not indicated, then the appropriate codes for selective catheterization and imaging should be reported in lieu of code 0075T or 0076T.)

0077T   Implanting and securing cerebral thermal perfusion probe, including twist drill or burr hole, to measure absolute cerebral tissue perfusion

➔ *CPT Assistant* May 05:7; *CPT Changes: An Insider's View* 2005

(0078T-0081T should be reported in accordance with the Endovascular Abdominal Aneurysm Repair guidelines established for 34800-34826)

0078T Endovascular repair using prosthesis of abdominal aortic aneurysm, pseudoaneurysm or dissection, abdominal aorta involving visceral branches (superior mesenteric, celiac and/or renal artery(s))

➲ *CPT Assistant* May 05:7, Jun 05:6; *CPT Changes: An Insider's View* 2005, 2006

➲ *Clinical Examples in Radiology* Winter 06:20

(Do not report 0078T in conjunction with 34800-34805, 35081, 35102, 35452, 35454, 35472, 37205-37208)

(Report 0078T in conjunction with 35454, 37205-37208 when these procedures are performed outside the target zone of the endoprosthesis)

+ 0079T Placement of visceral extension prosthesis for endovascular repair of abdominal aortic aneurysm involving visceral vessels, each visceral branch (List separately in addition to code for primary procedure)

➲ *CPT Assistant* May 05:7; *CPT Changes: An Insider's View* 2005

(Use 0079T in conjunction with 0078T)

(Do not report 0079T in conjunction with 34800-34805, 35081, 35102, 35452, 35454, 35472, 37205-37208)

(Report 0079T in conjunction with 35454, 37205-37208 when these procedures are performed outside the target zone of the endoprosthesis)

0080T Endovascular repair of abdominal aortic aneurysm, pseudoaneurysm or dissection, abdominal aorta involving visceral vessels (superior mesenteric, celiac or renal), using fenestrated modular bifurcated prosthesis (two docking limbs), radiological supervision and interpretation

➲ *CPT Assistant* May 05:7; *CPT Changes: An Insider's View* 2005

(Do not report 0080T in conjunction with 34800-34805, 35081, 35102, 35452, 35454, 35472, 37205-37208)

(Report 0080T in conjunction with 35454, 37205-37208 when these procedures are performed outside the target zone of the endoprosthesis)

+ 0081T Placement of visceral extension prosthesis for endovascular repair of abdominal aortic aneurysm involving visceral vessels, each visceral branch, radiological supervision and interpretation (List separately in addition to code for primary procedure)

➲ *CPT Assistant* May 05:7; *CPT Changes: An Insider's View* 2005

(Use 0081T in conjunction with 0080T)

(Do not report 0081T in conjunction with 34800-34805, 35081, 35102, 35452, 35454, 35472, 37205-37208)

(Report 0081T in conjunction with 35454, 37205-37208 when these procedures are performed outside the target zone of the endoprosthesis)

▶(0082T, 0083T have been deleted. To report, see 77373, 77435)◀

0084T Insertion of a temporary prostatic urethral stent

➲ *CPT Assistant* May 05:7; *CPT Changes: An Insider's View* 2005

0085T Breath test for heart transplant rejection

➲ *CPT Assistant* May 05:7; *CPT Changes: An Insider's View* 2005

0086T Left ventricular filling pressure indirect measurement by computerized calibration of the arterial waveform response to Valsalva maneuver

➲ *CPT Assistant* May 05:7; *CPT Changes: An Insider's View* 2005

▲ **0087T** Sperm evaluation, Hyaluronan sperm binding test

➲ *CPT Assistant* May 05:7, Dec 06:8; *CPT Changes: An Insider's View* 2005, 2008

0088T Submucosal radiofrequency tissue volume reduction of tongue base, one or more sites, per session (ie, for treatment of obstructive sleep apnea syndrome)

➲ *CPT Assistant* May 05:7, Sep 05:9; *CPT Changes: An Insider's View* 2005

0089T Actigraphy testing, recording, analysis and interpretation (minimum of three-day recording)

➲ *CPT Assistant* Jun 05:6, Feb 06:1; *CPT Changes: An Insider's View* 2006

0090T Total disc arthroplasty (artificial disc), anterior approach, including discectomy to prepare interspace (other than for decompression) cervical; single interspace

➲ *CPT Assistant* Jun 05:6, Feb 06:1; *CPT Changes: An Insider's View* 2006, 2007

(0091T has been deleted)

(To report total disc lumbar arthroplasty, use 22857)

+ 0092T each additional interspace (List separately in addition to code for primary procedure)

➲ *CPT Assistant* Jun 05:6, Feb 06:1; *CPT Changes: An Insider's View* 2006

(Use 0092T in conjunction with 0090T)

(For total disc lumbar arthroplasty of additional interspaces, use 0163T)

(Do not report 0092T in conjunction with 22857)

0093T Removal of total disc arthroplasty, anterior approach cervical; single interspace

➲ *CPT Assistant* Jun 05:6, Feb 06:1; *CPT Changes: An Insider's View* 2006, 2007

(0094T has been deleted)

(To report removal of total disc lumbar arthroplasty, use 22865)

+ 0095T each additional interspace (List separately in addition to code for primary procedure)

➲ *CPT Assistant* Jun 05:6, Feb 06:1; *CPT Changes: An Insider's View* 2006

(Use 0095T in conjunction with 0093T)

(For removal of total disc lumbar arthroplasty additional interspaces, use 0164T)

(Do not report 0095T in conjunction with 22865)

0096T Revision of total disc arthroplasty, anterior approach cervical; single interspace

➔ *CPT Assistant* Jun 05:6, Feb 06:1; *CPT Changes: An Insider's View* 2006, 2007

(Do not report 0096T in conjunction with 0093T)

(0097T has been deleted)

(To report revision of total disc lumbar arthroplasty, use 22862)

+ 0098T each additional interspace (List separately in addition to code for primary procedure)

➔ *CPT Assistant* Jun 05:6, Feb 06:1; *CPT Changes: An Insider's View* 2006

(Use 0098T in conjunction with 0096T)

(Do not report 0098T in conjunction with 22862, 0095T)

(0090T-0098T include fluoroscopy when performed)

(Do not report 0090T-0098T in conjunction with 22851, 49010, when performed at the same level)

(For revision of total disc lumbar arthroplasty additional interspaces, use 0165T)

(For decompression, see 63001-63048)

0099T Implantation of intrastromal corneal ring segments

➔ *CPT Assistant* Jun 05:6, Feb 06:1; *CPT Changes: An Insider's View* 2006

0100T Placement of a subconjunctival retinal prosthesis receiver and pulse generator, and implantation of intra-ocular retinal electrode array, with vitrectomy

➔ *CPT Assistant* Jun 05:6, Feb 06:1; *CPT Changes: An Insider's View* 2006

0101T Extracorporeal shock wave involving musculoskeletal system, not otherwise specified, high energy

➔ *CPT Assistant* Jun 05:6, Mar 06:1; *CPT Changes: An Insider's View* 2006

(For application of low energy musculoskeletal system extracorporeal shock wave, use 0019T)

0102T Extracorporeal shock wave, high energy, performed by a physician, requiring anesthesia other than local, involving lateral humeral epicondyle

➔ *CPT Assistant* Jun 05:6, Mar 06:1; *CPT Changes: An Insider's View* 2006

(For application of low energy musculoskeletal system extracorporeal shock wave, use 0019T)

0103T Holotranscobalamin, quantitative

➔ *CPT Assistant* Jun 05:6, Mar 06:1; *CPT Changes: An Insider's View* 2006

0104T Inert gas rebreathing for cardiac output measurement; during rest

➔ *CPT Assistant* Jun 05:6, Mar 06:1; *CPT Changes: An Insider's View* 2006

0105T during exercise

➔ *CPT Assistant* Jun 05:6, Mar 06:1; *CPT Changes: An Insider's View* 2006

0106T Quantitative sensory testing (QST), testing and interpretation per extremity; using touch pressure stimuli to assess large diameter sensation

➔ *CPT Assistant* Jun 05:6, Mar 06:1; *CPT Changes: An Insider's View* 2006

0107T using vibration stimuli to assess large diameter fiber sensation

➔ *CPT Assistant* Jun 05:6, Mar 06:1; *CPT Changes: An Insider's View* 2006

0108T using cooling stimuli to assess small nerve fiber sensation and hyperalgesia

➔ *CPT Assistant* Jun 05:6, Mar 06:1; *CPT Changes: An Insider's View* 2006

0109T using heat-pain stimuli to assess small nerve fiber sensation and hyperalgesia

➔ *CPT Assistant* Jun 05:6, Mar 06:1; *CPT Changes: An Insider's View* 2006

0110T using other stimuli to assess sensation

➔ *CPT Assistant* Jun 05:6, Mar 06:1; *CPT Changes: An Insider's View* 2006

0111T Long-chain (C20-22) omega-3 fatty acids in red blood cell (RBC) membranes

➔ *CPT Assistant* Jun 05:6, Mar 06:1; *CPT Changes: An Insider's View* 2006

(For very long chain fatty acids, use 82726)

▶(0115T-0117T have been deleted. To report, see 99605-99607)◀

(0120T has been deleted. To report, use 19105)

0123T Fistulization of sclera for glaucoma, through ciliary body

➔ *CPT Changes: An Insider's View* 2006

0124T Conjunctival incision with posterior juxtascleral placement of pharmacological agent (does not include supply of medication)

➔ *CPT Changes: An Insider's View* 2006

0126T Common carotid intima-media thickness (IMT) study for evaluation of atherosclerotic burden or coronary heart disease risk factor assessment

➔ *CPT Changes: An Insider's View* 2006

0130T Validated, statistically reliable, randomized, controlled, single-patient clinical investigation of FDA approved chronic care drugs, provided by a pharmacist, interpretation and report to the prescribing health care professional

➔ *CPT Changes: An Insider's View* 2006

▶(0133T has been deleted)◀

▶(0135T has been deleted. To report, use 50593)◀

0137T Biopsy, prostate, needle, saturation sampling for prostate mapping

➔ *CPT Changes: An Insider's View* 2006

(Do not report 0137T in conjunction with 76942)

0140T Exhaled breath condensate pH

➔ *CPT Changes: An Insider's View* 2006

Pancreatic islet cells are transplanted by infusion into the portal vein. The portal vein may be cannulated percutaneously with imaging guidance, by laparoscopy, or by laparotomy. Codes 0141T-0143T include infusion of islet cells with monitoring and management of portal and systemic hemodynamics, monitoring and management of blood glucose and insulin therapy, immunotherapy infusion, antibiotic infusion, analgesic and sedative administration and monitoring, and all other therapeutic injections and infusions administered during the islet infusion. Codes 0141T-0143T also include typical postprocedural care. When reporting 0141T, percutaneous portal vein catheterization is reported separately (see codes 36481, 75887). Code 0142T includes diagnostic laparotomy (49000, 49002). Code 0143T includes diagnostic laparoscopy (49320).

0141T Pancreatic islet cell transplantation through portal vein, percutaneous

> *CPT Changes: An Insider's View* 2007

(For open approach, use 0142T)

(For laparoscopic approach, use 0143T)

(For percutaneous portal vein catheterization, use 36481)

(For radiological supervision and interpretation, use 75887)

0142T Pancreatic islet cell transplantation through portal vein, open

> *CPT Changes: An Insider's View* 2007

(For percutaneous approach, use 0141T)

(For laparoscopic approach, use 0143T)

(Do not report 0142T in conjunction with 49000, 49002)

0143T Laparoscopy, surgical, pancreatic islet cell transplantation through portal vein

> *CPT Changes: An Insider's View* 2007

(For percutaneous approach, use 0141T)

(For open approach, use 0142T)

(Do not report 0143T in conjunction with 49320)

0144T Computed tomography, heart, without contrast material, including image postprocessing and quantitative evaluation of coronary calcium

> *CPT Changes: An Insider's View* 2007
> *Clinical Examples in Radiology* Winter 06:6, 18; Bulletin #1 05:1

(Do not report 0144T in conjunction with 0145T-0151T)

▲ **0145T** Computed tomography, heart, with contrast material(s), including noncontrast images, if performed, cardiac gating and 3D image postprocessing; cardiac structure and morphology

> *CPT Changes: An Insider's View* 2007, 2008
> *Clinical Examples in Radiology* Winter 06:6, 18; Bulletin #1 05:1

(For cardiac structure and morphology in congenital heart disease, use 0150T)

▲ **0146T** computed tomographic angiography of coronary arteries (including native and anomalous coronary arteries, coronary bypass grafts), without quantitative evaluation of coronary calcium

> *CPT Changes: An Insider's View* 2007, 2008
> *Clinical Examples in Radiology* Winter 06:4-6; Bulletin #1 05:2

▲ **0147T** computed tomographic angiography of coronary arteries (including native and anomalous coronary arteries, coronary bypass grafts), with quantitative evaluation of coronary calcium

> *CPT Changes: An Insider's View* 2007, 2008
> *Clinical Examples in Radiology* Winter 06:6, 18; Bulletin #1 05:2

(Do not report 0147T in conjunction with 0144T)

▲ **0148T** cardiac structure and morphology and computed tomographic angiography of coronary arteries (including native and anomalous coronary arteries, coronary bypass grafts), without quantitative evaluation of coronary calcium

> *CPT Changes: An Insider's View* 2007, 2008
> *Clinical Examples in Radiology* Winter 06:6, 18; Bulletin #1 05:2

▲ **0149T** cardiac structure and morphology and computed tomographic angiography of coronary arteries (including native and anomalous coronary arteries, coronary bypass grafts), with quantitative evaluation of coronary calcium

> *CPT Changes: An Insider's View* 2007, 2008
> *Clinical Examples in Radiology* Winter 06:6, 19; Bulletin #1 05:2

(Do not report 0149T in conjunction with 0144T)

▲ **0150T** cardiac structure and morphology in congenital heart disease

> *CPT Changes: An Insider's View* 2007, 2008
> *Clinical Examples in Radiology* Winter 06:6, 19; Bulletin #1 05:2

+▲ **0151T** Computed tomography, heart, with contrast material(s), including noncontrast images, if performed, cardiac gating and 3D image postprocessing, function evaluation (left and right ventricular function, ejection-fraction and segmental wall motion) (List separately in addition to code for primary procedure)

> *CPT Changes: An Insider's View* 2007, 2008
> *Clinical Examples in Radiology* Winter 06:4-6, 19; Bulletin #1 05:2

(Use 0151T in conjunction with 0145T-0150T)

(0152T has been deleted. To report, see 0174T, 0175T)

▶(0153T has been deleted. To report, use 34806)◀

▶(0154T has been deleted. To report, use 93982)◀

0155T   Laparoscopy, surgical; implantation or replacement of gastric stimulation electrodes, lesser curvature (ie, morbid obesity)

➔ *CPT Changes: An Insider's View* 2007

0156T   revision or removal of gastric stimulation electrodes, lesser curvature (ie, morbid obesity)

➔ *CPT Changes: An Insider's View* 2007

(For open approach, see 0157T, 0158T)

▶For laparoscopic or open insertion, revision or removal of antral gastric neurostimulator electrodes, see 43647, 43648, 43881, 43882)◀

▶(For insertion, revision or removal of gastric neurostimulator pulse generator, see 64590, 64595)◀

▶(For electronic analysis and programming of antral gastric neurostimulator pulse generator, see 95980-95982)◀

▶(For electronic analysis and programming of a gastric neurostimulator, lesser curvature, use 0162T)◀

0157T   Laparotomy, implantation or replacement of gastric stimulation electrodes, lesser curvature (ie, morbid obesity)

➔ *CPT Changes: An Insider's View* 2007

0158T   Laparotomy, revision or removal of gastric stimulation electrodes, lesser curvature (ie, morbid obesity)

➔ *CPT Changes: An Insider's View* 2007

(For laparoscopic approach, see 0155T, 0156T)

(For insertion of gastric neurostimulator pulse generator, use 64590)

(For revision or removal of gastric neurostimulator pulse generator, use 64595)

▶(For electronic analysis and programming of antral gastric neurostimulator pulse generator, see 95980-95982)◀

▶(For electronic analysis and programming of a gastric neurostimulator, lesser curvature, use 0162T)◀

+ 0159T   Computer-aided detection, including computer algorithm analysis of MRI image data for lesion detection/characterization, pharmacokinetic analysis, with further physician review for interpretation, breast MRI (List separately in addition to code for primary procedure)

➔ *CPT Changes: An Insider's View* 2007

(Use 0159T in conjunction with 77058, 77059)

▶(Do not report 0159T in conjunction with 76376, 76377)◀

0160T   Therapeutic repetitive transcranial magnetic stimulation treatment planning

➔ *CPT Changes: An Insider's View* 2007

(Pre-treatment determination of optimal magnetic field strength via titration, treatment location determination and stimulation parameter and protocol programming in the therapeutic use of high power, focal magnetic pulses for the direct, noninvasive modulation of cortical neurons)

0161T   Therapeutic repetitive transcranial magnetic stimulation treatment delivery and management, per session

➔ *CPT Changes: An Insider's View* 2007

(Treatment session using high power, focal magnetic pulses for the direct, noninvasive modulation of cortical neurons. Clinical evaluation, safety monitoring and treatment parameter review in the therapeutic use of high power, focal magnetic pulses for the direct, noninvasive modulation of cortical neurons)

0162T   Electronic analysis and programming, reprogramming of gastric neurostimulator (ie, morbid obesity)

➔ *CPT Changes: An Insider's View* 2007

+ 0163T   Total disc arthroplasty (artificial disc), anterior approach, including discectomy to prepare interspace (other than for decompression), lumbar, each additional interspace

➔ *CPT Changes: An Insider's View* 2007

(Use 0163T in conjunction with 22857)

+ 0164T   Removal of total disc arthroplasty, anterior approach, lumbar, each additional interspace

➔ *CPT Changes: An Insider's View* 2007

(Use 0164T in conjunction with 22865)

+ 0165T   Revision of total disc arthroplasty, anterior approach, lumbar, each additional interspace

➔ *CPT Changes: An Insider's View* 2007

(Use 0165T in conjunction with 22862)

(0163T-0165T include fluoroscopy when performed)

(Do not report 0163T-0165T in conjunction with 22851, 49010, when performed at the same level)

(For cervical total disc arthroplasty procedures, see 0090T-0098T)

(For decompression, see 63001-63048)

0166T   Transmyocardial transcatheter closure of ventricular septal defect, with implant; without cardiopulmonary bypass

➔ *CPT Changes: An Insider's View* 2007

0167T   with cardiopulmonary bypass

➔ *CPT Changes: An Insider's View* 2007

▶(Do not report 0166T, 0167T in conjunction with 32551, 33210, 33211)◀

(For ventricular septal defect closure via percutaneous transcatheter implant delivery, use 93581)

0168T   Rhinophototherapy, intranasal application of ultraviolet and visible light, bilateral

➔ *CPT Changes: An Insider's View* 2007

0169T Stereotactic placement of infusion catheter(s) in the brain for delivery of therapeutic agent(s), including computerized stereotactic planning and burr hole(s)
> *CPT Changes: An Insider's View* 2007

(Do not report code 0169T in conjunction with 20660, 61107, 61795)

0170T Repair of anorectal fistula with plug (eg, porcine small intestine submucosa [SIS])
> *CPT Changes: An Insider's View* 2007

(For repair of anal fistula using fibrin glue, use 46706)

(Do not report 0170T in conjunction with 15430, 15431)

● **0171T** Insertion of posterior spinous process distraction device (including necessary removal of bone or ligament for insertion and imaging guidance), lumbar; single level
> *CPT Changes: An Insider's View* 2008

+● **0172T** each additional level (List separately in addition to code for primary procedure)
> *CPT Changes: An Insider's View* 2008

▶(Use 0172T in conjunction with 0171T)◀

+● **0173T** Monitoring of intraocular pressure during vitrectomy surgery (List separately in addition to code for primary procedure)
> *CPT Changes: An Insider's View* 2008

▶(Use 0173T in conjunction with 67036, 67039-67043, 67108, 67112)◀

+● **0174T** Computer-aided detection (CAD) (computer algorithm analysis of digital image data for lesion detection) with further physician review for interpretation and report, with or without digitization of film radiographic images, chest radiograph(s), performed concurrent with primary interpretation (List separately in addition to code for primary procedure)
> *CPT Changes: An Insider's View* 2008

▶(Use 0174T in conjunction with 71010, 71020, 71021, 71022, 71030)◀

● **0175T** Computer-aided detection (CAD) (computer algorithm analysis of digital image data for lesion detection) with further physician review for interpretation and report, with or without digitization of film radiographic images, chest radiograph(s), performed remote from primary interpretation
> *CPT Changes: An Insider's View* 2008

▶(Do not report 0175T in conjunction with 71010, 71020, 71021, 71022, 71030)◀

● **0176T** Transluminal dilation of aqueous outflow canal; without retention of device or stent
> *CPT Changes: An Insider's View* 2008

● **0177T** with retention of device or stent
> *CPT Changes: An Insider's View* 2008

● **0178T** Electrocardiogram, 64 leads or greater, with graphic presentation and analysis; with interpretation and report
> *CPT Changes: An Insider's View* 2008

● **0179T** tracing and graphics only, without interpretation and report
> *CPT Changes: An Insider's View* 2008

● **0180T** interpretation and report only
> *CPT Changes: An Insider's View* 2008

▶(For electrocardiogram, routine, with at least 12 leads separately performed, see 93000-93010)◀

● **0181T** Corneal hysteresis determination, by air impulse stimulation, bilateral, with interpretation and report
> *CPT Changes: An Insider's View* 2008

● **0182T** High dose rate electronic brachytherapy, per fraction
> *CPT Changes: An Insider's View* 2008

▶(Do not report 0182T in conjunction with 77761-77763, 77776-77778, 77781-77784, 77789)◀

● **0183T** Low frequency, non-contact, non-thermal ultrasound, including topical application(s), when performed, wound assessment, and instruction(s) for ongoing care, per day
> *CPT Changes: An Insider's View* 2008

Appendix A

Modifiers

▶This list includes all of the modifiers applicable to *CPT 2008* codes.

A modifier provides the means to report or indicate that a service or procedure that has been performed has been altered by some specific circumstance but not changed in its definition or code. Modifiers also enable health care professionals to effectively respond to payment policy requirements established by other entities.◄

21 Prolonged Evaluation and Management Services: When the face-to-face or floor/unit service(s) provided is prolonged or otherwise greater than that usually required for the highest level of evaluation and management service within a given category, it may be identified by adding modifier 21 to the evaluation and management code number. A report may also be appropriate.

▶22 Increased Procedural Services: When the work required to provide a service is substantially greater than typically required, it may be identified by adding modifier 22 to the usual procedure code. Documentation must support the substantial additional work and the reason for the additional work (ie, increased intensity, time, technical difficulty of procedure, severity of patient's condition, physical and mental effort required). **Note:** This modifier should not be appended to an E/M service.◄

23 Unusual Anesthesia: Occasionally, a procedure, which usually requires either no anesthesia or local anesthesia, because of unusual circumstances must be done under general anesthesia. This circumstance may be reported by adding modifier 23 to the procedure code of the basic service.

24 Unrelated Evaluation and Management Service by the Same Physician During a Postoperative Period: The physician may need to indicate that an evaluation and management service was performed during a postoperative period for a reason(s) unrelated to the original procedure. This circumstance may be reported by adding modifier 24 to the appropriate level of E/M service.

▶25 Significant, Separately Identifiable Evaluation and Management Service by the Same Physician on the Same Day of the Procedure or Other Service: It may be necessary to indicate that on the day a procedure or service identified by a CPT code was performed, the patient's condition required a significant, separately identifiable E/M service above and beyond the other service provided or beyond the usual preoperative and postoperative care associated with the procedure that was performed. A significant, separately identifiable E/M service is defined or substantiated by documentation that satisfies the relevant criteria for the respective E/M service to be reported (see **Evaluation and Management Services Guidelines** for instructions on determining level of E/M service). The E/M service may be prompted by the symptom or condition for which the procedure and/or service was provided. As such, different diagnoses are not required for reporting of the E/M services on the same date. This circumstance may be reported by adding modifier 25 to the appropriate level of E/M service. **Note:** This modifier is not used to report an E/M service that resulted in a decision to perform surgery. See modifier 57. For significant, separately identifiable non-E/M services, see modifier 59.◄

26 Professional Component: Certain procedures are a combination of a physician component and a technical component. When the physician component is reported separately, the service may be identified by adding modifier 26 to the usual procedure number.

▶32 Mandated Services: Services related to *mandated* consultation and/or related services (eg, third-party payer, governmental, legislative or regulatory requirement) may be identified by adding modifier 32 to the basic procedure.◄

47 Anesthesia by Surgeon: Regional or general anesthesia provided by the surgeon may be reported by adding modifier 47 to the basic service. (This does not include local anesthesia.) **Note:** Modifier 47 would not be used as a modifier for the anesthesia procedures.

50 Bilateral Procedure: Unless otherwise identified in the listings, bilateral procedures that are performed at the same operative session, should be identified by adding modifier 50 to the appropriate five digit code.

▶51 Multiple Procedures: When multiple procedures, other than E/M services, physical medicine and rehabilitation services, or provision of supplies (eg, vaccines), are performed at the same session by the same provider, the primary procedure or service may be reported as listed. The additional procedure(s) or service(s) may be identified by appending modifier 51 to the additional procedure or service code(s). **Note:** This modifier should not be appended to designated add-on codes (see Appendix D).◄

52 Reduced Services: Under certain circumstances a service or procedure is partially reduced or eliminated at the physician's discretion. Under these circumstances the service provided can be identified by its usual procedure number and the addition of modifier 52, signifying that the service is reduced. This provides a means of reporting reduced services without disturbing the identification of the basic service. **Note:** For hospital outpatient reporting of a previously scheduled procedure/service that is partially reduced or cancelled as a result of extenuating circumstances or those that threaten the well-being of the patient prior to or after administration of anesthesia, see modifiers 73 and 74 (see modifiers approved for ASC hospital outpatient use).

53 Discontinued Procedure: Under certain circumstances, the physician may elect to terminate a surgical or diagnostic procedure. Due to extenuating circumstances or those that threaten the well being of the patient, it may be necessary to indicate that a surgical or diagnostic procedure was started but discontinued. This circumstance may be reported by adding modifier 53 to the code reported by the physician for the discontinued procedure. **Note:** This modifier is not used to report the elective cancellation of a procedure prior to the patient's anesthesia induction and/or surgical preparation in the operating suite. For outpatient hospital/ambulatory surgery center (ASC) reporting of a previously scheduled procedure or service that is partially reduced or cancelled as a result of extenuating circumstances or those that threaten the well being of the patient prior to or after administration of anesthesia, see modifiers 73 and 74 (see modifiers approved for ASC hospital outpatient use).

54 Surgical Care Only: When one physician performs a surgical procedure and another provides preoperative and/or postoperative management, surgical services may be identified by adding modifier 54 to the usual procedure number.

55 Postoperative Management Only: When one physician performed the postoperative management and another physician performed the surgical procedure, the postoperative component may be identified by adding modifier 55 to the usual procedure number.

56 Preoperative Management Only: When one physician performed the preoperative care and evaluation and another physician performed the surgical procedure, the preoperative component may be identified by adding modifier 56 to the usual procedure number.

57 Decision for Surgery: An evaluation and management service that resulted in the initial decision to perform the surgery may be identified by adding modifier 57 to the appropriate level of E/M service.

▶**58 Staged or Related Procedure or Service by the Same Physician During the Postoperative Period:** It may be necessary to indicate that the performance of a procedure or service during the postoperative period was (a) planned or anticipated (staged); (b) more extensive than the original procedure; or (c) for therapy following a surgical procedure. This circumstance may be reported by adding modifier 58 to the staged or related procedure. **Note:** For treatment of a problem that requires a return to the operating or procedure room (eg, unanticipated clinical condition), see modifier 78.◀

▶**59 Distinct Procedural Service:** Under certain circumstances, it may be necessary to indicate that a procedure or service was distinct or independent from other non-E/M services performed on the same day. Modifier 59 is used to identify procedures or services, other than E/M services, that are not normally reported together but are appropriate under the circumstances. Documentation must support a different session, different procedure or surgery, different site or organ system, separate incision or excision, separate lesion, or separate injury (or area of injury in extensive injuries) not ordinarily encountered or performed on the same day by the same individual. However, when another already established modifier is appropriate it should be used rather than modifier 59. Only if no more descriptive modifier is

available and the use of modifier 59 best explains the circumstances should modifier 59 be used. **Note:** Modifier 59 should not be appended to an E/M service. To report a separate and distinct E/M service with a non-E/M service performed on the same date, see modifier 25.◀

62 Two Surgeons: When two surgeons work together as primary surgeons performing distinct part(s) of a procedure, each surgeon should report his/her distinct operative work by adding modifier 62 to the procedure code and any associated add-on code(s) for that procedure as long as both surgeons continue to work together as primary surgeons. Each surgeon should report the co-surgery once using the same procedure code. If additional procedure(s) (including add-on procedure(s) are performed during the same surgical session, separate code(s) may also be reported with modifier 62 added. **Note:** If a co-surgeon acts as an assistant in the performance of additional procedure(s) during the same surgical session, those services may be reported using separate procedure code(s) with modifier 80 or modifier 82 added, as appropriate.

63 Procedure Performed on Infants less than 4 kg: Procedures performed on neonates and infants up to a present body weight of 4 kg may involve significantly increased complexity and physician work commonly associated with these patients. This circumstance may be reported by adding modifier 63 to the procedure number. **Note:** Unless otherwise designated, this modifier may only be appended to procedures/services listed in the 20000-69990 code series. Modifier 63 should not be appended to any CPT codes listed in the **Evaluation and Management Services, Anesthesia, Radiology, Pathology/Laboratory, or Medicine** sections.

66 Surgical Team: Under some circumstances, highly complex procedures (requiring the concomitant services of several physicians, often of different specialties, plus other highly skilled, specially trained personnel, various types of complex equipment) are carried out under the "surgical team" concept. Such circumstances may be identified by each participating physician with the addition of modifier 66 to the basic procedure number used for reporting services.

▶**76 Repeat Procedure or Service by Same Physician:** It may be necessary to indicate that a procedure or service was repeated subsequent to the original procedure or service. This circumstance may be reported by adding modifier 76 to the repeated procedure or service.◀

77 Repeat Procedure by Another Physician: The physician may need to indicate that a basic procedure or service performed by another physician had to be repeated. This situation may be reported by adding modifier 77 to the repeated procedure or service.

▶**78 Unplanned Return to the Operating/Procedure Room by the Same Physician Following Initial Procedure for a Related Procedure During the Postoperative Period:** It may be necessary to indicate that another procedure was performed during the postoperative period of the initial procedure (unplanned procedure following initial procedure). When this procedure is related to the first and requires the use of an operating or procedure room, it may be reported by adding modifier 78 to the related procedure. (For repeat procedures, see modifier 76.)◄

79 Unrelated Procedure or Service by the Same Physician During the Postoperative Period: The physician may need to indicate that the performance of a procedure or service during the postoperative period was unrelated to the original procedure. This circumstance may be reported by using modifier 79. (For repeat procedures on the same day, see modifier 76.)

80 Assistant Surgeon: Surgical assistant services may be identified by adding modifier 80 to the usual procedure number(s).

81 Minimum Assistant Surgeon: Minimum surgical assistant services are identified by adding modifier 81 to the usual procedure number.

82 Assistant Surgeon (when qualified resident surgeon not available): The unavailability of a qualified resident surgeon is a prerequisite for use of modifier 82 appended to the usual procedure code number(s).

90 Reference (Outside) Laboratory: When laboratory procedures are performed by a party other than the treating or reporting physician, the procedure may be identified by adding modifier 90 to the usual procedure number.

91 Repeat Clinical Diagnostic Laboratory Test: In the course of treatment of the patient, it may be necessary to repeat the same laboratory test on the same day to obtain subsequent (multiple) test results. Under these circumstances, the laboratory test performed can be identified by its usual procedure number and the addition of modifier 91. **Note:** This modifier may not be used when tests are rerun to confirm initial results; due to testing problems with specimens or equipment; or for any other reason when a normal, one-time, reportable result is all that is required. This modifier may not be used when other code(s) describe a series of test results (eg, glucose tolerance tests, evocative/suppression testing). This modifier may only be used for laboratory test(s) performed more than once on the same day on the same patient.

►92 Alternative Laboratory Platform Testing: When laboratory testing is being performed using a kit or transportable instrument that wholly or in part consists of a single use, disposable analytical chamber, the service may be identified by adding modifier 92 to the usual laboratory procedure code (HIV testing 86701-86703). The test does not require permanent dedicated space; hence by its design it may be hand carried or transported to the vicinity of the patient for immediate testing at that site, although location of the testing is not in itself determinative of the use of this modifier.◄

99 Multiple Modifiers: Under certain circumstances two or more modifiers may be necessary to completely delineate a service. In such situations modifier 99 should be added to the basic procedure, and other applicable modifiers may be listed as part of the description of the service.

Anesthesia Physical Status Modifiers

The Physical Status modifiers are consistent with the American Society of Anesthesiologists ranking of patient physical status, and distinguishing various levels of complexity of the anesthesia service provided. All anesthesia services are reported by use of the anesthesia five-digit procedure code (00100-01999) with the appropriate physical status modifier appended.

Example: 00100-P1

Under certain circumstances, when another established modifier(s) is appropriate, it should be used in addition to the physical status modifier.

Example: 00100-P4-53

Physical Status Modifier P1: A normal healthy patient

Physical Status Modifier P2: A patient with mild systemic disease

Physical Status Modifier P3: A patient with severe systemic disease

Physical Status Modifier P4: A patient with severe systemic disease that is a constant threat to life

Physical Status Modifier P5: A moribund patient who is not expected to survive without the operation

Physical Status Modifier P6: A declared brain-dead patient whose organs are being removed for donor purposes

Modifiers Approved for Ambulatory Surgery Center (ASC) Hospital Outpatient Use

CPT Level I Modifiers

►25 Significant, Separately Identifiable Evaluation and Management Service by the Same Physician on the Same Day of the Procedure or Other Service: It may be necessary to indicate that on the day a procedure or service identified by a CPT code was performed, the patient's condition required a significant, separately identifiable E/M service above and beyond the other service provided or beyond the usual preoperative and postoperative care associated with the procedure that was performed. A significant, separately identifiable E/M service is defined or substantiated by documentation that satisfies the relevant criteria for the respective E/M service to be reported (see **Evaluation and Management Services Guidelines** for instructions on determining level of E/M service). The E/M service may be prompted by the symptom or condition for which the procedure and/or service was provided. As such, different diagnoses are not required for reporting of the E/M services on the same date. This circumstance may be reported by adding modifier 25 to the appropriate level of E/M service. **Note:** This modifier is not used to report an E/M service that resulted in a decision to perform surgery. See modifier 57. For significant, separately identifiable non-E/M services, see modifier 59.◄

27 Multiple Outpatient Hospital E/M Encounters on the Same Date: For hospital outpatient reporting purposes, utilization of hospital resources related to separate and distinct E/M encounters performed in multiple outpatient hospital settings on the same date may be reported by adding modifier 27 to each appropriate level outpatient and/or emergency department E/M code(s). This modifier provides a means of reporting circumstances involving evaluation and management services provided by physician(s) in more than one (multiple) outpatient hospital setting(s) (eg, hospital emergency department, clinic). **Note:** This modifier is not to be used for physician reporting of multiple E/M services performed by the same physician on the same date. For physician reporting of all outpatient evaluation and management services provided by the same physician on the same date and performed in multiple outpatient setting(s) (eg, hospital emergency department, clinic), see **Evaluation and Management, Emergency Department, or Preventive Medicine Services** codes.

50 Bilateral Procedure: Unless otherwise identified in the listings, bilateral procedures that are performed at the same operative session should be identified by adding modifier 50 to the appropriate five digit code.

52 Reduced Services: Under certain circumstances a service or procedure is partially reduced or eliminated at the physician's discretion. Under these circumstances the service provided can be identified by its usual procedure number and the addition of modifier 52, signifying that the service is reduced. This provides a means of reporting reduced services without disturbing the identification of the basic service. **Note:** For hospital outpatient reporting of a previously scheduled procedure or service that is partially reduced or cancelled as a result of extenuating circumstances or those that threaten the well-being of the patient prior to or after administration of anesthesia, see modifiers 73 and 74.

▶**58 Staged or Related Procedure or Service by the Same Physician During the Postoperative Period:** It may be necessary to indicate that the performance of a procedure or service during the postoperative period was (a) planned or anticipated (staged); (b) more extensive than the original procedure; or (c) for therapy following a surgical procedure. This circumstance may be reported by adding modifier 58 to the staged or related procedure. **Note:** For treatment of a problem that requires a return to the operating or procedure room (eg, unanticipated clinical condition), see modifier 78.◀

▶**59 Distinct Procedural Service:** Under certain circumstances, it may be necessary to indicate that a procedure or service was distinct or independent from other non-E/M services performed on the same day. Modifier 59 is used to identify procedures or services other than E/M services, that are not normally reported together but are appropriate under the circumstances. Documentation must support a different session, different procedure or surgery, different site or organ system, separate incision or excision, separate lesion, or separate injury (or area of injury in extensive injuries) not ordinarily encountered or performed on the same day

by the same individual. However, when another already established modifier is appropriate, it should be used rather than modifier 59. Only if no more descriptive modifier is available and the use of modifier 59 best explains the circumstances should modifier 59 be used. **Note:** Modifier 59 should not be appended to an E/M service. To report a separate and distinct E/M service with a non-E/M service performed on the same date, see modifier 25.◀

73 Discontinued Out-Patient Hospital/Ambulatory Surgery Center (ASC) Procedure Prior to the Administration of Anesthesia: Due to extenuating circumstances or those that threaten the well being of the patient, the physician may cancel a surgical or diagnostic procedure subsequent to the patient's surgical preparation (including sedation when provided, and being taken to the room where the procedure is to be performed), but prior to the administration of anesthesia (local, regional block(s) or general). Under these circumstances, the intended service that is prepared for but cancelled can be reported by its usual procedure number and the addition of modifier 73. **Note:** The elective cancellation of a service prior to the administration of anesthesia and/or surgical preparation of the patient should not be reported. For physician reporting of a discontinued procedure, see modifier 53.

74 Discontinued Out-Patient Hospital/Ambulatory Surgery Center (ASC) Procedure After Administration of Anesthesia: Due to extenuating circumstances or those that threaten the well being of the patient, the physician may terminate a surgical or diagnostic procedure after the administration of anesthesia (local, regional block(s), general) or after the procedure was started (incision made, intubation started, scope inserted, etc). Under these circumstances, the procedure started but terminated can be reported by its usual procedure number and the addition of modifier 74. **Note:** The elective cancellation of a service prior to the administration of anesthesia and/or surgical preparation of the patient should not be reported. For physician reporting of a discontinued procedure, see modifier 53.

▶**76 Repeat Procedure or Service by Same Physician:** It may be necessary to indicate that a procedure or service was repeated subsequent to the original procedure or service. This circumstance may be reported by adding modifier 76 to the repeated procedure or service.◀

77 Repeat Procedure by Another Physician: The physician may need to indicate that a basic procedure or service performed by another physician had to be repeated. This situation may be reported by adding modifier 77 to the repeated procedure or service.

▶**78 Unplanned Return to the Operating/Procedure Room by the Same Physician Following Initial Procedure for a Related Procedure During the Postoperative Period:** It may be necessary to indicate that another procedure was performed during the postoperative period of the initial procedure (unplanned procedure following initial procedure). When this procedure is related to the first and requires the use of an operating or room, it may be reported by adding modifier 78 to the related procedure. (For repeat procedures on the same day, see 76.)◀

79 **Unrelated Procedure or Service by the Same Physician During the Postoperative Period:** The physician may need to indicate that the performance of a procedure or service during the postoperative period was unrelated to the original procedure. This circumstance may be reported by using modifier 79. (For repeat procedures on the same day, see 76.)

91 **Repeat Clinical Diagnostic Laboratory Test:** In the course of treatment of the patient, it may be necessary to repeat the same laboratory test on the same day to obtain subsequent (multiple) test results. Under these circumstances, the laboratory test performed can be identified by its usual procedure number and the addition of modifier 91. **Note:** This modifier may not be used when tests are rerun to confirm initial results; due to testing problems with specimens or equipment; or for any other reason when a normal, one-time, reportable result is all that is required. This modifier may not be used when other code(s) describe a series of test results (eg, glucose tolerance tests, evocative/suppression testing). This modifier may only be used for laboratory test(s) performed more than once on the same day on the same patient.

Level II (HCPCS/National) Modifiers

E1 Upper left, eyelid

E2 Lower left, eyelid

E3 Upper right, eyelid

E4 Lower right, eyelid

F1 Left hand, second digit

F2 Left hand, third digit

F3 Left hand, fourth digit

F4 Left hand, fifth digit

F5 Right hand, thumb

F6 Right hand, second digit

F7 Right hand, third digit

F8 Right hand, fourth digit

F9 Right hand, fifth digit

FA Left hand, thumb

GG Performance and payment of a screening mammogram and diagnostic mammogram on the same patient, same day

GH Diagnostic mammogram converted from screening mammogram on same day

LC Left circumflex coronary artery (Hospitals use with codes 92980-92984, 92995, 92996)

LD Left anterior descending coronary artery (Hospitals use with codes 92980-92984, 92995, 92996)

LT Left side (used to identify procedures performed on the left side of the body)

QM Ambulance service provided under arrangement by a provider of services

QN Ambulance service furnished directly by a provider of services

RC Right coronary artery (Hospitals use with codes 92980-92984, 92995, 92996)

RT Right side (used to identify procedures performed on the right side of the body)

T1 Left foot, second digit

T2 Left foot, third digit

T3 Left foot, fourth digit

T4 Left foot, fifth digit

T5 Right foot, great toe

T6 Right foot, second digit

T7 Right foot, third digit

T8 Right foot, fourth digit

T9 Right foot, fifth digit

TA Left foot, great toe

Appendix B

Summary of Additions, Deletions, and Revisions

Appendix B shows the actual changes that were made to the code descriptors. New codes appear with a bullet (●) and are indicated as "Code Added." Revised codes are preceded with a triangle (▲). Within revised codes, the deleted language appears with a ~~strikethrough~~, while new text appears underlined. Codes with which conscious sedation would not be separately reported when performed at the same session by the same provider are denoted with the bullseye (⊙). The symbol ⚲ is used to identify codes for vaccines that are pending FDA approval (see **Appendix K**).

Revisions to the headings, notes, introductory paragraphs, and cross-references are not included in this Appendix, but are identified in the main text of the book with the "► ◄" symbols and presented in green.

Evaluation and Management

▲ 99296   **Subsequent inpatient neonatal critical care,** per day, for the evaluation and management of a critically ill neonate, 28 days of age or less

▲ 99304   Initial nursing facility care, per day, for the evaluation and management of a patient, which requires these 3 key components:

■ **A detailed or comprehensive history;**

■ **A detailed or comprehensive examination; and**

■ **Medical decision making that is straightforward or of low complexity.**

Counseling and/or coordination of care with other providers or agencies are provided consistent with the nature of the problem(s) and the patientís and/or familyís needs.

Usually, the problem(s) requiring admission are of low severity. Physicians typically spend 25 minutes with the patient and/or family or caregiver.

▲ 99305   Initial nursing facility care, per day, for the evaluation and management of a patient, which requires these 3 key components:

■ **A comprehensive history;**

■ **A comprehensive examination; and**

■ **Medical decision making of moderate complexity.**

Counseling and/or coordination of care with other providers or agencies are provided consistent with the nature of the problem(s) and the patientís and/or familyís needs.

Usually, the problem(s) requiring admission are of moderate severity. Physicians typically spend 35 minutes with the patient and/or family or caregiver.

▲ 99306   Initial nursing facility care, per day, for the evaluation and management of a patient, which requires these 3 key components:

■ **A comprehensive history;**

■ **A comprehensive examination; and**

■ **Medical decision making of high complexity.**

Counseling and/or coordination of care with other providers or agencies are provided consistent with the nature of the problem(s) and the patientís and/or familyís needs.

Usually, the problem(s) requiring admission are of high severity. Physicians typically spend 45 minutes with the patient and/or family or caregiver.

▲ 99307   Subsequent nursing facility care, per day, for the evaluation and management of a patient, which requires at least 2 of these 3 key components:

■ **A problem focused interval history;**

■ **A problem focused examination;**

■ **Straightforward medical decision making.**

Counseling and/or coordination of care with other providers or agencies are provided consistent with the nature of the problem(s) and the patientís and/or familyís needs.

Usually, the patient is stable, recovering, or improving. Physicians typically spend 10 minutes with the patient and/or family or caregiver.

▲ 99308   Subsequent nursing facility care, per day, for the evaluation and management of a patient, which requires at least 2 of these 3 key components:

■ **An expanded problem focused interval history;**

■ **An expanded problem focused examination;**

■ **Medical decision making of low complexity.**

Counseling and/or coordination of care with other providers or agencies are provided consistent with the nature of the problem(s) and the patientís and/or familyís needs.

Usually, the patient is responding inadequately to therapy or has developed a minor complication. Physicians typically spend 15 minutes with the patient and/or family or caregiver.

▲ 99309   Subsequent nursing facility care, per day, for the evaluation and management of a patient, which requires at least 2 of these 3 key components:

■ **A detailed interval history;**

■ **A detailed examination;**

■ **Medical decision making of moderate complexity.**

Counseling and/or coordination of care with other providers or agencies are provided consistent with the nature of the problem(s) and the patientís and/or familyís needs.

Usually, the patient has developed a significant complication or a significant new problem. Physicians typically spend 25 minutes with the patient and/or family or caregiver.

▲ 99310　Subsequent nursing facility care, per day, for the evaluation and management of a patient, which requires at least 2 of these 3 key components:

- A comprehensive interval history;

- A comprehensive examination;

- Medical decision making of high complexity.

Counseling and/or coordination of care with other providers or agencies are provided consistent with the nature of the problem(s) and the patientís and/or familyís needs.

The patient may be unstable or may have developed a significant new problem requiring immediate physician attention. Physicians typically spend 35 minutes with the patient and/or family or caregiver.

▲ 99318　Evaluation and management of a patient involving an annual nursing facility assessment, which requires these 3 key components:

- A detailed interval history;

- A comprehensive examination; and

- Medical decision making that is of low to moderate complexity.

Counseling and/or coordination of care with other providers or agencies are provided consistent with the nature of the problem(s) and the patientís and/or familyís needs.

Usually, the patient is stable, recovering, or improving. Physicians typically spend 30 minutes with the patient and/or family or caregiver.

99361　Medical conference by a physician with interdisciplinary team of health professionals or representatives of community agencies to coordinate activities of patient care (patient not present); approximately 30 minutes

99362　approximately 60 minutes

● 99366　Code added

● 99367　Code added

● 99368　Code added

99371　Telephone call by a physician to patient or for consultation or medical management or for coordinating medical management with other health care professionals (eg, nurses, therapists, social workers, nutritionists, physicians, pharmacists); simple or brief (eg, to report on tests and/or laboratory results, to clarify or alter previous instructions, to integrate new information from other health professionals into the medical treatment plan, or to adjust therapy)

99372　intermediate (eg, to provide advice to an established patient on a new problem, to initiate therapy that can be handled by telephone, to discuss test results in detail, to coordinate medical management of a new problem in an established patient, to discuss and evaluate new information and details, or to initiate new plan of care)

99373　complex or lengthy (eg, lengthy counseling session with anxious or distraught patient, detailed or prolonged discussion with family members regarding seriously ill patient, lengthy communication necessary to coordinate complex services of several different health professionals working on different aspects of the total patient care plan)

● 99406　Code added

● 99407　Code added

● 99408　Code added

● 99409　Code added

● 99441　Code added

● 99442　Code added

● 99443　Code added

● 99444　Code added

● 99477　Code added

Anesthesia

01905　Anesthesia for myelography, discography, vertebroplasty

▲ 01931　intrahepatic or portal circulation (eg, transvenous intrahepatic portosystemic transcutaneous porto-caval shunt[s] [TIPS])

● 01935　Code added

● 01936　Code added

Surgery

+▲ 11008　Removal of prosthetic material or mesh, abdominal wall for infection (eg, for chronic or recurrent mesh infection or necrotizing soft tissue infection) (List separately in addition to code for primary procedure)

▲ 17110　Destruction (eg, laser surgery, electrosurgery, cryosurgery, chemosurgery, surgical curettement), of benign lesions other than skin tags or cutaneous vascular proliferative lesions; up to 14 lesions

● 20555　Code added

▲ 20660　Application of cranial tongs, caliper, or stereotactic frame, including removal (separate procedure)

▲ 20690　Application of a uniplane (pins or wires in one plane), unilateral, external fixation system

▲ 20692　Application of a multiplane (pins or wires in more than one plane), unilateral, external fixation system (eg, Ilizarov, Monticelli type)

▲ 20900　Bone graft, any donor area; minor or small (eg, dowel or button)

▲ 20902　major or large

▲ 20910　Cartilage graft; costochondral

▲ 20912　nasal septum

▲ 20920　Fascia lata graft; by stripper

▲ 20922　by incision and area exposure, complex or sheet

▲ 20924　Tendon graft, from a distance (eg, palmaris, toe extensor, plantaris)

▲ 20926　Tissue grafts, other (eg, paratenon, fat, dermis)

+▲ 20930　Allograft for spine surgery only; morselized (List separately in addition to code for primary procedure)

+▲ 20931　structural (List separately in addition to code for primary procedure)

+▲ 20936 Autograft for spine surgery only (includes harvesting the graft); local (eg, ribs, spinous process, or laminar fragments) obtained from same incision (List separately in addition to code for primary procedure)

+▲ 20937 morselized (through separate skin or fascial incision) (List separately in addition to code for primary procedure)

+▲ 20938 structural, bicortical or tricortical (through separate skin or fascial incision) (List separately in addition to code for primary procedure)

+● 20985 Code added

+● 20986 Code added

+● 20987 Code added

● 21073 Code added

● 22206 Code added

● 22207 Code added

+● 22208 Code added

+▲ 22840 Posterior non-segmental instrumentation (eg, Harrington rod technique, pedicle fixation across one interspace, atlantoaxial transarticular screw fixation, sublaminar wiring at C1, facet screw fixation) (List separately in addition to code for primary procedure)

+▲ 22841 Internal spinal fixation by wiring of spinous processes (List separately in addition to code for primary procedure)

+▲ 22842 Posterior segmental instrumentation (eg, pedicle fixation, dual rods with multiple hooks and sublaminar wires); 3 to 6 vertebral segments (List separately in addition to code for primary procedure)

+▲ 22843 7 to 12 vertebral segments (List separately in addition to code for primary procedure)

+▲ 22844 13 or more vertebral segments (List separately in addition to code for primary procedure)

+▲ 22845 Anterior instrumentation; 2 to 3 vertebral segments (List separately in addition to code for primary procedure)

+▲ 22846 4 to 7 vertebral segments (List separately in addition to code for primary procedure)

+▲ 22847 8 or more vertebral segments (List separately in addition to code for primary procedure)

+▲ 22848 Pelvic fixation (attachment of caudal end of instrumentation to pelvic bony structures) other than sacrum (List separately in addition to code for primary procedure)

+▲ 22851 Application of intervertebral biomechanical device(s) (eg, synthetic cage(s), threaded bone dowel(s), methylmethacrylate) to vertebral defect or interspace (List separately in addition to code for primary procedure)

▲ 23515 Open treatment of clavicular fracture, ~~with or without~~includes internal~~or external~~ fixation, when performed

▲ 23615 Open treatment of proximal humeral (surgical or anatomical neck) fracture, ~~with or without~~includes internal ~~or external~~fixation, when performed, ~~with or without~~includes repair of tuberosity(s), when performed;

▲ 23616 with proximal humeral prosthetic replacement

▲ 23630 Open treatment of greater humeral tuberosity fracture, ~~with or without~~ includes internal~~or external~~ fixation, when performed

▲ 23670 Open treatment of shoulder dislocation, with fracture of greater humeral tuberosity, ~~with or without~~includes internal ~~or external~~fixation, when performed

▲ 23680 Open treatment of shoulder dislocation, with surgical or anatomical neck fracture, ~~with or without~~includes internal ~~or external~~fixation, when performed

~~24350~~ ~~Fasciotomy, lateral or medial (eg, tennis elbow or epicondylitis);~~

~~24351~~ ~~with extensor origin detachment~~

~~24352~~ ~~with annular ligament resection~~

~~24354~~ ~~with stripping~~

~~24356~~ ~~with partial ostectomy~~

● 24357 Code added

● 24358 Code added

● 24359 Code added

▲ 24545 Open treatment of humeral supracondylar or transcondylar fracture, ~~with or without~~includes internal ~~or external~~fixation, when performed; without intercondylar extension

▲ 24546 with intercondylar extension

▲ 24575 Open treatment of humeral epicondylar fracture, medial or lateral, ~~with or without~~includes internal ~~or external~~fixation, when performed

▲ 24579 Open treatment of humeral condylar fracture, medial or lateral, ~~with or without~~includes internal ~~or external~~fixation, when performed

▲ 24635 Open treatment of Monteggia type of fracture dislocation at elbow (fracture proximal end of ulna with dislocation of radial head), ~~with or without~~includes internal ~~or external~~fixation, when performed

▲ 24665 Open treatment of radial head or neck fracture, ~~with or without~~includes internal fixation or radial head excision, when performed;

▲ 24666 with radial head prosthetic replacement

▲ 24670 Closed treatment of ulnar fracture, proximal end (eg, olecranon or coronoid process[es]); without manipulation

▲ 24675 with manipulation

▲ 24685 Open treatment of ulnar fracture, proximal end (eg, olecranon or coronoid process[es]), ~~with or without~~includes internal ~~or external~~fixation, when performed

▲ 25515 Open treatment of radial shaft fracture, ~~with or without~~includes internal ~~or external~~fixation, when performed

▲ 25525 Open treatment of radial shaft fracture, includes ~~with~~ internal ~~and/or external~~ fixation, when performed, and closed treatment ~~of dislocation~~of distal radioulnar joint dislocation (Galeazzi fracture/ dislocation), includes ~~with or without~~ percutaneous skeletal fixation, when performed

▲ 25526 Open treatment of radial shaft fracture, ~~with~~includes internal ~~and/or external~~fixation, when performed, and open treatment ~~with or without internal or external fixation~~of distal radioulnar joint dislocation (Galeazzi fracture/dislocation), includes internal fixation, when performed, includes repair of triangular fibrocartilage complex

▲ 25545 Open treatment of ulnar shaft fracture, ~~with or without~~includes internal ~~or external~~fixation, when performed

▲ 25574 Open treatment of radial AND ulnar shaft fractures, with internal ~~or external~~fixation, when performed; of radius OR ulna

▲ 25575 of radius AND ulna

▲ 25628 Open treatment of carpal scaphoid (navicular) fracture, ~~with or without~~includes internal ~~or external~~fixation, when performed

▲ 26615   Open treatment of metacarpal fracture, single, ~~with or without~~includes internal ~~or external~~fixation, when performed, each bone

▲ 26650   Percutaneous skeletal fixation of carpometacarpal fracture dislocation, thumb (Bennett fracture), with manipulation~~, with or without external fixation~~

▲ 26665   Open treatment of carpometacarpal fracture dislocation, thumb (Bennett fracture), ~~with or without~~includes internal ~~or externa~~ fixation, when performed

▲ 26685   Open treatment of carpometacarpal dislocation, other than thumb; ~~with or without~~includes internal ~~or external~~fixation, when performed, each joint

▲ 26715   Open treatment of metacarpophalangeal dislocation, single, ~~with or without~~includes internal ~~or external~~fixation, when performed

▲ 26735   Open treatment of phalangeal shaft fracture, proximal or middle phalanx, finger or thumb, ~~with or without~~includes internal ~~or external~~fixation, when performed, each

▲ 26746   Open treatment of articular fracture, involving metacarpophalangeal or interphalangeal joint, ~~with or without~~includes internal ~~or external~~fixation, when performed, each

▲ 26765   Open treatment of distal phalangeal fracture, finger or thumb, ~~with or without~~includes internal ~~or external~~fixation, when performed, each

▲ 26785   Open treatment of interphalangeal joint dislocation, ~~with or without~~includes internal ~~or external~~fixation, when performed, single

▲ 27248   Open treatment of greater trochanteric fracture, ~~with or without~~includes internal ~~or external~~fixation, when performed

● 27267   Code added

● 27268   Code added

● 27269   Code added

● 27416   Code added

▲ 27511   Open treatment of femoral supracondylar or transcondylar fracture without intercondylar extension, ~~with or without~~includes internal ~~or external~~fixation, when performed

▲ 27513   Open treatment of femoral supracondylar or transcondylar fracture with intercondylar extension, ~~with or without~~includes internal ~~or external~~fixation, when performed

▲ 27514   Open treatment of femoral fracture, distal end, medial or lateral condyle, ~~with or without~~includes internal ~~or external~~fixation, when performed

▲ 27519   Open treatment of distal femoral epiphyseal separation, ~~with or without~~includes internal ~~or external~~fixation, when performed

▲ 27535   Open treatment of tibial fracture, proximal (plateau); unicondylar, ~~with or without~~includes internal ~~or external~~fixation, when performed

▲ 27540   Open treatment of intercondylar spine(s) and/or tuberosity fracture(s) of the knee, ~~with or without~~includes internal ~~or external~~fixation, when performed

▲ 27556   Open treatment of knee dislocation, ~~with or without~~includes internal ~~or external~~fixation, when performed; without primary ligamentous repair or augmentation/reconstruction

▲ 27557   with primary ligamentous repair

▲ 27558   with primary ligamentous repair, with augmentation/reconstruction

● 27726   Code added

▲ 27766   Open treatment of medial malleolus fracture, ~~with or without~~includes internal ~~or external~~fixation, when performed

● 27767   Code added

● 27768   Code added

● 27769   Code added

▲ 27784   Open treatment of proximal fibula or shaft fracture, ~~with or without~~includes internal ~~or external~~fixation, when performed

▲ 27792   Open treatment of distal fibular fracture (lateral malleolus), ~~with or without~~includes internal ~~or external~~fixation, when performed

▲ 27808   Closed treatment of bimalleolar ankle fracture (~~including Potts~~eg, lateral and medial malleoli, or lateral and posterior malleoli or medial and posterior malleoli); without manipulation

▲ 27810   with manipulation

▲ 27814   Open treatment of bimalleolar ankle fracture (eg, lateral and medial malleoli, or lateral and posterior malleoli, or medial and posterior malleoli), ~~with or without~~includes internal ~~or external~~fixation, when performed

▲ 27822   Open treatment of trimalleolar ankle fracture, ~~with or without~~includes internal ~~or external~~fixation, when performed, medial and/or lateral malleolus; without fixation of posterior lip

▲ 27823   with fixation of posterior lip

▲ 27826   Open treatment of fracture of weight bearing articular surface/portion of distal tibia (eg, pilon or tibial plafond), with internal ~~or external~~fixation, when performed; of fibula only

▲ 27827   of tibia only

▲ 27828   of both tibia and fibula

▲ 27829   Open treatment of distal tibiofibular joint (syndesmosis) disruption, ~~with or without~~includes internal ~~or external~~fixation, when performed

▲ 27832   Open treatment of proximal tibiofibular joint dislocation, ~~with or without~~includes internal ~~or external~~fixation, when performed, or with excision of proximal fibula

▲ 28415   Open treatment of calcaneal fracture, ~~with or without~~includes internal ~~or external~~fixation, when performed;

▲ 28420   with primary iliac or other autogenous bone graft (includes obtaining graft)

▲ 28445   Open treatment of talus fracture, ~~with or without~~includes internal ~~or external~~fixation, when performed

● 28446   Code added

▲ 28465   Open treatment of tarsal bone fracture (except talus and calcaneus), ~~with or without~~includes internal ~~or external~~fixation, when performed, each

▲ 28485   Open treatment of metatarsal fracture, ~~with or without~~includes internal ~~or external~~fixation, when performed, each

▲ 28505   Open treatment of fracture, great toe, phalanx or phalanges, ~~with or without~~includes internal ~~or external~~fixation, when performed

▲ 28525   Open treatment of fracture, phalanx or phalanges, other than great toe, ~~with or without~~includes internal ~~or external~~fixation, when performed, each

▲ 28555   Open treatment of tarsal bone dislocation, ~~with or without~~includes internal ~~or external~~fixation, when performed

▲ 28585   Open treatment of talotarsal joint dislocation, ~~with or without~~includes internal ~~or external~~fixation, when performed

▲ 28615   Open treatment of tarsometatarsal joint dislocation, ~~with or without~~includes internal ~~or external~~fixation, when performed

▲ 28645   Open treatment of metatarsophalangeal joint dislocation, ~~with or without~~includes internal ~~or external~~fixation, when performed

▲ 28675   Open treatment of interphalangeal joint dislocation, ~~with or without~~includes internal ~~or external~~fixation, when performed

● 29828   Code added

▲ 29855   Arthroscopically aided treatment of tibial fracture, proximal (plateau); unicondylar, includes ~~with or without~~internal ~~or external~~fixation, when performed (includes arthroscopy)

▲ 29856   bicondylar, includes ~~with or without~~internal ~~or external~~fixation, when performed (includes arthroscopy)

▲ 29866   Arthroscopy, knee, surgical; osteochondral autograft(s) (eg, mosaicplasty) (includes harvesting of the autograft[s])

● 29904   Code added

● 29905   Code added

● 29906   Code added

● 29907   Code added

~~32000~~   ~~Thoracentesis, puncture of pleural cavity for aspiration, initial or subsequent~~

~~32002~~   ~~Thoracentesis with insertion of tube with or without water seal (eg, for pneumothorax) (separate procedure)~~

~~32005~~   ~~Chemical pleurodesis (eg, for recurrent or persistent pneumothorax)~~

~~32019~~   ~~Insertion of indwelling tunneled pleural catheter with cuff~~

~~32020~~   ~~Tube thoracostomy with or without water seal (eg, for abscess, hemothorax, empyema) (separate procedure)~~

● 32421   Code added

● 32422   Code added

⊙ ● 32550   Code added

⊙ ● 32551   Code added

● 32560   Code added

+ ● 33257   Code added

+ ● 33258   Code added

+ ● 33259   Code added

+ ▲ 33517   Coronary artery bypass, using venous graft(s) and arterial graft(s); single vein graft ~~(List separately in addition to code for arterial graft)~~(List separately in addition to code for primary procedure)

+ ▲ 33518   two venous grafts ~~(List separately in addition to code for arterial graft)~~(List separately in addition to code for primary procedure)

+ ▲ 33519   three venous grafts ~~(List separately in addition to code for arterial graft)~~(List separately in addition to code for primary procedure)

+ ▲ 33521   four venous grafts ~~(List separately in addition to code for arterial graft)~~(List separately in addition to code for primary procedure)

+ ▲ 33522   five venous grafts ~~(List separately in addition to code for arterial graft)~~(List separately in addition to code for primary procedure)

+ ▲ 33523   six or more venous grafts ~~(List separately in addition to code for arterial graft)~~(List separately in addition to code for primary procedure)

● 33864   Code added

+ ● 34806   Code added

● 35523   Code added

+ ▲ 35600   Harvest of upper extremity artery, one segment, for coronary artery bypass procedure (List separately in addition to code for primary procedure)

~~36540~~   ~~Collection of blood specimen from a completely implantable venous access device~~

~~36550~~   ~~Declotting by thrombolytic agent of implanted vascular access device or catheter~~

● 36591   Code added

● 36592   Code added

● 36593   Code added

▲ 36660   Catheterization, umbilical artery, newborn, for diagnosis or therapy

▲ 38792   for identification of sentinel node

● 41019   Code added

~~43750~~   ~~Percutaneous placement of gastrostomy tube, without imaging or endoscopic guidance~~

▲ 43760   Change of gastrostomy tube, percutaneous, without imaging or endoscopic guidance

▲ 43761   Repositioning of the gastric feeding tube, ~~any method,~~through the duodenum for enteric nutrition

▲ 43770   Laparoscopy, surgical, gastric restrictive procedure; placement of adjustable gastric ~~band~~restrictive device (eg, gastric band and subcutaneous port components)

▲ 43771   revision of adjustable gastric ~~band~~restrictive device component only

▲ 43772   removal of adjustable gastric ~~band~~restrictive device component only

▲ 43773   removal and replacement of adjustable gastric ~~band~~restrictive device component only

▲ 43774   removal of adjustable gastric ~~band~~restrictive device and subcutaneous port components

▲ 43848   Revision, open, of gastric restrictive procedure for morbid obesity, other than adjustable gastric ~~band~~restrictive device (separate procedure)

▲ 44300   Placement, enterostomy or cecostomy, tube open (eg, for feeding or decompression ~~or feeding~~) (separate procedure)

45190   Grammatical Change

~~47710~~   ~~Anastomosis, choledochal cyst, without excision~~

~~49200~~   ~~Excision or destruction, open, intra-abdominal or retroperitoneal tumors or cysts or endometriomas;~~

~~49201~~   ~~extensive~~

● 49203   Code added

● 49204   Code added

● 49205   Code added

⊙ ● 49440   Code added

⊙ ● 49441   Code added

⊙ ● 49442   Code added

⊙ ● 49446   Code added

● **49450**   Code added

● **49451**   Code added

● **49452**   Code added

● **49460**   Code added

● **49465**   Code added

+▲ **49568**   Implantation of mesh or other prosthesis for incisional or ventral hernia repair <u>or mesh for closure of debridement for necrotizing soft tissue infection</u> (List separately in addition to code for the incisional or ventral hernia repair)

⊙● **50385**   Code added

⊙● **50386**   Code added

⊙● **50593**   Code added

    ~~**51000**~~   ~~Aspiration of bladder by needle~~

    ~~**51005**~~   ~~Aspiration of bladder; by trocar or intracatheter~~

    ~~**51010**~~   ~~with insertion of suprapubic catheter~~

● **51100**   Code added

● **51101**   Code added

● **51102**   Code added

+▲ **51797**   intra-abdominal voiding pressure (AP) (rectal, gastric, intraperitoneal) <u>(List separately in addition to code for primary procedure)</u>

    ~~**52510**~~   ~~Transurethral balloon dilation of the prostatic urethra~~

● **52649**   Code added

● **55920**   Code added

▲ **57284**   Paravaginal defect repair (including repair of cystocele, ~~stress urinary incontinence, and/or incomplete vaginal prolapse~~ <u>if performed); open abdominal approach</u>

● **57285**   Code added

● **57423**   Code added

▲ **57500**   Biopsy <u>of cervix</u>, single or multiple, or local excision of lesion, with or without fulguration (separate procedure)

● **58570**   Code added

● **58571**   Code added

● **58572**   Code added

● **58573**   Code added

    ~~**60001**~~   ~~Aspiration and/or injection, thyroid cyst~~

● **60300**   Code added

▲ **61210**   for implanting ventricular catheter, reservoir, EEG electrode(s), pressure recording device, or other cerebral monitoring device (separate procedure)

▲ **62284**   Injection procedure for myelography and/or computed tomography, spinal (other than C1-C2 and posterior fossa)

▲ **64834**   Suture of one nerve~~;~~ hand or foot~~;~~ common sensory nerve

▲ **64835**   median motor thenar

▲ **64836**   ulnar motor

    ~~**67038**~~   ~~with epiretinal membrane stripping~~

● **67041**   Code added

● **67042**   Code added

● **67043**   Code added

● **67113**   Code added

▲ **67227**   Destruction of extensive or progressive retinopathy (eg, diabetic retinopathy), one or more sessions~~;~~<u>,</u> cryotherapy, diathermy

▲ **67228**   <u>Treatment of extensive or progressive retinopathy, one or more sessions; (eg, diabetic retinopathy),</u> photocoagulation ~~(laser or xenon arc) single session~~

● **67229**   Code added

● **68816**   Code added

Radiology

▲ **70496**   Computed tomographic angiography, head, ~~without contrast material(s), followed by~~ <u>with</u> contrast material(s) ~~and further sections~~, including <u>noncontrast images, if performed, and</u> image postprocessing

▲ **70498**   Computed tomographic angiography, neck, ~~without contrast material(s), followed by~~ <u>with</u> contrast material(s) ~~and further sections~~, including <u>noncontrast images, if performed, and</u> image postprocessing

▲ **71275**   Computed tomographic angiography, chest (noncoronary), ~~without contrast material(s), followed by~~<u>with</u> contrast material(s) ~~and further sections~~, including <u>noncontrast images, if performed, and</u> image postprocessing

▲ **72191**   Computed tomographic angiography, pelvis, ~~without contrast material(s), followed by~~<u>with</u> contrast material(s) ~~and further sections~~, including <u>noncontrast images, if performed, and</u> image postprocessing

▲ **73206**   Computed tomographic angiography, upper extremity, ~~without contrast material(s), followed by~~<u>with</u> contrast material(s) ~~and further sections~~, including <u>noncontrast images, if performed, and</u> image postprocessing

▲ **73706**   Computed tomographic angiography, lower extremity, ~~without contrast material(s), followed by~~<u>with</u> contrast material(s) ~~and further sections~~, including <u>noncontrast images, if performed, and</u> image postprocessing

▲ **74175**   Computed tomographic angiography, abdomen, ~~without contrast material(s), followed by~~<u>with</u> contrast material(s) ~~and further sections~~, including <u>noncontrast images, if performed, and</u> image postprocessing

    ~~**74350**~~   ~~Percutaneous placement of gastrostomy tube, radiological supervision and interpretation~~

    ~~**75552**~~   ~~Cardiac magnetic resonance imaging for morphology; without contrast material~~

    ~~**75553**~~   ~~with contrast material~~

    ~~**75554**~~   ~~Cardiac magnetic resonance imaging for function, with or without morphology; complete study~~

    ~~**75555**~~   ~~limited study~~

    ~~**75556**~~   ~~Cardiac magnetic resonance imaging for velocity flow mapping~~

● **75557**   Code added

● **75558**   Code added

● **75559**   Code added

● **75560**   Code added

● **75561** Code added

● **75562** Code added

● **75563** Code added

● **75564** Code added

▲ **75635** Computed tomographic angiography, abdominal aorta and bilateral iliofemoral lower extremity runoff, ~~radiological supervision and interpretation, without contrast material(s), followed by~~ with contrast material(s)~~and further sections,~~ including noncontrast images, if performed, and image postprocessing

▲ **75984** Change of percutaneous tube or drainage catheter with contrast monitoring (eg, ~~gastrointestinal system,~~ genitourinary system, abscess), radiological supervision and interpretation

▲ **76506** Echoencephalography, ~~B-scan and/or~~ real time with image documentation (gray scale) (for determination of ventricular size, delineation of cerebral contents, and detection of fluid masses or other intracranial abnormalities), including A-mode encephalography as secondary component where indicated

▲ **77371** Radiation treatment delivery, stereotactic radiosurgery (SRS), complete course of treatment of ~~cerebral~~ cranial lesion(s) consisting of 1 session; multi-source Cobalt 60 based

▲ **77372** Radiation treatment delivery, stereotactic radiosurgery (SRS), complete course of treatment of ~~cerebral~~ cranial lesion(s) consisting of 1 session; linear accelerator based

▲ **77432** Stereotactic radiation treatment management of ~~cerebral~~ cranial lesion(s) (complete course of treatment consisting of one session)

▲ **78600** Brain imaging, ~~limited procedure~~ less than 4 static views; ~~static~~

▲ **78601** with vascular flow

▲ **78605** Brain imaging, ~~complete study~~ minimum 4 static views; ~~static~~

▲ **78606** with vascular flow

▲ **78607** Brain imaging, tomographic (SPECT)

~~**78615** Cerebral vascular flow~~

▲ **78811** ~~Tumor imaging, p~~Positron emission tomography (PET) imaging; limited area (eg, chest, head/neck)

▲ **78812** skull base to mid-thigh

▲ **78813** whole body

▲ **78814** ~~Tumor imaging, p~~Positron emission tomography (PET) with concurrently acquired computed tomography (CT) for attenuation correction and anatomical localization imaging; limited area (eg, chest, head/neck)

▲ **78815** skull base to mid-thigh

▲ **78816** whole body

Pathology and Laboratory

● **80047** Code added

▲ **80048** Basic metabolic panel (Calcium, total)

This panel must include the following:

Calcium (**82310**)

Carbon dioxide (**82374**)

Chloride (**82435**)

Creatinine (**82565**)

Glucose (**82947**)

Potassium (**84132**)

Sodium (**84295**)

Urea nitrogen (BUN) (**84520**)

▲ **82272** Blood, occult, by peroxidase activity (eg, guaiac), qualitative, feces, ~~single specimen (eg, from digital rectal exam)~~1-3 simultaneous determinations, performed for other than colorectal neoplasm screening

● **82610** Code added

▲ **83898** amplification, target ~~of patient nucleic acid~~, each nucleic acid sequence

▲ **83900** amplification, target ~~of patient nucleic acid~~, multiplex, first two nucleic acid sequences

+▲ **83901** amplification, target ~~of patient nucleic acid~~, multiplex, each additional nucleic acid sequence beyond 2 (List separately in addition to code for primary procedure)

▲ **83908** ~~signal amplification of patient nucleic acid~~amplification, signal, each nucleic acid sequence

● **83993** Code added

● **84704** Code added

● **86356** Code added

● **86486** Code added

~~**86586** Unlisted antigen, each~~

▲ **86885** indirect, qualitative, each ~~antiserum~~reagent red cell

▲ **86886** indirect, ~~titer,~~ each ~~antiserum~~antibody titer

● **87500** Code added

● **87809** Code added

▲ **88380** Microdissection (ie, sample preparation of microscopically identified target)~~(eg, mechanical,;~~ laser capture~~)~~

● **88381** Code added

▲ **89320** ~~complete~~ ~~(volume, count, motility, and differential)~~

▲ **89321** ~~Semen analysis,~~ sperm presence and~~/or~~ motility of sperm, if performed ~~(not including Huhner test)~~

● **89322** Code added

● **89331** Code added

Medicine

▲ **90281** Immune globulin (Ig), human, for intramuscular use

▲ **90283** Immune globulin (IgIV), human, for intravenous use

● **90284** Code added

▲ **90287** Botulinum antitoxin, equine, any route

▲ **90288** Botulism immune globulin, human, for intravenous use

▲ 90291   Cytomegalovirus immune globulin (CMV-IgIV), human, for intravenous use

▲ 90296   Diphtheria antitoxin, equine, any route

▲ 90371   Hepatitis B immune globulin (HBIg), human, for intramuscular use

▲ 90375   Rabies immune globulin (RIg), human, for intramuscular and/or subcutaneous use

▲ 90376   Rabies immune globulin, heat-treated (RIg-HT), human, for intramuscular and/or subcutaneous use

▲ 90378   Respiratory syncytial virus immune globulin (RSV-IgIM), for intramuscular use, 50 mg, each

▲ 90379   Respiratory syncytial virus immune globulin (RSV-IgIV), human, for intravenous use

▲ 90384   Rho(D) immune globulin (RhIg), human, full-dose, for intramuscular use

▲ 90385   Rho(D) immune globulin (RhIg), human, mini-dose, for intramuscular use

▲ 90386   Rho(D) immune globulin (RhIgIV), human, for intravenous use

▲ 90389   Tetanus immune globulin (TIg), human, for intramuscular use

▲ 90393   Vaccinia immune globulin, human, for intramuscular use

▲ 90396   Varicella-zoster immune globulin, human, for intramuscular use

▲ 90399   Unlisted immune globulin

▲ 90476   Adenovirus vaccine, type 4, live, for oral use

▲ 90477   Adenovirus vaccine, type 7, live, for oral use

▲ 90581   Anthrax vaccine, for subcutaneous use

▲ 90585   Bacillus Calmette-Guerin vaccine (BCG) for tuberculosis, live, for percutaneous use

▲ 90586   Bacillus Calmette-Guerin vaccine (BCG) for bladder cancer, live, for intravesical use

▲ 90632   Hepatitis A vaccine, adult dosage, for intramuscular use

▲ 90633   Hepatitis A vaccine, pediatric/adolescent dosage-2 dose schedule, for intramuscular use

▲ 90634   Hepatitis A vaccine, pediatric/adolescent dosage-3 dose schedule, for intramuscular use

▲ 90636   Hepatitis A and hepatitis B vaccine (HepA-HepB), adult dosage, for intramuscular use

▲ 90645   Hemophilus influenza b vaccine (Hib), HbOC conjugate (4 dose schedule), for intramuscular use

▲ 90646   Hemophilus influenza b vaccine (Hib), PRP-D conjugate, for booster use only, intramuscular use

▲ 90647   Hemophilus influenza b vaccine (Hib), PRP-OMP conjugate (3 dose schedule), for intramuscular use

▲ 90648   Hemophilus influenza b vaccine (Hib), PRP-T conjugate (4 dose schedule), for intramuscular use

▲ 90649   Human Papilloma virus (HPV) vaccine, types 6, 11, 16, 18 (quadrivalent), 3 dose schedule, for intramuscular use

▲ 90655   Influenza virus vaccine, split virus, preservative free, when administered to children 6-35 months of age, for intramuscular use

▲ 90656   Influenza virus vaccine, split virus, preservative free, when administered to <u>individuals</u> 3 years and older, for intramuscular use

▲ 90657   Influenza virus vaccine, split virus, when administered to children 6-35 months of age, for intramuscular use

▲ 90658   Influenza virus vaccine, split virus, when administered to <u>individuals</u> 3 years of age and older, for intramuscular use

▲ 90660   Influenza virus vaccine, live, for intranasal use

✎ ● 90661   Code added

✎ ● 90662   Code added

✎ ● 90663   Code added

▲ 90665   Lyme disease vaccine, adult dosage, for intramuscular use

▲ 90669   Pneumococcal conjugate vaccine, polyvalent, when administered to children younger than 5 years, for intramuscular use

▲ 90675   Rabies vaccine, for intramuscular use

▲ 90676   Rabies vaccine, for intradermal use

▲ 90680   Rotavirus vaccine, pentavalent, 3 dose schedule, live, for oral use

▲ 90690   Typhoid vaccine, live, oral

▲ 90691   Typhoid vaccine, Vi capsular polysaccharide (ViCPs), for intramuscular use

▲ 90692   Typhoid vaccine, heat- and phenol-inactivated (H-P), for subcutaneous or intradermal use

▲ 90693   Typhoid vaccine, acetone-killed, dried (AKD), for subcutaneous use (U.S. military)

✎ ▲ 90698   Diphtheria, tetanus toxoids, acellular pertussis vaccine, haemophilus influenza Type B, and poliovirus vaccine, inactivated (DTaP - Hib - IPV), for intramuscular use

▲ 90700   Diphtheria, tetanus toxoids, and acellular pertussis vaccine (DTaP), when administered to <u>individuals</u> younger than 7 years, for intramuscular use

▲ 90701   Diphtheria, tetanus toxoids, and whole cell pertussis vaccine (DTP), for intramuscular use

▲ 90702   Diphtheria and tetanus toxoids (DT) adsorbed when administered to <u>individuals</u> younger than 7 years, for intramuscular use

▲ 90703   Tetanus toxoid adsorbed, for intramuscular use

▲ 90704   Mumps virus vaccine, live, for subcutaneous use

▲ 90705   Measles virus vaccine, live, for subcutaneous use

▲ 90706   Rubella virus vaccine, live, for subcutaneous use

▲ 90707   Measles, mumps and rubella virus vaccine (MMR), live, for subcutaneous use

▲ 90708   Measles and rubella virus vaccine, live, for subcutaneous use

▲ 90710   Measles, mumps, rubella, and varicella vaccine (MMRV), live, for subcutaneous use

▲ 90712   Poliovirus vaccine, (any type[s]) (OPV), live, for oral use

▲ 90713   Poliovirus vaccine, inactivated (IPV), for subcutaneous or intramuscular use

▲ 90714   Tetanus and diphtheria toxoids (Td) adsorbed, preservative free, when administered to <u>individuals</u> 7 years or older, for intramuscular use

▲ 90715   Tetanus, diphtheria toxoids and acellular pertussis vaccine (Tdap), when administered to <u>individuals</u> 7 years or older, for intramuscular use

▲ 90716   Varicella virus vaccine, live, for subcutaneous use

▲ 90717   Yellow fever vaccine, live, for subcutaneous use

▲ 90718   Tetanus and diphtheria toxoids (Td) adsorbed when administered to <u>individuals</u> 7 years or older, for intramuscular use

▲ 90719   Diphtheria toxoid, for intramuscular use

▲ **90720** Diphtheria, tetanus toxoids, and whole cell pertussis vaccine and Hemophilus influenza B vaccine (DTP-Hib), for intramuscular use

▲ **90721** Diphtheria, tetanus toxoids, and acellular pertussis vaccine and Hemophilus influenza B vaccine (DtaP-Hib), for intramuscular use

▲ **90723** Diphtheria, tetanus toxoids, acellular pertussis vaccine, Hepatitis B, and poliovirus vaccine, inactivated (DtaP-HepB-IPV), for intramuscular use

▲ **90725** Cholera vaccine for injectable use

▲ **90727** Plague vaccine, for intramuscular use

▲ **90732** Pneumococcal polysaccharide vaccine, 23-valent, adult or immunosuppressed patient dosage, when administered to <u>individuals </u>2 years or older, for subcutaneous or intramuscular use

▲ **90733** Meningococcal polysaccharide vaccine (any group(s)), for subcutaneous use

▲ **90734** Meningococcal conjugate vaccine, serogroups A, C, Y and W-135 (tetravalent), for intramuscular use

▲ **90735** Japanese encephalitis virus vaccine, for subcutaneous use

▲ **90736** Zoster (shingles) vaccine, live, for subcutaneous injection

▲ **90740** Hepatitis B vaccine, dialysis or immunosuppressed patient dosage (3 dose schedule), for intramuscular use

▲ **90743** Hepatitis B vaccine, adolescent (2 dose schedule), for intramuscular use

▲ **90744** Hepatitis B vaccine, pediatric/adolescent dosage (3 dose schedule), for intramuscular use

▲ **90746** Hepatitis B vaccine, adult dosage, for intramuscular use

▲ **90747** Hepatitis B vaccine, dialysis or immunosuppressed patient dosage (4 dose schedule), for intramuscular use

▲ **90748** Hepatitis B and Hemophilus influenza b vaccine (HepB-Hib), for intramuscular use

▲ **90749** Unlisted vaccine/toxoid

▲ **90760** Intravenous infusion, hydration; initial, ~~up to 1~~ 31 minutes to 1 hour

● **90769** Code added

+● **90770** Code added

+● **90771** Code added

+● **90776** Code added

▲ **92135** Scanning computerized ophthalmic diagnostic imaging<u>, posterior segment, </u>(eg, scanning laser) with interpretation and report, unilateral

⊙▲ **93501** Right heart catheterization

⊙▲ **93505** Endomyocardial biopsy

⊙▲ **93508** Catheter placement in coronary artery(s), arterial coronary conduit(s), and/or venous coronary bypass graft(s) for coronary angiography without concomitant left heart catheterization

⊙▲ **93510** Left heart catheterization, retrograde, from the brachial artery, axillary artery or femoral artery; percutaneous

⊙▲ **93511** by cutdown

⊙▲ **93514** Left heart catheterization by left ventricular puncture

⊙▲ **93524** Combined transseptal and retrograde left heart catheterization

⊙▲ **93526** Combined right heart catheterization and retrograde left heart catheterization

⊙▲ **93527** Combined right heart catheterization and transseptal left heart catheterization through intact septum (with or without retrograde left heart catheterization)

⊙▲ **93528** Combined right heart catheterization with left ventricular puncture (with or without retrograde left heart catheterization)

⊙▲ **93529** Combined right heart catheterization and left heart catheterization through existing septal opening (with or without retrograde left heart catheterization)

⊙▲ **93530** Right heart catheterization, for congenital cardiac anomalies

▲ **93531** Combined right heart catheterization and retrograde left heart catheterization, for congenital cardiac anomalies

▲ **93532** Combined right heart catheterization and transseptal left heart catheterization through intact septum with or without retrograde left heart catheterization, for congenital cardiac anomalies

▲ **93533** Combined right heart catheterization and transseptal left heart catheterization through existing septal opening, with or without retrograde left heart catheterization, for congenital cardiac anomalies

⊙▲ **93541** for pulmonary angiography

⊙▲ **93542** for selective right ventricular or right atrial angiography

⊙▲ **93543** for selective left ventricular or left atrial angiography

⊙▲ **93619** Comprehensive electrophysiologic evaluation with right atrial pacing and recording, right ventricular pacing and recording, His bundle recording, including insertion and repositioning of multiple electrode catheters, without induction or attempted induction of arrhythmia

⊙▲ **93620** Comprehensive electrophysiologic evaluation including insertion and repositioning of multiple electrode catheters with induction or attempted induction of arrhythmia; with right atrial pacing and recording, right ventricular pacing and recording, His bundle recording

⊙▲ **93624** Electrophysiologic follow-up study with pacing and recording to test effectiveness of therapy, including induction or attempted induction of arrhythmia

⊙▲ **93640** Electrophysiologic evaluation of single or dual chamber pacing cardioverter-defibrillator leads including defibrillation threshold evaluation (induction of arrhythmia, evaluation of sensing and pacing for arrhythmia termination) at time of initial implantation or replacement;

⊙▲ **93641** with testing of single or dual chamber pacing cardioverter-defibrillator pulse generator

⊙▲ **93642** Electrophysiologic evaluation of single or dual chamber pacing cardioverter-defibrillator (includes defibrillation threshold evaluation, induction of arrhythmia, evaluation of sensing and pacing for arrhythmia termination, and programming or reprogramming of sensing or therapeutic parameters)

⊙▲ **93650** Intracardiac catheter ablation of atrioventricular node function, atrioventricular conduction for creation of complete heart block, with or without temporary pacemaker placement

⊙▲ **93651** Intracardiac catheter ablation of arrhythmogenic focus; for treatment of supraventricular tachycardia by ablation of fast or slow atrioventricular pathways, accessory atrioventricular connections or other atrial foci, singly or in combination

⊙▲ **93652** for treatment of ventricular tachycardia

▲ **93660** Evaluation of cardiovascular function with tilt table evaluation, with continuous ECG monitoring and intermittent blood pressure monitoring, with or without pharmacological intervention

● 93982   Code added

▲ 95004   Percutaneous tests (scratch, puncture, prick) with allergenic extracts, immediate type reaction, <u>including test interpretation and report by a physician,</u> specify number of tests

▲ 95024   Intracutaneous (intradermal) tests with allergenic extracts, immediate type reaction, <u>including test interpretation and report by a physician,</u> specify number of tests

▲ 95027   Intracutaneous (intradermal) tests, sequential and incremental, with allergenic extracts for airborne allergens, immediate type reaction, <u>including test interpretation and report by a physician,</u> specify number of tests

● 95980   Code added

● 95981   Code added

● 95982   Code added

▲ 96101   Psychological testing (includes psychodiagnostic assessment of emotionality, intellectual abilities, personality and psychopathology, eg, MMPI, Rorschach, WAIS), per hour of the psychologist{RQ}s or physician{RQ}s time, both face-to-face time <u>administering tests to</u> ~~with~~ the patient and time interpreting <u>these</u> test results and preparing the report

▲ 96118   Neuropsychological testing (eg, Halstead-Reitan Neuropsychological Battery, Wechsler Memory Scales and Wisconsin Card Sorting Test), per hour of the psychologist{RQ}s or physician{RQ}s time, both face-to-face time <u>administering tests to</u> ~~with~~ the patient and time interpreting <u>these</u> test results and preparing the report

● 96125   Code added

● 98966   Code added

● 98967   Code added

● 98968   Code added

● 98969   Code added

▲ 99148   Moderate sedation services (other than those services described by codes 00100-01999), provided by a physician other than the health care professional performing the diagnostic or therapeutic service that the sedation supports; younger than 5 years of age, first 30 minutes intra-service time

▲ 99149   age 5 years or older, first 30 minutes intra-service time

● 99174   Code added

● 99605   Code added

● 99606   Code added

+● 99607   Code added

Category II Codes

● 0505F   Code added

● 0507F   Code added

● 0509F   Code added

● 1040F   Code added

● 1050F   Code added

● 1055F   Code added

● 1060F   Code added

● 1061F   Code added

● 1065F   Code added

● 1066F   Code added

● 1070F   Code added

● 1071F   Code added

● 1080F   Code added

● 1090F   Code added

● 1091F   Code added

● 1100F   Code added

● 1101F   Code added

● 1110F   Code added

● 1111F   Code added

▲ 2010F   Vital signs ~~recorded~~(temperature, pulse, respiratory rate, and blood pressure) documented and reviewed ~~(includes at minimum: temperature, pulse, respiration, and blood pressure)~~(CAP)[2] (EM)[5]

▲ 2014F   Mental status assessed ~~(normal/mildly impaired/severely impaired)~~(CAP)[1] (EM)[5]

● 2019F   Code added

● 2020F   Code added

● 2021F   Code added

● 2027F   Code added

● 2029F   Code added

● 2030F   Code added

● 2031F   Code added

● 3044F   Code added

● 3045F   Code added

~~3047F~~   ~~Most recent hemoglobin A1c level (LE) 9.0% (DM)⁴~~

● 3073F   Code added

● 3074F   Code added

● 3075F   Code added

~~3076F~~   ~~Most recent systolic blood pressure (LT) 140 mm Hg (HTN)⁴ (DM)⁴~~

● 3082F   Code added

● 3083F   Code added

● 3084F   Code added

● 3085F   Code added

● 3088F   Code added

● 3089F   Code added

● 3090F   Code added

● 3091F   Code added

● 3092F   Code added

● 3093F   Code added

● 3095F   Code added

● 3096F   Code added

●	**3100F**	Code added	●	**4070F**	Code added
	~~3101F~~	~~Internal carotid stenosis 30 — 99% range (STR)⁵~~	●	**4073F**	Code added
	~~3102F~~	~~Internal carotid stenosis below 30% (STR)⁵~~	●	**4075F**	Code added
●	**3110F**	Code added	●	**4077F**	Code added
●	**3111F**	Code added	●	**4079F**	Code added
●	**3112F**	Code added	●	**4084F**	Code added
●	**3120F**	Code added	●	**4090F**	Code added
●	**3130F**	Code added	●	**4095F**	Code added
●	**3132F**	Code added	●	**4100F**	Code added
●	**3140F**	Code added	●	**4110F**	Code added
●	**3141F**	Code added	●	**4115F**	Code added
●	**3142F**	Code added	●	**4120F**	Code added
	~~3143F~~	~~Documentation of order for barium swallow test (GERD)⁵~~	●	**4124F**	Code added
●	**3150F**	Code added	●	**5005F**	Code added
●	**3155F**	Code added	●	**5010F**	Code added
●	**3160F**	Code added	●	**5015F**	Code added
●	**3170F**	Code added	●	**6010F**	Code added
●	**3200F**	Code added	●	**6015F**	Code added
●	**3210F**	Code added	●	**6020F**	Code added

● **4005F** Code added

● **4007F** Code added

Category III Codes

● **4019F** Code added

● **4041F** Code added

~~0024T~~	~~Non-surgical septal reduction therapy (eg, alcohol ablation), for hypertrophic obstructive cardiomyopathy, with coronary arteriograms, with or without temporary pacemaker~~

● **4042F** Code added

~~0054T~~	~~Computer assisted musculoskeletal surgical navigational orthopedic procedure, with image guidance based on fluoroscopic images (List separately in addition to code for primary procedure)~~

● **4043F** Code added

● **4044F** Code added

~~0055T~~	~~Computer assisted musculoskeletal surgical navigational orthopedic procedure, with image guidance based on CT/MRI images (List separately in addition to code for primary procedure)~~

▲ **4045F** Appropriate empiric antibiotic prescribed ~~(See measure developer's Web site for definition of appropriate antibiotic)~~ (CAP)¹, (EM)⁵

~~0056T~~	~~Computer assisted musculoskeletal surgical navigational orthopedic procedure, image-less (List separately in addition to code for primary procedure)~~

● **4046F** Code added

● **4047F** Code added

~~0065T~~	~~Ocular photoscreening, with interpretation and report, bilateral~~

● **4048F** Code added

● **4049F** Code added

▲ **0068T** Acoustic heart sound recording and computer analysis; with interpretation and report ~~(List separately in addition to codes for electrocardiography)~~

● **4051F** Code added

● **4052F** Code added

● **4053F** Code added

▲ **0069T** acoustic heart sound recording and computer analysis only ~~(List separately in addition to codes for electrocardiography)~~

● **4054F** Code added

● **4055F** Code added

▲ **0070T** interpretation and report only ~~(List separately in addition to codes for electrocardiography)~~

● **4056F** Code added

● **4058F** Code added

~~0074T~~	~~Online evaluation and management service, per encounter, provided by a physician, using the Internet or similar electronic communications network, in response to a patient's request, established patient~~

● **4060F** Code added

● **4062F** Code added

▲ **0087T** Sperm evaluation, Hyaluronan sperm binding test~~assay~~

● **4064F** Code added

● **4065F** Code added

~~0115T~~	~~Medication therapy management service(s) provided by a pharmacist, individual, face-to-face with patient, initial 15 minutes, with assessment, and intervention if provided; initial encounter~~

● **4066F** Code added

● **4067F** Code added

~~0116T~~	~~subsequent encounter~~

~~0117T~~ ~~each additional 15 minutes (List separately in addition to code for primary service)~~

~~0133T~~ ~~Upper gastrointestinal endoscopy, including esophagus, stomach, and either the duodenum and/or jejunum as appropriate, with injection of implant material into and along the muscle of the lower esophageal sphincter (eg, for treatment of gastroesophageal reflux disease)~~

~~0135T~~ ~~Ablation, renal tumor(s), unilateral, percutaneous, cryotherapy~~

▲ 0145T Computed tomography, heart, ~~without contrast material followed by~~ with contrast material(s) ~~and further sections~~, including noncontrast images, if performed, cardiac gating and 3D image postprocessing; cardiac structure and morphology

▲ 0146T computed tomographic angiography of coronary arteries (including native and anomalous coronary arteries, coronary bypass grafts), without quantitative evaluation of coronary calcium

▲ 0147T computed tomographic angiography of coronary arteries (including native and anomalous coronary arteries, coronary bypass grafts), with quantitative evaluation of coronary calcium

▲ 0148T cardiac structure and morphology and computed tomographic angiography of coronary arteries (including native and anomalous coronary arteries, coronary bypass grafts), without quantitative evaluation of coronary calcium

▲ 0149T cardiac structure and morphology and computed tomographic angiography of coronary arteries (including native and anomalous coronary arteries, coronary bypass grafts), with quantitative evaluation of coronary calcium

▲ 0150T cardiac structure and morphology in congenital heart disease

+▲ 0151T Computed tomography, heart, ~~without contrast material followed by~~ with contrast material(s) ~~and further sections~~, including noncontrast images, if performed, cardiac gating and 3D image postprocessing, function evaluation (left and right ventricular function, ejection-fraction and segmental wall motion) (List separately in addition to code for primary procedure)

~~0153T~~ ~~Transcatheter placement of wireless physiologic sensor in aneurysmal sac during endovascular repair, including radiological supervision and interpretation and instrument calibration (List separately in addition to code for primary procedure)~~

~~0154T~~ ~~Noninvasive physiologic study of implanted wireless pressure sensor in aneurysmal sac following endovascular repair, complete study including recording, analysis of pressure and waveform tracings, interpretation and report~~

● 0171T Code added

+● 0172T Code added

+● 0173T Code added

+● 0174T Code added

● 0175T Code added

● 0176T Code added

● 0177T Code added

● 0178T Code added

● 0179T Code added

● 0180T Code added

● 0181T Code added

● 0182T Code added

● 0183T Code added

Appendix C

Clinical Examples

As described in *CPT 2008*, clinical examples of the CPT codes for Evaluation and Management (E/M) services are intended to be an important element of the coding system. The clinical examples, when used with the E/M descriptors contained in the full text of *CPT*, provide a comprehensive and powerful tool for physicians to report the services provided to their patients.

The American Medical Association is pleased to provide you with these clinical examples for *CPT 2008*. The clinical examples that are provided in this supplement are limited to Office or Other Outpatient Services, Hospital Inpatient Services, Consultations, Critical Care, Prolonged Services and Care Plan Oversight.

These clinical examples do not encompass the entire scope of medical practice. Inclusion or exclusion of any particular specialty group does not infer any judgment of importance or lack thereof; nor does it limit the applicability of the example to any particular specialty.

Of utmost importance is that these clinical examples are just that: examples. A particular patient encounter, depending on the specific circumstances, must be judged by the services provided by the physician for that particular patient. Simply because the patient's complaints, symptoms, or diagnoses match those of a particular clinical example, does not automatically assign that patient encounter to that particular level of service. The three components (history, examination, and medical decision making) must be met and documented in the medical record to report a particular level of service.

New Patient

Office or Other Outpatient Service

99201   Initial office visit for a 50-year-old male from out-of-town who needs a prescription refill for a nonsteroidal anti-inflammatory drug. (Anesthesiology)

Initial office visit for a 40-year-old female, new patient, requesting information about local pain clinics. (Anesthesioogy/Pain Medicine)

Initial office visit for a 10-year-old girl for determination of visual acuity as part of a summer camp physical (does not include determination of refractive error). (Ophthalmology)

Initial office visit for an out-of-town patient requiring topical refill. (Dermatology)

Initial office visit for a 65-year-old male for reassurance about an isolated seborrheic keratosis on upper back. (Plastic Surgery)

Initial office visit for an out-of-state visitor who needs refill of topical steroid to treat lichen planus. (Dermatology)

Initial office visit for an 86-year-old male, out-of-town visitor, who needs prescription refilled for an anal skin preparation that he forgot. (General Surgery/Colon & Rectal Surgery)

Initial office visit for a patient with alveolar osteitis for repacking. (Oral & Maxillofacial Surgery)

Initial office visit for a patient with a pedunculated lesion of the neck which is unsightly. (Dermatology)

Initial office visit for a 10-year-old male, for limited subungual hematoma not requiring drainage. (Internal Medicine)

Initial office visit with an out-of-town visitor who needs a prescription refilled because she forgot her hay fever medication. (Allergy & Immunology/Internal Medicine)

Initial office visit with a 9-month-old female with diaper rash. (Pediatrics)

Initial office visit with a 10-year-old male with severe rash and itching for the past 24 hours, positive history for contact with poison oak 48 hours prior to the visit. (Family Medicine)

Initial office visit with a 5-year-old female to remove sutures from simple wound placed by another physician. (Plastic Surgery)

Initial office visit for a 22-year-old male with a smal area of sunburn requiring first aid. (Dermatology/Family Medicine/Internal Medicine)

Initial office visit for the evaluation and management of a contusion of a finger. (Orthopaedic Surgery)

99202   Initial office visit for a 13-year-old patient with comedopapular acne of the face unresponsive to over-the-counter medications. (Family Medicine)

Initial office visit for a patient with a clinically benign lesion or nodule of the lower leg which has been present for many years. (Dermatology)

Initial office visit for a patient with a circumscribed patch of dermatitis of the leg. (Dermatology)

Initial office visit for a patient with papulosquamous eruption of elbows. (Dermatology)

Initial office visit for a 9-year-old patient with erythematous grouped, vesicular eruption of the lip of three day's duration. (Pediatrics)

Initial office visit for an 18-year-old male referred by an orthodontist for advice regarding removal of four wisdom teeth. (Oral & Maxillofacial Surgery)

Initial office visit for a 14-year-old male, who was referred by his orthodontist, for advice on the exposure of impacted maxillary cuspids. (Oral & Maxillofacial Surgery)

Initial office visit for a patient presenting with itching patches on the wrists and ankles. (Dermatology)

Initial office visit for a 30-year-old male for evaluation and discussion of treatment of rhinophyma. (Plastic Surgery)

Initial office visit for a 16-year-old male with severe cystic acne, new patient. (Dermatology)

Initial office evaluation for gradual hearing loss, 58-year-old male, history and physical examination, with interpretation of complete audiogram, air bone, etc. (Otolaryngology)

Initial evaluation and management of recurrent urinary infection in female. (Internal Medicine)

Initial office visit with a 10-year-old girl with history of chronic otitis media and a draining ear. (Pediatrics)

Initial office visit for a 10-year-old female with acute maxillary sinusitis. (Family Medicine)

Initial office visit for a patient with recurring episodes of herpes simplex who has developed a clustering of vesicles on the upper lip. (Internal Medicine)

Initial office visit for a 25-year-old patient with a single season allergic rhinitis. (Allergy & Immunology)

99203 Initial office visit of a 76-year-old male with a stasis ulcer of three month's duration. (Dermatology)

Initial office visit for a 30-year-old female with pain in the lateral aspect of the forearm. (Physical Medicine & Rehabilitation)

Initial office visit for a 15-year-old patient with a four-year history of moderate comedopapular acne of the face, chest, and back with early scarring. Discussion of use of systemic medication. (Dermatology)

Initial office visit for a patient with papulosquamous eruption of the elbow with pitting of nails and itchy scalp. (Dermatology)

Initial office visit for a 57-year-old female who complains of painful parotid swelling for one week's duration. (Oral & Maxillofacial Surgery)

Initial office visit for a patient with an ulcerated non-healing lesion or nodule on the tip of the nose. (Dermatology)

Initial office visit for a patient with dermatitis of the antecubital and popliteal fossae. (Dermatology)

Initial office visit for a 22-year-old female with irregular menses. (Family Medicine)

Initial office visit for a 50-year-old female with dyspepsia and nausea. (Family Medicine)

Initial office visit for a 53-year-old laborer with degenerative joint disease of the knee with no prior treatment. (Orthopaedic Surgery)

Initial office visit for a 60-year-old male with Dupuytren's contracture of one hand with multiple digit involvement. (Orthopaedic Surgery)

Initial office visit for a 33-year-old male with painless gross hematuria without cystoscopy. (Internal Medicine)

Initial office visit for a 55-year-old female with chronic blepharitis. There is a history of use of many medications. (Ophthalmology)

Initial office visit for an 18-year-old female with a two-day history of acute conjunctivitis. Extensive history of possible exposures, prior normal ocular history, and medication use is obtained. (Ophthalmology)

Initial office visit for a 14-year-old male with unilateral anterior knee pain. (Physical Medicine & Rehabilitation)

Initial office visit of an adult who presents with symptoms of an upper-respiratory infection that has progressed to unilateral purulent nasal discharge and discomfort in the right maxillary teeth. (Otolaryngology, Head & Neck Surgery)

Initial office visit of a 40-year-old female with symptoms of atopic allergies including eye and sinus congestion, often associated with infections. She would like to be tested for allergies. (Otolaryngology, Head & Neck Surgery)

Initial office visit of a 65-year-old with nasal stuffiness. (Otolaryngology, Head & Neck Surgery)

Initial office visit for initial evaluation of a 48-year-old man with recurrent low back pain radiating to the leg. (General Surgery)

Initial office visit for evaluation, diagnosis, and management of painless gross hematuria in a new patient, without cystoscopy. (Internal Medicine)

Initial office visit with couple for counseling concerning voluntary vasectomy for sterility. Spent 30 minutes discussing procedure, risks and benefits, and answering questions. (Urology)

Initial office visit of a 49-year-old male with nasal obstruction. Detailed exam with topical anesthesia. (Plastic Surgery)

Initial office visit for evaluation of a 13-year-old female with progressive scoliosis. (Physical Medicine & Rehabilitation)

Initial office visit for a 21-year-old female desiring counseling and evaluation of initiation of contraception. (Family Practice/Internal Medicine/Obstetrics & Gynecology)

Initial office visit for a 49-year-old male presenting with painless blood per rectum associated with bowel movement. (Colon & Rectal Surgery)

Initial office visit for a 19-year-old football player with three-day-old acute knee injury; now with swelling and pain. (Orthopaedic Surgery)

99204 Initial office visit for a 13-year-old female with progressive scoliosis. (Orthopaedic Surgery)

Initial office visit for a 34-year-old female with primary infertility for evaluation and counseling. (Obstetrics & Gynecology)

Initial office visit for a 6-year-old male with multiple upper respiratory infections. (Allergy & Immunology)

Initial office visit for a patient with generalized dermatitis of 80 percent of the body surface area. (Dermatology)

Initial office visit for an adolescent who was referred by school counselor because of repeated skipping school. (Psychiatry)

Initial office visit for a 50-year-old machinist with a generalized eruption. (Dermatology)

Initial office visit for a 45-year-old female who has been abstinent from alcohol and benzodiazepines for three months but complains of headaches, insomnia, and anxiety. (Psychiatry)

Initial office visit for a 60-year-old male with recent change in bowel habits, weight loss, and abdominal pain. (Abdominal Surgery/General Surgery)

Initial office visit for a 50-year-old male with an aortic aneurysm who is considering surgery. (General Surgery)

Initial office visit for a 17-year-old female with depression. (Internal Medicine)

Initial office visit of a 40-year-old with chronic draining ear, imbalance, and probable cholesteatoma. (Otolaryngology, Head & Neck Surgery)

Initial office visit for initial evaluation of a 63-year-old male with chest pain on exertion. (Cardiology/Internal Medicine)

Initial office visit for evaluation of a 70-year-old patient with recent onset of episodic confusion. (Internal Medicine)

Initial office visit for a 7-year-old female with juvenile diabetes mellitus, new to area, past history of hospitalization times three. (Pediatrics)

Initial office visit of a 50-year-old female with progressive solid food dysphagia. (Gastroenterology)

Initial office visit for a 34-year-old patient with primary infertility, including counseling. (Obstetrics & Gynecology)

Initial office visit for evaluation of a 70-year-old female with polyarthralgia. (Rheumatology)

Initial office visit for a patient with papulosquamous eruption involving 60 percent of the cutaneous surface with joint pain. Combinations of topical and systemic treatments discussed. (Dermatology)

99205 Initial office visit for a patient with disseminated lupus erythematosus with kidney disease, edema, purpura, and scarring lesions on the extremities plus cardiac symptoms. (Dermatology/General Surgery/Internal Medicine)

Initial office visit for a 25-year-old female with systemic lupus erythematosus, fever, seizures, and profound thrombodytopenia. (Rheumatology/Allergy & Immunology)

Initial office visit for an adult with multiple cutaneous blisters, denuded secondarily infected ulcerations, oral lesions, weight loss, and increasing weakness refractory to high dose costicosteroid. Initiation of new immunosuppressive therapy. (Dermatology)

Initial office visit for a 28-year-old male with systemic vasculitis and compromised circulation to the limbs. (Rheumatology)

Initial office visit for a 41-year-old female new to the area requesting rheumatologic care, on disability due to scleroderma and recent hospitalization for malignant hypertension. (Rheumatology)

Initial office visit for a 52-year-old female with acute four extermity weakness and shortness of breath one week post-flu vaccination. (Physical Medicine & Rehabilitation)

Initial office visit for a 60-year-old male with previous back surgery; now presents with back and pelvic pain, two-month history of bilateral progressive calf and thigh tightness and weakness when walking, causing several falls. (Orthopaedic Surgery)

Initial office visit for an adolescent referred from emergency department after making suicide gesture. (Psychiatry)

Initial office visit for a 49-year-old female with a history of headaches and dependence on opioids. She reports weight loss, progressive headache, and depression. (Psychiatry)

Initial office visit for a 50-year-old female with symptoms of rash, swellings, recurrent arthritic complaints, and diarrhea and lymphadenopathy. Patient has had a 25 lb weight loss and was recently camping in the Amazon. (Allergy & Immunology)

Initial office visit for a 34-year-old uremic Type I diabetic patient referred for ESRD modality assessment and planning. (Nephrology)

Initial office visit for a 75-year-old female with neck and bilateral shoulder pain, brisk deep tendon reflexes, and stress incontinence. (Physical Medicine & Rehabilitation)

Initial office visit for an 8-year-old male with cerebral palsy and spastic quadriparesis. (Physical Medicine & Rehabilitation)

Initial office visit for a 73-year-old male with known prostate malignancy, who presents with severe back pain and a recent onset of lower extremity weakness. (Physical Medicine & Rehabilitation)

Initial office visit for a 38-year-old male with paranoid delusions and a history of alcohol abuse. (Psychiatry)

Initial office visit for a 12-week-old with bilateral hip dislocations and bilateral club feet. (Orthopaedic Surgery)

Initial office visit for a 29-year-old female with acute orbital congestion, eyelid retraction, and bilateral visual loss from optic neuropathy. (Ophthalmology)

Initial office visit for a 70-year-old diabetic patient with progressive visual field loss, advanced optic disc cupping and neovascularization of retina. (Ophthalmology)

Initial office visit for a newly diagnosed Type I diabetic patient. (Endocrinology)

Initial office evaluation of a 65-year-old female with exertional chest pain, intermittent claudication, syncope and a murmur of aortic stenosis. (Cardiology)

Initial office visit for a 73-year-old male with an unexplained 20 lb weight loss. (Hematology/Oncology)

Initial office evaluation, patient with systemic lupus erythematosus, fever, seizures and profound thrombocytopenia. (Allergy & Immunology/Internal Medicine/Rheumatology)

Initial office evaluation and management of patient with systemic vasculitis and compromised circulation to the limbs. (Rheumatology)

Initial office visit for a 24-year-old homosexual male who has a fever, a cough, and shortness of breath. (Infectious Disease)

Initial outpatient evaluation of a 69-year-old male with severe chronic obstructive pulmonary disease, congestive heart failure, and hypertension. (Family Medicine)

Initial office visit for a 17-year-old female, who is having school problems and has told a friend that she is considering suicide. The patient and her family are consulted in regard to treatment options. (Psychiatry)

Initial office visit for a female with severe hirsutism, amenorrhea, weight loss and a desire to have children. (Endocrinology/Obstetrics & Gynecology)

Established Patient

99211 Initial office visit for a 42-year-old male on hypertensive medication, newly arrived to the area, with diastolic blood pressure of 110, history of recurrent calculi, episodic headaches, intermittent chest pain and orthopnea. (Internal Medicine)

Office visit for an 82-year-old female, established patient, for a monthly B12 injection with documented Vitamin B12 deficiency. (Geriatrics/Internal Medicine/Family Medicine)

Office visit for a 50-year-old male, established patient, for removal of uncomplicated facial sutures. (Plastic Surgery)

Office visit for an established patient who lost prescription for lichen planus. Returned for new copy. (Dermatology)

Office visit for an established patient undergoing orthodontics who complains of a wire which is irritating his/her cheek and asks you to check it. (Oral & Maxillofacial Surgery)

Office visit for a 50-year-old female, established patient, seen for her gold injection by the nurse. (Rheumatology)

Office visit for a 73-year-old female, established patient, with pernicious anemia for weekly B12 injection. (Gastroenterology)

Office visit for an established patient for dressing change on a skin biopsy. (Dermatology)

Office visit for a 19-year-old, established patient, for removal of sutures from a two cm. laceration of forehead, which you placed four days ago in ER. (Plastic Surgery)

Office visit of a 20-year-old female, established patient, who receives an allergy vaccine injection and is observed for a reaction by the nurse. (Otolaryngology, Head & Neck Surgery)

Office visit for a 45-year-old male, established patient, with chronic renal failure for the administration of erythropoietin. (Nephrology)

Office visit for an established patient, a Peace Corps enlistee, who requests documentation that third molars have been removed. (Oral & Maxillofacial Surgery)

Office visit for a 69-year-old female, established patient, for partial removal of antibiotic gauze from an infected wound site. (Plastic Surgery)

Office visit for a 9-year-old, established patient, successfully treated for impetigo, requiring release to return to school. (Dermatology/Pediatrics)

Office visit for an established patient requesting a return-to-work certificate for resolving contact dermatitis. (Dermatology)

Office visit for an established patient who is performing glucose monitoring and wants to check accuracy of machine with lab blood glucose by technician who checks accuracy and function of patient machine. (Endocrinology)

Follow-up office visit for a 65-year-old female with a chronic indwelling percutaneous nephrostomy catheter seen for routine pericatheter skin care and dressing change. (Interventional Radiology)

Outpatient visit with 19-year-old male, established patient, for supervised drug screen. (Addiction Medicine)

Office visit with 12-year-old male, established patient, for cursory check of hematoma one day after venipuncture. (Internal Medicine)

Office visit with 31-year-old female, established patient, for return to work certificate. (Anesthesiology)

Office visit for a 42-year-old, established patient, to read tuberculin test results. (Allergy & Immunology)

Office visit for 14-year-old, established patient, to re-dress an abrasion. (Orthopaedic Surgery)

Office visit for a 45-year-old female, established patient, for a blood pressure check. (Obstetrics & Gynecology)

Office visit for a 23-year-old, established patient, for instruction in use of peak flow meter. (Allergy & Immunology)

Office visit for prescription refill for a 35-year-old female, established patient, with schizophrenia who is stable but has run out of neuroleptic and is scheduled to be seen in a week. (Psychiatry)

99212   Office visit for an 11-year-old, established patient, seen in follow-up for mild comedonal acne of the cheeks on topical desquamating agents. (Dermatology/Family Medicine/Pediatrics)

Office visit for a 10-year-old female, established patient, who has been swimming in a lake, now presents with a one-day history of left ear pain with purulent drainage. (Family Medicine)

Office visit for a child, established patient, with chronic secretory otitis media. (Otolaryngology, Head & Neck Surgery)

Office visit for an established patient seen in follow-up of clearing patch of localized contact dermatitis. (Family Medicine/Dermatology)

Office visit for an established patient returning for evaluation of response to treatment of lichen planus on wrists and ankles. (Dermatology)

Office visit for an established patient with tinea pedis being treated with topical therapy. (Dermatology)

Office visit for an established patient with localized erythematous plaque of psoriasis with topical hydration. (Dermatology)

Office visit for a 50-year-old male, established patient, recently seen for acute neck pain, diagnosis of spondylosis, responding to physical therapy and intermittent cervical traction. Returns for evaluation for return to work. (Neurology)

Office visit for an established patient with recurring episodes of herpes simplex who has developed a clustering of vesicles on the upper lip. (Oral & Maxillofacial Surgery)

Evaluation fo a 50-year-old male, established patient, who has experienced a recurrence of knee pain after he discontinued NSAID. (Anesthesiology/Pain Medicine)

Office visit for an established patient with an irritated skin tag for reassurance. (Dermatology)

Office visit for a 40-year-old, established patient, who has experienced a systemic allergic reaction following administration of immunotherapy. The dose must be readjusted. (Allergy & Immunology)

Office visit for a 33-year-old, established patient, for contusion and abrasion of lower extremity. (Orthopaedic Surgery)

Office visit for a 22-year-old male, established patient, one month after I & D of "wrestler's ear." (Plastic Surgery)

Office visit for a 21-year-old, established patient, who is seen in follow-up after antibiotic therapy for acute bacterial tonsilitis. (Otolaryngology, Head & Neck Surgery)

Office visit for a 4-year-old, established patient, with tympanostomy tubes, check-up. (Otolaryngology, Head & Neck Surgery)

Office visit for an established patient who has had needle aspiration of a peritonsillar abscess. (Otolaryngology, Head & Neck Surgery)

Follow-up office examination for evaluation and treatment of acute draining ear in a 5-year-old with tympanotomy tubes. (Otolaryngology, Head & Neck Surgery)

Office visit, established patient, 6-year-old with sore throat and headache. (Family Medicine/Pediatrics)

Office evaluation for possible purulent bacterial conjunctivitis with one- to two-day history of redness and discharge, 16-year-old female, established patient. (Pediatrics/Internal Medicine/Family Medicine)

Office visit for a 65-year-old female, established patient, returns for three-week follow-up for resolving severe ankle sprain. (Orthopaedic Surgery)

Office visit, sore throat, fever, and fatigue in a 19-year-old college student, established patient. (Internal Medicine)

Office visit with a 33-year-old female, established patient, recently started on treatment for hemorrhoidal complaints, for re-evaluation. (Colon & Rectal Surgery)

Office visit with a 36-year-old male, established patient, for follow-up on effectiveness of medicine management of oral candidiasis. (Oral & Maxillofacial Surgery)

Office visit for a 27-year-old female, established patient, with complaints of vaginal itching. (Obstetrics & Gynecology)

Office visit for a 65-year-old, established patient, with eruptions on both arms from poison oak exposure. (Allergy & Immunology/Internal Medicine)

99213 Office visit for an established patient with new lesions of lichen planus in spite of topical therapies. (Dermatology)

Office visit for the quarterly follow-up of a 45-year-old male with stable chronic asthma requiring regular drug therapy. (Allergy & Immunology)

Office visit for a 13-year-old, established patient, with comedopapular acne of the face which has shown poor response to topical medication. Discussion of use of systemic medication. (Dermatology)

Office visit for a 62-year-old female, established patient, for follow-up for stable cirrhosis of the liver. (Internal Medicine/Family Medicine)

Office visit for a 3-year-old, established patient, with atopic dermatitis and food hypersensitivity for quarterly follow-up evaluation. The patient is on topical lotions and steroid creams as well as oral antihistamines. (Allergy & Immunology)

Office visit for an 80-year-old female, established patient, to evaluate medical management of osteoarthritis of the temporomandibular joint. (Rheumatology)

Office visit for a 70-year-old female, established patient, one year post excision of basal cell carcinoma of nose with nasolabial flap. Now presents with new suspicious recurrent lesion and suspicious lesion of the back. (Plastic Surgery)

Office visit for a 68-year-old female, established patient, with polymyalgia rheumatic, maintained on chronic low-dose corticosteroid, with no new complaints. (Rheumatology)

Office visit for a 3-year-old female, established patient, for earache and dyshidrosis of feet. (Pediatrics/Family Medicine)

Office visit for an established patient for 18-months post-operative follow-up of TMJ repair. (Oral & Maxillofacial Surgery)

Office visit for a 45-year-old male, established patient, being re-evaluated for recurrent acute prostatitis. (Urology)

Office visit for a 43-year-old male, established patient, with known reflex sympathetic dystrophy. (Anesthesiology)

Office visit for an established patient with an evenly pigmented superficial nodule of leg which is symptomatic. (Dermatology)

Office visit for an established patient with psoriasis involvement of the elbows, pitting of the nails, and itchy scalp. (Dermatology)

Office visit for a 27-year-old male, established patient, with deep follicular and perifollicular inflammation unable to tolerate systemic antibiotics due to GI upset, requires change of systemic medication. (Dermatology)

Office visit for a 16-year-old male, established patient, who is on medication for exercise-induced bronchospasm. (Allergy & Immunology)

Office visit for a 60-year-old, established patient, with chronic essential hypertension on multiple drug regimen, for blood pressure check. (Family Medicine)

Office visit for a 20-year-old male, established patient, for removal of sutures in hand. (Family Medicine)

Office visit for a 58-year-old female, established patient, with unilateral painful bunion. (Orthopaedic Surgery)

Office visit for a 45-year-old female, established patient, with known osteoarthritis and painful swollen knees. (Rheumatology)

Office visit for a 25-year-old female, established patient, complaining of bleeding and heavy menses. (Obstetrics & Gynecology)

Office visit for a 55-year-old male, established patient, with hypertension managed by a beta blocker/thiazide regime; now experiencing mild fatigue. (Nephrology)

Office visit for a 65-year-old female, established patient, with primary glaucoma for interval determination of intraocular pressure and possible adjustment of medication. (Ophthalmology)

Office visit for a 56-year-old male, established patient, with stable exertional angina who complains of new onset of calf pain while walking. (Cardiology)

Office visit for a 63-year-old female, established patient, with rheumatoid arthritis on auranofin and ibuprofen, seen for routine follow-up visit. (Rheumatology)

Office visit for an established patient with Graves' disease, three months post I-131 therapy, who presents with lassitude and malaise. (Endocrinology)

Office visit for the quarterly follow-up of a 63-year-old male, established patient, with chronic myofascial pain syndrome, effectively managed by doxepin, who presents with new onset urinary hesitancy. (Pain Medicine)

Office visit for the biannual follow-up of an established patient with migraine variant having infrequent, intermittent, moderate to severe headaches with nausea and vomiting, which are sometimes effectively managed by ergotamine tartrate and an antiemetic, but occasionally requiring visits to an emergency department. (Pain Medicine)

Office visit for an established patient after discharge from a pain rehabilitation program to review and adjust medication dosage. (Pain Medicine)

Office visit with 55-year-old male, established patient, for management of hypertension, mild fatigue, on beta blocker/thiazide regimen. (Family Medicine/Internal Medicine)

Outpatient visit with 37-year-old male, established patient, who is three years post total colectomy for chronic ulcerative colitis, presents for increased irritation at his stoma. (General Surgery)

Office visit for a 70-year-old diabetic hypertensive established patient with recent change in insulin requirement. (Internal Medicine/Nephrology)

Office visit with 80-year-old female, established patient, for follow-up osteoporosis, status-post compression fractures. (Rheumatology)

Office visit for an established patient with stable cirrhosis of the liver. (Gastroenterology)

Routine, follow-up office evaluation at a three-month interval for a 77-year-old female, established patient, with nodular small cleaved-cell lymphoma. (Hematology/Oncology)

Quarterly follow-up office visit for a 45-year-old male, established patient, with stable chronic asthma, on steroid and bronchodilator therapy. (Pulmonary Medicine)

Office visit for a 50-year-old female, established patient, with insulin-dependent diabetes mellitus and stable coronary artery disease, for monitoring. (Family Medicine/Internal Medicine)

99214 Office visit for an established patient now presenting with generalized dermatitis of 80% of the body surface area. (Dermatology)

Office visit for a 32-year-old female, established patient, with new onset right lower quadrant pain. (Family Medicine)

Office visit for reassessment and reassurance/counseling of a 40-year-old female, established patient, who is experiencing increased symptoms while on a pain management treatment program. (Pain Medicine)

Office visit for a 30-year-old, established patient, under management for intractable low back pain, who now presents with new onset right posterior thigh pain. (Pain Medicine)

Office visit for an established patient with frequent intermittent, moderate to severe headaches requiring beta blocker or tricyclic antidepressant prophylaxis, as well as four symptomatic treatments, but who is still experiencing headaches at a frequency of several times a month that are unresponsive to treatment. (Pain Medicine)

Office visit for an established patient with psoriasis with extensive involvement of scalp, trunk, palms, and soles with joint pain. Combinations of topical and systemic treatments discussed and instituted. (Dermatology)

Office visit for a 55-year-old male, established patient, with increasing night pain, limp, and progressive varus of both knees. (Orthopaedic Surgery)

Follow-up visit for a 15-year-old withdrawn patient with four-year history of papulocystic acne of the face, chest, and back with early scarring and poor response to past treatment. Discussion of use of systemic medication. (Dermatology)

Office visit for a 28-year-old male, established patient, with regional enteritis, diarrhea, and low-grade fever. (Internal Medicine)

Office visit for a 25-year-old female, established patient, following recent arthrogram and MR imaging for TMJ pain. (Oral & Maxillofacial Surgery)

Office visit for a 32-year-old female, established patient, with large obstructing stone in left mid-ureter, to discuss management options including urethroscopy with extraction or ESWL. (Urology)

Evaluation for a 28-year-old male, established patient, with new onset of low back pain. (Anesthesiology/Pain Medicine)

Office visit for a 28-year-old female, established patient, with right lower quadrant abdominal pain, fever, and anorexia. (Internal Medicine/Family Medicine)

Office visit for a 45-year-old male, established patient, four months follow-up of L4-5 discectomy, with persistent incapacitating low back and leg pain. (Orthopaedic Surgery)

Outpatient visit for a 77-year-old male, established patient, with hypertension, presenting with a three-month history of episodic substernal chest pain on exertion. (Cardiology)

Office visit for a 25-year-old female, established patient, for evaluation of progressive saddle nose deformity of unknown etiology. (Plastic Surgery)

Office visit for a 65-year-old male, established patient, with BPH and severe bladder outlet obstruction, to discuss management options such as TURP. (Urology)

Office visit for an adult diabetic established patient with a past history of recurrent sinusitis who presents with a one-week history of double vision. (Otolaryngology, Head & Neck Surgery)

Office visit for an established patient with lichen planus and 60% of the cutaneous surface involved, not responsive to systemic steroids, as well as developing symptoms of progressive heartburn and paranoid ideation. (Dermatology)

Office visit for a 52-year-old male, established patient, with a 12-year history of bipolar disorder responding to lithium carbonate and brief psychotherapy. Psychotherapy and prescription provided. (Psychiatry)

Office visit for a 63-year-old female, established patient, with a history of familial polyposis, status post-colectomy with sphincter sparing procedure, who now presents with rectal bleeding and increase in stooling frequency. (General Surgery)

Office visit for a 68-year-old male, established patient, with the sudden onset of multiple flashes and floaters in the right eye due to a posterior vitreous detachment. (Ophthalmology)

Office visit for a 55-year-old female, established patient, on cyclosporin for treatment of resistant, small vessel vasculitis. (Rheumatology)

Follow-up office visit for a 55-year-old male, two months after iliac angioplasty with new onset of contralateral extremity claudication. (Interventional Radiology)

Office visit for a 68-year-old male, established patient, with stable angina, two months post myocardial infarction, who is not tolerating one of his medications. (Cardiology)

Weekly office visit for 5FU therapy for an ambulatory established patient with metastatic colon cancer and increasing shortness of breath. (Hematology/Oncology)

Follow-up office visit for a 60-year-old male, established patient, whose post-traumatic seizures have disappeared on medication and who now raises the question of stopping the medication. (Neurology)

Office evaluation on new onset RLQ pain in a 32-year-old female, established patient. (Urology/General Surgery/Internal Medicine/Family Medicine)

Office evaluation of 28-year-old, established patient, with regional enteritis, diarrhea, and low-grade fever. (Family Medicine/Internal Medicine)

Office visit with 50-year-old female, established patient, diabetic, blood sugar controlled by diet. She now complains of frequency of urination and weight loss, blood sugar of 320, and negative ketones on dipstick. (Internal Medicine)

Follow-up office visit for a 45-year-old, established patient, with rheumatoid arthritis on gold, methotrexate, or immunosuppressive therapy. (Rheumatology)

Office visit for a 60-year-old male, established patient, two years post-removal of intracranial meningioma, now with new headaches and visual disturbance. (Neurosurgery)

Office visit for a 68-year-old female, established patient, for routine review and follow-up of non-insulin dependent diabetes, obesity, hypertension, and congestive heart failure. Complains of vision difficulties and admits dietary noncompliance. Patient is counseled concerning diet and current medications adjusted. (Family Medicine)

99215 Office visit for an established patient who developed persistent cough, rectal bleeding, weakness, and diarrhea plus pustular infection on skin. Patient on immunosuppressive therapy. (Dermatology)

Office visit for an established patient with disseminated lupus erythematosus, extensive edema of extremities, kidney disease, and weakness requiring monitored course on azathioprene, corticosteroid and complicated by acute depression. (Dermatology/Internal Medicine/Rheumatology)

Office visit for an established patient with progressive dermatomyositis and recent onset of fever, nasal speech, and regurgitation of fluids through the nose. (Dermatology)

Office visit for a 28-year-old female, established patient, who is abstinent from previous cocaine dependence, but reports progressive panic attacks and chest pains. (Psychiatry)

Office visit for an established adolescent patient with history of bipolar disorder treated with lithium; seen on urgent basis at family's request because of severe depressive symptoms. (Psychiatry)

Office visit for an established patient having acute migraine with new onset neurological symptoms and whose headaches are unresponsive to previous attempts at management with a combination of preventive and abortive medication. (Pain Medicine)

Office visit for an established patient with exfoliative lichen planus with daily fever spikes, disorientation, and shortness of breath. (Dermatology)

Office visit for a 25-year-old, established patient, two years post-burn with bilateral ectropion, hypertrophic facial burn scars, near absence of left breast, and burn syndactyly of both hands. Discussion of treatment options following examination. (Plastic Surgery)

Office visit for a 6-year-old, established patient, to review newly diagnosed immune deficiency with recommendations for therapy including IV immunoglobulin and chronic antibiotics. (Allergy & Immunology)

Office visit for a 36-year-old, established patient, three months status post-transplant, with new onset of peripheral edema, increased blood pressure, and progressive fatigue. (Nephrology)

Office visit for an established patient with Kaposi's sarcoma who presents with fever and widespread vesicles. (Dermatology)

Office visit for a 27-year-old female, established patient, with bipolar disorder who was stable on lithium carbonate and monthly supportive psychotherapy but now has developed symptoms of hypomania. (Psychiatry)

Office visit for a 25-year-old male, established patient with a history of schizophrenia who has been seen bi-monthly but is complaining of auditory hallucinations. (Psychiatry)

Office visit for a 62-year-old male, established patient, three years postoperative abdominal perineal resection, now with a rising carcinoembryonic antigen, weight loss, and pelvic pain. (Abdominal Surgery)

Office visit for a 42-year-old male, established patient, nine months postoperative emergency vena cava shunt for variceal bleeding, now presents with complaints of one episode of "dark" bowel movement, weight gain, tightness in abdomen, whites of eyes seem "yellow" and occasional drowsiness after eating hamburgers. (Abdominal Surgery)

Office visit for a 68-year-old male, established patient, with biopsy-proven rectal carcinoma, for evaluation and discussion of treatment options. (General Surgery)

Office visit for a 60-year-old, established patient, with diabetic nephropathy with increasing edema and dyspnea. (Endocrinology)

Office visit with 30-year-old male, established patient for three-month history of fatigue, weight loss, intermittent fever, and presenting with diffuse adenopathy and splenomegaly. (Family Medicine)

Office visit for restaging of an established patient with new lymphadenopathy one year post-therapy for lymphoma. (Hematology/Oncology)

Office visit for evaluation of recent onset syncopal attacks in a 70-year-old female, established patient. (Internal Medicine)

Follow-up visit, 40-year-old mother of three, established patient, with acute rheumatoid arthritis, anatomical Stage 3, ARA function Class 3 rheumatoid arthritis, and deteriorating function. (Rheumatology)

Follow-up office visit for a 65-year-old male, established patient, with a fever of recent onset while on outpatient antibiotic therapy for endocarditis. (Infectious Disease)

Office visit for a 75-year-old, established patient, with ALS (amyotrophic lateral sclerosis), who is no longer able to swallow. (Neurology)

Office visit for a 70-year-old female, established patient, with diabetes mellitus and hypertension, presenting with a two-month history of increasing confusion, agitation and short-term memory loss. (Family Medicine/Internal Medicine)

Hospital Inpatient Services

Initial Hospital Care

New or Established Patient

99221 Initial hospital visit following admission for a 42-year-old male for observation following an uncomplicated mandible fracture. (Plastic Surgery/Oral & Maxillofacial Surgery)

Initial hospital visit for a 40-year-old patient with a thrombosed synthetic arteriovenous conduit. (Nephrology)

Initial hospital visit for a healthy 24-year-old male with an acute onset of low back pain following a lifting injury. (Internal Medicine/Anesthesiology/Pain Medicine)

Initial hospital visit for a 69-year-old female with controlled hypertension, scheduled for surgery. (Internal Medicine/Cardiology)

Initial hospital visit for a 24-year-old healthy female with benign tumor of palate. (Oral & Maxillofacial Surgery)

Initial hospital visit for a 14-year-old female with infectious mononucleosis and dehydration. (Internal Medicine)

Initial hospital visit for a 62-year-old female with stable rheumatoid arthritis, admitted for total joint replacement. (Rheumatology)

Initial hospital visit for a 12-year-old patient with a laceration of the upper eyelid, involving the lid margin and superior canaliculus, admitted prior to surgery for IV antibiotic therapy. (Plastic Surgery)

Initial hospital visit for a 69-year-old female with controlled hypertension, scheduled for surgery. (Cardiology)

Hospital admission, examination, and initiation of treatment program for a 67-year-old male with uncomplicated pneumonia who requires IV antibiotic therapy. (Internal Medicine)

Hospital admission for an 18-month-old with 10% dehydration. (Pediatrics)

Hospital admission for a 12-year-old with a laceration of the upper eyelid involving the lid margin and superior canaliculus, admitted prior to surgery for IV antibiotic therapy. (Ophthalmology)

Hospital admission for a 32-year-old female with severe flank pain, hematuria and presumed diagnosis of ureteral calculus as determined by Emergency Department physician. (Urology)

Initial hospital visit for a patient with several large venous stasis ulcers not responding to outpatient therapy. (Dermatology)

Initial hospital visit for 21-year-old pregnant patient (nine-weeks gestation) with hyperemesis gravidarum. (Obstetrics & Gynecology)

Initial hospital visit for a 73-year-old female with acute pyelonephritis who is otherwise generally healthy. (Geriatrics)

Initial hospital visit for 62-year-old patient with cellulitis of the foot requiring bedrest and intravenous antibiotics. (Orthopaedic Surgery)

99222 Initial hospital visit for a 50-year-old patient with lower quadrant abdominal pain and increased temperature, but without septic picture. (General Surgery/Abdominal Surgery/Colon & Rectal Surgery)

Initial hospital visit for airway management, due to a benign laryngeal mass. (Otolaryngology, Head & Neck Surgery)

Initial hospital visit for a 66-year-old female with an L-2 vertebral compression fracture with acute onset of paralytic ileus; seen in the office two days previously. (Orthopaedic Surgery)

Initial hospital visit and evaluation of a 15-year-old male admitted with peritonsillar abscess or cellulitis requiring intravenous antibiotic therapy. (Otolaryngology, Head & Neck Surgery)

Initial hospital visit for a 42-year-old male with vertebral compression fracture following a motor vehicle accident. (Orthopaedic Surgery)

Initial hospital visit for a patient with generalized atopic dermatitis and secondary infection. (Dermatology)

Initial hospital visit for a 3-year-old patient with high temperature, limp, and painful hip motion of 18 hours' duration. (Pediatrics/Orthopaedic Surgery)

Initial hospital visit for a young adult, presenting with an acute asthma attack unresponsive to outpatient therapy. (Allergy & Immunology)

Initial hospital visit for an 18-year-old male who has suppurative sialoadenitis and dehydration. (Oral & Maxillofacial Surgery)

Initial hospital visit for a 65-year-old female for acute onset of thrombotic cerebrovascular accident with contralateral paralysis and aphasia. (Neurology)

Initial hospital visit for a 50-year-old male chronic paraplegic patient with pain and spasm below the lesion. (Anesthesiology)

Partial hospital admission for an adolescent patient from chaotic blended family, transferred from inpatient setting, for continued treatment to control symptomatic expressions of hostility and depression. (Psychiatry)

Initial hospital visit for a 15-year-old male with acute status asthmaticus, unresponsive to outpatient therapy. (Internal Medicine)

Initial hospital visit for a 61-year-old male with history of previous myocardial infarction, who now complains of chest pain. (Internal Medicine)

Initial hospital visit of a 15-year-old on medications for a sore throat over the last two weeks. The sore throat has worsened and patient now has dysphagia. The exam shows large necrotic tonsils with an adequate airway and small palpable nodes. The initial mono test was negative. (Otolaryngology, Head & Neck Surgery)

Initial hospital evaluation of a 23-year-old allergy patient admitted with eyelid edema and pain on fifth day of oral antibiotic therapy. (Otolaryngology, Head & Neck Surgery)

Hospital admission, young adult patient, failed previous therapy and now presents in acute asthmatic attack. (Family Medicine/Allergy & Immunology)

Hospital admission of a 62-year-old smoker, established patient, with bronchitis in acute respiratory distress. (Internal Medicine/Pulmonary Medicine)

Hospital admission, examination, and initiation of a treatment program for a 65-year-old female with new onset of right-sided paralysis and aphasia. (Neurology)

Hospital admission, examination, and initiation of treatment program for a 66-year-old chronic hemodialysis patient with fever and a new pulmonary infiltrate. (Nephrology)

Hospital admission for an 8-year-old febrile patient with chronic sinusitis and severe headache, unresponsive to oral antibiotics. (Allergy & Immunology)

Hospital admission for a 40-year-old male with submaxillary cellulitis and trismus from infected lower molar. (Oral & Maxillofacial Surgery)

99223 Initial hospital visit for a 45-year-old female, who has a history of rheumatic fever as a child and now has anemia, fever, and congestive heart failure. (Cardiology)

Initial hospital visit for a 50-year-old male with acute chest pain and diagnostic electrocardiographic changes of an acute anterior myocardial infarction. (Cardiology/Family Medicine/Internal Medicine)

Initial hospital visit of a 75-year-old with progressive stridor and dysphagia with history of cancer of the larynx treated by radiation therapy in the past. Exam shows a large recurrent tumor of the glottis with a mass in the neck. (Otolaryngology, Head & Neck Surgery)

Initial hospital visit for a 70-year-old male admitted with chest pain, complete heart block, and congestive heart failure. (Cardiology)

Initial hospital visit for an 82-year-old male who presents with syncope, chest pain, and ventricular arrhythmias. (Cardiology)

Initial hospital visit for a 75-year-old male with history of arteriosclerotic coronary vascular disease, who is severely dehydrated, disoriented, and experiencing auditory hallucinations. (Psychiatry)

Initial hospital visit for a 70-year-old male with alcohol and sedative-hypnotic dependence, admitted by family for severe withdrawal, hypertension, and diabetes mellitus. (Psychiatry)

Initial hospital visit for a persistently suicidal latency-aged child whose parents have requested admission to provide safety during evaluation, but are anxious about separation from her. (Psychiatry)

Initial psychiatric visit for an adolescent patient without previous psychiatric history, who was transferred from the medical ICU after a significant overdose. (Psychiatry)

Initial hospital visit for a 35-year-old female with severe systemic lupus erythematosus on corticosteroid and cyclophosphamide, with new onset of fever, chills, rash, and chest pain. (Rheumatology)

Initial hospital visit for a 52-year-old male with known rheumatic heart disease who presents with anasarca, hypertension, and history of alcohol abuse. (Cardiology)

Initial hospital visit for a 55-year-old female with a history of congenital heart disease; now presents with cyanosis. (Cardiology)

Initial hospital visit for a psychotic, hostile, violently combative adolescent, involuntarily committed, for seclusion and restraint in order to provide for safety on unit. (Psychiatry)

Initial hospital visit for a now subdued and sullen teenage male with six-month history of declining school performance, increasing self-endangerment, and resistance of parental expectations, including running away past weekend after physical fight with father. (Psychiatry)

Initial partial hospital admission for a 17-year-old female with history of borderline mental retardation who has developed auditory hallucinations. Parents are known to abuse alcohol, and Child Protective Services is investigating allegations of sexual abuse of a younger sibling. (Psychiatry)

Initial hospital visit of a 67-year-old male admitted with a large neck mass, dysphagia, and history of myocardial infarction three months before. (Otolaryngology, Head & Neck Surgery)

Initial hospital visit for a patient with suspected cerebrospinal fluid rhinorrhea which developed two weeks after head injury. (Otolaryngology, Head & Neck Surgery)

Initial hospital visit for a 25-year-old female with history of poly-substance abuse and psychiatric disorder. The patient appears to be psychotic with markedly elevated vital signs. (Psychiatry)

Initial hospital visit for a 70-year-old male with cutaneous T-cell lymphoma who has developed fever and lymphadenopathy. (Internal Medicine)

Initial hospital visit for a 62-year-old female with known coronary artery disease, for evaluation of increasing edema, dyspnea on exertion, confusion, and sudden onset of fever with productive cough. (Internal Medicine)

Initial hospital visit for a 3-year-old female with 36-hour history of sore throat and high fever; now with sudden onset of lethargy, irritability, photophobia, and nuchal rigidity. (Pediatrics)

Initial hospital visit for a 26-year-old female for evaluation of severe facial fractures (LeFort's II/III). (Plastic Surgery)

Initial hospital visit for a 55-year-old female for bilateral mandibular fractures resulting in flail mandible and airway obstruction. (Plastic Surgery)

Initial hospital visit for a 71-year-old patient with a red painful eye four days following uncomplicated cataract surgery due to endophthalmitis. (Ophthalmology)

Initial hospital visit for a 45-year-old patient involved in a motor vehicle accident who suffered a perforating corneoscleral laceration with loss of vision. (Ophthalmology)

Initial hospital visit for a 58-year-old male who has Ludwig's angina and progressive airway compromise. (Oral & Maxillofacial Surgery)

Initial hospital visit for a patient with generalized systemic sclerosis, receiving immunosuppressive therapy because of recent onset of cough, fever, and inability to swallow. (Dermatology)

Initial hospital visit for an 82-year-old male who presents with syncope, chest pain, and ventricular arrhythmias. (Cardiology)

Initial hospital visit for a 62-year-old male with history of previous myocardial infarction, comes in with recurrent, sustained ventricular tachycardia. (Cardiology)

Initial hospital visit for a chronic dialysis patient with infected PTFE fistula, septicemia, and shock. (Nephrology)

Initial hospital visit for a 1-year-old male, victim of child abuse, with central nervous system depression, skull fracture, and retinal hemorrhage. (Family Medicine/Neurology)

Initial hospital visit for a 25-year-old female with recent C4-5 quadriplegia, admitted for rehabilitation. (Physical Medicine & Rehabilitation)

Initial hospital visit for an 18-year-old male, post-traumatic brain injury with multiple impairment. (Physical Medicine & Rehabilitation)

Initial partial hospital admission for 16-year-old male, sullen and subdued, with six-month history of declining school performance, increasing self-endangerment, and resistance to parental expectations. (Psychiatry)

Initial hospital visit for a 16-year-old primigravida at 32-weeks gestation with severe hypertension (200/110), thrombocytopenia, and headache. (Obstetrics & Gynecology)

Initial hospital visit for a 49-year-old male with cirrhosis of liver with hematemesis, hepatic encephalopathy, and fever. (Gastroenterology)

Initial hospital visit for a 55-year-old female in chronic pain who has attempted suicide. (Psychiatry)

Initial hospital visit for a 70-year-old male, with multiple organ system disease, admitted with history of being aneuric and septic for 24 hours prior to admission. (Urology)

Initial hospital visit for a 3-year-old female with 36-hour history of sore throat and high fever, now with sudden onset of lethargy, irritability, photophobia, and nuchal rigidity. (Internal Medicine)

Initial hospital visit for a 78-year-old male, transfers from nursing home with dysuria and pyuria, increasing confusion, and high fever. (Internal Medicine)

Initial hospital visit for a 1-day-old male with cyanosis, respiratory distress, and tachypnea. (Cardiology)

Initial hospital visit for a 3-year-old female with recurrent tachycardia and syncope. (Cardiology)

Initial hospital visit for a thyrotoxic patient who presents with fever, atrial fibrillation, and delirium. (Endocrinology)

Initial hospital visit for a 50-year-old Type I diabetic who presents with diabetic ketoacidosis with fever and obtundation. (Endocrinology)

Initial hospital visit for a 40-year-old female with anatomical stage 3, ARA functional class 3 rheumatoid arthritis on methotrexate, corticosteroid, and nonsteroidal anti-inflammatory drugs. Patient presents with severe arthritis flare, new oral ulcers, abdominal pain, and leukopenia. (Rheumatology)

Initial hospital exam of a pediatric patient with high fever and proptosis. (Otolaryngology, Head & Neck Surgery)

Initial hospital visit for a 25-year-old patient admitted for the first time to the rehab unit, with recent C-4-5 quadriplegia. (Physical Medicine & Rehabilitation)

Hospital admission, examination, and initiation of treatment program for a previously unknown 58-year-old male who presents with acute chest pain. (Cardiology)

Hospital admission, examination, and initiation of induction chemotherapy for a 42-year-old patient with newly diagnosed acute myelogenous leukemia. (Hematology/Oncology)

Hospital admission following a motor vehicle accident of a 24-year-old male with fracture dislocation of C5-6; neurologically intact. (Neurosurgery)

Hospital admission for a 78-year-old female with left lower lobe pneumonia and a history of coronary artery disease, congestive heart failure, osteoarthritis and gout. (Family Medicine)

Hospital admission, examination, and initiation of treatment program for a 65-year-old immunosuppressed male with confusion, fever, and a headache. (Infectious Disease)

Hospital admission for a 9-year-old with vomiting, dehydration, fever, tachypnea, and an admitting diagnosis of diabetic ketoacidosis. (Pediatrics)

Initial hospital visit for a 65-year-old male who presents with acute myocardial infarction, oliguria, hypotension, and altered state of consciousness. (Cardiology)

Initial hospital visit for a hostile/resistant adolescent patient who is severely depressed and involved in poly-substance abuse. Patient is experiencing significant conflict in his chaotic family situation and was suspended from school following an attack on a teacher with a baseball bat. (Psychiatry)

Initial hospital visit for 89-year-old female with fulminant hepatic failure and encephalopathy. (Gastroenterology)

Initial hospital visit for a 42-year-old female with rapidly progressing scleroderma, malignant hypertension, digital infarcts, and oligurea. (Rheumatology)

Subsequent Hospital Care

99231 Subsequent hospital visit for a 65-year-old female, post-open reduction and internal fixation of a fracture. (Physical Medicine & Rehabilitation)

Subsequent hospital visit for a 33-year-old patient with pelvic pain who is responding to pain medication and observation. (Obstetrics & Gynecology)

Subsequent hospital visit for a 21-year-old female with hyperemesis who has responded well to intravenous fluids. (Obstetrics & Gynecology)

Subsequent hospital visit to re-evaluate postoperative pain and titrate patient-controlled analgesia for a 27-year-old female. (Anesthesiology)

Follow-up hospital visit for a 35-year-old female, status post-epidural analgesia. (Anesthesiology/Pain Medicine)

Subsequent hospital visit for a 56-year-old male, post-gastrectomy, for maintenance of analgesia using an intravenous dilaudid infusion. (Anesthesiology)

Subsequent hospital visit for a 4-year-old on day three receiving medication for uncomplicated pneumonia. (Allergy & Immunology)

Subsequent hospital visit for a 30-year-old female with urticaria which has stabilized with medication. (Allergy & Immunology)

Subsequent hospital visit for a 76-year-old male with venous stasis ulcers. (Dermatology)

Subsequent hospital visit for a 24-year-old female with otitis externa, seen two days before in consultation, now to have otic wick removal. (Otolaryngology, Head & Neck Surgery)

Subsequent hospital visit for a 27-year-old with acute labyrinthitis. (Otolaryngology, Head & Neck Surgery)

Subsequent hospital visit for a 10-year-old male admitted for lobar pneumonia with vomiting and dehydration; is becoming afebrile and tolerating oral fluids. (Family Medicine/Pediatrics)

Subsequent hospital visit for a 62-year-old patient with resolving cellulitis of the foot. (Orthopaedic Surgery)

Subsequent hospital visit for a 25-year-old male admitted for supra-ventricular tachycardia and converted on medical therapy. (Cardiology)

Subsequent hospital visit for a 27-year-old male two days after open reduction and internal fixation for malar complex fracture. (Plastic Surgery)

Subsequent hospital visit for a 76-year-old male with venous stasis ulcers. (Geriatrics)

Subsequent hospital visit for a 67-year-old female admitted three days ago with bleeding gastric ulcer; now stable. (Gastroenterology)

Subsequent hospital visit for stable 33-year-old male, status post-lower gastrointestinal bleeding. (General Surgery/Gastroenterology)

Subsequent hospital visit for a 29-year-old auto mechanic with effort thrombosis of left upper extremity. (General Surgery)

Subsequent hospital visit for a 14-year-old female in middle phase of inpatient treatment, who is now behaviorally stable and making satisfactory progress in treatment. (Psychiatry)

Subsequent hospital visit for an 18-year-old male with uncomplicated asthma who is clinically stable. (Allergy & Immunology)

Subsequent hospital visit for a 55-year-old male with rheumatoid arthritis, two days following an uncomplicated total joint replacement. (Rheumatology)

Subsequent hospital visit for a 60-year-old dialysis patient with an access infection, now afebrile on antibiotic. (Nephrology)

Subsequent hospital visit for a 36-year-old female with stable post-rhinoplasty epistaxis. (Plastic Surgery)

Subsequent hospital visit for a 66-year-old female with L-2 vertebral compression fracture with resolving ileus. (Orthopaedic Surgery)

Subsequent hospital visit for a patient with peritonsillar abscess. (Otolaryngology, Head & Neck Surgery)

Subsequent hospital visit for an 18-year-old female responding to intravenous antibiotic therapy for ear or sinus infection. (Otolaryngology, Head & Neck Surgery)

Subsequent hospital visit for a 70-year-old male admitted with congestive heart failure who has responded to therapy. (Cardiology)

Follow-up hospital visit for a 32-year-old female with left ureteral calculus; being followed in anticipation of spontaneous passage. (Urology)

Subsequent hospital visit for a 4-year-old female, admitted for acute gastroenteritis and dehydration, requiring IV hydration; now stable. (Family Medicine)

Subsequent hospital visit for a 50-year-old Type II diabetic who is clinically stable and without complications requiring regulation of a single dose of insulin daily. (Endocrinology)

Subsequent hospital visit to reassesses the status of a 65-year-old patient post-open reduction and internal fixation of hip fracture, on the rehab unit. (Physical Medicine & Rehabilitation)

Subsequent hospital visit for a 78-year-old male with cholangiocarcinoma managed by biliary drainage. (Interventional Radiology)

Subsequent hospital visit for a 50-year-old male with uncomplicated myocardial infarction who is clinically stable and without chest pain. (Family Medicine/Cardiology/Internal Medicine)

Subsequent hospital visit for a stable 72-year-old lung cancer patient undergoing a five-day course of infusion chemotherapy. (Hematology/Oncology)

Subsequent hospital visit, two days post admission for a 65-year-old male with a CVA (cerebral vascular accident) and left hemiparesis, who is clinically stable. (Neurology/Physical Medicine and Rehabilitation)

Subsequent hospital visit for now stable, 33-year-old male, status post lower gastrointestinal bleeding. (General Surgery)

Subsequent visit on third day of hospitalization for a 60-year-old female recovering from an uncomplicated pneumonia. (Infectious Disease/Internal Medicine/Pulmonary Medicine)

Subsequent hospital visit for a 3-year-old patient in traction for a congenital dislocation of the hip. (Orthopaedic Surgery)

Subsequent hospital visit for a 4-year-old female, admitted for acute gastroenteritis and dehydration, requiring IV hydration; now stable. (Family Medicine/Internal Medicine)

Subsequent hospital visit for 50-year-old female with resolving uncomplicated acute pancreatitis. (Gastroenterology)

99232 Subsequent hospital visit for a patient with venous stasis ulcers who developed fever and red streaks adjacent to the ulcer. (Dermatology/Internal Medicine/Family Medicine)

Subsequent hospital visit for a 66-year-old male for dressing changes and observation. Patient has had a myocutaneous flap to close a pharyngeal fistula and now has a low-grade fever. (Plastic Surgery)

Subsequent hospital visit for a 54-year-old female admitted for myocardial infarction, but who is now having frequent premature ventricular contractions. (Internal Medicine)

Subsequent hospital visit for an 80-year-old patient with a pelvic rim fracture, inability to walk, and severe pain; now 36 hours post-injury, experiencing urinary retention. (Orthopaedic Surgery)

Subsequent hospital visit for a 17-year-old female with fever, pharyngitis, and airway obstruction, who after 48 hours develops a maculopapular rash. (Pediatrics/Family Medicine)

Follow-up hospital visit for a 32-year-old patient admitted the previous day for corneal ulcer. (Dermatology)

Follow-up visit for a 67-year-old male with congestive heart failure who has responded to antibiotics and diuretics, and has now developed a monoarthropathy. (Internal Medicine)

Follow-up hospital visit for a 58-year-old male receiving continuous opioids who is experiencing severe nausea and vomiting. (Pain Medicine)

Subsequent hospital visit for a patient after an auto accident who is slow to respond to ambulation training. (Physical Medicine & Rehabilitation)

Subsequent hospital visit for a 14-year-old with unstable bronchial asthma complicated by pneumonia. (Allergy & Immunology)

Subsequent hospital visit for a 50-year-old diabetic, hypertensive male with back pain not responding to conservative inpatient management with continued radiation of pain to the lower left extremity. (Orthopaedic Surgery)

Subsequent hospital visit for a 37-year-old female on day five of antibiotics for bacterial endocarditis, who still has low-grade fever. (Cardiology)

Subsequent hospital visit for a 54-year-old patient, post MI (myocardial infarction), who is out of the CCU (coronary care unit) but is now having frequent premature ventricular contractions on telemetry. (Cardiology/Internal Medicine)

Subsequent hospital visit for a patient with neutropenia, a fever responding to antibiotics, and continued slow gastrointestinal bleeding on platelet support. (Hematology/Oncology)

Subsequent hospital visit for a 50-year-old male admitted two days ago for sub-acute renal allograft rejection. (Nephrology)

Subsequent hospital visit for a 35-year-old drug addict, not responding to initial antibiotic therapy for pyelonephritis. (Urology)

Subsequent hospital visit of an 81-year-old male with abdominal distention, nausea, and vomiting. (General Surgery)

Subsequent hospital care for a 62-year-old female with congestive heart failure, who remains dyspneic and febrile. (Internal Medicine)

Subsequent hospital visit for a 73-year-old female with recently diagnosed lung cancer, who complains of unsteady gait. (Pulmonary Medicine)

Subsequent hospital visit for a 20-month-old male with bacterial meningitis treated one week with antibiotic therapy; has now developed a temperature of 101.0. (Pediatrics)

Subsequent hospital visit for 13-year-old male admitted with left lower quadrant abdominal pain and fever, not responding to therapy. (General Surgery)

Subsequent hospital visit for a 65-year-old male with hemiplegia and painful paretic shoulder. (Physical Medicine & Rehabilitation)

99233   Subsequent hospital visit for a 38-year-old male, quadriplegic with acute autonomic hyperreflexia, who is not responsive to initial care. (Physical Medicine & Rehabilitation)

Follow-up hospital visit for a teenage female who continues to experience severely disruptive, violent and life-threatening symptoms in a complicated multi-system illness. Family/social circumstances also a contributing factor. (Psychiatry)

Subsequent hospital visit for a 42-year-old female with progressive systemic sclerosis (scleroderma), renal failure on dialysis, congestive heart failure, cardiac arrhythmias, and digital ulcers. (Allergy & Immunology)

Subsequent hospital visit for a 50-year-old diabetic, hypertensive male with nonresponding back pain and radiating pain to the lower left extremity, who develops chest pain, cough, and bloody sputum. (Orthopaedic Surgery)

Subsequent hospital visit for a 64-year-old female, status post-abdominal aortic aneurysm resection, with non-responsive coagulopathy, who has now developed lower GI bleeding. (Abdominal Surgery/Colon & Rectal Surgery/General Surgery)

Follow-up hospital care of a patient with pansinusitis infection complicated by a brain abscess and asthma; no response to current treatment. (Otolaryngology, Head & Neck Surgery)

Subsequent hospital visit for a patient with a laryngeal neoplasm who develops airway compromise, suspected metastasis. (Otolaryngology, Head & Neck Surgery)

Subsequent hospital visit for a 49-year-old male with significant rectal bleeding, etiology undetermined, not responding to treatment. (Abdominal Surgery/General Surgery/Colon & Rectal Surgery)

Subsequent hospital visit for a 50-year-old male, post-aortocoronary bypass surgery; now develops hypotension and oliguria. (Cardiology)

Subsequent hospital visit for an adolescent patient who is violent, unsafe, and noncompliant, with multiple expectations for participation in treatment plan and behavior on the treatment unit. (Psychiatry)

Subsequent hospital visit for an 18-year-old male being treated for presumed PCP psychosis. Patient is still moderately symptomatic with auditory hallucinations and is insisting on signing out against medical advice. (Psychiatry)

Subsequent hospital visit for an 8-year-old female with caustic ingestion, who now has fever, dyspnea, and dropping hemoglobin. (Gastroenterology)

Follow-up hospital visit for a chronic renal failure patient on dialysis who develops chest pain and shortness of breath and a new onset pericardial friction rub. (Nephrology)

Subsequent hospital visit for a 44-year-old patient with electrical burns to the left arm with ascending infection. (Orthopaedic Surgery)

Subsequent hospital visit for a patient with systemic sclerosis who has aspirated and is short of breath. (Dermatology)

Subsequent hospital visit for a 65-year-old female, status post-op resection of abdominal aortic aneurysm, with suspected ischemic bowel. (General Surgery)

Subsequent hospital visit for a 50-year-old male, post-aortocoronary bypass surgery, now develops hypotension and oliguria. (Cardiology)

Subsequent hospital visit for a 65-year-old male, following an acute myocardial infarction, who complains of shortness of breath and new chest pain. (Cardiology)

Subsequent hospital visit for a 65-year-old female with rheumatoid arthritis (stage 3, class 3) admitted for urosepsis. On the third hospital day, chest pain, dyspnea and fever develop. (Rheumatology)

Follow-up hospital care of a pediatric case with stridor, laryngomalacia, established tracheostomy, complicated by multiple medical problems in PICU. (Otolaryngology, Head & Neck Surgery)

Subsequent hospital visit for a 60-year-old female, four days post uncomplicated inferior myocardial infarction who has developed severe chest pain, dyspnea, diaphoresis and nausea. (Family Medicine)

Subsequent hospital visit for a patient with AML (acute myelogenous leukemia), fever, elevated white count and uric acid undergoing induction chemotherapy. (Hematology/Oncology)

Subsequent hospital visit for a 38-year-old quadriplegic male with acute autonomic hyperreflexia, who is not responsive to initial care. (Physical Medicine & Rehabilitation)

Subsequent hospital visit for a 65-year-old female postoperative resection of abdominal aortic aneurysm, with suspected ischemic bowel. (General Surgery)

Subsequent hospital visit for a 60-year-old female with persistent leukocytosis and a fever seven days after a sigmoid colon resection for carcinoma. (Infectious Disease)

Subsequent hospital visit for a chronic renal failure patient on dialysis, who develops chest pain, shortness of breath and new onset of pericardial friction rub. (Nephrology)

Subsequent hospital visit for a 65-year-old male with acute myocardial infarction who now demonstrates complete heart block and congestive heart failure. (Cardiology)

Subsequent hospital visit for a 25-year-old female with hypertension and systemic lupus erythematosus, admitted for fever and respiratory distress. On the third hospital day, the patient presented with purpuric skin lesions and acute renal failure. (Allergy & Immunology)

Subsequent hospital visit for a 55-year-old male with severe chronic obstructive pulmonary disease and bronchospasm; initially admitted for acute respiratory distress requiring ventilatory support in the ICU. The patient was stabilized, extubated and transferred to the floor, but has now developed acute fever, dyspnea, left lower lobe rhonchi and laboratory evidence of carbon dioxide retention and hypoxemia. (Family Medicine/Internal Medicine)

Subsequent hospital visit for 46-year-old female, known liver cirrhosis patient, with recent upper gastrointestinal hemorrhage from varices; now with worsening ascites and encephalopathy. (Gastroenterology)

Subsequent hospital visit for 62-year-old female admitted with acute subarachnoid hemorrhage, negative cerebral arteriogram, increased lethargy and hemiparesis with fever. (Neurosurgery)

Consultations

Office or Other Outpatient Consultations

New or Established Patient

99241 Initial office consultation for a 40-year-old female in pain from blister on lip following a cold. (Oral & Maxillofacial Surgery)

Initial office consultation for a 62-year-old construction worker with olecranon bursitis. (Orthopaedic Surgery)

Office consultation with 25-year-old postpartum female with severe symptomatic hemorrhoids. (Colon & Rectal Surgery)

Office consultation with 58-year-old male, referred for follow-up of creatinine level and evaluation of obstructive uropathy, relieved two months ago. (Nephrology)

Office consultation for 30-year-old female tennis player with sprain or contusion of the forearm. (Orthopaedic Surgery)

Office consultation for a 45-year-old male, requested by his internist, with asymptomatic torus palatinus requiring no further treatment. (Oral & Maxillofacial Surgery)

99242 Initial office consultation for a 20-year-old male with acute upper respiratory tract symptoms. (Allergy & Immunology)

Initial office consultation for a 29-year-old soccer player with painful proximal thigh/groin injury. (Orthopaedic Surgery)

Initial office consultation for a 66-year-old female with wrist and hand pain, numbness of finger tips, suspected median nerve compression by carpal tunnel syndrome. (Plastic Surgery)

Initial office consultation for a patient with a solitary lesion of discoid lupus erythematosus on left cheek to rule out malignancy or self-induced lesion. (Dermatology)

Office consultation for management of systolic hypertension in a 70-year-old male scheduled for elective prostate resection. (Geriatrics)

Office consultation with 27-year-old female, with old amputation, for evaluation of existing above-knee prosthesis. (Physical Medicine & Rehabilitation)

Office consultation with 66-year-old female with wrist and hand pain, and finger numbness, secondary to suspected carpal tunnel syndrome. (Orthopaedic Surgery)

Office consultation for 61-year-old female, recently on antibiotic therapy, now with diarrhea and leukocytosis. (Abdominal Surgery)

Office consultation for a patient with papulosquamous eruption of elbow with pitting of nails and itchy scalp. (Dermatology)

Office consultation for a 30-year-old female with single season allergic rhinitis. (Allergy & Immunology)

99243 Initial office consultation for a 60-year-old male with avascular necrosis of the left femoral head with increasing pain. (Orthopaedic Surgery)

Office consultation for a 31-year-old woman complaining of palpitations and chest pains. Her internist had described a mild systolic click. (Cardiology)

Office consultation for a 65-year-old female with persistent bronchitis. (Infectious Disease)

Office consultation for a 65-year-old man with chronic low-back pain radiating to the leg. (Neurosurgery)

Office consultation for 23-year-old female with Crohn's disease not responding to therapy. (Abdominal Surgery/Colon & Rectal Surgery)

Office consultation for 25-year-old patient with symptomatic knee pain and swelling, with torn anterior cruciate ligament and/or torn meniscus. (Orthopaedic Surgery)

Office consultation for a 67-year-old patient with osteoporosis and mandibular atrophy with regard to reconstructive alternatives. (Oral & Maxillofacial Surgery)

Office consultation for 39-year-old patient referred at a perimenopausal age for irregular menses and menopausal symptoms. (Obstetrics & Gynecology)

99244 Initial office consultation for a 28-year-old male, HIV+, with a recent change in visual acuity. (Ophthalmology)

Initial office consultation for a 15-year-old male with failing grades, suspected drug abuse. (Pediatrics)

Initial office consultation for a 36-year-old factory worker, status four months post-occupational low back injury and requires management of intractable low back pain. (Pain Medicine)

Initial office consultation for a 45-year-old female with a history of chronic arthralgia of TMJ and associated myalgia and sudden progressive symptomatology over last two to three months. (Oral & Maxillofacial Surgery)

Initial office consultation for evaluation of a 70-year-old male with appetite loss and diminished energy. (Psychiatry)

Initial office consultation for an elementary school-aged patient, referred by pediatrician, with multiple systematic complaints and recent onset of behavioral discontrol. (Psychiatry)

Initial office consultation for a 23-year-old female with developmental facial skeletal anomaly and subsequent abnormal relationship of jaw(s) to cranial base. (Oral & Maxillofacial Surgery)

Initial office consultation for a 45-year-old myopic patient with a one-week history of floaters and a partial retinal detachment. (Ophthalmology)

Initial office consultation for a 65-year-old female with moderate dementia, mild unsteadiness, back pain fatigue on ambulation, intermittent urinary incontinence. (Neurosurgery)

Initial office consultation for a 33-year-old female referred by endocrinologist with amenorrhea and galactorrhea, for evaluation of pituitary tumor. (Neurosurgery)

Initial office consultation for a 34-year-old male with new onset nephrotic syndrome. (Nephrology)

Initial office consultation for a 39-year-old female with intractable chest wall pain secondary to metastatic breast cancer. (Anesthesiology/Pain Medicine)

Initial office consultation for a patient with multiple giant tumors of jaws. (Oral & Maxillofacial Surgery)

Initial office consultation for a patient with a failed total hip replacement with loosening and pain upon walking. (Orthopaedic Surgery)

Initial office consultation for a 60-year-old female with three-year history of intermittent tic-like unilateral facial pain; now constant pain for six weeks without relief by adequate carbamazepine dosage. (Neurosurgery)

Initial office consultation for a 45-year-old male heavy construction worker with prior lumbar disc surgery two years earlier; now gradually recurring low back and unilateral leg pain for three months, unable to work for two weeks. (Neurosurgery)

Initial office consultation of a patient who presents with a 30-year history of smoking and right neck mass. (Otolaryngology, Head & Neck Surgery)

Office consultation with 38-year-old female, with inflammatory bowel disease, who now presents with right lower quadrant pain and suspected intra-abdominal abscess. (General Surgery/Colon & Rectal Surgery)

Office consultation with 72-year-old male with esophageal carcinoma, symptoms of dysphagia, and reflux. (Thoracic Surgery)

Office consultation for discussion of treatment options for a 40-year-old female with a 2-cm adenocarcinoma of the breast. (Radiation Oncology)

Office consultation for young patient referred by pediatrician because of patient's short attention span, easy distractibility and hyperactivity. (Psychiatry)

Office consultation for 66-year-old female, history of colon resection for adenocarcinoma six years earlier, now with severe mid-back pain; X rays showing osteoporosis and multiple vertebral compression fractures. (Neurosurgery)

Office consultation for a patient with chronic pelvic inflammatory disease who now has left lower quadrant pain with a palpable pelvic mass. (Obstetrics & Gynecology)

Office consultation for a patient with long-standing psoriasis with acute onset of erythroderma, pustular lesions, chills, and fever. Combinations of topical and systemic treatments discussed and instituted. (Dermatology)

99245 Initial office consultation for a 35-year-old multiple-trauma male patient with complex pelvic fractures, for evaluation and formulation of management plan. (Orthopaedic Surgery)

Initial emergency room consultation for 10-year-old male in status epilepticus, recent closed head injury, information about medication not available. (Neurosurgery)

Initial emergency room consultation for a 23-year-old patient with severe abdominal pain, guarding, febrile, and unstable vital signs. (Obstetrics & Gynecology)

Office consultation for a 67-year-old female longstanding uncontrolled diabetic who presents with retinopathy, nephropathy, and a foot ulcer. (Endocrinology)

Office consultation for a 37-year-old male for initial evaluation and management of Cushing's disease. (Endocrinology)

Office consultation for a 60-year-old male who presents with thyrotoxicosis, exophthalmos, frequent premature ventricular contractions and congestive heart failure. (Endocrinology)

Initial office consultation for a 36-year-old patient, one year status post occupational herniated cervical disk treated by laminectomy, requiring management of multiple sites of intractable pain, depression, and narcotic dependence. (Pain Medicine)

Office consultation for a 58-year-old man with a history of MI and CHF who complains of the recent onset of rest angina and shortness of breath. The patient has a systolic blood pressure of 90mmHG and is in Class IV heart failure. (Cardiology)

Emergency department consultation for a 1-year-old with a three-day history of fever with increasing respiratory distress who is thought to have cardiac tamponade by the ER physician. (Cardiology)

Office consultation in the emergency department for a 25-year-old male with severe, acute, closed head injury. (Neurosurgery)

Office consultation for a 23-year-old female with Stage II A Hodgkins disease with positive supraclavicular and mediastinal nodes. (Radiation Oncology)

Office consultation for a 27-year-old juvenile diabetic patient with severe diabetic retinopathy, gastric atony, nephrotic syndrome and progressive renal failure, now with a serum creatinine of 2.7, and a blood pressure of 170/114. (Nephrology)

Office consultation for independent medical evaluation of a patient with a history of complicated low back and neck problems with previous multiple failed back surgeries. (Orthopaedic Surgery)

Office consultation for an adolescent referred by pediatrician for recent onset of violent and self-injurious behavior. (Psychiatry)

Office consultation for a 6-year-old male for evaluation of severe muscle and joint pain and a diffuse rash. Patient well until 4-6 weeks earlier, when he developed arthralgia, myalgias, and a fever of 102 for one week. (Rheumatology)

Inpatient Consultations

New or Established Patient

99251 Initial hospital consultation for a 27-year-old female with fractured incisor post-intubation. (Oral & Maxillofacial Surgery)

Initial hospital consultation for an orthopaedic patient on IV antibiotics who has developed an apparent candida infection of the oral cavity. (Oral & Maxillofacial Surgery)

Initial inpatient consultation for a 30-year-old female complaining of vaginal itching, post orthopaedic surgery. (Obstetrics & Gynecology)

Initial inpatient consultation for a 36-year-old male on orthopaedic service with complaint of localized dental pain. (Oral & Maxillofacial Surgery)

99252 Initial hospital consultation for a 45-year-old male, previously abstinent alcoholic, who relapsed and was admitted for management of gastritis. The patient readily accepts the need for further treatment. (Addiction Medicine)

Initial hospital consultation for a 35-year-old dialysis patient with episodic oral ulcerations. (Oral & Maxillofacial Surgery)

Initial inpatient preoperative consultation for a 43-year-old female with cholecystitis and well-controlled hypertension. (Cardiology)

Initial inpatient consultation for recommendation of antibiotic prophylaxis for a patient with a synthetic heart valve who will undergo urologic surgery. (Internal Medicine)

Initial inpatient consultation for possible drug induced skin eruption in 50-year-old male. (Dermatology)

Preoperative inpatient consultation for evaluation of hypertension in a 60-year-old male who will undergo a cholecystectomy. Patient had a normal annual check-up in your office four months ago. (Internal Medicine)

Initial inpatient consultation for 66-year-old patient with wrist and hand pain and finger numbness, secondary to carpal tunnel syndrome. (Orthopaedic Surgery/Plastic Surgery)

Initial inpatient consultation for a 66-year-old male smoker referred for pain management immediately status post-biliary tract surgery done via sub-costal incision. (Anesthesiology/Pain Medicine)

99253 Initial hospital consultation for a 50-year-old female with incapacitating knee pain due to generalized rheumatoid arthritis. (Orthopaedic Surgery)

Initial hospital consultation for a 60-year-old male with avascular necrosis of the left femoral heel with increasing pain. (Orthopaedic Surgery)

Initial hospital consultation for a 45-year-old female with compound mandibular fracture and concurrent head, abdominal and/or orthopaedic injuries. (Oral & Maxillofacial Surgery)

Initial hospital consultation for a 22-year-old female, paraplegic, to evaluate wrist and hand pain. (Orthopaedic Surgery)

Initial hospital consultation for a 40-year-old male with 10-day history of incapacitating unilateral sciatica, unable to walk now, not improved by bed rest. (Neurosurgery)

Initial hospital consultation, requested by pediatrician, for treatment recommendations for a patient admitted with persistent inability to walk following soft tissue injury to ankle. (Physiatry)

Initial hospital consultation for a 27-year-old previously healthy male who vomited during IV sedation and may have aspirated gastric contents. (Anesthesiology)

Initial hospital consultation for a 33-year-old female, post-abdominal surgery, who now has a fever. (Internal Medicine)

Initial inpatient consultation for a 57-year-old male, post lower endoscopy, for evaluation of abdominal pain and fever. (General Surgery)

Initial inpatient consultation for rehabilitation of a 73-year-old female one week after surgical management of a hip fracture. (Physical Medicine & Rehabilitation)

Initial inpatient consultation for diagnosis/management of fever following abdominal surgery. (Internal Medicine)

Initial inpatient consultation for a 35-year-old female with a fever and pulmonary infiltrate following cesarean section. (Pulmonary Medicine)

Initial inpatient consultation for a 42-year-old nondiabetic patient, postop cholecystectomy, now with an acute urinary tract infection. (Nephrology)

Initial inpatient consultation for 53-year-old female with moderate uncomplicated pancreatitis. (Gastroenterology)

Initial inpatient consultation for 45-year-old patient with chronic neck pain with radicular pain of the left arm. (Orthopaedic Surgery)

Initial inpatient consultation for 8-year-old patient with new onset of seizures who has a normal examination and previous history. (Neurology)

99254 Initial hospital consultation for a 15-year-old patient with painless swelling of proximal humerus with lytic lesion by X ray. (Orthopaedic Surgery)

Initial hospital consultation for evaluation of a 29-year-old female with a diffusely positive medical review of systems and history of multiple surgeries. (Psychiatry)

Initial hospital consultation for a 70-year-old diabetic female with gangrene of the foot. (Orthopaedic Surgery)

Initial inpatient consultation for a 47-year-old female with progressive pulmonary infiltrate, hypoxemia, and diminished urine output. (Anesthesiology)

Initial hospital consultation for a 13-month-old with spasmodic cough, respiratory distress, and fever. (Allergy & Immunology)

Initial hospital consultation for a patient with failed total hip replacement with loosening and pain upon walking. (Orthopaedic Surgery)

Initial hospital consultation for a 62-year-old female with metastatic breast cancer to the femoral neck and thoracic vertebra. (Orthopaedic Surgery)

Initial hospital consultation for a 39-year-old female with nephrolithiasis requiring extensive opioid analgesics, whose vital signs are now elevated. She initially denied any drug use, but today gives history of multiple substance abuse, including opioids and prior treatment for a personality disorder. (Psychiatry)

Initial hospital consultation for a 70-year-old female without previous psychiatric history, who is now experiencing nocturnal confusion and visual hallucinations following hip replacement surgery. (Psychiatry)

Initial inpatient consultation for evaluation of a 63-year-old in the ICU with diabetes and chronic renal failure who develops acute respiratory distress syndrome 36 hours after a mitral valve replacement. (Anesthesiology)

Initial inpatient consultation for a 66-year-old female with enlarged supraclavicular lymph nodes, found on biopsy to be malignant. (Hematology/Oncology)

Initial inpatient consultation for a 43-year-old female for evaluation of sudden painful visual loss, optic neuritis and episodic paresthesia. (Ophthalmology)

Initial inpatient consultation for evaluation of a 71-year-old male with hyponatremia (serum sodium 114) who was admitted to the hospital with pneumonia. (Nephrology)

Initial inpatient consultation for a 72-year-old male with emergency admission for possible bowel obstruction. (Internal Medicine/General Surgery)

Initial inpatient consultation for a 35-year-old female with fever, swollen joints, and rash of one-week duration. (Rheumatology)

99255 Initial inpatient consultation for a 76-year-old female with massive, life-threatening gastrointestinal hemorrhage and chest pain. (Gastroenterology)

Initial inpatient consultation for a 75-year-old female, admitted to intensive care with acute respiratory distress syndrome, who is hypersensitive, has a moderate metabolic acidosis, and a rising serum creatinine. (Nephrology)

Initial hospital consultation for patient with a history of complicated low back pain and neck problems with previous multiple failed back surgeries. (Orthopaedic Surgery/Neurosurgery)

Initial hospital consultation for a 66-year-old female, two days post-abdominal aneurysm repair, with oliguria and hypertension of one-day duration. (Nephrology/Internal Medicine)

Initial hospital consultation for a patient with shotgun wound to face with massive facial trauma and airway obstruction. (Oral & Maxillofacial Surgery)

Initial hospital consultation for patient with severe pancreatitis complicated by respiratory insufficiency, acute renal failure, and abscess formation. (General Surgery/Colon & Rectal Surgery)

Initial hospital consultation for a 35-year-old multiple-trauma male patient with complex pelvic fractures to evaluate and formulate management plan. (Orthopaedic Surgery)

Initial inpatient consultation for adolescent patient with fractured femur and pelvis who pulled out IVs and disconnected traction in attempt to elope from hospital. (Psychiatry)

Initial hospital consultation for a 16-year-old primigravida at 32-weeks gestation requested by a family practitioner for evaluation of severe hypertension, thrombocytopenia, and headache. (Obstetrics & Gynecology)

Initial hospital consultation for a 58-year-old insulin-dependent diabetic with multiple antibiotic allergies, now with multiple fascial plane abscesses and airway obstruction. (Oral & Maxillofacial Surgery)

Initial inpatient consultation for a 55-year-old male with known cirrhosis and ascites, now with jaundice, encephalopathy, and massive hematemesis. (Gastroenterology)

Initial hospital consultation for a 25-year-old male, seen in emergency room with severe, closed head injury. (Neurosurgery)

Initial hospital consultation for a 2-day-old male with single ventricle physiology and subaortic obstruction. Family counseling following evaluation for multiple, staged surgical procedures. (Thoracic Surgery)

Initial hospital consultation for a 45-year-old male admitted with subarachnoid hemorrhage and intracranial aneurysm on angiogram. (Neurosurgery)

Initial inpatient consultation for myxedematous patient who is hypoventilating and obtunded. (Endocrinology)

Initial hospital consultation for a 45-year-old patient with widely metastatic lung carcinoma, intractable back pain, and a history that includes substance dependence, NSAID allergy, and two prior laminectomies with fusion for low back pain. (Pain Medicine)

Initial hospital consultation for evaluation of treatment options in a 50-year-old patient with cirrhosis, known peptic ulcer disease, hypotension, encephalopathy, and massive acute upper gastrointestinal bleeding which cannot be localized by endoscopy. (Interventional Radiology)

Initial inpatient consultation in the ICU for a 70-year-old male who experienced a cardiac arrest during surgery and was resuscitated. (Cardiology)

Initial inpatient consultation for a patient with severe pancreatitis complicated by respiratory insufficiency, acute renal failure and abscess formation. (Gastroenterology)

Initial inpatient consultation for a 70-year-old cirrhotic male admitted with ascites, jaundice, encephalopathy, and massive hematemesis. (Gastroenterology)

Initial inpatient consultation in the ICU for a 51-year-old patient who is on a ventilator and has a fever two weeks after a renal transplantation. (Infectious Disease)

Initial inpatient consultation for evaluation and formulation of plan for management of multiple trauma patient with complex pelvic fracture, 35-year-old male. (General Surgery/Orthopaedic Surgery)

Initial inpatient consultation for a 50-year-old male with a history of previous myocardial infarction, now with acute pulmonary edema and hypotension. (Cardiology)

Initial inpatient consultation for 45-year-old male with recent, acute subarachnoid hemorrhage, hesitant speech, mildly confused, drowsy. High risk group for HIV+ status. (Neurosurgery)

Initial inpatient consultation for 36-year-old female referred by her internist to evaluate a patient being followed for abdominal pain and fever. The patient has developed diffuse abdominal pain, guarding, rigidity and increased fever. (Obstetrics & Gynecology)

Emergency Department Services

New or Established Patient

99281   Emergency department visit for a patient for removal of sutures from a well-healed, uncomplicated laceration. (Emergency Medicine)

Emergency department visit for a patient for tetanus toxoid immunization. (Emergency Medicine)

Emergency department visit for a patient with several uncomplicated insect bites. (Emergency Medicine)

99282   Emergency department visit for a 20-year-old student who presents with a painful sunburn with blister formation on the back. (Emergency Medicine)

Emergency department visit for a child presenting with impetigo localized to the face. (Emergency Medicine)

Emergency department visit for a patient with a minor traumatic injury of an extremity with localized pain, swelling, and bruising. (Emergency Medicine)

Emergency department visit for an otherwise healthy patient whose chief complaint is a red, swollen cystic lesion on his/her back. (Emergency Medicine)

Emergency department visit for a patient presenting with a rash on both legs after exposure to poison ivy. (Emergency Medicine)

Emergency department visit for a young adult patient with infected sclera and purulent discharge from both eyes without pain, visual disturbance or history of foreign body in either eye. (Emergency Medicine)

99283   Emergency department visit for a sexually active female complaining of vaginal discharge who is afebrile and denies experiencing abdominal or back pain. (Emergency Medicine)

Emergency department visit for a well-appearing 8-year-old who has a fever, diarrhea, and abdominal cramps, is tolerating oral fluids and is not vomiting. (Emergency Medicine)

Emergency department visit for a patient with an inversion ankle injury, who is unable to bear weight on the injured foot and ankle. (Emergency Medicine)

Emergency department visit for a patient who has a complaint of acute pain associated with a suspected foreign body in the painful eye. (Emergency Medicine)

Emergency department visit for a healthy, young adult patient who sustained a blunt head injury with local swelling and bruising without subsequent confusion, loss of consciousness or memory deficit. (Emergency Medicine)

99284   Emergency department visit for a 4-year-old who fell off a bike sustaining a head injury with brief loss of consciousness. (Emergency Medicine)

Emergency department visit for an elderly female who has fallen and is now complaining of pain in her right hip and is unable to walk. (Emergency Medicine)

Emergency department visit for a patient with flank pain and hematuria. (Emergency Medicine)

Emergency department visit for a female presenting with lower abdominal pain and a vaginal discharge. (Emergency Medicine)

99285   Emergency department visit for a patient with a complicated overdose requiring aggressive management to prevent side effects from the ingested materials. (Emergency Medicine)

Emergency department visit for a patient with a new onset of rapid heart rate requiring IV drugs. (Emergency Medicine)

Emergency department visit for a patient exhibiting active, upper gastrointestinal bleeding. (Emergency Medicine)

Emergency department visit for a previously healthy young adult patient who is injured in an automobile accident and is brought to the emergency department immobilized and has symptoms compatible with intra-abdominal injuries or multiple extremity injuries. (Emergency Medicine)

Emergency department visit for a patient with an acute onset of chest pain compatible with symptoms of cardiac ischemia and/or pulmonary embolus. (Emergency Medicine)

Emergency department visit for a patient who presents with a sudden onset of "the worst headache of her life," and complains of a stiff neck, nausea, and inability to concentrate. (Emergency Medicine)

Emergency department visit for a patient with a new onset of a cerebral vascular accident. (Emergency Medicine)

Emergency department visit for acute febrile illness in an adult, associated with shortness of breath and an altered level of alertness. (Emergency Medicine)

Critical Care Services

99291   First hour of critical care of a 65-year-old male with septic shock following relief of ureteral obstruction caused by a stone.

First hour of critical care of a 15-year-old with acute respiratory failure from asthma.

First hour of critical care of a 45-year-old who sustained a liver laceration, cerebral hematoma, flailed chest, and pulmonary contusion after being struck by an automobile.

First hour of critical care of a 65-year-old female who, following a hysterectomy, suffered a cardiac arrest associated with a pulmonary embolus.

First hour of critical care of a 6-month-old with hypovolemic shock secondary to diarrhea and dehydration.

First hour of critical care of a 3-year-old with respiratory failure secondary to pneumocystis carinii pneumonia.

Prolonged Services

Prolonged Physician Service With Direct (Face-to-Face) Patient Contact

Office or Other Outpatient

99354/ 99355   A 20-year-old female with history of asthma presents with acute bronchospasm and moderate respiratory distress. Initial evaluation shows respiratory rate 30, labored breathing and wheezing heard in all lung fields. Office treatment is initiated, which includes intermittent bronchial dilation and subcutaneous epinephrine. Requires intermittent physician face-to-face time with patient over a period of 2-3 hours. (Family Medicine/Internal Medicine)

Inpatient

99356   A 34-year-old primigravida presents to hospital in early labor. Admission history and physical reveals severe preeclampsia. Physician supervises management of preeclampsia, IV magnesium initiation and maintenance, labor augmentation with pitocin, and close maternal-fetal monitoring. Physician face-to-face involvement includes 40 minutes of continuous bedside care until the patient is stable, then is intermittent over several hours until the delivery. (Family Medicine/Internal Medicine/Obstetrics & Gynecology)

Prolonged Physician Service Without Direct Patient (Face-to-Face) Contact

99358/ 99359   A 65-year-old new patient with multiple problems is seen and evaluated. After the visit, the physician requires extensive time to talk with the patient's daughter, to review complex, detailed medical records transferred from previous physicians and to complete a comprehensive treatment plan. This plan also requires the physician to personally initiate and coordinate the care plan with a local home health agency and a dietician. (Family Medicine/Internal Medicine)

Physician Standby Services

99360   A 24-year-old patient is admitted to OB unit attempting VBAC. Fetal monitoring shows increasing fetal distress. Patient's blood pressure is rising and labor progressing slowly. A primary care physician is requested by the OB/GYN to standby in the unit for possible cesarean delivery and neonatal resuscitation. (Family Medicine/Internal Medicine)

Care Plan Oversight Services

99375   First month of care plan oversight for terminal care of a 58-year-old female with advanced intraabdominal ovarian cancer. Care plan includes home oxygen, diuretics IV for edema and ascites control and pain control management involving IV morphine infusion when progressive ileus occurred. Physician phone contacts with nurse, family, and MSW. Discussion with MSW concerning plans to withdraw supportive measures per patient wishes. Documentation includes review and modification of care plan and certifications from nursing, MSW, pharmacy, and DME. (Family Medicine/Internal Medicine)

Appendix D

Summary of CPT Add-on Codes

This listing is a summary of CPT add-on codes for *CPT 2008*. The codes listed are identified in *CPT 2008* with a ✚ symbol.

01953	15366	22840	33961
01968	15401	22841	34806
01969	15421	22842	34808
11001	15431	22843	34813
11008	15787	22844	34826
11101	15847	22845	35306
11201	16036	22846	35390
11732	17003	22847	35400
11922	17312	22848	35500
13102	17314	22851	35572
13122	17315	26125	35600
13133	19001	26861	35681
13153	19126	26863	35682
15003	19291	27358	35683
15005	19295	27692	35685
15101	19297	31620	35686
15111	20930	31632	35697
15116	20931	31633	35700
15121	20936	31637	36218
15131	20937	32501	36248
15136	20938	33141	36476
15151	20985	33225	36479
15152	20986	33257	37185
15156	20987	33258	37186
15157	22103	33259	37206
15171	22116	33508	37208
15176	22208	33517	37250
15201	22216	33518	37251
15221	22226	33519	38102
15241	22328	33521	38746
15261	22522	33522	38747
15301	22525	33523	43635
15321	22527	33530	44015
15331	22534	33572	44121
15336	22585	33768	44128
15341	22614	33884	44139
15361	22632	33924	44203

44213	64484	88155
44701	64623	88185
44955	64627	88311
47001	64727	88312
47550	64778	88313
48400	64783	88314
49326	64787	90466
49435	64832	90468
49568	64837	90472
49905	64859	90474
51797	64872	90761
56606	64874	90766
57267	64876	90767
58110	64901	90768
58611	64902	90770
59525	66990	90771
60512	67225	90775
61316	67320	90776
61517	67331	92547
61609	67332	92608
61610	67334	92627
61611	67335	92973
61612	67340	92974
61641	69990	92978
61642	74301	92979
61795	75774	92981
61864	75946	92984
61868	75964	92996
62148	75968	92998
62160	75993	93320
63035	75996	93321
63043	76125	93325
63044	76802	93571
63048	76810	93572
63057	76812	93609
63066	76814	93613
63076	76937	93621
63078	77001	93622
63082	77051	93623
63086	77052	93662
63088	78020	94645
63091	78478	95873
63103	78480	95874
63295	78496	95920
63308	78730	95962
64472	83901	95967
64476	87187	95973
64480	87904	95975

95979
96411
96415
96417
96423
96570
96571
97546
97811
97814
99100
99116
99135
99140
99145
99150
99290
99292
99354
99355
99356
99357
99358
99359
99602
99607
0049T
0063T
0076T
0079T
0081T
0092T
0095T
0098T
0151T
0159T
0163T
0164T
0165T
0172T
0173T
0174T

Appendix E

Summary of CPT Codes Exempt From Modifier 51

►This listing is a summary of CPT codes that are exempt from the use of modifier 51. Procedures on this list are typically performed with another procedure but may be a stand-alone procedure and not always be performed with other specified procedures. For add-on codes, see Appendix D. This is not an exhaustive list of procedures that are typically exempt from multiple procedure reductions. The codes listed are identified in *CPT 2008* with a ⊘ symbol.◄

17004

20974

20975

31500

36620

44500

61107

93503

93539

93540

93544

93545

93555

93556

93600

93602

93603

93610

93612

93615

93616

93618

93631

94610

95900

95903

95904

99143

99144

Appendix F

Summary of CPT Codes Exempt From Modifier 63

This listing is a summary of CPT codes that are exempt from the use of modifier 63. The codes listed are additionally identified in *CPT 2008* with the parenthetical instruction "(Do not report modifier 63 in conjunction with…)"

30540	36660	63700
30545	39503	63702
31520	43313	63704
33401	43314	63706
33403	43520	65820
33470	43831	
33472	44055	
33502	44126	
33503	44127	
33505	44128	
33506	46070	
33610	46705	
33611	46715	
33619	46716	
33647	46730	
33670	46735	
33690	46740	
33694	46742	
33730	46744	
33732	47700	
33735	47701	
33736	49215	
33750	49491	
33755	49492	
33762	49495	
33778	49496	
33786	49600	
33922	49605	
33960	49606	
33961	49610	
36415	49611	
36420	53025	
36450	54000	
36460	54150	
36510	54160	

Appendix G

Summary of CPT Codes That Include Moderate (Conscious) Sedation

The following list of procedures includes conscious sedation as an inherent part of providing the procedure. These codes are identified in the CPT codebook with a ⊙ symbol.

Because these services include moderate sedation, it is not appropriate for the same physician to report both the service and the sedation codes 99143-99145. It is expected that if conscious sedation is provided to the patient as part of one of these services, it is provided by the same physician who is providing the service.

In the unusual event when a second physician other than the health care professional performing the diagnostic or therapeutic services provides moderate sedation in the facility setting (eg, hospital, outpatient hospital/ambulatory surgery center, skilled nursing facility) for the procedures listed in Appendix G, the second physician can report 99148-99150. However, for the circumstance in which these services are performed by the second physician in the nonfacility setting (eg, physician office, freestanding imaging center), codes 99148-99150 would not be reported. Moderate sedation does not include minimal sedation (anxiolysis), deep sedation, or monitored anesthesia care (00100-01999).

The inclusion of a procedure on this list does not prevent separate reporting of an associated anesthesia procedure or service (CPT codes 00100-01999) when performed by a physician other than the health care professional performing the diagnostic or therapeutic procedure. In such cases, the person providing anesthesia services shall be present for the purpose of continuously monitoring the patient and shall not act as a surgical assistant. When clinical conditions of the patient require such anesthesia services, or in the circumstances when the patient does not require sedation, the operating physician is not required to report the procedure as a reduced service using modifier 52.

19298	31624	31725	33208
20982	31625	32201	33210
22526	31628	32550	33211
22527	31629	32551	33212
31615	31635	33010	33213
31620	31645	33011	33214
31622	31646	33206	33216
31623	31656	33207	33217

33218	43202	43456
33220	43204	43458
33222	43205	43750
33223	43215	44360
33233	43216	44361
33234	43217	44363
33235	43219	44364
33240	43220	44365
33241	43226	44366
33244	43227	44369
33249	43228	44370
35470	43231	44372
35471	43232	44373
35472	43234	44376
35473	43235	44377
35474	43236	44378
35475	43237	44379
35476	43238	44380
36555	43239	44382
36557	43240	44383
36558	43241	44385
36560	43242	44386
36561	43243	44388
36563	43244	44389
36565	43245	44390
36566	43246	44391
36568	43247	44392
36570	43248	44393
36571	43249	44394
36576	43250	44397
36578	43251	44500
36581	43255	44901
36582	43256	45303
36583	43257	45305
36585	43258	45307
36590	43259	45308
36870	43260	45309
37184	43261	45315
37185	43262	45317
37186	43263	45320
37187	43264	45321
37188	43265	45327
37203	43267	45332
37210	43268	45333
37215	43269	45334
37216	43271	45335
43200	43272	45337
43201	43453	45338

45339	92978	93620
45340	92979	93621
45341	92980	93622
45342	92981	93624
45345	92982	93640
45355	92984	93641
45378	92986	93642
45379	92987	93650
45380	92995	93651
45381	92996	93652
45382	93312	
45383	93313	
45384	93314	
45385	93315	
45386	93316	
45387	93317	
45391	93318	
45392	93501	
47011	93505	
48511	93508	
49021	93510	
49041	93511	
49061	93514	
49440	93524	
49441	93526	
49442	93527	
49446	93528	
50021	93529	
50382	93530	
50384	93539	
50385	93540	
50386	93541	
50387	93542	
50592	93543	
50593	93544	
58823	93545	
66720	93555	
69300	93556	
77600	93561	
77605	93562	
77610	93571	
77615	93572	
92953	93609	
92960	93613	
92961	93615	
92973	93616	
92974	93618	
92975	93619	

Appendix H

Alphabetic Index of Performance Measures by Clinical Condition or Topic

Appendix H is an alphabetical listing of the diseases, **clinical conditions, and topics** with which the measures and codes are associated. It provides an overview of the performance measures, a listing of the CPT Category II codes that may be used with each measure, as well as any applicable reporting instructions. It is intended to be used as a crosswalk to the Category II code section allowing users an overview of the measures and the Category II codes that should be used with each measure, linking the Category II codes to the specific measures and measure sets from which these codes were derived. The clinical conditions or topics are listed in alphabetical order within this appendix to allow rapid access to the conditions or topics currently included in the CPT codebook. For the latest Appendix H information, visit the Web site at www.ama-assn .org/go/cpt.

In order for a patient to be included in the numerator for a particular performance measure, a patient must meet the denominator inclusion criteria for that measure. Prior to coding, users must review (1) the complete description of the code in the Category II section of the CPT codebook and Web site and (2) the specification documents of its associated performance measure as found on the measure developer's Web site. The superscripted numbers that follow the specific title for the performance measure direct users to footnotes at the bottom of each page of this appendix. The footnotes identify the measure developer and the developer's Web address.

In addition, the modifiers included within the Category II code section and Appendix H are only intended to be used when parenthetical notes, guidelines, or reporting language specifically allow their use.

Performance Measure Exclusion Modifier

Performance measurement exclusion modifiers may be used to indicate that a service specified by a performance measure was considered but, due to either medical, patient, or sytems reason(s) documented in the medical record, the service was not provided. These modifiers serve as denominator exclusions from the performance measure. Not all listed measures provide for exclusions. The modifiers currently available include the noted listing:

▶**Reporting Modifier**
Modifier 8P is intended to be used as a reporting modifier to allow the reporting of circumstances when an action described in a measure's numerator is not performed and the reason is not otherwise specified.◀

1P Performance measure exclusion modifier due to medical reasons
Includes:
- not indicated (absence of organ/limb, already received/performed, other)
- contraindicated (patient allergic history, potential adverse drug interaction, other)
- other medical reasons

2P Performance measure exclusion modifier due to patient reasons
Includes:
- Patient declined
- Economic, social, or religious reasons
- Other patient reasons

3P Performance measure exclusion modifier due to system reasons
Includes:
- Resources to perform the services not available (eg, equipment, supplies)
- Insurance coverage or payer-related limitations
- Other reasons attributable to health care delivery system

▶**8P Performance measure reporting modifier—action not performed, reason not otherwise specified◀**

▶[1]Physician Consortium for Performance Improvement: www.physicianconsortium.org◀
[2]National Committee on Quality Assurance (NCQA): Health Employer Data Information Set (HEDIS®), www.ncqa.org
[3]Joint Commission on Accreditation of Healthcare Organizations (JCAHO), ORYX Initiative Performance Measures: www.jcaho.org/pms
[4]National Diabetes Quality Improvement Alliance: www.nationaldiabetesalliance.org
▶[5]Joint measure from the Physician Consortium for Performance Improvement, www.physicianconsortium.org, and National Committee on Quality Assurance (NCQA), www.ncqa.org◀
▶[6]The Society of Thoracic Surgeons, www.sts.org, and National Quality Forum, www.qualityforum.org◀

Brief Description of Performance Measure & Source and Reporting Instructions	CPT Code(s)	Code Descriptor
Asthma		
Asthma Assessment[1]—Whether or not patient was evaluated during at least one office visit during the reporting year for the frequency (numeric) of daytime and nocturnal asthma symptoms **Numerator:** Patients who were evaluated during at least one office visit during the reporting year for the frequency (numeric) of daytime and nocturnal asthma symptoms **Denominator:** All patients aged 5-40 years with asthma **Percentage** of patients aged 5-40 years with asthma who were evaluated during at least one office visit during the reporting year for the frequency (numeric) of daytime and nocturnal asthma symptoms **Reporting Instructions:** To be counted in calculations of this measure, symptom frequency must be numerically quantified. Measure may also be met by physician documentation or patient completion of an asthma assessment tool/survey/questionnaire. Assessment tool may include the Quality Metric Asthma Control Test™, National Asthma Education & Prevention Program (NAEPP) Asthma Symptoms and Peak Flow Diary ▶There are no exclusions for this measure; modifiers 1P, 2P, and 3P may not be used.◀	1005F	Asthma symptoms evaluated (includes physician documentation of numeric frequency of symptoms or patient completion of an asthma assessment tool/survey/questionnaire)
Asthma Pharmacologic Therapy[1]—Whether or not patient with mild, moderate, or severe *persistent* asthma was prescribed *either* the preferred long-term control medication (inhaled corticosteroid) or an acceptable alternative treatment **Numerator:** Patients who were prescribed *either* the preferred[a] long-term control medication (inhaled corticosteroids) or an acceptable alternative treatment[b] (cromolyn sodium, leukotriene modifier, nedocromil, OR sustained release theophylline) **Denominator:** All patients aged 5-40 years with mild, moderate or severe persistent asthma **Exclusion(s):** Documentation of patient reason(s) (eg economic, social, religious) for not prescribing either the preferred long-term control medication (inhaled corticosteroids) or an acceptable alternative treatment. (There are no medical exclusion criteria.) **Percentage** of all patients with mild, moderate, or severe *persistent* asthma who were prescribed *either* the preferred long-term control medication (inhaled corticosteroids) or an acceptable alternative treatment **Reporting Instructions:** Report 1038F or 1039F for each asthma patient. If long-term control medication (or acceptable alternative treatment) prescribed, report 4015F. Report 4015F with 1038F. Report modifier 2P for patient who meets exclusion criteria. Modifier 1P may not be reported with 4015F. [a, b]Refer to complete description of measure developer's Web site for list of medications, treatment recommendations, dosages	4015F **Denominator Codes:** 1038F 1039F	Persistent asthma, preferred long-term control medication or acceptable alternative treatment, prescribed Persistent asthma (mild, moderate or severe) Intermittent asthma
Chronic Obstructive Pulmonary Disease (COPD)		
Smoking Assessment[1]—Whether or not patient with COPD was queried about smoking **Numerator:** All patients who were queried about smoking during one or more office visits each year **Denominator:** All patients with the diagnosis of COPD **Percentage** of patients who were queried about smoking at least annually **Reporting Instructions:** When reporting 1000F, it is required to report 1034F and/or 1035F or 1036F ▶There are no exclusions for this measure; modifiers 1P, 2P, and 3P may not be used◀	1000F 1034F 1035F 1036F	Tobacco use assessed Current tobacco smoker Current smokeless tobacco user (eg, chew, snuff) Tobacco non-user

▶[1]Physician Consortium for Performance Improvement: www.physicianconsortium.org◀
[2]National Committee on Quality Assurance (NCQA): Health Employer Data Information Set (HEDIS®), www.ncqa.org
[3]Joint Commission on Accreditation of Healthcare Organizations (JCAHO), ORYX Initiative Performance Measures: www.jcaho.org/pms
[4]National Diabetes Quality Improvement Alliance: www.nationaldiabetesalliance.org
▶[5]Joint measure from the Physician Consortium for Performance Improvement, www.physicianconsortium.org, and National Committee on Quality Assurance (NCQA), www.ncqa.org◀
▶[6]The Society of Thoracic Surgeons, www.sts.org, and National Quality Forum, www.qualityforum.org◀

Brief Description of Performance Measure & Source and Reporting Instructions	CPT Code(s)	Code Descriptor
Chronic Obstructive Pulmonary Disease (COPD), cont'd		
Assessment of Symptoms[1]—Whether or not patient had COPD symptoms assessed at least annually **Numerator:** All patients with COPD symptoms assessed during one or more office visits each year **Denominator:** All patients with the diagnosis of COPD **Percentage** of patients who were assessed for COPD symptoms at least annually ►There are no exclusions for this measure; modifiers 1P, 2P, and 3P may not be used◄	1015F	Chronic obstructive pulmonary disease (COPD) symptoms assessed (Includes assessment of at least one of the following: dyspnea, cough/sputum, wheezing), or respiratory symptom assessment tool completed
Spirometry Evaluation[1]—Whether or not patient spirometry results were documented **Numerator:** All patients with documented spirometry results on the medical record **Denominator:** All patients with the diagnosis of COPD **Exclusion Criteria:** Documentation of medical, patient, or system reason(s) for no spirometry evaluation **Percentage** of patients with COPD who had a spirometry evaluation documented **Reporting Instructions:** For patients with appropriate exclusion criteria, report 3023F with modifier 1P, 2P, or 3P	3023F	Spirometry results documented and reviewed
Smoking Cessation Intervention[1]—Whether or not the patient who is a smoker received a smoking cessation intervention **Numerator:** All smokers who received a smoking cessation intervention during one or more office visits each year **Denominator:** All patients with the diagnosis of COPD identified as smokers **Percentage** of smokers with COPD who received a smoking cessation intervention at least annually **Reporting Instructions:** Report 1034F for each cigarette smoker. Report either 1034F, 1035F, or 1036F for each patient. If patient is a smoker and received cessation intervention, report 4000F or 4001F, or both. Report 4000F or 4001F only if 1034F has been reported ►There are no exclusions for this measure; modifiers 1P, 2P, and 3P may not be used◄	4000F 4001F **Denominator Codes:** 1034F 1035F 1036F	Tobacco use cessation intervention, counseling Tobacco use cessation intervention, pharmacologic therapy Current tobacco smoker Current smokeless tobacco user (eg, chew, snuff) Current tobacco non-user
Inhaled Bronchodilator[1]—Whether or not the symptomatic patient was prescribed an inhaled bronchodilator **Numerator:** All symptomatic patients who were prescribed an inhaled bronchodilator **Denominator:** All patients with the diagnosis of COPD who have an $FEV_1/FVC < 70\%$ and have symptoms **Denominator Inclusions:** Documentation of COPD symptoms; Documentation of $FEV_1/FVC < 70\%$ **Denominator Exclusions:** Documentation of medical, patient, or system reason(s) for not prescribing an inhaled bronchodilator **Percentage** of symptomatic patients with COPD who were prescribed an inhaled bronchodilator **Reporting Instructions:** Report either 3025F or 3027F for all COPD patients. For patients with appropriate exclusion criteria, report 4025F with modifier 1P, 2P, or 3P	4025F **Denominator Codes:** 3025F 3027F	Inhaled bronchodilator prescribed Spirometry test results demonstrate $FEV_1/FVC < 70\%$ with COPD symptoms (eg, dyspnea, cough/sputum, wheezing) Spirometry test results demonstrate $FEV_1/FVC \geq 70\%$ or patient does not have COPD symptoms
Assessment of Oxygen Saturation[1]—Whether or not oxygen saturation was assessed at least annually **Numerator:** All patients with oxygen saturation assessed and documented **Denominator:** All patients with the diagnosis of COPD and a $FEV_1 > 40\%$ of predicted value <div align="center">(continued)</div>	3028F	Oxygen saturation results documented and reviewed (Includes assessment through pulse oximetry or arterial blood gas measurement)

►[1]Physician Consortium for Performance Improvement: www.physicianconsortium.org◄
[2]National Committee on Quality Assurance (NCQA): Health Employer Data Information Set (HEDIS®), www.ncqa.org
[3]Joint Commission on Accreditation of Healthcare Organizations (JCAHO), ORYX Initiative Performance Measures: www.jcaho.org/pms
[4]National Diabetes Quality Improvement Alliance: www.nationaldiabetesalliance.org
►[5]Joint measure from the Physician Consortium for Performance Improvement, www.physicianconsortium.org, and National Committee on Quality Assurance (NCQA), www.ncqa.org◄
►[6]The Society of Thoracic Surgeons, www.sts.org, and National Quality Forum, www.qualityforum.org◄

Brief Description of Performance Measure & Source and Reporting Instructions	CPT Code(s)	Code Descriptor
Chronic Obstructive Pulmonary Disease (COPD), cont'd		
Denominator Inclusion: Documentation of $FEV_1 < 40\%$ of predicted value **Denominator Exclusions:** Documentation of medical, patient, or system reason(s) for not assessing oxygen saturation **Percentage** of COPD patients with oxygen saturation assessed at least annually **Reporting Instructions:** Report 3040F or 3042F for all COPD patients. If oxygen saturation assessed, also report 3028F. For patients with appropriate exclusion criteria, report 3028F with modifier 1P, 2P, or 3P	**Denominator Codes:** **3040F** **3042F**	Functional expiratory volume $(FEV_1) < 40\%$ of predicted value Functional expiratory volume $(FEV_1) \geq 40\%$ of predicted value
Long-Term Oxygen Therapy[1]— Whether or not patient with COPD was prescribed long-term oxygen therapy **Numerator:** All patients who were prescribed long-term oxygen therapy **Denominator:** All patients with a diagnosis of COPD and an oxygen saturation $\leq 88\%$ or a $PaO_2 \leq 55$ mm Hg **Denominator Inclusion:** $PaO_2 \leq 55$ mm Hg or oxygen saturation $\leq 88\%$ **Denominator Exclusion:** Documentation of medical, patient, or system reason(s) for not prescribing long-term oxygen therapy **Percentage** of patients with COPD that were prescribed long-term oxygen therapy **Reporting Instructions:** Report 3035F or 3037F for all COPD patients. Report 4030F with 3035F if long-term oxygen therapy prescribed For patients with appropriate exclusion criteria, report 4030F with modifier 1P, 2P, or 3P	**4030F** **Denominator Codes:** **3035F** **3037F**	Long-term oxygen therapy prescribed (more than fifteen hours per day) Oxygen saturation $\leq 88\%$ or a $PaO_2 \leq 55$ mm Hg Oxygen saturation $> 88\%$ or $PaO_2 > 55$ mmHg
Recommendation of Influenza Immunization[1]—Whether or not COPD patient received recommendation for influenza immunization annually **Numerator:** All patients who were recommended to receive an influenza immunization during one or more office visits every year **Denominator:** All patients with the diagnosis of COPD **Denominator Exclusion:** Documentation of immunization given during the current flu season; documentation of medical or system reason(s) for not recommending an influenza immunization **Percentage** of patients with COPD who were recommended to receive an influenza immunization annually **Reporting Instructions:** Report only one code (4035F) for immunization recommended **or** immunization ordered or administrated (4037F) For patients with appropriate exclusion criteria, report 4035F with modifier 1P or 3P	**4035F** **4037F** **Category I Codes:** **90656** **90658** **90660**	Influenza immunization recommended Influenza immunization ordered or administered Influenza virus vaccine, split virus, preservative free, when administered children 6-35 months of age, for intramuscular use Influenza virus vaccine, split virus, when administered to 3 years of age and older, for intramuscular use Influenza virus vaccine, live virus, for intranasal use
Influenza Immunization Administered[1]—Whether or not influenza immunization was received during a current flu season **Numerator:** All patients who are administered an influenza immunization during the visit or who have already received an influenza immunization during the current flu season **Denominator:** All patients with the diagnosis of COPD **Denominator Inclusion:** Documentation of visit during flu season **Denominator Exclusion:** Documentation that patient is planning to receive influenza immunization during current flu season; documentation of medical, patient, or system reason(s) for not administering the influenza immunization **Percentage** of patients who received influenza immunization during the current flu season **Reporting Instructions:** Use 4037F with appropriate exclusion criteria (medical, patient, or system use 4037F with modifier 1P, 2P, or 3P). If patient planning to receive immunization use 1P modifier with order code (4037F). Report only one code.	**4037F** **Category I Codes:** **90656** **90658** **90660**	Influenza immunization ordered or administered Influenza virus vaccine, split virus, preservative free, when administered to children 6-35 months of age, for intramuscular use Influenza virus vaccine, split virus, when administered to 3 years of age and older, for intramuscular use Influenza virus vaccine, live virus, for intranasal use

▶[1]Physician Consortium for Performance Improvement: www.physicianconsortium.org◀

[2]National Committee on Quality Assurance (NCQA): Health Employer Data Information Set (HEDIS®), www.ncqa.org

[3]Joint Commission on Accreditation of Healthcare Organizations (JCAHO), ORYX Initiative Performance Measures: www.jcaho.org/pms

[4]National Diabetes Quality Improvement Alliance: www.nationaldiabetesalliance.org

▶[5]Joint measure from the Physician Consortium for Performance Improvement, www.physicianconsortium.org, and National Committee on Quality Assurance (NCQA), www.ncqa.org◀

▶[6]The Society of Thoracic Surgeons, www.sts.org, and National Quality Forum, www.qualityforum.org◀

Brief Description of Performance Measure & Source and Reporting Instructions	CPT Code(s)	Code Descriptor
Chronic Obstructive Pulmonary Disease (COPD), cont'd		
Assessment of Pneumococcus Immunization Status[1]—Whether or not pneumococcus immunization status was assessed **Numerator:** All patients who were assessed for pneumococcus immunization status **Denominator:** All patients with the diagnosis of COPD **Denominator Exclusion:** Documentation of medical, patient, or system reason(s) for not recommending pneumococcus immunization **Percentage** of patients with COPD that were assessed for pneumococcus immunization status **Reporting Instructions:** For patients with appropriate criteria documented for not assessing pneumococcus immunization status, report 1022F with modifier 1P, 2P, or 3P.	1022F	Pneumococcus immunization status assessed
Pneumococcus Immunization Administered[1]—Whether or not the patient was administered a pneumococcus immunization during a visit or had already received a pneumococcus immunization **Numerator:** All patients who are administered a pneumococcus immunization during a visit or who have already received a pneumoccus immunization status **Denominator:** All patients with the diagnosis of COPD **Denominator Exclusions:** Pneumococcus immunization recommended but not administered; documentation of medical, patient, system reason(s) for not administering the pneumococcus immunization **Percentage** of patients who were administered a pneumococcus immunization during a visit or who had already received a pneumcoccus immunization **Reporting Instructions:** Report only one code for ordered or administered. For patients with appropriate exclusion criteria, report 4040F with modifier 1P, 2P, or 3P. If patient planning to receive immunization use 1P modifier with order code (4040F). Report only one code.	4040F **Category I Codes:** 90669 90732	Pneumococcal immunization ordered or administered Pneumococcal conjugate vaccine, polyvalent, when adminstered to children younger than 5 years, for intramuscular use Pneumococcal polysaccharide vaccine, 23-valent, adult or immunosuppressed patient dosage, when adminstered to 2 years or older, for subcutaneous or intramuscular use
Pulmonary Rehabilitation: Exercise Training Recommended[1]—Whether or not patient exercise training was recommended **Numerator:** All patients for whom exercise training was recommended **Denominator:** All patients with the diagnosis of COPD and dyspnea **Denominator Inclusion:** Documentation of dyspnea (1019F) **Denominator Exclusion:** Documentation of medical or system reason(s) for not recommending exercise training **Percentage** of patients for whom exercise training was recommended **Reporting Instructions:** Report 1018F or 1019F for all COPD patients. For patients with appropriate exclusion criteria, report 4033F with modifier 1P or 3P. Report 4033F with 1019F.	4033F **Denominator Codes:** 1018F 1019F	Pulmonary rehabilitation exercise training recommended Dyspnea assessed, not present Dyspnea assessed, present
Community-Acquired Bacterial Pneumonia (CAP)		
Chest Radiograph[1]—Whether or not patient had a chest X ray performed **Numerator:** All patients with a chest X ray performed **Denominator:** All patients with the diagnosis of community-acquired bacterial pneumonia **Denominator Exclusion:** Documentation of medical, patient, or system reason(s) for not performing a chest X ray **Percentage** of community-acquired bacterial pneumonia patients ≥ 18 years of age with a chest X ray performed **Reporting Instructions:** For patients with appropriate exclusion criteria, report 3006F with modifier 1P, 2P, or 3P	3006F	Chest X-ray results documented and reviewed

▶[1]Physician Consortium for Performance Improvement: www.physicianconsortium.org◀

[2]National Committee on Quality Assurance (NCQA): Health Employer Data Information Set (HEDIS®), www.ncqa.org

[3]Joint Commission on Accreditation of Healthcare Organizations (JCAHO), ORYX Initiative Performance Measures: www.jcaho.org/pms

[4]National Diabetes Quality Improvement Alliance: www.nationaldiabetesalliance.org

▶[5]Joint measure from the Physician Consortium for Performance Improvement, www.physicianconsortium.org, and National Committee on Quality Assurance (NCQA), www.ncqa.org◀

▶[6]The Society of Thoracic Surgeons, www.sts.org, and National Quality Forum, www.qualityforum.org◀

Brief Description of Performance Measure & Source and Reporting Instructions	CPT Code(s)	Code Descriptor
Community-Acquired Bacterial Pneumonia (CAP), cont'd		
Composite Code: Community-Acquired Bacterial Pneumonia Assessment— See individual measures listed below for (includes all of the following components): Comorbid conditions assessed (1026F) Vital signs recorded (2010F) Mental status assessed (2014F) Hydration status assessed (2018F)	0012F	Community-acquired bacterial pneumonia assessment
Assessment of Comorbid Conditions[1]—Whether or not patient was assessed for comorbid conditions **Numerator:** All patients assessed for history of comorbid conditions **Denominator:** All patients with the diagnosis of community-acquired bacterial pneumonia **Percentage** of patients ≥ 18 years of age with community-acquired bacterial pneumonia who were assessed for comorbid conditions ▶**Reporting Instructions:** There are no exclusions for this measure; modifiers 1P, 2P, and 3P may not be used◀	1026F	Comorbid conditions assessed (eg, includes assessment for presence or absence of: malignancy, liver disease, congestive heart failure, cerebrovascular disease, renal disease, chronic obstructive pulmonary disease, asthma, diabetes, other comorbid conditions)
Vital Signs[1]—Whether or not patient had vital signs recorded **Numerator:** All patients with vital signs recorded **Denominator:** All patients with the diagnosis of community-acquired bacterial pneumonia **Percentage** of community-acquired bacterial pneumonia patients ≥ 18 years of age with vital signs recorded ▶**Reporting Instructions:** There are no exclusions for this measure; modifiers 1P, 2P, and 3P may not be used◀	2010F	Vital signs recorded (includes at minimum: temperature, pulse, respiration, and blood pressure)
Assessment of Oxygen Saturation[1]—Whether or not patient had oxygen saturation assessed **Numerator:** All patients with oxygen saturation assessed **Denominator:** All patients with the diagnosis of community-acquired bacterial pneumonia **Exclusion Criteria:** Documentation of medical, patient, or system reason(s) for not assessing oxygen saturation **Percentage** of patients ≥ 18 years of age with community-acquired bacterial pneumonia with oxygen saturation assessed **Reporting Instructions:** For patients with appropriate exclusion criteria, report 3028F with modifier 1P, 2P, or 3P	3028F	Oxygen saturation results documented and reviewed (Includes assessment through pulse oximetry or arterial blood gas measurement)
Assessment of Mental Status[1]—Whether or not patient had mental status assessed **Numerator:** All patients with mental status assessed **Denominator:** All patients with the diagnosis of community-acquired bacterial pneumonia **Percentage** of community-acquired bacterial pneumonia patients age ≥ 18 years of age with mental status assessed ▶**Reporting Instructions:** There are no exclusions for this measure; modifiers 1P, 2P, and 3P may not be used◀	2014F	Mental status assessed (normal/ mildly impaired/severely impaired)
Assessment of Hydration Status[1]—Whether or not the patient had hydration status assessed **Numerator:** All patients with hydration status assessed **Denominator:** All patients with the diagnosis of community-acquired bacterial pneumonia **Percentage** of community-acquired bacterail pneumonia patients age ≥ 18 years of age with hydration status assessed ▶**Reporting Instructions:** There are no exclusions for this measure; modifiers 1P, 2P, and 3P may not be used◀	2018F	Hydration status assessed (normal/ mildly dehydrated/severely dehydrated)

▶[1]Physician Consortium for Performance Improvement: www.physicianconsortium.org◀

[2]National Committee on Quality Assurance (NCQA): Health Employer Data Information Set (HEDIS®), www.ncqa.org

[3]Joint Commission on Accreditation of Healthcare Organizations (JCAHO), ORYX Initiative Performance Measures: www.jcaho.org/pms

[4]National Diabetes Quality Improvement Alliance: www.nationaldiabetesalliance.org

▶[5]Joint measure from the Physician Consortium for Performance Improvement, www.physicianconsortium.org, and National Committee on Quality Assurance (NCQA), www.ncqa.org◀

▶[6]The Society of Thoracic Surgeons, www.sts.org, and National Quality Forum, www.qualityforum.org◀

Brief Description of Performance Measure & Source and Reporting Instructions	CPT Code(s)	Code Descriptor
Community-Acquired Bacterial Pneumonia (CAP), cont'd		
Level of Care Rationale[1]—Whether or not an assessment was made to determine the level of care **Numerator:** All patients with documented rationale for level of care **Denominator:** All patients with the diagnosis of community-acquired bacterial pneumonia **Percentage** of community-acquired bacterial pneumonia patients ≥ 18 years of age who had a documented rationale for level of care based on severity of illness and safety of home care ▶**Reporting Instructions:** There are no exclusions for this measure; modifiers 1P, 2P, and 3P may not be used◀	6005F	Rationale (eg, severity of illness and safety) for level of care (eg, home, hospital) documented
Empiric Antibiotic[1]—Whether or not patient was prescribed an appropriate empiric antibiotic **Numerator:** All patients with an appropriate empiric antibiotic prescribed **Denominator:** All patients with the diagnosis of community-acquired bacterial pneumonia **Denominator Exclusion:** Documentation of medical, patient, or system reasons(s) for not prescribing an antibiotic **Percentage** of community-acquired bacterial pneumonia patients ≥ 18 years of age who were prescribed an appropriate empiric antibiotic **Reporting Instructions:** For patients with appropriate exclusion criteria, report 4045F with modifier 1P, 2P, or 3P	4045F	Appropriate empiric antibiotic prescribed (See measure developer's Web site for definition of appropriate antibiotic)
Smoking Assessment[1]—Whether or not patient was queried about smoking **Numerator:** All patients who were queried about smoking **Denominator:** All patients with the diagnosis of community-acquired bacterial pneumonia **Percentage** of patients with community-acquired bacterial pneumonia who were queried about smoking **Reporting Instructions:** When reporting 1000F, it is required to report 1034F, and/or 1035F, or 1036F ▶**Reporting Instructions:** There are no exclusions for this measure; modifiers 1P, 2P, and 3P may not be used◀	1000F 1034F 1035F 1036F	Tobacco use assessed Current tobacco smoker Current smokeless tobacco user (eg, chew, snuff) Current tobacco non-user
Smoking Cessation Intervention[1]—Whether or not patient received a smoking cessation intervention **Numerator:** All patients who received a smoking cessation intervention **Denominator:** All patients with the diagnosis with community-acquired bacterial pneumonia identified as smokers **Percentage** of patients ≥ 18 years of age with community-acquired bacterial pneumonia who received a smoking cessation intervention **Reporting Instructions:** Report 1034F for each cigarette smoker. Report either 1034F, 1035F, or 1036F for each patient. If patient is a smoker and received cessation intervention, report 4000F or 4001F, or both. Report 4000F or 4001F only if 1034F has been reported ▶**Reporting Instructions:** There are no exclusions for this measure; modifiers 1P, 2P, and 3P may not be used◀	4000F 4001F **Denominator Codes:** 1034F 1035F 1036F	Tobacco use cessation intervention, counseling Tobacco use cessation intervention, pharmacologic therapy Current tobacco smoker Current smokeless tobacco user (eg, chew, snuff) Current tobacco non-user
Assessment of Influenza Immunization Status[1, 2]—Whether or not patient was assessed for influenza immunization status **Numerator:** All patients who were assessed for influenza immunization status **Denominator:** All patients with the diagnosis of community-acquired bacterial pneumonia **Denominator Exclusion:** Documentation of medical, patient, or system reason(s) that immunization was not indicated (continued)	1030F	Influenza immunization status assessed

▶[1]Physician Consortium for Performance Improvement: www.physicianconsortium.org◀

[2]National Committee on Quality Assurance (NCQA): Health Employer Data Information Set (HEDIS®), www.ncqa.org

[3]Joint Commission on Accreditation of Healthcare Organizations (JCAHO), ORYX Initiative Performance Measures: www.jcaho.org/pms

[4]National Diabetes Quality Improvement Alliance: www.nationaldiabetesalliance.org

▶[5]Joint measure from the Physician Consortium for Performance Improvement, www.physicianconsortium.org, and National Committee on Quality Assurance (NCQA), www.ncqa.org◀

▶[6]The Society of Thoracic Surgeons, www.sts.org, and National Quality Forum, www.qualityforum.org◀

Brief Description of Performance Measure & Source and Reporting Instructions	CPT Code(s)	Code Descriptor
Community-Acquired Bacterial Pneumonia (CAP), cont'd		
Percentage of patients age ≥ 18 years of age with community-acquired bacterial pneumonia who were assessed for influenza immunization status **Reporting Instructions:** Use 1030F if documentation shows that influenza vaccine was administered. For patients with appropriate exclusion criteria, report 1030F with modifier 1P, 2P, or 3P		
Assessment of Pneumococcus Immunization Status[1,2]—Whether or not patient was assessed for pneumococcus immunization status **Numerator:** All patients who were assessed for pneumococcus immunization status **Denominator:** All patients with the diagnosis of community-acquired bacterial pneumonia **Denominator Exclusion:** Documentation that immunization was not indicated; documentation of medical, patient, or system reason that immunization was not indicated **Percentage** of patients ≥ 18 years of age with community-acquired bacterial pneumonia who were assessed for pneumococcus immunization status **Reporting Instructions:** Use 1022F if documentation shows that pneumococcus vaccine was administered. For patient with appropriate exclusion criteria, report 1022F with modifier 1P, 2P, or 3P	**1022F**	Pneumococcus immunization status assessed
►Coronary Artery Bypass Graft (CABG)◄		
►Use of Internal Mammary Artery (IMA) graft in primary, Isolated Coronary Artery Bypass Graft (CABG) Surgery[6]—Whether or not a patient received an IMA graft in the performance of a primary, isolated CABG procedure **Numerator:** All patients who received an IMA graft in isolated CABG procedures **Denominator:** All patients who received a primary isolated CABG procedure **Exclusion(s):** Medical reasons for not receiving an IMA graft in the performance of a primary, isolated CABG procedure **Reporting Instructions:** This measure is not intended for use with repeat CABG procedures. For patients with documented medical reasons for not receiving an IMA graft in the performance of a primary, isolated CABG procedure, report modifier 1P with code 4110F◄	►4110F◄	►Internal mammary artery graft performed for primary, isolated coronary artery bypass graft procedure◄
►Use of Beta Blocker in Isolated Coronary Artery Bypass Graft (CABG) Surgery[6]—Whether or not a patient was administered beta blocker within 24 hours prior to surgical incision for isolated CABG surgery **Numerator:** Patients who were administered beta blocker within 24 hours prior to surgical incision **Denominator:** All patients undergoing isolated CABG surgery **Exclusion(s):** Medical reasons for not administering beta blocker within 24 hours prior to surgical incision for isolated CABG surgery **Percentage** of patients who were administered beta blocker within 24 hours prior to surgical incision for isolated CABG surgery **Reporting Instructions:** For patients with medical reasons for not administering beta blocker within 24 hours prior to surgical incision for isolated CABG surgery, report modifier 1P with code 4115F◄	►4115F◄	►Beta blocker administered within 24 hours prior to surgical incision◄

►[1]Physician Consortium for Performance Improvement: www.physicianconsortium.org◄

[2]National Committee on Quality Assurance (NCQA): Health Employer Data Information Set (HEDIS®), www.ncqa.org

[3]Joint Commission on Accreditation of Healthcare Organizations (JCAHO), ORYX Initiative Performance Measures: www.jcaho.org/pms

[4]National Diabetes Quality Improvement Alliance: www.nationaldiabetesalliance.org

►[5]Joint measure from the Physician Consortium for Performance Improvement, www.physicianconsortium.org, and National Committee on Quality Assurance (NCQA), www.ncqa.org◄

►[6]The Society of Thoracic Surgeons, www.sts.org, and National Quality Forum, www.qualityforum.org◄

Brief Description of Performance Measure & Source and Reporting Instructions	CPT Code(s)	Code Descriptor
Coronary Artery Disease (CAD)		
Smoking Cessation Evaluation[1]—Whether or not patient with CAD was queried one or more times about cigarette smoking **Numerator:** Patients who were queried one or more times about cigarette smoking **Denominator:** All patients with CAD **Percentage** of patients who were queried one or more times about cigarette smoking **Reporting Instructions:** When reporting 1000F, it is required to report 1034F, and/or 1035F, or 1036F ▶There are no exclusions for this measure; modifiers 1P, 2P, and 3P may not be used◀	**1000F** **1034F** **1035F** **1036F**	Tobacco use assessed Current tobacco smoker Current smokeless tobacco user (eg, chew, snuff) Current tobacco non-user
Smoking Cessation Intervention[1]—Whether or not patient identified as a cigarette smoker received intervention for smoking cessation **Numerator:** Patients who were received smoking cessation intervention **Denominator:** All patients with CAD identified as cigarette smokers **Percentage** of patients identified as cigarette smokers who received intervention for smoking cessation **Reporting Instructions:** Report 1034F for each cigarette smoker. Report either 1034F, 1035F, or 1036F for each patient. If patient is a smoker and received cessation intervention, report 4000F or 4001F, or both. Report 4000F or 4001F only if 1034F has been reported ▶There are no exclusions for this measure; modifiers 1P, 2P, and 3P may not be used◀	**4000F** **4001F** **Denominator Codes:** **1034F** **1035F** **1036F**	Tobacco use cessation intervention, counseling Tobacco use cessation intervention, pharmacologic therapy Current tobacco smoker Current smokeless tobacco user (eg, chew, snuff) Current tobacco non-user
Symptom & Activity Assessment[1]—Whether or not patient's level of activity and anginal symptoms were evaluated during office visit **Numerator:** Patients evaluated for both level of activity and anginal symptoms during one or more office visits **Denominator:** All patients with CAD **Percentage** of patients who were evaluated for both level of activity and anginal symptoms during one or more office visits ▶**Reporting Instructions:** There are no exclusions for this measure; modifiers 1P, 2P, and 3P may not be used◀	**1002F**	Anginal symptoms and level of activity assessed
Blood Pressure Measurement[1]—Most recent systolic and diastolic blood pressure measurement **Numerator:** Patients who had a blood pressure measurement during the last office visit **Denominator:** All patients with CAD **Percentage** of patients who had a blood pressure measurement during the last office visit ▶**Reporting Instructions:** There are no exclusions for this measure; modifiers 1P, 2P, and 3P may not be used◀	**2000F**	Blood pressure measured
Lipid Profile[1]—Whether or not a lipid profile was obtained **Numerator:** Patients who received at least one lipid profile (or ALL component tests) **Denominator:** All patients with CAD **Percentage** of patients who received at least one lipid profile (or ALL component tests)	**3011F**	Lipid panel results documented and reviewed (must include total cholesterol, HDL-C, triglycerides and calculated LDL-C)
Drug Therapy for Lowering LDL-Cholesterol[1]—Whether or not patient was prescribed lipid-lowering therapy **Numerator:** Patients who were prescribed lipid-lowering therapy **Denominator:** All patients with CAD **Denominator Exclusion(s):** Documentation of medical, patient, or system reason(s) for not prescribing lipid-lowering therapy **Percentage** of patients who were prescribed a lipid-lowering therapy (based on current ACC/AHA guidelines) **Reporting Instructions:** For patients with appropriate exclusion criteria, report code 4002F with modifier 1P, 2P, or 3P	**4002F**	Statin therapy prescribed

▶[1]Physician Consortium for Performance Improvement: www.physicianconsortium.org◀

[2]National Committee on Quality Assurance (NCQA): Health Employer Data Information Set (HEDIS®), www.ncqa.org

[3]Joint Commission on Accreditation of Healthcare Organizations (JCAHO), ORYX Initiative Performance Measures: www.jcaho.org/pms

[4]National Diabetes Quality Improvement Alliance: www.nationaldiabetesalliance.org

▶[5]Joint measure from the Physician Consortium for Performance Improvement, www.physicianconsortium.org, and National Committee on Quality Assurance (NCQA), www.ncqa.org◀

▶[6]The Society of Thoracic Surgeons, www.sts.org, and National Quality Forum, www.qualityforum.org◀

Brief Description of Performance Measure & Source and Reporting Instructions	CPT Code(s)	Code Descriptor
Coronary Artery Disease (CAD), cont'd		
Beta-blocker Therapy-Prior Myocardial Infarction (MI)[1]—Whether or not CAD patient with prior MI at any time was prescribed beta-blocker therapy **Numerator:** Patients who were prescribed beta-blocker therapy **Denominator:** All patients with CAD who also have a prior MI at any time **Denominator Exclusion(s):** Documentation of medical, patient reason(s) for not prescribing beta-blocker therapy, or system reason **Percentage** of CAD patients who also have prior MI at any time who were prescribed beta-blocker therapy **Reporting Instructions:** For patients with appropriate exclusion criteria, report code 4006F with modifier 1P, 2P, or 3P	4006F	Beta-blocker therapy prescribed
Angiotensin Converting Enzyme (ACE) Inhibitor or Angiotensin Receptor Blocker (ARB) Therapy[1]—Whether or not CAD patient with diabetes and/or left ventricular systolic dysfunction (LVSD) was prescribed ACE inhibitor or ARB therapy **Numerator:** Patients who were prescribed ACE inhibitor or ARB therapy **Denominator:** All CAD patients aged ≥ 18 years of age with diabetes and/or left ventricular ejection fraction (LVEF) < 40% or moderately or severely depressed left ventricular systolic function. **Exclusion Criteria:** Documentation of medical, patient, or system reason(s) for not prescribing ACE or ARB therapy **Percentage** of CAD patients who also have diabetes and/or left ventricular systolic dysfunction (LVSD) who were prescribed ACE inhibitor or ARB therapy **Reporting Instructions:** Report either 3021F or 3022F or corresponding ICD-9 diagnosis code for diabetes for each CAD patient. For patient with appropriate exclusion criteria, report 4009F with modifier 1P, 2P, or 3P	4009F **Denominator Codes:** 3021F 3022F	Angiotensin converting enzyme (ACE) inhibitor or Angiotensin Receptor Blocker (ARB) therapy prescribed Left ventricular ejection fraction (LVEF) < 40% or documentation of moderately or severely depressed left ventricular systolic function Left ventricular ejection fraction (LVEF) ≥ 40% or documentation as normal or mildly depressed left ventricular systolic function
Antiplatelet Therapy[1]—Whether or not patient was prescribed antiplatelet therapy **Numerator:** Patients who were prescribed antiplatelet therapy **Denominator:** All patients with CAD **Denominator Exclusion(s):** Documentation of medical, patient, or system reason(s) for not prescribing antiplatelet therapy **Percentage** of patients who were prescribed antiplatelet therapy **Reporting Instructions:** For patients with appropriate exclusion criteria, report code 4011F with modifier 1P, 2P, or 3P	4011F	Oral antiplatelet therapy prescribed (eg, aspirin, clopidogrel/Plavix, or combination of aspirin and dipyridamole/Aggrenox)
Diabetes		
A1c Management[4] (Measure #1)—Whether or not patient received one or more A1c test(s) **Numerator:** Patients who received one or more A1c test(s) **Denominator:** Patients with diagnosed diabetes 18-75 years of age **Percentage** of patients with diagnosed diabetes aged 18-75 years with one or more A1c test(s) **Reporting Instructions:** In order to meet this measure, the date of test when it was performed and the corresponding result are required. For this reason, report one of the three Category II codes listed and use the date of service as the date of the test, not the date of the reporting of the Category II code. The measure may also be met by reporting the Category I code 83036, Hemoglobin; by copper sulfate method, non-automated, glycated, when performed ►To report most recent hemoglobin A1c level ≤ 9.0%, see codes 3044F-3045F◄	►3044F◄ ►3045F◄ 3046F **Category I Codes:** 83036	►Most recent hemoglobin A1c HbA1c level < 7.0%◄ ►Most recent hemoglobin A1c (HbA1c) level 7.0%-9.0%◄ Most recent hemoglobin A1c level > 9.0% Hemoglobin; glycosylated (A1C)

►[1]Physician Consortium for Performance Improvement: www.physicianconsortium.org◄
[2]National Committee on Quality Assurance (NCQA): Health Employer Data Information Set (HEDIS®), www.ncqa.org
[3]Joint Commission on Accreditation of Healthcare Organizations (JCAHO), ORYX Initiative Performance Measures: www.jcaho.org/pms
[4]National Diabetes Quality Improvement Alliance: www.nationaldiabetesalliance.org
►[5]Joint measure from the Physician Consortium for Performance Improvement, www.physicianconsortium.org, and National Committee on Quality Assurance (NCQA), www.ncqa.org◄
►[6]The Society of Thoracic Surgeons, www.sts.org, and National Quality Forum, www.qualityforum.org◄

Brief Description of Performance Measure & Source and Reporting Instructions	CPT Code(s)	Code Descriptor
Diabetes, cont'd		
A1c Management[4] (Measure #2)—Whether or not patient's most recent A1c level > 9.0% (poor control) **Numerator:** Patients with most recent A1c level > 9.0% (poor control) **Denominator:** Patients diagnosed with diabetes 18-75 years of age **Percentage** of patients with most recent A1c level > 9.0% (poor control) **Reporting Instructions:** In order to meet this measure, the date of test when it was performed and the corresponding result are required. For this reason, report one of the three Category II codes listed and use the date of service as the date of the test, not the date of the reporting of the category II code ▶To report most recent hemoglobin A1c level < 9.0%, see codes 3044F-3045F◀	▶3044F 3045F◀ 3046F	▶Most recent hemoglobin A1c HbA1c level < 7.0% Most recent hemoglobin A1c (HbA1c) level 7.0%-9.0%◀ Most recent hemoglobin A1c level > 9.0%
▶**A1c Management**[2] (Measure #3)—Whether or not patient's most recent A1c level < 7.0% (tight control) **Numerator:** Patients with most recent A1c level < 7.0% (tight control) **Denominator:** Patients diagnosed with diabetes 18-75 years of age **Exclusion(s):** Documentation of medical reasons for not pursuing tight control of A1c level **Percentage** of patients with most recent A1c level < 7.0% (tight control) **Reporting Instructions:** In order to meet this measure, the date of test when it was performed and the corresponding result are required. For this reason, report one of the three Category II codes listed and use the date of service as the date of the test, not the date of the reporting of the category II code For patients with appropriate exclusion criteria report 3044F, 3045F, or 3046F with 1P To report most recent hemoglobin A1c level ≤ 9.0%, see codes 3044F-3045F◀	▶3044F 3045F 3046F◀	▶Most recent hemoglobin HbA1c level < 7.0% Most recent hemoglobin HbA1c level 7.0%-9.0% Most recent hemoglobin A1c level > 9.0%◀
Lipid Management[4] (Measure #1)—Whether or not patient received at least one LDL-C test **Numerator:** Patients who received at least one LDL-C test **Denominator:** Patients diagnosed with diabetes 18-75 years of age **Percentage** of patients diagnosed with diabetes aged 18-75 years with at least one LDL-C test **Reporting Instructions:** In order to meet this measure, the date of test when it was performed and the corresponding result are required. For this reason, report one of the three Category II codes listed and use the date of service as the date of the test, not the date of the reporting of the Category II code. The measure may also be met by reporting the listed lipid test Category I codes, when performed ▶There are no exclusions for this measure; modifiers 1P, 2P, and 3P may not be used◀	3048F 3049F 3050F **Category I Codes:** 80061 82465 83700 83701 83704 83721	Most recent LDL-C < 100 mg/dL Most recent LDL-C 100-129 mg/dL Most recent LDL-C ≥ 130 mg/dL Lipid panel Cholesterol, serum or whole blood, total Lipoprotein, blood; electrophoretic separation and quantitation high resolution fractionation and quantitation of lipoproteins including lipoprotein subclasses when performed (eg, electrophoresis, ultracentrifugation) quantitation of lipoprotein particle numbers and lipoprotein particle subclasses (eg, by nuclear magnetic resonance spectroscopy) Lipoprotein, direct measurement, low density cholesterol

▶[1]Physician Consortium for Performance Improvement: www.physicianconsortium.org◀

[2]National Committee on Quality Assurance (NCQA): Health Employer Data Information Set (HEDIS®), www.ncqa.org

[3]Joint Commission on Accreditation of Healthcare Organizations (JCAHO), ORYX Initiative Performance Measures: www.jcaho.org/pms

[4]National Diabetes Quality Improvement Alliance: www.nationaldiabetesalliance.org

▶[5]Joint measure from the Physician Consortium for Performance Improvement, www.physicianconsortium.org, and National Committee on Quality Assurance (NCQA), www.ncqa.org◀

▶[6]The Society of Thoracic Surgeons, www.sts.org, and National Quality Forum, www.qualityforum.org◀

Brief Description of Performance Measure & Source and Reporting Instructions	CPT Code(s)	Code Descriptor
Diabetes, cont'd		
Lipid Management[4] (Measure #2)—Whether or not patient's most recent LDL-C < 130 mg/dL **Numerator:** Patients with most recent LDL-C < 130 mg/dL **Denominator:** Patients diagnosed with diabetes aged 18-75 years **Percentage** of patients diagnosed with diabetes aged 18-75 years with most recent LDL-C < 130 mg/dL **Reporting Instructions:** In order to meet this measure, the date of test, when it was performed, and the corresponding result are required. For this reason, report one of the three Category II codes listed and use the date of service as the date of the test, not the date of the reporting of the Category II code ▶There are no exclusions for this measure; modifiers 1P, 2P, and 3P may not be used◀	3048F 3049F 3050F	Most recent LDL-C < 100 mg/dL Most recent LDL-C 100-129 mg/dL Most recent LDL-C ≥ 130 mg/dL
Lipid Management[4] (Measure #3)—Whether or not patient's most recent LDL-C < 100 mg/dL **Numerator:** Patients whose most recent LDL-C is < 100 mg/dL **Denominator:** Patients diagnosed with diabetes 18-75 years of age **Percentage** of patients diagnosed with diabetes 18-75 years of age whose most recent LDL-C < 100 mg/dL **Reporting Instructions:** In order to meet this measure, the date of test when it was performed and the corresponding result are required. For this reason, report one of the three Category II codes listed and use the date of service as the date of the test, not the date of the reporting of the Category II code ▶There are no exclusions for this measure; modifiers 1P, 2P, and 3P may not be used◀	3048F 3049F 3050F	Most recent LDL-C < 100 mg/dL Most recent LDL-C 100-129 mg/dL Most recent LDL-C ≥ 130 mg/dL
Urine Protein Screening[4]—Whether or not a patient received at least one test for microalbumin during the measurement year **or** had evidence of medical attention for existing nephropathy **or** has documentation of microalbuminuria or albuminuria **or** is on an angiotensin converting enzyme (ACE) inhibitor or angiotensin receptor blocker (ARB) **Numerator:** Patients with at least one test for microalbumin during the measurement year; or who had evidence of medical attention for existing nephropathy or documentation of microalbuminuria or albuminuria or are on an ACE inhibitor or ARB therapy **Denominator:** Patients diagnosed with diabetes 18-75 years of age **Percentage** of patients diagnosed with diabetes 18-75 years of age with at least one test for microalbumin during the measurement year; or who had evidence of medical attention for existing nephropathy or documentation of microalbuminuria or albuminuria or are on an ACE inhibitor or ARB therapy **Reporting Instructions:** Report any one of the codes listed using the following: 1. Codes 3060F, 3061F, and 3062F may be used to indicate that a patient received at least one test for microalbuminuria 2. Code 3066F may be used if there is evidence of nephropathy **or** if there was a patient visit to a nephrologist 3. Code 3062F may be used to indicate that a patient had documentation of microalbuminuria or albuminuria 4. Code 4009F may be used if patient is on an ACE inhibitor or ARB therapy 5. Any CPT Category I code and corresponding result, when performed, and reported with any of the following ICD-9-CM diagnosis or procedure codes found in specifications: ICD-9-CM codes: 39.27, 39.42, 39.43, 39.53, 39.93-39.95, 54.98, 55.4-55.6, 250.4, 403, 404, 405.01, 405.11, 405.91, 581.81, 582.9, 583.81, 584-586, 588, 753.0, 753.1, 791.0; V codes: V42.0, V45.1, V56 (continued)	3060F 3061F 3062F 3066F 4009F **Category I Codes:** 82042, 82043,	Positive microalbuminuria test result documented and reviewed Negative microalbuminuria test result documented and reviewed Positive macroalbuminuria test result documented and reviewed Documentation of treatment for nephropathy (eg, patient receiving dialysis, patient being treated for ESRD, CRF, ARF, or renal insufficiency, any visit to a nephrologist) Angiotensin converting enzyme (ACE) inhibitor or Angiotensin Receptor Blocker (ARB) therapy prescribed

▶[1]Physician Consortium for Performance Improvement: www.physicianconsortium.org◀
[2]National Committee on Quality Assurance (NCQA): Health Employer Data Information Set (HEDIS®), www.ncqa.org
[3]Joint Commission on Accreditation of Healthcare Organizations (JCAHO), ORYX Initiative Performance Measures: www.jcaho.org/pms
[4]National Diabetes Quality Improvement Alliance: www.nationaldiabetesalliance.org
▶[5]Joint measure from the Physician Consortium for Performance Improvement, www.physicianconsortium.org, and National Committee on Quality Assurance (NCQA), www.ncqa.org◀
▶[6]The Society of Thoracic Surgeons, www.sts.org, and National Quality Forum, www.qualityforum.org◀

Brief Description of Performance Measure & Source and Reporting Instructions	CPT Code(s)	Code Descriptor
Diabetes, cont'd		
6. CPT Category I codes for microalbumin measurement or quantitative timed urine albumin measurement and corresponding result as follows: 82042, 82043, 82044, 83518, 84156, or (84160, 84165, 84166) with code 81050	82044, 83518, 84156, 84160, 84165, 84166, 81050, 90920, 90921, 90924, 90925, 90935, 90937, 90945, 90947, 90989, 90993, 90999	
Eye Examination[4]—Whether or not patient received a dilated eye exam or seven standard field stereoscopic photos with interpretation by an ophthalmologist or optometrist or imaging validated to match diagnosis from these photos during the reporting year or during the prior year if the patient is at low risk* for retinopathy **Numerator:** Patients who received a dilated eye exam or seven standard field stereoscopic photos with interpretation by an ophthalmologist or optometrist or imaging validated to match diagnosis from these photos during the reporting year, or during the prior year, if patient is at low risk* for retinopathy **Denominator:** Patients with diagnosed diabetes 18-75 years of age; Low risk patient (defined as a patient who had no evidence of retinopathy in the prior year) must have had an evaluation in the prior year **Percentage** of patients who received a dilated eye exam or seven standard field stereoscopic photos with interpretation by an ophthalmologist or optometrist or imaging validated to match diagnosis from these photos during the reporting year **Reporting Instructions:** Only one of these codes should be reported *A patient is considered low risk if the following criterion is met: has no evidence of retinopathy on one of the accepted examinations in the prior year	2022F OR 2024F OR 2026F OR 3072F Category I Codes: 99201 99212 99241 92002 92004 92012 92014 92225 92226	Dilated retinal eye exam with interpretation by an ophthalmologist or optometrist documented and reviewed OR Seven standard field stereoscopic photos with interpretation by an ophthalmologist or optometrist documented and reviewed OR Eye imaging validated to match diagnosis from seven standard field stereoscopic photos results documented and reviewed OR Low risk for retinopathy (no evidence of retinopathy in the prior year) Office/outpatient visit, new Office/outpatient visit, established pt. Office consultation Eye exam, new patient Eye exam, new patient Eye exam, established pt. Eye exam & treatment Special eye exam, initial Special eye exam, subsequent
Foot Examination[4]—Whether or not patient received at least one foot exam, defined in any manner **Numerator:** Patients who received at least one foot exam, defined in any manner **Denominator:** Patients diagnosed with diabetes 18-75 years of age **Denominator Exclusions:** Patients with bilateral foot/leg amputation **Percentage** of patients diagnosed with diabetes 18-75 years of age receiving at least one foot exam, defined in any manner **Reporting Instructions:** Report 2028F with modifier 1P for patients with bilateral foot/leg amputation	2028F	Foot examination performed (includes examination through visual inspection, sensory exam with monofilament, and pulse exam – report when any of the three components are completed)

▶[1]Physician Consortium for Performance Improvement: www.physicianconsortium.org◀

[2]National Committee on Quality Assurance (NCQA): Health Employer Data Information Set (HEDIS®), www.ncqa.org

[3]Joint Commission on Accreditation of Healthcare Organizations (JCAHO), ORYX Initiative Performance Measures: www.jcaho.org/pms

[4]National Diabetes Quality Improvement Alliance: www.nationaldiabetesalliance.org

▶[5]Joint measure from the Physician Consortium for Performance Improvement, www.physicianconsortium.org, and National Committee on Quality Assurance (NCQA), www.ncqa.org◀

▶[6]The Society of Thoracic Surgeons, www.sts.org, and National Quality Forum, www.qualityforum.org◀

Brief Description of Performance Measure & Source and Reporting Instructions	CPT Code(s)	Code Descriptor
Diabetes, cont'd		
▶**Blood Pressure Management**[2] (Measure #1)—Whether or not patient's most recent blood pressure is < 130 mm Hg systolic and < 80 mm Hg diastolic **Numerator:** Patients whose most recent blood pressure is < 130 mm Hg systolic and < 80 mm Hg diastolic **Denominator:** Patients diagnosed with diabetes 18-75 years of age **Exclusion(s):** Documentation of medical reasons that diastolic < 80 is not medically indicated. Documentation of medical reasons that systolic < 130 is not medically indicated. **Percentage** of patients diagnosed with diabetes 18-75 years of age with most recent blood pressure < 130 mm Hg systolic and < 80 mm Hg diastolic. **Reporting Instructions:** Two codes must be reported here. For the systolic blood pressure value, report one of the three systolic codes; for the diastolic blood pressure value, report one of the three diastolic codes. For patients in whom a goal of 130/80 is not medically indicated, report codes 3075F, 3077F, 3078F, 3079F, 3080F with modifier 1P◀	▶3074F 3075F 3077F 3078F 3079F 3080F◀	▶Most recent systolic blood pressure < 130 mm Hg Most recent systolic blood pressure 130-139 mm Hg Most recent systolic blood pressure ≥ 140 mm Hg Most recent diastolic blood pressure < 80 mm Hg Most recent diastolic blood pressure 80-89 mm Hg Most recent diastolic blood pressure ≥ 90 mm Hg◀
Blood Pressure Management[4] (Measure #2)—Whether or not patient's most recent blood pressure is < 140/80 mm Hg **Numerator:** Patients whose most recent blood pressure < 140/80 mm Hg **Denominator:** Patients diagnosed with diabetes 18-75 years of age **Percentage** of patients diagnosed with diabetes 18-75 years of age with most recent blood pressure < 140/80 mm Hg **Reporting Instructions:** Two codes must be reported here. For the systolic blood pressure value, report one of the two systolic codes; for the diastolic blood pressure value, report one of the three diastolic codes. To report most recent recent systolic blood pressure < 140 mm Hg, see codes 3074F-3075F. ▶There are no exclusions for this measure; modifiers 1P, 2P, and 3P may not be used◀	**Systolic Codes:** ▶3074F 3075F◀ 3077F **Diastolic Codes:** 3078F 3079F 3080F	 ▶Most recent systolic blood pressure < 130 mm Hg Most recent systolic blood pressure 130-139 mm Hg◀ Most recent systolic blood pressure ≥ 140 mm Hg Most recent diastolic blood pressure < 80 mm Hg Most recent diastolic blood pressure 80-89 mm Hg Most recent diastolic blood pressure ≥ 90 mm Hg
Smoking Cessation[4]—Whether or not patient's smoking status was ascertained and documented **Numerator:** Patients whose smoking status was ascertained and documented **Denominator:** Patients diagnosed with diabetes 18-75 years of age **Percentage** of patients diagnosed with diabetes 18-75 years of age whose smoking status was ascertained and documented **Reporting Instructions:** Report 1034F for each cigarette smoker. Report either 1034F, 1035F, or 1036F for each patient. If patient is a smoker and received cessation intervention, report 4000F or 4001F, or both. Report 4000F or 4001F only if 1034F has been reported ▶There are no exclusions for this measure; modifiers 1P, 2P, and 3P may not be used◀	4000F 4001F **Denominator Codes:** 1034F 1035F 1036F	Tobacco use cessation intervention, counseling Tobacco use cessation intervention, pharmacologic therapy Current tobacco smoker Smokeless tobacco user Current tobacco non-user

▶[1]Physician Consortium for Performance Improvement: www.physicianconsortium.org◀

[2]National Committee on Quality Assurance (NCQA): Health Employer Data Information Set (HEDIS®), www.ncqa.org

[3]Joint Commission on Accreditation of Healthcare Organizations (JCAHO), ORYX Initiative Performance Measures: www.jcaho.org/pms

[4]National Diabetes Quality Improvement Alliance: www.nationaldiabetesalliance.org

▶[5]Joint measure from the Physician Consortium for Performance Improvement, www.physicianconsortium.org, and National Committee on Quality Assurance (NCQA), www.ncqa.org◀

▶[6]The Society of Thoracic Surgeons, www.sts.org, and National Quality Forum, www.qualityforum.org◀

Brief Description of Performance Measure & Source and Reporting Instructions	CPT Code(s)	Code Descriptor
►Emergency Medicine (EM)◄		
►Electrocardiogram Performed for NonTraumatic Chest Pain[5] (Measure #1)— Whether or not the patient aged 40 years and older with an emergency department discharge diagnosis of nontraumatic chest pain had an ECG performed **Numerator:** Patients who had an ECG performed **Denominator:** All patients aged 40 years and older with an emergency department discharge diagnosis of nontraumatic chest pain **Exclusion(s):** Documentation of medical reason(s) for not performing an ECG; documentation of patient reason(s) for not performing an ECG **Percentage** of patients aged 40 years and older with an emergency department discharge diagnosis of nontraumatic chest pain who had an ECG performed **Reporting Instructions:** For patient with appropriate exclusion criteria, report 3120F with modifier 1P or 2P◄	►3120F Category I Codes: 93000, 93010◄	►12-Lead ECG performed◄
►Aspirin at Arrival for Acute Myocardial Infarction (AMI)[5] (Measure #2)—Whether or not the patient with an emergency department discharge diagnosis of AMI had documentation of receiving aspirin within 24 hours before emergency department arrival or during emergency department stay **Numerator:** Patients who had documentation of receiving aspirin within 24 hours before emergency department arrival or during emergency department stay **Denominator:** All patients with an emergency department discharge diagnosis of acute myocardial infarction **Exclusion(s):** Documentation of medical reason(s) for not receiving aspirin within 24 hours before emergency department arrival or during emergency department stay; documentation of patient reason(s) for not receiving aspirin within 24 hours before emergency department arrival or during emergency department stay **Percentage** of patients with AMI who had documentation of receiving aspirin within 24 hours before or after hospital arrival **Reporting Instructions:** For patient with appropriate exclusion criteria, report 4084F with modifier 1P or 2P◄	►4084F◄	►Aspirin received within 24 hours before emergency department arrival or during emergency department stay◄
►Electrocardiogram Performed for Syncope[5] (Measure #3)—Whether or not the patient aged 60 years and older with an emergency department discharge diagnosis of syncope had an ECG performed **Numerator:** Patients who had an ECG performed **Denominator:** All patients aged 60 years and older with an emergency department discharge diagnosis of syncope **Exclusion(s):** Documentation of medical reason(s) for not performing an ECG; documentation of patient reason(s) for not performing an ECG Percentage of patients aged 60 years and older with an emergency department discharge diagnosis of syncope who had an ECG performed **Reporting Instructions:** For patient with appropriate exclusion criteria, report 3120F with modifier 1P or 2P◄	►3120F Category I Codes: 93000 93010◄	►12-Lead ECG performed◄
►Vital Signs for Community-Acquired Bacterial Pneumonia[5] (Measure #4)— Whether or not the patient aged 18 years and older with the diagnosis of community-acquired pneumonia had vital signs documented and reviewed **Numerator:** Patients with vital signs (temperature, pulse, respiratory rate, and blood pressure) documented and reviewed **Denominator:** All patients aged 18 years and older with the diagnosis of community-acquired bacterial pneumonia (continued)	►2010F◄	►Vital signs (temperature, pulse, respiratory rate, and blood pressure) documented and reviewed◄

►[1]Physician Consortium for Performance Improvement: www.physicianconsortium.org◄

[2]National Committee on Quality Assurance (NCQA): Health Employer Data Information Set (HEDIS®), www.ncqa.org

[3]Joint Commission on Accreditation of Healthcare Organizations (JCAHO), ORYX Initiative Performance Measures: www.jcaho.org/pms

[4]National Diabetes Quality Improvement Alliance: www.nationaldiabetesalliance.org

►[5]Joint measure from the Physician Consortium for Performance Improvement, www.physicianconsortium.org, and National Committee on Quality Assurance (NCQA), www.ncqa.org◄

►[6]The Society of Thoracic Surgeons, www.sts.org, and National Quality Forum, www.qualityforum.org◄

Brief Description of Performance Measure & Source and Reporting Instructions	CPT Code(s)	Code Descriptor
▶Emergency Medicine (EM)◀, cont'd		
Exclusion(s): None **Percentage** of patients aged 18 years and older with the diagnosis of community-acquired bacterial pneumonia with vital signs documented and reviewed **Reporting Instructions:** There are no exclusions for this measure; modifiers 1P, 2P and 3P may not be used◀		
▶**Assessment of Oxygen Saturation for Community-Acquired Bacterial Pneumonia**[5] (Measure #5)—Whether or not the patient aged 18 years and older with the diagnosis of community-acquired bacterial pneumonia had oxygen saturation documented and reviewed **Numerator:** Patients with oxygen saturation documented and reviewed **Denominator:** All patients aged 18 years and older with the diagnosis of community-acquired bacterial pneumonia **Exclusion(s):** Documentation of medical, patient, or system reason(s) for not documenting and reviewing oxygen saturation **Percentage** of patients aged 18 years and older with the diagnosis of community-acquired bacterial pneumonia with oxygen saturation documented and reviewed **Reporting Instructions:** For patients with appropriate exclusion criteria, report 3028F with modifier 1P, 2P, or 3P◀	▶3028F◀	▶Oxygen saturation results documented and reviewed◀
▶**Assessment of Mental Status for Community-Acquired Bacterial Pneumonia**[5] (Measure #6)—Whether or not the patient aged 18 years and older with the diagnosis of community-acquired bacterial pneumonia had mental status assessed **Numerator:** Patients with mental status assessed **Denominator:** All patients aged 18 years and older with the diagnosis of community-acquired bacterial pneumonia with mental status assessed. **Exclusions:** None **Percentage** of patients aged 18 years and older with the diagnosis of community-acquired bacterial pneumonia with mental status assessed **Reporting Instructions:** There are no exclusions for this measure; modifiers 1P, 2P, and 3P may not be used◀	▶2014F◀	▶Mental status assessed◀
▶**Empiric Antibiotic for Community-Acquired Bacterial Pneumonia**[5] (Measure #7)—Whether or not the patient aged 18 years and older with a diagnosis of community-acquired bacterial pneumonia had an appropriate empiric antibiotic prescribed **Numerator:** Patients with an appropriate empiric antibiotic prescribed Appropriate empiric antibiotic for treatment of community-acquired bacterial pneumonia (CAP) should include any medication from one of the following four drug classes: Fluoroquinolones, Macrolides, Doxycycline, Beta Lactam with Macrolide or Doxycycline (as defined by current ATS/IDSA guidelines). **Denominator:** All patients 18 years and older with the diagnosis of community-acquired bacterial pneumonia **Exclusion(s):** Documentation of medical, patient, or system reason(s) for not prescribing an antibiotic **Percentage** of patients aged 18 years and older with the diagnosis of community-acquired bacterial pneumonia with an appropriate empiric antibiotic prescribed **Reporting Instructions:** For patients with appropriate exclusion criteria, report 4045F with modifier 1P, 2P, or 3P◀	▶4045F◀	▶Appropriate empiric antibiotic prescribed◀

▶[1]Physician Consortium for Performance Improvement: www.physicianconsortium.org◀

[2]National Committee on Quality Assurance (NCQA): Health Employer Data Information Set (HEDIS®), www.ncqa.org

[3]Joint Commission on Accreditation of Healthcare Organizations (JCAHO), ORYX Initiative Performance Measures: www.jcaho.org/pms

[4]National Diabetes Quality Improvement Alliance: www.nationaldiabetesalliance.org

▶[5]Joint measure from the Physician Consortium for Performance Improvement, www.physicianconsortium.org, and National Committee on Quality Assurance (NCQA), www.ncqa.org◀

▶[6]The Society of Thoracic Surgeons, www.sts.org, and National Quality Forum, www.qualityforum.org◀

Brief Description of Performance Measure & Source and Reporting Instructions	CPT Code(s)	Code Descriptor
►**End-Stage Renal Disease (ESRD)**◄		
►**Kt/V Measurement for Hemodialysis**[1]—Number of calendar months during the reporting year in which patient with a diagnosis of ESRD 18 years and older and receiving hemodialysis has a Kt/V measurement performed **Numerator:** Number of calendar months during the reporting year a Kt/V measurement was performed on a patient receiving hemodialysis **Denominator**: Number of calendar months where ESRD patient 18 years of age and older was receiving hemodialysis **Exclusion Criteria**: Documentation of medical or patient reason(s) for not having a Kt/V measurement performed during months when hemodialysis received **Percentage** of calendar months during the reporting year in which patients aged 18 years and older with a diagnosis of ESRD and receiving hemodialysis had a Kt/V measurement performed **Reporting Instructions:** Report 4052F or 4053F or 4054F for ESRD patient receiving hemodialysis. Report 3082F or 3083F or 3084F for the corresponding Kt/V measurement. Report during the calendar month when patient is receiving hemodialysis. For patient with appropriate exclusion criteria, report 3082F or 3083F or 3084F with modifier 1P or 2P◄	►3082F 3083F 3084F **Denominator Codes:** 4052F 4053F 4054F◄	►Kt/V < 1.2 (Clearance of urea [Kt]/volume [V]) Kt/V ≥ 1.2 and ≤ 1.7 (Clearance of urea [Kt]/volume [V]) Kt/V ≥ 1.7 (Clearance of urea [Kt]/volume [V]) Hemodialysis via functioning arterio-venous (AV) fistula Hemodialysis via functioning arterio-venous (AV) graft Hemodialysis via catheter◄
►**Plan of Care for Inadequate Hemodialysis**[1]—Whether or not there was a documented plan of care for each Kt/V < 1.2 for a patient aged 18 years and older with a diagnosis of ESRD and receiving hemodialysis during the reporting year **Numerator:** Documented plan of care for each episode of Kt/V < 1.2 during the reporting year Plan of care, for example, may include checking for adequacy of the AV access, increasing the blood flow, increasing the dialyzer size, or increasing the time of dialysis sessions **Denominator:** Every episode of Kt/V < 1.2 for all patients 18 years of age and older with a diagnosis of ESRD and receiving hemodialysis **Percentage** of episodes of Kt/V < 1.2 for patients aged 18 years and older with a diagnosis of ESRD receiving hemodialysis who had a documented plan of care during the reporting year **Reporting Instructions:** If Kt/V < 1.2, report 3082F. If plan of care is documented, also report 0505F. There are no exclusions for this measure; modifiers 1P, 2P, and 3P may not be used◄	►0505F **Denominator Codes:** 3082F◄	►Hemodialysis plan of care documented Kt/V < 1.2 (Clearance of urea [Kt]/volume [V])◄
►**AV Fistula**[1]—Whether or not a patient aged 18 years and older with a diagnosis of ESRD and receiving hemodialysis has a functioning AV fistula or is referred for an AV fistula at least once during the reporting year **Numerator:** Patients who have a functioning AV fistula or are referred for an AV fistula at least once during the reporting year **Denominator:** All patients aged 18 years and older with a diagnosis of ESRD and receiving hemodialysis **Exclusion Criteria**: Documentation of functioning AV graft; documentation of medical reason(s) for not having an AV fistula or not being referred for an AV fistula; documentation of patient reason(s) for not having an AV fistula or not being referred for an AV fistula	►4051F **Denominator Codes:** 4052F 4053F	►Referred for an arterio-venous (AV) fistula Hemodialysis via functioning arterio-venous (AV) fistula Hemodialysis via functioning arterio-venous (AV) graft

(continued)

►[1]Physician Consortium for Performance Improvement: www.physicianconsortium.org◄

[2]National Committee on Quality Assurance (NCQA): Health Employer Data Information Set (HEDIS®), www.ncqa.org

[3]Joint Commission on Accreditation of Healthcare Organizations (JCAHO), ORYX Initiative Performance Measures: www.jcaho.org/pms

[4]National Diabetes Quality Improvement Alliance: www.nationaldiabetesalliance.org

►[5]Joint measure from the Physician Consortium for Performance Improvement, www.physicianconsortium.org, and National Committee on Quality Assurance (NCQA), www.ncqa.org◄

►[6]The Society of Thoracic Surgeons, www.sts.org, and National Quality Forum, www.qualityforum.org◄

Brief Description of Performance Measure & Source and Reporting Instructions	CPT Code(s)	Code Descriptor
►End-Stage Renal Disease (ESRD)◄, cont'd		
Percentage of patients aged 18 years of age and older with a diagnosis of ESRD and receiving hemodialysis who have a functioning AV fistula or are referred for an AV fistula at least once during the reporting year **Reporting Instructions:** Report 4052F, 4053F or 4054F to specify the type of access for each patient receiving hemodialysis For patient receiving hemodialysis via a catheter, report 4051F if referred for an AV fistula For patient receiving hemodialysis via AV graft, reporting 4053F will exclude patient from measure, 1P or 2P is not required. For patient with medical or patient exclusion criteria, report 4051F with modifier 1P or 2P◄	4054F◄	Hemodialysis via catheter◄
►**Kt/V Measurement for Peritoneal Dialysis**[1]—Whether or not a patient aged 18 years and older with a diagnosis of ESRD and receiving peritoneal dialysis had a Kt/V measurement at least during the reporting year **Numerator:** Patients who had a Kt/V measurement at least twice during the reporting year **Denominator:** Patients aged 18 years and older with a diagnosis of ESRD and receiving peritoneal dialysis **Exclusion Criteria:** Documentation of medical reason(s) for not having a Kt/V measurement performed at least twice during the reporting year; documentation of patient reason(s) for not receiving a Kt/V measurement performed at least twice during the reporting year **Percentage** of patients aged 18 years and older with a diagnosis of ESRD and receiving peritoneal dialysis who had a Kt/V measurement at least twice during the reporting year **Reporting Instructions:** Report 4055F for patient receiving peritoneal dialysis. If Kt/V measurement performed, also report 3082F or 3083F or 3084F. For patient with appropriate exclusion criteria, report 3082F or 3083F or 3084F with modifier 1P or 2P◄	►3082F 3083F 3084F **Denominator Code:** 4055F◄	►Kt/V <1.2 (Clearance of urea [Kt]/volume [V]) Kt/V ≥ 1.2 and ≤ 1.7 (Clearance of urea [Kt]/volume [V]) Kt/V ≥ 1.7 (Clearance of urea [Kt]/volume [V]) Patient receiving peritoneal dialysis◄
►**Plan of Care for Inadequate Peritoneal Dialysis**[1]—Whether or not there was a documented plan of care for each episode of Kt/V < 1.7 for a patient aged 18 years and older with a diagnosis of ESRD and receiving peritoneal dialysis during the reporting year **Numerator:** Documented plan of care for each episode of Kt/V < 1.7 during the reporting year Plan of care may, for example, include assessing for non-adherence with the peritoneal prescription, sampling, and collection; assessing for error in the peritoneal dialysis prescription and/or inadequate monitoring of the delivered dose; performing peritoneal equilibrium testing; assessing for inadequate patient education; increasing the exchange volume; or increasing the number of exchanges per 24 hours **Denominator:** Every episode of Kt/V < 1.7 for all patients aged 18 years and older with a diagnosis of ESRD and receiving peritoneal dialysis **Percentage** of episodes of Kt/V < 1.7 for patients aged 18 years and older with a diagnosis of ESRD and receiving peritoneal dialysis who had a documented plan of care during the reporting year **Reporting Instructions:** If Kt/V < 1.7, report code 3082F or 3083F. If patient plan of care is documented, also report 0507F. There are no exclusions for this measure; modifiers 1P, 2P, and 3P may not be used.◄	►0507F **Denominator Codes:** 3082F 3083F◄	►Peritoneal dialysis plan of care documented Kt/V < 1.2 (Clearance of urea [Kt]/volume [V]) Kt/V ≥ 1.2 and ≤ 1.7 (Clearance of urea [Kt]/volume [V])◄

►[1]Physician Consortium for Performance Improvement: www.physicianconsortium.org◄
[2]National Committee on Quality Assurance (NCQA): Health Employer Data Information Set (HEDIS®), www.ncqa.org
[3]Joint Commission on Accreditation of Healthcare Organizations (JCAHO), ORYX Initiative Performance Measures: www.jcaho.org/pms
[4]National Diabetes Quality Improvement Alliance: www.nationaldiabetesalliance.org
►[5]Joint measure from the Physician Consortium for Performance Improvement, www.physicianconsortium.org, and National Committee on Quality Assurance (NCQA), www.ncqa.org◄
►[6]The Society of Thoracic Surgeons, www.sts.org, and National Quality Forum, www.qualityforum.org◄

Brief Description of Performance Measure & Source and Reporting Instructions	CPT Code(s)	Code Descriptor
►Eye Care (EC)◄		
►**Primary Open-Angle Glaucoma: Optic Nerve Evaluation**[5] (Measure #1)—Whether or not the patient aged 18 years and older with a diagnosis of primary open-angle glaucoma had an optic nerve head evaluation during one or more office visits within 12 months **Numerator:** Patients who have an optic nerve head evaluation during one or more office visits within 12 months **Denominator:** All patients aged 18 years and older with a diagnosis of primary open-angle glaucoma **Exclusion Criteria:** Documentation of medical reason(s) for not performing an optic nerve head evaluation **Percentage** of patients aged 18 years and older with a diagnosis of primary open-angle glaucoma who have an optic nerve head evaluation during one or more office visits within 12 months **Reporting Instructions:** For patients with appropriate exclusion criteria, report 2027F with modifier 1P. Modifier 1P may also be used if physician is asked to report on this measure but is not the physician providing the primary management of primary open angle glaucoma◄	►2027F◄	►Optic nerve head evaluation performed◄
►**Age-Related Eye Disease Study (AREDS): AREDS Formulation Prescribed/ Recommended**[5] (Measure #2)—Whether or not the patient aged 50 years and older with a diagnosis of age-related macular degeneration had the AREDS formulation prescribed/ recommended within 12 months **Numerator:** Patients who had the AREDS formulation prescribed/recommended within 12 months **Denominator:** All patients aged 50 years and older with a diagnosis of age-related macular degeneration **Exclusion Criteria:** Documentation of medical reason(s) for not prescribing/ recommending antioxidant vitamin or mineral supplements the AREDS formulation (eg, mild AMD, patient smokes, patient does not meet criteria for antioxidant vitamin or mineral supplements as outlined in the AREDS) **Percentage** of patients aged 50 years and older with a diagnosis of age-related macular degeneration who had the AREDS formulation prescribed/recommended within 12 months **Reporting Instructions:** For patients with appropriate exclusion criteria, report 4007F with modifier 1P. Report 4007F with 1P modifier for patient with mild AMD. Modifier 1P may be used if physician is asked to report on this measure but is not the physician providing the primary management of AMD◄	►4007F	►Age-Related Eye Disease Study (AREDS) formulation prescribed or recommended◄
►**Age-Related Macular Degeneration: Dilated Macular Examination**[5] (Measure #3)—Whether or not the patient aged 50 years and older with a diagnosis of age-related macular degeneration had a dilated macular examination performed which included documentation of the presence or absence of macular thickening or hemorrhage AND the level of macular degeneration severity during one or more office visits within 12 months **Numerator:** Patients who had a dilated macular examination performed which included documentation of the presence or absence of macular thickening or hemorrhage AND the level of macular degeneration severity during one or more office visits within 12 months **Denominator:** All patients aged 50 years and older with a diagnosis of age-related macular degeneration (continued)	►2019F◄	►Dilated macular exam performed, including documentation of the presence or absence of macular thickening or hemorrhage AND the level of macular degeneration severity◄

►[1]Physician Consortium for Performance Improvement: www.physicianconsortium.org◄

[2]National Committee on Quality Assurance (NCQA): Health Employer Data Information Set (HEDIS®), www.ncqa.org

[3]Joint Commission on Accreditation of Healthcare Organizations (JCAHO), ORYX Initiative Performance Measures: www.jcaho.org/pms

[4]National Diabetes Quality Improvement Alliance: www.nationaldiabetesalliance.org

►[5]Joint measure from the Physician Consortium for Performance Improvement, www.physicianconsortium.org, and National Committee on Quality Assurance (NCQA), www.ncqa.org◄

►[6]The Society of Thoracic Surgeons, www.sts.org, and National Quality Forum, www.qualityforum.org◄

Brief Description of Performance Measure & Source and Reporting Instructions	CPT Code(s)	Code Descriptor
►Eye Care (EC)◄, cont'd		
Exclusion Criteria: Documentation of medical or patient reason(s) for not performing a dilated macular examination **Percentage** of patients aged 50 years and older with a diagnosis of age-related macular degeneration who had a dilated macular examination performed which included documentation of the presence or absence of macular thickening or hemorrhage AND the level of macular degeneration severity during one or more office visits within 12 months **Reporting Instructions:** For patient with appropriate exclusion criteria, report 2019F with modifier 1P or 2P Modifier 1P may also be used if physician is asked to report on this measure but is not the physician providing the primary management of AMD◄		
►**Cataracts: Assessment of Visual Functional Status**[5] (Measure #4)—Whether or not the patient aged 18 years and older with a diagnosis of cataract(s) was assessed for visual functional status during one or more office visits within 12 months **Numerator:** Patients who were assessed for visual functional status during one or more office visits within 12 months Medical record must include: Documentation that patient is operating well with vision or not operating well with vision based on discussion with the patient OR Documentation of use of a standardized scale or completion of an assessment questionnaire (eg, VF-14, ADVS [Activities of Daily Vision Scale], or VFQ [Visual Function Questionnaire]) **Denominator:** All patients aged 18 years and older with a diagnosis of cataract(s) **Exclusion Criteria:** Documentation of medical reason(s) for not assessing for visual functional status **Percentage** of patients aged 18 years and older with a diagnosis of cataract(s) who were assessed for visual functional status during one or more office visits within 12 months **Reporting Instructions:** For patient with appropriate exclusion criteria, report 1055F with modifier 1P Modifier 1P may be used if physician is asked to report on this measure but is not the physician providing the primary management for cataract(s)◄	►1055F◄	►Visual functional status assessed◄
►**Cataracts: Documentation of Presurgical Axial Length, Corneal Power Measurement and Method of Intraocular Lens Power Calculation**[5] (Measure #5)—Whether or not the patient aged 18 years and older who had cataract surgery had documentation of presurgical axial length, corneal power measurement and method of intraocular lens power calculation performed and documented within six months prior to the procedure **Numerator:** Patients who had the presurgical axial length, corneal power measurement and method of intraocular lens power calculation performed and documented within six months prior to the procedure **Denominator:** All patients aged 18 years and older who had cataract surgery **Exclusion Criteria:** Documentation of medical reason(s) for not performing the pre-surgical axial length, corneal power measurement and method of intraocular lens power calculation (continued)	►3073F◄	►Pre-surgical (cataract) axial length, corneal power measurement and method of intraocular lens power calculation documented (must be performed within six months prior to surgery) ◄

►[1]Physician Consortium for Performance Improvement: www.physicianconsortium.org◄
[2]National Committee on Quality Assurance (NCQA): Health Employer Data Information Set (HEDIS®), www.ncqa.org
[3]Joint Commission on Accreditation of Healthcare Organizations (JCAHO), ORYX Initiative Performance Measures: www.jcaho.org/pms
[4]National Diabetes Quality Improvement Alliance: www.nationaldiabetesalliance.org
►[5]Joint measure from the Physician Consortium for Performance Improvement, www.physicianconsortium.org, and National Committee on Quality Assurance (NCQA), www.ncqa.org◄
►[6]The Society of Thoracic Surgeons, www.sts.org, and National Quality Forum, www.qualityforum.org◄

Brief Description of Performance Measure & Source and Reporting Instructions	CPT Code(s)	Code Descriptor
►Eye Care (EC)◄, cont'd		
Percentage of patients aged 18 years and older who had cataract surgery who had documentation of pre-surgical axial length, corneal power measurement and method of intraocular lens power calculation performed and documented within six months prior to the procedure **Reporting Instructions:** For patients with appropriate exclusion criteria, report 3073F with modifier 1P◄		
►**Cataracts: Presurgical Dilated Fundus Evaluation**[5] (Measure #6)—Whether or not the patient aged 18 years and older who had cataract surgery had a dilated fundus evaluation performed within six months prior to the procedure **Numerator:** Patients who had a dilated fundus evaluation performed within six months prior to the procedure **Denominator:** All patients aged 18 years and older who had cataract surgery **Exclusion Criteria:** Documentation of patient reason(s) for not performing a dilated fundus evaluation **Percentage** of patients aged 18 years and older who had cataract surgery who had a dilated fundus evaluation performed within six months prior to the procedure **Reporting Instructions:** Report 2020F when presurgical dilated fundus evaluation performed; for patients with appropriate exclusion criteria, report 2020F with modifier 2P◄	►2020F◄	►Dilated fundus evaluation performed within six months prior to cataract surgery◄
►**Diabetic Retinopathy: Documentation of Presence or Absence of Macular Edema and Level of Severity of Retinopathy**[5] (Measure #7)—Whether or not the patient aged 18 years and older with a diagnosis of diabetic retinopathy had a dilated macular or fundus exam performed which included documentation of the level of severity of retinopathy AND the presence or absence of macular edema during one or more office visits within 12 months **Numerator:** Patients who had a dilated macular or fundus exam performed which included documentation of the level of severity of retinopathy AND the presence or absence of macular edema during one or more office visits within 12 months Medical record must include: Documentation of the level of severity of retinopathy (eg background diabetic retinopathy, proliferative diabetic retinopathy, nonproliferative diabetic retinopathy) AND Documentation of whether macular edema was present or absent **Denominator:** All patients aged 18 years and older with a diagnosis of diabetic retinopathy **Exclusion Criteria:** Documentation of medical or patient reason(s) for not receiving a dilated macular or fundus examination **Percentage** of patients aged 18 years and older with a diagnosis of diabetic retinopathy who had a dilated macular or fundus exam performed which included documentation of the level of severity of retinopathy AND the presence or absence of macular edema during one or more office visits within 12 months **Reporting Instructions:** For patients with appropriate exclusion criteria, report 2021F with modifier 1P or 2P Modifier 1P may be used if physician is asked to report on this measure but is not the physician providing the primary management of diabetic retinopathy◄ <div align="center">(continued)</div>	►2021F◄	►Dilated macular or fundus exam performed, including documentation of the presence or absence of macular edema AND level of severity of retinopathy◄

►[1]Physician Consortium for Performance Improvement: www.physicianconsortium.org◄

[2]National Committee on Quality Assurance (NCQA): Health Employer Data Information Set (HEDIS®), www.ncqa.org

[3]Joint Commission on Accreditation of Healthcare Organizations (JCAHO), ORYX Initiative Performance Measures: www.jcaho.org/pms

[4]National Diabetes Quality Improvement Alliance: www.nationaldiabetesalliance.org

►[5]Joint measure from the Physician Consortium for Performance Improvement, www.physicianconsortium.org, and National Committee on Quality Assurance (NCQA), www.ncqa.org◄

►[6]The Society of Thoracic Surgeons, www.sts.org, and National Quality Forum, www.qualityforum.org◄

Brief Description of Performance Measure & Source and Reporting Instructions	CPT Code(s)	Code Descriptor
►**Eye Care (EC)◄, cont'd**		
►**Diabetic Retinopathy: Communication with the Physician Managing Ongoing Diabetes Care**[5] (Measure #8)—Whether or not the patient aged 18 years and older with a diagnosis of diabetic retinopathy who had a dilated macular or fundus exam performed had documented communication to the physician who manages the ongoing care of the patient with diabetes regarding the findings of the dilated macular or fundus exam at least once within 12 months **Numerator:** Patients with documentation, at least once within 12 months, of communication of the findings of the dilated macular or fundus exam to the physician who manages the patient's diabetic care Documentation in the medical record indicating that the results of the macular or fundus exam were communicated (eg, verbally, or by letter) with the physician managing the patient's diabetic care OR A copy of a letter in the medical record to the physician managing the patient's diabetic care outlining the findings of the dilated macular or fundus exam. **Denominator:** All patients aged 18 years and older with a diagnosis of diabetic retinopathy who had a dilated macular or fundus exam performed **Exclusion Criteria:** Documentation of medical reason(s) for not communicating the findings of the macular or fundus exam to the physician who manages the ongoing care of the patient with diabetes Documentation of patient reason(s) for not communicating the findings of the macular or fundus exam to the physician who manages the ongoing care of the patient with diabetes **Percentage** of patients aged 18 years and older with a diagnosis of diabetic retinopathy who had a dilated macular or fundus exam performed with documented communication to the physician who manages the ongoing care of the patient with diabetes regarding the findings of the dilated macular or fundus exam at least once within 12 months **Reporting Instructions:** Report 2021F for each patient who had a dilated macular or fundus exam performed meeting the denominator inclusion. Do not report 5010F without a modifier unless reporting 2021F. Also report 5010F where findings of dilated macular or fundus exam communicated to the physician managing the diabetes care; for patients with appropriate exclusion criteria, report 5010F with modifier 1P or 2P. Modifier 1P may be used if physician is asked to report on this measure but is not the physician providing the primary management of diabetic retinopathy.◄	►**5010F◄** **Denominator Code:** ►**2021F◄**	►Findings of dilated macular or fundus exam communicated to the physician managing the diabetes care Dilated macular or fundus exam performed, including documentation of the presence or absence of macular edema AND level of severity of retinopathy◄
►**Gastroesophageal Reflux Disease (GERD)◄**		
►**Assessment for Alarm Symptoms**[5] (Measure #1)—Whether or not the patient aged 18 years and older with diagnosis of GERD, seen for an initial evaluation, was assessed for the presence or absence of the following alarm symptoms: involuntary weight loss, dysphagia, and GI bleeding **Numerator:** Patients who were assessed for the presence or absence of the following alarm symptoms: involuntary weight loss, dysphagia, and GI bleeding **Denominator:** All patients aged 18 years and older with the diagnosis of GERD, seen for an initial evaluation **Exclusion(s):** Documentation of medical reason(s) for not assessing for alarm symptoms **Percentage** of patients aged 18 years and older with a diagnosis of GERD, seen for an initial evaluation, who were assessed for the presence or absence of the following alarm symptoms: involuntary weight loss, dysphagia, and GI bleeding **Reporting Instructions:** Report either 1070F or 1071F when alarm symptoms assessed. For patient with appropriate exclusion criteria, report 1070F with modifier 1P◄	►**1070F** **1071F◄**	►Alarm symptoms (involuntary weight loss, dysphagia, or gastrointestinal bleeding) assessed; none present Alarm symptoms (involuntary weight loss, dysphagia, or gastrointestinal bleeding) assessed; one or more present◄

►[1]Physician Consortium for Performance Improvement: www.physicianconsortium.org◄

[2]National Committee on Quality Assurance (NCQA): Health Employer Data Information Set (HEDIS®), www.ncqa.org

[3]Joint Commission on Accreditation of Healthcare Organizations (JCAHO), ORYX Initiative Performance Measures: www.jcaho.org/pms

[4]National Diabetes Quality Improvement Alliance: www.nationaldiabetesalliance.org

►[5]Joint measure from the Physician Consortium for Performance Improvement, www.physicianconsortium.org, and National Committee on Quality Assurance (NCQA), www.ncqa.org◄

►[6]The Society of Thoracic Surgeons, www.sts.org, and National Quality Forum, www.qualityforum.org◄

Brief Description of Performance Measure & Source and Reporting Instructions	CPT Code(s)	Code Descriptor
►Gastroesophageal Reflux Disease (GERD)◄, cont'd		
►**Upper endoscopy for patients with alarm symptoms**[5] (Measure #2)—Whether or not the patient aged 18 years and older with a diagnosis of GERD, seen for an initial evaluation, with documentation of at least one alarm symptom was either referred for upper endoscopy or had an upper endoscopy performed **Numerator:** Patients who were either referred for an upper endoscopy or had an upper endoscopy performed **Denominator:** All patients aged 18 years and older with a diagnosis of GERD, seen for an initial evaluation, with documentation of at least one alarm symptom (*involuntary weight loss, dysphagia, or GI bleeding*) **Exclusion(s):** Documentation of medical, patient, or system reason(s) for not referring for or not performing an upper endoscopy **Percentage** of patients aged 18 years and older with a diagnosis of GERD, seen for an initial evaluation, with at least one alarm symptom, who were either referred for an upper endoscopy or had an upper endoscopy performed **Reporting Instructions:** Report 1070F or 1071F for each patient. If patient had documentation of at least one GERD alarm symptom and had upper endoscopy performed, report 3130F or the corresponding Category I code. If patient had documentation of at least one GERD alarm symptom and was referred for upper endoscopy, report 3132F. For patient with appropriate exclusion criteria, report either 3130F or 3132F with modifier 1P, 2P, or 3P◄	►**3130F** 3132F **Category I Codes:** **43234, 43235, 43236, 43250, 43251, 43258** **Denominator Codes:** 1070F 1071F◄	►Upper gastrointestinal endoscopy performed Documentation of referral for upper gastrointestinal endoscopy Alarm symptoms (involuntary weight loss, dysphagia, or gastrointestinal bleeding) assessed; none present Alarm symptoms (involuntary weight loss, dysphagia, or gastrointestinal bleeding) assessed; one or more present◄
►**Biopsy for Barrett's Esophagus**[5] (Measure #3)—Whether or not the patient aged 18 years and older with a diagnosis of GERD or heartburn whose endoscopy report indicates a suspicion of Barrett's esophagus had a forceps esophageal biopsy performed **Numerator:** Patients who had a forceps esophageal biopsy performed **Denominator:** All patients aged 18 years and older with a diagnosis of GERD or heartburn whose endoscopy report indicates a suspicion of Barrett's esophagus **Exclusion(s):** Documentation of medical reason(s) for not performing a forceps esophageal biopsy **Percentage** of patients aged 18 years and older with a diagnosis of GERD or heartburn whose endoscopy report indicates a suspicion of Barrett's esophagus who had a forceps esophageal biopsy performed **Reporting Instructions:** This measure should be reported by the physician performing the endoscopy. Report 3140F or 3141F for each patient. If endoscopy report included documentation that Barrett's esophagus was suspected, also report 3150F if patient had esophageal biopsy performed. For patient with appropriate exclusion criteria, report 3150F with modifier 1P◄	►**3150F** **Denominator Codes:** 3140F 3141F◄	►Forceps esophageal biopsy performed Upper gastrointestinal endoscopy report indicates suspicion of Barrett's esophagus Upper gastrointestinal endoscopy report indicates no suspicion of Barrett's esophagus◄
►**Barium swallow – inappropriate use**[5] (Measure #5)—Whether or not the patient aged 18 years and older seen for an initial evaluation of GERD did not have a Barium swallow test ordered **Numerator:** Patients who did not have Barium swallow test ordered **Denominator:** All patients aged 18 years and older seen for an initial evaluation of GERD **Exclusion(s):** Documentation of medical reason(s) for ordering a Barium swallow test (continued)	►**3142F** 3200F◄	►Barium swallow test ordered Barium swallow test not ordered◄

►[1]Physician Consortium for Performance Improvement: www.physicianconsortium.org◄

[2]National Committee on Quality Assurance (NCQA): Health Employer Data Information Set (HEDIS®), www.ncqa.org

[3]Joint Commission on Accreditation of Healthcare Organizations (JCAHO), ORYX Initiative Performance Measures: www.jcaho.org/pms

[4]National Diabetes Quality Improvement Alliance: www.nationaldiabetesalliance.org

►[5]Joint measure from the Physician Consortium for Performance Improvement, www.physicianconsortium.org, and National Committee on Quality Assurance (NCQA), www.ncqa.org◄

►[6]The Society of Thoracic Surgeons, www.sts.org, and National Quality Forum, www.qualityforum.org◄

Brief Description of Performance Measure & Source and Reporting Instructions	CPT Code(s)	Code Descriptor
►**Gastroesophageal Reflux Disease (GERD)◄, cont'd**		
Percentage of patients aged 18 years and older seen for an initial evaluation of GERD who did not have a Barium swallow test ordered **Reporting Instructions:** If barium swallow test was ordered at initial evaluation for GERD, report 3142F. If barium swallow was not ordered at initial evaluation, report 3200F. If there is documentation that supports the reason for ordering a barium swallow, report 3142F with modifier 1P◄		
►**Geriatrics (GER)◄**		
►**Medication Reconciliation**[5] (Measure #1)—Whether or not the patient aged 65 years and older discharged from any inpatient facility (eg, hospital, skilled nursing facility, or rehabilitation facility) and seen within 60 days following discharge in the office by the physician providing on-going care had a reconciliation of the discharge medications with the current medication list in the outpatient medical record documented **Numerator:** Patients who had a reconciliation of the discharge medications with the current medication list in the outpatient medical record documented **Denominator:** All patients aged 65 years and older discharged from any inpatient facility (eg, hospital, skilled nursing facility, or rehabilitation facility) and seen within 60 days following discharge in the office by the physician providing on-going care **Exclusion(s):** None **Percentage** of patients aged 65 years and older discharged from any inpatient facility (eg, hospital, skilled nursing facility, or rehabilitation facility) and seen within 60 days following discharge in the office by the physician providing on-going care who had a reconciliation of the discharge medications with the current medication list in the medical record documented **Reporting Instructions:** Report only for patients who were discharged from an inpatient facility (eg hospital, skilled nursing facility, or rehabilitation facility) within the last 60 days. If there is documentation of reconcilation of discharge medications with the current medication list, report 1111F. There are no exclusions; modifiers 1P, 2P, and 3P may not be used◄	►**1111F** **Denominator Code:** **1110F◄**	►Discharge medications reconciled with the current medication list in outpatient medical record Patient discharged from an inpatient facility (eg hospital, skilled nursing facility, or rehabilitation facility) within the last 60 days◄
►**Advance Care Plan**[5] (Measure #2)—Whether or not the patient aged 65 years and older had documentation of a surrogate decision maker or advance care plan in the medical record **Numerator:** Patients with documentation of a surrogate decision maker or advance care plan in the medical record **Denominator:** All patients aged 65 years and older **Exclusion(s):** Documentation of patient reason(s) for not documenting a surrogate decision maker or advance care plan in the medical record (eg, patient does not wish to discuss advance care planning) **Percentage** of patients aged 65 years and older with documentation of a surrogate decision maker or advance directive in the medical record **Reporting Instructions:** For patient with appropriate exclusion criteria, report 1080F with modifier 2P◄	►**1080F◄**	►Surrogate decision maker or advance care plan documented in the medical record◄

►[1]Physician Consortium for Performance Improvement: www.physicianconsortium.org◄

[2]National Committee on Quality Assurance (NCQA): Health Employer Data Information Set (HEDIS®), www.ncqa.org

[3]Joint Commission on Accreditation of Healthcare Organizations (JCAHO), ORYX Initiative Performance Measures: www.jcaho.org/pms

[4]National Diabetes Quality Improvement Alliance: www.nationaldiabetesalliance.org

►[5]Joint measure from the Physician Consortium for Performance Improvement, www.physicianconsortium.org, and National Committee on Quality Assurance (NCQA), www.ncqa.org◄

►[6]The Society of Thoracic Surgeons, www.sts.org, and National Quality Forum, www.qualityforum.org◄

Brief Description of Performance Measure & Source and Reporting Instructions	CPT Code(s)	Code Descriptor
►Geriatrics (GER)◄, cont'd		
►**Assessment of Presence or Absence of Urinary Incontinence in Women Aged 65 Years and Older**[5] (Measure #3)—Whether or not the female patient aged 65 years and older was assessed for the presence or absence of urinary incontinence within 12 months **Numerator:** Patients who were assessed for the presence or absence of urinary incontinence within 12 months Urinary incontinence is defined as any involuntary leakage of urine **Denominator:** All female patients aged 65 years and older **Exclusion(s):** Documentation of medical reason(s) for not assessing for the presence or absence of urinary incontinence **Percentage** of female patients aged 65 years and older who were assessed for the presence or absence of urinary incontinence within 12 months **Reporting Instructions:** For patient with appropriate exclusion criteria, report 1090F with modifier 1P.◄	►1090F◄	►Presence or absence of urinary incontinence assessed◄
►**Characterization of Urinary Incontinence in Women Aged 65 Years and Older**[5] (Measure #4)—Whether or not the female patient aged 65 years and older with a diagnosis of urinary incontinence whose urinary incontinence was characterized at least once within 12 months **Numerator:** Patients whose urinary incontinence was characterized (may include one or more of the following: frequency, volume, timing, type of symptoms or how bothersome to the patient) at least once within 12 months **Denominator:** All female patients aged 65 years and older with a diagnosis of urinary incontinence **Exclusion(s):** None **Percentage** of female patients aged 65 years and older with a diagnosis of urinary incontinence whose urinary incontinence was characterized at least once within 12 months **Reporting Instructions:** There are no exclusions for this measure; modifiers 1P, 2P, and 3P may not be used.◄	►1091F◄	►Urinary incontinence characterized (eg frequency, volume, timing, type of symptoms, how bothersome)◄
►**Plan of Care for Urinary Incontinence in Women Aged 65 Years and Older**[5] (Measure #5)—Whether or not the female patient aged 65 years and older with a diagnosis of urinary incontinence had a documented plan of care for urinary incontinence at least once within 12 months **Numerator:** Patients with a documented plan of care for urinary incontinence at least once within 12 months **Definition:** Plan of care may include behavioral interventions (eg, bladder training, pelvic floor muscle training, prompted voiding), referral to specialist, surgical treatment, re-assess at follow-up visit, lifestyle interventions, addressing comorbid factors, modifications or discontinuation of medications contributing to urinary incontinence, or pharmacologic therapy **Denominator:** All female patients aged 65 years and older with a diagnosis of urinary incontinence **Exclusion(s):** None **Percentage** of female patients aged 65 years and older with a diagnosis of urinary incontinence with a documented plan of care for urinary incontinence at least once within 12 months **Reporting Instructions:** There are no exclusions for this measure. Modifiers 1P, 2P, and 3P may not be used.◄	►0509F◄	►Urinary incontinence plan of care documented◄

►[1]Physician Consortium for Performance Improvement: www.physicianconsortium.org◄

[2]National Committee on Quality Assurance (NCQA): Health Employer Data Information Set (HEDIS®), www.ncqa.org

[3]Joint Commission on Accreditation of Healthcare Organizations (JCAHO), ORYX Initiative Performance Measures: www.jcaho.org/pms

[4]National Diabetes Quality Improvement Alliance: www.nationaldiabetesalliance.org

►[5]Joint measure from the Physician Consortium for Performance Improvement, www.physicianconsortium.org, and National Committee on Quality Assurance (NCQA), www.ncqa.org◄

►[6]The Society of Thoracic Surgeons, www.sts.org, and National Quality Forum, www.qualityforum.org◄

Brief Description of Performance Measure & Source and Reporting Instructions	CPT Code(s)	Code Descriptor
►Geriatrics (GER)◄, cont'd		
►**Screening for Future Fall Risk**[5] (Measure #6)—Whether or not the patient aged 65 years and older was screened for future fall risk (two or more falls in the past year or any fall with injury in the past year) at least once within 12 months **Numerator:** Patients who were screened for future fall risk (patients are considered at risk for future falls if they have had two or more falls in the past year or any fall with injury in the past year) at least once within 12 months **Denominator:** All patients aged 65 years and older **Exclusion(s):** Documentation of medical reason(s) for not screening for future fall risk (eg, patient is not ambulatory) **Percentage** of patients aged 65 years and older who were screened for future fall risk at least once within 12 months **Reporting Instructions:** For patient with appropriate exclusion criteria, report either 1100F or 1101F with modifier 1P◄	►**1100F** **1101F**◄	►Patient screened for future fall risk; documentation of two or more falls in the past year or any fall with injury in the past year Patient screened for future fall risk; documentation of no falls in the past year or only one fall without injury in the past year◄
Heart Failure (HF)		
Composite Measure: Heart Failure Assessment[1] See individual measures listed below for the following: Level of activity assessed (1003F) Clinical symptoms of volume overload (excess) assessed (1004F) Blood pressure measured (2000F) Weight recorded (2001F) Clinical signs of volume overload (excess) assessed (2002F)	**0001F**	►Heart failure assessed◄
Assessment of Activity Level[1]—Number of visits with assessment of activity level per number of visits **Numerator:** Patient visits with assessment of current level of activity OR documentation of standardized scale OR completion of assessment tool (May include use of New York Heart Association Functional Classification of Congestive Heart Failure, Kansas City Cardiomyopathy Questionnaire; Minnesota™ Living with Heart Failure Questionnaire, or Guyatt's Chronic Heart Failure Questionnaire) **Denominator:** All patient visits for patients aged ≥ 18 years with heart failure **Percentage** of patient visits with assessment of activity level ►**Reporting Instructions:** There are no exclusions for this measure; modifiers 1P, 2P, and 3P may not be used◄	**1003F**	Level of activity assessed
Assessment of Clinical Symptoms of Volume Overload (Excess)[1]—Number of patient visits with assessment of clinical symptoms of volume overload (excess) per number of visits **Numerator:** Patient visits with assessment of clinical *symptoms* of volume overload (excess) Assessment for absence or presence of symptoms of volume overload must include dyspnea, orthopnea, or documentation of standardized scale or completion of assessment tool (may include New York Heart Association Functional Classification of Congestive Heart Failure, Kansas City Cardiomyopathy Questionnaire; Minnesota™ Living with Heart Failure Questionnaire, or Guyatt's Chronic Heart Failure Questionnaire) **Denominator:** All patient visits for patients aged ≥ 18 years with heart failure **Percentage** of patient visits with assessment of clinical symptoms of volume overload (excess) ►**Reporting Instructions:** There are no exclusions for this measure; modifiers 1P, 2P, and 3P may not be used◄	**1004F**	Clinical symptoms of volume overload (excess) assessed

►[1]Physician Consortium for Performance Improvement: www.physicianconsortium.org◄

[2]National Committee on Quality Assurance (NCQA): Health Employer Data Information Set (HEDIS®), www.ncqa.org

[3]Joint Commission on Accreditation of Healthcare Organizations (JCAHO), ORYX Initiative Performance Measures: www.jcaho.org/pms

[4]National Diabetes Quality Improvement Alliance: www.nationaldiabetesalliance.org

►[5]Joint measure from the Physician Consortium for Performance Improvement, www.physicianconsortium.org, and National Committee on Quality Assurance (NCQA), www.ncqa.org◄

►[6]The Society of Thoracic Surgeons, www.sts.org, and National Quality Forum, www.qualityforum.org◄

Brief Description of Performance Measure & Source and Reporting Instructions	CPT Code(s)	Code Descriptor
Heart Failure (HF), cont'd		
Blood Pressure Measurement[1]—Number of visits with blood pressure measurement recorded per number of visits **Numerator:** Patient visits with blood pressure measurement recorded **Denominator:** All patient visits for patients aged ≥ 18 years with HF **Percentage** of patient visits with a blood pressure measurement recorded ▶**Reporting Instructions:** There are no exclusions for this measure; modifiers 1P, 2P, and 3P may not be used◀	**2000F**	Blood pressure measure
Weight Measurement[1]—Number of visits with weight measurement recorded per number of visits **Numerator:** Patient visits with weight measurement recorded **Denominator:** All patient visits for patients aged ≥ 18 years with heart failure **Percentage** of patient visits with weight measurement recorded ▶**Reporting Instructions:** There are no exclusions for this measure; modifiers 1P, 2P, and 3P may not be used◀	**2001F**	Weight recorded
Assessment of Clinical Signs of Volume Overload (Excess)[1]—Number of visits with assessment of clinical *signs* of volume overload (excess) per number of visits **Numerator:** Patient visits with assessment of clinical *signs* of volume overload (excess) Assessment for presence or absence of signs of volume overload must include: peripheral edema OR Rales OR Hepatomegaly OR Ascites OR Assessment of jugular venous pressure OR S3 or S4 gallop **Denominator:** All patient visits for patients aged ≥ 18 years with heart failure **Percentage** of patient visits with assessment of clinical signs of volume overload (excess) ▶**Reporting Instructions:** There are no exclusions for this measure; modifiers 1P, 2P, and 3P may not be used◀	**2002F**	Clinical signs volume overload (excess) assessed
Left Ventricular Function (LVF) Assessment[1]—Whether or not patient has quantitative or qualitative results of LVF assessment recorded **Numerator:** Patients with quantitative or qualitative results of LVF assessment recorded **Denominator:** All patients aged ≥ 18 years with heart failure **Percentage** of patients with quantitative or qualitative results of LVF assessment recorded ▶**Reporting Instructions:** There are no exclusions for this measure; modifiers 1P, 2P, and 3P may not be used◀	**3020F**	Left ventricular function (LVF) assessment (eg, echocardiography, nuclear test, or ventriculography) documented in the medical record (Includes: Quantitative or qualitative assessment results)
Patient Education[1]—Whether or not patient education was provided **Numerator:** Patients provided with patient education at one or more visit(s) Patient education should include one or more of the following: weight monitoring; diet (sodium restriction); symptom management; physical activity; smoking cessation; medication instruction; minimizing or avoiding use of NSAIDs; referral for visiting nurse; referral for specific educational or management programs; or prognosis/end-of-life issues **Denominator:** All patients aged ≥ 18 years with heart failure and with one or more visit(s) **Denominator Inclusion(s):** Patients with one or more visit(s) **Percentage** of heart failure patients who were provided with patient education on disease management and health behavior changes during one or more visit(s) ▶**Reporting Instructions:** There are no exclusions for this measure; modifiers 1P, 2P, and 3P may not be used◀	**4003F**	Patient education, written/oral, appropriate for patients with heart failure performed

▶[1]Physician Consortium for Performance Improvement: www.physicianconsortium.org◀

[2]National Committee on Quality Assurance (NCQA): Health Employer Data Information Set (HEDIS®), www.ncqa.org

[3]Joint Commission on Accreditation of Healthcare Organizations (JCAHO), ORYX Initiative Performance Measures: www.jcaho.org/pms

[4]National Diabetes Quality Improvement Alliance: www.nationaldiabetesalliance.org

▶[5]Joint measure from the Physician Consortium for Performance Improvement, www.physicianconsortium.org, and National Committee on Quality Assurance (NCQA), www.ncqa.org◀

▶[6]The Society of Thoracic Surgeons, www.sts.org, and National Quality Forum, www.qualityforum.org◀

Brief Description of Performance Measure & Source and Reporting Instructions	CPT Code(s)	Code Descriptor
Heart Failure (HF), cont'd		
Beta-Blocker Therapy[1]—Whether or not HF patient with LVSD was prescribed beta-blocker therapy **Numerator:** Patients who were prescribed beta-blocker therapy **Denominator:** All heart failure patients ≥ 18 years of age with left ventricular ejection fraction (LVEF) < 40% or with moderately or severely depressed left ventricular systolic function **Denominator Inclusion(s):** Patients with heart failure and left ventricular systolic dysfunction (LVSD) (LVEF < 40% or with moderately or severely depressed left ventricular systolic function) **Denominator Exclusion(s):** Documentation of medical, patient, or system reason(s) for not prescribing beta-blocker therapy. **Percentage** of heart failure patients with LVSD who were prescribed beta-blocker therapy **Reporting Instructions:** Report either 3021F or 3022F for each heart failure patient. For patient with appropriate exclusion criteria, report 4006F with modifier 1P, 2P, or 3P	4006F **Denominator Codes:** 3021F 3022F	Beta-blocker therapy prescribed Left ventricular ejection fraction (LVEF) < 40% or documentation of moderately or severely depressed left ventricular systolic function Left ventricular ejection fraction (LVEF) ≥ 40% or documentation as normal or mildly depressed left ventricular systolic function
Angiotensin Converting Enzyme (ACE) Inhibitor or Angiotensin Receptor Blocker (ARB) Therapy for left ventricular systolic dysfunction (LVSD)[1]—Whether or not heart failure patients who also have LVSD were prescribed ACE inhibitor or ARB therapy **Numerator:** Patients who were prescribed ACE inhibitor or ARB therapy **Denominator Inclusion:** All heart failure patients aged ≥ 18 years with left ventricular ejection fraction (LVEF < 40% or with moderately or severely depressed left ventricular systolic function) **Denominator Exclusion(s):** Documentation of medical, patient, or system reasons for not prescribing ACE inhibitor or ARB therapy **Percentage** of heart failure patients who also have LVSD and who were prescribed ACE or ARB inhibitor **Reporting Instructions:** Report either 3021F or 3022F for each heart failure patient. For patients with appropriate exclusion criteria, report 4009F with modifier 1P, 2P, or 3P	4009F **Denominator Codes:** 3021F 3022F	Angiotensin converting enzyme (ACE) inhibitor or Angiotensin Receptor Blocker (ARB) therapy prescribed Left ventricular ejection fraction (LVEF) < 40% or documentation of moderately or severely depressed left ventricular systolic function Left ventricular ejection fraction (LVEF) ≥ 40% or documentation as normal or mildly depressed left ventricular systolic function
Warfarin Therapy for Patients With Atrial Fibrillation[1]—Whether or not heart failure patient who also has paroxysmal or chronic atrial fibrillation was prescribed warfarin therapy **Numerator:** Patients who were prescribed warfarin therapy **Denominator:** All heart failure patients aged ≥ 18 years with paroxysmal or chronic atrial fibrillation **Denominator Inclusion:** Patients with heart failure and paroxysmal or chronic atrial fibrillation **Denominator Exclusion(s):** Documentation of medical, patient, or system reason(s) for not prescribing warfarin therapy **Percentage** of heart failure patients who also have paroxysmal or chronic atrial fibrillation who were prescribed warfarin therapy **Reporting Instructions:** For patients with appropriate exclusion criteria, report 4012F with modifier 1P, 2P, or 3P	4012F	Warfarin therapy prescribed

▶[1]Physician Consortium for Performance Improvement: www.physicianconsortium.org◀

[2]National Committee on Quality Assurance (NCQA): Health Employer Data Information Set (HEDIS®), www.ncqa.org

[3]Joint Commission on Accreditation of Healthcare Organizations (JCAHO), ORYX Initiative Performance Measures: www.jcaho.org/pms

[4]National Diabetes Quality Improvement Alliance: www.nationaldiabetesalliance.org

▶[5]Joint measure from the Physician Consortium for Performance Improvement, www.physicianconsortium.org, and National Committee on Quality Assurance (NCQA), www.ncqa.org◀

▶[6]The Society of Thoracic Surgeons, www.sts.org, and National Quality Forum, www.qualityforum.org◀

Brief Description of Performance Measure & Source and Reporting Instructions	CPT Code(s)	Code Descriptor
Heart Failure (HF), cont'd		
Heart Failure Discharge Instructions[3] **Numerator:** Heart failure patients with documentation that they or their caregivers were given written discharge instructions or other educational material addressing all of the following: activity level, diet, discharge medications, follow-up appointment, weight monitoring, what to do if symptoms worsen **Denominator:** Heart failure patients discharged home **Exclusion(s):** Patients less than 18 years of age **Percentage** of hospitalized heart failure patients in the denominator who received written discharge instructions ►**Reporting Instructions:** There are no exclusions for this measure; modifiers 1P, 2P, and 3P may not be used◄	4014F	Written discharge instructions provided
Hypertension (HTN)		
Blood Pressure Measurement[1]—Number of visits with blood pressure measurement recorded per number of visits **Numerator:** Patient visits with blood pressure measurement recorded **Denominator:** All patient visits for patients aged ≥ 18 years with hypertension **Percentage** of patient visits with blood pressure recorded for patients aged ≥ 18 years ►**Reporting Instructions:** There are no exclusions for this measure; modifiers 1P, 2P, and 3P may not be used◄	2000F	Blood pressure measure
Plan of Care[1]—Number of visits with documented plan of care for hypertension per number of visits during which either systolic blood pressure ≥140 mm Hg or diastolic blood pressure ≥ 90 mm Hg **Numerator:** Patient visits with documented plan of care for hypertension Plan of care should include one or more of the following: Recheck blood pressure at specified future date, initiate or alter pharmacologic therapy, initiate or alter non-pharmacologic therapy **Denominator:** All patient visits during which patients ≥ 18 years of age diagnosed with hypertension have either systolic blood pressure ≥ 140 mm Hg or diastolic blood pressure ≥ 90 mm Hg **Percentage** of patient visits during which either systolic blood pressure ≥ 140 mm Hg or diastolic blood pressure ≥ 90 mm Hg, with documented plan of care for hypertension **Reporting Instructions:** For this measure to be met, three codes must be reported: one code for systolic blood pressure, one code for diastolic blood pressure, and the code for hypertension plan of care (4050F). If no documentation of plan of care, or patient does not have elevated blood pressure at the visit, report only two codes for corresponding systolic and diastolic blood pressure values To report most recent systolic blood pressure < 140 mmHg, see codes 3074F-3075F ►There are no exclusions for this measure; modifiers 1P, 2P, and 3P may not be used◄	4050F **Denominator Codes:** **Systolic Codes:** ►3074F 3075F◄ 3077F **Diastolic Codes:** 3078F 3079F 3080F	Hypertension plan of care documented as appropriate ►Most recent systolic blood pressure < 130 mm Hg Most recent systolic blood pressure pressure 130-139 mm Hg◄ Most recent systolic blood pressure ≥ 140 mm HG Most recent diastolic blood pressure < 80 mm Hg Most recent diastolic blood pressure 80-89 mm Hg Most recent diastolic blood pressure ≥ 90 mm Hg
►**Major Depressive Disorder (MDD)**◄		
►**Suicide Risk Assessment**[1]—Whether or not a patient aged 18 years and older with a new diagnosis or recurrent episode of MDD was assessed for suicide risk at each visit during the reporting year (continued)	►3085F	►Suicide risk assessed

►[1]Physician Consortium for Performance Improvement: www.physicianconsortium.org◄
[2]National Committee on Quality Assurance (NCQA): Health Employer Data Information Set (HEDIS®), www.ncqa.org
[3]Joint Commission on Accreditation of Healthcare Organizations (JCAHO), ORYX Initiative Performance Measures: www.jcaho.org/pms
[4]National Diabetes Quality Improvement Alliance: www.nationaldiabetesalliance.org
►[5]Joint measure from the Physician Consortium for Performance Improvement, www.physicianconsortium.org, and National Committee on Quality Assurance (NCQA), www.ncqa.org◄
►[6]The Society of Thoracic Surgeons, www.sts.org, and National Quality Forum, www.qualityforum.org◄

Brief Description of Performance Measure & Source and Reporting Instructions	CPT Code(s)	Code Descriptor
▶Major Depressive Disorder (MDD)◀, cont'd		
Numerator: Patients who had a suicide risk assessment at each visit during the reporting year **Denominator:** Patients aged 18 years and older with a new diagnosis of an initial or recurrent episode of MDD **Exclusion:** Documentation that patient is in remission (no longer meeting DSM-IV™ criteria) **Percentage** of patients aged 18 years and older with a new diagnosis or recurrent episode of MDD who had a suicide risk assessment completed at each visit during the reporting year **Reporting Instructions:** Report 3093F for each patient with a new, confirmed diagnosis of MDD. Report 3085F for assessment of suicide risk. For patient with appropriate exclusion criteria, report 3092F.◀	**Denominator Codes:** 3093F **Exclusion Code:** 3092F◀	Documentation of new diagnosis of initial or recurrent episode of major depressive disorder Major depressive disorder, in remission◀
▶**Severity Classification at Initial Visit**[1]—Whether or not a patient aged 18 years and older was classified for severity of his/her MDD during the visit in which the new diagnosis or recurrent episode was identified during the reporting year **Numerator:** Patients whose severity of MDD was classified during the visit in which the new diagnosis or recurrent episode was identified during the reporting year **Denominator:** All patients aged 18 years and older with a new diagnosis of an initial or recurrent episode of MDD **Exclusion:** None **Percentage** of patients aged 18 years and older with a new diagnosis or recurrent episode of MDD whose severity of MDD was classified during the visit in which the new diagnosis or recurrent episode was identified during the reporting year **Reporting Instructions:** Report 3093F for each patient with a new diagnosis of an initial or recurrent episode of MDD during the reporting year. Also report 3088F or 3089F or 3090F or 3091F or 3092F for the corresponding severity classification. There are no exclusions for this measure; modifiers 1P, 2P, and 3P may not be used.◀	▶**Severity Classification Codes:** 3088F 3089F 3090F 3091F 3092F **Denominator Code:** 3093F◀	 ▶Major depressive disorder, mild Major depressive disorder, moderate Major depressive disorder, severe without psychotic features Major depressive disorder, severe with psychotic features Major depressive disorder, in remission Documentation of new diagnosis of initial or recurrent episode of major depressive disorder◀
▶**Treatment: Psychotherapy, Medication Management, and/or Electroconvulsive Therapy (ECT)**[1]—Whether or not the patient aged 18 years and older with a new diagnosis or recurrent episode of MDD received therapy appropriate to his/her classification during the reporting year **Numerator:** Patients who received therapy appropriate to their classification during the reporting year *Appropriate treatment for corresponding severity classification:* **Mild MDD:** Psychotherapy OR Antidepressant medication **Moderate MDD:** Psychotherapy OR Antidepressant medication OR Psychotherapy and antidepressant medication (continued)	▶**Treatment Codes:** 4060F 4062F 4064F 4065F	 ▶Psychotherapy services provided Patient referral for psychotherapy documented Antidepressant pharmacotherapy prescribed Antipsychotic pharmacotherapy prescribed

▶[1]Physician Consortium for Performance Improvement: www.physicianconsortium.org◀
[2]National Committee on Quality Assurance (NCQA): Health Employer Data Information Set (HEDIS®), www.ncqa.org
[3]Joint Commission on Accreditation of Healthcare Organizations (JCAHO), ORYX Initiative Performance Measures: www.jcaho.org/pms
[4]National Diabetes Quality Improvement Alliance: www.nationaldiabetesalliance.org
▶[5]Joint measure from the Physician Consortium for Performance Improvement, www.physicianconsortium.org, and National Committee on Quality Assurance (NCQA), www.ncqa.org◀
▶[6]The Society of Thoracic Surgeons, www.sts.org, and National Quality Forum, www.qualityforum.org◀

Brief Description of Performance Measure & Source and Reporting Instructions	CPT Code(s)	Code Descriptor
►Major Depressive Disorder (MDD)◄, cont'd		
Severe MDD without psychotic features: Antidepressant medications OR Psychotherapy and antidepressant medications	4066F	Electroconvulsive Therapy (ECT) provided
Severe MDD with psychotic features: Antidepressant medication and antipsychotic medication OR ECT	4067F	Patient referral for electroconvulsive therapy (ECT) documented
Denominator: All patients aged 18 years and older with a new diagnosis of an initial or recurrent episode of MDD	90870	Electroconvulsive therapy
Exclusion Criteria: Documentation of medical, patient, or system reason(s) for not prescribing treatment.	**Severity Classification Codes:**	
Percentage of patients aged 18 years and older with a new diagnosis or recurrent episode of MDD who received therapy appropriate to their severity classification during the reporting year		
Reporting Instructions: Report 3093F for each patient with a new diagnosis of an initial or recurrent episode of MDD. Report one code from severity classification codes for each patient. Report all treatment codes that apply. For patient with appropriate exclusion criteria, report an appropriate treatment code with modifier 1P, 2P, or 3P.	3088F	Major depressive disorder, mild
	3089F	Major depressive disorder, moderate
Mild MDD: Report 3088F and: (a) Psychotherapy—4060F or 4062F (b) Antidepressant medication—4064F	3090F	Major depressive disorder, severe without psychotic features
Moderate MDD: Report 3089F and: (c) Psychotherapy—4060F or 4062F (d) Antidepressant medication—4064F (e) Psychotherapy and antidepressant medication—4060F or 4062F AND 4064F	3091F	Major depressive disorder, severe with psychotic features
Severe MDD without psychotic features: Report 3090F and: (f) Antidepressant medications—4064F (g) Psychotherapy and antidepressant medications—4060F or 4062F AND 4064F	3092F	Major depressive disorder, in remission
Severe MDD with psychotic features: Report 3091F and: (h) Antidepressant medication and antipsychotic medication—4064F and 4065F	**Denominator Code:**	
(i) ECT—4066F or 4067F or 90870◄	3093F◄	Documentation of new diagnosis of initial or recurrent episode of major depressive disorder◄
►Melanoma (ML)◄		
►**Patient Medical History**[5] (Measure #1)—Whether or not the patient with either a current diagnosis of cutaneous melanoma or a history of cutaneous melanoma has a medical history taken that included being asked if they have any new or changing moles at one or more office visits within 12 months **Numerator:** Patients who had a medical history taken that included being asked if they have any new or changing moles at least once within 12 months **Denominator:** All patients with a current diagnosis of cutaneous melanoma or a history of cutaneous melanoma **Exclusion(s):** Documentation of medical, patient, or system reason(s) for not asking about presence of any new or changing moles **Percentage** of patients with either a current diagnosis of cutaneous melanoma or a history of cutaneous melanoma who had a medical history taken that included being asked if they have any new or changing moles at least once within 12 months **Reporting Instructions:** For patient with appropriate exclusion criteria report 1050F with modifier 1P, 2P, or 3P◄	►1050F◄	►History obtained regarding new or changing moles◄

►[1]Physician Consortium for Performance Improvement: www.physicianconsortium.org◄
[2]National Committee on Quality Assurance (NCQA): Health Employer Data Information Set (HEDIS®), www.ncqa.org
[3]Joint Commission on Accreditation of Healthcare Organizations (JCAHO), ORYX Initiative Performance Measures: www.jcaho.org/pms
[4]National Diabetes Quality Improvement Alliance: www.nationaldiabetesalliance.org
►[5]Joint measure from the Physician Consortium for Performance Improvement, www.physicianconsortium.org, and National Committee on Quality Assurance (NCQA), www.ncqa.org◄
►[6]The Society of Thoracic Surgeons, www.sts.org, and National Quality Forum, www.qualityforum.org◄

Brief Description of Performance Measure & Source and Reporting Instructions	CPT Code(s)	Code Descriptor
▶Melanoma (ML)◀, cont'd		
▶**Complete Physical Skin Examination**[5] (Measure #2)—Whether or not the patient with either a current diagnosis of cutaneous melanoma or a history of cutaneous melanoma had a complete physical skin exam performed at one or more office visits within 12 months **Numerator:** Patients who had a complete physical skin exam performed at least once within 12 months **Denominator:** All patients with a current diagnosis of cutaneous melanoma or a history of cutaneous melanoma **Exclusion(s):** Documentation of medical, patient, or system reason(s) for not performing a complete skin exam **Percentage** of patients with either a current diagnosis of cutaneous melanoma or a history of cutaneous melanoma who had a complete physical skin exam performed at one or more office visits within 12 months **Reporting Instructions:** For patient with appropriate exclusion criteria report 2029F with modifier 1P, 2P, or 3P◀	▶2029F◀	▶Complete physical skin exam performed◀
▶**Counseling on Self-Examination**[5] (Measure #3)—Whether or not the patient with either a current diagnosis of cutaneous melanoma or a history of cutaneous melanoma was counseled at least once within 12 months to perform a self-examination for new or changing moles **Numerator:** Patients who were counseled at least once within 12 months to perform a self-examination for new or changing moles **Denominator:** All patients with a current diagnosis of cutaneous melanoma or a history of cutaneous melanoma **Exclusion(s):** Documentation of medical, patient, or system reason(s) for not counseling the patient to perform a self-examination for new or changing moles **Percentage** of patients with either a current diagnosis of cutaneous melanoma or a history of cutaneous melanoma who were counseled, at least once within 12 months, to perform a self-examination for new or changing moles **Reporting Instructions:** For patient with appropriate exclusion criteria report 5005F with modifier 1P, 2P, or 3P◀	▶5005F◀	▶Patient counseled on self-examination for new or changing moles◀
Osteoarthritis (Adult)		
Composite Measure: Osteoarthritis Assessment—See individual measures listed below for: Osteoarthritis symptoms and functional status assessed (1006F) Use of anti-inflammatory or over-the-counter (OTC) analgesic medications assessed (1007F) Initial examination of the involved joint(s) (includes visual inspection, palpation, range of motion) (2004F)	0005F	Osteoarthritis assessed
▶**Symptom and Functional Assessment**[1]—Patient visits with assessment for function and pain/number of visits **Numerator:** Patient visits with assessment for level of function and pain documented during the reporting year◀ **Denominator:** All visits for patients aged ≥ 21 years with osteoarthritis ▶**Exclusion:** None **Percentage** of osteoarthritis patient visits with assessment for function and pain during the reporting year◀ **Reporting Instructions:** Use when osteoarthritis is addressed during the patient encounter ▶There are no exclusions for this measure; modifiers 1P, 2P, and 3P may not be used◀	1006F	Osteoarthritis symptoms and functional status assessed (may include the use of a standardized scale or the completion of an assessment questionnaire, such as the SF-36, AAOS Hip & Knee Questionnaire)

▶[1]Physician Consortium for Performance Improvement: www.physicianconsortium.org◀
[2]National Committee on Quality Assurance (NCQA): Health Employer Data Information Set (HEDIS®), www.ncqa.org
[3]Joint Commission on Accreditation of Healthcare Organizations (JCAHO), ORYX Initiative Performance Measures: www.jcaho.org/pms
[4]National Diabetes Quality Improvement Alliance: www.nationaldiabetesalliance.org
▶[5]Joint measure from the Physician Consortium for Performance Improvement, www.physicianconsortium.org, and National Committee on Quality Assurance (NCQA), www.ncqa.org◀
▶[6]The Society of Thoracic Surgeons, www.sts.org, and National Quality Forum, www.qualityforum.org◀

Brief Description of Performance Measure & Source and Reporting Instructions	CPT Code(s)	Code Descriptor
Osteoarthritis (Adult), cont'd		
Assessment for Use of Anti-inflammatory or Analgesic OTC Medications[1]— Patient visits with assessment for use of anti-inflammatory or analgesic OTC medications per number of visits during the reporting year **Numerator:** Patient visits with assessment for use of anti-inflammatory or analgesic OTC medications **Denominator:** All patient visits for patients aged ≥ 21 years with osteoarthritis **Percentage** of osteoarthritis patient visits with assessment for use of anti-inflammatory or analgesic over-the-counter (OTC) medications **Reporting Instructions:** Use when osteoarthritis is addressed during the patient encounter ►There are no exclusions for this measure; modifiers 1P, 2P, and 3P may not be used◄	1007F	Use of anti-inflammatory or analgesic over-the-counter (OTC) medications for symptom relief assessed
Nonsteroidal Anti-inflammatory Drug (NSAID) Risk Assessment[1]—Whether or not patient on prescribed or OTC NSAIDs was assessed for GI/renal risk factors during the reporting year **Numerator:** Patients who were assessed for *all* of the following GI and Renal risk factors during the reporting year: • GI bleed • History of peptic ulcer disease (PUD) • Concomitant use of glucocorticoids or anticoagulants • Smoking • Significant alcohol use • Age > 65 years • Renal disease (Cr > 2.0 mg/dl) • Hypertension • Heart failure • Concomitant use of diuretic or angiotensin-converting enzyme (ACE) inhibitor **Denominator:** All patients ≥ 21 years of age with osteoarthritis on a prescribed or OTC NSAID **Percentage** of patients ≥ 21 years of age with osteoarthritis on prescribed or OTC NSAIDs who were assessed for gastrointestinal and renal risk factors during the reporting year ►**Reporting Instructions:** There are no exclusions for this measure; modifiers 1P, 2P, and 3P may not be used◄	1008F	Gastrointestinal and renal risk factors assessed for patients on prescribed or OTC non-steroidal anti-inflammatory drug (NSAID)
Physical Examination of the Involved Joint[1]—Whether or not a physical examination of the involved joint was performed during the initial visit during the reporting year **Numerator:** Patients for whom a physical examination of the involved joint was performed during the initial visit during the reporting year **Denominator:** All patients aged ≥ 21 years of age with osteoarthritis **Percentage** of patients ≥ 21 years of age with osteoarthritis for whom a physical examination of the involved joint was performed during the initial visit during the reporting year **Reporting Instructions:** Use only for initial osteoarthritis visit or for visits for new joint involvement ►There are no exclusions for this measure; modifiers 1P, 2P, and 3P may not be used◄	2004F	Initial examination of the involved joint(s) (includes visual inspection, palpation, range of motion)

►[1]Physician Consortium for Performance Improvement: www.physicianconsortium.org◄
[2]National Committee on Quality Assurance (NCQA): Health Employer Data Information Set (HEDIS®), www.ncqa.org
[3]Joint Commission on Accreditation of Healthcare Organizations (JCAHO), ORYX Initiative Performance Measures: www.jcaho.org/pms
[4]National Diabetes Quality Improvement Alliance: www.nationaldiabetesalliance.org
►[5]Joint measure from the Physician Consortium for Performance Improvement, www.physicianconsortium.org, and National Committee on Quality Assurance (NCQA), www.ncqa.org◄
►[6]The Society of Thoracic Surgeons, www.sts.org, and National Quality Forum, www.qualityforum.org◄

Brief Description of Performance Measure & Source and Reporting Instructions	CPT Code(s)	Code Descriptor
Osteoarthritis (Adult), cont'd		
Anti-inflammatory/Analgesic Therapy[1]—Patient visits during which an anti-inflammatory agent or analgesic was considered/Number of visits during the reporting year **Numerator:** Patient visits during which an anti-inflammatory agent or analgesic was considered during the reporting year **Denominator:** All patient visits for patients aged ≥ 21 years of age with osteoarthritis **Numerator Inclusion(s):** Documentation that an anti-inflammatory agent or analgesic was prescribed; Documentation of medical or patient reasons(s) for not prescribing an anti-inflammatory agent or analgesic ▶**Percentage** of visits for patients ≥21 years of age with osteoarthritis during which an anti-inflammatory agent or analgesic was considered during the reporting year◀ **Reporting Instructions:** Report 4016F alone or with modifier (1P if medical reason for not prescribing an anti-inflammatory or analgesic was documented or 2P modifier if patient reason for not prescribing an anti-inflammatory or analgesic was documented.) For this measure, the modifiers do not act as denominator exclusions, but rather demonstrate that therapy was considered and are included in the numerator when calculating the measure	**4016F**	Anti-inflammatory/analgesic agent prescribed
Gastrointestinal Prophylaxis[1]—Patient visits during which GI prophylaxis was considered/Number of visits during the reporting year **Numerator:** Patient visits during which GI prophylaxis was considered during the reporting year **Denominator:** All visits for patients aged ≥ 21 years of age with osteoarthritis on a prescribed or OTC NSAID **Numerator Inclusion(s):** Documentation that GI prophylaxis was prescribed; documentation of medical or patient reason(s) for not prescribing GI prophylaxis **Percentage** of visits for patients aged ≥ 21 years of age with osteoarthritis during which GI prophylaxis was considered during the reporting year **Reporting Instructions:** Report 4017F alone or with modifier (1P if medical reason for not prescribing GI prophylaxis was documented or 2P modifier if patient reason for not prescribing GI prophylaxis was documented). For this measure, the modifiers do not act as denominator exclusions, but rather demonstrate that therapy was considered and are included in the numerator when calculating the measure	**4017F**	Gastrointestinal prophylaxis for NSAID use prescribed
▶**Therapeutic Exercise for the Involved Joint**[1]—Patient visits during which therapeutic exercise for the hip or knee was considered/Number of visits during the reporting year◀ **Numerator:** Patient visits during which therapeutic exercise for the knee or hip was considered during the reporting year **Denominator:** All patient visits for patients ≥ 21 years of age with osteoarthritis of the hip or knee **Numerator Inclusion(s):** Documentation of medical or patient reason(s) for not instructing therapeutic exercise or prescribing physical therapy for the hip or knee; documentation that therapeutic exercise for the hip or knee was instructed; documentation that physical therapy for the hip or knee was prescribed **Percentage** of visits for patients ≥ 21 years of age with osteoarthritis of the hip or knee during which therapeutic exercise for the hip or knee (therapeutic exercise instructed or physical therapy prescribed) was considered during the reporting year (continued)	**4018F**	Therapeutic exercise for the involved joint(s) instructed or physical or occupational therapy prescribed

▶[1]Physician Consortium for Performance Improvement: www.physicianconsortium.org◀

[2]National Committee on Quality Assurance (NCQA): Health Employer Data Information Set (HEDIS®), www.ncqa.org

[3]Joint Commission on Accreditation of Healthcare Organizations (JCAHO), ORYX Initiative Performance Measures: www.jcaho.org/pms

[4]National Diabetes Quality Improvement Alliance: www.nationaldiabetesalliance.org

▶[5]Joint measure from the Physician Consortium for Performance Improvement, www.physicianconsortium.org, and National Committee on Quality Assurance (NCQA), www.ncqa.org◀

▶[6]The Society of Thoracic Surgeons, www.sts.org, and National Quality Forum, www.qualityforum.org◀

Brief Description of Performance Measure & Source and Reporting Instructions	CPT Code(s)	Code Descriptor
Osteoarthritis (Adult), cont'd		
Reporting Instructions: Report 4018F alone or or with modifier (1P if medical reason for not instructing therapeutic exercise or prescribing physical therapy was documented; 2P if patient reason for not instructing therapeutic exercise or prescribing physical therapy was documented.) For this measure, the modifiers do not act as denominator exclusions, but rather demonstrate that therapy was considered and are included in the numerator when calculating the measure		
▶Osteoporosis (OP)◀		
▶**Communication with the Physician Managing On-going Care Post Fracture**[5] (Measure #1)—Whether or not the patient aged 50 years and older treated for a hip, spine or distal radial fracture had documentation of communication to the physician managing the patient's on-going care that a fracture occurred and that the patient was or should be tested or treated for osteoporosis **Numerator:** Patients with documentation of communication with the physician managing the patient's on-going care that a fracture occurred and that the patient was or should be tested or treated for osteoporosis Communication may include: Documentation in the medical record indicating that the physician treating the fracture communicated (eg, verbally, by letter, DEXA report was sent with the physician managing the patient's on-going care OR A copy of a letter in the medical record outlining whether the patient was or should be treated for osteoporosis. **Denominator:** All patients aged 50 years and older treated for hip, spine or distal radial fracture **Exclusion Criteria:** Documentation of medical or patient reason(s) for not communicating with the physician managing the patient's on-going care that a fracture occurred and that the patient was or should be tested or treated for osteoporosis **Percentage** of patients aged 50 years and older treated for a hip, spine or distal radial fracture with documentation of communication with the physician managing the patient's on-going care that a fracture occurred and that the patient was or should be tested or treated for osteoporosis **Reporting Instructions:** If the physician treating the fracture is the same physician who is providing the ongoing care, report 5015F. For patient with appropriate exclusion criteria report 5015F with modifier 1P or 2P. Communication to the physician managing the ongoing care of the patient must occur within 3 months of treatment for the fracture to allow reporting of 5015◀	▶5015F◀	▶Documentation of communication that a fracture occurred and that the patient was or should be tested or treated for osteoporosis◀
▶**Screening or Therapy for Women Aged 65 Years and Older**[5] (Measure #2)—Whether or not the female patient aged 65 years and older who had a central DXA measurement ordered or performed at least once since age 60 or pharmacologic therapy prescribed within 12 months **Numerator:** Patients who had a central DXA measurement ordered or results documented at least once since age 60 or pharmacologic therapy prescribed within 12 months **Denominator:** All female patients aged 65 years and older (continued)	▶3095F 3096F	▶Central Dual-energy X-ray Absorptiometry (DXA) results documented Central Dual-energy X-ray Absorptiometry (DXA) ordered

▶[1]Physician Consortium for Performance Improvement: www.physicianconsortium.org◀
[2]National Committee on Quality Assurance (NCQA): Health Employer Data Information Set (HEDIS®), www.ncqa.org
[3]Joint Commission on Accreditation of Healthcare Organizations (JCAHO), ORYX Initiative Performance Measures: www.jcaho.org/pms
[4]National Diabetes Quality Improvement Alliance: www.nationaldiabetesalliance.org
▶[5]Joint measure from the Physician Consortium for Performance Improvement, www.physicianconsortium.org, and National Committee on Quality Assurance (NCQA), www.ncqa.org◀
▶[6]The Society of Thoracic Surgeons, www.sts.org, and National Quality Forum, www.qualityforum.org◀

Brief Description of Performance Measure & Source and Reporting Instructions	CPT Code(s)	Code Descriptor
▶Osteoporosis (OP)◀, cont'd		
Exclusion Criteria: Documentation of medical, patient, or system reason(s) for not ordering or performing a central DXA measurement or not prescribing pharmacologic therapy **Percentage** of female patients aged 65 years and older who have a central DXA measurement ordered or results documented at least once since age 60 or pharmacologic therapy prescribed within 12 months **Reporting Instructions:** Report 3095F if patient has documentation of being tested since age 60. Report 3096F If Central DXA was ordered. Report 4005F if patient was treated using pharmacologic agents for osteoporosis. For patient with appropriate exclusion criteria report either 3095F, 3096F, or 4005F with modifier 1P, 2P, or 3P◀	4005F◀	Pharmacologic therapy (other than minerals/vitamins) for osteoporosis prescribed◀
▶**Management Following Fracture**[5] (Measure #3)—Whether or not the patient aged 50 years and older with a fracture of the hip, spine or distal radius had a central DXA measurement ordered or results documented or pharmacologic therapy prescribed **Numerator:** Patients who had a central DXA measurement ordered or results documented or pharmacologic therapy prescribed **Denominator:** All patients aged 50 years and older with a fracture of the hip, spine or distal radius **Exclusion Criteria:** Documentation of medical, patient, or system reason(s) for not ordering or performing a central DXA measurement or not prescribing pharmacologic therapy **Percentage** of patients aged 50 years and older with a fracture of the hip, spine or distal radius who had a central DXA measurement ordered or performed or pharmacologic therapy prescribed **Reporting Instructions:** Report either 3095F or 4005F if patient has documentation of being tested or treated for osteoporosis. Report 3096F if Central DXA was ordered. For patient with appropriate exclusion criteria report either 3095F, 3096F or 4005F with modifier 1P, 2P, or 3P. The management (DXA ordered or performed or pharmacologic therapy prescribe) should occur within 3 months of notification of the fracture from the physician treating the fracture◀	▶3095F 3096F 4005F 76075◀	▶Central Dual-energy X-ray Absorptiometry (DXA) results documented Central Dual-energy X-ray Absorptiometry (DXA) ordered Pharmacologic therapy (other than minerals/vitamins) for osteoporosis prescribed Dual energy X-ray absorptiometry (DXA), bone density study, one or more sites; axial skeleton (eg, hips, pelvis, spine)◀
▶**Pharmacologic Therapy**[5] (Measure #4)—Whether or not the patient aged 50 years and older with a diagnosis of osteoporosis was prescribed pharmacologic therapy within 12 months **Numerator:** Patients who were prescribed pharmacologic therapy* within 12 months **Denominator:** All patients aged 50 years and older with the diagnosis of osteoporosis **Exclusion Criteria:** Documentation of medical, patient, or system reason(s) for not prescribing pharmacologic therapy **Percentage** of patients aged 50 years and older with a diagnosis of osteoporosis who were prescribed pharmacologic therapy within 12 months (continued)	▶4005F◀	▶Pharmacologic therapy (other than minerals/vitamins) for osteoporosis prescribed◀

▶[1]Physician Consortium for Performance Improvement: www.physicianconsortium.org◀
[2]National Committee on Quality Assurance (NCQA): Health Employer Data Information Set (HEDIS®), www.ncqa.org
[3]Joint Commission on Accreditation of Healthcare Organizations (JCAHO), ORYX Initiative Performance Measures: www.jcaho.org/pms
[4]National Diabetes Quality Improvement Alliance: www.nationaldiabetesalliance.org
▶[5]Joint measure from the Physician Consortium for Performance Improvement, www.physicianconsortium.org, and National Committee on Quality Assurance (NCQA), www.ncqa.org◀
▶[6]The Society of Thoracic Surgeons, www.sts.org, and National Quality Forum, www.qualityforum.org◀

Brief Description of Performance Measure & Source and Reporting Instructions	CPT Code(s)	Code Descriptor
►Osteoporosis (OP)◄, cont'd		
Reporting Instructions: For patient with appropriate exclusion criteria report 4005F with modifier 1P, 2P, or 3P.◄ *US Food and Drug Administration approved pharmacologic options for osteoporosis prevention and/or treatment of postmenopausal osteoporosis include, in alphabetical order: bisphosphonates (alendronate, ibandronate, and risedronate), calcitonin, estrogens (estrogens and/or hormone therapy), parathyroid hormone [PTH (1-34), teriparatide], and selective estrogen receptor modules or SERMS (raloxifene).		
►**Counseling for Vitamin D and Calcium Intake and Exercise**[5] (Measure #5)— Whether or not the patient, regardless of age, with a diagnosis of osteoporosis is either receiving both calcium and vitamin D or had documented counseling regarding both calcium and vitamin D intake, and exercise at least once within 12 months **Numerator:** Patients who are either receiving both calcium and vitamin D or have been counseled regarding both calcium and vitamin D intake, and exercise at least once within 12 months **Denominator:** All patients, regardless of age, with the diagnosis of osteoporosis **Exclusion Criteria:** Documentation of medical reason(s) for patient not receiving both calcium and vitamin D and not needing counseling regarding both calcium and vitamin D intake, and exercise (eg, patient has dementia and is unable to receive counseling) **Percentage** of patients, regardless of age, with a diagnosis of osteoporosis who either received both calcium and vitamin D or had documented counseling regarding both calcium and vitamin D intake, and exercise at least once within 12 months **Reporting Instructions:** Report 4019F if there is documentation that patient is either receiving both calcium and vitamin D or was counseled regarding calcium and vitamin D use; and also counseled on exercise within 12 months For patient with appropriate exclusion criteria report 4019F with modifier 1P◄	►4019F◄	►Documentation of receipt of counseling on exercise AND either both calcium and vitamin D use or counseling regarding both calcium and vitamin D use◄
►Pediatric Acute Gastroenteritis (PAG)◄		
►**Documentation of Hydration Status**[1]—Whether or not a patient 1 month through 5 years of age with a diagnosis of acute gastroenteritis had a documented hydration status **Numerator:** Patients with documented hydration status **Denominator:** Patients 1 month through 5 years of age with the diagnosis of acute gastroenteritis **Exclusions:** None **Percentage** of patients 1 month through 5 years of age with a diagnosis of acute gastroenteritis who had hydration status documented **Reporting Instructions:** There are no exclusions for this measure; modifiers 1P, 2P, and 3P may not be used◄	►2030F 2031F◄	►Hydration status documented, normally hydrated Hydration status documented, dehydrated◄
►**Weight Measurement**[1]—Whether or not patient 1 month through 5 years of age with a diagnosis of acute gastroenteritis had weight measurement recorded **Numerator:** Patients who had their weight measurement recorded **Denominator:** Patients 1 month through 5 years of age with a diagnosis of acute gastroenteritis **Percentage** of patients 1 month through 5 years of age with a diagnosis of acute gastroenteritis who had weight measurement recorded **Reporting Instructions:** There are no exclusions for this measure; modifiers 1P, 2P, and 3P may not be used◄	►2001F◄	►Weight recorded◄

►[1]Physician Consortium for Performance Improvement: www.physicianconsortium.org◄
[2]National Committee on Quality Assurance (NCQA): Health Employer Data Information Set (HEDIS®), www.ncqa.org
[3]Joint Commission on Accreditation of Healthcare Organizations (JCAHO), ORYX Initiative Performance Measures: www.jcaho.org/pms
[4]National Diabetes Quality Improvement Alliance: www.nationaldiabetesalliance.org
►[5]Joint measure from the Physician Consortium for Performance Improvement, www.physicianconsortium.org, and National Committee on Quality Assurance (NCQA), www.ncqa.org◄
►[6]The Society of Thoracic Surgeons, www.sts.org, and National Quality Forum, www.qualityforum.org◄

Brief Description of Performance Measure & Source and Reporting Instructions	CPT Code(s)	Code Descriptor
►Pediatric Acute Gastroenteritis (PAG)◄, cont'd		
►**Recommendation of Appropriate Oral Rehydration Solution**[1]—Whether or not an appropriate oral rehydration solution was recommended for the patient 1 month through 5 years of age with a diagnosis of acute gastroenteritis **Numerator:** Patients for whom an appropriate oral rehydration solution was recommended **Denominator:** Patients 1 month through 5 years of age with the diagnosis of acute gastroenteritis, treated in ambulatory settings (eg, physician office or treated in the emergency department and discharged to home) **Percentage** of patients 1 month through 5 years of age with the diagnosis of acute gastroenteritis for whom an appropriate oral rehydration solution was recommended **Reporting Instructions:** Report 2030F or 2031F for all patients. Report 4056F with 2031F. There are no exclusions for this measure; modifiers 1P, 2P, and 3P may not be used◄	►**4056F** **Denominator Codes:** **2030F** **2031F**◄	►Appropriate oral rehydration solution recommended Hydration status documented, normally hydrated Hydration status documented, dehydrated◄
►**Education**[1]—Whether or not a patient's caregiver received education on diet and on when to contact the physician for a patient 1 month through 5 years of age with a diagnosis of acute gastroenteritis **Numerator:** Patients whose caregiver received education regarding diet and when to contact the physician **Denominator:** All patients 1 month through 5 years of age with the diagnosis of acute gastroenteritis, treated in ambulatory settings (physician office or treated in the emergency room and discharged to home) **Percentage** of patients 1 month through 5 years of age with a diagnosis of acute gastroenteritis whose caregiver received education regarding diet and on when to contact the physician **Reporting Instructions:** There are no exclusions for this measure; modifiers 1P, 2P, and 3P may not be used◄	►**4058F**◄	►Pediatric gastroenteritis education provided to caregiver◄
►Pediatric Pharyngitis (PHAR)◄		
►**Appropriate Testing for Children with Pharyngitis**[2]—Whether or not children 2-18 years of age (inclusive) who were diagnosed with pharyngitis and dispensed or prescribed an antibiotic received a group A strep test. **Numerator:** Patients who received a group A streptococcus (strep) test **Denominator:** All patients aged 2-18 years with the diagnosis of pharyngitis who were dispensed or prescribed antibiotic treatment **Exclusion(s):** Medical or patient reasons for not performing Group A Strep Tests **Percentage** of children 2-18 years of age (inclusive) diagnosed with pharyngitis and dispensed or prescribed an antibiotic who received a group A strep test for the visit **Reporting Instructions:** Note: Because this measure is being specified for physician reporting, the instructions request physicians to report prescribing or dispensing of medication. For Medical or patient reasons for not performing a Group A Strep Test, report code 3210F with modifier 1P or 2P. There are no performance measure exclusions for codes 4120F and 4124F for children with pharyngitis. Do not report modifiers 1P, 2P, or 3P with these codes for this condition◄	►**3210F** **Category I Codes:** **87070, 87071, 87081, 87430, 87650-87652, 87880** **Denominator Codes:** **4120F** **4124F**◄	►Group A strep test performed Antibiotic prescribed or dispensed Antibiotic neither prescribed nor dispensed◄

►[1]Physician Consortium for Performance Improvement: www.physicianconsortium.org◄

[2]National Committee on Quality Assurance (NCQA): Health Employer Data Information Set (HEDIS®), www.ncqa.org

[3]Joint Commission on Accreditation of Healthcare Organizations (JCAHO), ORYX Initiative Performance Measures: www.jcaho.org/pms

[4]National Diabetes Quality Improvement Alliance: www.nationaldiabetesalliance.org

►[5]Joint measure from the Physician Consortium for Performance Improvement, www.physicianconsortium.org, and National Committee on Quality Assurance (NCQA), www.ncqa.org◄

►[6]The Society of Thoracic Surgeons, www.sts.org, and National Quality Forum, www.qualityforum.org◄

Brief Description of Performance Measure & Source and Reporting Instructions	CPT Code(s)	Code Descriptor
►Perioperative Care 2 (PERI 2)◄		
►**Timing of Prophylactic Antibiotics–Ordering Physician**[5] (Measure #1)—Whether or not the surgical patient aged 18 years and older undergoing a procedure with the indications for prophylactic parenteral antibiotics had an order for an antibiotic to be given within one hour (if vancomycin, two hours) prior to the surgical incision (or start of procedure when no incision is required) **Numerator:** Surgical patients who have an order for an antibiotic to be given within one hour (if vancomycin, two hours) prior to the surgical incision (or start of procedure when no incision is required) **Denominator:** All surgical patients aged 18 years and older undergoing procedures with the indications for prophylactic parenteral antibiotics (List of procedures is available in measure specifications) **Exclusion Criteria:** Documentation of medical reason(s) for not ordering an antibiotic to be given within one hour (if vancomycin, two hours) prior to the surgical incision (or start of procedure when no incision is required) **Percentage** of surgical patients aged 18 years and older undergoing procedures with the indications for prophylactic parenteral antibiotics who have an order for an antibiotic to be given within one hour (if vancomycin, two hours) prior to the surgical incision (or start of procedure when no incision is required) **Reporting Instructions:** It is anticipated that this measure will be reported by the physician performing the procedure • There must be documentation of an order (written, verbal, or standing order/protocol) specifying that antibiotic is to be given within the specified timeframe OR documentation that antibiotic has been given within the specified timeframe • Report 4047F if prophylactic antibiotic was ordered or 4048F if antibiotic has been given • For patient meeting exclusion criteria, report 4047F with modifier 1P◄	►4047F 4048F◄	►Documentation of order for prophylactic antibiotics to be given within one hour (if fluoroquinolone or vancomycin, two hours) prior to surgical incision (or start of procedure when no incision is required) Documentation that prophylactic antibiotic was given within one hour (if fluoroquinolone or vancomycin, two hours) prior to surgical incision (or start of procedure when no incision is required)◄
►**Timing of Prophylactic Antibiotics – Administering Physician**[5] (Measure #2)—Whether or not administration of prophylactic parenteral antibiotic was initiated within one hour (if fluoroquinolone or vancomycin, two hours) prior to the surgical incision (or start of procedure when no incision is required) for the surgical patient aged 18 years and older who had an order for a prophylactic parenteral antibiotic to be given within one hour (if fluoroquinolone or vancomycin, two hours) prior to the surgical incision (or start of procedure when no incision is required) **Numerator:** Surgical patients for whom administration of a prophylactic antibiotic has been initiated within one hour (if fluoroquinolone or vancomycin, two hours) prior to the surgical incision (or start of procedure when no incision is required) **Denominator:** All surgical patients aged 18 years and older who have an order for a parenteral antibiotic to be given within one hour (if fluoroquinolone or vancomycin, two hours) prior to the surgical incision (or start of procedure when no incision is required) **Exclusion Criteria:** None **Percentage** of surgical patients aged 18 years and older who have an order for a parenteral antibiotic to be given within one hour (if fluoroquinolone or vancomycin, two hours) prior to the surgical incision (or start of procedure when no incision is required) for whom administration of a prophylactic antibiotic has been initiated within one hour (if fluoroquinolone or vancomycin, two hours) prior to the surgical incision (or start of procedure when no incision is required) (continued)	►4048F **Denominator Code:** 4047F◄	►Documentation that prophylactic antibiotic was given within one hour (if fluoroquinolone or vancomycin, two hours) prior to surgical incision (or start of procedure when no incision is required) Documentation of order for prophylactic antibiotic to be given within one hour (if fluoroquinolone or vancomycin, two hours) prior to surgical incision (or start of procedure when no incision is required)◄

►[1]Physician Consortium for Performance Improvement: www.physicianconsortium.org◄
[2]National Committee on Quality Assurance (NCQA): Health Employer Data Information Set (HEDIS®), www.ncqa.org
[3]Joint Commission on Accreditation of Healthcare Organizations (JCAHO), ORYX Initiative Performance Measures: www.jcaho.org/pms
[4]National Diabetes Quality Improvement Alliance: www.nationaldiabetesalliance.org
►[5]Joint measure from the Physician Consortium for Performance Improvement, www.physicianconsortium.org, and National Committee on Quality Assurance (NCQA), www.ncqa.org◄
►[6]The Society of Thoracic Surgeons, www.sts.org, and National Quality Forum, www.qualityforum.org◄

Brief Description of Performance Measure & Source and Reporting Instructions	CPT Code(s)	Code Descriptor
►Perioperative Care 2 (PERI 2)◄, cont'd		
Reporting Instructions: • It is anticipated that the physician administering or responsible for the administering the prophylactic antibiotic will report this measure. The identification of patients for the denominator of this measure is exclusively dependent on the presence of an order for prophylactic antibiotics to be given. A surgical procedure list is not used to identify these patients • There must be documentation of an order (written, verbal, or standing order/protocol) specifying that antibiotic is to be given within the specified timeframe • Report 4047F where there is documentation of an order for prophylactic antibiotics to be given within one hour of surgical incision. If antibiotics were not given within the appropriate timeframe as ordered, report only 4047F • Also report 4048F when prophylactic antibiotic was given within the specified timeframe. • There are no exclusions for this measure; modifiers 1P, 2P, and 3P may not be used◄		
►**Selection of Prophylactic Antibiotic—First OR Second Generation Cephalosporin**[5] (Measure #3)—Whether or not the surgical patient aged 18 years and older undergoing a procedure with the indications for a first OR second generation cephalosporin had an order for cefazolin OR cefuroxime for antimicrobial prophylaxis **Numerator:** Surgical patients who had an order for cefazolin OR cefuroxime for antimicrobial prophylaxis **Denominator:** All surgical patients aged 18 years and older undergoing procedures with the indications for a first OR second generation cephalosporin prophylactic antibiotic (List of procedures is available in measure specifications) **Exclusion Criteria:** Documentation of medical reason(s) for not ordering cefazolin OR cefuroxime for antimicrobial prophylaxis **Percentage** of surgical patients aged 18 years and older undergoing procedures with the indications for a first OR second generation cephalosporin prophylactic antibiotic who had an order for cefazolin OR cefuroxime for antimicrobial prophylaxis **Reporting Instructions:** • It is anticipated that this measure will be reported by the physician performing the procedure • There must be documentation of an *order* (written, verbal, or standing order/protocol) for cefazolin or cefuroxime for antimicrobial prophylaxis OR documentation that cefazolin or cefuroxime was *given* • Report 4041F if cefazolin or cefuroxime was ordered. • If either cefazolin or cefuroxime was administered, there is a presumption that an order existed for that administration. In this case, 4041F should be reported • For patient with appropriate exclusion criteria report 4041F with modifier 1P◄	►4041F◄	►Documentation of order for cefazolin OR cefuroxime for antimicrobial prophylaxis◄
►**Discontinuation of Prophylactic Antibiotics (Noncardiac Procedures)**[5] (Measure #4)—Whether or not the non-cardiac surgical patient aged 18 years and older undergoing a procedure with the indications for prophylactic antibiotics AND who received a prophylactic antibiotic, has an order for discontinuation of prophylactic antibiotics within 24 hours of surgical end time **Numerator:** Noncardiac surgical patients who have an order for discontinuation of prophylactic antibiotics within 24 hours of surgical end time **Denominator:** All noncardiac surgical patients 18 years and older undergoing procedures with the indications for prophylactic antibiotics AND who received a prophylactic antibiotic (List of procedures is available in measure specifications) (continued)	►4049F **Denominator Codes:** 4046F	►Documentation that order was given to discontinue prophylactic antibiotics within 24 hours of surgical end time, noncardiac procedure Documentation that prophylactic antibiotics were given within 4

►[1]Physician Consortium for Performance Improvement: www.physicianconsortium.org◄

[2]National Committee on Quality Assurance (NCQA): Health Employer Data Information Set (HEDIS®), www.ncqa.org

[3]Joint Commission on Accreditation of Healthcare Organizations (JCAHO), ORYX Initiative Performance Measures: www.jcaho.org/pms

[4]National Diabetes Quality Improvement Alliance: www.nationaldiabetesalliance.org

►[5]Joint measure from the Physician Consortium for Performance Improvement, www.physicianconsortium.org, and National Committee on Quality Assurance (NCQA), www.ncqa.org◄

►[6]The Society of Thoracic Surgeons, www.sts.org, and National Quality Forum, www.qualityforum.org◄

Brief Description of Performance Measure & Source and Reporting Instructions	CPT Code(s)	Code Descriptor
►Perioperative Care 2 (PERI 2)◄, cont'd		
Exclusion Criteria: Documentation of medical reason(s) for not discontinuing prophylactic antibiotics within 24 hours of surgical end time **Percentage** of non-cardiac surgical patients aged 18 years and older undergoing procedures with the indications for prophylactic antibiotics AND who received a prophylactic antibiotic, who have an order for discontinuation of prophylactic antibiotics within 24 hours of surgical end time **Reporting Instructions:** • It is anticipated that this measure will be reported by the physician performing the procedure • Patients may be counted as having "received a prophylactic antibiotic" if the antibiotic was received within 4 hours prior to the surgical incision (or start of procedure when no incision is required) or intraoperatively • There must be documentation of an *order* (written, verbal or standing order/protocol) specifying that prophylactic antibiotic is to be discontinued within 24 hours of surgical end time **OR** specifying a course of antibiotic administration limited to that 24-hour period (eg, to be given every 8 hours for three doses) **OR** documentation that prophylactic antibiotic *was* discontinued within 24 hours of surgical end time • Report either 4046F or 4042F for each patient. If patient received prophylactic antibiotics and there was an order for discontinuation within 24 hours after surgical end time, also report 4049F. For patient with appropriate exclusion criteria, report 4049F with modifier 1P◄	4042F◄	hours prior to surgical incision or given intraoperatively Documentation that prophylactic antibiotics were neither given within 4 hours prior to surgical incision nor given intraoperatively◄
►**Discontinuation of Prophylactic Antibiotics (Cardiac Procedures)**[5] (Measure #5)—Whether or not the cardiac surgical patient aged 18 years and older undergoing a procedure with the indications for prophylactic antibiotics AND who received prophylactic antibiotics, has an order for discontinuation of prophylactic antibiotics within 48 hours of surgical end time **Numerator:** Cardiac surgical patients who have an order for discontinuation of prophylactic antibiotics within 48 hours of surgical end time **Denominator:** All cardiac surgical patients 18 years and older undergoing procedures with the indications for prophylactic antibiotics AND who received a prophylactic antibiotic (List of procedures available in measure specifications) **Exclusion Criteria:** Documentation of medical reason(s) for not discontinuing prophylactic antibiotics within 48 hours of surgical end time **Percentage** of cardiac surgical patients aged 18 years and older undergoing procedures with the indications for prophylactic antibiotics AND who received a prophylactic antibiotic, who have an order for discontinuation of prophylactic antibiotics within 48 hours of surgical end time **Reporting Instructions:** • It is anticipated that this measure will be reported by the physician performing the procedure • Patients may be counted as having "received a prophylactic antibiotic" if the antibiotic was received within 4 hours prior to the surgical incision (or start of procedure when no incision is required) or intraoperatively • There must be documentation of an *order* (written, verbal or standing order/protocol) specifying that prophylactic antibiotic is to be discontinued within 48 hours of surgical end time **OR** specifying a course of antibiotic administration limited to that 48-hour (continued)	►4043F **Denominator Codes:** 4046F 4042F◄	►Documentation that an order was given to discontinue prophylactic antibiotics within 48 hours of surgical end time, cardiac procedure Documentation that prophylactic antibiotics were given within 4 hours prior to surgical incision or given intraoperatively Documentation that prophylactic antibiotics were neither given within 4 hours prior to surgical incision nor given intraoperatively◄

►[1]Physician Consortium for Performance Improvement: www.physicianconsortium.org◄

[2]National Committee on Quality Assurance (NCQA): Health Employer Data Information Set (HEDIS®), www.ncqa.org

[3]Joint Commission on Accreditation of Healthcare Organizations (JCAHO), ORYX Initiative Performance Measures: www.jcaho.org/pms

[4]National Diabetes Quality Improvement Alliance: www.nationaldiabetesalliance.org

►[5]Joint measure from the Physician Consortium for Performance Improvement, www.physicianconsortium.org, and National Committee on Quality Assurance (NCQA), www.ncqa.org◄

►[6]The Society of Thoracic Surgeons, www.sts.org, and National Quality Forum, www.qualityforum.org◄

Brief Description of Performance Measure & Source and Reporting Instructions	CPT Code(s)	Code Descriptor
▶**Perioperative Care 2 (PERI 2)◀, cont'd**		
period (eg, to be given every 8 hours for three doses") **OR** documentation that prophylactic antibiotic *was* discontinued within 48 hours of surgical end time • Report either 4046F or 4042F for each patient. If patient received prophylactic antibiotics and there was an order for discontinuation within 48 hours after surgical end time, also report 4043F. For patient with appropriate exclusion criteria, report 4043F with modifier 1P◀		
▶**Perioperative Care 2 (PERI)◀**		
▶**Venous Thromboembolism (VTE) Prophylaxis**[5] (Measure #6)—Whether or not the surgical patient aged 18 years and older undergoing a procedure for which VTE prophylaxis is indicated in all patients had an order for LMWH, LDUH, adjusted-dose warfarin, fondaparinux, or mechanical prophylaxis to be given within 24 hours prior to incision time or within 24 hours after surgery end time LMWH-Low molecular weight heparin LDUH-Low-dose unfractionated heparin **Numerator:** Surgical patients who had an order for LMWH, LDUH, adjusted-dose warfarin, fondaparinux or mechanical prophylaxis to be given within 24 hours prior to incision time or within 24 hours after surgery end time **Denominator:** All surgical patients aged 18 years and older undergoing procedures for which VTE prophylaxis is indicated in all patients (List of procedures available in measure specifications) **Exclusion Criteria:** Documentation of medical reason(s) for patient not receiving LMWH, LDUH, adjusted-dose warfarin, fondaparinux, or mechanical prophylaxis within 24 hours prior to incision time or 24 hours after surgery end time **Percentage** of surgical patients aged 18 years and older undergoing procedures for which VTE prophylaxis is indicated in all patients who had an order for LMWH, LDUH, adjusted-dose warfarin, fondaparinux or mechanical prophylaxis to be given within 24 hours prior to incision time or within 24 hours after surgery end time **Reporting Instructions:** • There must be documentation of an order (written, verbal or standing order/protocol) for VTE prophylaxis OR documentation that VTE prophylaxis was received • Report 4044F where there is documentation of an order for VTE prophylaxis or where it was given within the specified timeframe • For patient with appropriate exclusion criteria, report 4044F with modifier 1P◀	▶4044F◀	▶Documentation that an order was given for venous thromboembolism (VTE) prophylaxis to be given within 24 hrs prior to incision time or 24 hours after surgery end time◀
Prenatal-Postpartum Care		
Timeliness of Prenatal Care[2] **Numerator:** Number of women who received a prenatal care visit as a member of the managed care organization (MCO) in the first trimester or within 42 days of enrollment in the MCO **Denominator:** Women who had live births between November 6 of the year prior to the measurement year and November 5 of the measurement year, who were continuously enrolled at least 43 days prior to delivery through 56 days after delivery **Percentage** of patients in the denominator who received prenatal care ▶**Reporting Instructions:** There are no exclusions for this measure; modifiers 1P, 2P, and 3P may not be used◀	0500F	Initial prenatal care visit (report at first prenatal encounter with health care professional providing obstetrical care. Report also date of visit and, in a separate field, the date of the last menstrual period – LMP)

▶[1]Physician Consortium for Performance Improvement: www.physicianconsortium.org◀

[2]National Committee on Quality Assurance (NCQA): Health Employer Data Information Set (HEDIS®), www.ncqa.org

[3]Joint Commission on Accreditation of Healthcare Organizations (JCAHO), ORYX Initiative Performance Measures: www.jcaho.org/pms

[4]National Diabetes Quality Improvement Alliance: www.nationaldiabetesalliance.org

▶[5]Joint measure from the Physician Consortium for Performance Improvement, www.physicianconsortium.org, and National Committee on Quality Assurance (NCQA), www.ncqa.org◀

▶[6]The Society of Thoracic Surgeons, www.sts.org, and National Quality Forum, www.qualityforum.org◀

Brief Description of Performance Measure & Source and Reporting Instructions	CPT Code(s)	Code Descriptor
Prenatal-Postpartum Care, cont'd		
Prenatal Flow Sheet[1]—Whether or not patient has a prenatal flowsheet in use by the date of the first physician visit **Numerator:** Number of patients with a flow sheet in use by the date of the first physician visit, which contains at a minimum: blood pressure, weight, urine protein, uterine size, fetal heart tones, and estimated date of delivery **Denominator:** Pregnant women seen for prenatal care **Exclusion(s):** Patients seen for consultation only, not for continuing care **Percentage** of patients in the denominator with a prenatal flow sheet in use by the first physician visit ▶**Reporting Instructions:** There are no exclusions for this measure; modifiers 1P, 2P, and 3P may not be used◀	0501F	Prenatal flow sheet documented in medical record by first prenatal visit (documentation includes at mininum blood pressure, weight, urine protein, uterine size, fetal heart tones, and estimated date of delivery). Report also date of visit and, in a separate field, the date of the last menstrual period – LMP (Note: If reporting 0501F, Prenatal flow sheet, it is not necessary to report 0500F, Initial prenatal care visit)
Frequency of Ongoing Prenatal Care[2] **Numerator:** Number of women in the denominator who had an unduplicated count of less than 21%, 21%-40%, 41%-60%, 61%-80%, or greater than or equal to 81% of the expected number of prenatal care visits, adjusted for the month of pregnancy at time of enrollment and gestational age **Denominator:** Women who had live births during the measurement year **Exclusion(s):** MCOs must exclude members for whom a prenatal visit is not indicated **Percentage** of patients in the denominator with expected number of prenatal visits ▶**Reporting Instructions:** There are no exclusions for this measure; modifiers 1P, 2P, and 3P may not be used◀	0502F	Subsequent prenatal care visit
Postpartum Care[2] **Numerator:** Number of women in the denominator who had a postpartum visit on or between 21 days and 56 days after delivery **Denominator:** Women who had live births between November 6 of the year prior to the measurement year and November 5 of the measurement year, who were continuously enrolled at least 43 days prior to delivery through 56 days after delivery **Percentage** of patients in the denominator who had a postpartum visit between 21 and 56 days after delivery ▶**Reporting Instructions:** There are no exclusions for this measure; modifiers 1P, 2P, and 3P may not be used◀	0503F	Postpartum care visit
Preventive Care & Screening (PV)		
Adult Influenza Immunization[1]—Whether or not patient received an influenza immunization **Numerator:** Patients who received an influenza immunization **Denominator:** All patients greater than or equal to 50 years of age **Exclusion Criteria:** Documentation of medical, patient, or system reason(s) for declining immunization **Percentage** of patients who received an influenza immunization **Reporting Instructions:** For patients with appropriate exclusion criteria use 4037F with modifier 1P, 2P, or 3P. Use 4037F with modifier 1P if previously immunized for current season	4037F	Influenza immunization ordered or administered
	90656	Influenza virus vaccine, split virus, preservative free, when administered to 3 years and older, for intramuscular use
	90658	Influenza virus vaccine, split virus, when administered to 3 years of age and older, for intramuscular use
	90660	Influenza virus vaccine, live, for intranasal use

▶[1]Physician Consortium for Performance Improvement: www.physicianconsortium.org◀

[2]National Committee on Quality Assurance (NCQA): Health Employer Data Information Set (HEDIS®), www.ncqa.org

[3]Joint Commission on Accreditation of Healthcare Organizations (JCAHO), ORYX Initiative Performance Measures: www.jcaho.org/pms

[4]National Diabetes Quality Improvement Alliance: www.nationaldiabetesalliance.org

▶[5]Joint measure from the Physician Consortium for Performance Improvement, www.physicianconsortium.org, and National Committee on Quality Assurance (NCQA), www.ncqa.org◀

▶[6]The Society of Thoracic Surgeons, www.sts.org, and National Quality Forum, www.qualityforum.org◀

Brief Description of Performance Measure & Source and Reporting Instructions	CPT Code(s)	Code Descriptor
Preventive Care & Screening (PV), cont'd		
Adult Colorectal Cancer Screening[1]—Whether or not patient was screened for colorectal cancer during the one-year measurement period **Numerator:** Patients with any of the recommended colorectal cancer screening test(s) performed (fecal occult blood testing annually; flexible sigmoidoscopy every five years; annual fecal occult blood testing plus flexible sigmoidoscopy every five years; double contrast barium enema every five years; colonoscopy every ten years) **Denominator:** All patients aged greater than or equal to 50 years **Denominator Exclusion:** Documentation of medical, patient, or system reason(s) for not providing colorectal cancer screening **Percentage** of patients screened for colorectal cancer **Reporting Instructions:** For patients with appropriate exclusion criteria, report 3017F with modifier 1P, 2P, or 3P	3017F	Colorectal cancer screening results documented and reviewed
Screening Mammography[1]—Whether or not female patient had a mammogram performed during the two-year measurement period **Numerator:** Female patients who had a mammogram performed **Denominator:** All female patients aged 50-69 years **Exclusion criteria:** Documentation of medical, patient, or system reason(s) for declining or not performing screening mammography **Percentage** of female patients who had a mammogram performed during the two-year measurement period **Reporting Instructions:** For patients with appropriate exclusion criteria use 3014F with modifier 1P, 2P, or 3P	3014F	Screening mammography results documented and reviewed
Tobacco Use[1]—Whether or not patient was queried about tobacco use one or more times **Numerator:** Patients who were queried about tobacco use one or more times **Denominator:** All patients aged ≥ 18 years at the beginning of the two-year measurement period **Percentage** of patients queried about tobacco use one or more times during the two-year measurement period **Reporting Instructions:** When reporting 1000F, it is required to report 1034F, and/or 1035F, or 1036F ▶There are no exclusions for this measure; modifiers 1P, 2P, and 3P may not be used◀	1000F 1034F 1035F 1036F	Tobacco use, smoking, assess Current tobacco smoker Smokeless tobacco user Tobacco non-user
Tobacco Use Intervention[1]—Whether or not patient identified as a tobacco user received cessation intervention **Numerator:** Patients identified as tobacco users who received cessation intervention **Denominator:** All patients ≥ 18 years at the beginning of the two-year measurement period identified as tobacco users **Percentage** of patients identified as tobacco users who received cessation intervention during the two year measurement period **Reporting Instructions:** Report 1034F, 1035F or 1036F for each patient. If patient is a tobacco user (1034F or 1035F) and received cessation intervention, report 4000F or 4001F or both ▶There are no exclusions for this measure; modifiers 1P, 2P, and 3P may not be used◀	4000F 4001F **Denominator Codes:** 1034F 1035F 1036F	Tobacco use cessation intervention, counseling Tobacco use cessation intervention, pharmacologic therapy Current tobacco smoker Smokeless tobacco user Tobacco non-user

▶[1]Physician Consortium for Performance Improvement: www.physicianconsortium.org◀

[2]National Committee on Quality Assurance (NCQA): Health Employer Data Information Set (HEDIS®), www.ncqa.org

[3]Joint Commission on Accreditation of Healthcare Organizations (JCAHO), ORYX Initiative Performance Measures: www.jcaho.org/pms

[4]National Diabetes Quality Improvement Alliance: www.nationaldiabetesalliance.org

▶[5]Joint measure from the Physician Consortium for Performance Improvement, www.physicianconsortium.org, and National Committee on Quality Assurance (NCQA), www.ncqa.org◀

▶[6]The Society of Thoracic Surgeons, www.sts.org, and National Quality Forum, www.qualityforum.org◀

Brief Description of Performance Measure & Source and Reporting Instructions	CPT Code(s)	Code Descriptor
►Stroke and Stroke Rehabilitation (STR)◄		
►**Deep Vein Thrombosis Prophylaxis (DVT) for Ischemic Stroke or Intracranial Hemorrhage**[5] (Measure #1)—Whether or not the patient aged 18 years and older with the diagnosis of *ischemic* stroke OR *intracranial hemorrhage* received DVT prophylaxis by end of hospital day 2 **Numerator:** Patients who received Deep Vein Thrombosis (DVT) prophylaxis by end of hospital day 2 **Definition:** For purposes of this measure, DVT prophylaxis can include Low Molecular Weight Heparin (LMWH), Low-Dose Unfractionated Heparin (LDUH), intravenous heparin, low-dose subcutaneous heparin, or intermittent pneumatic compression devices **Denominator:** All patients aged 18 years and older with the diagnosis of *ischemic* stroke OR intracranial hemorrhage **Exclusion(s):** Documentation of medical reason(s) (including physician documentation that patient is ambulatory) for not receiving DVT prophylaxis by end of hospital day 2; documentation of patient reason(s) for not receiving DVT prophylaxis by end of hospital day 2 **Percentage** of patients aged 18 years and older with the diagnosis of *ischemic* stroke OR intracranial hemorrhage who received DVT prophylaxis by end of hospital day 2 **Reporting Instructions:** For patient with appropriate exclusion criteria report 4070F with modifier 1P or 2P.◄	►4070F◄	►Deep Vein Thrombosis (DVT) prophylaxis received by end of hospital day 2◄
►**Discharged on Antiplatelet Therapy**[5] (Measure #2)—Whether or not the patient aged 18 years and older with the diagnosis of *ischemic stroke* or *TIA* was prescribed antiplatelet therapy at discharge **Numerator:** Patients who were prescribed antiplatelet therapy at discharge **Definition:** Antiplatelet therapy: aspirin, combination of aspirin and extended-release dipyridamole, clopidogrel, ticlopidine **Denominator:** All patients aged 18 years and older with a diagnosis of *ischemic stroke* or *TIA* **Exclusion(s):** Documentation of medical reason(s) (including documentation that patient is on anticoagulation therapy) for not prescribing antiplatelet therapy at discharge; documentation of patient reason(s) for not prescribing antiplatelet therapy at discharge **Percentage** of patients aged 18 years and older with a diagnosis of *ischemic stroke* or *TIA* who were prescribed antiplatelet therapy at discharge **Reporting Instructions:** For patient with appropriate exclusion criteria report 4073F with modifier 1P or 2P.◄	►4073F◄	►Oral antiplatelet therapy prescribed at discharge◄
►**Anticoagulant Therapy Prescribed for Atrial Fibrillation at Discharge**[5] (Measure #3)—Whether or not the patient aged 18 years and older with the diagnosis of *ischemic stroke* or *TIA* with documented permanent, persistent, or paroxysmal atrial fibrillation was prescribed an anticoagulant at discharge **Numerator:** Patients who were prescribed an anticoagulant at discharge **Denominator:** All patients aged 18 years and older with the diagnosis of *ischemic stroke* or *TIA* with documented permanent, persistent, or paroxysmal atrial fibrillation **Exclusion(s):** Documentation of medical or patient reason(s) for not prescribing an anticoagulant at discharge **Percentage** of patients aged 18 years and older with the diagnosis of *ischemic stroke* or *TIA* with documented permanent, persistent, or paroxysmal atrial fibrillation who were prescribed an anticoagulant at discharge (continued)	►4075F **Denominator Codes:** 1060F 1061F◄	►Anticoagulant therapy prescribed at discharge Documentation of permanent OR persistent OR paroxysmal atrial fibrillation Documentation of absence of permanent AND persistent AND paroxysmal atrial fibrillation◄

►[1]Physician Consortium for Performance Improvement: www.physicianconsortium.org◄

[2]National Committee on Quality Assurance (NCQA): Health Employer Data Information Set (HEDIS®), www.ncqa.org

[3]Joint Commission on Accreditation of Healthcare Organizations (JCAHO), ORYX Initiative Performance Measures: www.jcaho.org/pms

[4]National Diabetes Quality Improvement Alliance: www.nationaldiabetesalliance.org

►[5]Joint measure from the Physician Consortium for Performance Improvement, www.physicianconsortium.org, and National Committee on Quality Assurance (NCQA), www.ncqa.org◄

►[6]The Society of Thoracic Surgeons, www.sts.org, and National Quality Forum, www.qualityforum.org◄

Brief Description of Performance Measure & Source and Reporting Instructions	CPT Code(s)	Code Descriptor
►Stroke and Stroke Rehabilitation (STR)◄, cont'd		
Reporting Instructions: Report 1060F or 1061F for each patient. If anticoagulant therapy prescribed at discharge, also report 4075F. For patient with appropriate exclusion criteria report 4075F with modifier 1P or 2P◄		
►**Tissue Plasminogen Activator (t-PA) Considered**[5] (Measure #4)—Whether or not the patient aged 18 years and older with the diagnosis of *ischemic* stroke whose time from symptom onset to arrival is less than 3 hours was considered for t-PA administration **Numerator:** Patients who were considered for t-PA administration(given t-PA or documented reasons for patient not being a candidate for therapy) **Denominator:** All patients aged 18 years and older with the diagnosis of *ischemic* stroke whose time from symptom onset to arrival is less than 3 hours **Exclusion(s):** None **Percentage** of patients aged 18 years and older with the diagnosis of *ischemic* stroke whose time from symptom onset to arrival is less than 3 hours who were considered for t-PA administration **Reporting Instructions:** Report either 1065F or 1066F for each patient. If time from symptom onset to arrival is less than 3 hours, and t-PA was considered, also report 4077F◄	►4077F Denominator Codes: 1065F 1066F◄	►Documentation that tissue plasminogen activator (t-PA) administration was considered Ischemic stroke symptom onset of < 3 hours prior to arrival Ischemic stroke symptom onset ≥ 3 hours prior to arrival◄
►**Screening for Dysphagia**[5] (Measure #5)—Whether or not the patient aged 18 years and older with the diagnosis of *ischemic stroke* or *intracranial hemorrhage* underwent a dysphagia screening process before taking any foods, fluids or medication by mouth **Numerator:** Patients who underwent a dysphagia screening process before taking any foods, fluids or medication by mouth **Denominator:** All patients aged 18 years and older with the diagnosis of *ischemic stroke* or *intracranial hemorrhage* who receive any food, fluids, or medication by mouth **Exclusion(s):** Documentation of medical reason(s) for not screening for dysphagia before taking any foods, fluids or medication by mouth **Percentage** of patients aged 18 years and older with the diagnosis of *ischemic stroke* or *intracranial hemorrhage* who underwent a dysphagia screening process before taking any foods, fluids, or medication by mouth **Reporting Instructions:** • Report 6015F or 6020F for each patient • If dysphagia screening was conducted prior to receiving food, fluid or medication by mouth or prior to ordering food, fluid, or medication by mouth, also report 6010F • If patient is NPO, only report 6020F • For patient with appropriate exclusion criteria, report 6010F with modifier 1P◄	►6010F Denominator Codes: 6015F 6020F◄	►Dysphagia screening conducted prior to order for or receipt of any foods, fluids or medication by mouth Patient receiving or eligible to receive food, fluids or medication by mouth NPO (nothing by mouth) ordered◄
►**Consideration of Rehabilitation Services**[5] (Measure #6)—Whether or not consideration of rehabilitation services is documented for patients aged 18 years and older with the diagnosis of *ischemic stroke* or *intracranial hemorrhage* **Numerator:** Patients for whom consideration of rehabilitation services (ordered rehabilitation or documented that rehabilitation was not indicated) is documented **Denominator:** All patients aged 18 years and older with the diagnosis of *ischemic stroke* or *intracranial hemorrhage* **Exclusion(s):** None **Percentage** of patients aged 18 years and older with the diagnosis of *ischemic stroke* or *intracranial hemorrhage* for whom consideration of rehabilitation services is documented **Reporting Instructions:** Report 4079F if rehabilitation services considered (ordered or not indicated with documented reasons). There are no exclusions for this measure; modifiers 1P, 2P, and 3P may not be used. When 4079F is not reported, it indicates rehabilitation services were not considered◄	►4079F◄	►Documentation that rehabilitation services were considered◄

►[1]Physician Consortium for Performance Improvement: www.physicianconsortium.org◄

[2]National Committee on Quality Assurance (NCQA): Health Employer Data Information Set (HEDIS®), www.ncqa.org

[3]Joint Commission on Accreditation of Healthcare Organizations (JCAHO), ORYX Initiative Performance Measures: www.jcaho.org/pms

[4]National Diabetes Quality Improvement Alliance: www.nationaldiabetesalliance.org

►[5]Joint measure from the Physician Consortium for Performance Improvement, www.physicianconsortium.org, and National Committee on Quality Assurance (NCQA), www.ncqa.org◄

►[6]The Society of Thoracic Surgeons, www.sts.org, and National Quality Forum, www.qualityforum.org◄

Brief Description of Performance Measure & Source and Reporting Instructions	CPT Code(s)	Code Descriptor
►Stroke and Stroke Rehabilitation (STR)◄, cont'd		
►**Carotid Imaging Reports**[5] (Measure #7)—Whether or not the final report of a carotid imaging study (neck MR angiography [MRA], neck CT angiography [CTA], neck duplex ultrasound, carotid angiogram) for a patient aged 18 years and older with a diagnosis of *ischemic stroke* or *TIA* includes direct or indirect reference to measurements of distal internal carotid diameter as the denominator for stenosis measurement **Numerator:** Final carotid imaging study reports that include direct or indirect reference to measurements of distal internal carotid diameter as the denominator for stenosis measurement **Definition:** "Direct or indirect reference to measurements of distal internal carotid diameter as the denominator for stenosis measurement" includes direct angiographic stenosis calculations based on the distal lumen as the denominator for stenosis measurement OR an equivalent validated method referenced to the above method (eg, for duplex ultrasound studies, velocity parameters that correlate the *residual* internal carotid lumen with methods based on the *distal* internal carotid lumen) **Denominator:** All final reports for carotid imaging studies (neck MR angiography [MRA], neck CT angiography [CTA], neck duplex ultrasound, carotid angiogram) performed for patients aged 18 years and older with a diagnosis of *ischemic stroke* or *TIA* **Exclusion(s):** Documentation of medical reason(s) for not including direct or indirect reference to measurements of distal internal carotid diameter **Percentage** of final reports for carotid imaging studies (neck MR angiography [MRA], neck CT angiography [CTA], neck duplex ultrasound, carotid angiogram) performed for patients aged 18 years and older with the diagnosis of *ischemic stroke* or *TIA* that include direct or indirect reference to measurements of distal internal carotid diameter as the denominator for stenosis measurement **Reporting Instructions:** For patient with appropriate exclusion criteria report 3100F with modifier 1P.◄	► ▲3100F◄	►Carotid image study report includes direct or indirect reference to measurements of distal internal carotid diameter as the denominator for stenosis measurement◄
►**Computed Tomography (CT) or Magnetic Resonance Imaging (MRI) Reports** (Measure #8)—Whether or not the final report of a CT or MRI study of the brain performed within 24 hours of arrival to the hospital for a patient aged 18 years and older with a diagnosis of *ischemic stroke* or *TIA* or *intracranial hemorrhage* includes documentation of the presence or absence of each of the following: hemorrhage **and** mass lesion **and** acute infarction **Numerator:** Final reports of the initial CT or MRI that include documentation of the presence or absence of each of the following: hemorrhage **and** mass lesion **and** acute infarction **Denominator:** All final reports for CT or MRI studies of the brain performed within 24 hours of arrival to the hospital for patients aged 18 years and older with an admitting diagnosis of *ischemic stroke* or *TIA* or *intracranial hemorrhage* **Exclusion(s):** None **Percentage** of final reports for CT or MRI studies of the brain performed within 24 hours of arrival to the hospital for patients aged 18 years and older with the diagnosis of *ischemic stroke* or *TIA* or *intracranial hemorrhage* that include documentation of the presence or absence of each of the following: hemorrhage **and** mass lesion **and** acute infarction (continued)	►3110F **Denominator Codes:** **3111F** **3112F**◄	►Presence or absence of hemorrhage and mass lesion and acute infarction documented in final CT or MRI report CT or MRI of the brain performed within 24 hours of arrival to the hospital CT or MRI of the brain performed greater than 24 hours after arrival to the hospital◄

►[1]Physician Consortium for Performance Improvement: www.physicianconsortium.org◄

[2]National Committee on Quality Assurance (NCQA): Health Employer Data Information Set (HEDIS®), www.ncqa.org

[3]Joint Commission on Accreditation of Healthcare Organizations (JCAHO), ORYX Initiative Performance Measures: www.jcaho.org/pms

[4]National Diabetes Quality Improvement Alliance: www.nationaldiabetesalliance.org

►[5]Joint measure from the Physician Consortium for Performance Improvement, www.physicianconsortium.org, and National Committee on Quality Assurance (NCQA), www.ncqa.org◄

►[6]The Society of Thoracic Surgeons, www.sts.org, and National Quality Forum, www.qualityforum.org◄

Brief Description of Performance Measure & Source and Reporting Instructions	CPT Code(s)	Code Descriptor
►Stroke and Stroke Rehabilitation (STR)◄, cont'd		
Reporting Instructions: It is intended that this measure be reported during an inpatient stay for ischemic stroke, TIA or intracranial hemorrhage. Report 3111F or 3112F for each patient. If CT or MRI of brain was performed within 24 hours of arrival to the hospital and final CT or MRI report included documentation of presence or absence of hemorrhage **and** mass lesion **and** acute infarction, also report 3110F. There are no exclusions for this measure; modifiers 1P, 2P, and 3P may not be used◄		
►Upper Respiratory Infection in Children (URI)◄		
►**Appropriate Treatment for Children with Upper Respiratory Infection**[2]—Whether or not children 3 months to 18 years of age (inclusive) who were seen for a visit with a diagnosis of only upper respiratory infection (URI) were appropriately NOT prescribed or dispensed an antibiotic. **Numerator:** Patients who were not prescribed or dispensed an antibiotic on the visit. **Denominator:** All patients aged 3 months to 18 years (inclusive) with only a diagnosis of upper respiratory infection **Exclusion(s):** Documentation of Medical Reason(s) for prescribing antibiotic. **Percentage** of children 3 months to 18 years of age (inclusive) who were seen for a visit with a diagnosis of only upper respiratory infection (URI) and were appropriately not prescribed or dispensed an antibiotic. **Reporting Instructions:** Measure note: This measure is being specified for physician reporting. Antibiotic dispensing from claims data is not the denominator criteria (see NCQA HEDIS®2007 health plan measure) • For URI patients with documented medical reasons for prescribing or dispensing an antibiotic, report modifier 1P with code 4124F • There are no performance measure exclusions for 4120F. Do not report modifiers 1P, 2P, or 3P with this code◄	►**4120F** **4124F**◄	►Antibiotic prescribed or dispensed Antibiotic neither prescribed nor dispensed◄

►[1]Physician Consortium for Performance Improvement: www.physicianconsortium.org◄

[2]National Committee on Quality Assurance (NCQA): Health Employer Data Information Set (HEDIS®), www.ncqa.org

[3]Joint Commission on Accreditation of Healthcare Organizations (JCAHO), ORYX Initiative Performance Measures: www.jcaho.org/pms

[4]National Diabetes Quality Improvement Alliance: www.nationaldiabetesalliance.org

►[5]Joint measure from the Physician Consortium for Performance Improvement, www.physicianconsortium.org, and National Committee on Quality Assurance (NCQA), www.ncqa.org◄

►[6]The Society of Thoracic Surgeons, www.sts.org, and National Quality Forum, www.qualityforum.org◄

Appendix I

Genetic Testing Code Modifiers

This listing of modifiers is intended for reporting with molecular laboratory procedures related to genetic testing. Genetic testing modifiers should be used in conjunction with CPT and HCPCS codes to provide diagnostic granularity of service to enable providers to submit complete and precise genetic testing information without altering test descriptors. These two-character modifiers are categorized by mutation. The first (numeric) character indicates the disease category and the second (alpha) character denotes gene type. Introductory guidelines in the molecular diagnostic and molecular cytogenetic code sections of the CPT codebook provide further guidance in interpretation and application of genetic testing modifiers.

Neoplasia (Solid Tumor, Excluding Sarcoma and Lymphoma)

0A	BRCA1 (hereditary breast/ovarian cancer)
0B	BRCA2 (hereditary breast cancer)
0C	Neurofibromin (neurofibromatosis, type 1)
0D	Merlin (neurofibromatosis, type 2)
0E	c-RET (multiple endocrine neoplasia, types 2A/B, familial medullary thyroid carcinoma)
0F	VHL (Von Hippel Lindau disease, renal carcinoma)
0G	SDHD (hereditary paraganglioma)
0H	SDHB (hereditary paraganglioma)
0I	ERRB2, commonly called Her-2/neu
0J	MLH1 (HNPCC, mismatch repair genes)
0K	MSH2, MSH6, or PMS2 (HNPCC, mismatch repair genes)
0L	APC (hereditary polyposis coli)
0M	Rb (retinoblastoma)
0N	TP53, commonly called p53
0O	PTEN (Cowden's syndrome)
0P	KIT, also called CD117 (gastrointestinal stromal tumor)
0Z	Solid tumor gene, not otherwise specified

Neoplasia (Sarcoma)

1A	WT1 or WT2 (Wilm's tumor)
1B	PAX3, PAX7, or FOXO1A (alveolar rhabdomyosarcoma)
1C	FLI1, ERG, ETV1, or EWSR1 (Ewing's sarcoma, desmoplastic round cell)
1D	DDIT3 or FUS (myxoid liposarcoma)
1E	NR4A3, RBF56, or TCF12 (myxoid chondrosarcoma)
1F	SSX1, SSX2, or SYT (synovial sarcoma)
1G	MYCN (neuroblastoma)
1H	COL1A1 or PDGFB (dermatofibrosarcoma protruberans)
1I	TFE3 or ASPSCR1 (alveolar soft parts sarcoma)
1J	JAZF1 or JJAZ1 (endometrial stromal sarcoma)
1Z	Sarcoma gene, not otherwise specified

Neoplasia (Lymphoid/Hematopoietic)

2A	RUNX1 or CBFA2T1, commonly called AML1 or ETO, genes associated with t(8;21) AML1—also ETO (acute myelogenous leukemia)
2B	BCR or ABL1, genes associated with t(9;22) (chronic myelogenous or acute leukemia) BCR—also ABL (chronic myeloid, acute lymphoid leukemia)
2C	PBX1 or TCF3, genes associated with t(1;19) (acute lymphoblastic leukemia) CGF1
2D	CBFB or MYH11, genes associated with inv 16 (acute myelogenous leukemia) CBF beta (leukemia)
2E	MLL (acute leukemia)
2F	PML or RARA, genes associated with t(15;17) (acute promyelocytic leukemia) PML/RAR alpha (promyelocytic leukemia)
2G	ETV6, commonly called TEL, gene associated with t(12;21) (acute leukemia) TEL (Leukemia)
2H	BCL2 (B cell lymphoma, follicle center cell origin) bcl-2 (Lymphoma)
2I	CCND1, commonly called BCL1, cyclin D1 (Mantle cell lymphoma, myeloma) bcl-1 (lymphoma)
2J	MYC (Burkitt lymphoma) c-myc (lymphoma)
2K	IgH (lymphoma/leukemia)
2L	IGK (lymphoma/leukemia)
2M	TRB, T cell receptor beta (lymphoma/leukemia)
2N	TRG, T cell receptor gamma (lymphoma/leukemia)

2O   SIL or TAL1 (T cell leukemia)

2T   BCL6 (B cell lymphoma)

2Q   API1 or MALT1 (MALT lymphoma)

2R   NPM or ALK, genes associated with t(2;5) (anaplastic large cell lymphoma)

2S   FLT3 (Acute myelogenous leukemia)

2Z   Lymphoid/hematopoietic neoplasia, not otherwise specified

Non-Neoplastic Hematology/Coagulation

3A   F5, commonly called Factor V (Leiden, others) (hypercoagulable state)

3B   FACC (Fanconi anemia)

3C   FACD (Fanconi anemia)

3D   HBB, beta globin (thalassemia, sickle cell anemia, other hemoglobinopathies)

3E   HBA, commonly called alpha globin (thalassemia)

3F   MTHFR (elevated homocystinemia)

3G   F2, commonly called prothrombin (20210, others) (hypercoagulable state) prothrombin (factor II, 20210A) (hypercoagulable state)

3H   F8, commonly called factor VIII (hemophilia A/VWF)

3I   F9, commonly called factor IX (hemophilia B)

3K   F13, commonly called factor XIII (bleeding or hypercoagulable state) beta globin

3Z   Non-neoplastic hematology/coagulation, not otherwise specified

Histocompatiblity/Blood Typing/Identity/Microsatellite

4A   HLA-A

4B   HLA-B

4C   HLA-C

4D   HLA-D

4E   HLA-DR

4F   HLA-DQ

4G   HLA-DP

4H   Kell

4I   Fingerprint for engraftment (post allogeneic progenitor cell transplant)

4J   Fingerprint for donor allelotype (allogeneic transplant)

4K   Fingerprint for recipient allelotype (allogeneic transplant)

4L   Fingerprint for leukocyte chimerism (allogeneic solid organ transplant)

4M   Fingerprint for maternal versus fetal origin

4N   Microsatellite instability

4O   Microsatellite loss (loss of heterozygosity)

4Z   Histocompatiblity/blood typing, not otherwise specified

Neurologic, Non-Neoplastic

5A   ASPA, commonly called Aspartoacylase A (Canavan disease)

5B   FMR-1 (fragile X, FRAXA, syndrome)

5C   FRDA, commonly called Frataxin (Freidreich ataxia)

5D   HD, commonly called Huntington (Huntington's disease)

5E   GABRA5, NIPA1, UBE3A, or ANCR GABRA (Prader Willi-Angelman syndrome)

5F   GJB2, commonly called Connexin-26 (hereditary hearing loss) Connexin-32 (GJB2) (hereditary deafness)

5G   GJB1, commonly called Connexin-32 (X-linked Charcot-Marie-Tooth disease)

5H   SNRPN (Prader Willi-Angelman syndrome)

5I   SCA1, commonly called Ataxin-1 (spinocerebellar ataxia, type 1)

5J   SCA2, commonly called Ataxin-2 (spinocerebellar ataxia, type 2)

5K   MJD, commonly called Ataxin-3 (spinocerebellar ataxia, type 3, Machado-Joseph disease)

5L   CACNA1A (spinocerebellar ataxia, type 6)

5M   ATXN7 Ataxin-7 (spinocerebellar ataxia, type 7)

5N   PMP-22 (Charcot-Marie-Tooth disease, type 1A)

5O   MECP2 (Rett syndrome)

5Z   Neurologic, non-neoplastic, not otherwise specified

Muscular, Non-Neoplastic

6A DMD, commonly called dystrophin (Duchenne/Becker muscular dystrophy)

6B DMPK (myotonic dystrophy, type 1)

6C ZNF-9 (myotonic dystrophy, type 2)

6D SMN1/SMN2 (autosomal recessive spinal muscular atrophy)

6E MTTK, commonly called tRNAlys (myotonic epilepsy, MERRF)

6F MTTL1, commonly called tRNAleu (mitochondrial encephalomyopathy, MELAS)

6Z Muscular, not otherwise specified

Metabolic, Other

7A APOE, commonly called apolipoprotein E (cardiovascular disease or Alzheimer's disease)

7B NPC1 or NPC2, commonly called sphingomyelin phosphodiesterase (Nieman-Pick disease)

7C GBA, commonly called acid beta glucosidase (Gaucher disease)

7D HFE (hemochromatosis)

7E HEXA, commonly called hexosaminidase A (Tay-Sachs disease)

7F ACADM (medium chain acyl CoA dehydrogenase deficiency)

7Z Metabolic, other, not otherwise specified

Metabolic, Transport

8A CFTR (cystic fibrosis)

8B PRSS1 (hereditary pancreatitis)

8C Long QT syndrome, KCN (Jervell and Lange-Nielsen syndromes, types 1, 2, 5, and 6) and SCN (Brugada syndrome, SIDS and type 3)

8Z Metabolic, transport, not otherwise specified

Metabolic-Pharmacogenetics

9A TPMT, commonly called (thiopurine methyltransferase) (patients on antimetabolite therapy)

9B CYP2 genes, commonly called cytochrome p450 (drug metabolism)

9C ABCB1, commonly called MDR1 or p-glycoprotein (drug transport)

9D NAT2 (drug metabolism)

9L Metabolic-pharmacogenetics, not otherwise specified

Dysmorphology

9M FGFR1 (Pfeiffer and Kallman syndromes)

9N FGFR2 (Crouzon, Jackson-Weiss, Apert, Saethre-Chotzen syndromes)

9O FGFR3 (achondroplasia, hypochondroplasia, thanatophoric dysplasia, types I and II, Crouzon syndrome with acanthosis nigricans, Muencke syndromes)

9P TWIST (Saethre-Chotzen syndrome)

9Q DGCR, commonly called CATCH-22 (DiGeorge and 22q11 deletion syndromes)

9Z Dysmorphology, not otherwise specified

Appendix J

Electrodiagnostic Medicine Listing of Sensory, Motor, and Mixed Nerves

This summary assigns each sensory, motor, and mixed nerve with its appropriate nerve conduction study code in order to enhance accurate reporting of codes 95900, 95903, and 95904. Each nerve constitutes one unit of service.

Motor Nerves Assigned to Codes 95900 and 95903

I. Upper extremity, cervical plexus, and brachial plexus motor nerves
  A. Axillary motor nerve to the deltoid
  B. Long thoracic motor nerve to the serratus anterior
  C. Median nerve
     1. Median motor nerve to the abductor pollicis brevis
     2. Median motor nerve, anterior interosseous branch, to the flexor pollicis longus
     3. Median motor nerve, anterior interosseous branch, to the pronator quadratus
     4. Median motor nerve to the first lumbrical
     5. Median motor nerve to the second lumbrical
  D. Musculocutaneous motor nerve to the biceps brachii
  E. Radial nerve
     1. Radial motor nerve to the extensor carpi ulnaris
     2. Radial motor nerve to the extensor digitorum communis
     3. Radial motor nerve to the extensor indicis proprius
     4. Radial motor nerve to the brachioradialis
  F. Suprascapular nerve
     1. Suprascapular motor nerve to the supraspinatus
     2. Suprascapular motor nerve to the infraspinatus
  G. Thoracodorsal motor nerve to the latissimus dorsi
  H. Ulnar nerve
     1. Ulnar motor nerve to the abductor digiti minimi
     2. Ulnar motor nerve to the palmar interosseous
     3. Ulnar motor nerve to the first dorsal interosseous
     4. Ulnar motor nerve to the flexor carpi ulnaris
  I. Other
II. Lower extremity motor nerves
  A. Femoral motor nerve to the quadriceps
     1. Femoral motor nerve to vastus medialis
     2. Femoral motor nerve to vastus lateralis
     3. Femoral motor nerve to vastus intermedialis
     4. Femoral motor nerve to rectus femoris
  B. Ilioinguinal motor nerve
  C. Peroneal (fibular) nerve
     1. Peroneal motor nerve to the extensor digitorum brevis
     2. Peroneal motor nerve to the peroneus brevis
     3. Peroneal motor nerve to the peroneus longus
     4. Peroneal motor nerve to the tibialis anterior
  D. Plantar motor nerve
  E. Sciatic nerve
  F. Tibial nerve
     1. Tibial motor nerve, inferior calcaneal branch, to the abductor digiti minimi
     2. Tibial motor nerve, medial plantar branch, to the abductor hallucis
     3. Tibial motor nerve, lateral plantar branch, to the flexor digiti minimi brevis
  G. Other

III. Cranial nerves and trunk
    A. Cranial nerve VII (facial motor nerve)
        1. Facial nerve to the frontalis
        2. Facial nerve to the nasalis
        3. Facial nerve to the orbicularis oculi
        4. Facial nerve to the orbicularis oris
    B. Cranial nerve XI (spinal accessory motor nerve)
    C. Cranial nerve XII (hypoglossal motor nerve)
    D. Intercostal motor nerve
    E. Phrenic motor nerve to the diaphragm
    F. Recurrent laryngeal nerve
    G. Other
IV. Nerve Roots
    A. Cervical nerve root stimulation
        1. Cervical level 5 (CT)
        2. Cervical level 6 (C6)
        3. Cervical level 7 (C7)
        4. Cervical level 8 (C8)
    B. Thoracic nerve root stimulation
        1. Thoracic level 1 (T1)
        2. Thoracic level 2 (T2)
        3. Thoracic level 3 (T3)
        4. Thoracic level 4 (T4)
        5. Thoracic level 5 (T5)
        6. Thoracic level 6 (T6)
        7. Thoracic level 7 (T7)
        8. Thoracic level 8 (T8)
        9. Thoracic level 9 (T9)
      10. Thoracic level 10 (T10)
      11. Thoracic level 11 (T11)
      12. Thoracic level 12 (T12)

C. Lumbar nerve root stimulation
        1. Lumbar level 1 (L1)
        2. Lumbar level 2 (L2)
        3. Lumbar level 3 (L3)
        4. Lumbar level 4 (L4)
        5. Lumbar level 5 (L5)
D. Sacral nerve root stimulation
        1. Sacral level 1 (S1)
        2. Sacral level 2 (S2)
        3. Sacral level 3 (S3)
        4. Sacral level 4 (S4)

Sensory and Mixed Nerves Assigned to Code 95904

I. Upper extremity sensory and mixed nerves
    A. Lateral antebrachial cutaneous sensory nerve
    B. Medial antebrachial cutaneous sensory nerve
    C. Medial brachial cutaneous sensory nerve
    D. Median nerve
        1. Median sensory nerve to the first digit
        2. Median sensory nerve to the second digit
        3. Median sensory nerve to the third digit
        4. Median sensory nerve to the fourth digit
        5. Median palmar cutaneous sensory nerve
        6. Median palmar mixed nerve
    E. Posterior antebrachial cutaneous sensory nerve
    F. Radial sensory nerve
        1. Radial sensory nerve to the base of the thumb
        2. Radial sensory nerve to digit 1

G. Ulnar nerve
   1. Ulnar dorsal cutaneous sensory nerve
   2. Ulnar sensory nerve to the fourth digit
   3. Ulnar sensory nerve to the fifth digit
   4. Ulnar palmar mixed nerve
H. Intercostal sensory nerve
I. Other

II. Lower extremity sensory and mixed nerves
   A. Lateral femoral cutaneous sensory nerve
   B. Medial calcaneal sensory nerve
   C. Medial femoral cutaneous sensory nerve
   D. Peroneal nerve
      1. Deep peroneal sensory nerve
      2. Superficial peroneal sensory nerve, medial dorsal cutaneous branch
      3. Superficial peroneal sensory nerve, intermediate dorsal cutaneous branch
   E. Posterior femoral cutaneous sensory nerve
   F. Saphenous nerve
      1. Saphenous sensory nerve (distal technique)
      2. Saphenous sensory nerve (proximal technique)
   G. Sural nerve
      1. Sural sensory nerve, lateral dorsal cutaneous branch
      2. Sural sensory nerve
   H. Tibial sensory nerve (digital nerve to toe 1)
   I. Tibial sensory nerve (medial plantar nerve)
   J. Tibial sensory nerve (lateral plantar nerve)
   K. Other

III. Head and trunk sensory nerves
   A. Dorsal nerve of the penis
   B. Greater auricular nerve
   C. Ophthalmic branch of the trigeminal nerve
   D. Pudendal sensory nerve
   E. Suprascapular sensory nerves
   F. Other

The following table provides a reasonable maximum number of studies performed per diagnostic category necessary for a physician to arrive at a diagnosis in 90% of patients with that final diagnosis. The numbers in each column represent the number of studies recommended. The appropriate number of studies to be performed is based upon the physician's discretion.

| Indication | Needle EMG (95860-95864, 95867-95870) | Type of Study/Maximum Number of Studies | | | |
| | | Nerve Conduction Studies (95900, 95903, 95904) | | Other EMG Studies (95934, 95936, 95937) | |
		Motor NCS With and/or Without F wave	Sensory NCS	H-Reflex	Neuromuscular Junction Testing (Repetitive Stimulation)
Carpal Tunnel (Unilateral)	1	3	4	—	—
Carpal Tunnel (Bilateral)	2	4	6	—	—
Radiculopathy	2	3	2	2	—
Mononeuropathy	1	3	3	2	—
Polyneuropathy/Mononeuropathy Multiplex	3	4	4	2	—
Myopathy	2	2	2	—	2
Motor Neuronopathy (eg, ALS)	4	4	2	—	2
Plexopathy	2	4	6	2	—
Neuromuscular Junction	2	2	2	—	3
Tarsal Tunnel Syndrome (Unilateral)	1	4	4	—	—
Tarsal Tunnel Syndrome (Bilateral)	2	5	6	—	—
Weakness, Fatigue, Cramps, or Twitching (Focal)	2	3	4	—	2
Weakness, Fatigue, Cramps, or Twitching (General)	4	4	4	—	2
Pain, Numbness, or Tingling (Unilateral)	1	3	4	2	—
Pain, Numbness, or Tingling (Bilateral)	2	4	6	2	—

Appendix K

Product Pending FDA Approval

Some vaccine products have been assigned a CPT Category I code in anticipation of future approval from the Food and Drug Administration (FDA). The following is a list of the vaccine product codes pending FDA approval status that are identified in the CPT codebook with the ⋌ symbol. Upon revision of the approval status by the FDA, notation of this revision will be provided via the AMA CPT Category I Vaccine Codes Internet listing (www.ama-assn.org/ama/pub/category/10902.html) and in subsequent publications of the CPT codebook.

90661

90662

90663

90698

Appendix L

Vascular Families

Assignment of branches to first, second, and third order in this table of vascular families makes the assumption that the starting point is catheterization of the aorta. This categorization would not be accurate, for instance, if a femoral or carotid artery were catheterized directly in an antegrade direction. Arteries highlighted in bold are those more commonly reported during arteriographic procedures.

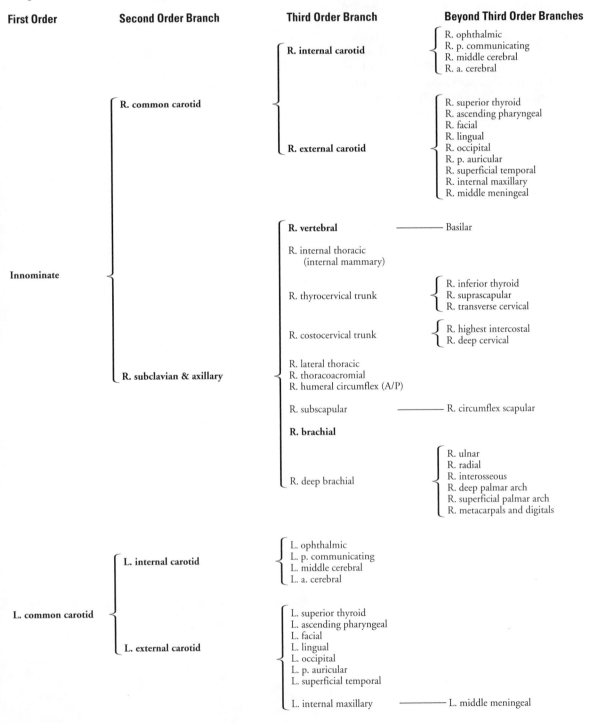

First Order	Second Order Branch	Third Order Branch	Beyond Third Order Branches

Innominate

R. common carotid
- **R. internal carotid** — R. ophthalmic / R. p. communicating / R. middle cerebral / R. a. cerebral
- **R. external carotid** — R. superior thyroid / R. ascending pharyngeal / R. facial / R. lingual / R. occipital / R. p. auricular / R. superficial temporal / R. internal maxillary / R. middle meningeal

R. subclavian & axillary
- **R. vertebral** — Basilar
- R. internal thoracic (internal mammary)
- R. thyrocervical trunk — R. inferior thyroid / R. suprascapular / R. transverse cervical
- R. costocervical trunk — R. highest intercostal / R. deep cervical
- R. lateral thoracic / R. thoracoacromial / R. humeral circumflex (A/P)
- R. subscapular — R. circumflex scapular
- **R. brachial**
- R. deep brachial — R. ulnar / R. radial / R. interosseous / R. deep palmar arch / R. superficial palmar arch / R. metacarpals and digitals

L. common carotid
- **L. internal carotid** — L. ophthalmic / L. p. communicating / L. middle cerebral / L. a. cerebral
- **L. external carotid** — L. superior thyroid / L. ascending pharyngeal / L. facial / L. lingual / L. occipital / L. p. auricular / L. superficial temporal / L. internal maxillary — L. middle meningeal

R = right, L = left, A = anterior, P = posterior

First Order	Second Order Branch	Third Order Branch	Beyond Third Order Branches

L. subclavian & axillary
- **L. vertebral**
- L. internal thoracic (internal mammary)
- L. thyrocervical trunk
  - L. inferior thyroid
  - L. suprascapular
  - L. transverse cervical
- L. costocervical trunk
  - L. highest intercostal
  - L. deep cervical
- L. lateral thoracic
- L. thoracoacromial
- L. humeral circumflex (A/P)
- L. subscapular — L. circumflex scapular
- **L. brachial**
- L. deep brachial
  - L. ulnar
  - L. radial
  - L. interosseous
    - L. deep palmar arch
    - L. superficial palmar arch
    - L. metacarpals and digitals

Intercostals

Bronchials

Recurrent esophageal

Inferior phrenic —— Superior suprarenal

Celiac trunk
- L. gastric —— Esophageal branch
- Splenic
  - Dorsal pancreatic —— Inferior transverse pancreatic
  - Great pancreatic
  - Caudal pancreatic
  - Gastroepiploic
  - Short gastrics
- Common hepatic
  - Gastroduodenal
    - P. superior pancreaticoduodenal
    - A. superior pancreaticoduodenal
  - Proper Hepatic
    - L. hepatic
    - R. hepatic
    - Cystic
    - Gastroepiploic
    - Supraduodenal
    - Intermediate hepatic

Middle suprarenal

Superior mesenteric
- Middle colic
- Inferior pancreaticoduodenal
  - P. inferior pancreaticoduodenal
  - A. inferior pancreaticoduodenal
- Jejunal
- Ileocolic
- Appendicular
- P. cecal
- A. cecal
- Marginal
- R. colic

R = right, L = left, A = anterior, P = posterior

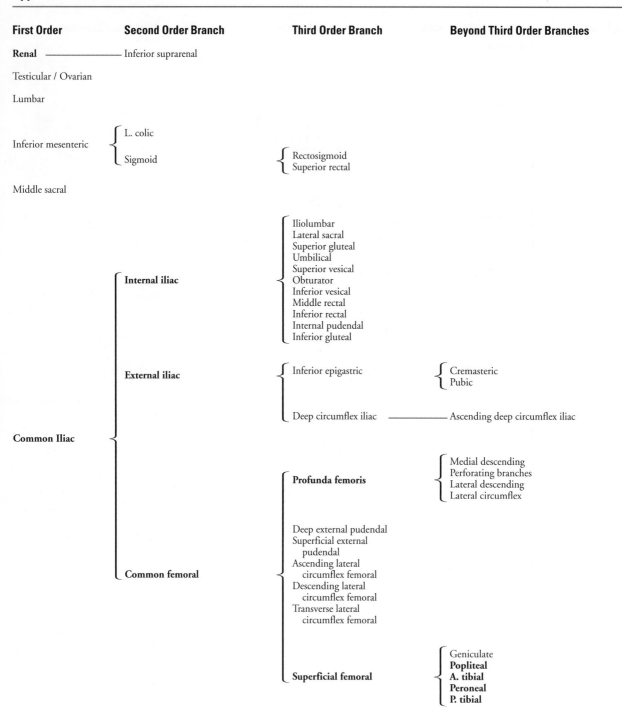

First Order	Second Order Branch	Third Order Branch	Beyond Third Order Branches

Renal —————— Inferior suprarenal

Testicular / Ovarian

Lumbar

Inferior mesenteric
- L. colic
- Sigmoid —— Rectosigmoid / Superior rectal

Middle sacral

Common Iliac

Internal iliac
- Iliolumbar
- Lateral sacral
- Superior gluteal
- Umbilical
- Superior vesical
- Obturator
- Inferior vesical
- Middle rectal
- Inferior rectal
- Internal pudendal
- Inferior gluteal

External iliac
- Inferior epigastric — Cremasteric / Pubic
- Deep circumflex iliac ————— Ascending deep circumflex iliac

Profunda femoris
- Medial descending
- Perforating branches
- Lateral descending
- Lateral circumflex

Common femoral
- Deep external pudendal
- Superficial external pudendal
- Ascending lateral circumflex femoral
- Descending lateral circumflex femoral
- Transverse lateral circumflex femoral

Superficial femoral
- Geniculate
- **Popliteal**
- **A. tibial**
- **Peroneal**
- **P. tibial**

R. & L. main pulmonary arteries (venous selective)

Reference: Kadir S. *Atlas of Normal and Variant Angiographic Anatomy.* Philadephia, Pa: WB Saunders Co; 1991.
R = right, L = left, A = anterior, P = posterior

Appendix M

Crosswalk to Deleted CPT Codes

This listing is a summary of the deleted *CPT 2007* codes and descriptors that have been crosswalked to *CPT 2008* codes.

Deleted CPT 2007 Code	CPT 2008 Code	CPT 2007 Code Descriptor
01905	01935, 01936	Anesthesia for myelography, discography, vertebroplasty
24350	24357-24359	Fasciotomy, lateral or medial (eg, tennis elbow or epicondylitis);
24351	24357-24359	Fasciotomy, lateral or medial (eg, tennis elbow or epicondylitis); with extensor origin detachment
24352	24357-24359	Fasciotomy, lateral or medial (eg, tennis elbow or epicondylitis); with annular ligament resection
24354	24357-24359	Fasciotomy, lateral or medial (eg, tennis elbow or epicondylitis); with stripping
24356	24357-24359	Fasciotomy, lateral or medial (eg, tennis elbow or epicondylitis); with partial ostectomy
32000	32421	Thoracentesis, puncture of pleural cavity for aspiration, initial or subsequent
32002	32422	Thoracentesis with insertion of tube with or without water seal (eg, for pneumothorax) (separate procedure)
32005	32560	Chemical pleurodesis (eg, for recurrent or persistent pneumothorax)
32019	32550	Insertion of indwelling tunneled pleural catheter with cuff
32020	32551	Tube thoracostomy with or without water seal (eg, for abscess, hemothorax, empyema) (separate procedure)
36540	36591	Collection of blood specimen from a completely implantable venous access device
36550	36593	Declotting by thrombolytic agent of implanted vascular access device or catheter
43750	43246	Percutaneous placement of gastrostomy tube
49200	49203-49205, 58957, 58958	Excision or destruction, open, intra-abdominal or retroperitoneal tumors or cysts or endometriomas;
49201	49203-49205, 58957, 58958	Excision or destruction, open, intra-abdominal or retroperitoneal tumors or cysts or endometriomas; extensive
51000	51100	Aspiration of bladder by needle
51005	51101	Aspiration of bladder; by trocar or intracatheter
51010	51102	Aspiration of bladder; with insertion of suprapubic catheter
60001	60300	Aspiration and/or injection, thyroid cyst
67038	67041, 67042, 67043	Vitrectomy, mechanical, pars plana approach; with epiretinal membrane stripping
75552	75557-75564	Cardiac magnetic resonance imaging for morphology; without contrast material
75553	75557-75564	Cardiac magnetic resonance imaging for morphology; with contrast material
75554	75557-75564	Cardiac magnetic resonance imaging for function, with or without morphology; complete study
75555	75557-75564	Cardiac magnetic resonance imaging for function, with or without morphology; limited study
75556	75557-75564	Cardiac magnetic resonance imaging for velocity flow mapping
78615	78610	Cerebral vascular flow
86586	86356, 86486	Unlisted antigen, each
99361	99365-99368	Medical conference by a physician with interdisciplinary team of health professionals or representatives of community agencies to coordinate activities of patient care (patient not present); approximately 30 minutes

Deleted CPT 2007 Code	CPT 2008 Code	CPT 2007 Code Descriptor
99362	99366-99368	Medical conference by a physician with interdisciplinary team of health professionals or representatives of community agencies to coordinate activities of patient care (patient not present); approximately 60 minutes
99371	99441-99443	Telephone call by a physician to patient or for consultation or medical management or for coordinating medical management with other health care professionals (eg, nurses, therapists, social workers, nutritionists, physicians, pharmacists); simple or brief (eg, to report on tests and/or laboratory results, to clarify or alter previous instructions, to integrate new information from other health professionals into the medical treatment plan, or to adjust therapy)
99372	99441-99443	Telephone call by a physician to patient or for consultation or medical management or for coordinating medical management with other health care professionals (eg, nurses, therapists, social workers, nutritionists, physicians, pharmacists); intermediate (eg, to provide advice to an established patient on a new problem, to initiate therapy that can be handled by telephone, to discuss test results in detail, to coordinate medical management of a new problem in an established patient, to discuss and evaluate new information and details, or to initiate new plan of care)
99373	99441-99443	Telephone call by a physician to patient or for consultation or medical management or for coordinating medical management with other health care professionals (eg, nurses, therapists, social workers, nutritionists, physicians, pharmacists); complex or lengthy (eg, lengthy counseling session with anxious or distraught patient, detailed or prolonged discussion with family members regarding seriously ill patient, lengthy communication necessary to coordinate complex services of several different health professionals working on different aspects of the total patient care plan)
3047F	3044F, 3045F	Most recent hemoglobin A1c level $\leq$ 9.0% (DM)
3076F	3074F, 3075F	Most recent systolic blood pressure < 140 mm Hg (HTN) (DM)
3143F	3142F	Documentation of order for barium swallow test (GERD)
0054T	20985-20987	Computer-assisted musculoskeletal surgical navigational orthopedic procedure, with image-guidance based on fluoroscopic images (List separately in addition to code for primary procedure)
0055T	20985-20987	Computer-assisted musculoskeletal surgical navigational orthopedic procedure, with image-guidance based on CT/MRI images (List separately in addition to code for primary procedure)
0056T	20985-20987	Computer-assisted musculoskeletal surgical navigational orthopedic procedure, image-less (List separately in addition to code for primary procedure)
0065T	99174	Ocular photoscreening, with interpretation and report, bilateral
0074T	98969, 99444	Online evaluation and management service, per encounter, provided by a physician, using the Internet or similar electronic communications network, in response to a patient's request, established patient
0115T	99605-99607	Medication therapy management service(s) provided by a pharmacist, individual, face-to-face with patient, initial 15 minutes, with assessment, and intervention if provided; initial encounter
0116T	99605-99607	Medication therapy management service(s) provided by a pharmacist, individual, face-to-face with patient, initial 15 minutes, with assessment, and intervention if provided; subsequent encounter
0117T	99605-99607	Medication therapy management service(s) provided by a pharmacist, individual, face-to-face with patient, initial 15 minutes, with assessment, and intervention if provided; each additional 15 minutes (List separately in addition to code for primary service)
0135T	50593	Ablation, renal tumor(s), unilateral, percutaneous, cryotherapy
0153T	34806	Transcatheter placement of wireless physiologic sensor in aneurysmal sac during endovascular repair, including radiological supervision and interpretation and instrument calibration (List separately in addition to code for primary procedure)
0154T	93982	Noninvasive physiologic study of implanted wireless pressure sensor in aneurysmal sac following endovascular repair, complete study including recording, analysis of pressure and waveform tracings, interpretation and report

Index

Instructions for the Use of the CPT Index

Main Terms

The index is organized by main terms. Each main term can stand alone, or be followed by up to three modifying terms. There are four primary classes of main entries:

1. Procedure or service.
   For example: Endoscopy; Anastomosis; Splint

2. Organ or other anatomic site.
   For example: Tibia; Colon; Salivary Gland

3. Condition.
   For example: Abscess; Entropion; Tetralogy of Fallot

4. Synonyms, Eponyms and Abbreviations.
   For example: EEG; Bricker Operation; Clagett Procedure

Modifying Terms

A main term may be followed by a series of up to three indented terms that modify the main term. When modifying terms appear, one should review the list, as these subterms do have an effect on the selection of the appropriate code for the procedure.

Code Ranges

Whenever more than one code applies to a given index entry, a code range is listed. If several non-sequential codes apply, they will be separated by a comma. For example:

Esophagus
   Reconstruction 43300, 43310, 43313

If two or more sequential codes apply, they will be separated by a hyphen. For example:

Debridement
   Burns 01951-01953, 16020-16030

Conventions

As a space saving convention, certain words infer some meaning. This convention is primarily used when a procedure or service is listed as a subterm. For example:

Knee
   Incision (of)

In this example, the word in parentheses (of) does not appear in the index, but it is inferred. As another example:

Pancreas
   Anesthesia (for procedures on)

In this example, as there is no such entity as pancreas anesthesia, the words in parentheses are inferred. That is, anesthesia for procedures on the pancreas.

The alphabetic index is NOT a substitute for the main text of *CPT*. Even if only one code appears, the user must refer to the main text to ensure that the code selection is accurate.

A

A Vitamin
See Vitamin, A

A-II
See Angiotensin II

Abbe-Estlander Procedure
See Reconstruction; Repair, Cleft Lip

Abdomen
Abdominal Aorta
  Angiography 75635
Abdominal Wall
  Removal
    Mesh 11008
    Prosthesis .11008
  Repair
    Hernia 49491-49496, 49501,
                49507, 49521, 49590
  Tumor
    Excision 22900
    Unlisted Services and Procedures 22999
Abscess
  Incision and Drainage 49020, 49040
  Open 49040
  Percutaneous 49021
Angiography 74175, 75635
Artery
  Ligation 37617
Biopsy 49000
Bypass Graft 35907
Cannula/Catheter
  Removal 49422
Celiotomy
  for Staging .49220
CT Scan 74150-74175, 75635
Cyst
  Destruction/Excision 49203-49205
Drainage
  Fluid 49080-49081
Ectopic Pregnancy 59130
Endometrioma
  Destruction/Excision 49203-49205
Exploration 49000-49002
  Blood Vessel 35840
  Staging 58960
Incision 49000
  Staging 58960
Incision and Drainage
  Pancreatitis 48000
Infraumbilical Panniculectomy 15830
Injection
  Air 49400
  Contrast Material 49400
Insertion
  Catheter 49419-49421, 49324
  Venous Shunt 49425
Intraperitoneal
  Catheter Exit Site 49436
  Catheter Insertion 49324, 49435
  Catheter Removal 49422
  Catheter Revision 49325
  Shunt
    Ligation .49428

Removal 49429
Laparotomy
  Staging 49220
Magnetic Resonance Imaging
(MRI) .74181-74183
Needle Biopsy
  Mass 49180
Peritoneocentesis 49080-49081
Radical Resection 51597
Repair
  Blood Vessel 35221
    with Other Graft 35281
    with Vein Graft 35251
  Hernia 49491-49525, 49560-49587
  Suture 49900
Revision
  Venous Shunt 49426
Suture 49900
Tumor
  Destruction/Excision 49203-49205
Ultrasound 76700-76705
Unlisted Services and Procedures 49999
Wound Exploration
  Penetrating 20102
X-Ray 74000-74022

Abdominal
Aorta
  See Abdomen, Abdominal Aorta; Aorta,
  Abdominal
Aortic Aneurysm
  See Aorta, Abdominal, Aneurysm
Deliveries
  See Caesarean Delivery
Hysterectomy
  See Hysterectomy, Abdominal
Lymphangiogram
  See Lymphangiography, Abdomen
Paracentesis
  See Abdomen, Drainage
Radiographies
  See Abdomen, X-Ray
Wall
  See Abdomen, Abdominal Wall
  Debridement
    Infected 11005-11006
    Reconstruction 49905
  Removal
    Mesh 11008
    Prosthesis 11008
  Surgery 22999
  Tumor
    Excision .22900

Abdominohysterectomy
See Hysterectomy, Abdominal

Abdominopelvic Amputation
See Amputation, Interpelviabdominal

Abdominoplasty 15830, 15847
See Panniculectomy
Excision 15847

Ablation
Anal
  Polyp 46615
  Tumor 46615
Bone
  Tumor 20982

Colon
  Tumor 45339
Cryosurgical
  Fibroadenoma 19105
  Renal Mass 50250
  Renal Tumor
    Percutaneous 50593
CT Scan Guidance 77013
Endometrial 58353-58356, 58563
Endometrium
  Ultrasound Guidance 58356
Heart
  Arrhythmogenic Focus 93650-93652
    See Cardiology; Diagnostic, Intracardiac
    Pacing and Mapping
  Atrioventricular Node Function 93650
Liver
  Tumor
    Laparoscopic 47370-47371
    Open 47380-47382
Lung
  Tumor
    Radiofrequency 32998
Magnetic Resonance Guidance 77022
Parenchymal Tissue
  CT Scan Guidance 77013
Prostate 55873
Pulmonary Tumor 32998
Radiofrequency 32998
Renal Cyst 50541
Renal Mass 50542
  Radiofrequency 50592
Renal Tumor
  Cryotherapy
    Percutaneous 50593
Turbinate Mucosa 30801-30802
Ultrasound
  Guidance .76940
  Uterine Tumor 0071T-0072T
Uterine Tumor
  Ultrasound, Focused 0071T-0072T
Vein
  Endovenous 36475-36479

Abortion
See Obstetrical Care
Incomplete 59812
Induced
  by Dilation and Curettage 59840
  by Dilation and Evacuation 59841
  by Saline 59850-59851
  by Vaginal Suppositories 59855-59856
  with Hysterectomy 59100, 59852, 59857
Missed
  First Trimester 59820
  Second Trimester 59821
Septic 59830
Spontaneous 59812
Therapeutic
  by Saline .59850
    with Dilation and Curettage 59851
    with Hysterectomy 59852

Abrasion
Skin
  Chemical Peel 15788-15793
  Dermabrasion 15780-15783
  Lesion 15786-15787

Abscess

Abdomen 49040-49041
  Incision and Drainage
    Open 49040
    Percutaneous 49021
Anal
  Incision and Drainage 46045-46050
Ankle 27603
Appendix
  Incision and Drainage 44900
    Open 44900
    Percutaneous 44901
Arm, Lower 25028
  Excision 25145
  Incision and Drainage 25035
Arm, Upper
  Incision and Drainage 23930-23935
Auditory Canal, External 69020
Bartholin's Gland
  Incision and Drainage 56420
Bladder
  Incision and Drainage 51080
Brain
  Drainage 61150-61151
  Excision 61514, 61522
  Incision and Drainage 61320-61321
Breast
  Incision and Drainage 19020
Carpals
  Incision, Deep 25035
Clavicle
  Sequestrectomy 23170
Drainage
  with X-Ray 75989
Ear, External
  Complicated 69005
  Simple 69000
Elbow
  Incision and Drainage 23930-23935
Epididymis
  Incision and Drainage 54700
Excision
  Olecranon Process 24138
  Radius 24136
  Ulna 24138
Eyelid
  Incision and Drainage 67700
Facial Bones
  Excision 21026
Finger 26010-26011
  Incision and Drainage 26034
Foot
  Incision 28005
Gums
  Incision and Drainage 41800
Hand
  Incision and Drainage 26034
Hematoma
  Incision and Drainage 27603
Hip
  Incision and Drainage 26990-26992
Humeral Head 23174
Humerus
  Excision 24134
  Incision and Drainage 23935
Kidney
  Incision and Drainage 50020
    Open 50020

    Percutaneous 50021
Leg, Lower
  Incision and Drainage 27603
Liver 47010
  Drainage
    Open 47010
    Injection 47015
    Repair 47300
  Localization
    Nuclear Medicine 78806-78807
Lung
  Percutaneous Drainage 32200-32201
Lymph Node
  Incision and Drainage 38300-38305
Lymphocele Drainage 49062
Mandible
  Excision 21025
Mouth
  Incision and Drainage 40800-40801,
    41005-41009, 41015-41018
Nasal Septum
  Incision and Drainage 30020
Neck
  Incision and Drainage 21501-21502
Ovarian
  Incision and Drainage 58820-58822
    Abdominal Approach 58822
    Vaginal Approach 58820
Ovary
  Drainage
    Percutaneous 58823
Palate
  Incision and Drainage 42000
Paraurethral Gland
  Incision and Drainage 53060
Parotid Gland Drainage 42300-42305
Pelvic
  Drainage
    Percutaneous 58823
Pelvis
  Incision and Drainage 26990-26992,
    45000
Pericolic
  Drainage
    Percutaneous 58823
Perineum
  Incision and Drainage 56405
Perirenal or Renal
  Drainage 50020-50021
    Percutaneous 50021
Peritoneum
  Incision and Drainage
    Open 49020
    Percutaneous 49021
Prostate
  Incision and Drainage 55720-55725
  Transurethral Drainage 52700
Radius
  Incision, Deep 25035
Rectum
  Incision and Drainage ..45005-45020, 46040,
    46060
Retroperitoneal 49060-49061
  Drainage
    Open 49060
    Percutaneous 49061

Salivary Gland
  Drainage 42300-42320
Scapula
  Sequestrectomy 23172
Scrotum
  Incision and Drainage 54700, 55100
Shoulder
  Drainage 23030
Skene's Gland
  Incision and Drainage 53060
Skin
  Incision and Drainage 10060-10061
  Puncture Aspiration 10160
Soft Tissue
  Incision 20000-20005
Spine
  Incision and Drainage 22010-22015
Subdiaphragmatic 49040-49041
Sublingual Gland
  Drainage 42310-42320
Submaxillary Gland
  Drainage 42310-42320
Subphrenic 49040-49041
Testis
  Incision and Drainage 54700
Thoracostomy 32551
Thorax
  Incision and Drainage 21501-21502
Throat
  Incision and Drainage 42700-42725
Tongue
  Incision and Drainage 41000-41006
Tonsil
  Incision and Drainage 42700
Ulna
  Incision, Deep 25035
Urethra
  Incision and Drainage 53040
Uvula
  Incision and Drainage 42000
Vagina
  Incision and Drainage 57010
Vulva
  Incision and Drainage 56405
Wrist
  Excision 25145
  Incision and Drainage 25028, 25035
X-Ray 76080

Abscess, Nasal
See Nose, Abscess

Abscess, Parotid Gland
See Parotid Gland, Abscess

Absorptiometry
Dual Energy 3095F-3096F
  Body Composition 0028T
  Bone
    Appendicular 77081
    Axial Skeleton 77080
    Vertebral 77082
Dual Photon
  Bone 78351
Radiographic
  Photodensity 77083
Single Photon
  Bone 78350

Adductor Tenotomy of Hip
See Tenotomy, Hip, Adductor

Adenoidectomy
See Adenoids, Excision

Adenoids
Excision 42830-42836
    with Tonsils 42820-42821
Unlisted Services and Procedures 42999

Adenoma
Pancreas
    Excision 48120
Thyroid Gland Excision 60200

Adenosine 3'5' Monophosphate
See Cyclic AMP

Adenosine Diphosphate
Blood 82030

Adenosine Monophosphate (AMP)
Blood 82030

Adenovirus
Antibody 86603
Antigen Detection
    Enzyme Immunoassay 87301
    Immunofluorescense 87260

Adenovirus Vaccine
See Vaccines

Adenylic Acid
See Adenosine Monophosphate (AMP)

ADH
See Antidiuretic Hormone

Adhesions
Epidural 0027T, 62263-62264
Eye
    Corneovitreal 65880
    Incision
        Anterior Segment 65860-65870
        Posterior Segment 65875
Intermarginal
    Construction 67880
        Transposition of Tarsal Plate 67882
Intestinal
    Enterolysis .44005
        Laparoscopic 44180
Intracranial
    Lysis 62161
Intrauterine
    Lysis 58559
Labial
    Lysis 56441
Lungs
    Lysis 32124
Pelvic
    Lysis 58660, 58662, 58740
Penile
    Lysis
        Post-circumcision 54162
Preputial
    Lysis 54450
Urethral
    Lysis 53500

Adipectomy
See Lipectomy

ADL
See Activities of Daily Living

Administration
Immunization
    Each Additional Vaccine/Toxoid 90472, 90474
        with Counseling 90466, 90468
    One Vaccine/Toxoid 90471, 90473
        with Counseling 90465, 90467

ADP
See Adenosine Diphosphate

ADP Phosphocreatine Phosphotransferase
See CPK

Adrenal Cortex Hormone
See Corticosteroids

Adrenal Gland
Biopsy 60540-60545
Excision
    Laparoscopy 60650
    Retroperitoneal Tumor 60545
Exploration 60540-60545
Nuclear Medicine
    Imaging 78075

Adrenal Medulla
See Medulla

Adrenalectomy 60540
Anesthesia 00866
Laparoscopic .50545

Adrenalin
See Catecholamines
Blood 82383
Urine 82384

Adrenaline-Noradrenaline
Testing .82382-82384

Adrenocorticotropic Hormone (ACTH) . . .80400-80406, 80412, 80418, 82024
Blood or Urine .82024
Stimulation Panel 80400-80406

Adrenogenital Syndrome .56805, 57335

Adult T Cell Leukemia Lymphoma Virus I
See HTLV I

Advanced Life Support
See Emergency Department Services
Physician Direction 99288

Advancement
Genioglossus 21199
Tendon
    Foot 28238

Advancement Flap
See Skin, Adjacent Tissue Transfer

Aerosol Inhalation
See Pulmonology, Therapeutic
Pentamidine 94642

AFB
See Acid Fast Bacilli (AFB)

Afferent Nerve
See Sensory Nerve

AFP
See Alpha-Fetoprotein

After Hours Medical Services .99050

Agents, Anticoagulant
See Clotting Inhibitors

Agglutinin
Cold 86156-86157
Febrile 86000

Aggregation
Platelet 85576

AHG
See Clotting Factor

AICD (Pacing Cardioverter-Defibrillator)
See Defibrillator, Heart; Pacemaker, Heart

Aid, Hearing
See Hearing Aid

AIDS Antibodies
See Antibody, HIV

AIDS Virus
See HIV-1

Akin Operation
See Bunion Repair

ALA
See Aminolevulinic Acid (ALA)

Alanine 2 Oxoglutarate Aminotransferase
See Transaminase, Glutamic Pyruvic

Alanine Amino (ALT) 84460

Alanine Transaminase
See Transaminase, Glutamic Pyruvic

Albarran Test
See Water Load Test

Albumin
Ischemia modified 82045
Serum 82040
Urine 82042-82044

Alcohol
Breath 82075
Ethyl
    Blood 82055
    Urine 82055
Ethylene Glycol 82693

Alcohol Dehydrogenase
See Antidiuretic Hormone

Alcohol, Isopropyl
See Isopropyl Alcohol

Alcohol, Methyl
See Methanol

Aldolase
Blood 82085

Aldosterone
Blood 82088
Suppression Evaluation 80408
Urine 82088

Alimentary Canal
See Gastrointestinal Tract

Alkaline Phosphatase 84075-84080
Leukocyte 85540
WBC 85540

Alkaloids
See Specific Drug
Urine 82101

Allergen Bronchial Provocation Tests
See Allergy Tests; Bronchial Challenge Test

Allergen Challenge, Endobronchial
See Bronchial Challenge Test

Allergen Immunotherapy
Allergen
      Prescription/Supply/Injection . .95120-95125
            with Extract Supply 95144
                  Injection 95115-95117
Antigens 95144
IgE 86003-86005
IgG 86001
Insect Venom
      Prescription/Supply 95145-95149
      Prescription/Supply/Injection . .95130-95134
Prescription/Supply 95165
      Insect, Whole Body 95170
Rapid Desensitization 95180

Allergy Services/Procedures
See Office and/or Other Outpatient Services;
Allergen and Immunotherapy
Education and Counseling 99201-99215
Unlisted Services and Procedures 95199

Allergy Tests
Challenge Test
      Bronchial 95070-95071
      Ingestion 95075
Eye Allergy 95060
Food Allergy .95075
Intradermal
      Allergen Extract 95024-95028
      Biologicals 95015
      Drugs 95015
      Incremental 95027
      Venoms .95015
Nasal Mucous Membrane Test 95065
Nose Allergy .95065
Patch
      Application Tests 95044
      Photo Patch 95052
Photosensitivity 95056
Provocative Testing 95078

Skin Tests
      Allergen Extract 95004, 95024, 95027
      Biologicals 95010
      Drugs 95010
      Venoms .95010

Allogeneic Donor
Lymphocyte Infusion 38242

Allogeneic Transplantation
See Homograft

Allograft
Aortic Valve 33406, 33413
Bone
      Structural 20931
Cartilage
      Knee 27415
Lung Transplant 32850
Skin 15300-15336
Spine Surgery
      Morselized 20930
      Structural 20931

Allograft Preparation
Heart 33933, 33944
Intestines 44715-44721
Kidney 50323-50329
Liver 47143-47147
Lung 32855-32856, 33933
Pancreas 48551-48552
Renal 50323-50329

Allotransplantation
Intestines 44135-44136
Renal 50360-50365
      Removal 50370

Almen Test
See Blood, Feces

Alpha-1 Antitrypsin 82103-82104

Alpha-2 Antiplasmin 85410

Alpha-Fetoprotein
Amniotic Fluid 82106
Serum .82105, 82107

Alphatocopherol 84446

ALT
See Transaminase, Glutamic Pyruvic

Altemeier Procedure
See Anus; Rectum, Prolapse, Excision

Aluminum
Blood 82108

Alveola
Fracture
      Closed Treatment 21421
      Open Treatment 21422-21423

Alveolar Cleft
Ungrafted Bilateral 21147
Ungrafted Unilateral 21146

Alveolar Nerve
Avulsion 64738
Incision 64738
Transection .64738

Alveolar Ridge
Fracture
      Closed Treatment 21440
      Open Treatment 21445

Alveolectomy 41830

Alveoloplasty 41874

Alveolus
Excision 41830

Amide, Procaine
See Procainamide

Amikacin
Assay 80150

Amine
Vaginal Fluid 82120

Amino Acids 82127-82139

Aminolevulinic Acid (ALA)
Blood or Urine 82135

Aminotransferase
See Transaminase

Aminotransferase, Alanine
See Transaminase, Glutamic Pyruvic

Aminotransferase, Aspartate
See Transaminase, Glutamic Oxaloacetic

Amitriptyline
Assay 80152

Ammonia
Blood 82140
Urine 82140

Amniocenteses
See Amniocentesis

Amniocentesis 59000
See Chromosome Analysis
Induced Abortion 59850
      with Dilation and Curettage 59851
      with Dilation and Evacuation 59851
      with Hysterectomy 59852
Urine
      with Amniotic Fluid Reduction 59001

Amnioinfusion
Transabdominal 59070

Amnion
Amniocentesis 59000
      with Amniotic Fluid Reduction 59001
Amnioinfusion
      Transabdominal 59070

Amniotic Fluid
Alpha-Fetoprotein 82106
Scan 82143
Testing 83661, 83663-83664

Amniotic Membrane
See Amnion

Amobarbital 82205

AMP
See Adenosine Monophosphate (AMP)

AMP, Cyclic
See Cyclic AMP

Amphetamine
Blood or Urine 82145

Amputation
See Radical Resection; Replantation
Ankle 27888
Arm, Lower 25900-25905, 25915
    Revision 25907-25909
Arm, Upper 24900-24920
    and Shoulder 23900-23921
    Revision 24925-24930
    with Implant 24931-24935
Cervix
    Total 57530
Ear
    Partial 69110
    Total 69120
Finger 26910-26952
Foot 28800-28805
Hand at Metacarpal 25927
    at Wrist .25920
        Revision 25922
    Revision 25924, 25929-25931
Interpelviabdominal 27290
Interthoracoscapular 23900
Leg, Lower 27598, 27880-27882
    Revision 27884-27886
Leg, Upper 27590-27592
    at Hip 27290-27295
    Revision 27594-27596
Metacarpal 26910
Metatarsal 28810
Penis
    Partial 54120
    Radical 54130-54135
    Total 54125
Thumb 26910-26952
Toe 28810-28825
Tuft of Distal Phalanx 11752
Upper Extremity 24940
    Cineplasty 24940

Amputation through Hand
See Hand, Amputation

Amputation, Nose
See Resection, Nose

Amylase
Blood 82150
Urine 82150

ANA
See Antinuclear Antibodies (ANA)

Anabolic Steroid
See Androstenedione

Anal Abscess
See Abscess, Anal

Anal Bleeding
See Anus, Hemorrhage

Anal Fistula
See Fistula, Anal

Anal Fistulectomy
See Excision, Fistula, Anal

Anal Fistulotomy
See Fistulotomy, Anal

Anal Sphincter
Dilation 45905
Incision 46080

Anal Ulceration
See Anus, Fissure

Analgesia
See Anesthesia; Sedation

Analgesic Cutaneous Electrostimulation
See Application, Neurostimulation

Analysis
Computer Data 99090
Electroencephalogram
    Digital 95957
Electronic
    Drug Infusion Pump 62367-62368
    Pacing Cardioverter-Defibrillator 93640-
             93642, 93741-93744
      See Pacemaker, Heart
    Pulse Generator 0162T, 95970-95971,
             95980-95982
Physiologic Data, Remote 99091
Protein
    Tissue
        Western Blot 88372
Semen 89320-89322
    Sperm Isolation 89260-89261

Analysis, Spectrum
See Spectrophotometry

Anaspadias
See Epispadias

Anastomosis
Arteriovenous Fistula
    Direct 36821
    with Bypass Graft 35686
    with Graft 36825-36830, 36832
Artery
    to Aorta .33606
    to Artery
        Cranial 61711
Bile Duct
    to Bile Duct 47800
    to Intestines 47760, 47780
Bile Duct to Gastrointestinal 47785
Broncho-Bronchial 32486
Caval to Mesenteric 37160
Cavopulmonary 33768
Colorectal 44620
Epididymis
    to Vas Deferens
        Bilateral 54901
        Unilateral 54900
Excision
    Trachea 31780-31781

Fallopian Tube 58750
Gallbladder to Intestines 47720-47740
Hepatic Duct to Intestines 47765, 47802
Ileo-Anal 45113
Intestine to Intestine 44130
Intestines
    Colo-anal 45119
    Cystectomy 51590
    Enterocystoplasty 51960
    Ileoanal 44157-44158
    Resection
        Laparoscopic 44202-44205
Intrahepatic Portosystemic 37182-37183
Jejunum 43825
Microvascular
    Free Transfer
        Jejunum 43496
Nerve
    Facial to Hypoglossal 64868
    Facial to Phrenic 64870
Oviduct 58750
Pancreas to Intestines 48520-48540, 48548
Portocaval 37140
Pulmonary 33606
Renoportal 37145
Splenorenal 37180-37181
Stomach 43825
    to Duodenum 43810, 43855
        Revision 43850
    to Jejunum 43820, 43860-43865
Tubotubal 58750
Ureter
    to Bladder 50780-50785
    to Colon 50810-50815
        Removal 50830
    to Intestine 50800, 50820-50825
        Removal 50830
    to Kidney 50727-50750
    to Ureter 50727, 50760-50770
Vein
    Saphenopopliteal 34530
Vein to Vein 37140-37160, 37182-37183

Anastomosis of Lacrimal Sac to Conjunctival Sac
See Conjunctivorhinostomy

Anastomosis of Pancreas
See Pancreas, Anastomosis

Anastomosis, Aorta-Pulmonary Artery
See Aorta, Anastomosis, to Pulmonary Artery

Anastomosis, Bladder, to Intestine
See Enterocystoplasty

Anastomosis, Hepatic Duct
See Hepatic Duct, Anastomosis

Anderson Tibial Lengthening . .27715
See Ankle; Tibia, Osteoplasty, Lengthening

Androstanediol Glucuronide . . .82154

Androstanolone
See Dihydrotestosterone

Androstenedione
Blood or Urine 82157

Anesthesia Local
See Anesthesia, Local

Aneurysm Repair
See Aorta; Artery

Angel Dust
See Phencyclidine

Angina Assessment
See Performance Measure

Angiocardiographies
See Heart, Angiography

Angiography
See Aortography

Angioma
See Lesion, Skin

Angioplasties, Coronary Balloon
See Percutaneous Transluminal Angioplasty

Angioplasty

Angioscopy

Angiotensin Converting Enzyme (ACE)
See Performance Measures

Angiotensin Forming Enzyme
See Renin

Angiotensin I 84244
Riboflavin 84252

Angiotensin II
Blood or Urine 82163

Angle Deformity
Reconstruction
   Toe 28313

Anhydride, Carbonic
See Carbon Dioxide

Anhydrides, Acetic
See Acetic Anhydrides

Animal
Inoculation 87001-87003, 87250

Ankle
See Fibula; Leg, Lower; Tibia; Tibiofibular Joint
Abscess
   Incision and Drainage 27603
Amputation 27888
Arthrocentesis 20605
Arthrodesis 27870
Arthrography 73615
Arthroplasty 27700-27703
Arthroscopy
   Surgical 29891-29899
Arthrotomy 27610-27612, 27620-27626
Biopsy 27613-27614, 27620
Bursa
   Incision and Drainage 27604
Disarticulation 27889
Dislocation
   Closed Treatment 27840-27842
   Open Treatment 27846-27848
Exploration 27610, 27620
Fracture
   Bimalleolar 27808-27814
   Lateral 27786-27814, 27792
   Medial 27760-27766, 27808-27814
   Posterior 27767-27769, 27808-27814
   Trimalleolar 27816-27823
Fusion 27870
Hematoma
   Incision and Drainage 27603
Incision 27607
Injection
   Radiologic 27648
Lesion
   Excision 27630
Magnetic Resonance Imaging
(MRI) 73721-73723
Manipulation 27860
Removal
   Foreign Body 27610, 27620
   Implant 27704
   Loose Body 27620
Repair
   Achilles Tendon 27650-27654
   Ligament 27695-27698
   Tendon 27612, 27680-27687
Strapping 29540
Synovium
   Excision 27625-27626

Tenotomy 27605-27606
Tumor
   Excision 27615-27619
Unlisted Services and Procedures 27899
X ray 73600-73610
   with Contrast 73615

Ankylosis (Surgical)
See Arthrodesis

Annuloplasty
Percutaneous, Intradiscal 0062T, 0063T,
               22526-22527

Anogenital Region
See Perineum

Anoplasty
Stricture 46700-46705

Anorectal
Biofeedback 90911
Repair
   Fistula 0170T, 46706

Anorectal Exam (Surgical) 45990

Anorectal Myectomy
See Myomectomy, Anorectal

Anorectovaginoplasty 46744-46746

Anoscopy
Ablation
   Polyp 46615
   Tumor 46615
Biopsy 46606
Dilation 46604
Exploration 46600
Hemorrhage 46614
Removal
   Foreign Body 46608
   Polyp 46610-46612
   Tumor 46610-46612

Antebrachium
See Forearm

Antecedent, Plasma Thromboplastin
See Plasma Thromboplastin, Antecedent

Antepartum Care
Cesarean Delivery 59510
   Previous 59610, 59618
Vaginal Delivery 59425-59426

Anterior Ramus of Thoracic Nerve
See Intercostal Nerve

Anthrax Vaccine
See Vaccines

Anthrogon
See Follicle Stimulating Hormone (FSH)

Anti Australia Antigens
See Antibody, Hepatitis B

Anti D Immunoglobulin
See Immune Globulins, Rho (D)

Anti-Human Globulin Consumption Test
See Coombs Test

Anti-Phospholipid Antibody
See Antibody, Phospholipid

Antiactivator, Plasmin
See Alpha-2 Antiplasmin

Antibiotic Administration
Injection 90772
Prescribed or Dispensed 4120F-4124F

Antibiotic Sensitivity 87181-87184,
                            87188
Enzyme Detection 87185
Minimum Bactericidal Concentration 87187
Minimum Inhibitory Concentration 87186

Antibodies, Thyroid-Stimulating
See Immunoglobulin, Thyroid Stimulating

Antibodies, Viral
See Viral Antibodies

Antibody
See Antibody Identification; Microsomal Antibody
Actinomyces 86602
Adenovirus 86603
Antinuclear 86038-86039
Antiphosphatidylserine (Phospholipid) 86148
Antiprothrombin 0030T
Antistreptolysin O 86060-86063
Aspergillus 86606
Bacterium 86609
Bartonella 86611
Beta 2 Glycoprotein I 86146
Blastomyces 86612
Blood Crossmatch 86920-86923
Bordetella 86615
Borrelia 86618-86619
Brucella 86622
Campylobacter 86625
Candida 86628
Cardiolipin 86147
Chlamydia 86631-86632
Coccidioides 86635
Coxiella Burnetii 86638
Cryptococcus 86641
Cyclic Citrullinated Peptide (CCP) 86200
Cytomegalovirus 86644-86645
Cytotoxic Screen 86807-86808
Deoxyribonuclease 86215
Deoxyribonucleic Acid (DNA) ...86225-86226
Diphtheria 86648
Ehrlichia 86666
Encephalitis 86651-86654
Enterovirus 86658
Epstein-Barr Virus 86663-86665
Fluorescent 86255-86256
Francisella Tularensis 86668
Fungus 86671
Giardia Lamblia 86674
Growth Hormone 86277
Helicobacter Pylori 86677
Helminth 86682
Hemophilus Influenza 86684
Hepatitis
   Delta Agent 86692

Arteriotomy
See Incision, Artery; Transection, Artery

Arteriovenous Anastomosis ...36818-
36820

Arteriovenous Fistula
Cannulization
    Vein 36815
Hemodialysis via Fistula 4052F
Referral 4051F
Repair
    Abdomen 35182
      Acquired or Traumatic 35189
    Head 35180
      Acquired or Traumatic 35188
    Lower Extremity 35184
      Acquired or Traumatic 35190
    Neck 35180
      Acquired or Traumatic 35188
    Thorax 35182
      Acquired or Traumatic 35189
    Upper Extremity 35184
      Acquired or Traumatic 35190
Revision
    with Thrombectomy 36833
    without Thrombectomy 36832
Thrombectomy
    Dialysis Graft
      without Revision 36831
    Graft 36870

Arteriovenous Malformation
Cranial
    Repair 61680-61692, 61705-61708
Spinal
    Excision 63250-63252
    Injection 62294
    Repair 63250-63252

Arteriovenous Shunt
Angiography 75790
Catheterization 36145

Artery
Abdomen
    Angiography 75726
    Catheterization 36245-36248
    Ligation 37617
Adrenal
    Angiography 75731-75733
Anastomosis
    Cranial 61711
Angioplasty 75962-75968
Aorta
    Angioplasty 35452
    Atherectomy 35481, 35491
Aortobi-iliac
    Bypass Graft 35538, 35638
Aortobifemoral
    Bypass Graft 35540
Aortofemoral
    Bypass Graft 35539
Aortoiliac
    Bypass Graft 35537, 35637
    Embolectomy 34151-34201
    Thrombectomy 34151-34201
Aortoiliofemoral 35363

Arm
    Angiography 75710-75716
    Harvest 35600
Atherectomy
    Open 35480-35485
    Percutaneous 35490-35495
Axillary
    Aneurysm 35011-35013
    Angioplasty 35458
    Embolectomy 34101
    Thrombectomy 34101
    Thromboendarterectomy 35321
Basilar
    Aneurysm 61698, 61702
Biopsy
    Transcatheter 75970
Brachial
    Aneurysm 35011-35013
    Angiography 75658
    Bypass Graft 35510, 35512, 35522-35525
    Catheterization 36120
    Embolectomy 34101
    Exploration 24495
    Exposure 34834
    Thrombectomy 34101
    Thromboendarterectomy 35321
Brachiocephalic
    Angioplasty 35458
    Atherectomy 35484, 35494
    Catheterization 36215-36218
Bypass Graft
    with Composite Graft 35681-35683
Cannulization
    for Extra Corporeal Circulation 36823
    to Vein 36810-36815
Carotid
    Aneurysm 35001-35002, 61697-61705
    Vascular Malformation or Carotid
      Cavernous Fistula 61710
    Angiography 75660-75680
    Bypass Graft ...33891, 35501-35510, 35526,
             35601-35606, 35626, 35642
    Catheterization 36100
    Decompression 61590-61591,
              61595-61596
    Embolectomy 34001
    Exploration 35701
    Ligation 37600-37606, 61611-61612
    Stenosis
      Imaging Study Measurement 3100F
    Thrombectomy 34001
    Thromboendarterectomy 35301, 35390
    Transection 61611-61612
    Transposition 33889
Carotid, Common
    Intima-Media Thickness (IMT) Study ..0126T
Celiac
    Aneurysm 35121-35122
    Bypass Graft 35531, 35631
    Embolectomy 34151
    Thrombectomy 34151
    Thromboendarterectomy 35341
Chest
    Ligation 37616
Coronary
    Angiography 93556
    Atherectomy 92995-92996

Bypass 33517-33519
    Arterial 33533-33536
    Bypass Venous Graft ...33510-33517, 35523
      Internal Mammary Artery Graft 4110F
    Graft 33503-33505
    Ligation 33502
    Repair 33500-33507
    Thrombectomy
      Percutaneous 92973
Digital
    Sympathectomy 64820
Ethmoidal
    Ligation 30915
Extra Corporeal Circulation
    for Regional Chemotherapy
      of Extremity 36823
Extracranial
    Vascular Studies
      Non-Invasive, Physiologic 93875
Extremities
    Vascular Studies 93922-93923
Extremity
    Bypass Graft Revision 35879-35884
    Catheterization 36140
    Ligation 37618
Femoral
    Aneurysm 35141-35142
    Angioplasty 35456
    Atherectomy 35483, 35493
    Bypass Graft ...35521, 35533, 35551-35558,
          35566, 35621, 35646-35647,
          35651-35661, 35666, 35700
    Bypass Graft Revision 35883-35884
    Bypass In-Situ 35583-35585
    Embolectomy 34201
    Exploration 35721
    Exposure 34812-34813
    Thrombectomy 34201
    Thromboendarterectomy 35371-35372
Great Vessel
    Repair 33770-33781
Head
    Angiography 75650
Hepatic
    Aneurysm 35121-35122
Iliac
    Aneurysm 35131-35132, 75954
    Angioplasty 35454
    Atherectomy 35482, 35492
    Bypass Graft 35563, 35663
    Embolectomy 34151-34201
    Exposure 34820, 34833
    Graft 34900
    Occulsion Device 34808
    Thrombectomy 34151-34201
    Thromboendarterectomy 35351,
             35361-35363
Iliofemoral
    Bypass Graft 35548-35549, 35565
    Thromboendarterectomy ...35355, 35363
    X ray with Contrast 75630
Innominate
    Aneurysm 35021-35022
    Embolectomy 34001-34101
    Thrombectomy 34001-34101
    Thromboendarterectomy 35311

Body of Vertebra
See Vertebral Body

Body Section
X ray 76100
   Motion 76101-76102

Body System, Neurologic
See Nervous System

Boil
See Furuncle

Boil, Vulva
See Abscess, Vulva

Bone
See Specific Bone
Ablation
   Tumor 20982
Biopsy 20220-20245
Carpal
   See Carpal Bone
Cheek
   See Cheekbone
CT Scan
   Density Study 77078-77079
Cyst
   Drainage 20615
   Injection 20615
Dual Energy X-ray Absorptiometry ..77080-77081
Excision
   Epyphyseal Bar 20150
   Facial Bones 21026
   Mandible 21025
Facial
   See Facial Bone
Fixation
   Caliper 20660
   Cranial Tong 20660
   Halo 20661-20663, 21100
   Interdental 21110
   Multiplane 20692
   Pin/Wire 20650
   Skeletal
     Humeral Epicondyle
       Percutaneous 24566
   Stereotactic Frame 20660
   Uniplane 20690
Fracture
   Osteoporosis Screening 5015F
Hyoid
   See Hyoid Bone
Insertion
   Needle 36680
   Osseointegrated Implant
     for External Speech Processor/
     CochlearStimulator 69714-69718
Marrow
   Cytogenic Testing 3155F
Metatarsal
   See Metatarsal Bone
Nasal
   See Nasal Bone
Navicular
   See Navicular
Nuclear Medicine
   Density Study 78350-78351
   Imaging 78300-78320

   SPECT 78320
   Unlisted Services and Procedures 78399
Osteoporosis
   Pharmacologic Therapy 4005F
Protein 83937
Removal
   Fixation Device 20670-20680
Replacement
   Osseointegrated Implant
     for External Speech Processor/
     CochlearStimulator 69717-69718
Scan
   See Bone, Nuclear Medicine; Nuclear
   Medicine Imaging
Semilunar
   See Lunate
Sesamoid
   See Sesamoid Bone
Spur
   See Exostosis
Tarsal
   See Ankle Bone
Temporal
   See Temporal Bone
X ray
   Age Study 77072
   Dual Energy Absorptiometry ...77080-77081
   Length Study 77073
   Osseous Survey 77074-77077

Bone 4-Carboxyglutamic Protein
See Osteocalcin

Bone Conduction Hearing Device, Electromagnetic
Implantation/Replacement 69710
Removal/Repair 69711

Bone Density Study
Appendicular Skeleton 77079, 77081
Axial Skeleton 77078, 77080
Ultrasound 76977
Vertebral Fracture Assessment 77082

Bone Graft
Any Donor Area 20900-20902
Augmentation
   Mandibular Body 21127
Femur 27170
Fracture
   Orbit 21408
Harvesting 20900-20902
Malar Area 21210
Mandible 21215
Mandibular Ramus 21194
Maxilla 21210
Microvascular Anastomosis
   Fibula 20955
   Other 20962
Nasal Area 21210
Nasomaxillary Complex Fracture 21348
Open Treatment
   Craniofacial Separation 21436
Osteocutaneous Flap 20969-20973
Reconstruction
   Mandibular Rami 21194
   Midface 21145-21160
Skull 61316
   Excision 62148

Spine Surgery
   Allograft
     Morselized 20930
     Structural 20931
   Autograft
     Local 20936
     Morselized 20937
     Structural 20938
   Vascular Pedicle 25430

Bone Healing
Electrical Stimulation
   Invasive 20975
   Noninvasive 20974
Ultrasound Stimulation 20979

Bone Infection
See Osteomyelitis

Bone Marrow
Aspiration 38220
Harvesting 38230
Magnetic Resonance Imaging (MRI) 77084
Needle Biopsy 38221
Nuclear Medicine
   Imaging 78102-78104
Smear 85097
T-Cell Transplantation 38240-38242
Trocar Biopsy 38221

Bone Plate
Mandible 21244

Bone Wedge Reversal
Osteotomy 21122

Bordetella
Antibody 86615
Antigen Detection
   Direct Fluorescence 87265

Borrelia
Antibody 86618-86619

Borrelia burgdorferi ab
See Antibody, Lyme Disease

Borreliosis, Lyme
See Lyme Disease

Bost Fusion
See Arthrodesis, Wrist

Bosworth Operation
See Acromioclavicular Joint, Dislocation;
Arthrodesis, Vertebrae;Fasciotomy,

Bottle Type Procedure 55060

Botulinum Toxin
See Chemodenervation

Boutonniere Deformity 26426-26428

Bowel
See Intestine

Bowleg Repair 27455-27457

Boyd Hip Disarticulation
See Amputation, Leg, Upper; Radical Resection;
Replantation

Bronkodyl
See Theophylline

Brow Ptosis
Repair 67900

Brucella 86000
Antibody 86622

Bruise
See Hematoma

Brunschwig Operation 58240
See Hip; Pelvis, Exenteration

Brush Biopsy
See Biopsy; Needle Biopsy
Bronchi 31717

Brush Border ab
See Antibody, Heterophile

Bucca
See Cheek

Buccal Mucosa
See Mouth, Mucosa

Bulbourethral Gland
Excision 53250

Bulla
Incision and Drainage
   Puncture Aspiration 10160
Lung
   Excision-Plication 32141
      Endoscopic 32655

BUN
See Blood Urea Nitrogen; Urea Nitrogen

Bunion Repair 28296-28299
Chevron Procedure 28296
Concentric Procedure 28296
Joplin Procedure 28294
Keller Procedure 28292
Lapidus Procedure 28297
Mayo Procedure 28292
McBride Procedure 28292
Mitchell Procedure 28296
Silver Procedure 28290
with Implant 28293

Burgess Amputation
See Disarticulation, Ankle

Burkitt Herpesvirus
See Epstein-Barr Virus

Burns
Allograft .15300-15336
Debridement 01951-01953,
               15002-15005, 16020-16030
Dressings 16020-16030
Escharotomy 16035-16036
Excision .01951-01953
Initial Treatment 16000
Tissue Culture Skin Grafts 15100-15157
Xenograft 15400-15431

Burr Hole
Anesthesia 00214

Skull
   Biopsy Brain 61140
   Catheterization 61210
   Drainage
      Abscess 61150-61151
      Cyst 61150-61151
      Hematoma 61154-61156
   Exploration
      Infratentorial 61253
      Supratentorial 61250
   for Implant of Neurostimulator
   Array 61863-61868
   Injection, Contrast Media 61120
   Insertion
      Catheter 61210
      Reservoir 61210

Burrow's Operation
See Skin, Adjacent Tissue Transfer

Bursa
Ankle 27604
Arm, Lower 25031
Elbow
   Excision 24105
   Incision and Drainage 23931
Femur
   Excision 27062
Foot
   Incision and Drainage 28001
Hip
   Incision and Drainage 26991
Injection 20600-20610
Ischial
   Excision 27060
Joint
   Aspiration 20600-20610
   Drainage 20600-20610
   Injection 20600-20610
Knee
   Excision 27340
Leg, Lower 27604
Palm
   Incision and Drainage 26025-26030
Pelvis
   Incision and Drainage 26991
Shoulder
   Drainage .23031
Wrist 25031
   Excision 25115-25116

Bursectomy
See Excision, Bursa

Bursitis, Radiohumeral
See Tennis Elbow

Bursocentesis
See Aspiration, Bursa

Button
Nasal Septal Prosthesis
   Insertion 30220

Butyrylcholine Esterase
See Cholinesterase

Bypass Graft
Aortobi-iliac 35538, 35638
Aortobifemoral 35540
Aortofemoral .35539

Aortoiliac 35537, 35637
Axillary Artery 35516-35522, 35533,
             35616-35623, 35650, 35654
Brachial Artery 35510, 35512, 35522-35525
Carotid Artery 33891, 35501-35510, 35526,
             35601-35606, 35626, 35642
Celiac Artery 35531, 35631
Coronary Artery
   Angiography 93556
   Arterial 33533-33536
   Venous Graft 33510-33516
Excision
   Abdomen .35907
   Extremity .35903
   Neck 35901
   Thorax 35905
Femoral Artery 35521, 35533, 35551-35558,
            35566, 35621, 35646-35647,
            35651-35661, 35666, 35700
Harvest
   Endoscopic 33508
   Upper Extremity Vein 35500
Iliac Artery 35563
Iliofemoral Artery . . .35548-35549, 35565, 35665
Mesenteric Artery 35531, 35631
Peroneal Artery 35566-35571, 35666-35671
Placement
   Vein Patch 35685
Popliteal Artery 35551-35558, 35571, 35623,
            35651, 35656, 35671, 35700
Renal Artery 35536, 35560, 35631-35636
Reoperation .35700
Repair
   Abdomen .35907
   Extremity .35903
   Lower Extremity
      with Composite Graft 35681-35683
   Neck 35901
   Thorax 35905
Revascularization
   Extremity .35903
   Neck 35901
   Thorax 35905
Revision
   Lower Extremity
      Femoral Artery 35883-35884
      with Angioplasty 35879
      with Vein Interposition 35881
Secondary Repair 35870
Splenic Artery 35536, 35636
Subclavian Artery . . .35506, 35511-35516, 35526,
            35606-35616, 35626, 35645
Thrombectomy 37184-37186
   Other Than Hemodialysis Graft or
   Fistula 35875-35876
Tibial Artery . .35566-35571, 35623, 35666-35671
Vertebral Artery 35508, 35515, 35642-35645
with Composite Graft 35681

Bypass In-Situ
Femoral Artery 35583-35585
Peroneal Artery 35585-35587
Popliteal Artery 35583, 35587
Tibial Artery 35585-35587
Ventricular Restoration 33548

Bypass, Cardiopulmonary
See Cardiopulmonary Bypass

C

C-13
Urea Breath Test 83013-83014
Urease Activity 83013-83014

C-14
Urea Breath Test 78267-78268
Urease Activity 83013-83014

C-Peptide 80432, 84681

C-Reactive Protein 86140-86141

C-Section
See Cesarean Delivery

C Vitamin
See Ascorbic Acid

CABG
See Coronary Artery Bypass Graft (CABG)

Cadmium
Urine 82300

**Caffeine Halothane Contracture
Test (CHCT)** 89049

Calcaneal Spur
See Heel Spur

Calcaneus
Craterization 28120
Cyst
    Excision 28100-28103
Diaphysectomy 28120
Excision 28118-28120
Fracture
    Open Treatment 28415-28420
    Percutaneous Fixation 28406
    with Manipulation 28405-28406
    without Manipulation 28400
Repair
    Osteotomy 28300
Saucerization 28120
Tumor
    Excision 27647, 28100-28103
X ray 73650

Calcareous Deposits
Subdeltoid
    Removal 23000

Calcifediol
Blood or Urine 82306

Calcifediol Assay
See Calciferol

Calciferol
Blood or Urine 82307

Calcification
See Calcium, Deposits

Calciol
See Vitamin, D-3

Calcitonin
Blood or Urine 82308
Stimulation Panel 80410

Calcium
Blood
    Infusion Test 82331
Deposits
    See Removal, Calculi(Stone); Removal, Foreign
    Bodies
Ionized 82330
Total 82310
Urine 82340

**Calcium-Binding Protein, Vitamin
K-Dependent**
See Osteocalcin

Calcium-Pentagastrin Stimulation .
                                    80410

Calculus
Analysis 82355-82370
Destruction
    Bile Duct 43265
    Pancreatic Duct 43265
Removal
    Bile Duct 43264, 47554, 74327
    Bladder 51050, 52310-52318, 52352
    Kidney 50060-50081, 50130,
                    50561, 50580, 52352
    Pancreatic Duct 43264
    Ureter 50610-50630, 50961, 50980,
                51060-51065, 52320-52325, 52352
    Urethra 52310-52315, 52352

Calculus of Kidney
See Calculus, Removal, Kidney

Caldwell-Luc Procedure
See Sinus/Sinuses, Maxillary; Sinusotomy;
Sternum, Fracture
Orbital Floor Blowout Fracture 21385
Sinusotomy 31030-31032

Caliper
Application/Removal 20660

Callander Knee Disarticulation
See Disarticulation, Knee

Callosum, Corpus
See Corpus Callosum

Calmette Guerin Bacillus Vaccine
See BCG Vaccine

Caloric Vestibular Test 92533

Calprotectin
Fecal 83993

Calycoplasty 50405

Camey Enterocystoplasty 50825

CAMP
See Cyclic AMP

Campbell Procedure 27422

Campylobacter
Antibody 86625

Campylobacter Pylori
See Helicobacter Pylori

Canal, Ear
See Auditory Canal

Canal, Semicircular
See Semicircular Canal

Canaloplasty 69631, 69635

Candida
Antibody 86628
Skin Test 86485

Cannulation 36821
Arterial 36620-36625
Sinus
    Maxillary 31000
    Sphenoid 31002
Thoracic Duct 38794

Cannulation, Renoportal
See Anastomosis, Renoportal

Cannulization
See Catheterization
Arteriovenous 36145, 36810-36815
Declotting 36593, 36860-36861
ECMO 36822
External
    Declotting 36860-36861
Vas Deferens 55200
Vein to Vein 36800

Canthocystostomy
See Conjunctivorhinostomy

Canthopexy
Lateral 21282
Medial 21280

Canthoplasty 67950

Canthorrhaphy 67880-67882

Canthotomy 67715

Canthus
Reconstruction 67950

Cap, Cervical
See Cervical Cap

Capsule
See Capsulodesis
Elbow
    Arthrotomy 24006
    Excision 24006
Foot 28264
Interphalangeal Joint
    Excision 26525
    Incision 26525
Knee 27435
Metacarpophalangeal Joint
    Excision 26520
    Incision 26520
Metatarsophalangeal Joint
    Release 28289
Shoulder
    Incision 23020
Wrist
    Excision 25320

Capsulectomy
Breast
 Periprosthetic 19371

Capsulodesis
Metacarpophalangeal Joint 26516-26518

Capsulorrhaphy
Anterior 23450-23462
Multi-Directional Instability 23466
Posterior 23465
Wrist 25320

Capsulotomy
Breast
 Periprosthetic 19370
Foot 28260-28262
Hip
 with Release, Flexor Muscles 27036
Interphalangeal Joint 28272
Knee 27435
Metacarpophalangeal Joint 26520
Metatarsophalangeal Joint 28270
Toe 28270-28272
Wrist 25085

Captopril 80416-80417

Carbamazepine
Assay 80156-80157

Carbazepin
See Carbamazepine

Carbinol
See Methanol

**Carbohydrate Deficient
Transferrin** 82373

Carbon Dioxide
Blood or Urine 82374

Carbon Monoxide
Blood 82375-82376

Carbon Tetrachloride 84600

Carboxycathepsin
See Angiotensin Converting Enzyme (ACE)

Carboxyhemoglobin 82375-82376

Carbuncle
Incision and Drainage 10060-10061

Carcinoembryonal Antigen
See Antigen, Carcinoembryonic

Carcinoembryonic Antigen 82378

Cardiac
See Coronary
Muscle
 See Myocardium
Neoplasm
 See Heart, Tumor
Pacemaker
 See Heart, Pacemaker
Septal Defect
 See Septal Defect

Cardiac Arrhythmia, Tachycardia
See Tachycardia

Cardiac Atria
See Atria

Cardiac Catheterization
Combined Left and Right Heart 93526-93529
Combined Right and Retrograde Left
 Congenital Cardiac Anomalies 93531
Combined Right and Transseptal Left
 Congenital Cardiac Anomalies ..93532-93533
for Angiography 93508, 93541-93543
for Biopsy 93505
for Dilution Studies 93561-93562
Imaging 93555-93556
Injection 93539-93545
 See Catheterization, Cardiac
Left Heart 93510-93524
Pacemaker 33210
Right
 Congenital Cardiac Anomalies 93530
Right Heart 93501-93503

Cardiac Electroversion
See Cardioversion

Cardiac Event Recorder
Implantation 33282
Removal 33284

**Cardiac Magnetic Resonance
Imaging (CMRI)**
Complete Study 75554
Limited Study 75555
Morphology 75553
Velocity Flow Mapping 75556

Cardiac Massage
Thoracotomy......................32160

Cardiac Output
Indicator Dilution 93561-93562
Inert Gas Rebreathing 0104T-0105T

Cardiac Rehabilitation 93797-93798

Cardiac Transplantation
See Heart, Transplantation

Cardiectomy
Donor 33930, 33940

Cardioassist 0049T, 92970-92971

Cardiolipin Antibody 86147

Cardiology
See Defibrillator, Heart; Electrocardiography;
Pacemaker, Heart
Pacemaker Testing
 Antitachycardia System 93724
 Dual Chamber 93731-93733
 Leads 93640-93641
 Single Chamber ..93734-93735, 93741-93742
 Single/Dual Chamber 93641-93642
  Wearable Device ...93741-93742, 93745
Diagnostic
 Acoustic Recording with Computer Analysis
  Heart Sounds 0068T-0069T, 0070T
 Atrial Electrogram
  Esophageal Recording 93615-93616

Cardio-Defibrillator
 Evaluation and Testing 93640-93642,
          93741-93744
Echocardiography
 Doppler 93303-93321, 93662
 Intracardiac 93662
 Transesophageal 93318
 Transthoracic 93303-93317, 93350
Electrocardiogram
 Evaluation 93000, 93010, 93014,
        93660, 0178T-0180T
 Microvolt T-wave Alternans 93025
 Monitoring 93224-93237
 Patient-Demand 93268-93272
 Rhythm 93040-93042
 Tracing 93005
 Transmission 93012
Ergonovine Provocation Test 93024
Hemodynamic Monitoring
Non-invasive 0086T
Implantable Loop Recorder System ...93727
Intracardiac Pacing and Mapping 93631
 3-D Mapping 93613
 Follow-up Study 93624
 Stimulation and Pacing 93623
Intracardiac Pacing and Recording
 Arrhythmia Induction 93618-93624
 Bundle of His 93600, 93619-93620
 Comprehensive 93619-93622
 Intra-Atrial 93602, 93610
 Right Ventricle 93603
 Tachycardia Sites 93609
 Ventricular 93612
Intravascular Ultrasound 92978-92979
Left Ventricular Pressure
Measurement 0086T
Pacemaker Testing 93642
 Antitachycardia System 93724
 Dual Chamber 93731-93733
 Leads 93641
 Single Chamber 93734-93736
 Single/Dual Chamber 93641-93642
Perfusion Imaging 78460-78461
 See Nuclear Medicine
Stress Tests
 Cardiovascular 93015-93018
 Drug Induced 93024
 Multiple Gated Acquisition (MUGA) .78473
Tilt Table Evaluation 93660
Therapeutic
Cardio-Defibrillator
 Initial Set-up and Programming 93745
Cardioassist 92970-92971
Cardioversion 92960-92961
Intravascular Ultrasound 92978-92979
Pacing
 Transcutaneous, Temporary 92953
Thrombolysis 92975-92977
Thrombolysis, Coronary 92977
Valvuloplasty
 Percutaneous 92986-92990

Cardiomyotomy
See Esophagomyotomy

Cardioplasty 43320

Cardiopulmonary Bypass 33926
See Heart; Lung, Transplantation

Cell-Stimulating Hormone, Interstitial
See Luteinizing Hormone (LH)

Cellobiase
See Beta Glucosidase

Cellular Inclusion
See Inclusion Bodies

Central Shunt .33764

Central Venous Catheter Placement
Insertion
    Central .36555-36558
    Peripheral 36568-36569
Repair 36575
Replacement 36580-36585
Repositioning 36597

Central Venous Catheter Removal . .
                                      36589

Cephalic Version
of Fetus
    External 59412

Cephalocele
See Encephalocele

Cephalogram, Orthodontic
See Orthodontic Cephalogram

Cerclage
Cervix 57700
    Abdominal 59325
    Removal Under Anesthesia 59871
    Vaginal 59320

Cerebellopontine Angle Tumor
See Brain, Tumor, Excision; Brainstem;
Mesencephalon; Skull BaseSurgery

Cerebral Cortex Decortication
See Decortication

Cerebral Death
See Brain Death

Cerebral Hernia
See Encephalocele

Cerebral Perfusion Analysis . . .0042T

Cerebral Thermography
See Thermogram, Cephalic

Cerebral Ventriculographies
See Ventriculography

Cerebral Vessels
Angioplasty 61630
Dilation
    Intracranial Vasospasm 61640-61642
Occlusion 61623
Placement
    Stent 61635

Cerebrose
See Galactose

Cerebrospinal Fluid 86325
Nuclear Imaging 78630-78650

Cerebrospinal Fluid Leak 63744
Brain
    Repair 61618-61619, 62100
Nasal/Sinus Endoscopy
    Repair .31290-31291
Spinal Cord
    Repair .63707-63709

Cerebrospinal Fluid Shunt 63740,
                                       63746
Creation 62180-62192, 62200-62223
Irrigation 62194
Removal .62256-62258
Replacement 62160, 62194, 62225-62230
Reprogramming .62252

Ceruloplasmin 82390

Cerumen
Removal 69210

Cervical Cap .57170

Cervical Lymphadenectomy 38720-38724

Cervical Mucus Penetration Test 89330

Cervical Plexus
Injection
    Anesthetic 64413

Cervical Pregnancy 59140

Cervical Puncture 61050-61055

Cervical Smears 88141, 88155,
                      88164-88167, 88174-88175
See Cytopathology

Cervical Spine
See Vertebra, Cervical

Cervical Sympathectomy
See Sympathectomy, Cervical

Cervicectomy 57530

Cervicoplasty 15819

Cervicothoracic Ganglia
See Stellate Ganglion

Cervix
See Cytopathology
Amputation
    Total 57530
Biopsy 57500, 57520
    Colposcopy 57454-57455, 57460
Cauterization 57522
    Cryocautery 57511
    Electro or Thermal 57510
    Laser Ablation 57513
Cerclage 57700
    Abdominal 59325
    Removal Under Anesthesia 59871
    Vaginal 59320
Colposcopy 57452-57461
Conization 57461, 57520-57522
Curettage
    Endocervical 57454, 57456, 57505

Dilation
    Canal 57800
    Stump 57558
        and Curettage 57558
Ectopic Pregnancy 59140
Excision
    Radical 57531
    Stump
        Abdominal Approach 57540-57545
        Vaginal Approach 57550-57556
    Total 57530
Exploration
    Endoscopy 57452
Insertion
    Dilation 59200
    Laminaria 59200
    Prostaglandin 59200
Repair
    Cerclage 57700
    Abdominal 59325
    Suture 57720
    Vaginal 59320
Unlisted Services and Procedures 58999

Cesarean Delivery
Antepartum Care 59610, 59618
Delivery
    after Attempted Vaginal Delivery 59618
        Delivery Only 59620
        Postpartum Care 59622
        Routine Care 59610, 59618
Delivery Only 59514
Postpartum Care 59515
Routine Care 59510
Tubal Ligation at Time Of 58611
with Hysterectomy 59525

CGMP
See Cyclic GMP

Chalazion
Excision 67805
    Multiple
        Different Lids 67805
        Same Lid .67801
    Single 67800
    Under Anesthesia 67808

Challenge Tests
Bronchial Ingestion 95070-95075

Chambers Procedure 28300

Change
Catheter
    Genitourinary 75984
Fetal Position
    by Manipulation 59412
Tube or Stent
    Endoscopic
        Bile or Pancreatic Duct 43269

Change of, Dressing
See Dressings, Change

CHCT
See Caffeine Halothane Contracture Test

Cholecystectomy 47562-47564, 47600-47620
Any Method 47562-47564
   with Cholangiography ..47563, 47605, 47620
   with Exploration Common
   Duct 47564, 47610

Cholecystenterostomy 47570, 47720-47741

Cholecystography 74290-74291

Cholecystotomy 47480, 48001
Percutaneous 47490

Choledochoplasty
See Bile Duct, Repair

Choledochoscopy 47550

Choledochostomy 47420-47425

Choledochotomy 47420-47425

Choledochus, Cyst
See Cyst, Choledochal

Cholera Vaccine
Injectable 90725

Cholesterol
Measurement 83721
Serum 82465
Testing 83718-83719

Choline Esterase I
See Acetylcholinesterase

Choline Esterase II
See Cholinesterase

Cholinesterase
Blood 82480-82482

Cholylglycine
Blood 82240

Chondroitin Sulfate 82485

Chondromalacia Patella
Repair 27418

Chondropathia Patellae
See Chondromalacia Patella

Chondrosteoma
See Exostosis

Chopart Procedure 28800-28805
See Amputation, Foot; Radical Resection;
Replantation

Chordotomies
See Cordotomy

Chorioangioma
See Lesion, Skin

Choriogonadotropin
See Chorionic Gonadotropin

Choriomeningitides, Lymphocytic
See Lymphocytic Choriomeningitis

Chorionic Gonadotropin 80414, 84702-84703
Stimulation 80414-80415

Chorionic Growth Hormone
See Lactogen, Human Placental

Chorionic Tumor
See Hydatidiform Mole

Chorionic Villi
See Biopsy, Chorionic Villus

Chorionic Villus
Biopsy 59015

Choroid
Destruction
   Lesion 0016T, 67220-67225

Choroid Plexus
Excision 61544

Christmas Factor 85250

Chromaffinoma, Medullary
See Pheochromocytoma

Chromatin, Sex
See Barr Bodies

Chromatography
Column/Mass Spectrometry 82541-82544
Gas Liquid or HPLC 82486, 82491-82492
Paper 82487-82488
Thin-Layer 82489

Chromium 82495

Chromogenic Substrate Assay ..85130

Chromosome Analysis
See Amniocentesis
Added Study 88280-88289
Amniotic Fluid 88267-88269
   Culture 88235
Biopsy Culture
   Tissue 88233
Bone Marrow Culture 88237
Chorionic Villus 88267
   5 Cells 88261
   15-20 Cells 88262
   20-25 Cells 88264
   45 Cells 88263
   Culture 88235
for Breakage Syndromes 88245-88249
Fragile-X 88248
Lymphocyte Culture 88230
Pregnancy Associated Plasma Protein-A ...84163
Skin Culture
   Tissue 88233
Tissue Culture 88239
Unlisted Services and Procedures 88299

Chromotubation 58350
Oviduct 58350

Chronic Erection
See Priapism

Chronic Interstitial Cystitides
See Cystitis, Interstitial

Ciliary Body
Cyst
   Destruction
     Cryotherapy 66720
     Cyclodialysis 66740
     Cyclophotocoagulation 66710-66711
     Diathermy 66700
     Nonexcisional 66770
Destruction
   Cyclophotocoagulation 66710-66711
   Endoscopic 66711
Lesion
   Destruction 66770
Repair 66680

Cimino Type Procedure 36821

Cinefluorographies
See Cineradiography

Cineplasty
Arm, Lower or Upper 24940

Cineradiography
Esophagus 74230
Pharynx 70371, 74230
Speech Evaluation 70371
Swallowing Evaluation 74230
Unlisted Services and Procedures ..76120-76125

Circulation Assist
Aortic 33967, 33970
Balloon 33967, 33970
External 33960-33961

Circulation, Extracorporeal
See Extracorporeal Circulation

Circulatory Assist
See Circulation Assist

Circumcision
Repair 54163
Surgical Excision 54161
   Newborn 54160
with Clamp or Other Device 54152
   Newborn 54150

Cisternal Puncture 61050-61055

Cisternography 70015
Nuclear 78630

Citrate
Blood or Urine 82507

Clagett Procedure
See Chest Wall, Repair, Closure

Clavicle
Craterization 23180
Cyst
   Excision 23140
     with Allograft 23146
     with Autograft 23145
Diaphysectomy 23180
Dislocation
   Acromioclavicular Joint
     Closed Treatment 23540-23545
     Open Treatment 23550-23552

Coagulopathy 85390
Assay 85130

Cocaine
Blood or Urine 82520
Screen 82486

Coccidioides
Antibody 86635

Coccidioidin Test
See Streptokinase, Antibody

Coccidioidomycosis
Skin Test 86490

Coccygeal Spine Fracture
See Coccyx, Fracture

Coccygectomy 15920-15922, 27080

Coccyx
Excision 27080
Fracture
   Closed Treatment 27200
   Open Treatment 27202
Tumor
   Excision 49215
X ray 72220

Cochlear Device
Insertion 69930
Programming 92601-92604

Codeine
Alkaloid Screening 82101

Codeine Screen 82486

Cofactor Protein S
See Protein S

Coffey Operation
See Uterus, Repair, Suspension

Cognitive Function Tests ..96101-96120
See Neurology, Diagnostic

Cognitive Skills Development ..97532
See Physical Medicine/Therapy/Occupational
Therapy

Cold Agglutinin 86156-86157

Cold Pack Treatment 97010

Cold Preservation
See Cryopreservation

Cold Therapies
See Cryotherapy

Colectomy
Partial 44140
   Laparoscopic 44213
   with Anastomosis 44140
      Laparoscopic ...44204, 44207-44208
   with Coloproctostomy 44145-44146
   with Colostomy 44141-44144
      Laparoscopic 44206, 44208
   with Ileocolostomy
      Laparoscopic 44205
   with Ileostomy 44144

   with Ileum Removal 44160
   with Transcanal Approach 44147
Total
 · Laparoscopic 44210-44212
    with Proctectomy and Ileostomy ..44210-44212
    without Proctectomy 44210
  Open
    with Complete Proctectomy 45121
    with Ileostomy 44150-44151
    with Proctectomy 44155-44158

Collagen Cross Links 82523

Collagen Injection 11950-11954

Collar Bone
See Clavicle

Collateral Ligament
Ankle
   Repair 27695-27698
Interphalangeal Joint 26545
Knee Joint
   Repair 27409
Knee Repair 27405
Metacarpophalangeal Joint 26540-26542
Repair
   Ankle 27695-27698

Collection and Processing
Allogenic Blood
   Harvesting of Stem Cells 38205
Autologous Blood
   Harvesting of Stem Cells 38206
   Intraoperative 86891
   Preoperative 86890
Specimen
   Capillary Blood 36416
   Venous Access Device 36591
   Venous Blood 36415, 36591-36592
   Venous Catheter 36592
Washings
   Esophagus 91000
   Stomach 91055

Colles Fracture 25600-25605

Colles Fracture Reversed
See Smith Fracture

Collins Syndrome, Treacher
See Treacher-Collins Syndrome

Collis Procedure
See Gastroplasty with Esophagogastric
Fundoplasty

Colon
See Colon-Sigmoid
Biopsy 44025, 44100, 44322
   Endoscopic 44389, 45380, 45391-45392
Colostomy
   Revision 44340-44346
Colotomy 44322
   Colostomy 44320
CT Scan
   Colonography 0066T, 0067T
   Virtual Colonoscopy 0066T, 0067T

Destruction
   Lesion 44393, 45383
   Tumor 44393, 45383
Endoscopy
   Biopsy 44389, 45380, 45391-45392
   Destruction
    Lesion 44393
    Tumor 44393, 45383
   Dilation 45386
   Exploration 44388, 45378, 45381, 45386
   Hemorrhage 44391, 45382
   Injection, Submucosal 45381
   Placement
    Stent 45387
   Removal
    Foreign Body 44390, 45379
    Polyp 44392, 45384-45385
    Tumor 45384-45385
   Specimen Collection 45380
   Ultrasound 45391-45392
   via Colotomy 45355
   via Stoma 44388-44397
   Virtual 0066T, 0067T
Excision
   Partial 44140-44147, 44160
    Laparoscopic 44204-44208
   Total 44150-44158
    Laparoscopic 44210-44212
Exploration 44025
   Endoscopy 44388, 45378, 45381, 45386
Hemorrhage
   Endoscopic Control 44391, 45382
Hernia 44050
Incision
   Creation
    Stoma 44320-44322
   Exploration 44025
   Revision
    Stoma 44340-44346
Lavage
   Intraoperative 44701
Lesion
   Destruction 45383
   Excision 44110-44111
Lysis
   Adhesions 44005
Obstruction 44025-44050
Reconstruction
   Bladder from 50810
Removal
   Foreign Body 44025, 44390, 45379
   Polyp 44392
Repair
   Diverticula 44605
   Fistula 44650-44661
   Hernia 44050
   Malrotation 44055
   Obstruction 44050
   Ulcer 44605
   Volvulus 44050
   Wound 44605
Splenic Flexure
   Mobilization
    Laparoscopic 44213
Stoma Closure 44620-44625
Suture
   Diverticula 44605
   Fistula 44650-44661

Complement

Antigen 86160
Fixation Test 86171
Functional Activity 86161
Hemolytic
  Total 86162
Total 86162

Complete Blood Count (CBC) 85025-85027
See Blood Cell Count

Complete Colectomy
See Colectomy, Total

Complete Pneumonectomy
See Pneumonectomy, Completion

Complete Transposition of Great Vessels
See Transposition, Great Arteries

Complex, Factor IX
See Christmas Factor

Complex, Vitamin B
See B Complex Vitamins

Component Removal, Blood
See Apheresis

Composite Graft 15760-15770,
        35681-35683

Compound B
See Corticosterone

Compound F
See Cortisol

Compression, Nerve, Median
See Carpal Tunnel Syndrome

Computed Tomographic Scintigraphy
See Emission Computerized Tomography

Computed Tomography (CT)
See CT Scan; Specific Anatomic Site

Computer Analysis
Acoustic Recording
 Heart Sounds
  with Computer Analysis 0068T-0069T,
         0070T

Computer-Aided Detection
Chest X ray 0152T
Lesion
 Chest Radiograph 0174T-0175T
Mammography 77051-77052
 Magnetic Resonance Imaging (MRI) ...0159T

Computer-Assisted Navigation 20985-20987

Computer-Assisted Surgical Navigation
Imageless 20985
Image Guidance
 Intraoperative 20986
 Preoperative 20987

Computer-Assisted Testing
Neuropsychological 96120
Psychological 96103

Computer Data Analysis 99090

Computerized Emission Tomography
See Emission Computerized Tomography

Concentration of Specimen 87015

Concentration, Hydrogen-Ion
See pH

Concentration, Minimum Inhibitory
See Minimum Inhibitory Concentration

Concentric Procedure 28296

Concha Bullosa Resection
with Nasal/Sinus Endoscopy 31240

Conchae Nasale
See Nasal Turbinate

Conduction, Nerve
See Nerve Conduction

Conduit, Ileal
See Ileal Conduit

Condyle
Humerus
 Fracture
  Closed Treatment 24576-24577
  Open Treatment 24579
  Percutaneous 24582
Metatarsal
 Excision 28288
Phalanges
 Toe
  Excision 28126

Condyle, Mandibular
See Mandibular Condyle

Condylectomy
Temporomandibular Joint 21050
with Skull Base Surgery 61596-61597

Condyloma
Destruction 54050-54065

Conference
Medical
 with Interdisciplinary Team 99366-99368

Confirmation
Drug 80102

Congenital Arteriovenous Malformation
See Arteriovenous Malformation

Congenital Elevation of Scapula
See Sprengel's Deformity

Congenital Heart Septum Defect
See Septal Defect

Congenital Kidney Abnormality
Nephrolithotomy 50070
Pyeloplasty 50405
Pyelotomy 50135

Congenital Laryngocele
See Laryngocele

Congenital Vascular Anomaly
See Vascular Malformation

Conisation
See Cervix, Conization

Conization
Cervix 57461, 57520-57522

Conjoint Psychotherapy 90847
See Psychiatric Treatment, Family

Conjunctiva
Biopsy 68100
Cyst
 Incision and Drainage 68020
Fistulize for Drainage
 with Tube 68750
 without Tube 68745
Graft 65782
 Harvesting 68371
Harvesting 68371
Incision 0124T
Insertion Stent 68750
Lesion
 Destruction 68135
 Excision 68110-68130
  More than 1 cm 68115
  with Adjacent Sclera 68130
Reconstruction 68320-68335
 Symblepharon
  with Graft 68335
 with Flap
  Bridge or Partial 68360
  Total 68362
Repair
 Symblepharon
  Division 68340
  with Graft 68335
  without Graft 68330
 Wound
  Direct Closure 65270
  Mobilization and Rearrangement ...65272-
        65273
Unlisted Services and Procedures 68399

Conjunctivo-Tarso-Muller Resection 67908

Conjunctivocystorhinostomy
See Conjunctivorhinostomy

Conjunctivodacryocystostomy
See Conjunctivorhinostomy

Conjunctivoplasty 68320-68330
Reconstruction Cul de Sac
 with Extensive Rearrangement 68326
 with Graft 68326
  Buccal Mucous Membrane 68328
with Extensive Rearrangement 68320
with Graft 68320
 Buccal Mucous Membrane 68325

Internal Mammary Artery Graft 4110F
Reoperation 33530
Venous......................33510-33516

Coronary Endarterectomy 33572

Coroner's Exam 88045

Coronoidectomy
Temporomandibular Joint 21070

Corpectomy 63101-63103

Corpora Cavernosa
Corpus Spongiosum Shunt 54430
Glans Penis Fistulization 54435
Injection 54235
Irrigation
    Priapism 54220
Saphenous Vein Shunt 54420
X ray With Contrast 74445

Corpora Cavernosa, Plastic Induration
See Peyronie Disease

Corpora Cavernosography 74445

Corpus Callosum
Transection.......................61541

Corpus Vertebrae (Vertebrale)
See Vertebral Body

Correction of Cleft Palate
See Cleft Palate, Repair

Correction of Lid Retraction
See Repair, Eyelid, Retraction

Correction of Malrotation of Duodenum
See Ladd Procedure

Correction of Syndactyly
See Syndactyly, Repair

Correction of Ureteropelvic Junction
See Pyeloplasty

Cortex Decortication, Cerebral
See Decortication

Cortical Mapping
Transection
    by Electric Stimulation 95961-95962

Corticoids
See Corticosteroids

Corticoliberin
See Corticotropic Releasing Hormone (CRH)

Corticosteroid Binding Globulin
See Transcortin

Corticosteroid Binding Protein
See Transcortin

Corticosteroids
Blood 83491
Urine 83491

Corticosterone
Blood or Urine 82528

Corticotropic Releasing Hormone (CRH) 80412

Cortisol ..80400-80406, 80418-80420, 80436,
82530
Stimulation 80412
Total 82533

Cortisol Binding Globulin 84449

Costectomy
See Resection, Ribs

Costen Syndrome
See Temporomandibular Joint (TMJ)

Costotransversectomy 21610

Cothromboplastin
See Proconvertin

Cotte Operation 58400-58410
See Repair, Uterus, Suspension; Revision

Cotton Procedure
Bohler Procedure 28405

Counseling
See Preventive Medicine
Smoking and Tobacco Use
Cessation 99406-99407

Counseling and/or Risk Factor Reduction Intervention, Preventive Medicine, Individual Counseling
See Preventive Medicine, Counseling and/or Risk
Factor Reduction Intervention, Individual
Counseling

Count
Blood Cell
    See Blood Cell Count
Blood Platelet
    See Blood, Platelet,Count
Cell
    See Cell Count
Complete Blood
    See Complete Blood Count (CBC)
Erythrocyte
    See Red Blood Cell (RBC), Count
Leukocyte
    See White Blood Cell, Count
Reticulocyte
    See Reticulocyte, Count

Counterimmuno-Electrophoresis 86185

Counters, Cell
See Cell Count

Countershock, Electric
See Cardioversion

Coventry Tibial Wedge Osteotomy
See Osteotomy, Tibia

Cowper's Gland
Excision 53250

Coxa
See Hip

Coxiella Burnetii
Antibody 86638

Coxsackie
Antibody 86658

CPAP
See Continuous Positive Airway Pressure

CPK
Blood 82550-82552

CPR (Cardiopulmonary Resuscitation) 92950

Cranial Bone
Halo
    Thin Skull Osteology 20664
Reconstruction
    Extracranial 21181-21184
Tumor
    Excision 61563-61564

Cranial Halo 20661

Cranial Nerve
Avulsion 64732-64760, 64771
Cranial Nerve II
    See Optic Nerve
Cranial Nerve V
    See Trigeminal Nerve
Cranial Nerve VII
    See Facial Nerve
Cranial Nerve X
    See Vagus Nerve
Cranial Nerve XI
    See Accessory Nerve
Cranial Nerve XII
    See Hypoglossal Nerve
Decompression 61458, 64716
Implantation
    Electrode 64553, 64573
Incision 64732-64752, 64760, 65771
Injection
    Anesthetic 64400-64408, 64412
    Neurolytic 64600-64610
Insertion
    Electrode 64553, 64573
Neuroplasty 64716
Release 64716
Repair
    Suture, With or Without Graft ..64864-64865
Section 61460
Transection 64732-64760, 64771
Transposition 64716

Cranial Tongs
Application/Removal 20660
Removal 20665

Craniectomy 61501
See Craniotomy
Decompression 61322-61323, 61340-61343
Exploratory 61304-61305
Extensive, for Multiple Suture Craniosynostosis ..
61558-61559
for Electrode 61860-61875
Release Stenosis 61550-61552

Cutaneous Tissue
See Integumentary System

Cutaneous-Vesicostomy
See Vesicostomy, Cutaneous

CVS
See Biopsy, Chorionic Villus

Cyanacobalamin
See Cyanocobalamin

Cyanide
Blood 82600
Tissue 82600

Cyanocobalamin 82607-82608

Cyclic AMP .82030

Cyclic GMP .83008

Cyclic Somatostatin
See Somatostatin

Cyclocryotherapy
See Cryotherapy, Destruction, Ciliary Body

Cyclodialysis
Destruction
    Ciliary Body 66740

Cyclophotocoagulation
Destruction
    Ciliary Body 66710-66711

Cyclosporine
Assay 80158

Cyst
Abdomen
    Destruction/Excision 49203-49205
Ankle
    Capsule 27630
    Tendon Sheath 27630
Bartholin's Gland
    Excision 56740
    Repair 56440
Bile Duct 47715
Bladder
    Excision 51500
Bone
    Drainage .20615
    Injection 20615
Brain
    Drainage 61150-61151,
                        61156, 62161-62162
    Excision 61516, 61524, 62162
Branchial Cleft
    Excision 42810-42815
Breast
    Incision and Drainage 19020
    Puncture Aspiration 19000-19001
Calcaneus 28100-28103
Carpal 25130-25136
Choledochal .47715
Ciliary Body
    Destruction 66770
Clavicle
    Excision 23140-23146
Conjunctiva 68020

Dermoid
    Nose
        Excision 30124-30125
Drainage
    Contrast Injection 49424
        with X ray 76080
Excision
    Cheekbone 21030
    Clavicle 23140
        with Allograft 23146
        with Autograft 23145
    Femur 27355-27358
    Ganglion
        See Ganglion
    Humerus
        with Allograft 23156
        with Autograft 23155
    Hydatid
        See Echinococcosis
    Lymphatic
        See Lymphocele
    Maxilla 21030
    Mediastinum 32662
    Olecranon Process
        with Allograft 24126
        with Autograft 24125
    Pericardial 32661
    Pilonidal 11770-11772
    Radius
        with Allograft 24126
        with Autograft 24125
    Scapula 23140
        with Allograft 23146
        with Autograft 23145
    Ulna
        with Allograft 24126
        with Autograft 24125
    Zygoma 21030
Facial Bones
    Excision 21030
Femur 27065-27067
Fibula 27635-27638
Ganglion
    Aspiration/Injection 20612
Gums
    Incision and Drainage 41800
Hip 27065-27067
Humerus
    Excision 23150-23156, 24110
        with Allograft 24116
        with Autograft 24115
Ileum 27065-27067
Incision and Drainage 10060-10061
    Pilonidal 10080-10081
Iris
    Destruction 66770
Kidney
    Ablation 50541
    Aspiration 50390
    Excision 50280-50290
    Injection 50390
    X ray 74470
Knee
    Baker's 27345
    Excision 27347
Leg, Lower
    Capsule 27630
    Tendon Sheath 27630

Liver 47010
    Drainage .47010
        Open 47010
    Repair 47300
Lung
    Incision and Drainage 32200
    Removal 32140
Lymph Node
    Axillary/Cervical
        Excision 38550-38555
Mandible
    Excision 21040, 21046-21047
Maxilla
    Excision 21030, 21048-21049
Mediastinal
    Excision 39200
Metacarpal 26200-26205
Metatarsal 28104-28107
Mouth 41005-41009, 41015-41018
    Incision and Drainage 40800-40801
Mullerian Duct
    Excision 55680
Nose
    Excision 30124-30125
Olecranon 24120
Ovarian
    Excision 58925
    Incision and Drainage 58800-58805
Pancreas 48500
    Anastomosis 48520-48540
    Excision 48120
Pelvis
    Aspiration 50390
    Injection 50390
Pericardial
    Excision 33050
Phalanges
    Finger 26210-26215
    Toe 28108
Pilonidal
    Excision 11770-11772
    Incision and Drainage 10080-10081
Pubis 27065-27067
Radius 24120, 25120-25126
Rathke's Pouch
    See Craniopharyngioma
Removal
    Skin 10040
Retroperitoneal
    Destruction/Excision 49203-49205
Salivary Gland Creation
    Destruction/Excision
    Drainage .42409
    Excision 42408
Scapula
    Excision 23140-23146
Seminal Vesicle
    Excision 55680
Skin
    Puncture Aspiration 10160
Spinal Cord
    Aspiration 62268
    Incision and Drainage 63172-63173
Sublingual Gland Drainage 42409
    Excision 42408
Talus 28100-28103
Tarsal 28104-28107

D

D & C Yellow No. 7
See Fluorescein

D 2, Vitamin
See Calciferol

D and C
See Dilation and Curettage

D and E
See Dilation and Evacuation

D Galactose
See Galactose

D Glucose
See Glucose

D Vitamin
See Vitamin, D

D-Xylose Absorption Test 84620

Dacryoadenectomy
Partial 68505
Total 68500

Dacryocystectomy 68520

Dacryocystogram
See Dacryocystography

Dacryocystography 68850, 70170
Nuclear Imaging 78660

Dacryocystorhinostomy 68720
Total
    with Nasal/Sinus Endoscopy 31239

Dacryocystostomies
See Dacryocystotomy

Dacryocystotomy 68420

Daily Living Activities
See Activities of Daily Living

Damus-Kaye-Stansel Procedure
See Anastomosis, Pulmonary

Dana Operation
See Rhizotomy

Dandy Operation
See Ventriculocisternostomy

Dark Adaptation Examination ..92284

Dark Field Examination ...87164-87166

Darkroom Test
See Glaucoma, Provocative Test

Darrach Procedure
See Excision, Ulna, Partial

David Procedure
See Aorta, Ascending, Graft

Day Test
See Blood, Feces

de Quervain's Disease
Treatment 25000

Death, Brain
See Brain Death

Debridement
Brain 62010
Burns 01951-01953, 16020-16030
Mastoid Cavity
    Complex 69222
    Simple 69220
Metatarsophalangeal Joint 28289
Muscle
    Infected 11004-11006
Nails 11720-11721
Nose
    Endoscopic 31237
Pancreatic Tissue 48105
Skin
    Eczematous 11000-11001
    Full Thickness 11041
    Infected 11000-11006
    Partial Thickness 11040
    Subcutaneous Tissue 11042-11044
        Infected 11004-11006
    with Open Fracture and/or
    Dislocation 11010-11012
Sternum 21627
Wound
    Non-Selective 97602
    Selective 97597-97598

Debulking Procedure
Ovary/Pelvis 58952-58958

Decompression
See Section
Arm, Lower 24495, 25020-25025
Auditory Canal, Internal 69960
Brainstem 61575-61576
Cauda Equina 63011, 63017, 63047-63048,
           63056-63057, 63087-63091
Cranial Nerve 61458
Esophagogastric Varices 37181
Facial Nerve 61590
    Intratemporal
        Lateral to Geniculate Ganglion 69720,
                        69740
        Medial to Geniculate Ganglion 69725,
                        69745
        Total 69955
Finger 26035
Gasserian Ganglion
    Sensory Root 61450
Hand 26035-26037
Intestines
    Small 44021
Jejunostomy
    Laparoscopic 44186
Leg
    Fasciotomy 27600-27602
Nerve 64702-64727
    Root 63020-63048, 63055-63103
Nucleus of Disc
    Lumbar 62287

Optic Nerve 67570
Orbit 61330
    Removal of Bone 67414, 67445
Skull 61322-61323, 61340-61345
Spinal Cord 63001-63017, 63045-63103
    Cauda Equina 63005
Tarsal Tunnel Release 28035
Volvulus 45321, 45337
with Nasal/Sinus Endoscopy
    Optic Nerve 31294
    Orbit Wall 31292-31293
Wrist 25020-25025

Decortication
Lung
    Endoscopic 32651-32652
    Partial 32225
    Total 32220
    with Parietal Pleurectomy 32320

Decubiti
See Pressure Ulcer (Decubitus)

Decubitus Ulcers
See Debridement; Pressure Ulcer (Decubitus);
Skin Graft and Flap

Deetjeen's Body
See Blood, Platelet

Defect, Coagulation
See Coagulopathy

Defect, Heart Septal
See Septal Defect

Defect, Septal Closure, Atrial
See Heart, Repair, Atrial Septum

Deferens, Ductus
See Vas Deferens

Defibrillation
See Cardioversion

Defibrillator, Heart
See Pacemaker, Heart
Evaluation and Testing 93640-93642,
                      93741-93744
Insertion Single/Dual Chamber
    Electrodes 33216-33217, 33224-33225, 33249
    Pulse Generator 33240
Removal Single/Dual Chamber
    Electrodes 33243-33244
    Pulse Generator 33241
Repair 33218-33220
Repositioning Single/Dual Chamber
    Electrodes 33215, 33226
Revise Pocket Chest 33223
Wearable Device 93741-93742, 93745

Deformity, Boutonniere
See Boutonniere Deformity

Deformity, Sprengel's
See Sprengel's Deformity

Degenerative, Articular Cartilage, Patella
See Chondromalacia Patella

Degradation Products, Fibrin
See Fibrin Degradation Products

Dehydroepiandrosterone 82626

**Dehydroepiandrosterone
Sulfate** 82627

**Dehydrogenase,
6-Phosphogluconate**
See Phosphogluconate-6, Dehydrogenase

Dehydrogenase, Alcohol
See Antidiuretic Hormone

**Dehydrogenase,
Glucose-6-Phosphate**
See Glucose-6-Phosphate, Dehydrogenase

Dehydrogenase, Glutamate
See Glutamate Dehydrogenase

Dehydrogenase, Isocitrate
See Isocitric Dehydrogenase

Dehydrogenase, Lactate
See Lactic Dehydrogenase

Dehydrogenase, Malate
See Malate Dehydrogenase

Dehydroisoandrosterone Sulfate
See Dehydroepiandrosterone Sulfate

Delay of Flap
Skin Graft .15600-15630

Deligation
Ureter 50940

Deliveries, Abdominal
See Cesarean Delivery

Delivery
See Cesarean Delivery; Vaginal Delivery

Delorme Operation
See Pericardiectomy

Denervation
Hip
　Femoral 27035
　Obturator 27035
　Sciatic 27035

Denervation, Sympathetic
See Excision, Nerve, Sympathetic

Denis-Browne Splint 29590

Dens Axis
See Odontoid Process

**Denver Developmental
Screening Test** 96101-96103

Denver Krupic Procedure
See Aqueous Shunt, to Extraocular Reservoir

Denver Shunt
Patency Test 78291

Denver-Krupin Procedure 66180

Deoxycorticosterone
See Desoxycorticosterone

Deoxycortisol 80436, 82634

Deoxyephedrine
See Methamphetamine

Deoxyribonuclease
Antibody 86215

Deoxyribonuclease I
See DNAse

Deoxyribonucleic Acid
Antibody .86225-86226

Depilation
See Removal, Hair

Depletion
Plasma 38214
Platelet 38213
T-Cell 38210
Tumor Cell 38211

Deposit Calcium
See Calcium, Deposits

Depth Electrode
Insertion 61760

Derma-Fat-Fascia Graft 15770

Dermabrasion 15780-15783

Dermatology
Actinotherapy 96900
Examination of Hair
　Microscopic 96902
Ultraviolet A Treatment 96912
Ultraviolet B Treatment 96910
Ultraviolet Light Treatment 96900, 96913
Unlisted Services and Procedures 96999

Dermatoplasty
Septal 30620

Dermoid
See Cyst, Dermoid

Derrick-Burnet Disease
See Q Fever

Descending Abdominal Aorta
See Aorta, Abdominal

Desipramine
Assay 80160

Desmotomy
See Ligament, Release

Desoxycorticosterone 82633

Desoxycortone
See Desoxycorticosterone

Desoxyephedrine
See Methamphetamine

Desoxynorephedrin
See Amphetamine

Desoxyphenobarbital
See Primidone

Desquamation
See Exfoliation

Destruction
Acne 17340-17360
　Cryotherapy .17340
Arrhythmogenic Focus
　Heart 33250-33251, 33261
Bladder 51020, 52214-52224, 52354
Calculus
　Bile Duct 43265
　Kidney 50590
　Pancreatic Duct 43265
Chemical Cauterization
　Granulation Tissue 17250
Chemosurgery 17110-17111
Ciliary Body
　Cryotherapy .66720
　Cyclodialysis 66740
　Cyclophotocoagulation 66710-66711
　Diathermy 66700
　Endoscopic .66711
Cryosurgery 17110-17111
Curettement 17110-17111
Cyst
　Abdomen 49203-49205
　Ciliary Body .66770
　Iris 66770
Electrosurgery 17110-17111
Endometrial Ablation 58356
Endometriomas
　Abdomen 49203-49205
Fissure
　Anal .46940-46942
Hemorrhoids 46934-46936
Kidney 52354
　Endoscopic 50557, 50576
Laser Surgery 17110-17111
Lesion
　Anal 46900-46917, 46924
　Bladder 51030
　Breast 0061T
　Choroid 0016T, 67220-67225
　Ciliary Body .66770
　Colon 45383
　Conjunctiva .68135
　Cornea 65450
　Eyelid 67850
　Facial 17000-17004, 17280-17286
　Gastrointestinal, Upper 43258
　Gums 41850
　Intestines
　　Large 44393
　　Small 44369
　Iris 66770
　Mouth 40820
　Nose
　　Intranasal 30117-30118
　Palate 42160
　Penis
　　Cryosurgery 54056
　　Electrodesiccation 54055
　　Extensive .54065
　　Laser Surgery 54057
　　Simple 54050-54060
　　Surgical Excision 54060
　Pharynx 42808
　Prostate 45320

Diastase
See Amylase

Diastasis
See Separation

Diathermy 97024
See Physical Medicine/Therapy/Occupational
Therapy
Destruction
    Ciliary Body 66700
Lesion
    Retina 67208, 67227
Retinal Detachment
    Prophylaxis 67141
    Repair 67101

Diathermy, Surgical
See Electrocautery

Dibucaine Number 82638

Dichloride, Methylene
See Dichloromethane

Dichlorides, Ethylene
See Dichloroethane

Dichloroethane 84600

Dichloromethane 84600

Diethylamide, Lysergic Acid
See Lysergic Acid Diethylamide

Diethylether 84600

Differential Count
See White Blood Cell Count

Differentiation Reversal Factor
See Prothrombin

Diffusion Test, Gel
See Immunodiffusion

Digestive Tract
See Gastrointestinal Tract

Digit
See Finger; Toe
Replantation 20816-20822

Digital Artery Sympathectomy 64820

Digital Slit-Beam Radiograph
See Scanogram

Digits
Pinch Graft 15050

Digoxin
Assay 80162

Dihydrocodeinone 82646

Dihydrocodeinone Screen 82486

Dihydroepitestosterone
See Dihydrotestosterone

Dihydrohydroxycodeinone
See Oxycodinone

Dihydromorphinone 82486, 82649

Dihydrotestosterone 82651

Dihydroxyethanes
See Ethylene Glycol

Dihydroxyvitamin D 82652

Dilatation, Transluminal Arterial
See Angioplasty, Transluminal

Dilation
See Dilation and Curettage
Anal
    Endoscopy 46604
    Sphincter 45905
Bile Duct
    Endoscopy 43271, 47555-47556
    Stricture 74363
Bladder
    Cystourethroscopy 52260-52265
Bronchi
    Endoscopy 31630, 31636-31638
Cerebral Vessels
    Intracranial Vasospasm 61640-61642
Cervix
    Canal 57800
    Stump 57558
Colon
    Endoscopy 45386
Colon-Sigmoid
    Endoscopy 45340
Esophagus 43450-43458
    Balloon 43220, 43249
    Endoscopy 43220-43226, 43249
    Surgical 43510
Intestines, Small
    Endoscopy 44370
Kidney 50395
    Intra-Renal Stricture 52343, 52346
Lacrimal Punctum 68801
Larynx
    Endoscopy 31528-31529
Nasolacrimal Duct
    Balloon Catheter 68816
Pancreatic Duct
    Endoscopy 43271
Rectum
    Endoscopy 45303
    Sphincter 45910
Salivary Duct 42650-42660
Trachea
    Endoscopy 31630-31631, 31636-31638
Transluminal
    Aqueous Outflow Canal 0176T-0177T
Ureter 50395, 52341-52342, 52344-52345
    Endoscopy 50553, 50572, 50953, 50972
Urethra 52260-52265
    General 53665
    Suppository and/or Instillation .53660-53661
Urethral
    Stenosis 52281
    Stricture 52281, 53600-53621
Vagina 57400

Dilation and Curettage 59840
See Curettage; Dilation
Cervical Stump 57558
Cervix 57558, 57800

Corpus Uteri 58120
Hysteroscopy 58558
Postpartum 59160
with Amniotic Injections 59851
with Vaginal Suppositories 59856

Dilation and Evacuation 59841
with Amniotic Injections 59851

Dimethadione 82654

Dioxide, Carbon
See Carbon Dioxide

Dioxide, Silicon
See Silica

Dipeptidyl Peptidase A
See Angiotensin Converting Enzyme (ACE)

Diphenylhydantoin
See Phenytoin

Diphosphate, Adenosine
See Adenosine Diphosphate

Diphtheria
See Vaccines
Antibody 86648

Dipropylacetic Acid
Assay 80164

Direct Pedicle Flap
Formation 15570-15576

Disability Evaluation Services
Basic Life and/or Disability Evaluation 99450
Work-Related or Medical Disability
Evaluation 99455-99456

Disarticulation
Ankle 27889
Hip 27295
Knee 27598
Wrist 25920, 25924
    Revision 25922

Disarticulation of Shoulder
See Shoulder, Disarticulation

Disc Chemolyses, Intervertebral
See Chemonucleolysis

Disc, Intervertebral
See Intervertebral Disc

Discectomies
See Discectomy

Discectomies, Percutaneous
See Discectomy, Percutaneous

Discectomy 63075-63078
Additional Segment 22226
Arthrodesis
    Additional Interspace 22534, 22585
    Cervical 22554
    Lumbar 22533, 22558, 22630
    Thoracic 22532, 22556
Cervical 22220
Lumbar 22224, 22630
Percutaneous 62287
Thoracic 22222

with Fracture
    Closed Treatment 25680
    Open Treatment 25685
with Manipulation 25660, 25675, 25680

Dislocation, Radiocarpal Joint
See Radiocarpal Joint, Dislocation

Disorder
Blood Coagulation
    See Coagulopathy
Penis
    See Penis
Retinal
    See Retina

Displacement Therapy
Nose 30210

Dissection
Hygroma, Cystic
    Axillary/Cervical 38550-38555
Lymph Nodes 38542

Dissection, Neck, Radical
See Radical Neck Dissection

Distention
See Dilation

Diverticula, Meckel's
See Diverticulum, Meckel's

Diverticulectomy 44800
Esophagus 43130-43135

Diverticulectomy, Meckel's
See Meckel's Diverticulum, Excision

Diverticulum
Bladder
    See Bladder, Diverticulum
Meckel's
    Excision 44800
Repair
    Urethra 53400-53405

Division
Muscle
    Foot 28250
Plantar Fascia
    Foot 28250

Division, Isthmus, Horseshoe Kidney
See Symphysiotomy, Horseshoe Kidney

Division, Scalenus Anticus Muscle
See Muscle Division, Scalenus Anticus

Dl-Amphetamine
See Amphetamine

DMO
See Dimethadione

DNA
Antibody 86225-86226

DNA Endonuclease
See DNAse

DNA Probe
See Cytogenetics Studies; Nucleic Acid Probe

DNAse
Antibody 86215

Domiciliary Services
See Nursing Facility Services
Assisted Living 99339-99340
Discharge Services 99315-99316
Established Patient 99334-99337
New Patient 99324-99328

Donor Procedures
Conjunctival Graft 68371
Heart Excision 33940
Heart/Lung Excision 33930
Liver Segment 47140-47142
Stem Cells
    Donor Search 38204

Dopamine
See Catecholamines
Blood 82383-82384
Urine .82382, 82384

Doppler Echocardiography 76827-
    76828, 93307-93308, 93320-93350
Extracranial .93875
Intracardiac .93662
Transesophageal 93318
Transthoracic 93303-93317

Doppler Scan
Arterial Studies
    Extremities 93922-93924
    Fetal
        Middle Cerebral Artery 76821
        Umbilical Artery 76820
Extremities .93965
Intracranial Arteries 93886-93893

Dorsal Vertebra
See Vertebra, Thoracic

Dose Plan
See Dosimetry

Dosimetry
Radiation Therapy 77300, 77331
    Brachytherapy 77326-77328
    Intensity Modulation 77301
    Teletherapy 77305-77321

Double-Stranded DNA
See Deoxyribonucleic Acid

Doxepin
Assay 80166

DPH
See Phenytoin

Drainage
See Excision; Incision; Incision and Drainage; Paracentesis
Abdomen
    Abdomen Fluid 49080-49081
Abscess
    Appendix 44900-44901
        Percutaneous 44901
    Brain 61150-61151
    Eyelid 67700
    Liver 47010-47011

Ovary
    Percutaneous 58823
Pelvic
    Percutaneous 58823
Pericolic
    Percutaneous 58823
Perirenal or Renal 50020-50021
    Percutaneous 50021
Prostate 52700
Retroperitoneal 49060-49061
    Percutaneous 49061
Subdiaphragmatic or
Subphrenic 49040-49041
    Percutaneous 49040-49041
with X-Ray .75989
Amniotic Fluid
    Diagnostic Aspiration 59000
    Therapeutic Aspiration 59001
Bile Duct
    Transhepatic 75980
Brain Fluid .61070
Bursa 20600-20610
Cerebrospinal Fluid 61000-61020, 61050,
    61070, 62272
Cervical Fluid 61050
Cisternal Fluid 61050
Cyst
    Bone 20615
    Brain 61150-61151, 62161-62162
    Breast 19000-19001
    Ganglion .20612
    Liver 47010-47011
        Percutaneous 47011
    Salivary Gland 42409
    Sublingual Gland 42409
Extraperitoneal Lymphocele
    Laparoscopic 49323
    Open 49062
Eye
    Paracentesis
        with Aqueous Aspiration 65800
        with Aqueous-Release 65805
    with Removal
        Blood 65815
        Discission of Anterior Hyaloid
        Membrane 65810
        Vitreous 65810
Fetal Fluid .59074
Ganglion Cyst 20612
Hematoma
    Brain 61154-61156
    Vagina 57022-57023
Hematoma, Subungual 11740
Joint .20600-20610
Liver
    Abscess or Cyst 47010-47011
        Percutaneous 47011
Lymphocele
    Endoscopic 49323
Onychia 10060-10061
Orbit 67405, 67440
Pancreas
    See Anastomosis, Pancreas to Intestines
    Pseudocyst 48510-48511
        Percutaneous 48511
Paronychia 10060-10061
Pericardial Sac 32659

Endosteal Implant

Endothelioma, Dural

See Meningioma

Endotracheal Intubation
See Insertion, Endotracheal Tube

Endotracheal Tube
Intubation 31500

Endovascular Repair 0078T, 0079T,
0080T, 0081T, 33880-33891,
34800-34805, 34812-34826, 34833-34900
Angiography 75952-75959

Endovascular Therapy
Ablation
   Vein 36475-36479
Occlusion 61623

Enema
Home Visit for Fecal Impaction 99511
Intussusception 74283
Therapeutic
   for Intussusception 74283

Energies, Electromagnetic
See Irradiation

ENT
See Ear, Nose, and Throat; Otorhinolaryngology,
Diagnostic
Therapeutic
   See Otorhinolaryngology

Entamoeba Histolytica
Antigen Detection
   Enzyme Immunoassay 87336-87337

Enterectomy 44120-44121,
44126-44128, 44137, 44202
Donor .44132-44133
with Enterostomy 44125

Enterocele
Repair 57556
Hysterectomy
   with Colpectomy 58280

Enterocystoplasty 51960
Camey 50825

Enteroenterostomy
See Anastomosis, Intestines

Enterolysis 44005
Laparoscopic 44180

Enteropancreatostomy
See Anastomosis, Pancreas to Intestines

Enterorrhaphy 44602-44603, 44615

Enterostomy 44300
Closure 44625-44626
with Enterectomy
   Intestine, Small 44125

Enterotomy 44615

Enterovirus
Antibody 86658

Entropion
Repair 67921-67924
   Excision Tarsal Wedge 67923
   Suture 67921
   Thermocauterization 67922

Enucleation
Eye
   with Implant 65103
     Muscles Attached 65105
   without Implant 65101
Pleural 32540

Enucleation, Cyst, Ovarian
See Cystectomy, Ovarian

Enucleation, Prostate
See Prostate, Enucleation

Environmental Intervention
for Psychiatric Patients 90882

Enzyme Activity 82657
Radioactive Substrate 82658

Enzyme, Angiotensin Converting
See Angiotensin Converting Enzyme (ACE)

Enzyme, Angiotensin-Forming
See Renin

EOG
See Electro-oculography

Eosinocyte
See Eosinophils

Eosinophils
Nasal Smear .89190

Epiandrosterone 82666

Epicondylitides, Lateral Humeral
See Tennis Elbow

Epicondylitis, Radiohumeral
See Tennis Elbow

Epidemic Parotitis
See Mumps

Epididymectomy
Bilateral 54861
Unilateral 54860

Epididymis
Abscess
   Incision and Drainage 54700
Anastomosis
   to Vas Deferens
     Bilateral 54901
     Unilateral 54900
Biopsy 54800, 54865
Epididymography 74440
Excision
   Bilateral .54861
   Unilateral 54860
Exploration
   Biopsy 54865
Hematoma
   Incision and Drainage 54700
Lesion
   Excision
     Local .54830
     Spermatocele 54840
Needle Biopsy 54800
Spermatocele
   Excision .54840

Unlisted Services and Procedures 55899
X-Ray with Contrast 74440

Epididymograms 55300

Epididymography 74440

Epididymoplasty
See Repair, Epididymis

Epididymovasostomy
Bilateral 54901
Unilateral 54900

Epidural
Electrode
   Insertion .61531
   Removal .61535
Injection 62281-62282, 62310-62319,
64479-64484
Lysis 0027T, 62263-62264

Epidural Anesthesia
See Anesthesia, Epidural

Epidurography 72275

Epigastric
Hernia Repair 49572

Epiglottidectomy 31420

Epiglottis
Excision 31420

Epikeratoplasty 65767

Epilation
See Removal, Hair

Epinephrine
See Catecholamines
Blood 82383-82384
Urine 82384

Epiphyseal Arrest
Femur 20150, 27185, 27475, 27479-27485, 27742
Fibula 20150, 27477-27485, 27730-27742
Radius 20150, 25450-25455
Tibia . .20150, 27477-27485, 27730, 27734-27742
Ulna 20150, 25450-25455

Epiphyseal Separation
Radius
   Closed Treatment 25600
   Open Treatment 25607-25609

Epiphysiodesis
See Epiphyseal Arrest

Epiphysis
See Bone; Specific Bone

Epiploectomy 49255

Episiotomy 59300

Epispadias
Penis
   Reconstruction 54385
Repair 54380-54390
   with Exstrophy of Bladder 54390
   with Incontinence 54380-54390

Epistaxis 30901-30906
with Nasal/Sinus Endoscopy 31238

EPO
See Erythropoietin

Epstein-Barr Virus
Antibody 86663-86665

Equina, Cauda
See Cauda Equina

ERCP
See Bile Duct; Cholangiopancreatography;
Pancreatic Duct

ERG
See Electroretinography

Ergocalciferol
See Calciferol

Ergocalciferols
See Calciferol

Ergonovine Provocation Test ...93024

Erythrocyte
See Red Blood Cell (RBC)

Erythrocyte ab
See Antibody, Red Blood Cell

Erythrocyte Count
See Red Blood Cell (RBC), Count

Erythropoietin 82668

Escharotomy
Burns 16035-16036

Escherichia coli 0157
Antigen Detection
    Enzyme Immunoassay 87335

ESD
See Endoscopy, Gastrointestinal, Upper

Esophageal Acid Infusion Test
See Acid Perfusion Test

Esophageal Polyp
See Polyp, Esophagus

Esophageal Tumor
See Tumor, Esophagus

Esophageal Varices
Ligation 43205, 43400
Transection/Repair 43401

Esophagectomy
Partial 43116-43124
Total 43107-43113, 43124

Esophagoenterostomy
with Total Gastrectomy 43620

Esophagogastroduodenoscopies
See Endoscopy, Gastrointestinal, Upper

Esophagogastromyotomy
See Esophagomyotomy

Esophagogastrostomy 43320

Esophagojejunostomy 43340-43341

Esophagomyotomy ..32665, 43330-43331

Esophagorrhaphy
See Esophagus, Suture

Esophagoscopies
See Endoscopy, Esophagus

Esophagostomy 43350-43352
Closure 43420-43425

Esophagotomy 43020, 43045

Esophagotracheal Fistula
See Fistula, Tracheoesophageal

Esophagus
Acid Perfusion Test 91030
Acid Reflux Tests 91034-91038
Balloon Distension
    Provocation Study 91040
Biopsy
    Endoscopy 43202
    Forceps 3150F
Cineradiography 74230
Dilation 43450-43458
    Endoscopic 43220-43226, 43248-43249
    Surgical 43510
Endoscopy
    Biopsy 43202
    Dilation 43220-43226
    Exploration 43200
    Hemorrhage 43227
    Injection 43201, 43204
    Insertion Stent 43219
    Needle Biopsy 43232
    Removal
        Foreign Body 43215
        Polyp 43216-43217, 43228
        Tumor 43216, 43228
    Ultrasound 43231-43232
    Vein Ligation 43205
Excision
    Diverticula 43130-43135
    Partial 43116-43124
    Total 43107-43113, 43124
Exploration
    Endoscopy 43200
Hemorrhage 43227
Incision 43020, 43045
    Muscle 43030
Injection
    Sclerosing Agent 43204
    Submucosal 43201
Insertion
    Stent 43219
    Tamponade 43460
    Tube 43510
Intubation with Specimen Collection 91000
Lesion
    Excision 43100-43101
Ligation 43405
Motility Study 78258, 91010-91012
Needle Biopsy
    Endoscopy 43232
Nuclear Medicine
    Imaging (Motility) 78258
    Reflux Study 78262

Reconstruction 43300, 43310, 43313
Creation
    Stoma 43350-43352
    Esophagostomy 43350
    Fistula 43305, 43312, 43314
    Gastrointestinal 43360-43361
Removal
    Foreign Bodies ..43020, 43045, 43215, 74235
    Lesion 43216
    Polyp 43216-43217, 43228
Repair 43300, 43310, 43313
    Esophagogastric Fundoplasty ..43324-43325
        Laparoscopic 43280
    Esophagogastrostomy 43320
    Esophagojejunostomy 43340-43341
    Fistula ...43305, 43312, 43314, 43420-43425
    Muscle 43330-43331
    Pre-existing Perforation 43405
    Varices 43401
    Wound 43410-43415
Suture 43405
    Wound 43410-43415
Ultrasound
    Endoscopy 43231-43232
Unlisted Services and Procedures ..43289, 43499
Vein
    Ligation 43205, 43400
Video 74230
X-Ray 74220

Esophagus Neoplasm
See Tumor, Esophagus

Esophagus, Varix
See Esophageal Varices

Established Patient
Domiciliary or Rest Home Visit 99334-99337
Emergency Department Services ..99281-99285
Home Services 99347-99350
Hospital Inpatient Services 99221-99239
Hospital Observation Services ..99217-99220
Inpatient Consultations 99251-99255
Office and/or Other Outpatient
Consultations 99241-99245
Office Visit 99211-99215
Online Medical Evaluation 98969, 99444
Outpatient Visit 99211-99215
Telephone Services ..98966-98968, 99441-99443

Establishment
Colostomy
    Abdominal 50810
    Perineal 50810

Estes Operation
See Ovary, Transposition

Estlander Procedure 40525

Estradiol 82670
Response 80414

Estriol
Blood or Urine 82677

Estrogen
Blood or Urine 82671-82672
Receptor 84233

Adenoma
   Thyroid Gland 60200
Adrenal Gland 60540
   Laparoscopic 60650
   with Excision Retroperitoneal Tumor ..60545
Alveolus 41830
Anal Crypt 46210-46211
Anal Fissure 46200
Anal Tag 46220, 46230
Aorta
   Coarctation 33840-33851
Appendix 44950-44960
Arteriovenous Malformation
   Spinal 63250-63252
Arytenoid Cartilage 31400
   Endoscopic 31560-31561
Atrial Septum 33735-33737
Bartholin's Gland 56740
Bladder
   Diverticulum 51525
   Neck 51520
   Partial 51550-51565
   Total 51570, 51580, 51590-51597
      with Nodes 51575, 51585, 51595
   Transurethral 52640
   Tumor 51530
Bladder Neck Contracture
   Postoperative 52640
Bone
   Facial 21026
   Mandible 21025
   Postoperative
      Femur 20150
      Fibula 20150
      Radius 20150
      Tibia 20150
      Ulna 20150
Bone Abscess
   Facial 21026
   Mandible 21025
Brain
   Amygdala 61566
   Epileptogenic Focus 61536
   Hemisphere 61542-61543
   Hippocampus 61566
   Other Lobe 61323, 61539-61540
   Temporal Lobe 61537-61538
Brain Lobe
   See Lobectomy, Brain
Breast
   Biopsy 19100-19103
   Chest Wall Tumor 19260-19272
   Cyst 19120-19126
   Lactiferous Duct Fistula 19112
   Lesion 19120-19126
      by Needle Localization 19125-19126
   Mastectomy 19300-19307
   Nipple Exploration 19110
Bulbourethral Gland 53250
Bullae
   Lung 32141
      Endoscopic 32655
Burns 01951-01953, 15002-15005
Bursa
   Elbow 24105
   Femur 27062
   Ischial 27060

Knee 27340
Wrist 25115-25116
Bypass Graft 35901-35907
Calcaneus 28118-28120
Calculi (Stone)
   Parotid Gland 42330, 42340
   Salivary Gland 42330-42340
   Sublingual Gland 42330
   Submandibular Gland 42330-42335
Carotid Artery 60605
Carpal 25145, 25210-25215
Cartilage
   Knee Joint 27332-27333
   Shoulder Joint 23101
   Temporomandibular Joint 21060
   Wrist 25107
Caruncle
   Urethra 53265
Cataract
   Secondary 66830
Cervix
   Radical 57531
   Stump
      Abdominal Approach 57540-57545
      Vaginal Approach 57550-57556
   Total 57530
Chalazion
   Multiple
      Different Lids 67805
      Same Lid 67801
   Single 67800
   with Anesthesia 67808
Chest Wall
   Tumor 19260-19272
Choroid Plexus 61544
Clavicle
   Partial 23120, 23180
   Sequestrectomy 23170
   Total 23125
   Tumor
      Radical Resection 23200
Coccyx 27080
Colon
   Excision
      Partial 44140-44147, 44160
      with Anastomosis 44140
      Total 44150-44158
   Laparoscopic
      with Anastomosis ...44204, 44207-44208
      with Colostomy 44206, 44208
      with Ileocolostomy 44205
Condyle
   Temporomandibular Joint 21050
Constricting Ring
   Finger 26596
Cornea
   Epithelium 65435
      with Chelating Agent 65436
   Scraping 65430
Coronoidectomy 21070
Cowper's Gland 53250
Cranial Bone
   Tumor 61563-61564
Cyst
   See Ganglion Cyst
   Bile Duct 47715
   Bladder 51500

Brain 61516, 61524, 62162
Branchial 42810-42815
Calcaneus 28100-28103
Carpal 25130-25136
Cheekbone 21030
Clavicle 23140
   with Allograft 23146
   with Autograft 23145
Facial Bones 21030
Femur 27065-27067, 27355-27358
Fibula 27635-27638
Finger 26160
Foot 28090
Hand 26160
Hip 27065-27067
Humerus 23150, 24110
   with Allograft 23156, 24116
   with Autograft 23155, 24115
Ileum 27065-27067
Kidney 50280-50290
Knee 27345-27347
Lung 32140
Mandible 21040, 21046-21047
Maxilla 21030, 21048-21049
Mediastinal 39200
Mediastinum 32662
Metacarpal 26200-26205
Metatarsal 28104-28107
Mullerian Duct 55680
Nose 30124-30125
Olecranon 24120
Olecranon Process
   with Allograft 24126
   with Autograft 24125
Ovarian 58925
   See Cystectomy, Ovarian
Pericardial 33050
   Endoscopic 32661
Phalanges 26210-26215
   Toe 28108
Pilonidal 11770-11772
Pubis 27066-27067
Radius 24120, 25120-25126
   with Allograft 24126
   with Autograft 24125
Salivary Gland 42408
Scapula 23140
   with Allograft 23146
   with Autograft 23145
Seminal Vesicle 55680
Sublingual Gland 42408
Talus 28100-28103
Tarsal 28104-28107
Thyroglossal Duct 60280-60281
Thyroid Gland 60200
Tibia 27635-27638
Toe 28092
Ulna 24120, 25120-25126
   with Allograft 24126
   with Autograft 24125
Urachal
   Bladder 51500
Vaginal 57135
Destruction of the Vestibule of the Mouth
   See Mouth, Vestibule of, Excision, Destruction
Diverticulum, Meckel's
   See Meckel's Diverticulum, Excision

F

Face

CT Scan 70486-70488
Lesion
    Destruction 17000-17004, 17280-17286
Magnetic Resonance Imaging
(MRI) 70540-70543
Tumor Resection 21015

Face Lift 15824-15828

Facial Asymmetries
See Hemifacial Microsomia

Facial Bone
See Mandible; Maxilla
Tumor
    Excision 21034

Facial Bones
Abscess
    Excision 21026
Reconstruction
    Secondary 21275
Repair 21208-21209
Tumor
    Excision 21029-21030
    Resection
        Radical 21015
X-Ray 70140-70150

Facial Nerve
Anastomosis
    to Hypoglossal 64868
    to Phrenic Nerve 64870
    to Spinal Accessory 64866
Avulsion 64742
Decompression 61590, 61596
    Intratemporal
      Lateral to Geniculate Ganglion 69720,
                             69740
      Medial to Geniculate Ganglion 69725,
                             69745
    Total 69955
Function Study .92516
Incision 64742
Injection
    Anesthetic 64402
Mobilization 61590
Repair
    Lateral to Geniculate Ganglion 69740
    Medial to Geniculate Ganglion 69745
Repair/Suture
    with or without Graft 64864-64865
Suture
    Lateral to Geniculate Ganglion 69740
    Medial to Geniculate Ganglion 69745
Transection 64742

Facial Nerve Paralysis
Graft 15840-15845
Repair 15840-15845

Facial Prosthesis
Impression 21088

Facial Rhytidectomy
See Face Lift

Factor, ACTH-Releasing
See Corticotropic Releasing Hormone (CRH)

Factor, Antinuclear
See Antinuclear Antibodies (ANA)

Factor, Blood Coagulation
See Clotting Factor
Factor I
    See Fibrinogen
Factor II
    See Prothrombin
Factor III
    See Thromboplastin
Factor IV
    See Calcium
Factor VII
    See Proconvertin
Factor VIII
    See Clotting Factor
Factor IX
    See Christmas Factor
Factor X
    See Stuart-Prower Factor
Factor X, Activated
    See Thrombokinase
Factor Xa Inhibitor
    See Antithrombin III
Factor XI
    See PlasmaThromboplastin, Antecedent
Factor XII
    See Hageman Factor
Factor XIII
    See Fibrin Stabilizing Factor

Factor, Fitzgerald
See Fitzgerald Factor

Factor, Fletcher
See Fletcher Factor

Factor, Hyperglycemic-Glycogenolytic
See Glucagon

Factor Inhibitor Test 85335

Factor, Intrinsic
See Intrinsic Factor

Factor, Rheumatoid
See Rheumatoid Factor

Factor, Sulfation
See Somatomedin

Fallopian Tube
Anastomosis 58750
Catheterization 58345, 74742
Destruction
    Endoscopy .58670
Ectopic Pregnancy 59121
    with Salpingectomy and/or
    Oophorectomy 59120
Excision 58700-58720
Ligation 58600-58611
Lysis
    Adhesions 58740

Occlusion 58615
    Endoscopy .58671
Placement
    Implant for Occlusion 58565
Repair 58752
    Anastomosis 58750
    Create Stoma 58770
Tumor
    Resection 58950, 58952-58958
Unlisted Services and Procedures 58999
X-Ray 74742

Fallopian Tube Pregnancy
See Ectopic Pregnancy, Tubal

Fallot, Tetralogy of
See Tetralogy of Fallot

Family Psychotherapy
See Psychotherapy, Family

Fanconi Anemia
Chromosome Analysis 88248

Farnsworth-Munsell Color Test
See Color Vision Examination

Farr Test
See Gammaglobulin, Blood

Fasanella-Servat Procedure . . .67908

Fascia Graft 15840

Fascia Lata Graft
Harvesting 20920-20922

Fascial Defect
Repair 50728

Fascial Graft
Free
    Microvascular Anastomosis 15758
Open Treatment
    Sternoclavicular Dislocation 23532

Fasciectomy
Foot 28060
    Radical 28060-28062
Palm 26121-26125

Fasciocutaneous Flaps . . .15731-15738

Fasciotomy
Arm, Lower 24495, 25020-25025
Foot 28008
Hand Decompression 26037
Hip 27025
Knee 27305, 27496-27499
Leg, Lower 27600-27602, 27892-27894
Leg, Upper . . .27305, 27496-27499, 27892-27894
Palm 26040-26045
Plantar
    Endoscopic .29893
Thigh 27025
Toe 28008
Wrist 25020-25025

FAST
See Allergen Immunotherapy

Fat
Feces 82705-82715

Removal
    Lipectomy 15876-15879

Fat Stain
Feces 89125
Respiratory Secretions 89125
Sputum 89125
Urine 89125

Fatty Acid
Blood 82725
Long-Chain Omega-3
    Red Blood Cell (RBC) Membranes 0111T
Very Long Chain 82726

Favre-Durand Disease
See Lymphogranuloma Venereum

FC Receptor 86243

FDP
See Fibrin Degradation Products

Feedback, Psychophysiologic
See Biofeedback; Training, Biofeedback

Female Castration
See Oophorectomy

Female Gonad
See Ovary

Femoral Arteries
See Artery, Femoral

Femoral Nerve
Injection
    Anesthetic 64447-64448

Femoral Stem Prosthesis
See Arthroplasty, Hip

Femoral Vein
See Vein, Femoral

Femur
See Hip; Knee; Leg, Upper
Abscess
    Incision 27303
Bursa
    Excision 27062
Craterization 27070, 27360
Cyst
    Excision 27065-27067, 27355-27358
Diaphysectomy .27360
Drainage 27303
Excision 27070, 27360
    Epiphyseal Bar 20150
    Neurectomy
        Hamstring 27325
        Popliteal 27326
Fracture 27244
    Closed Treatment 27501-27503,
                            27267-27268
    Distal 27508, 27510, 27514
    Distal, Medial or Lateral Condyle 27509
        Open Treatment 27514
    Epiphysis 27516-27519
        Open Treatment 27519
    Intertrochanteric 27244
        Closed Treatment 27238

Treatment with Implant 27244
    with Implant 27245
    with Manipulation 27240
Neck
    Closed Treatment 27230-27232
    Open Treatment 27236
    Percutaneous Fixation 27235
Open Treatment 27245, 27269,
            27506-27507, 27511-27513
Percutaneous Fixation 27509
Peritrochanteric 27244
    Closed Treatment 27238
    Treatment with Implant 27244
    with Implant 27245
    with Manipulation 27240
Proximal End, Head
    Closed Treatment 27267-27268
    Open Treatment 27269
Shaft 27500, 27502, 27506-27507
Subtrochanteric 27244
    Closed Treatment 27238
    Treatment with Implant 27244
    with Implant 27245
    with Manipulation 27240
Supracondylar 27501-27503,
              27509, 27511-27513
    Open Treatment 27511, 27513
Transcondylar 27501-27503, 27509,
                   27511-27513
    Open Treatment 27511, 27513
Trochanteric
    Closed Treatment 27246
    Open Treatment 27248
    with Manipulation 27503
    without Manipulation 27501
Halo 20663
Lesion
    Excision 27062
Osteoplasty
    Lengthening 27466-27468
    Shortening 27465, 27468
Osteotomy
    without Fixation 27448
Prophylactic Treatment 27187, 27495
Realignment .27454
Reconstruction 27468
    at Knee 27442-27443, 27446
    Lengthening 27466-27468
    Shortening 27465, 27468
Repair 27470-27472
    Epiphysis 27181, 27475, 27742
    Arrest 27185
    Muscle Transfer 27110
    Osteotomy 27140, 27151-27156,
            27161-27165, 27450-27454
    with Graft 27170
Saucerization 27070, 27360
Tumor
    Excision . .27065-27067, 27355-27358, 27365
X-Ray 73550

Fenestration Procedure
Semicircular Canal 69820
    Revision 69840
Tracheostomy .31610

Fenestration, Pericardium
See Pericardiostomy

Fern Test 89060
See Smear and Stain, Wet Mount

Ferric Chloride
Urine 81005

Ferrihemoglobin
See Methemoglobin

Ferritin
Blood or Urine .82728

Ferroxidase
See Ceruloplasmin

Fertility Control
See Contraception

Fertility Test
Semen Analysis 89300-89322
Sperm Analysis 89331
    Cervical Mucus Penetration Test 89330
    Hamster Penetration 89329
Sperm Evaluation 89331

Fertilization
Assisted
    Oocyte
        Microtechnique 89280-89281
Oocyte
    with Co-Culture 89251

Fertilization in Vitro
See In Vitro Fertilization

Fetal Biophysical Profile .76818-76819

Fetal Contraction Stress Test ..59020

Fetal Hemoglobin 85461

Fetal Lung Maturity Assessment; LecithinSphingomyelin Ratio ..83661

Fetal Monitoring
See Monitoring, Fetal

Fetal Non-Stress Test 59025
Ultrasound 76818

Fetal Procedure
Amnioinfusion 59070
Cord Occlusion 59072
Fluid Drainage 59074
Shunt Placement 59076
Unlisted Fetal Invasive Procedure 59897
Unlisted Laparoscopy Procedure 59898
Unlisted Procedure, Maternity Care
and Delivery .59899

Fetal Testing
Amniotic Fluid
    Lung Maturity 83661, 83663-83664
Heart .76825-76826
    Doppler
        Complete 76827
        Follow-up or Repeat Study 76828
Hemoglobin 83030-83033, 85460
Ultrasound 76801-76828
    Heart 76825
    Middle Cerebral Artery 76821
    Umbilical Artery 76820

Nose
    Repair 30580-30600
Oval Window 69666
Postauricular 69700
Rectovaginal
    Abdominal Approach 57305
    Transperineal Approach 57308
    with Concomitant Colostomy 57307
Round Window .69667
Sclera
    Iridencleisis or Iridotasis 66165
    Sclerectomy with Punch or Scissors
    with Iridectomy 66160
    Thermocauterization with Iridectomy . .66155
    Trabeculectomy ab Externo in Absence
    Previous Surgery 66170
    Trabeculectomy ab Externo with
    Scarring 66172
    Trephination with Iridectomy 66150
Suture
    Kidney 50520-50526
    Ureter 50920-50930
Trachea 31755
Tracheoesophageal
    Repair 43305, 43312, 43314
    Speech Prosthesis 31611
Ureter 50920-50930
Urethra .53400-53405
Urethrovaginal .57310
    with Bulbocavernosus Transplant 57311
Vesicouterine
    Closure 51920-51925
Vesicovaginal
    Closure 51900
    Transvesical and Vaginal Approach . . .57330
    Vaginal Approach 57320
X-Ray 76080

Fistula Arteriovenous
See Arteriovenous Fistula

Fistulectomy
Anal 46060, 46270-46285
    See Hemorrhoids

Fistulization
Conjunction
    to Nasal Cavity 68745
Esophagus 43350-43352
Intestines 44300-44346
Lacrimal Sac
    to Nasal Cavity 68720
Penis 54435
Pharynx 42955
Sclera
    for Glaucoma 0123T
Tracheopharyngeal 31755

Fistulization, Interatrial
See Septostomy, Atrial

Fistulotomy
Anal 46270, 46280

Fitting
Cervical Cap 57170
Contact Lens 92070, 92310-92313
    See Contact LensServices
Diaphragm 57170

Low Vision Aid 92354-92355
    See SpectacleServices
Spectacle Prosthesis 92352-92353
Spectacles 92340-92342

Fitzgerald Factor 85293

Fixation
Interdental
    without Fracture 21497

Fixation (Device)
See Application; Bone, Fixation; Spinal
Instrumentation
Application
    External 20690-20692
Pelvic
    Insertion .22848
Removal
    External 20694
    Internal 20670-20680
Sacrospinous Ligament
    Vaginal Prolapse 57282
Shoulder 23700
Skeletal
    Humeral Epycondyle
      Percutaneous 24566
Spinal
    Insertion 22841-22847
    Prosthetic .22851
    Reinsertion 22849

Fixation Test, Complement
See Complement, Fixation Test

Fixation, External
See External Fixation

Fixation, Kidney
See Nephropexy

Fixation, Rectum
See Proctopexy

Fixation, Tongue
See Tongue, Fixation

Flank
See Back/Flank

Flap
See Skin Graft and Flap
Free
    Breast Reconstruction 19364
Grafts 15570-15738, 15842
Latissimus Dorsi
    Breast Reconstruction 19361
Omentum 49905
    Free
      with Microvascular Anastomosis . . .49906
Transverse Rectus Abdominis Myocutaneous
    Breast Reconstruction 19367-19369

Flatfoot Correction 28735

Flea Typhus
See Murine Typhus

Fletcher Factor 85292

Flow Cytometry 88182-88189
Diagnostic/Pretreatment 3170F

Flow-Volume Loop
See Pulmonology, Diagnostic
Pulmonary 94375

Flu Vaccines . . .90645-90648, 90655-90663

Fluid Collection
Incision and Drainage
    Skin 10140

Fluid, Amniotic
See Amniotic Fluid

Fluid, Body
See Body Fluid

Fluid, Cerebrospinal
See Cerebrospinal Fluid

Fluorescein
Angiography, Ocular 92287
Intravenous Injection
    Vascular Flow Check, Graft 15860

Fluorescein Angiography
See Angiography, Fluorescein

**Fluorescent In Situ
Hybridization** 88365

Fluoride
Blood 82735
Urine 82735

Fluoroscopy
Bile Duct
    Calculus Removal 74327
    Guide Catheter 74328, 74330
Chest
    Bronchoscopy 31622-31640
    Complete (Four Views) 71034
    Partial (Two Views) 71023
Drain Abscess .75989
GI Tract
    Guide Intubation 74340
Hourly 76000-76001
Introduction
    GI Tube 74340
Larynx 70370
Nasogastric 43752
Needle Biopsy .77002
Orogastric 43752
Pancreatic Duct
    Guide Catheter 74329-74330
Pharynx 70370
Renal
    Guide Catheter 74475
Spine/Paraspinous
    Guide Catheter/Needle 77003
Unlisted Services and Procedures 76496
Ureter
    Guide Catheter 74480
Venous Access Device 36598, 77001
Vertebra
    Osteoplasty 77291

Flurazepam
Blood or Urine .82742

Flush Aortogram 75722-75724

Frost Suture 67875

**Frozen Blood
Preparation** 86930-86932

Fructose 84375
Semen 82757

**Fructose Intolerance
Breath Test** 91065

Fruit Sugar
See Fructose

FSF 85290-85291

FSH
See Follicle Stimulating Hormone (FSH)

FSP
See Fibrin Degradation Products

FT-4 84439

Fulguration
See Destruction
Bladder 51020
Cystourethroscopy with 52214
    Lesion 52224
    Tumor 52234-52240
Ureter 50957, 50976
Ureterocele
    Ectopic 52301
    Orthotopic 52300

Fulguration, Endocavitary
See Electrocautery

Full Thickness Graft 15200-15261

Function Test, Lung
See Pulmonology, Diagnostic

Function Test, Vestibular
See Vestibular Function Tests

Function, Study, Nasal
See Nasal Function Study

Functional Ability
See Activities of Daily Living

Fundoplasty
Esophagogastric 43324-43325
    Laparoscopic 43280
    with Gastroplasty 43326

Fundoplication
See Fundoplasty, Esophagogastric

Fungus
Antibody 86671
Culture
    Blood 87103
    Hair 87101
    Identification 87106
    Nail 87101
    Other 87102
    Skin 87101
Tissue Exam 87220

Funnel Chest
See Pectus Excavatum

Furuncle
Incision and Drainage 10060-10061

Furuncle, Vulva
See Abscess, Vulva

Fusion
See Arthrodesis
Pleural Cavity 32560
Thumb
    in Opposition 26820

Fusion, Epiphyseal-Diaphyseal
See Epiphyseal Arrest

Fusion, Joint
See Arthrodesis

Fusion, Joint, Ankle
See Ankle, Arthrodesis

**Fusion, Joint, Interphalangeal,
Finger**
See Arthrodesis, Finger Joint, Interphalangeal

G

Gait Training 97116
See Physical Medicine/Therapy/Occupational
Therapy

Galactogram 77053-77054
Injection 19030

Galactokinase
Blood 82759

Galactose
Blood 82760
Urine 82760

Galactose-1-Phosphate
Uridyl Transferase 82775-82776

**Galeazzi Fracture/
Dislocation** 25525-25526

Gall Bladder
See Gallbladder

Gallbladder
See Bile Duct
Anastomosis
    with Intestines 47720-47741
Excision 47562-47564, 47600-47620
Exploration 47480
Incision 47490
Incision and Drainage 47480
Nuclear Medicine
    Imaging 78223
Removal
    Calculi (Stone) 47480
Repair
    with Gastroenterostomy 47741
    with Intestines 47720-47740
Unlisted Services and Procedures 47999
X-Ray with Contrast 74290-74291

Galvanocautery
See Electrocautery

Galvanoionization
See Iontophoresis

**Gamete Intrafallopian Transfer
(GIFT)** 58976

Gamete Transfer
In Vitro Fertilization 58976

Gamma Camera Imaging
See Nuclear Medicine

Gamma Glutamyl Transferase ..82977

Gamma Seminoprotein
See Antigen, Prostate Specific

Gammacorten
See Dexamethasone

Gammaglobulin
Blood 82784-82787

Gamulin Rh
See Immune Globulins, Rho (D)

Ganglia, Trigeminal
See Gasserian Ganglion

Ganglion
See Gasserian Ganglion
Cyst
    Aspiration/Injection 20612
    Drainage 20612
    Wrist
        Excision 25111-25112
Injection
    Anesthetic 64505, 64510

Ganglion Cervicothoracicum
See Stellate Ganglion

Ganglion Pterygopalatinum
See Sphenopalatine Ganglion

Ganglion, Gasser's
See Gasserian Ganglion

Gardner Operation
See Meningocele Repair

**Gardnerella Vaginalis
Detection** 87510-87512

Gasser Ganglion
See Gasserian Ganglion

Gasserian Ganglion
Sensory Root
    Decompression 61450
    Section 61450
Stereotactic 61790

Gastrectomy
Partial 43631-43635, 43845
    with Gastrojejunostomy 43632
Total 43621-43622
    with Esophagoenterostomy 43620
with Gastroduodenostomy 43631

Gastric Acid 82926-82928

Genioplasty 21120-21123
Augmentation 21120, 21123
Osteotomy 21121-21123

Genitourinary Sphincter, Artificial
See Prosthesis, Urethral Sphincter

Genotype Analysis
by Nucleic Acid
    Infectious Agent
        Hepatitis C Virus 87902
        HIV-1 Protease/Reverse
        Transcriptase 87901
        Vancomycin Resistance 87500

Gentamicin 80170
Assay 80170

Gentamycin Level
See Gentamicin

Gentiobiase
See Beta Glucosidase

Genus: Human Cytomegalovirus Group
See Cytomegalovirus

GERD
See Gastroesophageal Reflux Test

German Measles
See Rubella

Gestational Trophoblastic Tumor
See Hydatidiform Mole

GGT
See Gamma Glutamyl Transferase

GI Tract
See Gastrointestinal Tract

Giardia
Antigen Detection
    Enzyme Immunoassay 87329
    Immunofluorescence 87269

Giardia Lamblia
Antibody 86674

Gibbons Stent 52332

GIF
See Somatostatin

GIFT
See Gamete Intrafallopian Transfer

Gill Operation 63012

Gillies Approach
Fracture
    Zygomatic Arch 21356

Gingiva
See Gums

Gingiva, Abscess
See Abscess
Fracture
  See Abscess, Gums; Gums
    Zygomatic Arch
      See Abscess, Gums; Gums, Abscess

Gingivectomy 41820

Gingivoplasty 41872

Girdlestone Laminectomy
See Laminectomy

Girdlestone Procedure
See Acetabulum, Reconstruction

Gla Protein (Bone)
See Osteocalcin

Gland
See Specific Gland

Gland, Adrenal
See Adrenal Gland

Gland, Bartholin's
See Bartholin's Gland

Gland, Bulbourethral
See Bulbourethral Gland

Gland, Lacrimal
See Lacrimal Gland

Gland, Mammary
See Breast

Gland, Parathyroid
See Parathyroid Gland

Gland, Parotid
See Parotid Gland

Gland, Pituitary
See Pituitary Gland

Gland, Salivary
See Salivary Glands

Gland, Sublingual
See Sublingual Gland

Gland, Sweat
See Sweat Glands

Gland, Thymus
See Thymus Gland

Gland, Thyroid
See Thyroid Gland

Glasses
See Spectacle Services

Glaucoma
Cryotherapy 66720
Cyclophotocoagulation 66710-66711
Diathermy .66700
Fistulization of Sclera 66150
Provocative Test 92140

Glaucoma Drainage Implant
See Aqueous Shunt

Glenn Procedure 33766-33767

Glenohumeral Joint
Arthrotomy 23040
    with Biopsy 23100
    with Synovectomy 23105
Exploration 23107

Removal
    Foreign or Loose Body 23107

Glenoid Fossa
Reconstruction 21255

GLN
See Glutamine

Globulin
Antihuman 86880-86886
Immune 90281-90399
Sex Hormone Binding 84270

Globulin, Corticosteroid-Binding
See Transcortin

Globulin, Rh Immune
See Immune Globulins, Rho (D)

Globulin, Thyroxine-Binding
See Thyroxine Binding Globulin

Glomerular Procoagulant Activity
See Thromboplastin

Glomus Caroticum
See Carotid Body

Glossectomies
See Excision, Tongue

Glossopexy
See Tongue, Fixation

Glossorrhaphy
See Suture, Tongue

Glucagon 82943
Tolerance Panel 80422-80424
Tolerance Test 82946

Glucose 80422-80424,
                80430-80435, 95250-95251
Blood Test 82947-82950, 82962
Body Fluid .82945
Interstitial Fluid
    Continuous Monitoring 95250-95251
Tolerance Test 82951-82952
    with Tolbutamide 82953

Glucose Phosphate Isomerase
See Phosphohexose Isomerase

Glucose Phosphate Isomerase Measurement
See Phosphohexose Isomerase

Glucose-6-Phosphate
Dehydrogenase 82955-82960

Glucosidase 82963

Glucuronide Androstanediol . . .82154

Glue
Cornea Wound 65286
Sclera Wound 65286

Glukagon
See Glucagon

Glutamate Dehydrogenase
Blood 82965

Greater Vestibular Gland
See Bartholin's Gland

Green Operation
See Scapulopexy

Gridley Stain 88312

Grippe, Balkan
See Q Fever

Gritti Operation
See Amputation, Leg, Upper; Radical Resection;
Replantation

Groin Area
Repair
　　Hernia 49550-49557

Group Health Education . .98961-98962,
　　　　　　　　　　　　　　　　　　　99078

Grouping, Blood
See Blood Typing

Growth Factors, Insulin-Like
See Somatomedin

Growth Hormone 83003
Human 80418, 80428-80430, 86277

**Growth Hormone Release
Inhibiting Factor**
See Somatostatin

GTT
See Hydatidiform Mole

Guaiac Test
See Blood, Feces

Guanosine Monophosphate 83008

Guanosine Monophosphate, Cyclic
See Cyclic GMP

Guanylic Acids
See Guanosine Monophosphate

Guard Stain 88313

Gullet
See Esophagus

Gums
Abscess
　　Incision and Drainage 41800
Alveolus
　　Excision 41830
Cyst
　　Incision and Drainage 41800
Excision
　　Gingiva 41820
　　Operculum .41821
Graft
　　Mucosa 41870
Hematoma
　　Incision and Drainage 41800
Lesion
　　Destruction .41850
　　Excision 41822-41828
Mucosa
　　Excision 41828

Reconstruction
　　Alveolus 41874
　　Gingiva 41872
Removal
　　Foreign Body 41805
Tumor
　　Excision 41825-41827
Unlisted Services and Procedures 41899

Gunning-Lieben Test
See Acetone, Blood or Urine

Guthrie Test 84030

H

H Flu
See Hemophilus Influenza

H-Reflex Study 95934-95936

**HAA (Hepatitis Associated
Antigen)**
See Hepatitis Antigen, B Surface

HAAb
See Antibody, Hepatitis

Haemoglobin F
See Fetal Hemoglobin

Haemorrhage
See Hemorrhage

Haemorrhage Rectum
See Hemorrhage, Rectum

Hageman Factor 85280

HAI Test
See Hemagglutination Inhibition Test

Hair
Electrolysis 17380
KOH Examination 87220
Microscopic Evaluation 96902
Transplant
　　Punch Graft 15775-15776
　　Strip Graft 15220-15221

Hair Removal
See Removal, Hair

Hallux
See Great Toe

Halo
Body Cast 29000
Cranial 20661
　　for Thin Skull Osteology 20664
Femur 20663
Maxillofacial 21100
Pelvic 20662
Removal 20665

Haloperidol
Assay 80173

**Halstead-Reitan
Neurospychological Battery** . . .96118

Halsted Mastectomy
See Mastectomy, Radical

Halsted Repair
See Hernia, Repair, Inguinal

Ham Test
See Hemolysins

Hammertoe Repair 28285-28286

Hamster Penetration Test 89329

Hand
See Carpometacarpal Joint; Intercarpal Joint
Amputation
　　at Metacarpal 25927
　　at Wrist 25920
　　　　Revision 25922
　　Revision 25924, 25929-25931
Arthrodesis
　　Carpometacarpal Joint 26843-26844
　　Intercarpal Joint 25820-25825
Bone
　　Incision and Drainage 26034
Cast 29085
Decompression 26035-26037
Fracture
　　Carpometacarpal 26641-26650
　　Interphalangeal 26740-26746
　　Metacarpal 26600-26615
　　Metacarpophalangeal 26740-26746
　　Phalangeal 26720-26735, 26750-26765
Insertion
　　Tendon Graft 26392
Magnetic Resonance Imaging (MRI) 73218-73223
Reconstruction
　　Tendon Pulley 26500-26502
Removal
　　Implantation 26320
　　　　Tube/Rod 26390-26392, 26416
Repair
　　Blood Vessel 35207
　　Cleft Hand .26580
　　Muscle 26591-26593
　　Tendon
　　　　Extensor 26410-26416, 26426-26428,
　　　　　　　　　　　　　　　　26433-26437
　　　　Flexor 26350-26358, 26440
　　　　Profundus 26370-26373
Replantation 20808
Strapping 29280
Tendon
　　Excision 26390
　　　　Extensor 26415
Tenotomy 26450, 26460
Tumor
　　Excision 26115-26117
Unlisted Services and Procedures 26989
X-Ray 73120-73130

Hand Abscess
See Abscess, Hand

Hand Phalange
See Finger, Bone

Hand(s) Dupuytrens Contracture(s)
See Dupuytren's Contracture

Handling
Device .... .99002
Radioelement .... .77790
Specimen 99000-99001

Hanganutziu Deicher Antibodies
See Antibody, Heterophile

Haptoglobin 83010-83012

Hard Palate
See Palate

Harelip Operation
See Cleft Lip, Repair

Harii Procedure .... .25430

Harrington Rod
Insertion .... .22840
Removal .... .22850

Hartmann Procedure
Laparoscopic .... .44206
Open .... .44143

Harvest of Upper Extremity Artery for Coronary Artery Bypass 35600

Harvesting
Bone Graft 20900-20902
Bone Marrow .... .38230
Cartilage Graft 20910-20912
Conjunctival Graft .... .68371
Eggs
　In Vitro Fertilization .... .58970
Endoscopic
　Vein for Bypass Graft .... .33508
Fascia Lata Graft 20920-20922
Intestines 44132-44133
Kidney 50300-50320, 50547
Liver .... .47133, 47140-47142
Lower Extremity Vein
　for Vascular Reconstruction 35572
Skin
　for Tissue Culture .... .15040
Stem Cell 38205-38206
Tendon Graft .... .20924
Tissue Grafts .... .20926
Upper Extremity Artery
　for Coronary Artery Bypass Graft .... .35600
Upper Extremity Vein
　for Bypass Graft .... .35500

Hauser Procedure .... .27420

Hayem's Elementary Corpuscle
See Blood, Platelet

Haygroves Procedure
See Reconstruction, Acetabulum; Revision

HBcAb
See Antibody, Hepatitis

HBeAb
See Antibody, Hepatitis

HBeAg
See Hepatitis Antigen, Be

HBsAb
See Antibody, Hepatitis

HBsAg (Hepatitis B Surface Antigen)
See Hepatitis Antigen, B Surface

HCG
See Chorionic Gonadotropin

HCO3
See Bicarbonate

HCV Antibodies
See Antibody, Hepatitis C

HDL
See Lipoprotein

Head
Angiography .... .70496, 70544-70546
CT Scan 70450-70470, 70496
Excision 21015-21070
Fracture and/or Dislocation 21310-21497
Incision .... .21010, 61316, 62148
Introduction or Removal 21076-21116
Lipectomy, Suction Assisted .... .15876
Magnetic Resonance Angiography
(MRA) 70544-70546
Nerve
　Graft 64885-64886
Other Procedures .... .21299, 21499
Repair/Revision and/or
Reconstruction 21120-21296
Ultrasound Exam .... .76506, 76536
Unlisted Services and Procedures .... .21499
X-Ray .... .70350

Head Rings, Stereotactic
See Stereotactic Frame

Headbrace
Application .... .21100
Application/Removal .... .20661

Heaf Test
See TB Test

Health Behavior
See Evaluation and Management, Health
Behavior

Health Risk Assessment Instrument
See Preventive Medicine

Hearing Aid
Bone Conduction
　Implantation .... .69710
　Removal .... .69711
　Repair .... .69711
　Replacement .... .69710

Hearing Aid Check 92592-92593

Hearing Aid Services
Electroacoustic Test 92594-92595
Examination 92590-92591

Hearing Tests
See Audiologic Function Tests; Hearing
Evaluation

Hearing Therapy 92507-92508,
　　　　　　　　　　　　　　　.92601-92604

Heart
Ablation 33250-33266
Allograft Preparation .... .33933
Angiography
　Injection 93542-93543
　　See Cardiac Catheterization; Injection
Aortic Arch
　with Cardiopulmonary Bypass .... .33853
　without Cardiopulmonary Bypass ..... .33852
Aortic Valve
　Repair
　　Left Ventricle .... .33414
　Replacement 33405-33413
Arrhythmogenic Focus
　Catheter Ablation 93650-93652
　Destruction 33250-33251, 33261
Atria
　See Atria
Biopsy .... .93505
　Imaging Guidance .... .76932
　Ultrasound
　　Imaging Guidance .... .76932
Blood Vessel
　Repair 33320-33322
Cardiac Output Measurements ... .0104T-0105T,
　　　　　　　　　　　　　　.93561-93562
Cardiac Rehabilitation 93797-93798
Cardioassist 92970-92971
　Ventricular Assist Device
　　Extracorporeal .... .0049T
Cardiopulmonary Bypass
　with Lung Transplant .... .32852, 32854
Catheterization .... .93501, 93510-93533
　Combined Right and Retrograde Left
　　for Congenital Cardiac Anomalies ...93531
　Combined Right and Transseptal Left for
　　Congenital Cardiac
　　Anomalies 93532-93533
　Flow Directed .... .93503
　Right
　　for Congenital Cardiac Anomalies ...93530
　　See Catheterization, Cardiac
Closure
　Septal Defect .... .33615
　Ventricular 33675-33677, 33681-33688
　Valve
　　Atrioventricular .... .33600
　　Semilunar .... .33602
Commissurotomy
　Right Ventricle 33476-33478
Computed Tomography .... .0144T-0151T
CT Scan .... .0144T-0151T
Destruction
　Arrhythmogenic Focus .... .33250, 33261
Electrical Recording
　3-D Mapping .... .93613
　Acoustic Heart Sound .... .0068T-0069T,
　　　　　　　　　　　　.0070T, 33202-33203
　Atria .... .93602
　Atrial Electrogram, Esophageal
　　(or Trans-esophageal) 93615-93616
　Bundle of His .... .93600
　Comprehensive 93619-93622

Heart Sounds

Heart Vessels

Heat Unstable Haemoglobin

Heavy Lipoproteins

Heavy Metal

Heel

Heel Bone

Gastrointestinal, Upper
   Endoscopic Control 43255
Intestines, Small
   Endoscopic Control 44366, 44378
Liver
   Control 47350
Lung 32110
Nasal
   Cauterization 30901-30906
   Endoscopic Control 31238
Nasopharynx 42970-42972
Oropharynx 42960-42962
Rectum
   Endoscopic Control 45317
Throat 42960-42962
Uterus
   Postpartum 59160
Vagina 57180

Hemorrhoidectomy
Complex 46260
   with Fissurectomy 46261-46262
External Complete 46250
Ligature 46221
Simple 46255
   with Fissurectomy 46257-46258

Hemorrhoidopexy 46947

Hemorrhoids
Destruction 46934-46936
Incision
   External .46083
Injection
   Sclerosing Solution 46500
Ligation 46945-46946
Stapling 46947
Suture 46945-46946

Hemosiderin 83070-83071

Hemothorax
Thoracostomy 32551

Heparin 85520
See Clotting Inhibitors
Neutralization 85525
Protamine Tolerance Test 85530

Heparin Cofactor I
See Antithrombin III

Hepatectomy
Extensive .47122
Left Lobe 47125
Partial
   Donor 47140-47142
   Lobe 47120
Right Lobe .47130
Total
   Donor 47133

Hepatic Abscess
See Abscess, Liver

Hepatic Arteries
See Artery, Hepatic

Hepatic Artery Aneurysm
See Artery, Hepatic, Aneurysm

Hepatic Duct
Anastomosis
   with Intestines 47765, 47802
Exploration .47400
Incision and Drainage 47400
Nuclear Medicine
   Imaging 78223
Removal
   Calculi (Stone) 47400
Repair
   with Intestines 47765, 47802
Unlisted Services and Procedures 47999

Hepatic Haemorrhage
See Hemorrhage, Liver

Hepatic Portal Vein
See Vein, Hepatic Portal

Hepatic Portoenterostomies
See Hepaticoenterostomy

Hepatic Transplantation
See Liver, Transplantation

Hepaticodochotomy
See Hepaticostomy

Hepaticoenterostomy 47802

Hepaticostomy 47400

Hepaticotomy 47400

Hepatitis A and Hepatitis B . . .90636

Hepatitis A Vaccine
Adolescent/Pediatric
   2 Dose Schedule 90633
   3 Dose Schedule 90634
Adult Dosage 90632

Hepatitis Antibody
A 86708-86709
B
   B Core 86704-86705
   B Surface 86706
   Be 86707
C 86803-86804
Delta Agent 86692
IgG 86704, 86708
IgM 86704-86705, 86708-86709

Hepatitis Antigen
B 87515-87517
B Surface 87340-87341
Be 87350
C 87520-87522
Delta Agent 87380
G 87525-87527

Hepatitis B and Hib 90748

Hepatitis B Vaccine
Dosage
   Adolescent 90743
   Adult 90746
   Immunosuppressed 90740, 90747
   Pediatric/Adolescent 90744
and Hepatitis A Vaccine 90636

Hepatitis B Virus E Antibody
See Antibody, Hepatitis

Hepatitis B Virus Surface ab
See Antibody, Hepatitis B, Surface

Hepatorrhaphy
See Liver, Repair

Hepatotomy
Abscess 47010-47011
   Percutaneous 47011
Cyst .47010-47011
   Percutaneous 47011

Hernia Repair
Abdominal .49590
   Incisional 49560
   Recurrent 49565
Diaphragmatic 39502-39541
Epigastric .49570
   Incarcerated 49572
Femoral 49550
   Incarcerated 49553
   Recurrent 49555
   Recurrent Incarcerated 49557
Incisional
   Incarcerated 49561
Inguinal 49491, 49495-49500, 49505
   Incarcerated 49492, 49496,
                     49501, 49507, 49521
   Laparoscopic 49650-49651
   Recurrent 49520
   Sliding .49525
   Strangulated 49492
Lumbar 49540
Lung 32800
Orchiopexy 54640
Recurrent Incisional
   Incarcerated 49566
   Reducible 49565
Umbilicus
   Incarcerated 49582, 49587
   Reducible 49580, 49585
with Spermatic Cord 55540
   Spigelian 49590

Hernia, Cerebral
See Encephalocele

Hernia, Rectovaginal
See Rectocele

Hernia, Umbilical
See Omphalocele

Heroin Screen 82486

Heroin, Alkaloid Screening 82101

Herpes Simplex
Antibody 86696
Antigen Detection
   Immunofluorescence 87273-87274
   Nucleic Acid 87528-87530
Identification
   Smear and Stain 87207

Herpes Smear and Stain 87207

Herpes Virus-4 (Gamma), Human
See Epstein-Barr Virus

Herpes Virus-6
Detection 87531-87533

HIV-2
Antigen Detection
     Enzyme Immunoassay 87391

HK3 Kallikrein
See Antigen, Prostate Specific

HLA Typing 86812-86817

HMRK
See Fitzgerald Factor

HMW Kininogen
See Fitzgerald Factor

Hoffman Apparatus 20690

Hofmeister Operation
See Gastrectomy, Total

Holotranscobalamin 0103T

Holten Test
See Creatinine, Urine, Clearance

Home Services
Activities of Daily Living 99509
Anticoagulant Management 99363-99364
Apnea Monitoring 94774-94777
Catheter Care 99507
Enema Administration 99511
Established Patient 99347-99350
Hemodialysis 99512
Home Infusion Procedures 99601-99602
Individual or Family Counseling 99510
Intramuscular Injections 99506
Mechanical Ventilation 99504
New Patient 99341-99345
Newborn Care 99502
Postnatal Assessment 99501
Prenatal Monitoring 99500
Respiratory Therapy 99503
Sleep Studies 95805-95811
Stoma Care 99505
Unlisted Services and Procedures 99600
Ventilation Assist 94005

Home Visit
See House Calls

Homocyst(e)ine 83090
Urine 82615

Homogenization, Tissue 87176

Homograft
Skin 15300-15336

Homologous Grafts
See Graft

Homologous Transplantation
See Homograft

Homovanillic Acid
Urine 83150

Hormone Assay
ACTH 82024
Aldosterone
     Blood or Urine 82088
Androstenedione
     Blood or Urine 82157

Androsterone
     Blood or Urine 82160
Angiotensin II 82163
Corticosterone .82528
Cortisol
     Total 82533
Dehydroepiandrosterone 82626
Dihydroelestosterone 82651
Dihydrotestosterone 82651
Epiandrosterone 82666
Estradiol 82670
Estriol 82677
Estrogen 82671-82672
Estrone 82679
Follicle Stimulating Hormone 83001
Growth Hormone 83003
Hydroxyprogesterone 83498-83499
Luteinizing Hormone 83002
Somatotropin 83003
Testosterone 84403
Vasopressin 84588

Hormone Pellet Implantation . .11980

Hormone, Adrenocorticotrophic
See Adrenocorticotropic Hormone (ACTH)

Hormone, Corticotropin-Releasing
See Corticotropic Releasing Hormone (CRH)

Hormone, Growth
See Growth Hormone

Hormone, Human Growth
See Growth Hormone, Human

Hormone, Interstitial Cell-Stimulating
See Luteinizing Hormone (LH)

Hormone, Parathyroid
See Parathormone

Hormone, Pituitary Lactogenic
See Prolactin

Hormone, Placental Lactogen
See Lactogen, Human Placental

Hormone, Somatotropin Release-Inhibiting
See Somatostatin

Hormone, Thyroid-Stimulating
See Thyroid Stimulating Hormone (TSH)

Hormone-Binding Globulin, Sex
See Globulin, Sex Hormone Binding

Hormones, Adrenal Cortex
See Corticosteroids

Hormones, Antidiuretic
See Antidiuretic Hormone

Hospital Discharge Services
See Discharge Services, Hospital

Hospital Services
Inpatient Services 99238-99239
     Discharge Services 99238-99239,
                              1110F-1111F

Initial Care
     New or Established Patient . .99221-99233
     Initial Hospital Care 99221-99223
     Newborn 99431-99433, 99477
     Prolonged Services 99356-99357
     Subsequent Hospital Care 99231-99233
Observation
     Discharge Services 99234-99236
     Initial Care 99218-99220
     New or Established Patient . .99218-99220
Same Day Admission
     Discharge Services 99234-99236
Subsequent Newborn Care 99433

Hot Pack Treatment 97010
See Physical Medicine and Rehabilitation

House Calls 99341-99350

HPL
See Lactogen, Human Placental

HTLV I
Antibody
     Confirmatory Test 86689
     Detection 86687

HTLV II
Antibody 86688

HTLV III
See HIV

HTLV III Antibodies
See Antibody, HIV

HTLV IV
See HIV-2

Hubbard Tank Therapy 97036
See Physical Medicine/Therapy/Occupational Therapy

Hue Test 92283

Huggin Operation
See Orchiectomy, Simple

Huhner Test 89300, 89320

Human Chorionic Gonadotropin
See Chorionic Gonadotropin

Human Chorionic Somatomammotropin
See Lactogen, Human Placental

Human Cytomegalovirus Group
See Cytomegalovirus

Human Growth Hormone (HGH) 80418, 80428-80430

Human Herpes Virus 4
See Epstein-Barr Virus

Human Immunodeficiency Virus
See HIV

Human Immunodeficiency Virus 1
See HIV-1

Human Immunodeficiency Virus 2
See HIV-2

Hypnotherapy 90880

Hypodermis
See Subcutaneous Tissue

Hypogastric Plexus
Destruction 64681
Injection
    Anesthetic 64517
    Neurolytic 64681

Hypoglossal Nerve
Anastomosis
    to Facial Nerve 64868

Hypoglossal-Facial Anastomosis
See Anastomosis, Nerve, Facial to Hypoglossal

Hypopharynges
See Hypopharynx

Hypopharynx
Biopsy 42802

Hypophysectomy 61546-61548, 62165

Hypophysis
See Pituitary Gland

Hypopyrexia
See Hypothermia

Hypospadias
Repair 54300, 54352
    Complications 54340-54348
    First Stage 54304
        Proximal Penile or Penoscrotal 54332
    One Stage
        Meatal Advancement 54322
        Perineal 54336
    Urethroplasty
        Local Skin Flaps 54324
        Local Skin Flaps and Mobilization of
        Urethra 54326
        Local Skin Flaps, Skin Graft Patch
        and/or Island Flap 54328
        Urethroplasty for Second Stage .54308-54316
        Free Skin Graft 54316
        Urethroplasty for Third Stage 54318

Hypothermia 99185-99186

Hypoxia
Breathing Response 94450
High Altitude Simulation Test 94452-94453

Hysterectomy
Abdominal
    Radical 58210
    Resection of Ovarian Malignancy 58951,
                      58953-58956
    Supracervical 58180
    Total 58150, 58200, 58956
        with Colpo-Urethrocystopexy 58152
        with Omentectomy 58956
        with Partial Vaginectomy 58200
Cesarean
    after Cesarean Delivery 59525
    with Closure of Vesicouterine Fistula ..51925
Laparoscopic 58541-58544
    Radical 58548
    Total 58570-58573

Removal
    Lesion 59100
Supracervical
    Laparoscopic 58541-58544
Vaginal 58260-58270,
             58290-58294, 58550-58554
    Laparoscopic 58550, 58570-58573
    Radical 58285
    Removal Tubes/Ovaries 58262-58263,
           58291-58292, 58552, 58554
    Repair of Enterocele .58263, 58292, 58294
    with Colpectomy 58275-58280
    with Colpo-Urethrocystopexy ..58267, 58293

Hysterolysis
See Lysis, Adhesions, Uterus

Hysteroplasty 58540

Hysterorrhaphy 58520, 59350

Hysterosalpingography 74740
Catheterization 58345
Injection Procedure 58340

Hysterosalpingostomy
See Implantation, Tubouterine

Hysteroscopy
Ablation
    Endometrial 58563
Diagnostic 58555
Lysis
    Adhesions 58559
Placement
    Fallopian Tube Implants 58565
Removal
    Impacted Foreign Body 58562
    Leiomyomata 58561
Resection
    of Intrauterine Septum 58560
Surgical with Biopsy 58558
Unlisted Services and Procedures ..58578-58579

Hysterosonography
See Ultrasound; Sonohysterography

Hysterotomy 59100
See Ligation, Uterus
Induced Abortion
    with Amniotic Injections 59852
    with Vaginal Suppositories 59857

Hysterotrachelectomy
See Amputation, Cervix

I Antibodies, HTLV
See Antibody, HTLV-I

I, Angiotensin
See Angiotensin I

I, Coagulation Factor
See Fibrinogen

I, Heparin Co-Factor
See Antithrombin III

ICCE
See Extraction, Lens, Intracapsular

Ichthyosis, Sex Linked
See Syphilis Test

ICSH
See Luteinizing Hormone (LH)

Identification
Oocyte
    from Follicular Fluid 89254
Sperm
    from Aspiration 89257
    from Tissue 89264

IDH
See Isocitric Dehydrogenase, Blood

IG
See Immune Globulins

IgE 86003-86005

IgG 86001

II, Coagulation Factor
See Prothrombin

II, Cranial Nerve
See Optic Nerve

Ileal Conduit
Visualization 50690

Ileoscopy
via Stoma 44383

Ileostomy 44310, 45136
Continent (Kock Procedure) 44316
Laparoscopic 44186-44187
Non-Tube 44187
Revision 44312-44314

Iliac Arteries
See Artery, Iliac

Iliac Crest
Free Osteocutaneous Flap with Microvascular
Anastomosis 20970

Iliohypogastric Nerve
Injection
    Anesthetic 64425

Ilioinguinal Nerve
Injection
    Anesthetic 64425

Ilium
Craterization 27070
Cyst
    Excision 27065-27067
Excision 27070
Fracture
    Open Treatment 27215, 27218
Saucerization 27070
Tumor
    Excision 27065-27067

Mesencephalic Tract 61480
Metacarpophalangeal Joint
  Capsule 26520
Mitral Valve 33420-33422
Muscle
  See Myotomy
Nerve 64573-64580,
    64585, 64595, 64702-64772
  Foot 28035
  Root 63185-63190
  Sacral 64581
  Vagus 43640-43641
Nose
  See Rhinotomy
Orbit
  See Orbitotomy
Palm
  Fasciotomy 26040-26045
Pancreas
  Sphincter 43262
Penis
  Prepuce 54000-54001
    Newborn 54000
Pericardium
  with Clot Removal 33020
  with Foreign Body Removal 33020
  with Tube 33015
Pharynx
  Stoma 42955
Pleura
  Biopsy 32095-32100
Pleural Cavity
  Empyema 32035-32036
  Pneumothorax 32551
Prostate
  Exposure
    Bilateral Pelvic Lymphadenectomy .55865
    Insertion Radioactive Substance ...55860
    Lymph Node Biopsy 55862
    Transurethral 52450
Pterygomaxillary Fossa 31040
Pulmonary Valve 33470-33474
Pyloric Sphincter 43520
Retina
  Encircling Material 67115
Sclera
  Fistulization
    Iridencleisis or Iridotasis 66165
    Sclerectomy with Punch or Scissors
    with Iridectomy 66160
    Thermocauterization with
    Iridectomy 66155
    Trabeculectomy ab Externo in
    AbsencePrevious Surgery 66170
    Trephination with Iridectomy 66150
Semicircular Canal
  Fenestration 69820
  Revision 69840
Seminal Vesicle 55600-55605
  Complicated 55605
Shoulder
  Bone 23035
  Capsular Contracture Release 23020
  Removal
    Calcareous Deposits 23000
  Tenomyotomy 23405-23406
Shoulder Joint 23040-23044

Sinus
  Frontal 31070-31087
  Maxillary 31020-31032
    Endoscopic 31256-31267
    Multiple 31090
  Sphenoid
    Sinusotomy 31050-31051
Skin 10040, 10060-10061,
    10080-10081, 10120-10180
Skull 61316, 62148
  Suture 61550-61552
Spinal Cord 63200
  Tract 63170, 63194-63199
Stomach
  Creation
    Stoma 43830-43832
  Exploration 43500
  Pyloric Sphincter 43520
Synovectomy 26140
Temporomandibular Joint 21010
Tendon
  Arm, Upper 24310
Thigh
  Fasciotomy 27025
Thorax
  Empyema 32035-32036
  Pneumothorax 32551
Thyroid Gland
  See Thyrotomy
Tibia 27607
Toe
  Capsule 28270-28272
  Fasciotomy 28008
  Tendon 28232-28234
  Tenotomy 28010-28011
Tongue
  Frenum 41010
Trachea
  Emergency 31603-31605
  Planned 31600-31601
  with Flaps 31610
Tympanic Membrane 69420
  with Anesthesia 69421
Ureter 50600
Ureterocele 51535
Urethra 53000-53010
  Meatus 53020-53025
Uterus
  Remove Lesion 59100
Vagina
  Exploration 57000
Vas Deferens 55200
  for X-Ray 55300
Vestibule of the Mouth
  See Mouth, Vestibuleof, Incision
Vitreous Strands
  Laser Surgery 67031
  Pars Plana Approach 67030
Wrist 25100-25105
  Capsule 25085
  Decompression 25020-25025
  Tendon Sheath 25000-25001

Incision and Drainage

See Drainage; Incision
Abdomen
  Fluid 49080-49081
  Pancreatitis 48000

Abscess
  Abdomen 49020, 49040
    Open 49040
    Percutaneous 49021
  Anal 46045-46050
  Ankle 27603
  Appendix 44900
    Open 44900
    Percutaneous 44901
  Arm, Lower 25028
  Arm, Upper 23930-23931
  Auditory Canal, External 69020
  Bartholin's Gland 56420
  Bladder 51080
  Brain 61320-61321
  Breast 19020
  Ear, External
    Complicated 69005
    Simple 69000
  Elbow 23930
  Epididymis 54700
  Eyelid 67700
  Finger 26010-26011
  Gums 41800
  Hip 26990
  Kidney 50020
    Open 50020
    Percutaneous 50021
  Knee 27301
  Leg, Lower 27603
  Leg, Upper 27301
  Liver 47010
    Open 47010
    Percutaneous 47011
  Lung 32200
    Percutaneous 32201
  Lymph Node 38300-38305
  Mouth 40800-40801, 41005-41009,
    41015-41018
  Nasal Septum 30020
  Neck 21501-21502
  Nose 30000-30020
  Ovary 58820-58822
    Abdominal Approach 58822
  Palate 42000
  Paraurethral Gland 53060
  Parotid Gland 42300-42305
  Pelvis 26990, 45000
  Perineum 56405
  Peritoneum 49020
    Percutaneous 49021
  Prostate .45720-55725
  Rectum ..45005-45020, 46040, 46050-46060
  Retroperitoneal 49060
    Open 49060
  Salivary Gland 42300-42320
  Scrotum 54700, 55100
  Skene's Gland 53060
  Skin 10060-10061
  Subdiaphragmatic
    Percutaneous 49040-49041
  Sublingual Gland 42310-42320
  Submaxillary Gland 42310-42320
  Subphrenic
    Percutaneous 49040-49041
  Testis 54700
  Thorax 21501-21502
  Throat 42700-42725

Oviduct
    Chromotubation 58350
    Hydrotubation 58350
Ovoid
    Vagina
        for Brachytherapy 57155
Pacemaker
    Fluoroscopy/Radiography 71090
    Heart 33206-33208, 33212-33213
Pacing Cardio-Defibrillator
    Leads 33216-33220,
        33224-33225, 33243-33244
    Pulse Generator Only 33240-33241
Packing
    Vagina 57180
Penile Prosthesis, Inflatable
    See Penile Prosthesis, Insertion, Inflatable
Pessary
    Vagina 57160
Pin
    Skeletal Traction 20650
Probe
    Brain 61770
Prostaglandin 59200
Prostate
    Radioactive Substance 55860
Prosthesis
    Knee .27438, 27445
    Nasal Septal 30220
    Palate 42281
    Pelvic Floor .57267
    Penis
        Inflatable 54401-54405
        Noninflatable 54400
    Speech 31611
    Testis 54660
    Urethral Sphincter 53444-53445
Pulse Generator
    Brain 61885-61886
    Heart 33212-33213
    Spinal Cord .63685
Radioactive Material
    Bladder 51020
    Cystourethroscopy 52250
Receiver
    Brain 61885-61886
    Spinal Cord .63685
Reservoir
    Brain 61210-61215
    Spinal Cord .62360
    Subcutaneous 49419
Shunt 36835
    Abdomen
        Vein 49425
        Venous .49426
    Intrahepatic Portosystemic 37182
Spinal Instrument 22849
    Spinous Process 0171T-0172T, 22841
Spinal Instrumentation
    Anterior 22845-22847
    Internal Spinal Fixation 22841
    Pelvic Fixation 22848
    Posterior Nonsegmental
        Harrington Rod Technique 22840
    Posterior Segmental 22842-22844
    Prosthetic Device 22851

Stent
    Bile Duct 43268, 47801
        Percutaneous 47511
    Bladder 51045
    Conjunctiva .68750
    Coronary 92980-92981
    Esophagus .43219
    Gastrointestinal, Upper 43256
    Ileum 44383
    Indwelling 50605
    Lacrimal Duct 68815
    Pancreatic Duct 43268
    Small Intestines 44370, 44379
    Ureter 50688
    Ureter via Kidney 50393
    Ureteral 50947, 52332
    Urethral 0084T, 52282
Tamponade
    Esophagus .43460
Tandem
    Uterus
        for Brachytherapy 57155
Tendon Graft
    Finger 26392
    Hand 26392
Testicular Prosthesis
    See Prosthesis, Testicular, Insertion
Tissue Expanders
    Skin .11960-11971
Tube
    Bile Duct 43268
    Esophagus .43510
    Gastrointestinal, Upper 43241
    Ileum 44383
    Kidney 50398
    Pancreatic Duct 43268
    Small Intestines 44379
    Trachea 31730
    Ureter 50688
Ureteral Guide Wire 52334
Vascular Pedicle
    Carpal Bone 25430
Venous Access Device
    Central 36560-36566
    Peripheral 36570-36571
Ventilating Tube 69433
Ventricular Assist Device 33975
Wire
    Skeletal Traction 20650

Inspiratory Positive Pressure Breathing
See Intermittent Positive Pressure Breathing (IPPB)

Instillation
Contrast Material
Drugs
    Bladder 51720
    Kidney 50391
    Ureter 50391

Instillation, Bladder
See Bladder, Instillation

Instrumentation
See Application; Bone, Fixation; Spinal Instrumentation

Spinal
    Insertion 22840-22848, 22851
    Reinsertion .22849
    Removal 22850, 22852-22855

Insufflation, Eustachian Tube
See Eustachian Tube, Inflation

Insulin 80422, 80432-80435
Antibody 86337
Blood 83525
Free 83527

Insulin C-Peptide Measurement
See C-Peptide

Insulin Like Growth Factors
See Somatomedin

Insurance
Basic Life and/or Disability
Evaluation Services 99450
Examination 99450-99456

Integumentary System
Ablation
    Breast 19105
Biopsy 11100-11101
Breast
    Ablation 19105
    Excision 19100-19103,
        19110-19272, 19300-19307
    Incision 19000-19030
    Metallic Localization Clip Placement . .19295
    Preoperative Placement of
    Needle Localization 19290-19291
    Reconstruction 19316-19396
    Repair 19316-19396
    Unlisted Services and Procedures 19499
Burns 15002-15005, 15100-15101,
    15120-15121, 15400-15401, 16000-16036
Debridement 11000-11006, 11010-11044
Destruction
    See Dermatology
    Actinotherapy 96900
    Benign Lesion 17000-17004
    Chemical Exfoliation 17360
    Cryotherapy 17340
    Electrolysis Epilation 17380
    Malignant Lesion 17260-17286
        by Photodynamic Therapy 96567
    Mohs Micrographic Surgery . . .17311-17315
    Photodynamic Therapy 96567-96571
    Premalignant Lesion 17000-17004
    Unlisted Services and Procedures 17999
Drainage 10040, 10060-10061,
    10080-10081, 10120-10180
Excision
    Benign Lesion 11400-11471
    Debridement 11000-11006, 11010-11044
    Malignant Lesion 11600-11646
Incision 10040, 10060-10061,
    10080-10081, 10120-10180
Introduction 11900-11977
    Drug Delivery Implant 11981, 11983
Nails 11720-11765
Paring 11055-11057
Photography 96904
Pressure Ulcers 15920-15999

Isocitrate Dehydrogenase
See Isocitric Dehydrogenase

Isocitric Dehydrogenase
Blood 83570

Isolation
Sperm 89260-89261

Isomerase, Glucose 6 Phosphate
See Phosphohexose Isomerase

Isopropanol
See Isopropyl Alcohol

Isopropyl Alcohol 84600

Isthmusectomy
Thyroid Gland 60210-60225

IUD
See Intrauterine Device (IUD)

IV
See Injection, Chemotherapy; Intravenous
Therapy

IV Infusion Therapy
See Allergen Immunotherapy; Chemotherapy;
Infusion; Injection,Chemotherapy

IV Injection
See Injection, Intravenous

IV, Coagulation Factor
See Calcium

IVC Filter
Placement 75940

IVF
See Artificial Insemination; In Vitro Fertilization

Ivy Bleeding Time 85002

IX Complex, Factor
See Christmas Factor

J

Jaboulay Operation
See Gastroduodenostomy

Jaboulay Operation Gastroduodenostomy
See Gastroduodenostomy

Jannetta Procedure
See Decompression, Cranial Nerve; Section

Japanese, River Fever
See Scrub Typhus

Jatene Type 33770-33781

Jaw Joint
See Facial Bones; Mandible; Maxilla

Jaws
Muscle Reduction 21295-21296
X-Ray
    for Orthodontics 70355

Jejunostomy
Catheterization 44015
Contrast 49465
Insertion
    Catheter 44015
    Percutaneous 49441
Laparoscopic 44186-44187
Non-Tube 44187, 44310
Obstructive Material Removal 49460
Replacement 49451
with Pancreatic Drain 48001

Jejunum
Creation
    Stoma
    Laparoscopic 44186
Transfer
    with Microvascular Anastomosis
        Free 43496

Johannsen Procedure 53400

Joint
See Specific Joint
Acromioclavicular
    See AcromioclavicularJoint
Arthrocentesis 20600-20610
Aspiration 20600-20610
Dislocation
    See Dislocation
Drainage .20600-20610
Finger
    See Intercarpal Joint
Fixation (Surgical)
    See Arthrodesis
Foot
    See Foot, Joint
Hip
    See Hip Joint
Injection .20600-20610
Intertarsal
    See Intertarsal Joint
Knee
    See Knee Joint
Ligament
    See Ligament
Metacarpophalangeal
    See MetacarpophalangealJoint
Metatarsophalangeal
    See MetatarsophalangealJoint
Nuclear Medicine
    Imaging 78300, 78315
Radiology
    Stress Views 77071
Sacroiliac
    See Sacroiliac Joint
Shoulder
    See GlenohumeralJoint
Sternoclavicular
    See SternoclavicularJoint
Survey 77077
Temporomandibular
    See TemporomandibularJoint (TMJ)

Dislocation Temporomandibular
    See Dislocation, Temporomandibular Joint
Implant
    See Prosthesis, Temporomandibular Joint
Wrist
    See Radiocarpal Joint

Joint Syndrome, Temporomandibular
See Temporomandibular Joint (TMJ)

Jones and Cantarow Test
See Blood Urea Nitrogen; Urea Nitrogen,
Clearance

Jones Procedure 28760

Joplin Procedure 28294

Jugal Bone
See Cheekbone

Jugular Vein
See Vein, Jugular

K

K-Wire Fixation
Tongue 41500

Kader Operation
See Incision, Stomach, Creation, Stoma; Incision
and Drainage

Kala Azar Smear 87207

Kallidin I /Kallidin 9
See Bradykinin

Kallikrein HK3
See Antigen, Prostate Specific

Kallikreinogen
See Fletcher Factor

Kasai Procedure 47701

Kedani Fever
See Scrub Typhus

Keel
Insertion/Removal
    Laryngoplasty 31580

Kelikian Procedure 28280

Keller Procedure 28292

Kelly Urethral Plication 57220

Keratectomy
Partial
    for Lesion 65400

Keratomileusis 65760

Keratophakia 65765

Retinacular
　　Release 27425
Strapping 29530
Suture
　　Tendon 27380-27381
Transplantation
　　Chondrocytes 27412
　　Meniscus 29868
　　Osteochondral
　　　　Allograft 27415, 29867
　　　　Autograft 27412, 29866
Tumor
　　Excision 27327-27329, 27365
Unlisted Services and Procedures 27599
X-Ray.......................73560-73564
　　Arthrography 73580
　　Bilateral 73565
X-Ray with Contrast
　　Arthrography 73580

Knee Joint
Arthroplasty 27446

Knee Prosthesis
See Prosthesis, Knee

Kneecap
Excision 27350
Repair
　　Instability 27420-27424

Knock-Knee Repair 27455-27457

Kocher Operation 23650-23680
See Clavicle; Scapula; Shoulder, Dislocation, Closed Treatment

Kocher Pylorectomy
See Gastrectomy, Partial

Kock Pouch 44316
Formation 50825

Kock Procedure 44316

KOH
See Hair, Nails, Tissue, Examination for Fungi

Kraske Procedure 45116

Kroenlein Procedure 67420

Krukenberg Procedure 25915

Kuhlmann Test 96101-96103

Kyphectomy
More than Two Segments 22819
Up to Two Segments 22818

Kyphoplasty...............22523-22525

L

L Ascorbic Acid
See Ascorbic Acid

L Aspartate 2 Oxoglutarate Aminotransferase
See Transaminase, Glutamic Oxaloacetic

L Glutamine
See Glutamine

L-Alanine
See Aminolevulinic Acid (ALA)

L-Leucylnaphthylamidase
See Leucine Aminopeptidase

L/S Ratio
Amniotic Fluid 83661

Labial Adhesions
Lysis 56441

Labyrinth
See Ear, Inner

Labyrinthectomy 69905
with Mastoidectomy 69910
with Skull Base Surgery 61596

Labyrinthotomy
with Mastoidectomy 69802
with/without Cryosurgery 69801

Laceration Repair
See Specific Site

Lacrimal Duct
Balloon 68816
Canaliculi
　　Repair 68700
Dilation 68816
Exploration 68810
　　Canaliculi 68840
　　Stent 68815
　　with Anesthesia 68811
Insertion
　　Stent 68815
Nasolacrimal Duct Probing 68816
Removal
　　Dacryolith 68530
　　Foreign Body 68530
X-Ray with Contrast 70170

Lacrimal Gland
Biopsy 68510
Close Fistula 68770
Excision
　　Partial 68505
　　Total 68500
Fistulization 68720
Incision and Drainage 68400
Injection
　　X-Ray 68850
Nuclear Medicine
　　Tear Flow 78660
Removal
　　Dacryolith 68530
　　Foreign Body 68530
Repair
　　Fistula 68770
Tumor
　　Excision
　　　　Frontal Approach 68540
　　　　with Osteotomy 68550
X-Ray 70170

Lacrimal Punctum
Closure
　　by Plug 68761
　　by Thermocauterization, Ligation or
　　Laser Surgery 68760
Dilation 68801
Incision 68440
Repair 68705

Lacrimal Sac
Biopsy 68525
Excision 68520
Incision and Drainage 68420

Lacrimal System
Unlisted Services and Procedures 68899

Lactase Deficiency Breath
Test 91065

Lactate 83605

Lactate Dehydrogenase ...83615-83625

Lactic Acid 83605

Lactic Cytochrome Reductase
See Lactate Dehydrogenase

Lactic Dehydrogenase
See Lactate Dehydrogenase

Lactiferous Duct
See Mammary Duct; Mammary Ductogram
Excision 19112
Exploration 19110

Lactoferrin
Fecal 83630-83631

Lactogen, Human Placental 83632

Lactogenic Hormone
See Prolactin

Lactose
Urine 83633-83634

Ladd Procedure 44055

Lagophthalmos
Repair 67912

Laki Lorand Factor
See Fibrin Stabilizing Factor

Lamblia Intestinalis
See Giardia Lamblia

Lambrinudi Operation
See Arthrodesis, Foot Joint

Lamellar Keratoplasties
See Keratoplasty, Lamellar

Laminaria
Insertion 59200

Laminectomy ..62351, 63001, 63005-63011,
　　　　　　　　63015-63044, 63180-63200,
　　　　　　　　63265-63290, 63300-63655
Lumbar 22630, 63012
Surgical 63170-63172
with Facetectomy 63045-63048

Newborn 31520
Operative 31530-31561

Laryngotomy 31300
Diagnostic 31320

Larynx
Aspiration
    Endoscopy .31515
Biopsy
    Endoscopy 31510, 31535-31536, 31576
Dilation
    Endoscopic 31528-31529
Electromyography
    Needle 95865
Endoscopy
    Direct 31515-31571
    Excision 31545-31546
    Exploration 31505, 31520-31526, 31575
    Fiberoptic 31575-31579
        with Stroboscopy 31579
    Indirect 31505-31513
    Operative 31530-31561
Excision
    Lesion 31512, 31578
        Endoscopic 31545-31546
    Partial 31367-31382
    Total 31360-31365
    with Pharynx 31390-31395
Exploration
    Endoscopic 31505, 31520-31526, 31575
Fracture 31584
Insertion
    Obturator .31527
Nerve
    Destruction 31595
Reconstruction
    Burns 31588
    Cricoid Split 31587
    Other 31588
    Stenosis 31582
    Web 31580
Removal
    Foreign Body
        Endoscopic . . .31511, 31530-31531, 31577
    Lesion
        Endoscopic . . .31512, 31545-31546, 31578
Repair
    Reinnervation Neuromuscular Pedicle .31590
Stroboscopy .31579
Tumor
    Excision 31300
    Endoscopic 31540-31541
Unlisted Services and Procedures 31599
Vocal Cord(s)
    Injection 31513, 31570-31571
X-Ray 70370
    with Contrast 70373

Laser Surgery
Anus 46614, 46917
Cautery
    Esophagus .43227
Lacrimal Punctum 68760
Lens, Posterior 66821
Lesion
    Mouth 40820
    Nose 30117-30118

Penis 54057
    Skin 17000-17111, 17260-17286
Myocardium 33140-33141
Prostate 52647-52648
Spine
    Diskectomy 62287
Tumors
    Urethra and Bladder 52234
Urethra and Bladder 52214

Laser
Treatment 17000-17286, 96920-96922
See Destruction

Lateral Epicondylitis
See Tennis Elbow

Latex Fixation 86403-86406

LATS
See Thyrotropin Releasing Hormone (TRH)

Latzko Operation
See Repair, Vagina, Fistula; Revision

LAV
See HIV

LAV Antibodies
See Antibody, HIV

LAV-2
See HIV-2

Lavage
Colon 44701
Lung
    Bronchial .31624
    Total 32997
Mammary Duct 0046T, 0047T
Peritoneal 49080

LCM
See Lymphocytic Choriomeningitis

LD
See Lactate Dehydrogenase

LDH 83615-83625

LDL
See Lipoprotein, LDL

Lead 83655

Leadbetter Procedure 53431

Lecithin-Sphingomyelin Ratio .83661

Lecithinase C
See Tissue Typing

Lee and White Test 85345

LEEP Procedure 57460

LeFort Procedure
Vagina 57120

LeFort I Procedure
Midface Reconstruction 21141-21147, 21155,
                                21160
Palatal or Maxillary Fracture 21421-21423

LeFort II Procedure
Midface Reconstruction 21150-21151
Nasomaxillary Complex Fracture . . .21345-21348

LeFort III Procedure
Craniofacial Separation 21431-21436
Midface Reconstruction 21154-21159

Left Atrioventricular Valve
See Mitral Valve

Left Heart Cardiac Catheterization
See Cardiac Catheterization, Left Heart

Leg
Cast
    Rigid Total Contact 29445
Lower
    See Ankle; Fibula;Knee; Tibia
    Abscess
        Incision and Drainage 27603
    Amputation 27598, 27880-27882
        Revision 27884-27886
    Angiography 73706
    Artery
        Ligation .37618
    Biopsy 27613-27614
    Bursa
        Incision and Drainage 27604
    Bypass Graft 35903
    Cast 29405-29435, 29450
    CT Scan 73700-73706
    Decompression 27600-27602
    Exploration
        Blood Vessel 35860
    Fasciotomy 27600-27602, 27892-27894
    Hematoma
        Incision and Drainage 27603
    Lesion
        Excision .27630
    Magnetic Resonance Imaging
    (MRI) 73718-73720
    Neurectomy 27325-27326
    Repair
        Blood Vessel 35226
        Blood Vessel with Other Graft . . .35286
        Blood Vessel with Vein Graft 35256
        Fascia 27656
        Tendon 27658-27692
    Splint 29515
    Strapping .29580
    Suture
        Tendon 27658-27665
    Tumor
        Excision 27615-27619
    Ultrasound 76880
    Unlisted Services and Procedures 27899
    Unna Boot .29580
    X-Ray 73592
Upper
    See Femur
    Abscess 27301
    Amputation 27590-27592
        at Hip 27290-27295
        Revision 27594-27596
    Angiography 73706, 75635
    Artery
        Ligation .37618
    Biopsy 27323-27324

Palate
　Destruction .42160
　Excision 42104-42120
Pancreas
　Excision 48120
Pelvis
　Destruction .58662
Penis
　Destruction
　　Cryosurgery 54056
　　Electrodesiccation 54055
　　Extensive 54065
　　Laser Surgery 54057
　　Simple 54050-54060
　　Surgical Excision 54060
　Excision 54060
　　Penile Plaque 54110-54112
Pharynx
　Destruction .42808
　Excision 42808
Rectum
　Excision 45108
Removal
　Larynx 31512, 31578
Resection 52354
Retina
　Destruction
　　Extensive 67227-67228
　　Localized 0017T, 67208-67210
　　Radiation by Implantation of Source . . .67218
Sciatic Nerve
　Excision 64786
Sclera
　Excision 66130
Skin
　Abrasion 15786-15787
　Biopsy 11100-11101
　Destruction
　　Benign 17110-17111, 17250
　　Malignant 17260-17286
　　　by Photodynamic Therapy 96567
　　Premalignant 17000-17004
　Excision
　　Benign 11400-11471
　　Malignant 11600-11646
　Injection 11900-11901
　Paring or Curettement 11055-11057
　Shaving 11300-11313
Skin Tags
　Removal 11200-11201
Skull
　Excision . .61500, 61600-61608, 61615-61616
Spermatic Cord
　Excision 55520
Spinal Cord
　Destruction 62280-62282
　Excision 63265-63273
Stomach
　Excision 43611
Testis
　Excision 54512
Toe
　Excision 28092
Tongue
　Excision 41110-41114
Uvula
　Destruction .42145
　Excision 42104-42107

Vagina
　Destruction 57061-57065
Vulva
　Destruction
　　Extensive 56515
　　Simple 56501
Wrist Tendon
　Excision 25110

Leu 2 Antigens
See CD8

Leucine Aminopeptidase 83670

**Leukemia Lymphoma Virus I
Antibodies, Human T Cell**
See Antibody, HTLV-I

**Leukemia Lymphoma Virus I,
Adult T Cell**
See HTLV I

**Leukemia Lymphoma Virus II
Antibodies, Human TCell**
See Antibody, HTLV-II

**Leukemia Virus II, Hairy Cell
Associated, Human TCell**
See HTLV II

Leukoagglutinins 86021

Leukocyte
See White Blood Cell
Alkaline Phosphatase 85540
Antibody 86021
Count 85032, 85048, 89055
Histamine Release Test 86343
Phagocytosis 86344
Transfusion 86950

Levarterenol
See Noradrenalin

Levator Muscle Repair
See Blepharoptosis, Repair

LeVeen Shunt
Insertion 49425
Patency Test 78291
Revision 49426

Levulose
See Fructose

LGV
See Lymphogranuloma Venereum

LH
See Luteinizing Hormone (LH)

LHR
See Leukocyte Histamine Release Test

Lid Suture
See Blepharoptosis, Repair

Lidocaine
Assay 80176

Lift, Face
See Face Lift

Ligament
See Specific Site
Collateral
　Repair
　　Knee
　　　with Cruciate Ligament 27409
Dentate
　Section 63180-63182
Injection 20550
Release
　Coracoacromial 23415
　Transverse Carpal 29848
Repair
　Elbow 24343-24346
　Knee Joint 27405-27409

Ligation
Artery
　Abdomen .37617
　Carotid 37600-37606
　Chest 37616
　Coronary .33502
　Ethmoidal .30915
　Extremity .37618
　Fistula 37607
　Maxillary .30920
　Neck 37615
　Temporal .37609
Esophageal Varices 43204, 43400
Fallopian Tube
　Oviduct 58600-58611, 58670
Gastroesophageal 43405
Hemorrhoids 46945-46946
Oviducts 59100
Salivary Duct .42665
Shunt
　Aorta
　　Pulmonary 33924
　Peritoneal
　　Venous 49428
Thoracic Duct .38380
　Abdominal Approach 38382
　Thoracic Approach 38381
Vas Deferens .55450
Vein
　Clusters 37785
　Esophagus 43205, 43244, 43400
　Femoral 37650
　Gastric 43244
　Iliac 37660
　Jugular, Internal 37565
　Perforate .37760
　Saphenous 37700-37735, 37780
　Vena Cava 37620

Ligature Strangulation
Skin Tags 11200-11201

Light Coagulation
See Photocoagulation

Light Scattering Measurement
See Nephelometry

Light Therapy, UV
See Actinotherapy

Limb
See Extremity

Limited Lymphadenectomy for Staging
See Lymphadenectomy, Limited, for Staging

Limited Neck Dissection
with Thyroidectomy 60252

Limited Resection Mastectomies
See Breast, Excision, Lesion

Lindholm Operation
See Tenoplasty

Lingual Bone
See Hyoid Bone

Lingual Frenectomy
See Excision, Tongue, Frenum

Lingual Nerve
Avulsion 64740
Incision 64740
Transection 64740

Lingual Tonsil
See Tonsils, Lingual

Linton Procedure 37760

Lip
Biopsy 40490
Excision .40500-40530
    Frenum 40819
Incision
    Frenum 40806
Reconstruction 40525-40527
Repair 40650-40654
    Cleft Lip 40700-40761
    Fistula 42260
Unlisted Services and Procedures 40799

Lip, Cleft
See Cleft Lip

Lipase 83690

Lipectomy
Excision 15830-15839
Suction Assisted 15876-15879

Lipectomy, Aspiration
See Liposuction

Lipids
Feces 82705-82710

Lipo-Lutin
See Progesterone

Lipolysis, Aspiration
See Liposuction

Lipophosphodiesterase I
See Tissue Typing

Lipoprotein
(a) 83695
Blood 0026T, 83695, 83700-83721
LDL 83700-83704, 83721
Phospholipase A2 83698

Lipoprotein, Alpha
See Lipoprotein

Lipoprotein, Pre-Beta
See Lipoprotein, Blood

Liposuction 15876-15879

Lisfranc Operation
See Amputation, Foot; Radical Resection; Replantation

Listeria Monocytogenes
Antibody 86723

Lithium
Assay 80178

Litholapaxy 52317-52318

Lithotripsy
See Extracorporeal Shock Wave Therapy
Bile Duct Calculi (Stone)
    Endoscopy 43265
Bladder 52353
Kidney 50590, 52353
Pancreatic Duct Calculi (Stone)
    Endoscopy 43265
Ureter 52353
Urethra 52353
with Cystourethroscopy 52353

Lithotrity
See Litholapaxy

Liver
See Hepatic Duct
Ablation
    Tumor 47380-47382
    Laparoscopic 47370-47371
Abscess
    Aspiration 47015
    Incision and Drainage
        Open 47010
        Percutaneous 47011
        Injection 47015
Aspiration 47015
Biopsy 47100
Cyst
    Aspiration 47015
    Incision and Drainage
        Open 47010
        Percutaneous 47011
Excision
    Extensive 47122
    Partial . . .47120, 47125-47130, 47140-47142
    Total 47133
Injection 47015
    Radiologic 47505
    X-Ray 47500
Lobectomy 47125-47130
    Partial 47120
Needle Biopsy 47000-47001
Nuclear Medicine
    Function Study 78220
    Imaging 78201-78216
    Vascular Flow 78206
Repair
    Abscess 47300
    Cyst 47300
    Wound 47350-47362
Suture
    Wound 47350-47362

Transplantation 47135-47136
    Allograft Preparation 47143-47147
Trisegmentectomy 47122
Unlisted Services and Procedures . .47379, 47399

Living Activities, Daily
See Activities of Daily Living

Lobectomy
Brain 61323, 61537-61540
Contralateral Subtotal
    Thyroid Gland 60212, 60225
Liver 47120-47130
Lung 32480-32482
    Sleeve 32486
Parotid Gland 42410-42415
Segmental 32663
Sleeve 32486
Temporal Lobe 61537-61538
Thyroid Gland Partial 60210-60212
    Total .60220-60225
Total 32663

Lobotomy
Frontal 61490

Local Excision Mastectomies
See Breast, Excision, Lesion

Local Excision of Lesion or Tissue of Femur
See Excision, Lesion, Femur

Localization of Nodule
Radiographic
    Breast 77032

Log Hydrogen Ion Concentration
See pH

Long Acting Thyroid Stimulator
See Thyrotropin Releasing Hormone (TRH)

Long-Term Care Facility Visits
See Nursing Facility Services

Longmire Operation
See Anastomosis, Hepatic Duct to Intestines

Loopogram
See Urography, Antegrade

Loose Body
Removal
    Ankle 27620
    Carpometacarpal Joint 26070
    Elbow 24101
    Interphalangeal Joint 28020
        Toe 28024
    Knee Joint .27331
    Metatarsophalangeal Joint 28022
    Tarsometatarsal Joint 28020
    Toe 28022
    Wrist 25101

Lord Procedure
See Anal Sphincter, Dilation

Louis Bar Syndrome
See Ataxia Telangiectasia

Low Birth Weight Intensive Care Services 99298-99300

Low Density Lipoprotein
See Lipoprotein, LDL

Low Frequency Ultrasound 0183T

Low Vision Aids
See Spectacle Services
Fitting 92354-92355

Lower Extremities
See Extremity, Lower

Lower GI Series
See Barium Enema

LRH
See Luteinizing Releasing Factor

LSD
See Lysergic Acid Diethylamide

LTH
See Prolactin

Lumbar
See Spine
Aspiration, Disc
    Percutaneous 62287

Lumbar Plexus
Decompression 64714
Injection
    Anesthetic 64449
Neuroplasty 64714
Release 64714
Repair/Suture 64862

Lumbar Puncture
See Spinal Tap

Lumbar Spine Fracture
See Fracture, Vertebra, Lumbar

Lumbar Sympathectomy
See Sympathectomy, Lumbar

Lumbar Vertebra
See Vertebra, Lumbar

Lumen Dilation 74360

Lumpectomy 19301-19302

Lunate
Arthroplasty
    with Implant 25444
Dislocation
    Closed Treatment 25690
    Open Treatment 25695

Lung
Ablation 32998
Abscess
    Incision and Drainage
        Open 32200
        Percutaneous 32200-32201
Aspiration 32420
Biopsy 32095-32100
Bullae
    Excision 32141
        Endoscopic 32655

Cyst
    Incision and Drainage
        Open 32200
        Removal 32140
Decortication
    Endoscopic 32651-32652
    Partial 32225
    Total 32220
    with Parietal Pleurectomy 32320
Empyema
    Excision 32540
Excision
    Bronchus Resection 32486
    Completion 32488
    Donor
        Heart-Lung 33930
        Lung 32850
    Emphysematous 32491
    Empyema 32540
    Lobe 32480-32482
    Segment 32484
    Total 32440-32445
    Tumor 32503-32504
    Wedge Resection 32500
        Endoscopic 32657
Foreign Body
    Removal 32151
Hemorrhage 32110
Lavage
    Bronchial 31624
    Total 32997
Lysis
    Adhesions 32124
Needle Biopsy 32405
Nuclear Medicine
    Imaging, Perfusion 78580-78585
    Imaging, Ventilation 78586-78594
    Unlisted Services and Procedures 78599
Pneumocentesis 32420
Pneumolysis 32940
Pneumothorax 32960
Puncture 32420
Removal
    Bronchoplasty 32501
    Completion Pneumonectomy 32488
    Extrapleural 32445
    Single Lobe 32480
    Single Segment 32484
    Sleeve Lobectomy 32486
    Sleeve Pneumonectomy 32442
    Total Pneumonectomy 32440-32445
    Two Lobes 32482
    Volume Reduction 32491
    Wedge Resection 32500
Repair
    Hernia 32800
Segmentectomy 32484
Tear
    Repair 32110
Thoracotomy
    Biopsy 32095-32100
    Cardiac Massage 32160
    for Post-Op Complications 32120
    Removal
        Bullae 32141
        Cyst 32140
        Intrapleural Foreign Body 32150

        Intrapulmonary Foreign Body 32151
    Repair 32110
        with Excision-Plication of Bullae 32141
        with Open Intrapleural Pneumonolysis .32124
Transplantation 32851-32854, 33935
    Allograft Preparation ..32855-32856, 33933
    Donor Pneumonectomy
        Heart-Lung 33930
        Lung 32850
Tumor
    Removal 32503-32504
Unlisted Services and Procedures 32999

Lung Function Tests
See Pulmonology, Diagnostic

Lung Volume Reduction
Emphysematous 32491

Lupus Anticoagulant Assay 85705

Lupus Band Test
See Immunofluorescent Study

Luteinizing Hormone (LH) 80418, 80426, 83002

Luteinizing Releasing Factor ...83727

Luteotropic Hormone
See Prolactin

Luteotropin
See Prolactin

Luteotropin, Placental
See Lactogen, Human Placental

Lyme Disease 86617-86618

Lyme Disease ab
See Antibody, Lyme Disease

Lyme Disease Vaccine
See Vaccination

Lymph Duct
Injection 38790

Lymph Nodes
Abscess
    Incision and Drainage 38300-38305
Biopsy 38500, 38510-38530, 38570
    Needle 38505
Dissection 38542
Excision 38500, 38510-38530
    Abdominal 38747
    Inguinofemoral 38760-38765
    Laparoscopic 38571-38572
    Limited, for Staging
        Para-Aortic 38562
        Pelvic 38562
        Retroperitoneal 38564
    Pelvic 38770
    Radical
        Axillary 38740-38745
        Cervical 38720-38724
        Suprahyoid 38720-38724
    Retroperitoneal Transabdominal 38780
    Thoracic 38746
Exploration 38542

Heel 28405-28406
Hip 27257
Hip Socket 27222
Humeral 23605, 24505, 24535, 24577
　　Epicondyle 24565
Intercarpal 25660
Interphalangeal Joint . . .26340, 26770-26776
Lunate 25690
Malar Area 21355
Mandibular 21451
Metacarpal 26605-26607
Metacarpophalangeal . .26700-26706, 26742
Metacarpophalangeal Joint 26340
Metatarsal 28475-28476
Nasal Bone 21315-21320
Orbit 21401
Phalangeal Shaft 26727
　　Distal, Finger or Thumb 26755
　　Phalanges, Finger/Thumb 26725
Phalanges
　　Finger 26742, 26755, 26770-26776
　　Finger/Thumb 26727
　　Great Toe 28495-28496
　　Toes 28515
Radial 24655, 25565
Radial Shaft 25505
Radiocarpal 25660
Radioulnar 25675
Scapular 23575
Shoulder 23650-23655
　　with Greater Tuberosity 23665
Sternoclavicular 23525
　　with Neck Fracture 23675
Talus .28435-28436
Tarsal .28455-28456
Thumb .26641-26650
Tibial 27532, 27752
Trans-Scaphoperilunar 25680
Ulnar 24675, 25535, 25565
Vertebral 22315
Wrist 25259, 25624, 25635,
　　　　　　　25660, 25675, 25680, 25690
Foreskin 54450
Globe .92018-92019
Hip 27275
Interphalangeal Joint, Proximal 26742
Knee 27570
Osteopathic 98925-98929
Shoulder
　　Application of Fixation Apparatus 23700
Spine
　　with Anesthesia 22505
Temporomandibular Joint(s) (TMJ) 21073
Tibial, Distal 27762

Manometric Studies
Kidney
　　Pressure 50396
Rectum/Anus 91122
Ureter
　　Pressure 50686
Ureterostomy 50686

Manometry
Rectum 90911

Mantoux Test
See TB Test, Skin Test

Manual Therapy 97140

Maquet Procedure 27418

Marcellation Operation
See Hysterectomy, Vaginal

Marrow, Bone
See Bone Marrow

Marshall-Marchetti-Krantz
Procedure 51840-51841,
　　　　　　　　　　　　58152, 58267, 58293

Marsupialization
Bartholin's Gland Cyst 56440
Cyst
　　Sublingual Salivary 42409
Liver
　　Cyst or Abscess 47300
Pancreatic Cyst 48500
Skin 10040
Urethral Diverticulum 53240

Mass
Kidney
　　Ablation 50542
　　　　Cryosurgical 50250

Mass Spectrometry and Tandem
Mass Spectrometry
Analyte
　　Qualitative .83788
　　Quantitative 83789

Massage
Cardiac 32160
Therapy 97124
　　See PhysicalMedicine/Therapy/Occupational
　　Therapy

Masseter Muscle/Bone
Reduction 21295-21296

Mastectomy
Gynecomastia 19300
Modified Radical 19307
Partial .19301-19302
Radical 19303-19306
Simple, Complete 19303
Subcutaneous .19304

Mastectomy, Halsted
See Mastectomy, Radical

Mastoid
Excision
　　Complete 69502
　　Radical 69511
　　　　Modified 69505
　　　　Petrous Apicectomy 69530
　　Simple 69501
Obliteration 69670
Repair
　　by Excision 69601-69603
　　Fistula 69700
　　with Apicectomy 69605
　　with Tympanoplasty 69604

Mastoid Cavity
Debridement 69220-69222

Mastoidectomy
Osseointegrated Implant
　　for External Speech Processor/
　　CochlearStimulator 69715, 69718
with Apicectomy 69605
with Skull Base Surgery 61590, 61597
　　Decompression 61595
　　Facial Nerve 61595
with Tympanoplasty 69604, 69641-69646
　　Cochlear Device Implantation 69930
　　Complete 69502
　　　　Revision 69601
　　Ossicular Chain Reconstruction 69605
　　Radical 69511
　　　　Modified 69505
　　　　Revision 69602-69603
　　Simple 69501
　　with Labyrinthectomy 69910
　　with Labyrinthotomy 69802
　　with Petrous Apicectomy 69530

Mastoidotomy 69635-69637
with Tympanoplasty 69635
　　Ossicular Chain Reconstruction 69636
　　and Synthetic Prosthesis 69636

Mastoids
Polytomography 76101-76102
X-Ray 70120-70130

Mastopexy 19316

Mastotomy 19020

Maternity Care
See Abortion; Cesarean Delivery; Ectopic
Pregnancy; Obstetrical Care

Maternity Care and
Delivery 59612-59622, 59898

Maxilla
See Facial Bones; Mandible
Bone Graft 21210
CT Scan 70486-70488
Cyst
　　Excision 21048-21049
Excision 21030, 21032-21034
Fracture
　　Closed Treatment 21345, 21421
　　Open Treatment . .21346-21348, 21422-21423
　　with Fixation 21345-21347
Osteotomy 21206
Reconstruction
　　with Implant 21245-21246, 21248-21249
Tumor
　　Excision 21048-21049

Maxillary Arteries
See Artery, Maxillary

Maxillary Sinus
See Sinus/Sinuses, Maxillary

Maxillary Torus Palatinus
Tumor Excision 21032

Maxillectomy 31225-31230

Maxillofacial Fixation
Application
　　Halo Type Appliance 21100

Maxillofacial Impressions
Auricular Prosthesis 21086
Definitive Obturator Prosthesis 21080
Facial Prosthesis 21088
Interim Obturator Prosthesis 21079
Mandibular Resection Prosthesis 21081
Nasal Prosthesis 21087
Oral Surgical Splint 21085
Orbital Prosthesis 21077
Palatal Augmentation Prosthesis 21082
Palatal Lift Prosthesis 21083
Speech Aid Prosthesis 21084
Surgical Obturator Prosthesis 21076

Maxillofacial Procedures
Unlisted Services and Procedures 21299

Maxillofacial Prosthetics 21076-21089
Unlisted Services and Procedures 21089

Maydl Operation 45563, 50810
See Colostomy

Mayo Hernia Repair
See Hernia, Repair, Umbilicus

Mayo Procedure 28292

Maze Procedure
Endoscopic 33265-33266
Open .33254-33256

McBride Procedure 28292

McBurney Operation
See Hernia, Repair, Inguinal

McCannel Procedure 66682

McKissock Surgery
See Breast, Reduction

McVay Operation
See Hernia, Repair, Inguinal

Measles Uncomplicated
See Rubeola

Measles Vaccine
See Vaccines

Measles, German
See Rubella

Meat Fibers
Feces 89160

Meatoplasty 69310

Meatotomy 53020-53025
Cystourethroscopy 52281
Infant 53025
Prostate
　Laser Coagulation 52647
　Laser Vaporization 52648

Transurethral ElectrosurgicalResection
　Prostate 52601
Ureter 52290
Ureteral
　Cystourethroscopy 52290-52305

Meckel's Diverticulum
Excision 44800
Unlisted Services and Procedures 44899

Median Nerve
Decompression 64721
Neuroplasty 64721
Release 64721
Repair/Suture
　Motor Thenar 64835
Transposition 64721

Median Nerve Compression
See Carpal Tunnel Syndrome

Mediastinal Cyst
See Cyst, Mediastinal; Mediastinum, Cyst

Mediastinoscopy 39400

Mediastinotomy
Cervical Approach 39000
Transthoracic Approach 39010

Mediastinum
See Chest; Thorax
Cyst
　Excision 32662, 39200
Endoscopy
　Biopsy 39400
　Exploration 39400
Exploration 39000-39010
Incision and Drainage 39000-39010
Needle Biopsy 32405
Removal
　Foreign Body 39000-39010
Tumor
　Excision 32662, 39220
Unlisted Procedures 39499

Medical Disability Evaluation Services 99455-99456

Medical Genetics 96040
Genetic Counseling 96040

Medical Team Conference . . .99366-99368

Medical Testimony 99075

Medication Therapy Management
Pharmacist Provided 99605-99607

Medicine, Preventive
See Preventive Medicine

Medicine, Pulmonary
See Pulmonology

Medulla
Tractotomy .61470

Medullary Tract
Incision 61470
Section 61470

Meibomian Cyst
See Chalazion

Membrane Oxygenation, Extracorporeal
See Extracorporeal Membrane Oxygenation

Membrane, Mucous
See Mucosa

Membrane, Tympanic
See Ear, Drum

Meninges
Tumor
　Excision 61512, 61519

Meningioma
Excision 61512, 61519
Tumor
　Excision 61512, 61519

Meningitis, Lymphocytic Benign
See Lymphocytic Choriomeningitis

Meningocele Repair 63700-63702

Meningococcal
See Vaccines

Meningococcal Vaccine
See Vaccines

Meningococcus
See Neisseria Meningitidis

Meningomyelocele
See Myelomeningocele

Meniscectomy
Knee Joint 27332-27333
Temporomandibular Joint 21060

Meniscus
Knee
　Excision 27332-27333
　Repair 27403
　Transplantation 29868

Mental Nerve
Avulsion 64736
Incision 64736
Transection .64736

Meprobamate 83805

Mercury 83015, 83825

Mesencephalic Tract
Incision 61480
Section 61480

Mesencephalon
Tractotomy .61480

Mesenteric Arteries
See Artery, Mesenteric

Mesentery
Lesion
　Excision 44820
Repair 44850
Suture 44850
Unlisted Services and Procedures 44899

Microsomia, Hemifacial
See Hemifacial Microsomia

Microsurgery
Operating Microscope 69990

Microvascular Anastomosis
Bone Graft
　　Fibula 20955
　　Other 20962
Fascial Flap, Free 15758
Muscle Flap, Free 15756
Osteocutaneous Flap with 20969-20973
Skin Flap, Free .15757

Microvite A
See Vitamin, A

Microwave Therapy 97024
See Physical Medicine/Therapy/Occupational Therapy

Midbrain
See Brain; Brainstem; Mesencephalon; Skull Base Surgery

Midcarpal Medioccipital Joint
Arthrotomy 25040

Middle Cerebral Artery Velocimetry 76821

Middle Ear
See Ear, Middle

Midface
Reconstruction
　　Forehead Advancement 21159-21160
　　with Bone Graft 21145-21160, 21188
　　without Bone Graft 21141-21143

Migration Inhibitory Factor (MIF) 86378

Mile Operation
See Colectomy, Total, with Proctectomy

Milia, Multiple
Removal 10040

Miller Procedure 28737

Miller-Abbott Intubation .44500, 74340

Minerva Cast 29035
Removal 29710

Minimum Inhibitory Concentration 87186

Minimum Lethal Concentration 87187

Minnesota Multiphasic Personality Inventory
See MMPI

Miscarriage
Incomplete Abortion 59812
Missed Abortion
　　First Trimester 59820
　　Second Trimester 59821
Septic Abortion .59830

Missed Abortion
See Abortion

Mitchell Procedure 28296

Mitogen Blastogenesis 86353

Mitral Valve
Incision 33420-33422
Repair .33420-33427
　　Incision 33420-33422
Replacement 33430

Mitrofanoff Operation 50845
See Appendico-Vesicostomy

Miyagawanella
See Chlamydia

MLC
See Lymphocyte, Culture

MMPI 96101-96103
Computer-Assisted 96103

MMR Shots 90707
See Vaccines

Mobilization
Splenic Flexure 44139
　　Laparoscopic 44213
Stapes 69650

Moderate Sedation
See Sedation

Modified Radical Mastectomy
See Mastectomy, Modified Radical

Mohs Micrographic Surgery 17311-17315

Molar Pregnancy
See Hydatidiform Mole

Mold
Culture 87107

Mole, Carneous
See Abortion

Mole, Hydatid
See Hydatidiform Mole

Molecular Cytogenetics . .88271-88275
Interpretation and Report 88291

Molecular Diagnostics . . .83890-83914
Amplification 83898-83901, 83908
Cell Lysis 83907
Dot/Slot Production 83893
Enzymatic Digestion 83892
Extraction 83890-83891
Interpretation 83912
Molecular Isolation (Extraction) 83890
Mutation Identification 83904-83906
　　Enzymatic Ligation 83914
Mutation Scanning 83903
Nucleic Acid Amplification . .83900-83901, 83908
Nucleic Acid Extraction 83907
Nucleic Acid Probe 83896
Nucleic Acid Transfer 83897
Polymerase Reaction Chain 83898

Reverse Transcription 83902
RNA Stabilization 83913
Separation 83894
Separation and Identification
　　High Resolution Technique 83909

Molecular Oxygen Saturation
See Oxygen Saturation

Molecular Probes 88384-88386
Multiple
　　Array-Based Evaluation 88384-88386

Molluscum Contagiosum
Destruction 17110-17111, 54050-54065

Molteno Procedure 66180

Monilia
See Candida

Monitoring
Blood Pressure, 24 Hour 93784-93790
Electrocardiogram 93224-93237
　　See Electrocardiography
Electroencephalogram 95812-95813,
　　　　　　　　　　　　95950-95953, 95956
　　with Drug Activation 95954
　　with Physical Activation 95954
　　with WADA Activation 95958
Fetal
　　During Labor 59050-59051, 99500
　　　　Interpretation Only 59051
Glucose
　　Interstitial Fluid 95250-95251
Interstitial Fluid Pressure 20950
Intraocular Pressure 0173T
Pediatric Apnea 94774-94777
Seizure .61531, 61760

Monitoring, Sleep
See Polysomnography

Monoethylene Glycol
See Ethylene Glycol

Mononuclear Cell Antigen 86356

Mononucleosis Virus, Infectious
See Epstein-Barr Virus

Monophosphate, Adenosine
See Adenosine Monophosphate (AMP)

Monophosphate, Adenosine Cyclic
See Cyclic AMP

Monophosphate, Guanosine
See Guanosine Monophosphate

Monophosphate, Guanosine Cyclic
See Cyclic GMP

Monospot Test
See Rapid Test for Infection

Monoxide, Carbon
See Carbon Monoxide

Monteggia Fracture 24620-24635

Monticelli Procedure
See Application, Bone Fixation Device

Muscle Division
Scalenus Anticus 21700-21705
Sternocleidomastoid 21720-21725

Muscle Flaps 15731-15738
Free 15756

Muscle Grafts 15841-15845

Muscle Testing
Dynamometry, Eye 92260
Extraocular Multiple Muscles 92265
Manual 95831-95834

Muscle, Oculomotor
See Eye Muscles

Muscles
Repair
    Extraocular 65290, 67346

Musculo-Skeletal System
See Musculoskeletal System

Musculoplasty
See Muscle, Repair

Musculoskeletal System
Computer-Assisted Surgical
Navigation Procedure 20985-20987
Unlisted Services and Procedures 20999,
    24999, 25999, 26989, 27299, 27599, 27899
Unlisted Services and Procedures, Head . . .21499

Musculotendinous (Rotator) Cuff
Repair 23410-23412

Mustard Procedure
See Repair, Great Arteries; Revision

Myasthenia Gravis
Tensilon Test .95857

Myasthenic, Gravis
See Myasthenia Gravis

Mycobacteria
Culture 87116
    Identification 87118
Detection 87550-87562
Sensitivity Studies 87190

Mycoplasma
Antibody 86738
Culture 87109
Detection 87580-87582

Mycota
See Fungus

Myectomy, Anorectal
See Myomectomy, Anorectal

Myelencephalon
See Medulla

Myelin Basic Protein
Cerebrospinal Fluid 83873

Myelography
Brain 70010
Spine
    Cervical 72240
    Lumbosacral 72265

Thoracic 72255
Total 72270

Myelomeningocele
Repair 63704-63706

Myelotomy 63170

Myocardial
Perfusion Imaging . . .78460-78465, 78478-78480
    See Nuclear Medicine
Positron Emission Tomography (PET) 78459

Myocardial Imaging 78466-78469
Positron Emission Tomography
    Perfusion Study 78491-78492
Repair
    Postinfarction 33542

Myocutaneous Flaps 15731-15738,
                                        15756

Myofascial Pain Dysfunction Syndrome
See Temporomandibular Joint (TMJ)

Myofibroma
See Leiomyomata

Myoglobin 83874

Myomectomy
Anorectal 45108
Uterus 58140-58146, 58545-58546

Myoplasty
See Muscle, Repair

Myotomy
Esophagus 43030
Hyoid 21685

Myringoplasty 69620

Myringostomy
See Myringotomy

Myringotomy 69420-69421

Myxoid Cyst
See Ganglion

N

N. Meningitidis
See Neisseria Meningitidis

Naffziger Operation
See Decompression, Orbit; Section

Nagel Test
See Color Vision Examination

Nail Bed
Reconstruction 11762
Repair 11760

Nail Fold
Excision
    Wedge 11765

Nail Plate Separation
See Nails, Avulsion

Nails
Avulsion 11730-11732
Biopsy 11755
Debridement 11720-11721
Drainage 10060-10061
Evacuation
    Hematoma, Subungual 11740
Excision 11750-11752
KOH Examination 87220
Removal 11730-11732, 11750-11752
Trimming 11719

Narcosynthesis
Diagnostic and Therapeutic 90865

Nasal Abscess
See Nose, Abscess

Nasal Area
Bone Graft 21210

Nasal Bleeding
See Epistaxis

Nasal Bone
Fracture
    Closed Treatment 21310-21320
    Open Treatment 21325-21335
    with Manipulation 21315-21320
    without Manipulation 21310
X-Ray 70160

Nasal Deformity
Repair 40700-40761

Nasal Function Study 92512

Nasal Polyp
See Nose, Polyp

Nasal Prosthesis
Impression 21087

Nasal Septum
Abscess
    Incision and Drainage 30020
Fracture
    Closed Treatment 21337
    Open Treatment 21336
Hematoma
    Incision and Drainage 30020
Repair 30630
Submucous Resection 30520

Nasal Sinuses
See Sinus/Sinuses

Nasal Smear
Eosinophils 89190

Nasal Turbinate
Fracture
    Therapeutic 30930

Nasoethmoid Complex
Fracture
    Open Treatment 21338-21339
    Percutaneous Treatment 21340
Reconstruction 21182-21184

Nephroscopy
See Endoscopy, Kidney

Nephrostogram 50394

Nephrostolithotomy
Percutaneous 50080-50081

Nephrostomy 50040
Change Tube 50398
Endoscopic 50562-50570
Percutaneous 52334
with Drainage 50040
X-Ray with Contrast
    Guide Dilation 74485

Nephrostomy Tract
Establishment 50395

Nephrotomogram
See Nephrotomography

Nephrotomography 74415

Nephrotomy 50040-50045
with Exploration 50045

Nerve
Cranial
    See Cranial Nerve
Facial
    See Facial Nerve
Intercostal
    See Intercostal Nerve
Lingual
    See Lingual Nerve
Median
    See Median Nerve
Obturator
    See Obturator Nerve
Peripheral
    See Peripheral Nerve
Phrenic
    See Phrenic Nerve
Sciatic
    See Sciatic Nerve
Spinal
    See Spinal Nerve
Tibial
    See Tibial Nerve
Ulnar
    See Ulnar Nerve
Vestibular
    See Vestibular Nerve

Nerve Conduction
Motor Nerve 95900-95903
Sensory Nerve or Mixed 95904

Nerve Root
See Cauda Equina; Spinal Cord
Decompression 63020-63048, 63055-63103
Incision 63185-63190
Section 63185-63190

Nerve Stimulation, Transcutaneous
See Application, Neurostimulation

Nerve Teasing 88362

Nerve II, Cranial
See Optic Nerve

Nerve V, Cranial
See Trigeminal Nerve

Nerve VII, Cranial
See Facial Nerve

Nerve X, Cranial
See Vagus Nerve

Nerve XI, Cranial
See Accessory Nerve

Nerve XII, Cranial
See Hypoglossal Nerve

Nerves
Anastomosis
    Facial to Hypoglossal 64868
    Facial to Phrenic 64870
    Facial to Spinal Accessory 64866
Avulsion 64732-64772
Biopsy 64795
Decompression 64702-64727
Destruction 64600-64681
    Laryngeal, Recurrent 31595
Foot
    Excision 28055
    Incision 28035
Graft 64885-64907
Implantation
    Electrode 64553-64581
    to Bone 64787
    to Muscle 64787
Incision 43640-43641, 64732-64772
Injection
    Anesthetic 01991-01992, 64400-64530
    Neurolytic Agent 64600-64681
Insertion
    Electrode 64553-64581
Lesion
    Excision 64774-64792
Neurofibroma
    Excision 64788-64792
Neurolemmoma
    Excision 64788-64792
Neurolytic
    Internal 64727
Neuroma
    Excision 64774-64786
Neuroplasty 64702-64721
Removal
    Electrode 64585
Repair
    Graft 64885-64911
    Microdissection 69990
    Suture 64831-64876
Spinal Accessory
    Incision 63191
    Section 63191
Suture 64831-64876
Sympathectomy
    Excision 64802-64818
Transection 43640-43641, 64732-64772
Transposition 64718-64721
Unlisted Services and Procedures 64999

Nervous System
Nuclear Medicine
    Unlisted Services and Procedures 78699

Nesidioblast
See Islet Cell

Neural Conduction
See Nerve Conduction

Neural Ganglion
See Ganglion

Neurectomy
Foot 28055
Gastrocnemius 27326
Hamstring Muscle 27325
Leg, Lower 27326
Leg, Upper 27325
Popliteal 27326
Tympanic 69676

Neuroendoscopy
Intracranial 62160-62165

Neurofibroma
Cutaneous Nerve
    Excision 64788
Extensive
    Excision 64792
Peripheral Nerve
    Excision 64790

Neurolemmoma
Cutaneous Nerve
    Excision 64788
Extensive
    Excision 64792
Peripheral Nerve
    Excision 64790

Neurologic System
See Nervous System

Neurology
Brain Cortex Magnetic Stimulation .0160T-0161T
Brain Mapping 96020
Brain Surface Electrode
Stimulation 95961-95962
Central Motor
    Transcranial Motor
    Stimulation 95928-95929
Cognitive Performance 96125
Diagnostic
    Anal Sphincter 51785
    Autonomic Nervous Function
        Heart Rate Response 95921-95923
        Pseudomotor Response 95921-95923
        Sympathetic Function 95921-95923
Electrocorticogram
    Intraoperative 95829
Electroencephalogram (EEG) 95812-95827,
                                    95855
    Brain Death 95824
    Electrode Placement 95830
    Intraoperative 95955
    Monitoring 95812-95813,
                95950-95953, 95956
    Physical or Drug Activation 95954
    Sleep 95822, 95827
    Standard 95819
    WADA Activation 95958
Electroencephalography (EEG)
    Digital Analysis 95957

Nodes
See Lymph Nodes

Non-Invasive Vascular Imaging
See Vascular Studies

Non-Office Medical Services .. 99056
Emergency Care 99060

Non-Stress Test, Fetal 59025

Nonunion Repair
Femur
    with Graft 27472
    without Graft 27470
Metatarsal 28322
Tarsal Joint 28320

Noradrenalin
Blood 82383-82384
Urine 82384

Norchlorimipramine
See Imipramine

Norepinephrine
See Catecholamines
Blood 82383-82384
Urine 82384

Nortriptyline
Assay 80182

Norwood Procedure 33611-33612,
                             33619

See Repair, Heart, Ventricle; Revision

Nose
Abscess
    Incision and Drainage 30000-30020
Actinotherapy
    Intranasal 0168T
Artery
    Incision 30915-30920
Biopsy
    Intranasal 30100
Dermoid Cyst
    Excision
        Complex 30125
        Simple 30124
Displacement Therapy 30210
Endoscopy
    Diagnostic 31231-31235
    Surgical 31237-31294
Excision
    Rhinectomy 30150-30160
Fracture
    Closed Treatment 21345
    Open Treatment 21325-21336,
          21338-21339, 21346-21347
    Percutaneous Treatment 21340
    with Fixation 21330, 21340, 21345-21347
Hematoma
    Incision and Drainage 30000-30020
Hemorrhage
    Cauterization 30901-30906
Insertion
    Septal Prosthesis 30220
Intranasal
    Actinotherapy 0168T

Lesion
    External Approach 30118
    Internal Approach 30117
    Phototherapy 0168T
Lysis of Adhesions 30560
Phototherapy
    Intranasal 0168T
Polyp
    Excision
        Extensive 30115
        Simple 30110
Reconstruction
    Cleft Lip/Cleft Palate 30460-30462
    Dermatoplasty 30620
    Primary 30400-30420
    Secondary 30430-30450
    Septum 30520
Removal
    Foreign Body 30300
        Anesthesia 30310
        Lateral Rhinotomy 30320
Repair
    Adhesions 30560
    Cleft Lip 40700-40761
    Fistula 30580-30600, 42260
    Rhinophyma 30120
    Septum 30540-30545, 30630
    Synechia 30560
    Vestibular Stenosis 30465
Skin
    Excision 30120
    Surgical Planing 30120
Submucous Resection Turbinate
    Excision 30140
Turbinate
    Excision 30130-30140
    Fracture 30930
    Injection 30200
Turbinate Mucosa
    Cauterization 30801-30802
Unlisted Services and Procedures 30999

Nose Bleed 30901-30906
See Hemorrhage, Nasal

NTD 86384
See Nitroblue Tetrazolium Dye Test

Nuclear Antigen
Antibody 86235

Nuclear Imaging
See Nuclear Medicine

Nuclear Magnetic Resonance Imaging
See Magnetic Resonance Imaging (MRI)

Nuclear Magnetic Resonance Spectroscopy
See Magnetic Resonance Spectroscopy

Nuclear Medicine
Adrenal Gland Imaging 78075
Automated Data 78890-78891
Bile Duct
    Imaging 78223
Bladder
    Residual Study 78730

Blood
    Bone
        Density Study 78350-78351
        Imaging 78300-78320
        SPECT 78320
        Ultrasound 76977
        Unlisted Services and Procedures ... 78399
    Flow Imaging 78445
    Iron
        Red Cells 78140
    Platelet Survival 78190-78191
    Red Cell Survival 78130-78135
    Red Cells 78120-78121
    Unlisted Services and Procedures ... 78199
    Whole Blood Volume 78122
Bone Marrow
    Imaging 78102-78104
Brain
    Blood Flow 78610
    Cerebrospinal Fluid 78630-78650
    Imaging 78600-78609
        Vascular Flow 78610
Endocrine System
    Unlisted Services and Procedures 78099
Esophagus
    Imaging (Motility) 78258
    Reflux Study 78262
Gallbladder
    Imaging 78223
Gastric Mucosa
    Imaging 78261
Gastrointestinal
    Blood Loss Study 78278
    Protein Loss Study 78282
    Shunt Testing 78291
    Unlisted Services and Procedures 78299
Genitourinary System
    Unlisted Services and Procedures 78799
Heart
    Blood Flow 78414
    Blood Pool Imaging 78472-78473,
          78481-78483, 78494-78496
    Myocardial Imaging 78459, 78466-78469
    Myocardial Perfusion 78460-78465,
               78478-78480
    Shunt Detection 78428
    Unlisted Services and Procedures 78499
Hepatic Duct
    Imaging 78223
Inflammatory Process 78805-78807
Intestines
    Imaging 78290
Kidney
    Function Study 78725
    Imaging 78700-78707, 78710
    Vascular Flow 78701-78709
Lacrimal Gland Tear Flow 78660
Liver
    Function Study 78220
    Imaging 78201-78216
    Vascular Flow 78206
Lung
    Imaging Perfusion 78580-78585
    Imaging Ventilation 78586-78594
    Unlisted Services and Procedures ... 78599
Lymph Nodes 78195
Lymphatics 78195
    Unlisted Services and Procedures 78199

Nucleases, DNA
See DNAse

Nucleic Acid Probe 83896

Nucleolysis, Intervertebral Disc
See Chemonucleolysis

Nucleotidase 83915

Nursemaid Elbow 24640

Nursing Facility Discharge Services
See Discharge Services, Nursing Facility

Nursing Facility Services

Nuss Procedure

Nutrition Therapy

Nystagmus Tests
See Vestibular Function Tests

O

O$_2$ Saturation
See Oxygen Saturation

Ober-Yount Procedure 27025
See Fasciotomy, Hip

Obliteration

Oblongata, Medulla
See Medulla

Observation 99234-99236
See Evaluation and Management; Hospital Services

Obstetrical Care
Abortion
Induced
by Amniocentesis Injection . .59850-59852
See Abortion; Cesarean Delivery;
Ectopic Pregnancy
by Dilation and Curettage 59840
by Dilation and Evaluation 59841
Missed
First Trimester 59820
Second Trimester 59821
Spontaneous 59812
Therapeutic 59840-59852
Antepartum Care 59425-59426
Cesarean Delivery 59618-59622
Only 59514
Postpartum Care 59515
Routine 59510
with Hysterectomy 59525
Curettage
Hydatidiform Mole 59870
Evacuation
Hydatidiform Mole 59870
External Cephalic Version 59412
Miscarriage
Surgical Completion 59812-59821
Placenta Delivery 59414
Postpartum Care 59430, 59514
Septic Abortion 59830
Total (Global) 59400, 59610, 59618
Unlisted Services and Procedures . .59898-59899
Vaginal
after Cesarean 59610-59614
Vaginal Delivery 59409-59410
Delivery after Cesarean 59610-59614

Obstruction
See Occlusion

Obstruction Clearance
Venous Access Device 36595-36596

Obstruction Colon
See Colon, Obstruction

Obturator Nerve
Avulsion .64763-64766
Incision 64763-64766
Transection 64763-64766

Obturator Prosthesis 21076
Definitive 21080
Insertion
Larynx 31527
Interim 21079

Occipital Nerve, Greater
Avulsion 64744
Incision 64744
Injection
Anesthetic .64405
Transection .64744

Occlusion
Extracranial
Intracranial .61623
Fallopian Tube
Oviduct 58565, 58615
Penis
Vein 37790

Umbilical Cord 59072

Occlusive Disease of Artery
See Repair, Artery; Revision

Occult Blood 82270-82272
by Hemoglobin Immunoassay 82274

Occupational Therapy
Evaluation 97003-97004

Ocular Implant
See Orbital Implant
Insertion
in Scleral Shell 65130
Muscles, Attached 65140
Muscles, Not Attached 65135
Modification 65125
Reinsertion 65150
with Foreign Material 65155
Removal 65175

Ocular Muscle
See Eye Muscles

Ocular Orbit
See Orbit

Ocular Photoscreening 99174

Ocular Prostheses
See Prosthesis, Ocular

Oculomotor Muscle
See Eye Muscles

Oddi Sphincter
See Sphincter of Oddi

Odontoid Dislocation
Open Treatment/Reduction 22318
with Grafting 22319

Odontoid Fracture
Open Treatment/Reduction 22318
with Grafting 22319

Odontoid Process
Excision 22548

Oesophageal Neoplasm
See Tumor, Esophagus

Oesophageal Varices
See Esophageal Varices

Oesophagus
See Esophagus

Oestradiol
See Estradiol

Office and/or Other Outpatient Services
See History and Physical
Consultation
Established Patient 99211-99215
New Patient 99201-99205
Normal Newborn 99432
Office Visit
Established Patient 99211-99215
New Patient 99201-99205
Outpatient Visit

Established Patient 99211-99215
New Patient 99201-99205
Prolonged Services 99354-99355

Office Medical Services
After Hours 99050
Emergency Care 99058
Extended Hours 99051

Office or Other Outpatient Consultations
See Consultation, Office and/or Other Outpatient

Olecranon
See Elbow; Humerus; Radius; Ulna
Bursa
Arthrocentesis 20605
Cyst
Excision 24125-24126
Tumor
Cyst 24120
Excision 24125-24126

Olecranon Process
Craterization 24147
Diaphysectomy .24147
Excision 24147
Abscess 24138
Fracture
See Elbow; Humerus; Radius
Closed Treatment 24670-24675
Open Treatment 24685
Osteomyelitis 24138, 24147
Saucerization 24147
Sequestrectomy 24138

Oligoclonal Immunoglobulins .83916

Omentectomy 49255, 58950-58958
Laparotomy 58960
Oophorectomy .58943
Resection Ovarian Malignancy 58950-58952
Resection Peritoneal Malignancy . .58950-58958
Resection Tubal Malignancy 58950-58958

Omentum
Excision 49255, 58950-58958
Flap 49904-49905
Free
with Microvascular Anastomosis . . .49906
Omentopexy 49326
Unlisted Services and Procedures 49999

Omphalectomy 49250

Omphalocele
Repair 49600-49611

Omphalomesenteric Duct
Excision 44800

Omphalomesenteric Duct, Persistent
See Diverticulum, Meckel's

Oncoprotein
HER-2/neu 83950

Online Internet Assessment and Management
Nonphysician 98969
Physician 99444

Oxidoreductase, Alcohol-Nad+
See Antidiuretic Hormone

Oximetry (Noninvasive)
See Pulmonology, Diagnostic
Blood O_2 Saturation
    Ear or Pulse 94760-94762

Oxoisomerase
See Phosphohexose Isomerase

Oxosteroids
See Ketosteroids

Oxycodinone 80102-80103, 83925

Oxygen Saturation 82805-82810

Oxygenation, Extracorporeal Membrane
See Extracorporeal Membrane Oxygenation

Oxyproline
See Hydroxyproline

Oxytocin Stress Test, Fetal 59020

P

P & P
See Proconvertin

P B Antibodies
See Antibody, Heterophile

P-Acetamidophenol
See Acetaminophen

Pacemaker, Heart
See Cardiology; Defibrillator, Heart;
Electrocardiography
Conversion 33214
Electronic Analysis
    Antitachycardia System 93724
    Dual Chamber . . .93731-93733, 93743-93744
    Leads 93640-93641
    Single Chamber .93734-93735, 93741-93742
    Single/Dual Chamber 93641-93642
    Wearable Device 93741-93742, 93745
Insertion 33206-33208
    Electrode 33210-33211,
        33216-33217, 33224-33225
    Pulse Generator Only 33212-33213
Removal 33233-33237
    via Thoracotomy 33236-33237
Repair
    Electrode 33218-33220
Replacement
    Catheter 33210
    Electrode 33210-33211
    Insertion 33206-33208
    Pulse Generator 33212-33213
Repositioning
    Electrode 33215, 33226
Revise Pocket
    Chest 33222

Telephonic Analysis 93733, 93736
Upgrade 33214

Pachymetry
Eye 76514

Packing
Nasal Hemorrhage 30901-30906

Pain Management
Epidural/Intrathecal 62350-62351,
        62360-62362, 99601-99602
Intravenous Therapy .90765-90768, 90774-90775

Palate
Abscess
    Incision and Drainage 42000
Biopsy 42100
Excision 42120, 42145
Fracture
    Closed Treatment 21421
    Open Treatment 21422-21423
Lesion
    Destruction 42160
    Excision 42104-42120
Prosthesis
    Augmentation 21082
    Impression 42280
    Insertion 42281
    Lift 21083
Reconstruction
    Lengthening 42226-42227
Repair
    Cleft Palate 42200-42225
    Laceration 42180-42182
    Vomer Flap 42235
Unlisted Services and Procedures 42299

Palate, Cleft
See Cleft Palate

Palatoplasty 42200-42225

Palatoschisis
See Cleft Palate

Palm
Bursa
    Incision and Drainage 26025-26030
Fasciectomy 26121-26125
Fasciotomy 26040-26045
Tendon
    Excision 26170
Tendon Sheath
    Excision 26145
    Incision and Drainage 26020

Palsy, Seventh Nerve
See Facial Nerve Paralysis

Pancreas
Anastomosis
    with Intestines 48520-48540, 48548
Anesthesia 00794
Biopsy 48100
    Needle Biopsy 48102
Cyst
    Anastomosis 48520-48540
    Repair 48500
Debridement
    Peripancreatic Tissue 48105

Excision
    Ampulla of Vater 48148
    Duct 48148
    Partial . . .48140-48146, 48150, 48154, 48160
    Peripancreatic Tissue 48105
    Total 48155-48160
Lesion
    Excision 48120
Needle Biopsy 48102
Placement
    Drainage 48000-48001
Pseudocyst
    Drainage
        Open 48510
        Percutaneous 48511
Removal
    Calculi (Stone) 48020
Removal Transplanted Allograft 48556
Repair
    Cyst 48500
Resection 48105
Suture 48545
Transplantation 48160, 48550, 48554-48556
    Allograft Preparation 48550-48552
    Islet Cell 0141T, 0142T, 0143T
Unlisted Services and Procedures 48999
X-Ray with Contrast 74300-74305
    Injection Procedure 48400

Pancreas, Endocrine Only
See Islet Cell

Pancreatectomy
Donor 48550
Partial 48140-48146, 48150-48154, 48160
Total .48155-48160
with Transplantation 48160

Pancreatic DNAse
See DNAse

Pancreatic Duct
Destruction
    Calculi (Stone) 43265
Dilation
    Endoscopy 43271
Endoscopy
    Collection
        Specimen 43260
    Destruction
        Calculi (Stone) 43265
        Tumor .43272
    Dilation 43271
    Removal (Endoscopic)
        Calculi (Stone) 43264
        Foreign Body 43269
        Stent .43269
    Sphincter Pressure 43263
    Sphincterotomy 43262
    Tube Placement 43267-43268
Incision
    Sphincter .43262
Removal
    Calculi (Stone) 43264
    Foreign Body 43269
    Stent 43269
Tube Placement
    Nasopancreatic 43267
    Stent 43268

Patella, Chondromalacia
See Chondromalacia Patella

Patellar Tendon Bearing (PTB) Cast 29435

Patellectomy
with Reconstruction 27424

Paternity Testing 86910-86911

Patey's Operation
See Mastectomy, Radical

Pathologic Dilatation
See Dilation

Pathology
Clinical
    Consultation 80500-80502
Surgical 88355
    Consultation 88321-88325
      Intraoperative 88329-88334
    Decalcification Procedure 88311
    Electron Microscopy 88348-88349
    Gross and Micro Exam
      Level II 88302
      Level III 88304
      Level IV 88305
      Level V 88307
      Level VI 88309
    Gross Exam
      Level I 88300
    Histochemistry 88318-88319
    Immunocytochemistry 88342
    Immunofluorescent Study 88346-88347
    Morphometry
      Nerve 88356
      Skeletal Muscle 88355
      Tumor 88358-88361
    Nerve Teasing 88362
    Special Stain 88312-88314
    Staining 88312-88314
    Tissue Hybridization 88365
    Unlisted Services and Procedures 88399, 89240

PBG
See Porphobilinogen

PCP
See Phencyclidine

PCR
See Polymerase Chain Reaction

Peans' Operation
See Amputation, Leg, Upper, at Hip; Radical Resection; Replantation

Pectoral Cavity
See Chest Cavity

Pectus Carinatum
Reconstructive Repair 21740-21742
    with Thoracoscopy 21743

Pectus Excavatum
Reconstructive Repair 21740-21742
    with Thoracoscopy 21743

Pediatric Critical Care 99293-99294

Pediatric Intensive Care 99293

Pedicle Fixation
Insertion 22842-22844

Pedicle Flap
Formation 15570-15576
Island 15740
Neurovascular 15750
Transfer 15650

PEEP
See Pressure Breathing, Positive

Pelvi-Ureteroplasty
See Pyeloplasty

Pelvic Adhesions
See Adhesions, Pelvic

Pelvic Exam 57410

Pelvic Exenteration 51597

Pelvic Fixation
Insertion 22848

Pelvic Lymphadenectomy 58210, 58958

Pelvimetry 74710

Pelviolithotomy 50130

Pelvis
See Hip
Abscess
    Incision and Drainage 26990, 45000
Angiography 72191
Biopsy 27040-27041
Bone
    Drainage 26992
Brace Application 20662
Bursa
    Incision and Drainage 26991
CT Scan 72191-72194
Cyst
    Aspiration 50390
    Injection 50390
Destruction
    Lesion 58662
Endoscopy
    Destruction of Lesion 58662
    Lysis of Adhesions 58660
    Oviduct Surgery 58670-58671
Exclusion
    Small Intestine 44700
Exenteration 45126, 58240
Halo 20662
Hematoma
    Incision and Drainage 26990
Lysis
    Adhesions 58660
Magnetic Resonance Angiography 72198
Magnetic Resonance Imaging (MRI) 72195-72197
Removal
    Foreign Body 27086-27087
Repair
    Osteotomy 27158
    Tendon 27098

Ring
Dislocation 27193-27194, 27216-27218
    Fracture 27216-27218
      Closed Treatment 27193-27194
Tumor
    Excision 27047-27049
Ultrasound 76856-76857
Unlisted Services and Procedures for Hips and Hip Joint 27299
X-Ray 72170-72190, 73540
    Manometry 74710

Pemberton Osteotomy of Pelvis
See Osteotomy, Pelvis

Penectomy
See Amputation, Penis

Penetrating Keratoplasties
See Keratoplasty, Penetrating

Penile Induration
See Peyronie Disease

Penile Prosthesis
Insertion
    Inflatable 54401-54405
    Noninflatable 54400
Removal
    Inflatable 54406, 54410-54417
    Semi-Rigid 54415-54417
Repair
    Inflatable 54408
Replacement
    Inflatable 54410-54411, 54416-54417
    Semi-Rigid 54416-54417

Penile Rigidity Test 54250

Penile Tumescence Test 54250

Penis
Amputation
    Partial 54120
    Radical 54130-54135
    Total 54125
Biopsy 54100-54105
Circumcision
    Repair 54163
    Surgical Excision
      Newborn 54150, 54160
Excision
    Partial 54120
    Prepuce 54150-54161, 54163
    Total 54125-54135
Frenulum
    Excision 54164
Incision
    Prepuce 54000-54001
Incision and Drainage 54015
Injection
    for Erection 54235
    Peyronie Disease 54200
      Surgical Exposure Plaque 54205
    Vasoactive Drugs 54231
    X-Ray 54230
Insertion
    Prosthesis
      Inflatable 54401-54405
      Noninflatable 54400

Lesion
    Cornea 65450
    Retina 0017T, 67210, 67227-67228
Retinal Detachment
    Prophylaxis 67145
    Repair 67105

Photodensity
Radiographic
    Absorptiometry 77083

Photodynamic Therapy
External 96567

Photography
Skin
    Diagnostic 96904

Photography, Ocular
See Ophthalmosocpy, Diagnostic

Photopheresis
Extracorporeal 36522
Photophoresis
    See Actinotherapy; Photochemotherapy

Photoradiation Therapies
See Actinotherapy

Photoscreen, Ocular 99174

Photosensitivity Testing 95056
See Allergy Tests

Phototherapies
See Actinotherapy

Phototherapy, Ultraviolet
See Actinotherapy

Phrenic Nerve
Anastomosis
    to Facial Nerve 64870
Avulsion 64746
Incision 64746
Injection
    Anesthetic 64410
Transection .64746

Physical Medicine/Therapy/Occupational Therapy
See Neurology, Diagnostic
Activities of Daily Living 97535, 99509
Aquatic Therapy
    with Exercises 97113
Athletic Training
    Evaluation 97005
    Re-Evaluation 97006
Check-Out
    Orthotic/Prosthetic 97762
Cognitive Skills Development 97532
Community/Work Reintegration 97537
Evaluation 97001-97002
Kinetic Therapy 97530
Manual Therapy 97140
Modalities
    Contrast Baths 97034
    Diathermy Treatment 97024
    Electric Stimulation
        Attended, Manual 97032
        Unattended 97014

Hot or Cold Pack 97010
Hydrotherapy (Hubbard Tank) 97036
Infrared Light Treatment 97026
Iontophoresis 97033
Microwave Therapy 97024
Paraffin Bath 97018
Traction 97012
Ultrasound .97035
Ultraviolet Light 97028
Unlisted Services and Procedures 97039
Vasopneumatic Device 97016
Whirlpool Therapy 97022
Orthotics Training 97760
Osteopathic Manipulation 98925-98929
Procedures
    Aquatic Therapy 97113
    Direct 97032-97039
    Gait Training 97116
    Group Therapeutic 97150
    Massage Therapy 97124
    Neuromuscular Reeducation 97112
    Physical Performance Test 97750
    Supervised 97010-97028
    Therapeutic Exercises 97110
    Traction Therapy 97140
    Work Hardening 97545-97546
Prosthetic Training 97761
Sensory Integration 97533
Therapeutic Activities 97530
Unlisted Services and Procedures . .97139, 97799
Wheelchair Management 97542
Work Reintegration 97537

Physical Therapy
See Physical Medicine/Therapy/Occupational Therapy

Physician Services
Care Plan Oversight Services 99339-99340, 99374-99380
    Documentation of Plan/Surrogate Decision
    Maker 1080F
    Domiciliary Facility 99339-99340
    Home Health Agency Care 99374
    Home or Rest Home Care 99339-99340
    Hospice 99377-99378
    Nursing Facility 99379-99380
Case Management Services 99366-99368
Direction, Advanced Life Support 99288
Online 99444
Prolonged
    with Direct Patient Contact 99354-99357
        Outpatient/Office 99354-99355
    with Direct Patient Services
        Inpatient 99356-99357
    without Direct Patient Contact . .99358-99359
Standby 99360
Supervision, Care Plan Oversight
Services 99339-99340, 99374-99380
    Documentation of Plan/Surrogate Decision
    Maker 1080F
Team Conference 99367
Telephone 99441-99443

Piercing of Ear Lobe 69090

Piles
See Hemorrhoids

Pilonidal Cyst
Excision 11770-11772
Incision and Drainage 10080-10081

Pin
See Wire
Insertion/Removal
    Skeletal Traction 20650
Prophylactic Treatment
    Femur 27187
    Humerus .24498
    Shoulder 23490-23491

Pinch Graft 15050

Pinna
See Ear, External

Pinworms
Examination .87172

Pirogoff Procedure 27888

Pituitary Epidermoid Tumor
See Craniopharyngioma

Pituitary Gland
Excision .61546-61548
Tumor
    Excision 61546-61548, 62165

Pituitary Growth Hormone
See Growth Hormone

Pituitary Lactogenic Hormone
See Prolactin

Pituitectomy
See Excision, Pituitary Gland

PKU
See Phenylalanine

Placement
Adjustable Gastric Restrictive Device 43770
Broncheal Stent 31636-31637
Catheter
    Aneurysm Sac
        Pressure Sensor 34806
        Complete Study 93982
    Brain
        for Chemotherapy 0169T
    Breast
        for Interstitial Radioelement
        Application . . .19296-19298, 20555, 41019
    Bronchus
        for Intracavitary Radioelement
        Application 31643
        See Catheterization
    Head
        Interstitial Radioelement
        Application 41019
    Neck
        Interstitial Radioelement
        Application 41019
    Pelvic Organs
        Interstitial Radioelement
        Application 55920
        Prostate .55875
Catheter, Cardiac 93503
    See Catheterization, Cardiac

Plication, Sphincter, Urinary Bladder
See Bladder, Repair, Neck

Pneumocentesis
Lung 32420

Pneumocisternogram
See Cisternography

Pneumococcal Vaccine
See Vaccines

Pneumocystis Carinii
Antigen Detection
　　Immunofluorescence 87281

Pneumogastric Nerve
See Vagus Nerve

Pneumogram
Pediatric 94772

Pneumolysis .32940

Pneumonectomy 32440-32500
Completion 32488
Donor 32850, 33930
Sleeve 32442
Total 32440-32445

Pneumonology
See Pulmonology

Pneumonolysis 32940
Intrapleural 32652
Open Intrapleural 32124

Pneumonostomy 32200-32201

Pneumonotomy
See Incision, Lung

Pneumoperitoneum 49400

Pneumoplethysmography
Ocular 93875

Pneumothorax
Chemical Pleurodesis 32560
Pleural Scarification for Repeat 32215
Therapeutic
　　Injection Intrapleural Air 32960
Thoracentesis with Tube Insertion 32422

Polio
Antibody 86658
Vaccine .90712-90713

Poliovirus Vaccine
See Vaccines

Pollicization
Digit 26550

Polya Gastrectomy
See Gastrectomy, Partial

Polydactylism
See Polydactyly; Supernumerary Digit

Polydactyly
Digit
　　Reconstruction 26587
　　Repair 26587
Toe 28344

Polymerase Chain Reaction 83898

Polyp
Antrochoanal
　　Removal 31032
Esophagus
　　Ablation 43228
Nose
　　Excision
　　　　Endoscopic 31237-31240
　　　　Extensive 30115
　　　　Simple .30110
Sphenoid Sinus
　　Removal 31051
Urethra
　　Excision 53260

Polypectomy
Nose
　　Endoscopic 31237
Uterus 58558

Polypeptide, Vasoactive Intestinal
See Vasoactive Intestinal Peptide

Polysomnography 95808-95811

Polyuria Test
See Water Load Test

Pomeroy's Operation
See Tubal Ligation

Pooling
Blood Products 86965

Popliteal Arteries
See Artery, Popliteal

Popliteal Synovial Cyst
See Baker's Cyst

Poradenitistras
See Lymphogranuloma Venereum

PORP (Partial Ossicular Replacement Prosthesis) .69633, 69637

Porphobilinogen
Urine 84106-84110

Porphyrin Precursors 82135

Porphyrins
Feces 84126-84127
Urine 84119-84120

Port Film 77417

Portal Vein
See Vein, Hepatic Portal

Portoenterostomies, Hepatic
See Hepaticoenterostomy

Portoenterostomy 47701

Positional Nystagmus Test
See Nystagmus Tests, Positional

Positive End Expiratory Pressure
See Pressure Breathing, Positive

Positive-Pressure Breathing, Inspiratory
See Intermittent Positive Pressure Breathing (IPPB)

Positron Emission Tomography (PET)
Brain 78608-78609
Heart 78459
Myocardial Imaging
　　Perfusion Study 78491-78492

Post-Op Visit 99024

Postauricular Fistula
See Fistula, Postauricular

Postcaval Ureter
See Retrocaval Ureter

Postmortem
See Autopsy

Postop Vas Reconstruction
See Vasovasorrhaphy

Postoperative Wound Infection
Incision and Drainage 10180

Postpartum Care
Cesarean Delivery 59515
　　after Attempted Vaginal Delivery 59622
　　Previous 59610, 59614-59618, 59622
Vaginal Delivery .59430
　　after Previous Cesarean Delivery 59614

Potassium .84132
Urine 84133

Potential, Auditory Evoked
See Auditory Evoked Potentials

Potential, Evoked
See Evoked Potential

Potts-Smith Procedure 33762

Pouch, Kock
See Kock Pouch

PPP
See Fibrin Degradation Products

PRA
See Cytotoxic Screen

Prealbumin 84134

Prebeta Lipoproteins
See Lipoprotein, Blood

Pregnancy
Abortion
　　Induced 59855-59857
　　　　by Amniocentesis Injection . .59850-59852
　　　　by Dilation and Curettage 59840
　　　　by Dilation and Evaluation 59841

Proctocele
See Rectocele

Proctopexy
Laparoscopic 45400-45402
　　with Sigmoid Resection 45402
Open 45540-45541
　　with Sigmoid Excision 45550

Proctoplasty 45500-45505

Proctorrhaphy
See Rectum, Suture

Proctoscopies
See Anoscopy

Proctosigmoidoscopy
Ablation
　　Polyp or Lesion 45320
Biopsy 45305
Destruction
　　Tumor 45320
Dilation 45303
Exploration 45300
Hemorrhage Control 45317
Placement
　　Stent 45327
Removal
　　Foreign Body 45307
　　Polyp 45308-45315
　　Tumor 45315
Volvulus Repair 45321

Products, Gene
See Protein

Proetz Therapy
Nose 30210

Profibrinolysin
See Plasminogen

Progenitor Cell
See Stem Cell

Progesterone 84144

Progesterone Receptors 84234

Progestin Receptors
See Progesterone Receptors

Proinsulin 84206

Projective Test 96101-96103

Prokallikrein
See Fletcher Factor

Prokallikrein, Plasma
See Fletcher Factor

Prokinogenase
See Fletcher Factor

Prolactin 80418, 80440, 84146

Prolapse
See Procidentia

Prolapse, Rectal
See Procidentia, Rectum

Prolastin
See Alpha-1 Antitrypsin

Prolonged Services . .99354-99357, 99360
without Direct Patient Contact 99358-99359

Prophylactic Treatment
See Preventive Medicine
Antibiotic 4045F, 4047F-4049F
Antimicrobial .4046F
　　Cefazolin or Cefuroxime 4041F-4043F
Femoral Neck and Proximal Femur
　　Nailing .27187
　　Pinning .27187
　　Wiring 27187
Femur 27495
　　Nailing .27495
　　Pinning .27495
　　Wiring 27495
Humerus
　　Pinning, Wiring 24498
Radius 25490, 25492
　　Nailing 25490, 25492
　　Pinning 25490, 25492
　　Plating 25490, 25492
　　Wiring 25490, 25492
Shoulder
　　Clavicle .23490
　　Humerus 23491
Tibia 27745
Ulna 25491-25492
　　Nailing 25491-25492
　　Pinning 25491-25492
　　Plating 25491-25492
　　Wiring 25491-25492
Venous Thromboembolism (VTE) 4044F

Prophylaxis
Anticoagulant Therapy 4075F
Deep Vein Thrombosis (DVT) 4070F
Retina
　　Detachment
　　　　Cryotherapy, Diathermy 67141
　　　　Photocoagulation 67145

Prostaglandin 84150
Insertion 59200

Prostanoids
See Prostaglandin

Prostate
Ablation
　　Cryosurgery 55873
Abscess
　　Drainage .52700
　　Incision and Drainage 55720-55725
Biopsy 0137T, 55700-55705
Brachytherapy
　　Needle Insertion 55875-55876
Coagulation
　　Laser 52647
Destruction
　　Cryosurgery 55873
　　Thermotherapy 53850-53853
　　　　Microwave 53850
　　　　Radio Frequency 53852
Enucleation
　　Laser 52649

Excision
　　Partial 55801, 55821-55831
　　Perineal 55801-55815
　　Radical 55810-55815, 55840-55845
　　Retropubic 55831-55845
　　Suprapubic 55821
　　Transurethral . . .52402, 52601, 52612-52614
Exploration
　　Exposure .55860
　　with Nodes 55862-55865
Incision
　　Exposure 55860-55865
　　Transurethral 52450
Insertion
　　Catheter .55875
　　Needle 55875
　　Radioactive Substance 55860
Needle Biopsy 0137T, 55700
Placement
　　Catheter .55875
　　Dosimeter 55876
　　Fiducial Marker 55876
　　Interstitial Device 55876
　　Needle 55875
Thermotherapy
　　Transurethral 53850-53853
Ultrasound 76872-76873
Unlisted Services and Procedures 55899
　　Urinary System 53899
Urethra
　　Stent Insertion 0084T
Vaporization
　　Laser 52648

Prostate Specific
Antigen 84152-84154

Prostatectomy 52601
Laparascopic .55866
Perineal
　　Partial 55801
　　Radical 55810-55815
Retropubic
　　Partial 55831
　　Radical 55840-55845, 55866
Suprapubic
　　Partial 55821
Transurethral 52612-52614

Prostatic Abscess
See Abscess, Prostate

Prostatotomy 55720-55725

Prosthesis
Augmentation
　　Mandibular Body 21125
Auricular 21086
Breast
　　Insertion 19340-19342
　　Removal 19328-19330
　　Supply 19396
Check-Out 97762
　　See PhysicalMedicine/Therapy/Occupational
　　Therapy
Cornea 65770
Endovascular
　　Thoracic Aorta 33883-33886
Facial 21088

Radical Vaginal Hysterectomy
See Hysterectomy, Vaginal, Radical

Radical Vulvectomy
See Vulvectomy, Radical

Radio-Cobalt B12 Schilling Test
See Vitamin, B12, Absorption Study

Radioactive Colloid Therapy ...79300

Radioactive Substance

Radiocarpal Joint

Radiocinematographies
See Cineradiography

Radioelement

Radioelement Substance

Radiography
See Radiology, Diagnostic; X-Ray

Radioimmunosorbent Test
See Gammaglobulin, Blood

Radioisotope Brachytherapy
See Brachytherapy

Radioisotope Scan
See Nuclear Medicine

Radiological Marker

Radiology
See Nuclear Medicine, Radiation Therapy, X-Ray, Ultrasound

Radionuclide CT Scan
See Emission Computerized Tomography

Radionuclide Imaging
See Nuclear Medicine

Radionuclide Therapy
See Radiopharmaceutical Therapy

Radionuclide Tomography, Single-PhotonEmission-Computed
See SPECT

Radiopharmaceutical Therapy

Radiotherapeutic
See Radiation Therapy

Radiotherapies
See Irradiation

Radiotherapy, Surface
See Application, Radioelement, Surface

Radioulnar Joint

Radius
See Arm, Lower; Elbow; Ulna

Jejunum
  Free Transfer
    with Microvascular Anastomosis . . .43496
Kidney
  Fistula .50520-50526
  Horseshoe 50540
  Renal Pelvis 50400-50405
  Wound 50500
Knee
  Cartilage 27403
  Instability 27420
  Ligament 27405-27409
    Collateral 27405
    Collateral and Cruciate 27409
    Cruciate 27407-27409
  Meniscus 27403
  Tendon 27380-27381
Larynx
  Fracture 31584
  Reinnervation
    Neuromuscular Pedicle 31590
Leg
  Lower
    Fascia 27656
    Tendon 27658-27692
  Upper
    Muscle 27385-27386, 27400, 27430
    Tendon 27393-27400
Ligament
  See Ligament, Repair
Lip 40650-40654
  Cleft Lip 40700-40761
  Fistula 42260
Liver
  Abscess 47300
  Cyst 47300
  Wound 47350-47361
Lung
  Hernia 32800
  Pneumolysis 32940
  Tear 32110
Mastoidectomy
  Complete 69601
  Modified Radical 69602
  Radical 69603
  with Apicectomy 69605
  with Tympanoplasty 69604
Maxilla
  Osteotomy .21206
Mesentery 44850
Metacarpal
  Lengthening 26568
  Nonunion 26546
  Osteotomy .26565
Metacarpophalangeal Joint
  Capsulodesis 26516-26518
  Collateral Ligament 26540-26542
  Fusion 26516-26518
Metatarsal 28322
  Osteotomy 28306-28309
Microsurgery 69990
Mitral Valve 33420-33427
Mouth
  Laceration 40830-40831
  Vestibule of 40830-40845
Musculotendinous Cuff 23410-23412
Nail Bed 11760

Nasal Deformity
  Cleft Lip 40700-40761
Nasal Septum 30630
Navicular 25440
Neck Muscles
  Scalenus Anticus 21700-21705
  Sternocleidomastoid 21720-21725
Nerve 64876
  Graft 64885-64911
  Microrepair 69990
  Suture 64831-64876
Nose
  Adhesions .30560
  Fistula 30580-30600, 42260
  Rhinophyma 30120
  Septum 30540-30545, 30630
  Synechia 30560
  Vestibular Stenosis 30465
Omphalocele 49600-49611
Osteotomy
  Femoral Neck 27161
  Radius
    and Ulna 25365
  Ulna
    and Radius 25365
  Vertebra
    Additional Segment 22216, 22226
    Cervical 22210, 22220
    Lumbar 22214, 22224
    Thoracic 22212, 22222
Oviduct 58752
  Create Stoma 58770
Pacemaker
  Heart
    Electrode 33218-33220
Palate
  Laceration 42180-42182
  Vomer Flap 42235
Pancreas
  Cyst 48500
  Pseudocyst 48510-48511
    Percutaneous 48511
Paravaginal Defect 57284-57285, 57423
Pectus Carinatum 21740-21742
  with Thoracoscopy 21743
Pectus Excavatum 21740-21742
  with Thoracoscopy 21743
Pelvic Floor
  Prosthetic Insertion 57267
Pelvis
  Osteotomy .27158
  Tendon 27098
Penis
  Fistulization 54435
  Injury 54440
  Priapism 54420-54435
  Shunt 54420-54430
Perineum 56810
Periorbital Region
  Osteotomy 21260-21263
Phalanx
  Finger
    Lengthening 26568
    Osteotomy 26567
    Nonunion 26546
  Toe
    Osteotomy 28310-28312

Pharynx
  with Esophagus 42953
Pleura 32215
Prosthesis
  Penis 54408
Pulmonary Artery 33917-33920, 33925-33926
  Reimplantation 33788
Pulmonary Valve 33470-33474
Pulmonary Venous Return 33724
Pulmonary Venous Stenosis 33726
Quadriceps
  See Quadriceps, Repair
Radius
  Epiphyseal 25450-25455
  Malunion or Nonunion 25400, 25415
  Osteotomy 25350-25355, 25370-25375
  with Graft 25405, 25420-25426
Rectocele
  See Rectocele, Repair
Rectovaginal Fistula 57308
Rectum
  Fistula 0170T, 45800-45825
  Injury 45562-45563
  Prolapse 45505-45541, 45900
  Rectocele .45560
  Stenosis 45500
  with Sigmoid Excision 45550
Retinal Detachment with Diathermy
  See Diathermy, Retinal Detachment, Repair
Rotator Cuff
  See Rotator Cuff, Repair
Salivary Duct 42500-42505
  Fistula 42600
Scapula
  Fixation 23400
  Scapulopexy 23400
Sclera
  See Sclera, Repair
Scrotum 55175-55180
Septal Defect 33813-33814
Shoulder
  Capsule 23450-23466
  Cuff 23410-23412
  Ligament Release 23415
  Muscle Transfer 23395-23397
  Musculotendinous Rotator
    Cuff 23415-23420
  Tendon 23410-23412, 23430-23440
  Tenomyotomy 23405-23406
Simple, Integumentary System
  See Integumentary System, Repair, Simple
Sinus
  Ethmoid
    Cerebrospinal Fluid Leak 31290
  Sphenoid
    Cerebrospinal Fluid Leak 31291
Sinus of Valsalva 33702-33722
Skin
  Wound
    Complex 13100-13160
    Intermediate 12031-12057
    Simple 12020-12021
Skull
  Cerebrospinal Fluid Leak 62100
  Encephalocele 62120
Spica Cast 29720

Rib
Antibody 86756
Antigen Detection
    by Immunoassay
        with Direct Optical Observation
        Direct Fluorescense 87280
        Enzyme Immunoassay 87420
Excision 21600-21616, 32900
Fracture
    Closed Treatment 21800
    External Fixation 21810
    Open Treatment 21805
Graft
    to Face 21230
Resection 19260-19272, 32900
X-Ray 71100-71111

Riboflavin 84252

Richardson Operation
Hysterectomy
See Hysterectomy, Abdominal, Total

Richardson Procedure 53460

Rickettsia
Antibody 86757

Ridell Operation
See Sinusotomy, Frontal

Ridge, Alveolar
See Alveolar Ridge

Right Atrioventricular Valve
See Tricuspid Valve

Right Heart Cardiac Catheterization
See Cardiac Catheterization, Right Heart

Ripstein Operation
See Proctopexy

Risk Factor Reduction Intervention
See Performance Measures, Preventive Medicine

Risser Jacket 29010-29015
Removal 29710

Rocky Mountain Spotted
Fever 86000

Roentgen Rays
See X-Ray

Roentgenographic
See X-Ray

Roentgenography
See Radiology, Diagnostic

Ropes Test .83872

Rorschach Test 96101

Ross Information Processing
Assessment 96125

Ross Procedure 33413

Rotation Flap
See Skin, Adjacent Tissue Transfer

Rotator Cuff
Repair 23410-23420

Rotavirus
Antibody 86759
Antigen Detection
    Enzyme Immunoassay 87425

Rotavirus Vaccine 90680

Round Window
Repair Fistula 69667

Round Window Fistula
See Fistula, Round Window

Roux-En-Y Procedure 43621,
43633-43634, 43644, 43846,
47740-47741, 47780-47785, 48540

RPR 86592-86593

RSV
See Immune Globulins; Respiratory Syncytial
Virus

RT3
See Triiodothyronine, Reverse

Rubbing Alcohol
See Isopropyl Alcohol

Rubella
Antibody 86762
Vaccine 90706-90710

Rubella HI Test
See Hemagglutination Inhibition Test

Rubella/Mumps
See Vaccines

Rubeola
Antibody 86765
Antigen Detection
    Immunofluorescence 87283

Rubeolla
See Rubeola

Russell Viper Venom
Time 85612-85613

S

Sac, Endolymphatic
See Endolymphatic Sac

Saccomanno Technique 88108

Sacral Nerve
Implantation
    Electrode 64561, 64581
Insertion
    Electrode 64561, 64581

Sacroiliac Joint
Arthrodesis .27280
Arthrotomy .27050
Biopsy 27050
Dislocation
    Open Treatment 27218
Fusion 27280
Injection for Arthrography 27096
X-Ray 72200-72202, 73542

Sacrum
Tumor
    Excision .49215
X-Ray 72220

Sahli Test
See Gastroenterology, Diagnostic, Stomach

Salicylate
Assay 80196

Saline-Solution Abortion
See Abortion, Induced, by Saline

Salivary Duct
Catheterization 42660
Dilation 42650-42660
Ligation 42665
Repair 42500-42505
    Fistula 42600

Salivary Gland Virus
See Cytomegalovirus

Salivary Glands
Abscess
    Incision and Drainage 42310-42320
Biopsy 42405
Calculi (Stone)
    Excision 42330-42340
Cyst
    Drainage .42409
    Excision .42408
Injection
    X-Ray 42550
Needle Biopsy 42400
Nuclear Medicine
    Function Study 78232
    Imaging 78230-78231
Parotid
    Abscess 42300-42305
Unlisted Services and Procedures 42699
X-Ray 70380-70390
    with Contrast 70390

Salmonella
Antibody 86768

Salpingectomy 58262-58263,
58291-58292, 58552, 58554, 58661, 58700
Ectopic Pregnancy
    Laparoscopic Treatment 59151
    Surgical Treatment 59120
Oophorectomy 58943

Salpingo-Oophorectomy 58720
Resection Ovarian Malignancy 58950-58958
Resection Peritoneal Malignancy . .58950-58958
Resection Tubal Malignancy 58950-58958

Scleral Buckling Operation
See Retina, Repair, Detachment

Scleral Ectasia
See Staphyloma, Sclera

Sclerectomy 66160

Sclerotherapy
Venous 36468-36471

Sclerotomy
See Incision, Sclera

Screening, Drug
See Drug Screen
Alcohol and/or Substance Abuse ... 99408-99409

Scribner Cannulization 36810

Scrotal Varices
See Varicocele

Scrotoplasty 55175-55180

Scrotum
Abscess
　　Incision and Drainage 54700, 55100
Excision 55150
Exploration 55110
Hematoma
　　Incision and Drainage 54700
Removal
　　Foreign Body 55120
Repair 55175-55180
Ultrasound 76870
Unlisted Services and Procedures 55899

Scrub Typhus 86000

Second Look Surgery
See Reoperation

Section
See Decompression
Cesarean
　　See Cesarean Delivery
Cranial Nerve 61460
　　Spinal Access 63191
Dentate Ligament 63180-63182
Gasserian Ganglion
　　Sensory Root 61450
Medullary Tract 61470
Mesencephalic Tract 61480
Nerve Root 63185-63190
Spinal Accessory Nerve 63191
Spinal Cord Tract 63194-63199
Tentorium Cerebelli 61440
Vestibular Nerve
　　Transcranial Approach 69950
　　Translabyrinthine Approach 69915

Sedation
Moderate 99143-99150
　　with Independent Observation .. 99143-99145

Seddon-Brookes Procedure ... 24320

Sedimentation Rate
Blood Cell
　　Automated 85652
　　Manual 85651

Segmentectomy
Breast 19301-19302
Lung 32484

Seidlitz Powder Test
See X-Ray, with Contrast

Selective Cellular Enhancement Technique 88112

Selenium 84255

Self Care
See Physical Medicine/Therapy/Occupational Therapy
Training 97535, 98960-98962, 99509

Sella Turcica
CT Scan 70480-70482
X-Ray 70240

Semen
See Sperm

Semen Analysis 89300-89322
Sperm Analysis 89331
　　Antibodies 89325
with Sperm Isolation 89260-89261

Semenogelase
See Antigen, Prostate Specific

Semicircular Canal
Incision
　　Fenestration 69820
　　　Revised 69840

Semilunar
Bone
　　See Lunate
Ganglion
　　See Gasserian Ganglion

Seminal Vesicle
Cyst
　　Excision 55680
Excision 55650
Incision 55600-55605
Mullerian Duct
　　Excision 55680
Unlisted Services and Procedures 55899

Seminal Vesicles
Vesiculography 74440
X-Ray with Contrast 74440

Seminin
See Antigen, Prostate Specific

Semiquantitative 81005

Sengstaaken Tamponade
Esophagus 43460

Senning Procedure 33774-33777
See Repair, Great Arteries; Revision

Senning Type 33774-33777

Sensitivity Study
Antibiotic
　　Agar 87181
　　Disc 87184

Enzyme Detection 87185
Macrobroth 87188
MIC 87186
Microtiter 87186
MLC 87187
Mycobacteria 87190
Antiviral Drugs
HIV-1
　　Tissue Culture 87904

Sensor, Transcatheter Placement 34806

Sensorimotor Exam 92060

Sensory Nerve
Common
　　Repair/Suture 64834

Sentinel Node
Injection Procedure 38792

Separation
Craniofacial
　　Closed Treatment 21431
　　Open Treatment 21432-21436

Septal Defect
Repair 33813-33814
Ventricular
　　Closure 33675-33688
　　Open 33675-33688
　　Percutaneous 93581
　　Transmyocardial 0166T-0167T

Septectomy
Atrial 33735-33737
　　Balloon (Rashkind Type) 92992
　　Blade Method (Park) 92993
Closed
　　See Septostomy, Atrial
Submucous Nasal
　　See Nasal Septum, Submucous Resection

Septic Abortion
See Abortion, Septic

Septoplasty 30520

Septostomy
Atrial 33735-33737
　　Balloon (Rashkind Type) 92992
　　Blade Method (Park) 92993

Septum, Nasal
See Nasal Septum

Sequestrectomy
Carpal 25145
Clavicle 23170
Humeral Head 23174
Humerus 24134
Olecranon Process 24138
Radius 24136, 25145
Scapula 23172
Skull 61501
Ulna 24138, 25145

Serialography
Aorta 75625

Aorta to Pulmonary Artery
    Ascending .33755
    Descending 33762
    Central 33764
    Subclavian Pulmonary Artery 33750
    Vena Cava to Pulmonary
    Artery 33766-33768
Intra-Atrial 33735-33737
LeVeen
    See LeVeen Shunt
Nonvascular
    X-Ray 75809
Peritoneal
    Venous
        Injection 49427
        Ligation 49428
        Removal 49429
    X-Ray 75809
Pulmonary Artery
    See Pulmonary Artery, Shunt
Revision
    Arteriovenous 36832
Spinal Cord
    Creation 63740-63741
    Irrigation .63744
    Removal 63746
    Replacement 63744
Superior Mesenteric-Caval
    See Anastomosis, Caval to Mesenteric
Ureter to Colon 50815
Ventriculocisternal with Valve
    See Ventriculocisternostomy

Shuntogram 75809

Sialic Acid 84275

Sialodochoplasty 42500-42505

Sialogram
See Sialography

Sialography 70390

Sickling
Electrophoresis 83020

Siderocytes 85536

Siderophilin
See Transferrin

Sigmoid
See Colon-Sigmoid

Sigmoid Bladder
Cystectomy 51590

Sigmoidoscopy
Ablation
    Polyp 45339
    Tumor 45339
Biopsy 45331
Collection
    Specimen 45331
Exploration 45330, 45335
Hemorrhage Control 45334
Injection
    Submucosal 45335
Needle Biopsy 45342

Placement
    Stent 45345
Removal
    Foreign Body 45332
    Polyp 45333, 45338
    Tumor 45333, 45338
Repair
    Volvulus .45337
Ultrasound 45341-45342

**Signal-Averaged
Electrocardiography**
See Electrocardiogram

Silica 84285

Silicon Dioxide
See Silica

Silicone
Contouring Injections 11950-11954

Silver Operation
See Keller Procedure

Silver Procedure 28290

Simple Mastectomies
See Mastectomy

Single Photon Absorptiometry
See Absorptiometry, Single Photon

**Single Photon Emission Computed
Tomography**
See SPECT

Sinu, Sphenoid
See Sinus/Sinuses, Sphenoid

Sinus/Sinuses
Ethmoid
    Excision 31200-31205
    with Nasal/Sinus
        Endoscopy 31254-31255
    Repair of Cerebrospinal Leak 31290
Ethmoidectomy
    Excision 31254
Frontal
    Destruction 31080-31085
    Exploration 31070-31075
    with Nasal/Sinus Endoscopy 31276
Fracture
    Open Treatment 21343-21344
    Incision 31070-31087
Injection 20500
    Diagnostic 20501
Maxillary
    Antrostomy 31256-31267
    Excision 31225-31230
    Exploration 31020-31032
    with Nasal/Sinus Endoscopy 31233
    Incision 31020-31032, 31256-31267
    Irrigation .31000
    Skull Base 61581
    Surgery 61581
Multiple
    Incision 31090
Paranasal
    Incision 31090

Pilonidal
    See Cyst, Pilonidal
Sinus of Valsalva
    Repair 33702-33722
Sinus Venosus
    Repair 33645
Sphenoid
    Biopsy 31050-31051
    Exploration 31050-31051
    with Nasal/Sinus Endoscopy 31235
    Incision 31050-31051
    with Nasal/Sinus
        Endoscopy 31287-31288
    Irrigation .31002
    Repair of Cerebrospinal Leak 31291
    Sinusotomy 31050-31051
    Skull Base Surgery 61580-61581
Unlisted Services and Procedures 31299
X-Ray 70210-70220

Sinusectomy, Ethmoid
See Sinus/Sinuses; Ethmoidectomy

Sinusoidal Rotational Testing
See Ear, Nose and Throat

Sinusoscopy
Sinus
    Maxillary .31233
    Sphenoid .31235

Sinusotomy
See Sinus/Sinuses, Multiple
Combined 31090
Frontal Sinus
    Exploratory 31070-31075
    Nonobliterative 31086-31087
    Obliterative 31080-31085
Maxillary 31020-31032
Multiple
    Paranasal 31090
Sphenoid Sinus 31050-31051

Sirolimus
Drug Assay 80195

SISI Test .92564

Sistrunk Operation
See Cyst, Thyroid Gland, Excision

Six Minute Walk Test 94620

Size Reduction, Breast
See Breast, Reduction

Skeletal Fixation
Humeral Epicondyle
    Percutaneous 24566

Skeletal Traction
Insertion/Removal
    Pin/Wire .20650

Skene's Gland
Abscess
    Incision and Drainage 53060
Destruction 53270
Excision 53270

Skilled Nursing Facilities (SNFs)
See Nursing Facility Services

Replacement
- Plate 62143
- Prosthesis 62143

Tumor
- Excision 61500

X-Ray 70250-70260

Skull Base Surgery

Anterior Cranial Fossa
- Bicoronal Approach 61586
- Craniofacial Approach 61580-61583
- Extradural 61600-61601
- LeFort I Osteotomy Approach 61586
- Orbitocranial Approach 61584-61585
- Transzygomatic Approach 61586

Carotid Aneurysm 61613

Carotid Artery 61610
- Transection/Ligation 61609-61612

Craniotomy 62121

Dura
- Repair of Cerebrospinal
  Fluid Leak 61618-61619

Middle Cranial Fossa
- Extradural 61605, 61607
- Infratemporal Approach 61590-61591
- Intradural 61606, 61608

Orbitocranial Zygomatic Approach 61592

Posterior Cranial Fossa
- Extradural 61615
- Intradural 61616
- Transcondylar Approach 61596-61597
- Transpetrosal Approach 61598
- Transtemporal Approach 61595

Sleep Study 95806-95807

Actigraphy 0089T

Sliding Inlay Graft, Tibia

See Ankle; Tibia, Repair

Sling Operation

Incontinence 53440
- Removal 53442

Stress Incontinence 51992, 57287

Vagina 57287-57288

Small Bowel

See Intestines, Small

Neoplasm
- *See* Tumor, Intestines, Small

SMAS Flap 15829

Smear

Cervical
- *See* Cervical Smears

Papanicolaou
- *See* Pap Smears

Smear and Stain

See Cytopathology, Smears

Cornea 65430

Fluorescent 87206

Gram or Giesma 87205

Ova/Parasites 87177, 87209

Parasites 87207-87209

Wet Mount 87210

Smith Fracture 25600-25605

Smith-Robinson Operation

See Arthrodesis, Vertebra

Smoking and Tobacco Use Cessation

Counseling 99406-99407

SO$_4$

See Sulfate

Soave Procedure 45120

Sodium 84295, 84302

Urine 84300

Sodium Glycinate, Theophylline

See Theophylline

Sofield Procedure 24410

Soft Tissue

See Tissue, Soft

Solar Plexus

See Celiac Plexus

Solitary Cyst

See Bone, Cyst

Somatomammotropin, Chorionic 83632

Somatomedin 84305

Somatosensory Testing

Lower Limbs 95926

Trunk or Head 95927

Upper Limbs 95925

Somatostatin 84307

Somatotropin 83003

Somatotropin Release Inhibiting Hormone

See Somatostatin

Somatropin

See Growth Hormone, Human

Somnographies

See Polysomnography

Somophyllin T

See Theophylline

Sonography

See Echography

Sonohysterography 76831

Saline Infusion
- Injection Procedure 58340

Sore, Bed

See Pressure Ulcer (Decubitus)

Spasm Eyelid

See Blepharospasm

Special Services

After Hours Medical Services 99050

Analysis
- Remote Physiologic Data 99091

Computer Data Analysis 99090

Device Handling 99002

Emergency Care In Office 99058

Emergency Care Out of Office 99060

Extended Hours Medical Services ..99051-99053

Group Education 99078
- Self-Management 98961-98962

Hyperbaric Oxygen 99183

Hypothermia 99185-99186

Individual Education
- Self-management 98960

Medical Testimony 99075

Non-Office Medical Services 99056

On Call Services 99026-99027

Phlebotomy 99199

Post-Op Visit 99024

Pump Services 99190-99192

Reports and Forms
- Medical, Extended 99080
- Psychiatric 90889

Specimen Handling 99000-99001

Supply of Materials 99070
- Educational 99071

Unlisted Services and Procedures 99199

Unusual Travel 99082

Specific Gravity

Body Fluid 84315

Specimen Collection

Intestines 89100-89105

Stomach 89130-89141

Specimen Concentration 87015

Specimen Handling 99000-99001

SPECT 78607

See Emission Computerized Tomography

Abscess Localization 78807

Bone 78320

Cerebrospinal Fluid 78647

Heart
- Multiple 78465
- Single 78464

Kidney 78710

Liver 78205

Tumor Localization 78803

Spectacle Services

Fitting
- Low Vision Aid 92354-92355
- Spectacle Prosthesis 92352-92353
- Spectacles 92340-92342

Repair 92370-92371

Spectrometry

Mass
- Analyte
  - Qualitative 83788
  - Quantitative 83789

Spectrophotometry 84311

Atomic Absorption
- *See* Atomic Absorption Spectroscopy

Spectroscopy

Atomic Absorption 82190

Expired Breath Analysis 0064T

Magnetic Resonance 76390

Eyelid .67880
   Closure of 67875
   with Transposition of Tarsal Plate 67882
   Wound
      Full Thickness 67935
      Partial Thickness 67930
Facial Nerve
   Intratemporal
      Lateral to Geniculate Ganglion 69740
      Medial to Geniculate Ganglion 69745
Foot
   Tendon 28200-28210
Gastroesophageal . . . ., 43405
Great Vessel 33320-33322
Hemorrhoids 46945-46946
Hepatic Duct
   See Hepatic Duct,Repair
Intestine
   Large
      Diverticula 44605
      Ulcer 44605
      Wound .44605
Intestines
   Large
      Diverticula 44604
      Ulcer 44604
      Wound .44604
   Small
      Diverticula 44602-44603
      Fistula 44640-44661
      Plication 44680
      Ulcer 44602-44603
      Wound 44602-44603
      Stoma 44620-44625
Iris
   with Ciliary Body 66682
Kidney
   Fistula 50520-50526
   Horseshoe 50540
   Wound 50500
Leg, Lower
   Tendon 27658-27665
Leg, Upper
   Muscle 27385-27386
Liver
   Wound 47350-47361
Mesentery 44850
Nerve .64831-64876
Pancreas 48545
Pharynx
   Wound 42900
Rectum
   Fistula 45800-45825
   Prolapse 45540-45541
Removal
   Anesthesia 15850-15851
Spleen
   See Splenorrhapy
Stomach
   Fistula 43880
   Laceration 43501-43502
   Stoma 43870
   Ulcer 43501, 43840
   Wound 43840
Tendon
   Foot 28200-28210
   Knee 27380-27381

Testis
   Injury 54670
   Suspension 54620-54640
Thoracic Duct
   Abdominal Approach 38382
   Cervical Approach 38380
   Thoracic Approach 38381
Throat
   Wound 42900
Tongue
   to Lip 41510
Trachea
   Fistula
      with Plastic Repair 31825
      without Plastic Repair 31820
   Stoma
      with Plastic Repair 31825
      without Plastic Repair 31820
   Wound
      Cervical 31800
      Intrathoracic 31805
Ulcer 44604-44605
Ureter 50900
   Deligation 50940
   Fistula 50920-50930
Urethra
   Fistula 45820-45825, 53520
   Stoma 53520
   to Bladder 51840-51841
   Wound 53502-53515
Uterus
   Fistula 51920-51925
   Rupture 58520, 59350
   Suspension 58400-58410
Vagina
   Cystocele 57240, 57260
   Enterocele 57265
   Fistula
      Rectovaginal 57300-57307
      Transvesical and Vaginal
      Approach 57330
      Urethrovaginal 57310-57311
      Vesicovaginal 51900, 57320-57330
   Rectocele 57250-57260
   Suspension 57280, 57283
   Wound 57200-57210
Vas Deferens 55400
Vein
   Femoral .37650
   Iliac 37660
   Vena Cava 37620
Wound 44604-44605

Swallowing
Evaluation 92610-92613, 92616-92617
Imaging 74230
Treatment 92526

Swanson Procedure 28309

Sweat Collection
Iontophoresis 89230

Sweat Glands
Excision
   Axillary 11450-11451
   Inguinal 11462-11463
   Perianal 11470-11471
   Perineal 11470-11471
   Umbilical 11470-11471

Sweat Test 82435
See Chloride, Blood

Swenson Procedure 45120

Syme Procedure 27888

Sympathectomy
Artery
   Digital 64820
   Radial 64821
   Superficial Palmar Arch 64823
   Ulnar 64822
Cervical 64802
Cervicothoracic 64804
Digital Artery
   with Magnification 64820
Lumbar 64818
Presacral 58410
Thoracic 32664
Thoracolumbar 64809
with Rib Excision 21616

Sympathetic Nerve
Excision 64802-64818
Injection
   Anesthetic 64508, 64520-64530

Sympathins
See Catecholamines

Symphysiotomy
Horseshoe Kidney 50540

Symphysis, Pubic
See Pubic Symphysis

Syncytial Virus, Respiratory
See Respiratory Syncytial Virus

Syndactylism, Toes
See Webbed, Toe

Syndactyly
Repair 26560-26562

Syndesmotomy
See Ligament, Release

Syndrome
Adrenogenital
   See Adrenogenital Syndrome
Ataxia-Telangiectasia
   See Ataxia Telangiectasia
Bloom
   See Bloom Syndrome
Carpal Tunnel
   See Carpal Tunnel Syndrome
Costen's
   See Temporomandibular Joint (TMJ)
Erb -Goldflam
   See Myasthenia Gravis
Ovarian Vein
   See Ovarian Vein Syndrome
Synechiae, Intrauterine
   See Adhesions, Intrauterine
Treacher Collins
   See Treacher-Collins Syndrome
Urethral
   See Urethral Syndrome

Testosterone 84402
Response 80414
   Stimulation 80414-80415
Total 84403

Testosterone Estradiol Binding Globulin
See Globulin, Sex Hormone Binding

Tetanus 86280
Antibody 86774
Immunoglobulin 90389
Vaccine 90703

Tetrachloride, Carbon
See Carbon Tetrachloride

Tetralogy of Fallot ...33692-33697, 33924

Thal-Nissen Procedure 43325

Thawing
See Frozen Blood Preparation
Cryopreserved
   Embryo 89352
   Oocytes 89356
   Reproductive Tissue 89354
   Sperm 89353
Previously Frozen Cells 38208-38209

Thawing and Expansion
of Frozen Cell 88241

THBR
See Thyroid Hormone Binding Ratio

Theleplasty
See Nipples, Reconstruction

Theophylline
Assay 80198

Therapeutic
Abortion
   See Abortion, Therapeutic
Apheresis
   See Apheresis, Therapeutic
Drug Assay
   See Drug Assay
Mobilization
   See Mobilization
Photopheresis
   See Photopheresis
Radiology
   See Radiology, Therapeutic

Therapies
Cold
   See Cryotherapy
Exercise
   See Exercise Therapy
Family
   See Psychotherapy, Family
Language
   See Language Therapy
Milieu
   See Environmental Intervention
Occupational
   See Occupational Therapy
Photodynamic
   See Photochemotherapy

Photoradiation
   See Actinotherapy
Physical
   See PhysicalMedicine/Therapy/Occupational Therapy
Speech
   See Speech Therapy
Tocolytic
   See Tocolysis
Ultraviolet
   See Actinotherapy

Therapy
ACE Inhibitor Therapy
   See Performance Measures
Beta Blocker Therapy
   See Performance Measures
Desensitization
   See Allergen Immunotherapy
Hemodialysis
   See Hemodialysis
Hot Pack
   See Hot Pack Treatment
Pharmacologic; for Cessation of Tobacco Use
   See Performance Measures
Radiation
   Brachytherapy 0182T
      See Irradiation
Speech
   See Speech Therapy
Statin Therapy, Prescribed
   See Performance Measures

Thermocauterization
Ectropion
   Repair 67922
Lesion
   Cornea 65450

Thermocoagulation
See Electrocautery

Thermogram
Cephalic 93760
Peripheral 93762

Thermographies
See Thermogram

Thermography, Cerebral
See Thermogram, Cephalic

Thermotherapy
Prostate 53850-53853
   Microwave 53850
   Radiofrequency 53852

Thiamine 84425

Thiersch Operation 15050
See Pinch Graft

Thiersch Procedure 46753

Thigh
Fasciotomy 27025
   See Femur; Leg, Upper

Thin Layer Chromatographies
See Chromatography, Thin-Layer

Thiocyanate 84430

Third Disease
See Rubella

Thompson Procedure 27430

Thoracectomy
See Thoracoplasty

Thoracentesis 32421-32422

Thoracic
Anterior Ramus
   See Intercostal Nerve
Arteries
   See Artery, Thoracic
Cavity
   See Chest Cavity
Duct
   See Lymphatics
   Cannulation 38794
   Ligation 38380
      Abdominal Approach 38382
      Thoracic Approach 38381
   Suture
      Abdominal Approach 38382
      Cervical Approach 38380
      Thoracic Approach 38381
Empyema
   See Abscess, Thorax
Surgery
   Video-Assisted
      See Thoracoscopy
Vertebra
   See Vertebra, Thoracic
Wall
   See Chest Wall

Thoracocentesis
See Thoracentesis

Thoracoplasty 32905
with Closure Bronchopleural Fistula 32906

Thoracoscopy
Diagnostic 32601-32606
   with Biopsy 32602, 32604, 32606
   without Biopsy 32601, 32603, 32605
Surgical 32650-32665
   with Control Traumatic Hemorrhage ...32654
   with Creation Pericardial Window 32659
   with Esophagomyotomy 32665
   with Excision Mediastinal Cyst, Tumor and/or Mass 32662
   with Excision Pericardial Cyst, Tumor and/or Mass 32661
   with Excision-Plication of Bullae 32655
   with Lobectomy 32663
   with Parietal Pleurectomy 32656
   with Partial Pulmonary Decortication ..32651
   with Pleurodesis 32650
   with Removal Intrapleural Foreign Body 32653
   with Removal of Clot/Foreign Body ...32658
   with Sternum Reconstruction 21743
   with Thoracic Sympathectomy 32664
   with Total Pericardiectomy 32660
   with Total Pulmonary Decortication ..32652
   with Wedge Resection of Lung 32657

Thyroglobulin 84432
Antibody 86800

Thyroglossal Duct
Cyst
    Excision 60280-60281

Thyroid Gland
Cyst
    Aspiration 60300
    Excision 60200
    Incision and Drainage 60000
    Injection 60300
Excision
    for Malignancy
      Limited Neck Dissection 60252
      Radical Neck Dissection 60254
    Partial 60210-60225
    Secondary 60260
    Total 60240, 60271
      Cervical Approach 60271
      Removal All Thyroid Tissue 60260
      Sternal Split/Transthoracic
      Approach 60270
      Transcervical Approach 60520
Metastatic Cancer
    Nuclear Imaging 78015-78018
Needle Biopsy 60100
Nuclear Medicine
    Imaging 78010
    Imaging for Metastases 78015-78018
    Imaging with Flow 78011
    Imaging with Uptake 78006-78007
    Metastases Uptake 78020
    Uptake 78000-78003
Tumor
    Excision 60200

**Thyroid Hormone Binding
Ratio** 84479

Thyroid Hormone Uptake 84479

**Thyroid Stimulating Hormone
(TSH)** 80418, 80438-80440, 84443

**Thyroid Stimulating Hormone
Receptor ab**
See Thyrotropin Releasing Hormone (TRH)

**Thyroid Stimulating Immune
Globulins** 84445

Thyroid Stimulator, Long Acting
See Thyrotropin Releasing Hormone (TRH)

Thyroid Suppression Test
See Nuclear Medicine, Thyroid, Uptake

Thyroidectomy
Partial 60210-60225
Secondary 60260
Total 60240, 60271
    Cervical Approach 60271
    for Malignancy
      Limited Neck Dissection 60252
      Radical Neck Dissection 60254
      Removal All Thyroid Tissue 60260
      Sternal Split/Transthoracic Approach ..60270

Thyrolingual Cyst
See Cyst, Thyroglossal Duct

Thyrotomy 31300

Thyrotropin Receptor Ab
See Thyrotropin Releasing Hormone (TRH)

**Thyrotropin Releasing Hormone
(TRH)** 80438-80439

Thyroxine
Free 84439
Neonatal 84437
Total 84436
True 84436

Thyroxine Binding Globulin 84442

Tibia
See Ankle
Arthroscopy Surgical 29891-29892
Craterization 27360, 27640
Cyst
    Excision 27635-27638
Diaphysectomy 27360, 27640
Excision 27360, 27640
    Epiphyseal Bar 20150
Fracture
    Arthroscopic Treatment 29855-29856
      Plafond 29892
    Closed Treatment 27824-27825
    Distal 27824-27828
    Intercondylar 27538-27540
    Malleolus 27760-27766, 27808-27814
    Open Treatment 27535-27536,
              27758-27759, 27826-27828
    Plateau 29855-29856
      Closed Treatment 27530-27536
    Shaft 27752-27759
    with Manipulation 27825
    without Manipulation 27824
Incision 27607
Osteoplasty
    Lengthening 27715
Prophylactic Treatment 27745
Reconstruction 27418
    at Knee 27440-27443, 27446
Repair 27720-27725
    Epiphysis 27477-27485, 27730-27742
    Osteochondritis Dissecans
    Arthroscopy 29892
    Osteotomy 27455-27457,
            27705, 27709-27712
    Pseudoarthrosis 27727
Saucerization 27360, 27640
Tumor
    Excision 27635-27638, 27645
X-Ray 73590

Tibial
Arteries
    See Artery, Tibial
Nerve
    Repair/Suture
      Posterior 64840

Tibiofibular Joint
Arthrodesis 27871
Dislocation 27830-27832
Disruption
    Open Treatment 27829
Fusion 27871

TIG
See Immune Globulins, Tetanus

Time
Bleeding
    See Bleeding Time
Prothrombin
    See Prothrombin Time
Reptilase
    See Thrombin Time

Tinnitus
Assessment 92625

Tissue
Crystal Identification 89060
Culture
    Chromosome Analysis 88230-88239
    Homogenization 87176
    Non-neoplastic Disorder 88230, 88237
    Skin Grafts 15100-15101, 15120-15121
      Harvesting 15040
    Solid Tumor 88239
    Toxin/Antitoxin 87230
    Virus 87252-87253
Enzyme Activity 82657
Examination for Ectoparasites 87220
Examination for Fungi 87220
Expander
    Breast Reconstruction with 19357
    Insertion
      Skin 11960
    Removal
      Skin 11971
    Replacement
      Skin 11970
Grafts
    Harvesting 20926
Granulation
    See Granulation Tissue
Homogenization 87176
Hybridization In Situ 88365-88368
Mucosal
    See Mucosa
Preparation
    Drug Analysis 80103
Skin Harvest for Culture 15040
Soft
    Abscess 20000-20005
Transfer
    Adjacent
      Eyelids 67961
      Skin 14000-14350
    Facial Muscles 15845
    Finger Flap 14350
    Toe Flap 14350
Typing
    HLA Antibodies 86812-86817
    Lymphocyte Culture 86821-86822

Tissue Culture
from Skin Harvest 15040
Skin Grafts 15150-15157, 15340-15366

Treponema Pallidum

Antibody
  Confirmation Test 86781
Antigen Detection
  Direct Fluorescence 87285

TRH

See Thyrotropin Releasing Hormone (TRH)

Triacylglycerol

See Triglycerides

Triacylglycerol Hydrolase

See Lipase

Tributyrinase

See Lipase

Trichiasis

Repair 67825
  Epilation, by Forceps 67820
  Epilation, by Other than Forceps 67825
  Incision of Lid Margin 67830
    with Free Mucous Membrane
    Graft 67835

Trichina

See Trichinella

Trichinella

Antibody 86784
Trichogram 96902

Trichomonas Vaginalis

Antigen Detection
  Nucleic Acid 87660
  by Immunoassay with Direct Optical
  Observation 87808

Trichrome Stain 88313

Tricuspid Valve

Excision 33460
Repair 33463-33465
Replacement 33465
Repositioning 33468

Tridymite

See Silica

Trigeminal Ganglia

See Gasserian Ganglion

Trigeminal Nerve

Destruction 64600-64610
Injection
  Anesthetic 64400
  Neurolytic 64600-64610

Trigeminal Tract

Stereotactic
  Create Lesion 61791

Trigger Finger Repair 26055

Trigger Point

Injection
  One or Two Muscles 20552
  Two or More Muscles 20553

Triglyceridase

See Lipase

Triglyceride Lipase

See Lipase

Triglycerides 84478

Trigonocephaly 21175

Triiodothyronine

Free 84481
Reverse 84482
Total 84480
True 84480

Triolean Hydrolase

See Lipase

Trioxopurine

See Uric Acid

Tripcellim

See Trypsin

Trisegmentectomy 47122

Trocar Biopsy

Bone Marrow 38221

Trochanteric Femur Fracture

See Femur, Fracture, Trochanteric

Trophoblastic Tumor GTT

See Hydatidiform Mole

Troponin 84484

Qualitative 84512
Quantitative 84484

Truncal Vagotomies

See Vagotomy, Truncal

Truncus Arteriosus

Repair 33786

Truncus Brachiocephalicus

See Artery, Brachiocephalic

Trunk, Brachiocephalic

See Artery, Brachiocephalic

Trypanosomiases

See Trypanosomiasis

Trypanosomiasis 86171, 86280

Trypsin

Duodenum 84485
Feces 84488-84490

Trypsin Inhibitor, Alpha 1-Antitrypsin

See Alpha-1 Antitrypsin

Trypure

See Trypsin

Tsalicylate Intoxication

See Salicylate

TSH

See Thyroid Stimulating Hormone

TSI

See Thyroid Stimulating Immunoglobulin

Tsutsugamushi Disease

See Scrub Typhus

TT

See Thrombin Time

TT-3

See Triiodothyronine, True

TT-4

See Thyroxine, True

Tuba Auditoria (Auditiva)

See Eustachian Tube

Tubal Embryo Stage Transfer

See Embryo Transfer

Tubal Ligation 58600

Laparoscopic 58670
with Cesarean Delivery 58611

Tubal Occlusion

See Fallopian Tube, Occlusion; Occlusion
Create Lesion

Tubal Pregnancy 59121

with Salpingectomy and/or
Oophorectomy 59120

Tube Change

Colonic 49450
Duodenostomy 49451
Gastro-Jejunostomy 49452
Gastrostomy 43760, 49446
Jejunostomy 49451
Tracheostomy 31502

Tube Placement

Cecostomy Tube 44300, 49442
Duodenostomy Tube 49441
Endoscopic
  Bile Duct, Pancreatic Duct 43268
  Jejunostomy Tube
    Percutaneous 49441
  Nasobiliary, Nasopancreatic
    for Drainage 43267
Enterostomy Tube 44300
Gastrostomy Tube 43246, 49440
Nasogastric Tube 43752
Orogastric Tube 43752

Tube, Fallopian

See Fallopian Tube

Tubectomy

See Excision, Fallopian Tube

Tubed Pedicle Flap

Formation 15570-15576

Tubercle Bacilli

Culture 87116

Tubercleplasty

Tibia
  Anterior 27418

Tuberculin Test

See Skin, Tests, Tuberculosis

Ulnar Arteries
See Artery, Ulnar

Ulnar Nerve

Ultrasonic
See Ultrasound

Ultrasonic Cardiography
See Echocardiography

Ultrasonic Procedure 52325

Ultrasonography
See Echography

Ultrasound
See Echocardiography; Echography

Ultraviolet Light Therapy

Umbilectomy 49250

Umbilical

Umbilical Cord

Umbilicus

Undescended Testicle
See Testis, Undescended

Unfertilized Egg
See Ova

Unguis
See Nails

Unilateral Simple Mastectomy
See Mastectomy

Unlisted Services and Procedures 99499, 99600

Unna Paste Boot .... .29580
Removal .... .29700

UPP
See Urethra Pressure Profile

Upper
Digestive System Endoscopy
    See Endoscopy, Gastrointestinal, Upper
Extremity
    See Arm, Upper; Elbow; Humerus
Gastrointestinal Bleeding
    See Gastrointestinal,Upper, Hemorrhage
Gastrointestinal Endoscopy, Biopsy
    See Biopsy
    Planning
        See Biopsy, Gastrointestinal, Upper
        Endoscopy; Endoscopy, Gastrointestinal
GI Tract
    See Gastrointestinal Tract, Upper

Urachal Cyst
See Cyst, Urachal

Urea Breath Test 78267-78268, 83014

Urea Nitrogen
See Blood Urea Nitrogen
Clearance .... .84545
Quantitative .... .84520
Semiquantitative .... .84525
Urine .... .84540

Urea Nitrogen, Blood
See Blood Urea Nitrogen

Urecholine Supersensitivity Test
See Cystometrogram

Vasotomy 55200, 55300
Transurethral
   Cystourethroscopic 52402

Vasovasorrhaphy 55400

Vasovasostomy 55400

VATS
See Thoracoscopy

VDRL 86592-86593

Vein
Ablation
   Endovenous 36475-36479
Adrenal
   Venography 75840-75842
Anastomosis
   Caval to Mesenteric 37160
   Intrahepatic Portosystemic 37182-37183
   Portocaval 37140
   Reniportal 37145
   Saphenopopliteal 34530
   Splenorenal 37180-37181
   to Vein 37140-37160, 37182-37183
Angioplasty 75978
   Transluminal 35460
Arm
   Harvest of Vein for Bypass Graft 35500
   Venography 75820-75822
Axillary
   Thrombectomy 34490
Biopsy
   Transcatheter 75970
Cannulization
   to Artery 36810-36815
   to Vein 36800
Catheterization
   Central Insertion 36555-36558
   Organ Blood 36500
   Peripheral Insertion 36568-36569
   Removal 36589
   Repair 36575
   Replacement 36578-36581, 36584
   Umbilical 36510
Division
   Saphenous 37718-37722
Endoscopic Harvest
   for Bypass Graft 33508
External Cannula
   Declotting 36860-36861
Extremity
   Non-Invasive Studies 93965-93971
Femoral
   Repair 34501
Femoropopliteal
   Thrombectomy 34421-34451
Guidance
   Fluoroscopic 77001
   Ultrasound 76937
Hepatic Portal
   Splenoportography 75810
   Venography 75885-75887
Iliac
   Thrombectomy 34401-34451
Injection
   Sclerosing Agent 36468-36471
Insertion
   IVC Filter 75940

Interrupt
   Femoral 37650
   Iliac 37660
   Vena Cava 37620
Jugular
   Venography 75860
Leg
   Harvest for Vascular Reconstruction ...35572
   Venography 75820-75822
Ligation
   Clusters 37785
   Esophagus 43205
   Jugular 37565
   Perforation 37760
   Saphenous 37700-37735, 37780
   Secondary 37785
Liver
   Venography 75889-75891
Neck
   Venography 75860
Nuclear Medicine
   Thrombosis Imaging 78456-78458
Orbit
   Venography 75880
Placement
   IVC Filter 75940
Portal
   Catheterization 36481
Pulmonary
   Repair 33730
Removal
   Clusters 37785
   Saphenous 37720, 37730-37735, 37780
   Varicose 37765-37766
Renal
   Venography 75831-75833
Repair
   Aneurysm 36834
   Angioplasty 75978
   Graft 34520
Sampling
   Venography 75893
Sinus
   Venography 75870
Skull
   Venography 75870-75872
Spermatic
   Excision 55530-55540
   Ligation 55550
Splenic
   Splenoportography 75810
Stripping
   Saphenous 37718-37735
Subclavian
   Thrombectomy 34471-34490
Thrombectomy 37187-37188
   Other than Hemodialysis Graft
   or Fistula 35875-35876
Unlisted Services and Procedures 37799
Valve Transposition 34510
Varicose
   See Varicose Vein
Vena Cava
   Thrombectomy 34401-34451
   Venography 75825-75827

Velpeau Cast 29058

Vena Cava
Catheterization 36010
Reconstruction 34502
Resection with Reconstruction 37799

Vena Caval
Thrombectomy 50230

Venereal Disease Research
Laboratory
See VDRL

Venesection
See Phlebotomy

Venipuncture
See Cannulation; Catheterization
Child/Adult
   Cutdown 36425
   Percutaneous 36410
Infant
   Cutdown 36420
   Percutaneous 36400-36406
Routine 36415

Venography
Adrenal 75840-75842
Arm 75820-75822
Epidural 75872
Hepatic Portal 75885-75887
Injection 36005
Jugular 75860
Leg 75820-75822
Liver 75889-75891
Neck 75860
Nuclear Medicine 78445, 78457-78458
Orbit 75880
Renal 75831-75833
Sagittal Sinus 75870
Vena Cava 75825-75827
Venous Sampling 75893

Venorrhaphy
See Suture, Vein

Venotomy
See Phlebotomy

Venous Access Device
Blood Collection 36591-36592
Declotting 36593
Fluoroscopic Guidance 77001
Insertion
   Central 36560-36566
   Peripheral 36570-36571
Irrigation 96523
Obstruction Clearance 36595-36596
   Guidance 75901-75902
Removal 36590
Repair 36576
Replacement 36582-36583, 36585
   Catheter Only 36578

Venous Blood Pressure
See Blood Pressure, Venous

Venovenostomy
See Anastomosis, Vein

Viral Antibodies
................86280

Viral Warts
See Warts

Virtual Colonoscopy
Diagnostic 0067T
Screening 0066T

Virus
AIDS
  See HIV-1
Burkitt Lymphoma
  See Epstein-Barr Virus
Human Immunodeficiency
  See HIV
Influenza
  See Influenza Virus
Respiratory Syncytial
  See Respiratory Syncytial Virus
Salivary Gland
  See Cytomegalovirus

Virus Identification
Immunofluorescence 87254

Virus Isolation
............87250-87255

Visceral Larval Migrans
........86280

Viscosities, Blood
See Blood, Viscosity

Visit, Home
See House Calls

Visual Acuity Screen
.....99172-99173

Visual Field Exam
........92081-92083

Visual Function Screen
...1055F, 99172

Visual Reinforcement Audiometry
....................92579
See Audiologic Function Tests

Visualization
Ileal Conduit 50690

Vital Capacity Measurement
...94150

Vitamin
.....................84591
A 84590
B Complex
  See B Complex Vitamins
B-1 84425
B-12 82607-82608
  Absorption Study 78270-78272
  Holotranscobalamin 0103T
B-2 84252
B-6 84207
B-6 Measurement
  See Pyridoxal Phosphate
BC
  See Folic Acid
C 82180
D 82307, 82652, 4019F
D, 25-Hydroxy Measurement
  See Calcifediol
D-2
  See Calciferol
D-3 82306
E 84446

K 84597
K Dependent Bone Protein
  See Osteocalcin
K-Dependent Protein S
  See Protein S

Vitelline Duct
See Omphalomesenteric Duct

Vitrectomy
Anterior Approach
  Partial 67005
for Retinal Detachment 67112-67113
Monitoring of Intraocular Pressure 0173T
Pars Plana Approach 67036-67043
Subtotal 67010
  with Endolaser Panretinal
    Photocoagulation 67040
with Focal Endolaser Photocoagulation 67039
with Implantation or Replacement
  Drug Delivery System 67027

Vitreous
Aspiration 67015
Excision
  Pars Planta Approach 67036-67043
  with Focal Endolaser
    Photocoagulation 67039
Implantation
  Drug Delivery System 67027
Incision
  Strands 67030-67031
Injection
  Fluid Substitute 67025
  Pharmacologic Agent 67028
Removal
  Anterior Approach 67005
  Subtotal 67010
Replacement
  Drug Delivery System 67027
Strands
  Discission 67030
  Severing 67031
Subtotal 67010

VLDL
See Lipoprotein, Blood

VMA
See Vanillylmandelic Acid

Vocal Cords
Injection
  Endoscopy 31513
    Therapeutic 31570-31571

Voice Box
See Larynx

Voice Button
.................31611

Voiding Pressure Studies
Abdominal 51797
Bladder 51795
Rectum 51797

Volatiles
.....................84600

Volhard's Test
See Water Load Test

Volkman Contracture
.....25315-25316

Volume Reduction
Blood Products 86960

Volume Reduction, Lung
See Lung Volume Reduction

Von Kraske Proctectomy
See Proctectomy, Partial

VP
See Voiding Pressure Studies

Vulva
Abscess
  Incision and Drainage 56405
Colposcopy 56820
  Biopsy 56821
Excision
  Complete 56625, 56633-56640
  Partial 56620, 56630-56632
  Radical 56630-56631, 56633-56640
    Complete 56633-56640
    Partial 56630-56632
  Simple
    Complete 56625
    Partial 56620
Lesion
  Destruction 56501-56515
Perineum
  Biopsy 56605-56606
  Incision and Drainage 56405
Repair
  Obstetric 59300

Vulvectomy
Complete 56625, 56633-56640
Partial 56620, 56630-56632
Radical 56630-56631, 56633-56640
  Complete
    with Bilateral Inguinofemoral
      Lymphadenectomy 56637
    with Inguinofemoral, Iliac, and
      Pelvic Lymphadenectomy 56640
    with Unilateral Inguinofemoral
      Lymphadenectomy 56634
  Partial
    with Bilateral Inguinofemoral
      Lymphadenectomy 56632
    with Unilateral Inguinofemoral
      Lymphadenectomy 56631
  Simple
    Complete 56625
    Partial 56620

VZIG
See Immune Globulins, Varicella-Zoster

W

W-Plasty
See Skin, Adjacent Tissue Transfer

WADA Activation Test
.........95958
See Electroencephalography

X

X, Coagulation Factor
See Stuart-Prower Factor

X, Cranial Nerve
See Vagus Nerve

X-Linked Ichthyoses
See Syphilis Test

X-Ray

X-Ray Tomography, Computed
See CT Scan

Xa, Coagulation Factor
See Thrombokinase

Xenoantibodies
See Antibody, Heterophile

Xenografts, Skin
See Heterograft, Skin

Xenotransplantation
See Heterograft

Xerography
See Xeroradiography

Xeroradiography 76150

XI, Coagulation Factor
See Plasma Thromboplastin, Antecedent

XI, Cranial Nerve
See Accessory Nerve

XII, Coagulation Factor
See Hageman Factor

XII, Cranial Nerve
See Hypoglossal Nerve

XIII, Coagulation Factor
See Fibrin Stabilizing Factor

Xylose Absorption Test

Y

Yacoub Procedure
See Ascending Aorta Graft

Yeast
Culture 87106

Yellow Fever Vaccine 90717

Yersinia
Antibody 86793

Z

Ziegler Procedure
Discission Secondary Membranous
Cataract 66820

Zinc 84630

Zinc Manganese Leucine Aminopeptidase
See Leucine Aminopeptidase

Zygoma
See Cheekbone

Zygomatic Arch
Fracture
  Open Treatment 21356-21366
  with Manipulation 21355

The Newest Coding and Documentation Resources
from "The Source" of CPT® – the AMA

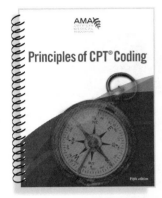

<< NEW >>

Principles of CPT® Coding, Fifth Edition

Updated and revised by the AMA, this resource provides the most in-depth review of the entire CPT® codebook available. Broad enough to educate the beginning coder, while serving as a useful tool for those with more experience, *Principles* explains the use of the codes and guidelines in a practical, easy-to-read style that addresses everyday coding challenges. Instructions on how to code from an operative report and coding tips with hints on codes assignment, bundling, and payer policies are included to increase coding understanding. This new edition contains: additional end-of-chapter exercises, expanded and revised chapter sections for the Surgery, Radiology, Pathology and Laboratory and Medicine.

Spiralbound, 8-1/2"x11", 580 pages
ISBN: 978-1-57947-967-1   Order #: OP501007
Price: $69.95   AMA member price: $49.95

<< NEW >>

Principles of CPT® Coding Workbook, Second Edition
(formerly CPT® Coding Workbook)

Revised and expanded, the second edition of *Principles of CPT® Coding Workbook* provides in-depth instruction on key coding concepts by CPT code section. Extensive coding scenarios and operative procedure exercises are given at the end of each chapter to test knowledge. New chapters on Category II codes and the appendixes in the CPT codebook are included as well as new illustrations, decision tree flow charts for selected specialties and expanded chapters on E/M, Medicine, Surgery, Anesthesiology and Radiology. Developed as a companion to the bestseller *Principles of CPT® Coding* to provide more coding instruction and exercises, this source can also be used as a stand-alone teaching tool.

Softbound, 8-1/2"x11", 300 pages
ISBN: 978-1-57947-883-4   Order #: OP570407
Price: $59.95   AMA member price: $44.95

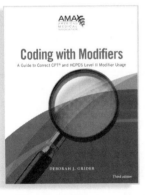

<< NEW >>

Coding with Modifiers: A Guide to Correct CPT® and HCPCS Level II Modifier Usage, Third Edition

The new third edition of *Coding with Modifiers* explains revisions made to modifiers in CPT® 2008, along with new tools to aid in modifier instruction. This edition contains updated CMS, third party payer, and AMA modifier guidelines to assist in coding accurately and avoiding payment delays. Coding tips and decision tree flow charts help clear up confusion surrounding modifier usage. A new test-taking tool is provided on CD-ROM, giving users a simulated test taking environment. New clinical examples and additional test-your-knowledge questions are also included.

Softbound, 8-1/2"x11", 500 pages
ISBN: 978-1-57947-889-6   Order #: OP322007
Price: $92.95   AMA member price: $69.95

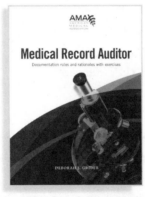

<< NEW >>

Medical Record Auditor, Second Edition

The new, second edition of *Medical Record Auditor* expands on the principles of medical record documentation and provides instructions on how to perform a medical record audit in the physician's or outpatient office. New to this edition: extensive coverage of E/M documentation and chart audits, guidelines for auditing radiology and operating room records, information on how to ensure medical records are compliant with current regulations, additional cases to test knowledge, exercises and expanded auditing tools. This invaluable reference also includes more than 110 auditing case examples and report templates, PowerPoint® presentations outlining each chapter and answer keys are included on CD-ROM.

Softbound, 8-1/2"x11", 458 pages
ISBN: 978-1-57947-884-1   Order #: OP301007
Price: $74.97   AMA member price: $54.95

AMERICAN MEDICAL ASSOCIATION

Order Today! Call toll-free (800) 621-8335 or order online at *www.amabookstore.com*

Time For a Practice Management Check-up?

The AMA offers a range of products to help your office run smooth and effectively

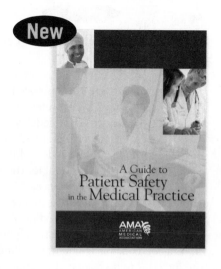

Maximizing Billing and Collections in the Medical Practice

Prevent undue financial losses in today's medical practice. Given the shrinking physician reimbursement environment, practices today need the tools and information necessary to maximize their billing and collections efforts; this book provides that and more. *Maximizing Billing and Collections in the Medical Practice* integrates the patient encounter with the billing and collections function to increase the likelihood of collecting every dollar the physician is entitled to receive.

Softbound with CD-ROM, 8-1/2"x11", 208 pages
Order #: OP318607
ISBN: I-57947-867-0
Price: $75.95   AMA member price: $56.95

A Guide to Patient Safety in the Medical Practice

Discover a greater understanding of the risks, consequences of errors and adverse events in the medical practice. This book is designed to stimulate the evolution of a patient safety culture in today's physician practice. Readers are provided with an in-depth review of the practical patient safety process and available tools for providers and business cases for a safer physician practice is also discussed.

Softbound, 7"x10" 300 pages
Order #: OP401006
ISBN: I-57947-674-0
Price: $59.95   AMA member price: $44.95

Other valuable practice management titles offered by the American Medical Association:
- Starting a Medical Practice
- Assessing the Value of the Medical Practice
- Managing the Medical Practice
- Buying, Selling and Owning a Medical Practice
- Financial Management of the Medical Practice
- Personnel Management in the Medical Practice

For more information on our practice success series or to review additional products and services visit *www.amabookstore.com* or call (800) 621-8335.

AMA
AMERICAN MEDICAL ASSOCIATION